Infectious Disease Epidemiology

Theory and Practice

Kenrad E. Nelson, MD
Professor
Departments of Epidemiology, International Health, and Medicine
Johns Hopkins Medical Institutions
Johns Hopkins University
Baltimore, Maryland

Carolyn Masters Williams, PhD, MPH
Epidemiology Branch, Basic Science Program
Division of AIDS
National Institute of Allergy and Infectious Diseases
Bethesda, Maryland

Neil M.H. Graham, MBBS, MD, MPH
Director
HIV Programs
Glaxo Wellcome, Inc.
Research Triangle Park, North Carolina

JONES AND BARTLETT PUBLISHERS
Sudbury, Massachusetts
BOSTON   TORONTO   LONDON   SINGAPORE

World Headquarters
Jones and Bartlett Publishers
40 Tall Pine Drive
Sudbury, MA 01776
978-443-5000
info@jbpub.com
www.jbpub.com

Jones and Bartlett Publishers Canada
2406 Nikanna Road
Mississauga, ON L5C 2W6
CANADA

Jones and Bartlett Publishers International
Barb House, Barb Mews
London W6 7PA
UK

The author has made every effort to ensure the accuracy of the information herein. However, appropriate information sources should be consulted, especially for new or unfamiliar procedures. It is the responsibility of every practitioner to evaluate the appropriateness of a particular opinion in the context of actual clinical situations and with due considerations to new developments. The author, editors, and the publisher cannot be held responsible for any typographical or other errors found in this book.

Cover design photograph of adult Ixodes tick is copyrighted by J. Stephen Dumler, MD, and is used with permission.

Cover design photograph of Ancylostoma duodenale is copyrighted by Gerhard A. Schad, PhD, and is used with permission.

Production Credits
Chief Executive Officer: Clayton Jones
Chief Operating Officer: Don W. Jones, Jr.
Executive V.P. & Publisher: Robert W. Holland, Jr.
V.P., Sales and Marketing: William J. Kane
V.P., Design and Production: Anne Spencer
V.P., Manufacturing and Inventory Control: Therese Bräuer
Publisher—Aspen: Michael Brown
Associate Editor: Chambers Moore
Production Assistant: Carolyn F. Rogers
Production Specialist: Anda Aquino-Eisenberg
Manufacturing and Inventory Coordinator: Amy Bacus
Printing and Binding: Edwards Brothers Ann Arbor

ISBN: 0-7637-1407-0

Printed in the United States of America
07 06 05 04 03   10 9 8 7 6 5 4 3

Table of Contents

Contributors

Joan L. Aron, PhD
President
Science Communication Studies
Columbia, Maryland
Associate, Department of Epidemiology
School of Hygiene and Public Health
Johns Hopkins University
Baltimore, Maryland

William R. Bishai, MD, PhD
Assistant Professor
Department of International Health
School of Hygiene and Public Health
Johns Hopkins University
Baltimore, Maryland

Robert E. Black, MD
Professor and Chair
Department of International Health
School of Hygiene and Public Health
Johns Hopkins University
Baltimore, Maryland

Richard E. Chaisson, MD
Professor
Departments of Medicine, Epidemiology, and
    International Health
Johns Hopkins Medical Institutions
Johns Hopkins University
Baltimore, Maryland

Rashid A. Chotani, MD, MPH
Research Associate
Division of Disease Control
Department of International Health
School of Hygiene and Public Health
Johns Hopkins University
Baltimore, Maryland

Jacqueline S. Coberly, PhD
Assistant Scientist
Department of International Health
Division of Disease Control
School of Hygiene and Public Health
Johns Hopkins University
Baltimore, Maryland

James Dick, PhD
Associate Professor
Department of Pathology
School of Medicine
W. Harry Feinstone Department of Molecular
    Microbiology and Immunology
School of Hygiene and Public Health
Johns Hopkins University
Baltimore, Maryland

Diane M. Dwyer, MD
Former Maryland State Epidemiologist and Director
Epidemiology and Disease Control Program
Maryland Department of Health and Mental Hygiene
Senior Associate
Department of Epidemiology
School of Hygiene and Public Health
Johns Hopkins University
Baltimore, Maryland

Gregory E. Glass, PhD
Associate Professor
W. Harry Feinstone Department of Molecular
    Microbiology and Immunology
School of Hygiene and Public Health
Johns Hopkins University
Baltimore, Maryland

Neil M.H. Graham, MBBS, MD, MPH
Director
HIV Programs
Glaxo Wellcome, Inc.
Research Triangle Park, North Carolina

Diane E. Griffin, MD, PhD
Professor and Chair
W. Harry Feinstone Department of Molecular
    Microbiology and Immunology
School of Hygiene and Public Health
Johns Hopkins University
Baltimore, Maryland

Carmela Groves, RN, MS
Chief, Division of Outbreak Investigation
Epidemiology and Disease Control Program
Maryland Department of Health and Mental Hygiene
Baltimore, Maryland

Susan M. Harrington, MT, MPH
Division of Microbiology
Department of Pathology
Johns Hopkins Hospital
Baltimore, Maryland

Anita M. Loughlin, MS
PhD Candidate
Department of Epidemiology
School of Hygiene and Public Health
Johns Hopkins University
Baltimore, Maryland

Richard H. Morrow, MD, MPH, FACP
Professor of International Health
School of Hygiene and Public Health
Johns Hopkins University
Baltimore, Maryland

Kenrad E. Nelson, MD
Professor
Departments of Epidemiology, International Health,
    and Medicine
Johns Hopkins Medical Institutions
Johns Hopkins University
Baltimore, Maryland
kenelson@jhsph.edu

Nikki M. Parrish, PhD
Department of Pathology
School of Medicine
Johns Hopkins University
Baltimore, Maryland

Trish M. Perl, MD, MSc
Hospital Epidemiologist
Assistant Professor
Departments of Medicine and Epidemiology
Johns Hopkins Medical Institutions
Johns Hopkins University
Baltimore, Maryland

Mary-Claire Roghmann, MD, MS
Hospital Epidemiologist
VA Maryland Health Care System
Assistant Professor
Departments of Medicine and Epidemiology and
    Preventive Medicine
University of Maryland School of Medicine
Baltimore, Maryland

Richard D. Semba, MD, MPH
Associate Professor
School of Medicine
Johns Hopkins University
Baltimore, Maryland

Clive Shiff, PhD, MSc
Associate Professor
W. Harry Feinstone Department of Molecular
    Microbiology and Immunology
School of Hygiene and Public Health
Johns Hopkins University
Baltimore, Maryland

Mark C. Steinhoff, MD
Professor
Departments of International Health and
    Epidemiology
School of Hygiene and Public Health
Department of Pediatrics
School of Medicine
Johns Hopkins University
Baltimore, Maryland

Steffanie A. Strathdee, PhD
Associate Professor
Department of Epidemiology
School of Hygiene and Public Health
Johns Hopkins University
Baltimore, Maryland

David L. Thomas, MD, MPH
Associate Professor of Medicine and Epidemiology
Johns Hopkins Medical Institutions
Johns Hopkins University
Baltimore, Maryland

Carolyn Masters Williams, PhD, MPH
Epidemiology Branch, Basic Science Program
Division of AIDS
National Institute of Allergy and Infectious
  Diseases
Bethesda, Maryland

Jonathan M. Zenilman, MD
Associate Professor
Departments of Medicine and Epidemiology
Johns Hopkins Medical Institutions
Johns Hopkins University
Baltimore, Maryland

Preface

The need for a book dealing specifically with infectious disease epidemiology has been clear to us for several years. No single book that covers the range of scientific conceptual material needed by an infectious disease epidemiologist is available. Organizing and teaching a course on the epidemiology of infectious diseases at the Johns Hopkins School of Hygiene and Public Health for the past 12 years has been an exciting and rewarding adventure.

The scope of infectious disease epidemiology has expanded substantially during the last decade. Important new pathogens have emerged and spread in human populations at an increasing rate. Organisms, such as *Sin nombe* virus, Human herpes virus type-8 (HHV-8), Cyclospora cayatenensis, and many others have been recognized very recently. It is important to note that the techniques for identifying, quantitating, and understanding the virulence factors of these new agents, as well as older infectious agents such as *Mycobacterium tuberculosis* and *Plasmodium falciparum* have advanced recently. New molecular techniques, such as the polymerase chain reaction, restriction fragment length polymorphism, and representational difference analysis have been developed and used to identify new infectious agents and to genotype or phenotype many human pathogens, prior to, or in the absence of their *in vitro* isolation using traditional microbiological methods. It has become essential that an infectious disease epidemiologist be familiar with these new methods in microbiology and molecular biology.

In addition, new scientific information has become available, which is very useful in an epidemiologist's effort to understand why new diseases have emerged. Techniques such as geographic mapping of environmental characteristics that influence vector populations, weather changes, and crop patterns can be applied to the distribution of disease, using geographic information system (GIS) analysis, in order to understand environmental factors promoting the emergence and re-emergence of infectious disease.

Also, new knowledge has become available recently about host susceptibility and resistance to infectious diseases. The discovery that certain individuals who are homozygous for a 32-base pair deletion in the chemokine receptor CXCR5 are resistant to infection with macrophage-tropic HIV-1 viruses and that persons, heterozygous for this mutation, progress more slowly after infection is a remarkable example of the contribution of studies of human genetics to our understanding of HIV pathogenesis. The ability of major epidemic diseases, such as malaria, to provide powerful genetic selection in human populations has been known for some time, since J.B.S. Haldane first proposed the idea of genetic polymorphism as a selective factor in human populations. The sequencing of the human genome is likely to provide further understanding of the relationship between human population genetics and important infections with microbial pathogens. The role of epidemic infectious diseases in the rise and fall of great civilizations and the outcome of major confrontations has been increasingly appreciated recently. The swine flu pandemic had a major effect in the outcome of World War I, as did smallpox in the European colonization of the Americas.

In addition, our understanding of the epidemiology of infectious disease has been advanced by the genetic sequencing and analysis of organisms such as the retroviruses (HIV-1, HIV-2, HTLV 1 and 2), hepatitis C virus, hepatitis B virus, influenza virus, *H influenzae, M tuberculosis,* and other pathogens. Detailed knowledge of the genetics of these pathogens has provided a clear understanding of the occurrence of epidemics or endemic infectious diseases in human populations.

Of course, some knowledge of the genetic characteristics of human pathogens remains elusive. For example, why was the H5/N1 influenza virus that emerged in Hong Kong in 1997 not transmitted between humans in spite of the remarkable virulence of this new human virus in the persons who acquired their infection directly from infected chickens? How can we predict the future of this new recombinant virus?

Another critically important knowledge base needed by the modern infectious disease epidemiologist is that of human behavior. Many of the modern emerging infectious diseases rely on human behavior for their persistence and spread. Certainly, HIV is a prime example. It has been remarkable that the HIV-1 virus has spread globally so rapidly, considering that it is not very infectious and its transmission relies on intimate sexual behavior or the injection of illicit drugs, which is a clandestine and illegal behavior in most societies. Control of the pandemic of AIDS has become the number one health priority for many countries as we enter the twenty-first century. Preventing the spread of AIDS has required a broader understanding of human behavior than most epidemiologists deemed necessary twenty years ago.

The understanding of the importance of the interspecies transmission of several viral agents has been appreciated by epidemiologists only recently. The spread of infection of primate retroviruses to humans has emphasized this risk. However, the emergence of other diseases, such as those due to Ebola virus, Arena viruses, Hantaviruses, influenza viruses, and others in recent years has emphasized the need for a better understanding of the critical role of human contact with other animals and the risk of zoonotic infections in the emergence of new diseases. With the advent and growth of xenotransplantation as an important new medical technology, the stakes may increase in the future. Time will tell us. But, at least for now, we should be forewarned of this potential risk.

It is, perhaps, obvious that an infectious disease epidemiologist needs to be fully versed in the basic methods of epidemiology. We have included chapters on modeling, study design, outbreak investigation, surveillance, and the evaluation of vaccines. The focus of these chapters in this book are the use of epidemiologic methods in dealing with infectious disease problems. These chapters may supplement, but certainly are not a substitute for, a course in basic epidemiology. At Johns Hopkins, students generally take a series of courses in epidemiology, of which, the course in infectious disease epidemiology focuses on the application of epidemiologic methods to infectious diseases. In the early chapters we have reviewed the history of the development of infectious disease concepts, given an overview of the field of microbiology, and reviewed some basic methods in molecular epidemiology.

These "methods chapters" are followed by current reviews of the epidemiology of many major infectious diseases. We have selected malaria, tuberculosis, hepatitis, sexually transmitted diseases (STDs), human immunodeficiency virus (HIV), acute respiratory infections (ARIs), diarrheal diseases, lyme disease, nosocomial infections, influenza, and selected parasitic diseases. Although this list of important infectious diseases is fairly comprehensive, it nevertheless is selective. We believe an infectious disease epidemiologist needs to be familiar with the features of important infectious diseases in addition to knowing the basic epidemiologic methods. Almost all of the chapters in this book have been written by our colleagues at Johns Hopkins. Indeed, most have taught in our course at one time or another. Their knowledge and expertise is obvious to us and the students who have taken the course. Their chapters focus on the epidemiology of the disease in the area of their expertise. In some instances, a clinical description or even a commonly used treatment is included when it is important to understand the epidemiology and prevention of a disease. However, this book primarily focuses on the epidemiology of infectious diseases. Detailed clinical descriptions and treatment options are covered in other texts. We hope the reader finds this book enlightening, interesting, and even pleasurable to read. We certainly enjoyed putting it together. We have learned a great deal in writing it, as we have over the years in teaching about the epidemiology of infectious diseases.

Acknowledgments

The routes the authors have taken to learn about the exciting scientific challenges in studying and teaching the epidemiology of infectious diseases have varied. However, they met at the Johns Hopkins School of Public Health about a decade ago, more or less. One of the greatest challenges and pleasures was to transmit the excitement involved in "doing" infectious disease epidemiology to their students and to each other. The high level of scientific and general intellectual curiosity that pervades the academic atmosphere at Johns Hopkins made the process very rewarding. The authors thank their students for often asking and sometimes answering the critical epidemiologic questions about infectious diseases. Also, the many talented and knowledgeable faculty colleagues at Johns Hopkins, several of whom have contributed to this book, have made the learning and teaching process a stimulating and rewarding adventure.

The authors' predecessors at Johns Hopkins have charted an interesting path for them to follow. Kenrad Nelson and Neil Graham are grateful to Frank Polk, who hired them to join the expanding research program in epidemiology at Johns Hopkins to meet the challenges of the HIV/AIDS pandemic. It has become increasingly clear since then that infectious diseases have not been "conquered" as was thought after the success of vaccine programs and antibiotics. For Kenrad Nelson, at Johns Hopkins, it was a pleasant surprise to learn that one of his first mentors in epidemiology, Dr. Alexander Langmuir, would come out of retirement and join the faculty at Johns Hopkins to teach epidemiology to a new generation of scientists. Dr. Nelson's two years in the EIS program at CDC, which was then under the leadership of Dr. Langmuir, changed the way he looked at medicine, science, and society forever. Other prominent epidemiologists have helped shape the atmosphere at the Johns Hopkins School of Hygiene and Public Health. In particular, Dr. Nelson acknowledges the influence of D.A. Henderson, who was first a colleague at CDC and then later returned to Hopkins after having successfully led the WHO smallpox eradication effort. Dr. Nelson also acknowledges George Comstock for his remarkable insight and experience in the epidemiology of infectious diseases; Jonathan Samet, an epidemiologist who has led the Department of Epidemiology into this new era of infectious diseases; and Richard Johnson and John Bartlett, who are clinicians/scientists with a keen understanding of the importance of epidemiology.

As a doctoral student at Johns Hopkins, Carolyn Williams keenly felt the lack of a comprehensive textbook dealing with infectious disease epidemiology. Working with Dr. Nelson, Dr. Graham, and the contributors to develop the materials for the course and the text has been a wonderful means to expand the breadth and depth of her knowledge in infectious disease epidemiology and she thanks them for the opportunity. Dr. Williams also thanks her classmates at Johns Hopkins for their contributions to the development of this text and their support throughout the writing of the book.

Coming from Adelaide, South Australia, to Johns Hopkins University was a great experience for Neil Graham. It fulfilled one of his dreams to work at one of the world's premiere medical and public health research institutions. It certainly lived up to its billing and Dr. Graham relished working in one of the great epidemiology departments. He has been delighted to continue his academic links since he joined Glaxo Wellcome in 1997. Dr. Graham thanks Dr. Nelson and Dr. Williams for their support during the transition. At Glaxo Wellcome, Dr. Graham has continued the fight against HIV at another of the world's premiere research institutions. His new colleagues have supported him greatly over the last three years, and he particularly thanks Gary Pakes, PharmD, for his tremendous help in pushing this book forward while he balanced other responsibilities.

The authors have also been extremely fortunate to have the very competent assistance of a remarkable administrative and secretarial staff, especially Barbara Gray and Clevetta Chandler, in the Infectious Disease Program in the Department of Epidemiology. It would be difficult to enumerate all of the problems they helped solve in creating this book. Also, Kathy Litzenberg at Aspen Publishers did a remarkably effective job of keeping the book moving.

Dr. Nelson thanks his wife, Karen, for being his companion all these years. He also thanks two of his grandsons, Jair and Jihar, for coloring all over a draft of a chapter on only one occasion.

Dr. Williams acknowledges her family for their support and comments. Many of the chapters were edited while she was at her parents' home in Connecticut. She treasures the hours she spent reading with her father during the last few months of his life. Dr. Williams is also, as always, thankful to her husband, Rick, and daughter, Katie, for their unflagging support and love.

Dr. Graham is indebted to his wife, Nicole Helen Graham, for allowing him to drag her and their three boys halfway around the world to answer the growing challenge offered by infectious diseases in the United States and around the world. The journey has been an exciting one; and, it is not finished yet!

PART I

Methods in Infectious Disease Epidemiology

Early History of Infectious Disease: Epidemiology and Control of Infectious Diseases

Kenrad E. Nelson

Epidemics of infectious diseases have been observed throughout recorded history. However, the explanatory theories offered for how epidemics have evolved are a result of the understanding of the natural forces and risk factors affecting the patterns of illness in society at the time. Many diseases, including smallpox, leprosy, tuberculosis, meningococcal infections, and diphtheria, were epidemic in ancient Greece and Egypt.[1] The Greek word *kynanche* was used to describe acute inflammation of the throat and larynx with dysphagia, which probably describes diphtheria.[1,2] Hippocrates, in *Airs, Water and Places*, described diseases that were always present in a population as endemic diseases, which is a term we still use. Other diseases that were not always present but sometimes occurred in large numbers were described as epidemic diseases in the Hippocratic writings. The factors leading to endemicity or epidemics of disease were felt to be climate, soil, water, mode of life, and nutrition.[2–5]

An epidemic that occurred in Athens in 430–427 B.C. had a profound effect on the civilization of ancient Greece.[6] This epidemic, which was described in detail by Thucydides, himself a victim, was analyzed recently by Langmuir et al.[7] They proposed that the epidemic was caused by influenza virus, complicated by infection with a toxin-producing strain of noninvasive staphylococcus and termed the epidemic the *Thucydides syndrome*. Another explanation for the "Plague of Athens" was proposed by Morrens and Chu,

namely, that the epidemic was due to Rift Valley Fever virus.[8] Holladay believes that the agent that caused this epidemic no longer exists because no current disease matches all of the described symptoms.[9] Nevertheless, the vivid description of the epidemic by Thucydides, which caused roughly 33% mortality of the population of ancient Athens, reminds us of the power of epidemics of infectious diseases to affect great civilizations profoundly.

During Roman times and throughout the Middle Ages, the theories of the Hippocratic writers dominated the thinking about the causes and mechanisms for the occurrence of epidemic diseases. Clearly, epidemics of infectious diseases had a major effect on European civilizations during the Middle Ages. The most dramatic example was the plague, which spread to Italy and Egypt in 1347 on merchant ships carrying rats and fleas infected with the plague bacillus.[1] During the next 5 years (1347–1351), plague, also known as the *Black Death*, had a major effect on the populations that it struck. Overall, it may have killed three Europeans out of ten, leaving some 24 million persons dead.[1,2,10,11] In the Middle East, the epidemics of plague killed about a quarter of the population. The control measures that were established focused primarily on quarantine and disposal of the bodies and (presumably contaminated) possessions of the victims. Although it was observed that large numbers of rats appeared during an epidemic of plague, the role of these rats and their fleas in these epidemics was not appreciated at the time. The pathogenic organism was not discovered until 1894, when Dr. Alexander Yersin and Dr. Shiba Sabuto Kitasato discovered the organism in both rats and humans who had died of plague during an epidemic in Hong Kong.[2,10] Two years later, in Bombay, Dr. Paul Lewis Simond of France established that the link between rats and humans was the rat flea, *Xenopsylla cheopis*.[2,10] Once a rat flea becomes infected with *Yersinia pestis*, the plague bacillus, it cannot digest its food, ie, rat blood. Therefore, it looks aggressively for another animal to feed on and, in so doing, passes the organism on to humans. After it is infected, the rat flea can hibernate for up to 50 days in grain, cloth, or other items and spread the disease to humans coming into contact with these items of commerce.

Another great epidemic disease, smallpox, had a major effect on human history. The first recorded epidemic was in 1350 B.C., during the Egyptian-Hittite war.[1] Typical smallpox scars have been seen on the faces of mummies from the time of the eighteenth and twentieth Egyptian dynasties (1570–1085 B.C.) and on the mummy of Ramses V, who died in 1157 B.C.[2]

Smallpox was disseminated during the Arabian expansion, the Crusades, the discovery of the West Indies, and the colonization of the Americas. The disease apparently was unknown in the New World prior to the appearance of the Spanish and Portuguese conquistadors. After smallpox was introduced, it decimated the Aztecs and Incas. Later on, smallpox had a devastating effect on native populations in eastern North America. There was a reasonable understanding of the means of spread of smallpox, however. At the least, it was appreciated that the skin lesions and scabs could transmit the disease. It was known that survivors of the infection were immune to reinfection after further exposure, although the mortality ranged from 10% to 50% in many epidemics. It was reported that smallpox accounted for 10% of the deaths in Europe during the eighteenth century.[1] Because of the immunity that was observed after an attack of smallpox, various methods were used to

inoculate or expose individuals to smallpox material, or scabs, in the hope that immunity could be established without the subject suffering the disease. This process was known as *variolation* and was advocated by Thomas Jefferson, Benjamin Franklin, and Cotton Mather. Napoleon reportedly variolated his army during the War of 1812. In 1796, Edward Jenner performed the first experiment in which he induced immunity to variola by intentionally inoculating an 8-year-old boy, James Phipps, with lesions containing cowpox (vaccinia virus) and later showed that the boy was immune to variolation, or challenge with variola virus.[12] Thus was born the science of vaccination, which led eventually (180 years later) to the eradication of smallpox.[12] This experiment grew out of the empiric observation that milk maids who had been infected with the cowpox (vaccinia) virus were relatively immune to smallpox. It is worthy of mention that other empiric attempts were proposed during the eighteenth century to induce protection against two other important diseases by intentional inoculation, ie, measles (called *morbillication*) and syphilis. Neither effort was successful.

Syphilis is another epidemic infectious disease of great historical importance. Syphilis became epidemic in the 1490s as a highly contagious venereal disease in Spain, Italy, and France. The origins of venereal syphilis are debated. One theory holds that it began as a tropical disease transmitted by direct (nonsexual) contact.[13] The organism, *Treponema pallidum*, has been isolated from patients with endemic (nonvenereal) syphilis (bejel) and yaws, also a nonvenereal treponemal disease. The name *syphilis* originated from a famous poem written in 1546 by Girolamo Fracastoro, entitled "Syphilis sive morbus Gallicus," which became very popular.[2,13] This poem recounts the legend of a handsome young shepherd named Syphilis, who, because of an insult to the god Apollo, was punished with a terrible disease, "the French Disease"—or syphilis. Syphilis spread rapidly through Europe and carried a high mortality. Also, the effect in the North American continent was quite dramatic. In Europe, by the 1530s, the venereal spread of syphilis was widely recognized.[13]

Fracastoro (1478–1553) was far ahead of his time in his revolutionary view of contagious infectious diseases. In a book published in 1546, *De contajione, contagiosis morbis et curatine (On contagion, contagious diseases and their treatment)*, he theorized that infectious diseases were transmitted from person to person by minute invisible particles.[2,14] This book is one of the great landmarks in the evolution of a scientific theory of communicable disease. Fracastoro conceived of the idea that infections were spread from person to person by minute invisible seeds, or "seminaria," that were specific for individual diseases, were self-replicating, and acted on the humors of the body to create disease. The seeds of a disease were probably not conceived of as microbes, because it would be another 100 years before Anton van Leeuwenhoek's invention of the microscope allowed microbes to be actually visualized for the first time. Finally, Fracastoro postulated three modes of transmission of contagious disease: by direct contact from one person to another, through contact with contaminated articles, such as fomites (a term that he coined and is still in use today), and through the air. He postulated that, under certain conditions, the environment becomes polluted with these seminaria and that epidemics occur in association with certain atmospheric and astrologic conditions.[2,15] He believed in astrology, as did most persons in his time. His theories were respected and certainly far ahead of their time; however, they remained unappreciated and unproven for the next 200 years. Nevertheless, he was able to persuade Pope Paul III to transfer the Council of Trent to Bologna because of the prevalence of contagious disease in Trent at the time and the risk to the participants of contact with contaminated fomites.[1]

Even before Fracastoro's theories, infectious diseases such as plague and leprosy were widely believed to be contagious and easily spread from one person to another. Indeed, in the Middle Ages, persons with leprosy or suspected leprosy were forced to carry a bell to warn others that they were coming. As far back as biblical times, the history of leprosy is rife with often irrational fear and stigmatization.

Malaria is another epidemic disease that has had a profound effect on human history and even on the selection of human genotypes.[16] The disease was present in Europe during the Middle Ages; a major European pandemic occurred in 1557 and 1558. In the period between 1630 and 1640,[17] Peruvian bark, or cinchona, was imported into Europe. Its active ingredient, quinine, was the first specific treatment for the disease. In 1717, Giovanni Maria Lancisi, an excellent clinician, published a book entitled *De noxiis palodum effloriis (on the noxious emanations of swamps)*. In this book, he speculated on the manner in which swamps produced malaria epidemics.[2] Lancisi theorized that swamps produced two kinds of emanations capable of producing disease, animate and inanimate. The animate emanations were mosquitoes, and these, he thought, could carry animalcules. His theories were close to the correct epidemiology of malaria. However, the epidemiology of malaria was not finally understood until the later part of the nineteenth century. The malaria parasite, *Plasmodium falciparum*, was originally discovered in 1880 by a French army surgeon, Alphonse Laveran. However, the mode of transmission was not proven until 1894, when Ronald Ross found the parasite in the stomach of an Anopheles mosquito. Subsequently, in 1898, he successfully transmitted avian malaria from an infected to an uninfected bird by the bite of a mosquito. In a letter to Patrick Manson (who had suggested the mosquito transmission theory to Ross) in July 1898, he described the results of his experiments.[18]

Anton van Leeuwenhoek (1632–1723) invented a microscope that was capable of visualizing microbes too small to be seen with the naked eye. He examined materials such as rainwater and human excretions, and described cocci, bacilli, and spirochetes, but he did not evaluate these organisms as agents of disease. Considerable controversy arose over the origin of these minute forms. Because they were often present in decaying or fermenting materials, some people maintained that they were spontaneously generated from inanimate material. However, Leeuwenhoek believed that they were derived from animate life. Indeed, Louis Pasteur demonstrated the dependence of fermentation on microorganisms in 1857 and, subsequently, showed that these organisms came from similar organisms present in the air.[19] It wasn't until the last two decades of the nineteenth century that numerous microorganisms were identified as the causative agents of important human diseases (Table 1–1). The demonstration that numerous microorganisms caused human and animal diseases followed after Robert Koch's demonstration in 1876 that he could reproducally transmit anthrax to mice by inoculating them with blood from sick cattle and that he could then recover the same rodlike bacteria from the sick mice as came from the cattle. Further, he could pass the disease from one mouse to another by inoculating them with these microorganisms.[2] These experiments resulted in the formulation of the "Henle-Koch postulates" for proof that a microorganism was the cause of an infectious disease.

The development of clinical medicine during the last two centuries probably played as important a role in the evolution of the principles of the epidemiology of infectious diseases as did microbiology. One of the earliest advocates of careful observation of patients' symptoms and their natural evolution or resolution was Thomas Sydenham, who lived in London from 1624 to 1689. He classified the different febrile illnesses plaguing London in the 1660s and 1670s in a book entitled *Observations Medicae*. His approach departed significantly from those of Galen and Hippocrates, who focused on illness and sick persons in general as unique events, rather than on trying carefully to differentiate specific diseases. The concepts initially proposed by Sydenham were advanced further by the efforts of Giovanni Morgagni, an eighteenth-century Italian physician. Morgagni inaugurated the method of clinicopathologic correlation, the association of particular signs and symptoms with pathologic changes in the tissues and or-

gans. This new way of thinking about diseases, requiring careful clinical observation, differentiation, and specific diagnosis, led naturally to the search for specific, as opposed to general, causes of illness.

About 10–20 years after the beginning of the profusion of research on bacteriology and the bacterial pathogenesis of human diseases, numerous scientists began to focus their investigations on vector-borne disease. The pioneering research of Ross in malaria, for which he was awarded the Nobel prize in medicine, has already been mentioned. The first proof that an animal disease was spread by an arthropod was the report in 1893 by Smith and Kilbourne of the transmission of Texas cattle fever (caused by a species of *Borrelia*) by a tick. Another group of landmark studies was organized in Cuba, which led to an understanding of the biology and epidemiology of yellow fever.[20] Although epidemics of yellow fever had been reported as far north as Philadelphia in the eighteenth and nineteenth centuries, the means of transmission of the disease were unclear. Some believed that the disease was spread directly from person to person. However, Stubbins Firth in 1804 observed that secondary cases among nurses or doctors caring for patients with the disease were unheard of. To prove that person-to-person transmission wasn't a risk, he undertook a remarkable series of self-experiments, in which he exposed himself orally and parenterally to the hemorrhagic vomitus, other excretions, and blood of patients dying of yellow fever. He was unable to transmit the infection in these experiments, and he concluded that yellow fever wasn't directly transmitted from person to person.[2] Early in the nineteenth century, it had been suggested by several physicians that yellow fever might be spread by mosquitoes.[2] The theory was restated by Carlos Finley, a Cuban physician, in 1881, but experimental proof was lacking.[2,21] When the United States occupied Cuba during the Spanish-American War, a yellow fever study commission with Walter Reed as its chairman was established to study the question further. The commission studied the transmission of yellow

Table 1–1 Discovery of Organisms of Human Diseases

Year	Disease or Organism	Scientist
1874	Leprosy	Hansen
1880	Malaria	Laveran
	Typhoid (organism seen in tissues)	Eberth
1882	Tuberculosis	Koch
	Glanders	Loeffler and Schutz
1883	Cholera	Koch
	Streptococcus (erysipelas)	Fehleisen
1884	Diphtheria	Klebs and Loeffler
	Typhoid (bacillia isolate)	Gaffky
	Staphylococcus	Rosenbach
	Streptococcus	Rosenbach
	Tetanus	Nicolaier
1885	*Escherichia coli*	Escherich
1886	Pneumococcus	A. Fraenkel
1887	Malta fever	Bruce
	Soft chancre	Ducrey
1892	Gas gangrene	Welch and Nuttall
1894	Plague	Yersin and Kitasato
	Botulism	Van Ermengen
1898	Dysentery bacillus	Shiga
1896	*Hemophilus influenzae*	Pfeiffer

fever by *Aedes aegypti* mosquitoes, using human volunteers (because there were no animal models). In the course of the investigation, one of the volunteers, who was a member of the committee, Jesse H. Lazear, contracted yellow fever following a mosquito bite and succumbed to the disease. After several definitive experiments, the commission was able to report that yellow fever was transmitted to humans by the bite of an infected mosquito. Subsequently, they were also able to show that the agent of yellow fever was present in blood that had been passed through a filter capable of retaining the smallest bacteria. They therefore concluded that the causative agent of yellow fever was a virus.[20] In 1898, Loeffler and Frosh had shown that hoof and mouth disease of cattle was caused by a filterable virus. However, the demonstration by Reed and co-workers that yellow fever could be transmitted by filtered blood was the first time that a specific human disease had been shown to be caused by a virus. Furthermore, their studies showed that yellow fever had an obligate insect cycle and was not transmitted directly from person to person.

Following this elegant demonstration that yellow fever was a vector-borne viral infection, several other arthropod diseases were studied by other scientists (Table 1–2). Also, many other human diseases caused by viruses were defined in the ensuing decades. The second human mosquito-borne viral infection to be identified was dengue, which is one of the re-emerging viral infections that have increased in importance in the last few decades. Dengue is spread by the same mosquitoes that transmit yellow fever, *A. aegypti*. The first clinical description of dengue is attributed to Benjamin Rush, a physician and signer of the U.S. Declaration of Independence, who lived in Philadelphia in 1780.[22] However, the means of transmission and the fact that the organism is a filterable virus were not appreciated until the experiments of Bancroft et al[2] in the Philippines in 1906. Rush's eloquent and accurate description of the clinical features of dengue in Philadelphia in 1780 is quoted below:

The pains which accompanied this fever were exquisitely severe in the head, back and limbs. The pains in the head were sometimes in the back parts of it, and at other times they occupied

Table 1–2 Discovery of Arthropod Vectors Responsible for the Transmission of Human Disease

Disease	Vector	Investigator	Year
Babesiosis (Texas cattle fever)	Deer tick	Smith and Kilbourne	1893
		(first human case of babesiosis)	1956
Yellow fever	Mosquito	Reed, Carroll, and Lazaer	1900
Dengue	Mosquito	Bancroft, Craig, and Asburn	1906
Rocky Mountain spotted fever	Wood tick	Ricketts, King	1906
Typhus, epidemic	Body louse	Nicolle	1909
Sandfly fever	Sandfly	Doerr, Franz, and Taussig	1909
Murine typhus	Rat louse	Mooser	1931
	Rat flea	Dyer	1931
Colorado tick fever	Wood tick	Topping, Cullyford, and Davis	1940
Rickettsial pox	Mite	Huebner, Jellison, and Pomerantz	1946
Lyme disease	Deer tick	Burgdorfer	1982
Cat scratch fever and bacillary angiomatosis	Cat flea	Koehler	1994
Human monocytic ehrlichiosis	Dog tick and lone star tick	Maedo et al	1986
Human granocytic ehrlichiosis	Deer tick	Chen et al	1994

only the eyeballs. In some people, the pains were so acute in their backs and hips, that they could not lie in bed. In others, the pains affected the neck and arms, so as to produce in one instance a difficulty of moving the fingers of the right hand. They all complained more or less of a soreness in the seats of these pains, particularly when they occupied the head and eyeballs. A few complained of their flesh being sore to the touch, in every part of the body. From these circumstances, the disease was sometimes believed to be a rheumatism. But its more general name among all classes of people was, the Break-bone fever.

Epidemiologic theories about the means of transmission of various infectious diseases often preceded the laboratory and clinical studies of the causative organisms. John Snow performed classic epidemiologic studies on the transmission of cholera in the mid-1850s, nearly 30 years prior to the identification of the causative organism.[23] Other examples exist. William Budd demonstrated the means of transmission of typhoid fever and the importance of the human carrier in transmission 35 years prior to the isolation of *Salmonella typhi*.[24] Ignatz Semmelweiss in Vienna in 1846 demonstrated with a retrospective record review that an epidemic of puerperal fever was related to transmission of infection on the hands of medical students and physicians (Figure 1–1). In contrast, the women

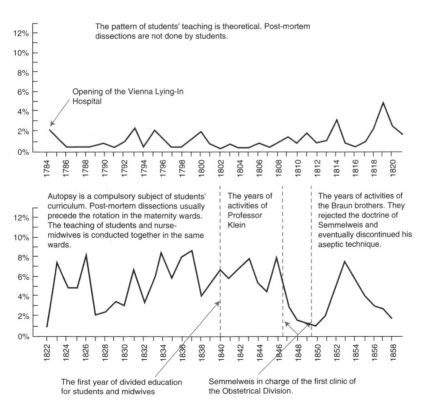

Figure 1–1 Maternal mortality statistics (predominantly from childbed fever) between 1784 and 1858 in the Vienna Lying-In Hospital, according to Semmelweis. Courtesy of Dr. L. Iffy, Newark, New Jersey.

who were delivered by midwives, who were using aseptic techniques (by immersing their hands in antiseptic solution prior to contact with the patient), had much lower rates of puerperal sepsis (Figure 1–2).[25]

The identification of the causative microorganisms of specific infections allowed for a much better understanding of their epidemiology, which proved useful for the development of more effective strategies for the prevention of infectious diseases. There is no doubt that the growth of microbiology, virology, and immunology paralleled and complemented the disciplines of epidemiology and public health in the prevention of infectious diseases.

Critical information about the epidemiologic characteristics of several infectious diseases has been obtained by careful observation of unusual epidemics and by self-experimentation. Peter Panum recorded his observation of an epidemic

of measles on the Faroe Islands in 1846.[26] Measles had not occurred in the population of these remote Scandinavian islands for a period of 65 years. Remarkably, attack rates among the exposed population were about 97%, but persons over age 65 were completely spared; thus demonstrating that immunity after an attack of natural measles persists for a lifetime. Further, Panum described the mean 14-day incubation period between cases.[26] Outbreaks of mumps and other contagious diseases in isolated populations also have contributed to our understanding of the epidemiology of these diseases.[27,28]

Human experimentation has provided critical knowledge about the epidemiology of several infectious diseases; the experiments of the yellow fever commission have already been described. Another example is provided by hookworm infection. Although human infections with hookworm were known since ancient times

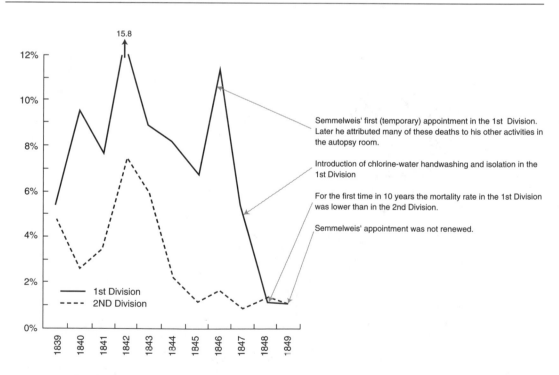

Figure 1–2 Mortality rates in first and second divisions of the Department of Obstetrics in the Vienna Lying-In Hospital between 1839 and 1849. Courtesy of Dr. L. Iffy, Newark, New Jersey.

and may have been the cause of the pallid appearance of Roman miners described by Lucretius in 50 B.C.,[2] the first specific published account of human hookworm disease was reported in 1843 by Angelo Dubini from Milan.[29] Later, he found hookworms in the intestines of nearly 20% of autopsies. However, the means of spread was commonly believed to be by the fecal-oral route until the observation of Arthur Looss in Cairo, Egypt, in 1898.[30] He was doing an experiment on *Stronglyloides stercoralis*, in which he swallowed several larvae of this organism to infect himself but, when he examined his stools, he found only hookworm eggs. Then he recalled that he had accidentally spilled a fecal inoculum on his hands. He had washed his hands carefully, although he recalled that a transitory red area had appeared on his skin, which itched before it spontaneously resolved. He then intentionally exposed his skin to another hookworm inoculum and, after a few minutes, was unable to find the organisms on his exposed skin. After several additional careful experiments, he reported the entrance of hookworms into humans by skin penetration of the parasites, rather than by ingestion.

Another physician who carried out several self-experiments on two different diseases was a Baptist missionary, Dr. Claude Herman Barlow. In his initial experiments, he infected himself with *Fasciolopsis buski* while in China and showed that the intestinal fluke, which infected many Chinese, existed in its larval form on the outer layer of water chestnuts, which were a staple of the Chinese diet.[31,32] In 1944, while working on a Rockefeller Foundation program in Cairo, Barlow intentionally infected himself with *Schistosoma haematobium*, a liver fluke that was endemic in Egypt.[33] The purpose of his experiment was to study carefully the natural history of the disease and to bring fully virulent parasites to the United States in order to evaluate whether snails present in the United States could transmit the organism. This was of considerable concern at the time because of the large number of U.S. servicemen who were about to return to the United States and who were infected with *S. haematobium* during their duty in Egypt in

World War II. Barlow found that U.S. snails were not capable of transmitting *S. haematobium*, although he nearly died from his infection.

One self-experimenter who did succumb was Daniel Carrion, a medical student in Lima, Peru, in 1895, who injected himself with the material from a chronic skin lesion called *Verraga peruana*. This self-experiment was designed to determine whether the same organism (later identified to be *Bartonella bacilliformis*) could also cause another disease, known as *Oroya fever*. Oroya fever was a more serious disease, involving the red blood cells. When Carrion developed Oroya fever, he proved that the two diseases were caused by the same infectious organism but the experiment cost him his life.

Another scientist, Dr. David Clyde, did several experiments on himself that made important contributions to the prospects for the development of a vaccine for the prevention of malaria. Because of the complex life cycle of malaria, involving major antigenic transformations of the organism with each stage of its life cycle, the development of a vaccine seemed a near impossibility for many years. However, Dr. Clyde performed several experiments in which he fed anopheline mosquitoes on patients with *P. falciparum* and *P. vivax* malaria, then irradiated the mosquitoes to kill the malaria sporozoites. However, the dose of radiation allowed for survival of the mosquitoes. He then allowed the irradiated mosquitoes to feed on himself. He found that, after bites by 350–1,000 infected mosquitoes, he had induced immunity to challenge with virulent malaria parasites.[34,35] His experiments spawned a major effort to develop a malaria sporozoite vaccine. This was deemed to be especially important because of the development of widespread resistance of anopheline mosquitoes to DDT and other insecticides, the only control measure in use at the time.

Another important contribution to the development of infectious disease epidemiology was the interest and emphasis during the middle and late eighteenth century and throughout the nineteenth century on "political arithmetic," or measurements of the vital statistics of causes of morbidity and mortality. One of the early leaders in the use of statistics to help understand the natural occurrence and epidemiology of infectious diseases was John Graunt, who lived in England and published *Natural and Political Observations—The Bills of Mortality* in 1662.[36] He published tables showing the number of deaths in London during the preceding third of a century. He used inductive reasoning to interpret the mortality trends and noted the ratio of male to female births and deaths, mortality by season, and mortality in persons living in rural versus urban locations. He examined several causes of deaths over time and constructed the first life tables. Subsequently, other observers used public health data for the study of epidemics of infectious diseases. A French mathematician, David Bernoullie, in 1760 analyzed smallpox mortality to estimate how the use of inoculation (ie, variolation) as a preventive measure might affect the life expectancy of the population.[2] Edwin Chadwick and William Farr in England made important contributions to the improvement and analytical use of public health statistical data. Civil registration of vital statistics was established in England in 1831.

In the late nineteenth and early twentieth century, rapid developments in the field of microbiology were paralleled by studies of the immunology and pathogenesis of infectious diseases. This research led to the development of treatments for diphtheria with antitoxin and the development of vaccines for rabies, anthrax, diphtheria, and tetanus. However, many of the antisera that were developed and antiseptics that were tried for the therapy of infectious diseases were of only limited effectiveness. In 1924, investigators at the Bayer pharmaceutical company in Germany synthesized a new antimalarial drug, pamaquine (Plasmoquine). Shortly thereafter, they synthesized other antimalarial compounds, including quinacrine (Atabrine).[37] The development of these new drugs gave some hope that specific effective antimicrobial treatments could be developed for infectious diseases. In 1932, Gerhardt Domagk did experiments on animals with some synthetic dyes to determine

whether they had antibacterial efficacy and found that a dye named *Prontosil* could cure mice that had been challenged with lethal doses of hemolytic streptococci.[37] This led to the development of several sulfa drugs. The sulfonamides were shown during World War II to be quite effective against a number of highly fatal infections, such as meningococcal meningitis. In the 1930s and 1940s, Alexander Fleming,

Table 1–3 Vaccine-Preventable Diseases, by Year of Vaccine Development or Licensure—United States, 1798–1998

Disease	Year
Smallpox*	1798[†]
Rabies	1885[†]
Typhoid	1896[†]
Cholera	1896[†]
Plague	1897[†]
Diphtheria*	1923[†]
Pertussis*	1926[†]
Tetanus*	1927[†]
Tuberculosis	1927[†]
Influenza	1945[§]
Yellow fever	1953[§]
Poliomyelitis*	1955[§]
Measles*	1963[§]
Mumps*	1967[§]
Rubella*	1969[§]
Anthrax	1970[§]
Meningitis	1975[§]
Pneumonia	1977[§]
Adenovirus	1980[§]
Hepatitis B*	1981[§]
Hemophilus influenzae type b*	1985[§]
Japanese encephalitis	1992[§]
Hepatitis A	1995[§]
Varicella*	1995[§]
Lyme disease	1998[§]
Rotavirus*	1998[§]

* Vaccine recommended for universal use in US children. For smallpox, routine vaccination was ended in 1971.
    [†] Vaccine developed (ie, first published results of vaccine usage).
    [§] Vaccine licensed for use in the United States.
    Source: Reprinted from *MMWR,* Centers for Disease Control and Prevention.

Howard Florey, and Ernst Chain at Oxford University conducted experiments that led to the demonstration that penicillin, a mold product, was effective against many pathogenic organisms.[37] Penicillin was shown to be effective against syphilis, gonorrhea, and pneumococcal infections. These landmark experiments gave birth to the search for new antibiotics produced by organisms in nature or synthesized in the laboratory. The better understanding of the epidemiology and pathogenesis of the classic infectious diseases, along with the development of effective vaccines for their prevention and strategies to discover or develop new antibiotics for their treatment, had a major impact on the incidence and mortality from many infectious diseases in the latter half of the twentieth century.

The Centers for Disease Control and Prevention recently published a review of the ten great public health achievements in the United States during the twentieth century.[38] At the top of its list is vaccination. During the last century, the average life span of persons in the United States was lengthened by about 30 years, and 25 years of this gain have been attributed to advances in public health. The vaccines developed and licensed to prevent vaccine-preventable diseases are shown in Table 1–3, and an estimate of their effect on reported infectious disease morbidity is shown in Table 1–4.

The public health actions to control infectious diseases in the twentieth century, which included marked improvements in sanitation, chlorination of nearly all public water supplies,

Table 1–4 Baseline Twentieth-Century Annual Morbidity and 1998 Provisional Morbidity from Nine Diseases with Vaccines Recommended before 1990 for Universal Use in Children—United States

Disease	Baseline 20th Century Annual Morbidity	1998 Provisional Morbidity	% Decrease
Smallpox	48,164*	0	100%
Diphtheria	175,885†	1	100%§
Pertussis	147,271¶	6,279	95.7%
Tetanus	1,314**	34	97.4%
Poliomyelitis (paralytic)	16,316††	0§§	100%
Measles	503,282¶¶	89	100%§
Mumps	152,209***	606	99.6%
Rubella	47,745†††	345	99.3%
Congenital rubella syndrome	823§§§	5	99.4%
Hemophilus influenzae type b	20,000¶¶¶	54****	99.7%

* Average annual number of cases during 1900–1904.
† Average annual number of reported cases during 1920–1922, 3 years before vaccine development.
§ Rounded to nearest tenth.
¶ Average annual number of reported cases during 1922–1925, 4 years before vaccine development.
** Estimated number of cases based on reported number of deaths during 1922–1926 assuming a case-fatality rate of 90%.
†† Average annual number of reported cases during 1951–1954, 4 years before vaccine licensure.
§§ Excludes one case of vaccine-associated polio reported in 1998.
¶¶ Average annual number of reported cases during 1958–1962, 5 years before vaccine licensure.
*** Number of reported cases in 1968, the first year reporting began and the first year after vaccine licensure.
††† Average annual number of reported cases during 1966–1968, 3 years before vaccine licensure.
§§§ Estimated number of cases based on seroprevalence data in the population and on the risk that women infected during a childbearing year would have a fetus with congenital rubella syndrome.[12]
¶¶¶ Estimated number of cases from population-based surveillance studies before vaccine licensure in 1985.[39]
**** Excludes 71 cases of *Hemophilus influenzae* disease of unknown serotype.
Source: Reprinted from *MMWR*, Centers for Disease Control and Prevention.

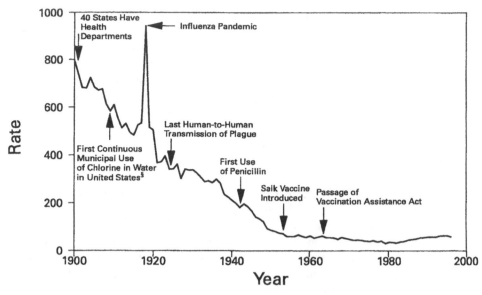

Note: Per 100,000 population per year. Adapted from Armstrong GL, Conn LA, Pinner RW. Trends in infectious disease mortality in the United States during the 20th century. *JAMA*. 1999;281:61–66.
§American Water Works Association. Water chlorination principles and practices: AWWA manual M20. Denver, Colorado: American Water Works Association; 1973.

Figure 1–3 Crude death rate for infectious diseases, United States, 1990–1996. *Source:* Reprinted with permission from *MMWR*, Vol. 48, No. 29, the Centers for Disease Control and Prevention.

development and use of vaccines to prevent infectious diseases and antibiotics for their treatment, along with improved methods for diagnosis were reviewed recently by the Centers for Disease Control and Infection (Figure 1–3). During the twentieth century, infectious disease mortality declined from about 800/100,000 population to under 50/100,000 and accounted for most of the improvement in life expectancy during the century in the United States. In 1900, 30.4% of all deaths occurred in children under 5 years of age. In 1997, the proportion of total mortality in this age group was only 1.4%.[39,40]

The dramatic changes in the incidence and epidemiology of important infectious diseases and the emergence of new infectious diseases during the twentieth century will be elucidated further in the following chapters of the book.

REFERENCES

1. Watts S. *Epidemics and History: Disease, Power and Imperialism*. New Haven, CT: Yale University Press; 1997.

2. Rosen G. *A History of Public Health*. Baltimore: Johns Hopkins University Press; 1993.

3. Temkin, O. *Hippocrates in a World of Pagans and Christians*. Baltimore: Johns Hopkins University Press; 1991.

4. Adams F, trans. *The Genuine Works of Hippocrates, Francis Adams Translation*. Baltimore: Williams & Wilkins; 1939.

5. Sigerist HE. *The Great Doctors*. New York: WW Norton & Company; 1933.

6. Poole JCF, Holladay AJ. Thucydides and the Plague of Athens. *Classic Q.* 1979;29:282–300.

7. Langmuir AD, Northern TD, Solomon J, Ray CG, Petersen E. The Thucydides syndrome. *N Engl J Med.* 1985; 313:1027–1030.

8. Morens DM, Chu MC. The plague of Athens. *N Engl J Med.* 1986;314:855.

9. Holladay AJ. The Thucydides syndrome: another view. *N Engl J Med.* 1986;315:1170–1173.

10. McNeill WH. *Plagues and Peoples.* New York: Doubleday; 1977.

11. Hirst LF. *The Conquest of Plague.* London: Oxford University Press; 1953.

12. Fenner F, Henderson DA, Anita I, Jezek Z, Ladnyl IR. *Smallpox and Its Eradication.* Geneva: World Health Organization; 1988.

13. Pusey EW. *The History and Epidemiology of Syphilis.* Springfield, IL: Charles C Thomas; 1933.

14. Hall MB. *The Scientific Renaissance, 1450–1630.* Mineola, NY: Dover Publications; 1994.

15. Fox JP, Hall CE, Elueback LR. *Epidemiology, Man and Disease.* London: MacMilyan; 1970:19–30.

16. Miller LH. Impact of malaria on genetic polymorphism and genetic diseases in Africans and African Americans. In: Roizman B, ed. *Infectious Diseases in an Age of Change.* Washington, DC: National Academy of Sciences, National Academy Press; 1995:99–111.

17. Bruce-Chwatt LJ, de Zulueta J. *The Rise and Fall of Malaria in Europe: A Historico-Epidemiological Study.* London: Oxford University Press; 1981.

18. Ronald R. *The Prevention of Malaria.* New York: EP Datton Company; 1910.

19. Pasteur L; Eliot CW, ed. *The Physiological Theory of Fermentation in Scientific Papers.* New York: PF Collier and Sons; 1910.

20. Reed W, Carroll J. The prevention of yellow fever. *Med Rec NY.* 1901;60:641–649.

21. Altman LK. *Who Goes First? The Story of Self-Experimentation in Medicine.* New York: Random House; 1986:134.

22. Rosh B. An account of the bilious remitting fever as it appeared in Philadelphia in the summer of 1780. In: *Medical Inquiries and Observations.* Philadelphia: Richard & Hall; 1789.

23. Snow. *On Cholera.* New York: Commonwealth Fund; 1936.

24. William B. *Typhoid Fever: Its Nature, Mode of Spreading and Prevention, London 1873.* New York: Delta Omega; 1931.

25. Semmelweiss IP; Murphy FP, trans-ed. *The Etiology, the Concept and the Prophylaxis of Childbed Fever. Med Classics.* Jan–Apr 1941:5.

26. Panum PL. *Observations Made during the Epidemic of Measles in the Faroe Island in the Year 1846.* Reprinted by the Delta Omega Society. New York, NY: FH Newton; 1940.

27. Nelson KE. Invited commentary on observations on a mumps epidemic in a "virgin" population. *Am J Epidemiol.* 1995;142:221–222.

28. Philips RN, Reinhardt R, Lackman DB. Observations on a mumps epidemic in a "virgin" population. *Am J Hyg.* 1959;69:91–111.

29. Dubini A. Nvove verme intestinalumano (*Ancylostoma duodenale*) constitutente un sestro gemere dei nematoide: proprii delluomo. *Aanali Universali de Medicina* 1843:106;5–13. In: Kean B, Mott KE, Russell AJ, trans. *Tropical Medicine and Parasitology.* Vol. 2. Ithaca, NY: Cornell University Press; 1978:287–291.

30. Looss A. Uber das Eindringen der Ankylostomalarrea in die Meatschliche Haut. *Zeatral blatt for Bakteriologic and Parisitenkunde.* 1898;24:441–448,483–488.

31. Barlow CH. The life cycle of the human intestinal fluke. *Fasciolopsis buski. Am J Hyg.* Monograph no. 4, July 1925.

32. Barlow CH. Experimental ingestion of the ova of *Fasciolopsi buski*; also the ingestion of adult *Fasciolopsis huski* for the purpose of artificial infestation. *J Parasitol.* 1921;8:40–44.

33. Barlow CH, Meleney HE. A voluntary infection with *Schistosoma hematobium. Am J Trop Med.* 1949;29:79–87.

34. Cyde DF, et al. Immunization of man against sporozoite-induced falciparum malaria. *Am J Med Sci.* 1973; 266:169–177.

35. Clyde DF, et al. Immunization of man against falciparum and vivax malaria by use of attenuated sporozoites. *Am J Trop Med Hyg.* 1975;24:397–401.

36. Wilcox WF, ed. *Natural and Political Observation Made upon the Bills of Mortality by John Graunt* (reprint of first ed., 1662). Baltimore: Johns Hopkins University Press; 1937.

37. Dowling HF. *Fighting Infection.* Cambridge, MA: Harvard University Press; 1977.

38. Centers for Disease Control and Prevention. Ten great public health achievements—United States, 1900–1999. *MMWR.* 1999;48:241–248.

39. Batelle Medical Technology Assessment and Policy Research Program, Center for Public Health Research and Evaluation. *A Cost Benefit Analysis of the Measles-Mumps-Rubella (MMR) Vaccine.* Arlington, VA: Batelle; 1994.

40. Centers for Disease Control and Prevention. Ten great public health achievements—United States, 1900–1999, Control of Infectious Diseases. *MMWR.* 1999;48:621–629.

CHAPTER 2

Epidemiology of Infectious Disease: General Principles

Kenrad E. Nelson

Studies of the epidemiology of infectious diseases include evaluation of the factors leading to infection with an organism, factors affecting the transmission of an organism, and those associated with clinically recognizable disease among those who are infected. Many epidemiologic concepts were originally developed in studies of infectious diseases. Some of these fundamental concepts were applied later to the study of noninfectious disease. Among these concepts are:

a. the incubation period, ie, that diseases caused by either an infectious agent or a noninfectious agent, eg, a toxin or carcinogen, have an intrinsic incubation period after contact with the agent before disease occurs, and

b. resistance, ie, that some individuals may have immunity or resistance to infection on a biological basis, ie, from previous infection, immunization, or because of host genetics, and remain uninfected after exposure.

When new epidemics of infectious diseases are described, they are usually first studied and described according to their epidemiologic characteristics. New infectious diseases can be classified according to their epidemiologic, clinical, or microbiologic features. Certainly, knowledge of all of these characteristics is important. However, the epidemiologic features of a disease are of paramount importance for a public health professional or an epidemiologist, who is concerned primarily with controlling or preventing the epidemic spread of an infection. On the other hand, a clinician whose primary role is to treat an individual patient may be more concerned with the clinical symptoms or pathophysiology of the disease. For example, an infectious agent that causes secretory diarrhea will be treated empirically with fluid replacement and symptomatic management of the pathophysiology, irrespective of how the infection was acquired or what the organism is. A microbiologist may be primarily interested in the characteristics of the organism and may ask, How can the organism be isolated or how can infection be diagnosed or confirmed in the laboratory? Is it possible to prepare a vaccine or treat the infection with an antibiotic? What are the essential growth requirements of the organism?

The control, treatment, and prevention of an epidemic usually involves the cooperative efforts of all three groups of specialists: epidemiologists, clinicians, and microbiologists. However, each has a unique orientation and contribution. This focus can best be appreciated by considering how infectious diseases are classified by each specialist.

THE CLASSIFICATION OF INFECTIOUS DISEASES

1. Clinicians tend to classify infectious diseases according to their most common or most important clinical manifestation or organ systems that are primarily affected. An example of a clinical classification is given in Table 2–1.

Table 2–1 Clinical Classification of Infections

Classification	Infection
a. Diarrheal Diseases	Secretory
	Invasive
b. Respiratory Diseases	Upper respiratory
	Lower respiratory
c. Central Nervous System Infection	Meningitis (bacterial vs. aseptic)
	Encephalitis
	Abscess
d. Cardiovascular Infection	Endocarditis
	Myocarditis
	Vasculitis
e. Sepsis	Disseminated

2. Microbiologists classify infectious diseases according to the characteristics of the causative organism. An example of a typical microbiologic classification of infectious diseases is shown in Table 2–2.

3. Epidemiologists usually classify infectious diseases according to two important epidemiologic characteristics—their means of transmission and the reservoir of the organism.

When a new disease appears on the scene, the detailed microbiologic characteristics of the organism usually are not known. The full range of symptoms that may occur after infection often is appreciated only later, after detailed clinical studies of many patients have been carried out. For example, the fact that infection with *Borrelia burgdorferii*, the cause of Lyme disease, was responsible not only for the classical skin lesion, erythema chronica migrans (ECM), but also for acute and chronic arthritis, vascular and cardiac disease, and neurologic symptoms, including Bell's palsy and encephalitis, was not appreciated initially. In fact, the full range of clinical manifestations of infection with *B. burgdorferii* is still being defined. Infectious diseases can be classified according to their means of transmis-sion into five distinct categories, as shown in Table 2–3.

The second means for the epidemiologic classification of infectious diseases is according to

Table 2–2 Microbiologic Classification of Infectious Diseases

Classification	Organism
a. Bacterial	Gram-negative
	Gram-positive
b. Viral	DNA virus
	RNA virus
	Enveloped vs. nonenveloped viruses
c. Fungal	Disseminated (biphasic)
	Localized
d. Parasitic	Protozoa
	Helminths
	Trematodes
	Cestodes
e. Prion	Protein

Table 2–3 Means of Transmission of Infectious Diseases and Their Characteristic Features

Transmission	Characteristics
1. Contact	Requires direct or indirect contact (eg, indirect = infected fomite, blood, or body fluid; direct = skin or sexual contact)
2. Food- or water-borne	Ingestion of contaminated food (outbreaks may be large and dispersed, depending on distribution of food)
3. Airborne	Inhalation of contaminated air
4. Vector-borne	Dependent on biology of the vector (mosquito, tick, snail, etc), as well as the infectivity of the organism
5. Perinatal	Similar to contact infection; however, the contact may occur in utero during pregnancy or at the time of delivery

their major reservoirs in nature. If one is aware of the reservoir of the agent, in addition to the means of transmission, it is generally possible to develop a strategy to prevent transmission, even when the microbiologic characteristics of the organism are not known. The demonstration of the water reservoir of cholera by John Snow in London in 1853 preceded the identification of the *Vibrio* cholera by Robert Koch in 1884.[1] The epidemiologic information alone was sufficient to develop public health strategies to limit exposure to contaminated water and prevent human infections. Similarly, the demonstration of the importance of human carriers of *Salmonella typhi* as the important reservoir in outbreaks of typhoid fever by Budd in 1858 antedated by 22 years the isolation of the organism in the laboratory by Eberth in 1880. Walter Reed succeeded in transmitting yellow fever by the bite of infected *Aedes aegypti* mosquitoes in 1901. It wasn't until 1928 that Stokes and colleagues isolated the causative virus in the laboratory. In more recent times, investigation of the epidemic at the American Legion convention in Philadelphia in 1976 demonstrated that the outbreak of Legionnaires' disease was due to airborne spread of microorganisms from a contaminated reservoir, the air conditioning system in the Bellevue-Stratford Hotel, and suggested that

further infections could be prevented by avoiding exposures to the air in the hotel.[2] The implicated organism, *Legionella pneumophila*, wasn't isolated and characterized in the laboratory until 1978 by McDade and Sheppard at the Centers for Disease Control and Prevention (CDC).

When organisms are classified according to their reservoirs in nature, four general categories are often considered:

1. human
2. animal (often called *zoonoses*)
3. soil
4. water

Some common examples of infectious diseases classified according to their reservoir are shown in Table 2–4.

Knowledge of the reservoir often is essential prior to devising rational and effective means of preventing transmission of infectious diseases. Prior to John Snow's demonstration that contaminated water was the reservoir of *Vibrio cholerae* in the outbreak in London in the 1850s, the predominant theories were that miasma, or exposure to foul or malodorous air, was the critical exposure leading to infection. However, there were no successful efforts to control the outbreak that were based on the miasma theory.

Table 2–4 Classification of Infectious Organisms by Their Reservoir in Nature

Reservoir	Some Typical Organisms
a. Human	*Treponema pallidum, Neisseria gonorrhoeae*, HIV, Hepatitis B and C virus, *Shigella, S. typhi*
b. Animals (zoonoses)	Rabies, *Yersinia pestis, Leptospira*, nontyphoid *Salmonella*, Brucella
c. Soil	*Histoplasma capsulatum* (and other systemic fungi), *Clostridium tetani, Clostridium botulinum*
d. Water	*Legionella, Pseudomonas aeruginosa, Mycobacterium marinum*

When Snow demonstrated that attack rates of cholera were highest in those receiving their water from one particular water company and subsequently terminated an epidemic by closing down the pump at one water source, the evidence was persuasive.[1]

In the Philadelphia outbreak of Legionnaires' disease, the critical exposure was to the contaminated air in the hotel. It was especially noteworthy in this epidemic that no secondary cases occurred among the household contacts of ill patients with pneumonia who did not visit or stay in the hotel.[2] Subsequent study of this outbreak and subsequent Legionellosis outbreaks have found that aerosolization of water contaminated with *L. pneumophila*, often from a cooling tower, was the critical exposure leading to infection and disease.[3-5] Studies of water from a variety of sources have found that contamination with various pathogenic species of *Legionella* is quite common, even in the absence of human illness.[6] Human infection usually requires inhalation of a contaminated droplet of a small particle-sized aerosol (less than 5 μ in diameter) so that the organism can reach the lower respiratory system. However, in the case of *Legionella*, procedures to disinfect the reservoir usually are only undertaken when aerosolization is posing a risk of infection and disease to humans. The water can be decontaminated by heating to temperatures above 120°F, and growth of the organism is inhibited below 70°F.[7]

Infectious Diseases Transmitted by More Than One Means

Some organisms may be spread by several different means, depending on the epidemiologic circumstances. Therefore, it is important for an epidemiologist to keep an open mind to detect unusual epidemiologic features of an infection. A few examples of infectious diseases that have been spread by multiple means are described below.

Tularemia

Perhaps a typical example of a disease that can be spread by more than one means is tularemia, which can be acquired by the bite of infected ticks or deer flies,[8] by contact with infected rabbits or other animals during the hunting season,[9,10] or by inhalation of an aerosol.[11,12] Also, nosocomial infection among microbiology laboratory workers has been reported from inhalation of infected aerosols of the causative organism, *Francisella tularensis.*[13] Curiously, none of the investigators who have studied epidemics of tularemia have found evidence that human-to-human transmission has occurred.[14]

Plague

Plague, the disease that has been associated with perhaps the most serious and extensive epidemic in human history, is caused by the plague bacillus, *Yersinia pestis*. The disease is a zoonotic disease of rodents that is transmitted to humans and other mammalian hosts from infected rodents by rat fleas. Percutaneous inoculation of the plague bacillus in humans initiates inflammation of lymph nodes draining the inoculation site, resulting in bubonic plague. Bloodstream invasion may lead to septicemic plague or to infection of other organ systems, such as the lung or meninges. Involvement of the lungs may result in pneumonic plague, which can then be transmitted from person to person via the respiratory route.

Historically, many epidemics of plague have spread rapidly through populations, causing very high mortality. The earliest description of plague occurred in the sixth century A.D. in Egypt, and the epidemic spread throughout North Africa and into Europe. Epidemic plague reappeared in the Far East in the fourteenth century and subsequently spread to Europe. During the "Great Plague" epidemic in London, which peaked in August and September 1665, 7,000 deaths per week were reported in a population of an estimated 500,000 persons. For unknown reasons, plague gradually disappeared from Europe in the eighteenth century, and the entire continent was free of plague by 1840.[15] Zinsser considers the disappearance of epidemics of plague from Europe to be one of the great mysteries of the epidemiology of infectious diseases.[16]

However, epidemics of plague have occurred in Asia in the late nineteenth century and more recently in Vietnam, during the war between 1962 and 1975.[17] An epidemic of plague was reported in India in 1994.[18] Sporadic cases of plague have occurred throughout the American Southwest for the past several decades, related to epizootics in infected prairie dogs.[19,20] The organism was first isolated by Yersin in Hong Kong in 1894.[21] A vaccine is available, but its efficacy in preventing pneumonic plague is unknown.

Anthrax

Anthrax is an infection with *Bacillus anthracis*, a gram-positive spore-forming organism that is a zoonotic disease in herbivorous animals. It can be transmitted to humans from contact with infected animals and has three clinical forms in humans: cutaneous, gastrointestinal, and inhalation anthrax.

The organisms from infected animals most often infect humans by contact with contaminated animal hides or pelts; this disease has been called *Woolsorter's disease*.[22] Infection can occur also by inoculation of organisms into the skin during butchering of an infected animal; this type of exposure usually leads to cutaneous anthrax, consisting of a black eschar on the skin with swelling and inflammation of the draining lymphatics. Consumption of meat from an infected animal leads to gastrointestinal anthrax, which has a much higher mortality than does cutaneous anthrax. Inhalation anthrax occurs when an infectious aerosol of *B. anthracis* spores is inhaled and germinates in the pulmonary lymphatic tissues. This form of anthrax is rare, which is fortunate because it usually is rapidly fatal.

An epidemic of inhalation anthrax occurred in persons living in Sverdlovsk, Union of Soviet Socialist Republics in April and May 1979. There were at least 96 cases and 66 deaths. The outbreak also affected cattle within 50 km of the city. Interestingly, Sverdlovsk was known to have a military facility that was suspected of manufacturing biologic weapons, including anthrax spores, for potential use in warfare. Initially, the Soviet authorities maintained that this outbreak was from gastrointestinal exposure due to the consumption of contaminated meat from cattle that had died of anthrax. However, in 1992, Meselson and colleagues visited the site of the epidemic and were able to conduct an epidemiologic investigation, together with Russian scientists. Their study found that all of the human cases were living or working in a narrow belt south of the city on the day the outbreak occurred.[23] Furthermore, the animal deaths also occurred in this belt, up to 50 km distant (Figure 2–1). The wind pattern on the day of the outbreak could explain the geographic distribution of cases. Subsequently, evidence was discov-

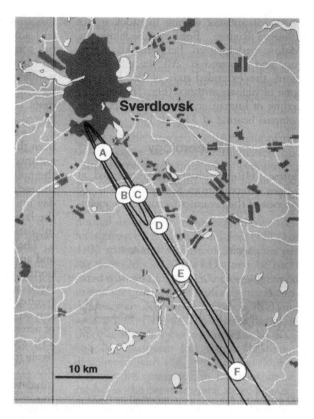

Figure 2–1 Russian villages with animal anthrax. Six villages where livestock died of anthrax in April 1979 are shown. Settled areas are shown in gray, roads in white, and calculated contours of constant dosage in black. *Source:* Reprinted with permission from M. Messelson et al., The Sverdlovsk Anthrax Outbreak of 1979, *Science*, Vol. 266, pp. 1202–1208, Copyright 1994, American Association for the Advancement of Science.

ered that many of the human cases had pneumonic anthrax. They concluded that this outbreak, the largest outbreak of human inhalation anthrax ever recorded, was due to an infectious aerosol emanating from the military facility. One very interesting finding in their study was that human cases continued to occur for up to 6 weeks after this point source exposure. Apparently, spores were inhaled and continued to germinate and cause disease for several weeks after they were inhaled. This outbreak has raised considerable concern among scientists and policy makers about the potential for the use of aerosolized *B. anthracis* spores as an agent of biologic terrorism.

Rabies

Rabies is a nearly uniformly fatal infection of the central nervous system that is almost always transmitted by a bite from an animal infected with the rabies virus. Historically, rabies has nearly always been acquired by a bite from an infected dog, skunk, fox, bat, or other animal. It has been regarded as a typical contact-transmitted infection, in that percutaneous inoculation of rabies virus by a bite is usually required. Nevertheless, a few persons have developed rabies from exposure to infected aerosols in caves harbored by many infected bats.[24] Also, rabies has occurred in a laboratory worker who was exposed to an infectious aerosol[25] and in persons who have received corneal transplants from a donor who died of undiagnosed rabies.[26] In recent years, in the United States, only 2–3 cases have occurred annually; however, reported bite exposures in these cases has been unusual. Of the 32 cases of rabies that were diagnosed in the United States between 1980 and 1996, 25 (78%) had no history of a bite exposure.[27] Some of these non–bite-transmitted cases in the United States have been in persons exposed in the same room (or closed space) to an infected bat; presumably, the transmission in these cases was by aerosol. Genetic analysis of the viruses has shown that 17 (53%) of these cases in the United States were related to rabies viruses found in insectivorous bats.

Brucellosis

Brucellosis is an infectious disease of humans acquired through contact with an infected animal, ie, a zoonosis. Four species of *Brucellae* have infected humans, *B. abortus* (from cattle), *B. melitensis* (from goats or sheep), *B. suis* (from pigs), and *B. canis* (from dogs); human infections with the two other known species, *B. ovis* (from sheep) and *B. neotomae* (from desert wood rats), have not been reported. Clinically, the most serious human infections are seen with *B. melitensis*. However, in the early decades of the twentieth century infections with *B. abortus* were common, and these infections often were acquired by the consumption of contaminated milk from infected cows. However, after World War II, the U.S. Department of Agriculture undertook a campaign to eliminate milk-borne brucellosis as a human health problem in the United States. The program included testing of cattle for *B. abortus* and slaughtering of infected animals or animals from infected herds, and pasteurization of all milk and dairy products.[28] This program was quite successful. More than 6,000 cases of human brucellosis were reported each year at the start of this program; the rate was 4.5 cases per 100,000 population in 1948. In the 1990s, only about 100 cases per year were reported; 0.05 cases per 100,000 population were

reported in 1993. Furthermore, in recent years, the cases usually had an occupation that directly exposed them to infected animals, such as slaughterhouse workers, farmers, or veterinarians. Brucellosis in these workers was acquired by direct contact with infected animals, not through consumption of infected milk. Also, *B. suis* infections from infected pigs have become proportionally more common, because the brucellosis control program was directed at eliminating the disease in cattle.

Transmission of Microbial Agents by Transfusions

There is evidence that several microbial agents can be transmitted by blood transfusion or contaminated injection, if exposure occurs during a time when the organisms are present in the blood stream. Hepatitis B virus, Hepatitis C vrius, and HIV are commonly transmitted by the transfusion of blood or blood products. *Trypanosoma cruzii*, a protozoan parasite that causes Chagas' disease, is usually transmitted to humans by the bite of a reduviid bug but can be transmitted by blood transfusion from a carrier.[29] Malaria usually is caused by the transmission of one of four species of *Plasmodium* parasites by the bite of an infected female *Anopheline* mosquito, but it can also be transmitted by blood transfusion or to an infant by perinatal transmission. Hepatitis A virus is generally transmitted by ingestion of contaminated food or water but can be transmitted by blood transfusion during the brief viremic stage early in the infection.

Perinatal Infections

Infections of an infant may be acquired from the mother in utero via placental transfer, during passage through the birth canal, or in the postpartum period.

Rubella

The dramatic effect of rubella infections during the first trimester of pregnancy in producing congenital anomalies in the infant was first reported by Sir Norman Gregg following an outbreak of rubella in Australia in 1940.[30] Gregg noted ocular defects and cardiac lesions in the affected infants. Subsequently, these findings were confirmed by studies during rubella outbreaks in Australia, the United States, and the United Kingdom. These studies further defined the congenital rubella syndrome (CRS) from intrauterine exposure to rubella during the first trimester of pregnancy, to include cataracts and other ocular abnormalities, cardiac defects, deafness, microcephaly, and mental retardation. Infants exposed during the first trimester of pregnancy carry a risk of the congenital rubella syndrome of nearly 90%; during the early second trimester, the risk of congenital abnormalities declines to 20–40% and often involves only deafness.

In 1962, the rubella virus was isolated by investigators at Harvard University[31] and independently by scientists at the Walter Reed Army Institute of Research.[32] Shortly thereafter, in 1964, a major epidemic of rubella and CRS occurred in the United States.[33] An attenuated live rubella virus vaccine was developed and licensed in the United States in 1969.[34] Subsequently, congenital rubella infections have become rare in the United States, due to routine immunization of infants and screening and selective immunization of susceptible women of child-bearing age.

Cytomegalovirus

Cytomegalovirus (CMV) infections during the first trimester of pregnancy are known to lead to congenital malformation, especially of the central nervous system. Cytomegalovirus was first isolated in human fibroblast cultures in 1956.[35–37] It is possible to screen pregnant women for susceptibility to infection during pregnancy. Epidemiologic studies suggest that CMV infection may occur in about 1% of all US births, or about 40,000 infants annually.[38] However, in most instances, these infections are asymptomatic. A national surveillance registry was established in the United States in 1990 by the CDC to monitor congenital CMV infec-

tions.[39] The most common clinical manifestation reported was petchiae, observed in 50% of cases, which was often accompanied by hepatosplenomegaly, intracranial calcification, and thrombocytopenia.

Herpes Simplex Virus

In contrast to CMV and rubella, in utero infection with herpes simplex virus (HSV) is rare, and when it does occur, it is most likely to lead to a miscarriage, rather than a congenital malformation. However, infants can be infected when passing through the birth canal if the mother has an active infection, especially with HSV type 2 (HSV-2), which causes recurrent genital tract infection. When the mother has an active HSV infection at the time of delivery, the infant can develop a generalized infection, which is quite serious. The risk to the newborn is higher when the mother has a primary HSV infection than when the HSV is a recurrence; the risk to the newborn is about 40% when exposed to a mother with primary infection, compared with 2–5% when the mother has a recurrent infection. In the latter situation, the infant's risk is modified by maternal passive transfer of antibodies to HSV-2 and by lower maternal viral load. Cesarean section is recommended to prevent neonatal herpes in children born to women with active HSV at the time of delivery. However, most cases of neonatal HSV occur where the mother was not identified as having active HSV infection. For example, during an 18-month hospital-based surveillance study, CDC identified 184 cases of neonatal herpes but only 22% of the mothers had a history of genital HSV infection, and only 9% had lesions at the time of delivery.[40]

Toxoplasmosis

Congenital infection with *Toxoplasma gondii* occurs when a pregnant woman develops infection, especially early in pregnancy. Clinical manifestations in the infant at birth include a

maculopapular rash, generalized lymphadenopathy, hepatomegaly, splenomegaly, jaundice,
or thrombocytopenia. Also, the infant can develop meningoencephalitis with cerebrospinal
fluid abnormalities, hydrocephalus, microcephaly, chorioretinitis, and/or convulsions. However, congenital infection is usually asymptomatic at birth, although sequelae can become
apparent several years later. Sequelae of congenital toxoplasma infection include mental retardation and learning disability. Also, ocular
toxoplasmosis most often results from reactivation of a congenital infection but it can occur
from an acquired infection, as well. Ocular toxoplasmosis usually occurs among adults.

Syphilis

Syphilis is caused by infection with the spirochete, *Treponema pallidum*. Syphilis is usually
transmitted sexually but can be transmitted by
the perinatal (congenital) route by infection
through the placenta, especially in the second
and third trimester, or, more rarely, transmission
can occur during delivery by contact of an infant
with the mucosa of a woman with primary or
secondary syphilis during the birth process.
Congenital syphilis can be asymptomatic or it
may manifest as multisystem involvement, including osteitis, hepatitis, lymphadenopathy,
pneumonitis, mucocutaneous lesions, anemia,
and hemorrhage. Late manifestation may involve the central nervous system, bones, teeth,
and/or eyes. Rates of congenital syphilis parallel
the rates of primary and secondary syphilis in
women and can be prevented by treatment of infected pregnant women with penicillin, to which
the organism is uniformly sensitive. Rates of
congenital syphilis have increased in the late
1980s and early 1990s, in part related to the epidemic of crack cocaine use in the United
States.[41]

Because newborns infected with each of these
agents have similar clinical symptoms, pediatri-
cians often consider all of them in the differential diagnosis of perinatal infections. The syndrome of congenital infection is often referred to
by the abbreviation *TORCHS* to signify the most
common etiologies, ie, toxoplasmosis, rubella,
CMV, HSV, syphilis.

Hepatitis B Virus

Women who are carriers of hepatitis B virus
(HBV) may transmit the virus to their infants in
utero or at the time of birth (peripartum). Infection of a newborn with HBV carries a very high
risk of chronic infection, with the possibility of
subsequent chronic active hepatitis, cirrhosis, or
liver cancer when carriage persists for decades.
Most perinatal transmission of HBV can be prevented by screening pregnant women for
HBsAg and administering hepatitis B immunoglobulin and a course of HBV vaccine to the infants of HBsAg carriers, beginning immediately
after birth.

Human Immunodeficiency Virus

Human immunodeficiency virus (HIV) is an
important viral infection that can be transmitted
perinatally from an infected woman to her newborn infant. Worldwide, the number of infected
infants born each year is estimated to be about
500,000. Recently, a clinical trial of zidovudine
given to infected women during pregnancy and
labor and to the newborn for the first 6 weeks of
life (ACTG trial 076) has shown a 74% reduction
in perinatal transmission associated with the use
of AZT during the second and third trimesters of
pregnancy, during labor and delivery, and in the
infant for the first six weeks of life.[42] A shorter
course of zidovudine starting at 34–36 weeks of
pregnancy and given only to HIV-infected pregnant women (not to the infants) in Thailand was
associated with a 51% reduction in the rate of
perinatal transmission.[43] Another study showed
that administration of nevaripine, a non-nucleo-
side reverse transcriptase inhibitor, to the mother
at the onset of labor and twice to the infant in the
first few days of life was associated with a reduction in HIV transmission.[44] The remarkable suc-

cess of the use of antiretroviral drugs given to infected women during pregnancy in reducing the perinatal transmission of HIV is one of the major recent advances in the prevention of acquired immune deficiency syndrome (AIDS). The epidemiology of HIV/AIDS is discussed further in the chapter on AIDS.

Other Infectious Agents

The most important infectious diseases that are transmitted by the perinatal route are discussed above; however, there is some evidence of transmission of several other agents, such as parvovirus B-19, varicella-zoster virus, and others. The most common agents incriminated in

perinatal infection and the effects of perinatal infection with these agents on the fetus and newborn infant are listed in Table 2–5.

EPIDEMIOLOGIC CHARACTERISTICS OF INFECTIOUS DISEASES

Incubation Period

The incubation period of an infectious disease is the time between exposure to an infectious agent and the onset of symptoms or signs of infection. Each infectious disease has a typical incubation period, which requires multiplication of the infectious agent to a threshold necessary

Table 2–5 Effects of Transplacental Fetal Infection

Organism or Disease	Prematurity	Effect of Infection on the Fetus and Newborn Infant			
		Intrauterine Growth Retardation and Low Birth Weight	Developmental Anomalies	Congenital Disease	Persistent Postnatal Infection
Viruses					
Rubella	–	+	–	+	+
Cytomegalovirus	+	+	+	+	–
Herpes simplex	+	–	–	+	+
Varicella-zoster	–	(+)	–	+	–
Mumps	–	–	–	(+)	–
Rubeola	+	–	–	+	–
Vaccinia	–	–	–	+	–
Smallpox	+	–	–	+	–
Coxsackieviruses B	–	–	(–)	+	–
Echoviruses	–	–	–	–	–
Polioviruses	–	–	–	–	–
Influenza	–	–	–	–	–
Hepatitis B	+	–	–	+	+
Human immuno- deficiency virus	(+)	(+)	(–)	+	+
Lymphocytic chorio- meningitis virus	–	–	–	+	–
Parvovirus	–	–	–	(+)	–

+, Evidence for effect; –, no evidence for effect; (–), association of effect with infection has been suggested and is under consideration.

Source: Reprinted with permission from Epidemiologic Concepts and Methods, in *Viral Infections of Humans,* 4th Ed., A.S. Evans & R.A. Kaslow, eds., p. 30, Copyright © 1997, Plenum Publishing Corporation.

to produce symptoms in the host. The incubation period for infectious diseases shows some variation, which occurs for a variety of reasons, including the dose or inoculum of the infectious agent, the route of inoculation, and the rate of replication of the organism. Even when numerous persons are exposed at the same time to a similar inoculum of the same strain of an infectious agent, such as consumption of food contaminated with *Salmonella* at a picnic, the length of the incubation period varies between individuals. A plot of the incubation period for persons exposed at the same time usually follows a log normal distribution. The antilogarithm of 1 standard deviation from the mean log incubation period has been referred to as the *dispersion factor* by Sartwell.[45] The dispersion factor multiplied by the mean log of the incubation period will define an interval above which 16% of the periods will fall, and the mean divided by the dispersion factor will define the period below which 16% will occur. Even diseases with very long incubation periods have been shown to follow similar patterns of distribution of their incubation periods. A recent study of the incubation periods of AIDS found that a log normal distribution reasonably described the incubation period of this disease, as well.[46]

The usual ranges of the incubation periods for a number of infectious diseases are shown in Figure 2–2. These incubation periods range from 6 to 12 hours for *B. cereus* and staphylococcal food poisoning to 5–10 years for AIDS and leprosy. The extrinsic incubation period applies to vector-borne infections; it is the time that a vector-borne agent requires for maturation to infectivity in the vector before it becomes infectious to humans. The extrinsic incubation period also has a medium and range that are unique to each organism. Also, the extrinsic incubation period can be affected by environmental conditions. For example, when *A. aegypti* mosquitoes were infected with dengue type 2 virus and held at 30° C, the mean extrinsic incubation period before they become infectious was 12 days, whereas at 32–35°C, they became infectious after only 7 days.[47] The extrinsic incubation periods for various species of *Plasmodium* are discussed in more detail in the chapter on Malaria.

Biologic Characteristics of the Organism

Infectivity

Infectivity is defined as the ability of an agent to cause infection in a susceptible host. The basic measure of infectivity is the minimum number of infectious particles required to establish infection. In diseases spread from person to person, the proportion of susceptible individuals who develop infection after exposure—the secondary attack rate—is a measure of the infectivity of an organism (Table 2–6).

Pathogenicity

Pathogenicity refers to the ability of a microbial agent to induce disease. Diseases such as rabies, smallpox, measles, chicken pox, and rhinovirus colds have high pathogenicity. Others, such as polio and arborvirus (mosquito-borne) infections, have low pathogenicity.

Virulence

Some dictionaries use the terms *virulence* and *pathogenicity* interchangeably. However, it is useful to consider them to be separate properties of an infectious agent. *Virulence* can be defined as the severity of the disease after infection occurs. Although smallpox and rhinoviruses both usually cause symptoms (both are pathogenic), smallpox infections are much more virulent. Virulence can best be measured by the case fatality rate or as the proportion of clinical cases that develop severe disease. It is possible to classify organisms based on their infectivity, pathogenicity, and virulence. Only a few diseases, eg, smallpox, airborne anthrax, and ebola virus, will be classified as ranking high in all three characteristics. Several diseases are ranked by these characteristics in Table 2–6. It is important to recognize that these properties of an infection may change over time under different circumstances. At one time, syphilis and streptococcal infections were highly virulent infections with

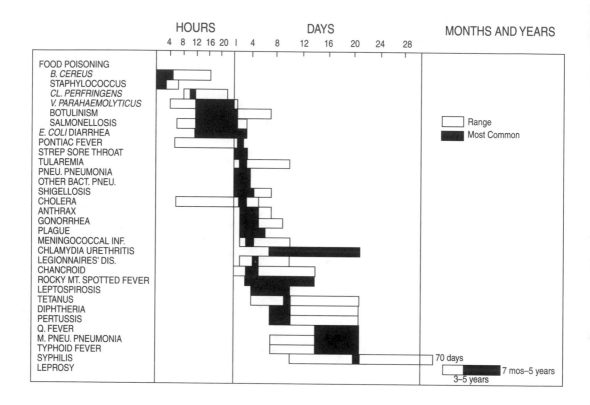

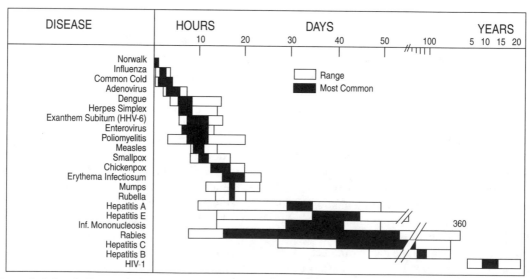

Figure 2–2 Incubation periods of common bacterial diseases (*top panel*) and viral diseases (*bottom panel*). *Source:* Reprinted with permission from *Viral Infections of Humans*, 4th Edition, A.S. Evans and R.A. Kaslow, eds., p. 20, Copyright © 1997, Plenum Publishing Corporation.

Table 2–6 Ranking of Infection by Infectivity, Pathogenicity, and Virulence

Severity*	Infectivity (Secondary Attack Rate = Ill/Number Exposed)	Pathogenicity (Illness Rate = Ill/Number Infected)	Virulence (Severe/Fatal Cases) / Total Cases
High	smallpox measles chicken pox	smallpox rabies measles chicken pox common cold	rabies smallpox tuberculosis leprosy
Intermediate	rubella mumps common cold	rubella mumps	poliomyelitis measles
Low	tuberculosis	poliomyelitis tuberculosis	measles chicken pox
Very low	leprosy	leprosy	rubella common cold

* The "severity" of an infection varies by how it is being measured.

Source: Reprinted with the permission of Simon & Schuster from *Epidemiology: Man and Disease* by John P. Fox, Carrie Hall & Lila R. Elveback. Copyright © 1970 Macmillan Publishing Company.

high mortality rates, but these diseases are now much less virulent. Changes in the epidemiologic characteristics of infectious diseases will be discussed in greater detail later in this chapter and elsewhere in this book.

Immunogenicity

Immunogenicity is the ability of an organism to produce an immune response after an infection that is capable of providing protection against reinfection with the same or a similar organism. Some organisms, such as measles, polio, HBV, or rubella, lead to solid, life-long immunity after an infection. Others, such as *Neisseria gonorrhoeae* or *Plasmodium falciparum,* are weakly immunogenic, and reinfection commonly occurs. Studies of the antigens that produce protective immunity after natural infections often have led to the development of effective vaccines. It should be noted that some microorganisms may provoke an immune response that is not protective from future infections. In a sense, they are immunogenic. However, sometimes these immune responses even may be deleterious to the host. Several types of

group A streptococci can provoke an immune response that leads to glomerulonephritis or acute rheumatic fever because of cross-reactive antibodies elicited in response to the streptococcal infection that react with endocardial or glomerular basement membrane antigens. In other instances, antibodies may occur that are markers of a previous or current infection but do not provide immunity to the organism or terminate an ongoing infection. These antibodies are often called *binding antibodies*, and they react to nonneutralizing antigens (or epitopes) of the organism. Examples of antibodies of this type are found in patients with hepatitis C virus infection, HIV infection, and HSV-2 infection. Persons with these antibodies have been or are infected with the virus and have antibodies but are not immune.

Inapparent Infections

An inapparent infection is an infection that can be documented by isolation of an organism by culture, demonstration of nucleic acid by polymerase chain reaction (PCR) amplification, or by demonstrating a specific immune response in a person who remains asymptomatic. The proportion of individuals with asymptomatic or clinically inapparent infections is a measure of the pathogenicity of the organism, as defined above. Inapparent infections are quite common in many infections and may play an important role in the propagation of an epidemic in some circumstances. The proportion of infected individuals who do not develop symptoms varies in different organisms. For example, most polio infections are inapparent. Also, inapparent nasopharyngeal carriage of meningococci is quite common during an epidemic due to this organism. Identification and treatment of carriers of meningococci or *Staphylococcus aureus* have been shown to help control epidemic transmission, because healthy carriers may play an important role in transmission. In the United States, persons who convert their tuberculin skin test and are infected but asymptomatic carriers of *Mycobacteriun tuberculosis* are often treated to prevent clinically active tuberculosis from de-

veloping later in their life and subsequent spread of infection to their contacts. On the other hand, inapparent infections with some organisms are quite rare. Most persons with measles, varicella, smallpox, or hanta virus infection are symptomatic. The proportion of infections that are symptomatic is of considerable importance in understanding the transmission during an epidemic and in designing methods to control epidemic or endemic transmission. The proportion of infections that are clinically inapparent among individuals infected with some important organisms is shown in Table 2–7.

The Carrier State

The epidemiologic importance of the asymptomatic carrier in the transmission of infectious diseases has been recognized for some time. An early classic example was an Irish cook in New York City in the early 1900s, Mary Mallon, who became known as "Typhoid Mary." She was quite healthy but had worked as a cook in many

Table 2–7 Subclinical/Clinical Ratio in Selected Viral Infections (Inapparent/Apparent Ratio)

Virus	Clinical Feature	Age at Infection (Years)	Estimated Subclinical/Clinical Ratio	Percentage of Infection with Clinical Features
Poliomyelitis	Paralysis	Child	±1000: 1	0.1–1
Epstein-Barr	Heterophil-positive infectious mononucleosis	1–5 6–15 16–25	>100: 1 10–100: 1 2–3: 1	1 1–10 35–50
Hepatitis A	Jaundice	<5 5–9 10–15 Adult	20: 1 11: 1 7: 1 2–3: 1	5 10 14 35–50
Rubella	Rash	5–20	2: 1	50
Influenza	Fever, cough	Young adult	1.5: 1	60
Measles	Rash, fever	5–20	1: 99	95
Rabies	CNS symptoms	Any age	0: 100	100

Source: Reprinted with permission from *Viral Infections of Humans*, 4th Ed., A.S. Evans & R.A. Kaslow, eds., p. 25, Copyright © 1997, Plenum Publishing Corporation.

homes where the residents developed typhoid fever after she was hired. Eventually, 53 cases of typhoid fever were traced to her. After she was located and cultures of her stool consistently grew *S. typhi*, she was confined and not allowed to work in food service between 1907 and 1910. After her release, she disappeared and changed her name. Two years later, outbreaks of typhoid fever involving over 200 persons were detected in hospitals in New York and New Jersey that were traced to her.[48] This remarkable story illustrates the potential importance of the carrier state in the transmission of typhoid fever. Patients infected with *S. typhi* may carry the organism in their gall bladders and excrete the organism in their stool for many years. Generally, antibiotic therapy is ineffective in curing their infections but many chronic carriers can be cured by cholecystectomy.[49]

Another, more modern example is that of "patient zero," who was at the center of a large cluster of men who developed Kaposi's sarcoma (KS), with or without *Pneumocystis carinii* pneumonia (PCP), in 1980–1981. This patient was a male homosexual flight attendant who had visited several large U.S. cities. He had sexual contact with all of the men who later became ill. This cluster of cases of KS and PCP was one of the early outbreaks of AIDS in the United States.[50] The carrier state may be of epidemiologic importance in any infectious disease that is transmitted from person to person. However, the average length of the carrier state, the site of replication and infectivity of the organism, and the usual means of spread determine the epidemiologic importance of asymptomatic carriers.

Outbreaks have been documented from chronic carriers in the respiratory tract, stool, genital tract, or blood. Nosocomial transmission from hospital workers to patients, from one patient to another, or from patients to health care workers is common. Currently, transmission of antibiotic-resistant staphylococci by healthy carriers of these organisms is of major concern in hospitals in the United States. Patients who are chronic carriers of Hepatitis B virus pose a significant risk to health care workers. As a result,

use of HBV vaccine is routinely recommended for health care professionals who are likely to be exposed. These issues are covered in more detail in the chapter on Nosocomial Infection.

Transfusion-Transmitted Infection

The transmission of infections by transfusion has received increasing attention in the last 20 years. Although transfusion-transmitted HBV was recognized for several decades, the introduction of screening of donors for HBsAg in 1973 reduced this risk. Subsequently, it became apparent that after screening of blood donors for hepatitis virus was introduced, posttransfusion hepatitis declined to about half of the previous rate but was not eliminated. The hepatitis C virus was identified and screening implemented in 1990. Also, the occurrence of HIV infection and AIDS among transfusion recipients and hemophiliacs has highlighted the risks of the transmission of infection by transfusion of blood or blood products from healthy carriers.

Currently, blood donors undergo extensive questioning about their risks to a variety of infectious agents, and they are screened for the presence of several pathogens. Pooled plasma products also undergo several viral inactivation steps and are heat-treated prior to their use. Nevertheless, the list of agents that may possibly be transmitted by the transfusion of blood or blood products continues to expand (Exhibit 2–1).

The Host–Parasite Relationship

Patterns of Natural History

After infection occurs, the subsequent course or natural history of an infection can be quite variable. Many infections are characterized by acute symptoms, some of which may be severe and even terminate fatally. In some infections, the proportion of patients with asymptomatic or clinically inapparent infections varies, but once the acute phase is over, the patient is immune to reinfection with the same agent. The common childhood contagious diseases, such as measles, mumps, and rubella, are characterized by this type of natural history.

Exhibit 2–1 Infections Transmitted by Transfusion

A. Viruses
  1. HIV, HTLVI/II
  2. HBV, HCV, HAV (rare)
  3. Parvovirus B-19
  4. CMV
  5. KSHV (HHV-8) (unproven)
  6. Others
B. Bacteria
  1. *T. pallidum* (rare)
  2. *Y. enterocolitica*
  3. Various gram-positive organisms by platelet transfusion (especially)
  4. *Ehrlichea* (rare)
C. Parasites
  1. *Trypanosoma cruzi*
  2. *Plasmodium* species
  3. *Babesia necrotica*
D. Other agents
  1. New variant Creutzfeldt-Jakob Disease prion (unproven)

In other infections, some patients may develop chronic or recurring infection, and others may recover and develop lasting immunity. Hepatitis B virus and herpes virus types 1 and 2 typify this type of natural history. Infection with some agents may lead to chronic sequelae, due to an autoimmune reaction or chronic tissue damage that occurs after the acute infection has subsided and without persistence of the organism or chronic infection. Poststreptococcal glomerulonephritis or rheumatic fever are typical of this type of natural history.

Some infectious agents may recur or relapse, even after the acute infection has resolved without sequelae. Typical of this pattern is HSV-1 and -2, varicella-zoster virus, and cytomegalovirus infections. Some infections may become chronic, with a variable proportion leading to progressive tissue damage at the primary site of the infection. Typical of this pattern is hepatitis C virus, HBV, and HIV.

Finally, some infections may become chronic and eventually lead to cancer in the target organ of the infection. Typical of this type of infection are human papillomavirus, HBV, and *Helicobacter pylori* infections. Infections that often exhibit each of these various natural history patterns are listed in Table 2–8.

It has been estimated by the World Health Organization (WHO) that over 15% of human cancers worldwide are caused by chronic infections. The proportion and types of human cancers associated with infectious agents are shown in Table 2–9.

The Immune Response to Infection

A detailed discussion of the immune responses to infection is well beyond the scope of this chapter. The topic is thoroughly covered in several textbooks. However, it might be useful to provide a very brief overview to introduce some concepts and nomenclature relative to the immune responses to infection.

Protection against infection consists of both specific immune responses against particular pathogens and nonspecific defenses directed against organisms or foreign antigens. Several compounds present in the normal intact skin, including lipids, lipoproteins, and peptides, are toxic to many organisms. Lysozyme in the tears and several proteins in the oral cavity have bactericidal activity. The acidic pH of the stomach is lethal to moderate doses of many enteric pathogens. The normal ciliary activity of the respiratory tract and the mucous layer coating the bronchus and bronchioles are an important first line of defense against respiratory organisms. The low pH of the vagina serves as a first line of defense against many sexually transmitted pathogens. Furthermore, natural killer (NK) cells and cells of the monocyte-macrophage lineage can provide some nonspecific defense against a pathogen. However, the immune responses generated by cells and antibodies that have been stimulated to respond to a specific pathogen usually are more effective.

The immune system consists of a few main classes of cells and a large variety of cell sub-

Table 2–8 Natural History Patterns of Some Important Infectious Diseases

Natural History	Disease
Acute with recovery and long-term immunity	Measles, Mumps, Rubella, Polio, Diphtheria
Acute with some chronic carriers	HBV, HSV-1 and -2, V2V, *Chlamydia trachomatis* Infections
Acute Disease, Chronic Sequelae without carrier state	Group A Streptococcal (ARF, AGN), Syphilis, Lyme Disease
Chronic Carriers common (or usual)	HIV, HBV, HSV-2, HPV, HCV, *Helicobacter pylori* Infections, Ophisthorchis viverini, Schistosoma infections
Chronic Carriers may develop cancer	HBV—Hepatocellular CA HCV—Hepatocellular CA HPV—Cervical or laryngeal CA *H. pylori*—Gastric CA HTLV-1—T cell leukemia EBV—Nasopharyngeal carcinoma HHV-8—Kaposi's sarcoma Ophisthorchis—Cholangiocarcinoma

Table 2–9 Infection and the Burden of Cancer Worldwide (1990)

Cancer	No. of Cases	Agent	% of Total Cancers
Stomach	504,928	*H. pylori*	5.3
Cervix, vulva	447,400	HPV	4.8
Liver	398,600	HBV, HCV	4.3
Lymphoma	46,779	EBV	0.5
Kaposi's sarcoma	43,525	HIV, HHV8	0.5
Bladder	10,249	*Schistosoma hematobium*	.1
Leukemia	2,662	HTLV-1	.1
Cholangiocarcinoma	808	Liver flukes (microns)	.1
Total infection-related cancers	1,454,951		15.6
Total no. of cancers	9,327,165		

Source: Data from WHO Web site.

sets. Lymphocytes provide direction for the main activities of the immune system and govern the nature of the immune response. Those that originate in the bone marrow are called *B lymphocytes*; those that originate in or traffic through the thymus are called *T lymphocytes*. Other cells of the immune system include circulating monocytes or macrophages, tissue macrophages, dendritic cells, langerhans cells, NK cells, mast cells, eosinophils, and basophils. Granulocytes are involved in phagocytosis of bacterial pathogens and eosinophils are involved in the reaction to parasitic pathogens and in allergic and autoimmune reactions.

B Lymphocytes and Humoral Immunity

The B lymphocytes are responsible for humoral immunity. These cells produce antibodies in the form of immunoglobulins that are reactive with foreign antigens. Five different isotypes of antibody are produced by B cells, namely, IgM, IgD, IgG, IgE, and IgA. Generally, the acute response to infection is characterized by a predominance of IgM antibodies that switch later to an IgG predominance. This pattern is useful in differentiating a recent, ie, within the past 3–6 months, from a more remote infection. For example, persons with IgM antibodies to hepatitis A virus (HAV) or the core antigen of HBV have had their primary HAV or HBV infections in the past 6 months. Persons with only IgG antibodies to HAV or HBV but no IgM antibodies were infected longer than 6 months ago. Antibodies of the IgA class may provide neutralization of pathogens on mucosal surfaces. IgE antibodies are often involved in the immune responses to parasites and in allergic reactions to foreign protein antigens.

Local Immunity—Mucosal Secretory IgA System

B lymphocytes secrete IgA antibodies, both in the blood and at the mucosal surfaces. These antibodies may be critical for resistance to infection in the respiratory, intestinal, and urogenital tracts. They are secreted after natural infection or following the administration of some whole virus vaccines. Vaccines given parenterally are less effective in inducing mucosal IgA. Therefore, some live virus vaccines, such as oral polio virus vaccines, may be more protective from infection than killed vaccines because they provide resistance to mucosal infection, as well as resistance to invasive infection.

T Lymphocytes and Cell-Mediated Immunity

T lymphocytes are important regulatory cells of the immune system. They interact with antigen presenting cells and secrete numerous cytokines, which activate effector cells and interact with cells through the major histocompatibility complex (MHC) proteins at the cell surface. T lymphocytes can be classified as helper cells if they have CD4$^+$ markers on their surface. The CD4$^+$ helper cells activate B cells, monocytes-macrophages, and other T helper cells by binding directly to these cells or by secreting specific cytokines that stimulate cell proliferation. The cells that have CD8$^+$ markers on their surface are cytotoxic T cells that lyse other cells that contain foreign proteins or viruses. Also, CD8$^+$ T cells can help modulate the immune response by suppressing the activation of effector cells, such as macrophages. Granuloma reactions to an infection with a mycobacteria consists of an organized cellular immune response with phagocytic effector cells, surrounded by CD4$^+$ cells and CD8$^+$ T suppressor cells on the periphery to provide a localized and controlled immune response to the organism. Natural killer cells resemble lymphocytes but have some distinctive properties, such as expression of a specific receptor for the Fc portion of IgG. In some circumstances, these NK cells can kill virus-infected or neoplastic cells by secretion of interferon gamma (IFN-G), especially when induced to do so by tumor necrosis factor and other cytokines produced by macrophages. Macrophages and monocytes function to process and deliver antigens for recognition by lymphocytes. Macrophages also can destroy intracellular virus-infected cells. These cells can respond to IFN-G secreted by the T cell, which activates the toxic oxygen and enzymatic pathways of the macrophage.

Granulocytes and Complement

Granulocytes are phagocytic cells that are involved in the protection against bacterial infections by ingesting and killing extracellular bacteria. The complement system is a set of enzymes and other proteins that attach to bacteria or foreign proteins and promote their destruction by phagocytosis. Persons who are deficient in some components of the complement system (especially C6, C7, or C8) have markedly increased susceptibility to recurrent infection with meningococci.[51]

Quantitation of Infectious Diseases

Epidemiologists use a variety of measurements to quantify the occurrence of disease. Fundamentally, these measurements are intended to estimate the burden of disease in a population or the incidence of disease—the rate at which the disease is spread among persons in the population. The prevalence of disease in a population is the number of people who are infected, divided by the number of people in the population. The numerator is those who are ill, those who have specific symptoms of the illness, or those who have microbiologic evidence of infection but do not exhibit symptoms. Each of these definitions yields different information, and each is a valid measure of the prevalence. However, it is critical that the definition of what constitutes infection be defined. The denominator in the prevalence equation is also defined by the epidemiologist. It may be the number of persons in the population, regardless of known exposure status, or it may be persons who were exposed. In the former case, the measurement of prevalence defines the burden of disease in the population overall; in the latter case, the definition gives the prevalence of disease among those exposed. Where exposure is common, age-specific population prevalence is commonly measured. Where exposure is rare, prevalence rates by exposure group are more frequently used.

The other commonly used measure is the incidence of disease. The incidence is the rate at which persons acquire the disease or the rate at which the infectious agent is being transmitted throughout the population. The incidence of disease always includes a unit of time—the number of cases of influenza in a given year, month, or week, for example.

The incidence and prevalence of disease are related to each other by the duration of disease. In cases where the duration of disease is short, the prevalence of disease will be approximately equal to the incidence of disease because most infections will be relatively recent. If, in contrast, the duration of the disease is long, the prevalence of disease will include both new and former cases of disease and will be larger than the incidence of disease. This relationship can be described by the equation:

$$Prevalence = Incidence \times Duration$$

At times, the incidence may be decreasing at the same time that prevalence is rising. Such may be the case with HIV infections in the United States and Western Europe at present, because combined antiretroviral therapy has prolonged survival and thereby increased the prevalence, but because of the effect of the drugs in reducing viral load, the transmission, or incidence of new cases, may be decreasing.

In other infectious diseases that have short duration but infected persons remain susceptible to reinfection, the incidence may exceed the point prevalence. Persons may have several episodes of diarrheal disease or rhinovirus respiratory infections per year that last only a few days. In these diseases, the point prevalence may be low but the annual incidence may be quite high. It may be preferable to measure the impact of these diseases with annual incidence rates. In contrast, in malaria hyperendemic areas, young children may receive hundreds of bites from infected mosquitoes every year. In this situation, the annual incidence of malaria is so high that it is difficult to measure. However, a blood film will allow determination of the point prevalence of infection, because the parasites persist in the blood for some time. Malaria prevalence data are more useful to differentiate populations at very high risk or of hyperendemic foci in an endemic area. These issues are discussed further in the chapters on Malaria, Diarrheal Infections, and Respiratory Infections.

SURVEILLANCE OF INFECTIOUS DISEASES

Surveillance of infectious diseases is essential to understand their epidemiology. *Surveillance* can be defined as the ongoing and systematic collection, collation, and analysis of data, and the dissemination of the results to those who need to know to avoid or prevent infections or epidemics.

In the United States, surveillance of infectious diseases is done by physicians and other health care workers, laboratories, clinics, and public health departments. Cases or outbreaks of selected infectious diseases are reported to the local health department by health care providers, laboratories, or hospitals. These reports are analyzed and forwarded to each state's Health Department, which reports the data to the CDC in Atlanta. Additional details of infectious disease surveillance are covered in Chapter 4.

TEMPORAL TRENDS OF INFECTIOUS DISEASES

Many infectious diseases undergo temporal variation in incidence. This temporal variability is sometimes easy to explain by changes in the exposure to the agent over time, such as in different seasons of the year or in different years.

Seasonal Variation

Vector-transmitted diseases, such as malaria, dengue, or St. Louis encephalitis (SLE), depend on exposure to infected mosquito vectors for their transmission. Therefore, these diseases are present only during the warm months of the year in temperate climates when the appropriate mosquito vectors are present. The seasonal distribution of SLE virus infections of the central nervous system in the United States that were reported to the CDC between 1988 and 1997 is shown in Figure 2–3. The marked and consistent seasonality of SLE is readily apparent and easily understood, because the transmission depends on bites of susceptible humans by infected *Culex pipiens* or other related mosquitoes. These mosquitoes breed only in the summer in temperate climates and must reach a certain density and level of infection with SLE virus before human infections occur. A description of the epidemiologic cycle of SLE in nature is shown in Figure 2–4. The important reservoir hosts for SLE are infected birds, both wild and domestic, which carry the virus without illness and develop high-level, persistent viremia with SLE virus after infection. These birds serve as the reservoir to infect mosquitoes. Because humans and other animals that may be bitten by SLE-infected mosquitoes have low levels of virus in the blood that is very transient, they are not effective as reservoir hosts to infect additional mosquitoes and maintain the epidemic. For this reason, they are termed *dead-end hosts*. In other mosquito-borne arboviral infections, such as Eastern equine encephalitis, Western equine encephalitis, or Venezuelan encephalitis, horses may commonly be infected when bitten by infected mosquitoes and develop symptomatic, even fatal, illness after infection. The rate of inapparent infections in humans may be 1,000 to 1 or higher; whereas, a much higher proportion of infected horses is symptomatic. Therefore, severe or fatal encephalitis in horses may serve as a harbinger that a subsequent human epidemic may follow. Substantial variations in the number of reported SLE infections by year are seen in the CDC data. Beyond the seasonal pattern, the year-to-year variation in the number of cases is not readily predictable. These mosquito-borne viral infections vary in relation to the number of mosquitoes, which may vary in density due to rainfall and temperature patterns, the number of reservoir hosts (espe-

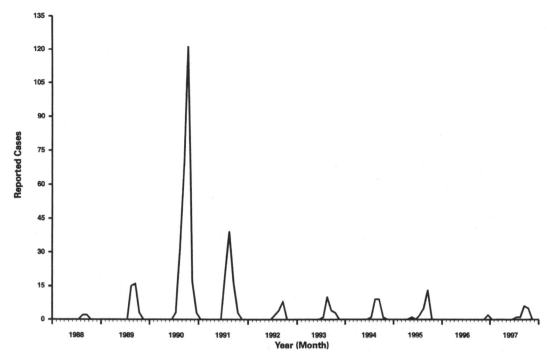

Figure 2–3 Arboviral infections (of the central nervous system)—reported laboratory-confirmed cases caused by St. Louis encephalitis virus, by month of onset, United States, 1988–1997. *Source:* Reprinted from *MMWR*, Summary of Notifiable Disease, 1997, Centers for Disease Control and Prevention.

cially wild birds) that are infected, and contact patterns between mosquitoes and birds and between infected mosquitoes and susceptible humans. Because of the interaction of these variables, it is difficult to predict from one year to the next whether an epidemic will occur. The important arthropod borne virus infections of humans are discussed further in Chapter 12.

Annual Variation

Prior to the development of effective vaccines for the prevention of many of the common childhood infections, such as measles, mumps, rubella, and varicella, these infections exhibited marked and repetitive cyclical trends, which depended largely on an epidemic exhausting susceptibles and another birth cohort replenishing them. For measles, the cycle for a major epidemic in an urban population in the United States repeated every other year, at which time, the number of cases roughly doubled, compared with the preceding and following years. With the widespread routine use of effective measles vaccine, the rates of measles have decreased dramatically, and the cyclical occurrence of cases has changed. However, cycles at 3- to 4-year intervals have persisted for reported cases of pertussis between 1967 and 1997 (Figure 2–5). This cyclical pattern indicates that persistent transmission of pertussis related to contact between an infected case and a susceptible host still occurs, despite the availability of a vaccine that has been used quite widely. In part, this persistence may relate to waning of the immunity induced by the whole-cell pertussis vaccine over time, the role of older children and adults in maintaining the transmission cycle of pertussis, and the

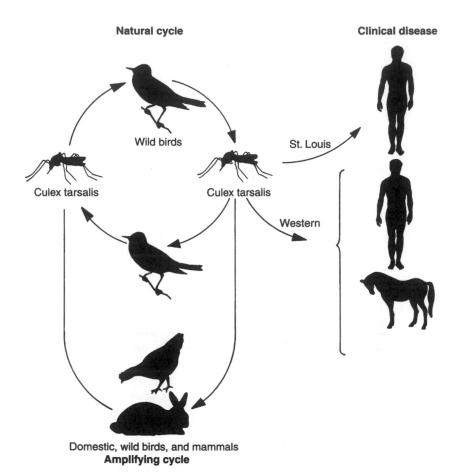

Figure 2–4 The sylvatic cycles of Western and St. Louis encephalitis viruses. The natural inapparent cycle is between *Culex tarsalis* and nestling and juvenile birds, but this cycle may be amplified by infection of domestic birds and wild and domestic mammals. Western encephalitis virus can replicate in mosquitoes at cooler temperatures, so epidemic disease in horses and humans may occur earlier in the summer and farther north into Canada. St. Louis encephalitis virus in the eastern United States involves *Culex pipiens* and other urban mosquitoes and causes urban epidemics. *Source:* Reprinted with permission from R.T. Johnson, *Viral Infections of the Nervous System*, © Lippincott Williams & Wilkins.

periodic replenishment of susceptibles. Most of the childhood infections are more common in the winter and early spring seasons. This seasonality has been postulated to be related to greater transmissability when populations spend more time indoors during the winter. Also, the low humidity of indoor air and the presence of other respiratory infections, which cause coughing and sneezing, may be critical factors in promoting the transmission during the winter.

Herd Immunity

Prior to the epidemiologic theories proposed by Kermack and McKendrick and by Reed and Frost from Johns Hopkins, the predominant theory was that epidemics occurred due to variation in the infectivity of the organism. Instead, these investigations showed that patterns of epidemics could be explained by the proportion and distribution of susceptible persons. In certain

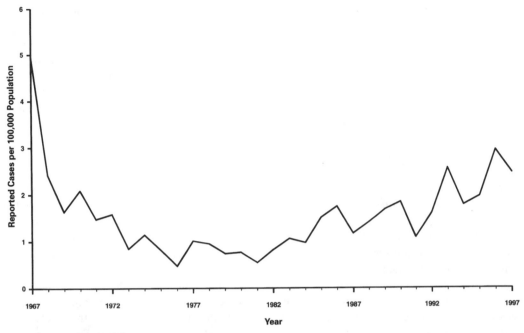

NOTE: DTP vaccine was licensed in 1940.

Figure 2–5 Pertussis (whooping cough) by year, United States, 1967–1997. *Source:* Reprinted from *MMWR*, Summary of Notifiable Disease, 1997, Centers for Disease Control and Prevention.

diseases that are spread from person to person, the level of immunity of the population may be critical in determining whether an epidemic will occur and, therefore, the risk of infection for a susceptible individual in the population. Because transmission is based on contact between an infected person and a susceptible person, if the number of immune persons is high enough that it is unlikely that a susceptible will have contact with an infected person, the population is said to have "herd immunity." Even though some susceptible persons remain in the population, epidemics are not sustained because the day-to-day contacts between persons do not result in contact between infected persons during the period that they are contagious and others who are still susceptible. The level of immunity required to attain herd immunity is dependent on the characteristics of the infectious disease. Those that are spread more readily will require a higher level of

immunity in the population than will those that are less infectious. The levels of herd immunity and individual susceptibility to infections are major epidemiologic factors that have influenced the periodicity and secular trends observed in many diseases, such as measles, rubella, varicella, and polio. A new epidemic of measles, prior to the era of widespread immunization, was dependent on the existence of a large cohort of susceptibles. A large enough pool of susceptibles to sustain an epidemic occurred every other year as new children were born. After an effective measles vaccine became available, epidemics were less common, less predictable, and often involved older individuals. Epidemics occurred even in immunized populations when clusters of susceptibles were exposed to an infectious case, such as on college campuses. The theoretical modeling of epidemics is covered more thoroughly in the chapter on Modeling.

Variations of Infectious Diseases over Decades

Tuberculosis

Many classic infectious diseases, such as tuberculosis, have decreased in incidence and mortality in the United States and Europe during the past century. Tuberculosis is still one of the most important infectious diseases globally. However, in the United States, the mortality rates from tuberculosis began to decline in the late nineteenth century. Between 1950 and 1985, tuberculosis morbidity declined at a rate of about 5% per year. Tuberculosis mortality by age in the United States is highest in older age groups.[52] However, the age-specific tuberculosis mortality data were studied in another way by Wade Hampton Frost. He examined the risk of tuberculosis death by birth cohort, rather than as cross-sectional age-specific mortality.[53] When the data are studied in this way, ie, as the risk of mortality from tuberculosis in a cohort of persons born in the same year, different conclusions are reached about the age-specific risk of mortality. In Figure 2–6, the mortality rates are depicted as age-specific mortality by birth cohort. The cohort analysis shows tuberculosis mortality. The reason for the higher mortality among older persons is that they were born at a time when the risk of tuberculosis was higher than it is at present. Their higher mortality reflects their elevated risk of infection due to subsequent activation of an infection that originally occurred when the incidence of tuberculosis was higher than more recent cohorts.[53,54]

Changes in Infectious Disease Morbidity and Mortality during the Nineteenth and Twentieth Centuries

During the eighteenth, nineteenth, and early twentieth centuries, infectious diseases were the major cause of morbidity and mortality. Reliable mortality data are available from the United Kingdom from the nineteenth century because early leaders, such as John Gaunt and William Farr, recognized the importance of surveillance

data to evaluate improvements in public health and promoted routine reporting of infectious disease mortality. The mortality rates from whooping cough, enteric fevers, and tuberculosis decreased over 100-fold between 1900 and 1960 in persons living in the United Kingdom. The mortality rates from these diseases decreased in the United States and other developed countries in Europe in a parallel fashion to those reported from the United Kingdom. In 1900, the death ratio from 10 of the most common infectious diseases varied from 202.2 per 100,000 population for influenza and pneumonia to 6.8 per 100,000 population for meningococcal infections. By 1970, only influenza and pneumonia infections were associated with mortality rates above 3 per 100,000 (Table 2–10).

A recent analysis of the trends in infectious disease mortality in the United States during the twentieth century documented the effect of the control of infectious diseases. The overall mortality from infectious diseases, which was 797 deaths per 100,000 in 1900, declined to 36 deaths per 100,000 in 1980.[55] However, the decline in mortality was reversed between 1980 and 1995, when the death rate increased to 63 deaths per 100,000 persons.[56] The trend of a steady decline was interrupted by a sharp spike of increased mortality during the 1918 influenza epidemic. Between 1938 and 1952, the decline was particularly rapid, with mortality decreasing by 8.2% per year. Pneumonia and influenza were responsible for the largest number of infectious disease deaths throughout the century. Tuberculosis caused a large number of deaths early in the century but tuberculosis mortality declined sharply after 1945. Although the crude mortality rate for infectious diseases has undergone dramatic reductions during the first eight decades of the twentieth century, the mortality from all noninfectious diseases has not shown a similar change (Figure 2–7). In fact, most of the decline in mortality during the twentieth century can be attributed to the dramatic reduction in infectious disease mortality. In the past few decades of the twentieth century, the mortality from coronary heart disease has declined sub-

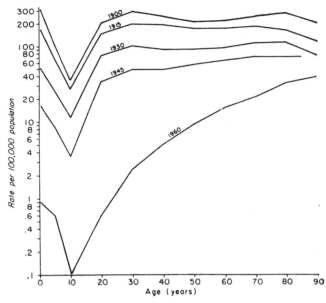

a

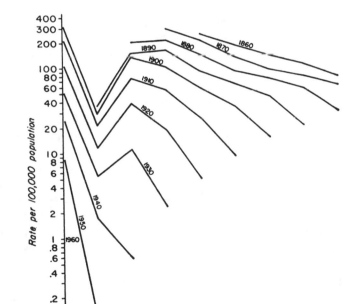

b

Figure 2–6 (a) Death rates from tuberculosis by age group for selected years; **(b)** Cohort analysis of death rates from tuberculosis by age group, 1860–1960. The line associated with each year indicates death rates by age group for persons born in that year. *Source:* Reprinted with permission from T.G. Doege, Tuberculosis Mortality in the United States, 1900 to 1960, *JAMA*, Vol. 192, pp. 1045–1048, © 1965, American Medical Association.

Table 2–10 Death Rates for Common Infectious Diseases in the United States in 1900, 1935, and 1970

Infectious Disease	Mortality Rate per 100,000 Population		
	1900	*1935*	*1970*
Influenza and pneumonia	202.2	103.9	30.9
Tuberculosis	194.4	55.1	2.6
Gastroenteritis	142.7	14.1	1.3
Diphtheria	40.3	3.1	0.0
Typhoid fever	31.3	2.7	0.0
Measles	13.3	3.1	0.0
Dysentery	12.0	1.9	0.0
Whooping cough	12.0	3.7	0.0
Scarlet fever (including streptococcal	9.6	2.1	0.0
sore throat)	6.8	2.1	0.3
Meningococcal infections			

Source: Reprinted from National Office of Vital Statistics, USPHS and Centers for Disease Control and Prevention.

stantially; however, this has been offset by increasing mortality for lung cancer and other diseases. Clearly, the decline in mortality from infectious diseases during the twentieth century stands as a tribute to the advances in public health and safer lifestyles, compared with that in previous centuries.

What caused these remarkable reductions in the mortality from the common infectious diseases? One might surmise that the development of modern microbiology with the understanding the discipline provided about the pathogenesis of specific infections led to the development of vaccines and effective antibiotics to prevent or treat infections. However, for most of these infections, the evidence suggests a more complex scenario. The decline in the annual death rates for tuberculosis in England and Wales antedated the identification of the tuberculosis bacillus; however, the slope of the declining mortality increased after 1948, with the availability of streptomycin, isoniazide, and other chemotherapeutic agents (Figure 2–8). Similarly, death rates from scarlet fever, diphtheria, and whooping cough (pertussis) in children under age 15 in England and Wales began to decline well before these or-

ganisms were identified in the laboratory, and the availability of effective antibiotics had a small effect on the overall mortality decline (Figure 2–9).[57] Also, dramatic declines in the death rates from measles and pertussis were seen among children in England and Wales decades prior to the identification of these organisms and the availability of vaccines or antibiotics to treat infected persons. What, then, can account for these declines in mortality? Recent experience with some of these diseases in poor and often malnourished children from developing countries in Africa has shown that some of these diseases still have high mortality in certain populations. For example, measles, which is rarely fatal when it occurs in children in the United States, is still associated with a 15–20% mortality in infants and children in Sub-Saharan Africa. Hypotheses to explain this difference have included poorer nutritional status, earlier ages at exposure, other concomitant infections, higher infectious dose, and greater crowding during epidemic spread among infants in Africa.[58,59] All of these factors may play a role but it is difficult to evaluate their independent contribution. Clearly, the complex changes that have occurred in society, hygiene, and lifestyle in the United States and in Europe during the late nineteenth and early twentieth centuries have had a profound effect on these diseases.

RECENT TRENDS IN INFECTIOUS DISEASE MORBIDITY AND MORTALITY IN THE UNITED STATES

Although the mortality from the classical infectious diseases declined dramatically in the late nineteenth century and the first 80 years of the twentieth century, several cultural and environmental changes occurred that fostered the emergence of a number of new infections and the re-emergence of older, well-recognized in-

fections. Indeed, it has been estimated that a larger number of new infections have emerged in the last decade or so than in the hundred years previously.

The most heralded, of course, is the HIV/ AIDS epidemic, which probably originated as a mutant or recombinant primate retrovirus that was spread to humans from chimpanzees in Africa in the 1950s or 1960s. The ensuing pandemic of AIDS has led to the emergence of many new and previously recognized but rare human pathogens, such as *P. carinii, Mycobacteria avium, Cryptosporidia parvum, Microsporidia, Bartonella rochelimea*, and *Penicillium marneffei*. The epidemic of AIDS is covered in more detail in the chapter on AIDS. In addition to HIV and AIDS, modern chemo-

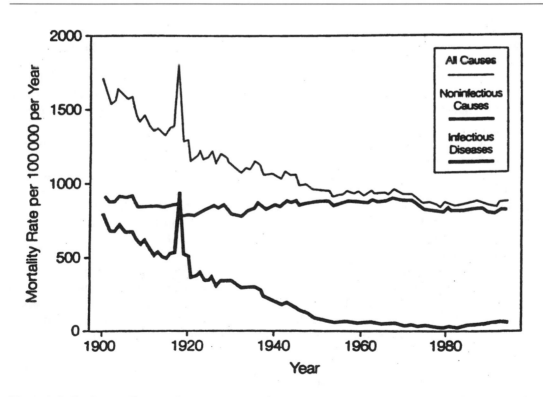

Figure 2–7 Crude mortality rates for all causes, noninfectious causes, and infectious diseases. *Source:* Reprinted from G.L. Armstrong, L.A. Conn, and R.W. Pinner, Trends in Infectious Disease Mortality in the United States during the 20th Century, *JAMA*, Vol. 281, pp. 61–66, 1999.

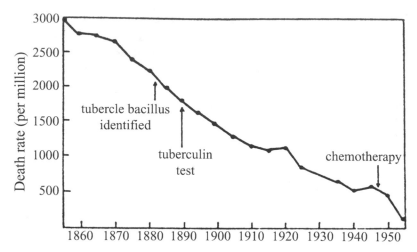

Figure 2–8 Mean annual death rate from respiratory tuberculosis, England and Wales. *Source:* Reprinted from E. Kass, Infectious Diseases and Social Change, *Journal of Infectious Diseases*, Vol. 23, No. 1, p. 111, © 1971, University of Chicago Press.

therapy of neoplasms, aging of the population, increased invasive therapeutic procedures in hospitalized patients, crowding of elderly patients in nursing homes and infants and children in day care centers, widespread use of broad spectrum antibiotics, environmental pollution, and other factors have led to the emergence of infectious diseases. These issues are covered in detail in Chapter 12.

An analysis was done by investigators for the CDC of all deaths in the United States between 1980 and 1992.[56] In this interval, the death rate due to infectious diseases as the underlying cause of death increased 58%, from 41 to 65 deaths per 100,000 population in the United States. Age-adjusted mortality from infectious diseases increased 39% during the same period. Infectious disease mortality increased 25% among those aged 65 years or older, from 271 to 338 per 100,000 population, and 5.5 times among 25- to 44-year-olds, from 6.9 to 38 deaths per 100,000 population. Mortality due to respiratory tract infections increased 20%, the death rate from septicemia increased 83%, and AIDS emerged as a major cause of death. These

national data are quite sobering because they clearly demonstrate that an increased infectious disease mortality has occurred recently in the U.S. population, which is not limited to newly emerging diseases, such as AIDS. The 10 leading underlying causes of mortality caused by infectious diseases in the United States in 1980 and 1992 are listed in Table 2–11.

RECENT WORLDWIDE TRENDS IN INFECTIOUS DISEASE MORBIDITY AND MORTALITY

Infectious diseases play a leading role in mortality and morbidity globally, due in large part to the continued importance of infectious diseases in Sub-Saharan Africa, Asia, and Latin America. Data were published recently from the Global Burden of Disease Study, which was initiated in 1992, in collaboration with the World Bank and the WHO. The goals of this study were to make reasonable estimates from the available data of the impact of various diseases as causes of disability, to develop unbiased assessments for major disorders, and to quantify the burden of disease with a measure that could be used for cost-effectiveness analysis. This study found that 98% of all deaths in children younger than 15 years of age are in the developing world and that 50% of deaths between ages 15 and 59 years of age were in the developing world.[60] The probability of death between birth and 15 years of age ranges from 22% in Sub-Saharan Africa to 1.1% in the established market economics. Probabilities of death between 15 and 50 years of age range from 7.2% for women in established market economics to 39.1% in Sub-Saharan Africa. Worldwide in 1990, communicable, maternal, perinatal, and nutritional disorders accounted for 17.2 million deaths, noncommunicable diseases for 28.1 million deaths, and injuries for 5.1 million deaths. The leading causes of death in 1990 were ischemic heart disease (6.3 million deaths), cerebrovascular accidents (4.4 million deaths), lower

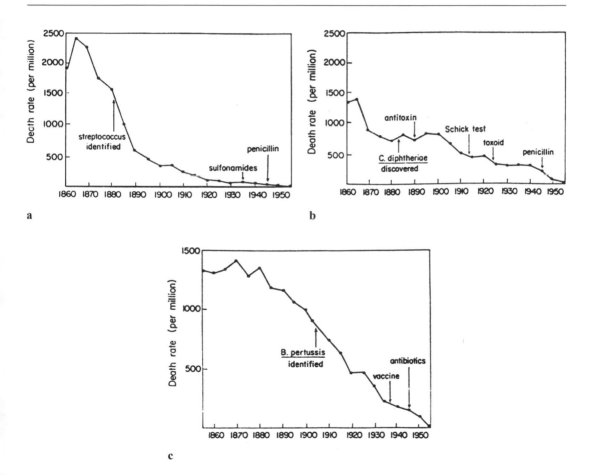

Figure 2–9 **(a)** Mean annual death rate from scarlet fever in children under 15 years of age, England and Wales; **(b)** Mean annual death rate from diphtheria in children under 15 years of age, England and Wales; and **(c)** Mean annual death rate from whooping cough in children under 15 years of age, England and Wales. *Source:* Reprinted with permission from E. Kass, Infectious Diseases and Social Change, *The Journal of Infectious Diseases*, Vol. 23, No. 1, pp. 110–114, © 1971, University of Chicago Press.

Table 2–11 Leading Underlying Causes of Mortality Caused by Infectious Diseases in the United States, 1980 and 1992

Rank	1980 Infectious Disease Group	No. of Deaths	Mortality per 100,000	1992 Infectious Disease Group	No. of Deaths	Mortality per 100,000
1	Respiratory tract infections	56,966	25.1	Respiratory tract infections	77,336	30.3
2	Septicemia	9,438	4.2	HIV/AIDS	33,581	13.2
3	Infections of kidney/urinary tract	8,006	3.5	Septicemia	19,667	7.7
4	Infections of the heart	2,486	1.1	Infections of kidney/urinary tract	12,399	4.9
5	Tuberculosis	2,333	1.0	Infections of the heart	3,950	1.5
6	Bacterial meningitis	1,402	0.6	Hepatobiliary disease	2,494	1.0
7	Gastrointestinal tract infections	1,377	0.6	Mycoses	2,298	0.9
8	Hepatobiliary disease	1,227	0.5	Tuberculosis	1,851	0.7
9	Perinatal infections	1,035	0.5	Gastrointestinal tract infections	985	0.4
10	Mycoses	680	0.3	Perinatal infections	965	0.4
Total infectious diseases		93,407	41.1		166,047	65.1
All deaths		1,989,841	878.0		2,175,613	852.7

Source: Reprinted with permission from Pinner, *The Journal of the American Medical Association*, Vol. 275, No. 3, pp. 189–193, Copyright 1996, The American Medical Association.

respiratory infections (4.3 million deaths), diarrheal diseases (2.9 million), perinatal disorders (2.4 million), chronic obstructive pulmonary disease (2.2 million), tuberculosis (2.0 million), measles (1.1 million), road traffic accidents (1.0 million), and lung cancer (0.9 million).

This WHO, World Bank study also concluded that effective treatment of tuberculosis is the most cost-effective health measure that could be implemented in developing countries in terms of prevention of mortality and increasing disability-adjusted life years (DALY).[61] The analysis of tuberculosis programs in Malawi, Mozambique and Tanzania has shown that treating smear-positive tuberculosis costs $20–52 per death averted. The cost per discounted year of life saved, therefore, is $1–3. There are few other interventions that are as cost-effective as is tuberculosis case treatment. This WHO analysis estimated that $150 million would be needed to treat 65% of smear-positive cases in low-income countries and 85% of middle-income countries with short-course chemotherapy. Clearly, the interaction between HIV and tuberculosis has made the tuberculosis problem more acute and intractable. The rapid and extensive spread of AIDS in countries in the developing world, where a high proportion of the population has latent tuberculosis, indicates that a public health strategy that is limited to treating active cases is unlikely to control the emerging tuberculosis epidemic effectively. However, recent research has shown that active tuberculosis generally is treatable with current chemotherapeutic regimes, even in the face of HIV infection. This issue is reviewed in greater detail in the chapter on Tuberculosis.

Other health interventions are cost-effective for the prevention of infectious disease morbidity and mortality, including effective sexually transmitted disease (STD) treatment; oral rehydration therapy for diarrhea; immunization for childhood diseases, including HBV; ivermectin for the treatment and prevention of onchocerchiasis and schistosomiasis; and zidovudine for the prevention of the perinatal transmission of HIV. The chemotherapy and chemoprophylaxis of malaria and antibiotic prophylaxis for the prevention of postsurgical infections are also cost-effective; these issues are reviewed in the chapters on Malaria and Nosocomial Infections.

Currently, the world's population is in a very delicate balance, with respect to infectious diseases. The continual emergence of new infectious diseases and the re-emergence of old infections, together with the potential for their global spread, underline the need for accurate surveillance and the development of newer strategies for their control and prevention. However, the successes of the last century should provide hope that infectious diseases can be controlled with the proper understanding and effort.

REFERENCES

1. Snow. *On Cholera*. New York: Commonwealth Fund; 1996.
2. Fraser DW, Tsai TR, Orenstein W, et al. Legionnaire's disease. Description of an epidemic of pneumonia. *N Engl J Med*. 1977;297:1189–1197.
3. Dondero TJ, Rentdorff RL, Mallison GF, et al. An outbreak of Legionnaire's disease associated with a contaminated air-conditioning cooling tower. *N Engl J Med*. 1980;302:365–370.
4. Cords LG, Fraser DW, Skailly P, et al. Legionnaire's disease outbreak at an Atlanta, Georgia country club: evidence for spread from an evaporative condenser. *Am J Epidemiol*. 1980;111:425–431.
5. Garbe PL, Davis BJ, Weisfeld JS, et al. Nosocomial Legionnaire's disease: epidemiologic demonstration of cooling towers as a source. *JAMA*. 1985;254:521–524.
6. Morris GK, Patton CM, Feeley JC, et al. Isolation of the Legionnaire's disease bacterium from environmental samples. *Ann Intern Med*. 1979;90:664–666.
7. Moraca E, Yu VC, Goetz A. Disinfection of water distribution system for Legionnella: a review of applicator procedures and methodologies. *Infect Control Hosp Epidemiol*. 1990;11:79–88.
8. Francis E. Deer-fly fever: a disease of man of hitherto unknown etiology. *Public Health Rep*. 1991;34:2061–2062.
9. Waring WB, Ruffin JJ. A tick-borne epidemic of tularemia. *N Engl J Med*. 1946;234:137.

10. Young LS, Bickewell DS, Archer BG, et al. Tularemia epidemic: Vermont 1968: forty-seven cases linked to contact with muskrats. *N Engl J Med.* 1969;280:1253–1260.

11. Teutsch SM, Martone WJ, Brink EW, et al. Pneumonic tularemia on Martha's Vineyard. *N Engl J Med.* 1979; 301:826–828.

12. Dahlstrand S, Ringertz O, Zetterberg B. Airborne tularemia in Sweden. *J Infect Dis.* 1971;3:7–16.

13. Barbeito MS, Alg RL, Wedum AG. Infectious bacterial aerosol from dropped Petri disk cultures. *Am J Med Technol.* 1961;27:318–322.

14. Hornick RB. Tularemia. In: Evans A, Brachman PS, eds. *Bacterial Infections of Humans: Epidemiology and Control.* 3rd ed. New York: Plenum Publishing; 1998: 823–837.

15. Hirst CF. *The Conquest of Plague.* London: Oxford University Press; 1953.

16. Zinsser H. *Rats, Lice and History.* Boston: Little, Brown; 1934.

17. Marshall JD Jr, Joy RJT, Ai NY, et al. Plague in Vietnam 1965–1966. *Am J Epidemiol.* 1967;86:603–616.

18. Campbell GL, Hughes JM. Plague in India: a new warning from an old nemesis. *Am Int Med.* 1995;122:151–153.

19. Eskey CR, Haas V. Plague in the western part of the United States. *Public Health Bull.* 1940;254:1–82.

20. Mann JM, Martone WJ, Myoce JM, et al. Endemic human plague in New Mexico: risk factors associated with infections. *J Infect Dis.* 1979;140:397–401.

21. Butler T. *Plague and Other Yersinia Infections.* New York: Plenum Publishing; 1983.

22. Laforce FM. Woolsorter's disease. *Acad Med.* 1978; 54:956–963.

23. Meselson M, Guillemin J, Hugh-Jones M, et al. The Sverdlousk anthrax outbreak of 1979. *Science.* 1994; 266:1202–1208.

24. Constantine DG. Rabies transmission by non-bite route. *Public Health Rep.* 1963;77:287–289.

25. Winkler WG, Fashinell TR, Leffingwell C, Howard P, Conomy JP. Airborne rabies transmission in a laboratory worker. *JAMA.* 1973;226:1219–1221.

26. Hooff SA, Burton RC, Wilson RW, et al. Human-to-human transmission of rabies by a corneal transplant. *N Engl J Med.* 1979;300:603–604.

27. Noah DC, Drenzik CL, Smith JS, et al. Epidemiology of human rabies in the United States, 1980 to 1996. *Ann Intern Med.* 1998;128:922–930.

28. Brown GM. The history of the brucellosis eradication program in the United States. *Ann Selavo.* 1977;19:20–34.

29. Grant IH, Gold JW, Witner M, et al. Transfusion-associated Chagas' disease acquired in the United States. *Ann Intern Med.* 1989;111:849–851.

30. Gregg NM. Congenital cataract following German measles in the mother. *Trans Ophthalmol Soc.* 1941; 3:35–46.

31. Weller TH, Neva FA. Propagation in tissue culture of cytopathic agents from patients with rubella-like illness. *Proc Soc Exp Biol Med.* 1962;11:215–225.

32. Parkman PD, Bueschler EL, Artenstein MS. Recovery of rubella virus from army recruits. *Proc Soc Exp Biol Med.* 1962;111:225–230.

33. Krugman S, ed. Rubella symposium. *Am J Dis Child.* 1965;110:345–476.

34. Krugman S, ed. International conference on rubella immunization. *Am J Dis Child.* 1969;118:2–410.

35. Smith MG. Propagation in tissue culture of a cytopathic virus from human salivary gland virus (SGV) disease. *Proc Soc Exp Biol Med.* 1956;92:424–430.

36. Rowe WP, Hartley JW, Waterman S, Turnan HC, Huebner RJ. Cytopathic agent resembling human salivary gland virus recovered from tissue culture of human adenoids. *Proc Soc Exp Biol Med.* 1956;92:418–424.

37. Weller TH, MaCaulay JC, Craig JM, Wirth P. Isolation of intranuclear inclusion producing agents from infants with illness resembling cytomegalic inclusion disease. *Pro Soc Exp Biol Med.* 1957;94:4–12.

38. Gershon AH, Gold E, Nankervis GA. Cytomegalovirus. In: Evans AS, Kaslow RA, eds. *Viral Infections of Humans, Epidemiology and Control.* New York: Plenum Publishing; 1997:229–251.

39. Dobbins JG, Stewart JAS. Surveillance of congenital cytomegalovirus disease 1990–1991. *MMWR.* 1992;41: SS-2.

40. Stone KM, Brooks CA, Guinan ME, Alexander ER. National surveillance for neonatal herpes virus infections. *Sex Transm Dis.* 1989;16:152–156.

41. Mcllinger AK, Goldberg M, Wade A, et al. Alternative case-finding in a crack-related syphilis epidemic—Philadelphia. *MMWR.* 1991;40:77–80.

42. Conner EM, Sperling RS, Gelber R, et al. Reduction of maternal–infant transmission of human immunodeficiency virus type 1 without zidovudine treatment. *N Engl J Med.* 1997;31:1173–1180.

43. Shaffer N, Chunchoonong R, Mock PA, et al. Short-course zidovudine for perinatal HIV-1 transmission in Bangkok, Thailand. *Lancet.* 1999;353:773–780.

44. Guay CA, Musoke P, Fleming T, et al. Intrapartum and neonatal single-dose nevirapine compared with zidovudine for prevention of mother-to-child transmission of HIV-1 in Kampala, Uganda: HIVNST o/z randomized trial. *Lancet.* 1999;254:795–802.

45. Sartwell PE. The distribution of incubation of disease. *Am J Epidemiol.* 1950;51:310–318.

46. Muñoz A, Kirby AJ, He DY, et al. Long-term survivors with HIV-1 longitudinal patterns of CD4⁺ lymphocytes. *J Acquir Immunodeficiency Syndr*. 1995;8:496–505.

47. Watts DM, Burke DS, Harrison BA, et al. Effect of temperature on the vector efficiency of *Aedes aegypti* for dengue 2 virus. *Am J Trop Med Hyg*. 1987;36:143–152.

48. Soper GA. The curious case of typhoid Mary. *Acad Med*. 1939;15:698–712.

49. Anders W, Conde F, Stephen W. Surgical treatment of the chronic typhoid carrier: report of 102 operated cases. *Dtsch Med Wochenschr*. 1955;89:1637–1648.

50. Shilts R. *And the Band Played On*. New York: St. Mortons Press; 1987.

51. Peterson BH, Lee TJ, Snyderman, Brooks GF. *Neisseria meningitidis* and *Neisseria gonorrhoeae* bacteremia associated with C6, C7, C8 deficiency. *Ann Intern Med*. 1979;90:917–920.

52. Rieder HL, Cauthen GM, Kelly GD, et al. Tuberculosis in the United States. *JAMA*. 1989;262:385–389.

53. Frost WH. The age selection of mortality from tuberculosis in successive decades. *Am J Hyg*. 1939 (Section A);30:91–96.

54. Doege TG. Tuberculosis mortality in the United States, 1900 to 1960. *JAMA*. 1965;192:1045–1048.

55. Armstrong GL, Conn LA, Pinner RW. Trends in infectious disease mortality in the United States during the 20th century. *JAMA*. 1999;281:61–66.

56. Pinner RW, Teutsch SM, Simonsen L, et al. Trends in infectious diseases mortality in the United States. *JAMA*. 1996;225:189–193.

57. Kass EM. Infectious disease and social change. *J Infect Dis*. 1971;123:110–114.

58. Aaby P, Bakh J, Lisse IM, Snits AJ. Measles mortality, state of nutrition, and family structure: a community study on Guinea-Bissau. *J Infect Dis*. 1983;147:693–701.

59. Aaby P. Malnutrition and overcrowding-exposure in severe measles infection: a review of community studies. *Rev Infect Dis*. 1988;10:478–491.

60. Murray CJ, Lopez AD. Alternative projections of mortality and disability by course, 1990–2020: global burden of disease study. *Lancet*. 1997;349:1498–1504.

61. Murray CJ, Lopez AD. Mortality by cause for eight regions of the world: global burden of disease study. *Lancet*. 1997;349:1269–1276.

CHAPTER 3

Study Design

Carolyn Masters Williams and Kenrad E. Nelson

Epidemiology is based on two fundamental tenets. The first is the observation that human disease does not occur at random. The second is that there are causal, and possibly preventable, factors that influence the development of disease. Studies of infectious disease epidemiology evaluate the contribution of different factors responsible for the transmission and acquisition of infections and those favoring endemic transmission and epidemics. Epidemiologic studies can also be used to evaluate the effects of interventions, eg, HIV protease inhibitors on AIDS mortality or the protective effect of bed nets in malaria prevention. How to structure the processes of observing study design is a critical step in the science of epidemiology. The study design must optimize the researcher's ability to evaluate and measure accurately the relationship between risk factors and disease in the study population, which can then be applied to the population as a whole.

Epidemiologic studies of an infectious disease can be designed to explore landmarks along the entire temporal process during which an individual is at risk, acquires infection, develops an infectious disease, or succumbs to it. Several chronic infectious diseases, such as tuberculosis or AIDS, may have different risk factors that are important for acquiring infection and development of disease. In addition to understanding disease among individuals, epidemiologists attempt to understand the burden of disease at a population level and the factors leading to epidemics. From these studies, measurements of the prevalence and incidence of disease and correlates and risk factors for infection are evaluated.

GOALS OF EPIDEMIOLOGIC RESEARCH

The Epidemiologic Triangle (Host-Agent and Environment)

The *epidemiologic triangle* is used to describe the relationship between the host (ie, the diseased person), the agent (ie, the infecting virus/bacteria/parasite/fungi), and the environment (ie, the setting in which transmission occurs) (Figure 3–1). This conceptual framework is useful in modeling the transmission dynamics of an infectious disease. Human hosts differ in susceptibility to infections, due to genetic, environmental, behavioral, and other characteristics. Infections differ in some respects from other diseases of humans, in that genetic and phenotypic variability of both the agent and the host can impact on its ability to cause disease and its epidemiology. Humans have interacted with infectious agents throughout evolutionary history, and changes in both the host and the agent have resulted from this selective interaction. Major epidemic diseases, such as malaria, tuberculosis, smallpox, and plague, have led to selective genetic changes in human populations. The evolution of several mutations among Africans and

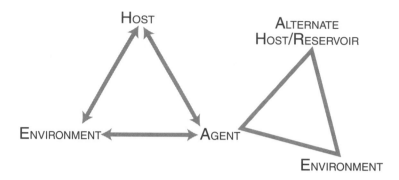

Figure 3–1 The Epidemiologic Triangle. For some diseases, the interaction may be described by the interaction between the host, environment, and agent. For other diseases, the interaction must also include a second triangle to describe the extrinsic life cycle of the agent outside of the human host.

Asians has resulted primarily from the selective pressure of hyperendemic malaria. Sickle hemoglobin, glucose-6-phosphate dehydrogenase deficiency, thalassemia, hemoglobin C, and hemoglobin E may be disadvantageous in homozygous individuals, but they have evolved in certain populations because they confer significant protection from malaria in heterozygous individuals.[1] In fact, it is possible to estimate the mortality rates from malaria that would have been necessary in previous generations to account for the current sickle cell hemoglobin gene frequency using the Hardy-Weinberg equation. On the agent side, escape mechanisms—techniques used by parasites to evade the host's immune system—may require a large portion of the parasite's genome but are effective enough that they are retained in the genome.

The environment also plays a significant role in infectious disease epidemiology. It is important to understand and characterize the environment in which transmission occurs and to be aware of environmental factors that facilitate the agent's survival or infectivity. It is straightforward to envision the role of environment for agents that have an extrinsic cycle, such as hookworm. For example, soil humidity, temperature, and other soil characteristics can influence the development of infectious *Ancylostoma duodenalae* larvae. After the development of infectious larvae, human behavior will result in infection and maintenance of the cycle. However, the environment is also important in the transmission of airborne viruses, such as influenza and varicella, because it affects the length of time that the viral particles remain infectious as an aerosol. The winter environment in temperate climates also facilitates transmission of influenza by bringing people indoors. However, influenza epidemics have been interrupted by extreme cold weather that has forced schools to close, thereby interrupting transmission among children and introduction of the virus into the home.

Epidemiologic studies are used to evaluate these relationships and efforts to alter them to our advantage, be they preventive or therapeutic in nature. Several designs have been used, including ecologic and surveillance studies, cohort studies (parallel and pre/postintervention designs), and traditional randomized clinical trials. In this chapter, we review several important and frequently used epidemiologic study designs and illustrate their use in evaluating infectious diseases.

CHOOSING A STUDY DESIGN

The optimal study design for a research question is a function of the hypothesis under investigation and the information that is available at the time of analysis. Prior to initiating an epidemiologic study, it is useful to consider several questions, namely, Who is to be studied (sampling)? What data are going to be collected (data collection)? and, How are these data going to be analyzed (analysis)? These issues may influence the design of an epidemiologic study.

Sampling

The design of epidemiologic studies requires the successful translation of an idea to a hypothesis that can be tested by measurable observations in a relevant study population. It is rarely possible to study the entire population at risk for a disease. Therefore, an epidemiologic study must first define the study sample—those persons who will be included in the study. Epidemiologists must "sample" from the population to have a manageable study. The study sample must be at risk for the disease and representative of the populations to which the study results will be applied. Also, the sample size must be large enough to ensure sufficient statistical power to evaluate the study hypothesis. Finally, the researchers must take into account other considerations of the sampling protocol. Issues such as cost, quality of data, degree of cooperation that can be expected from a given population, and the accessibility of the population for enrollment and follow-up can influence sampling protocols. Practical issues, such as the reliability and validity of data obtained by questionnaire or other means, confidentiality of the data, and effects of the study process on data gathering, may influence the study results.

Data Collection

Infectious disease epidemiology shares many of the considerations common to epidemiologic studies of other diseases. Data collection must ensure meaningful, reliable data. Data collection itself may involve the use of employment or medical record review, personal interviews, medical exams, environmental measurements, and other relevant information. Interviews may be conducted in person, by phone, by mail, or by computer. The participant may complete the questionnaire or may be asked the questions by a trained interviewer. Each of these methods has its advantages and disadvantages in reliability, reduction in response bias, and expense.

To conduct an epidemiologic study of an infectious disease, it must be possible to measure the occurrence of infection or disease. Although this may seem obvious, in practice, the occurrence of disease may be difficult or costly to determine (Exhibit 3–1). The study design must take into account what methods are available to ascertain whether an infection is present or has occurred, as well as their reliability and appropriateness in answering the research question. Depending on the study question, data may be collected as self-reports, abstracted from medical charts or laboratory reports, or the study may do the testing. Despite the expense, conducting testing within the study protocol can have a number of advantages, including standardized specimen collection and assay, and the development of a specimen archive for future studies.

Analysis

Evaluation of the study results includes evaluation of the conduct of the study as well as the data. Was the study performed in the manner in which it was designed? Did any deviations from design alter the quality of the results? Evaluation of the success of sampling procedures should be conducted. Who was ultimately studied? Also, the study should be evaluated with respect to any potential biases. Were biases introduced into the study by the manner in which it was conducted? Comparisons should be made between the actual study sample and the population targeted for study, the response rate of subgroups, and the composition of the population from which the sample was drawn. Data should be compared with studies of the research question in other populations by other investigators. Researchers may then determine whether the observed data are valid. Key questions that an epidemiologist should address are: How much of the measured

Exhibit 3–1 Issues in Determining the Occurrence of an Infectious Disease

Many infectious diseases result in the formation of antibodies. Antibodies are generally long-lasting and indicate that a person has been exposed to a disease. However, the presence or absence of antibodies leads to a number of questions.

1. **When was the person exposed?** Antibodies to mumps are long-lasting and could indicate infection in the distant past or a recent infection. Immunoglobulin type M (IgM) antibodies are the first to form, and high levels of these antibodies indicate that the infection is recent. IgG antibodies form later in the course of infection. Variation in the timing (but not the sequence) of the different antibody classes is seen among individuals.

2. **Has immunity waned or never formed?** Antibodies are not long-lasting for some infectious agents. Antibodies form several months after exposure to *B. burgdorferi* (the agent of Lyme disease) and may either wane or not form at all in persons who are treated early.

3. **Was the person exposed or vaccinated?** It may not be possible to differentiate those who are vaccinated from those who had disease. Vaccination against polio with the inactivated injection and oral inoculation will generate immunity that cannot be differentiated from immunity generated by polio disease. In contrast, the hepatitis-B vaccine results in antibodies against only one viral protein (HBs Ag). An infected individual will have antibodies to other viral proteins not included in the vaccine.

4. **Did the person have disease or just infection?** Antibody formation can occur in those who suffered severe disease and in those with subclinical symptoms. The presence of antibodies only demonstrates infection, not disease status. Cholera has low rates of clinical disease, and the prevalence of antibodies to cholera would overestimate the mortality and morbidity of a cholera epidemic.

effect may be explained by bias? Is there a dose-response effect? How do the results compare with other data available on this subject?

Specific study designs and the analysis of the data are reviewed briefly, and examples of their application to infectious diseases are described below. The reader should consult other sources for a more detailed description. Recommended references include Rothman and Greenland[2] and Diggle, Liang, and Zeger.[3]

TYPES OF EPIDEMIOLOGIC STUDY DESIGN

Descriptive Studies

Epidemiologic studies of infectious diseases are designed for several purposes. When a new disease is recognized, the main purpose may be to describe the nature of the disease and to evaluate the probable means of transmission, reservoir, and natural history. Sometimes, a new disease is known to be caused by a specific or-

ganism, eg, staphylococcal toxic shock syndrome; often, it is not, eg, Hantavirus pulmonary syndrome, Legionnaires' disease, and AIDS. Early studies may consist of descriptions of cases or groups of cases, which sometimes can be linked by a possible transmission route or exposure to a reservoir. These studies do not necessarily compare cases of an infectious disease with controls but only describe the disease and the exposures in the cases. At times, case reports or case series provide considerable understanding about the epidemiology of an infectious disease.

Case Reports

Case reports are a careful evaluation of a single case of disease in which the epidemiologist may describe the transmission, natural history, and/or treatment. Although case reports are based on an infection in a single patient, they may yield important new epidemiologic information regarding the disease. Four examples of illustrative case reports follow, two of rabies and two of HIV infection.

Rabies

Rabies is a zoonotic viral infection that is spread to humans by the bite of an infected animal. Although rabies vaccine can be given after exposure to prevent infection of the central nervous system (CNS), and such postexposure prophylaxis is usually successful, it is widely believed that the disease is universally fatal once the virus infects the CNS and signs and symptoms of CNS infection occur. Infection of the CNS is preventable, even after exposure, because there is no initial viremia, and the brain becomes infected from perineural transmission of the virus from the site of inoculation. Early treatment can prevent perineural transmission by neutralization of the rabies virus.

In October 1970, a 6-year-old boy was bitten by a rabid bat. He was given 14 doses of duck embryo rabies vaccine but developed rabies 21 days later. He eventually recovered completely after treatment with intensive care for nearly 2 months. This case report challenged the belief that rabies is always fatal after the onset of symptoms in humans.[4]

A second case report of rabies that influenced epidemiologic thinking about the means of transmission of the virus was the description of a cave explorer, a spelunker, who developed rabies after exploring a cave inhabited by large numbers of bats in Frio, Texas.[5] In this case, there was no history of a bite. Epidemiologic thinking until that time was that rabies could be transmitted only by the direct inoculation of virus by a bite from a rabid animal. This case was followed by a series of experiments in which animals were placed in the cave and protected from bites and even insect transmission but were exposed to the air in the infected cave. After several animals developed rabies during this exposure, the classic concepts of rabies transmission were challenged.[5] Additional studies showed that rodents could be infected by the aerosol route.[6,7] A review of case reports of rabies in the United States in the last 20 years has found that the majority of human cases has not had a history of a bite, and many of these have been acquired from bats.[8] The control of rabies in domestic animals in the United States has resulted in fewer human cases but those that occur from exposure to wild animals often had nonbite exposures.

HIV/AIDS: Efficacy of Bone Marrow Transplant in an HIV-Infected Patient

The natural history of HIV infection has been studied extensively. The HIV virus undergoes a life cycle in which the viral RNA is reverse transcribed to DNA, the proviral DNA message is incorporated into the host genome of the cell, usually a lymphocyte or macrophage, finally viral proteins are synthesized and new virus is assembled and released. Most retrovirologists believe that cure of an HIV infection would be difficult or impossible because the viral message is incorporated into long-lived host cells that can transmit viral DNA to daughter cells when they divide. The concept of HIV as an incurable infection was challenged several years ago with a report of a patient with HIV infection and non-Hodgkin's lymphoma.[9] The patient was given high doses of zidovudine, cyclophosphamide, and whole body irradiation prior to a bone marrow transplant. He recovered, but died 47 days after the transplantation. At autopsy, the investigators could not find evidence of HIV in his tissues by culture, in vitro hybridization, or polymerase chain reaction (PCR) amplification. The authors believed that the patient had been "cured" of his HIV infection by the marrow ablation and transplantation. Unfortunately, the patient died soon after transplantation, so long-term cure of the HIV infection was not proven. However, this case provoked extensive discussion and debate about the possibility of curing HIV infection by ablation of infected immune cells and reconstitution of bone marrow by transplantation. This debate has recently been reopened with the development of multiple new antiretroviral drugs and the use of highly active antiretroviral therapy (HAART), which can reduce the viral load in the blood to undetectable levels. Some investigators have hypothesized that a cure for AIDS might be possible if the cells in which proviral HIV DNA is integrated could be identified and killed or if they died without producing progeny.[10]

HIV/AIDS: Spontaneous Cure of HIV

A second case report challenged the concept that HIV is inevitably a chronic persistent infection. Bryceson and her colleagues from the University of California at Los Angeles reported a case of an infant who was born after 36 weeks' gestation to an asymptomatic HIV-positive woman.[11] She reported a history of sex with a former injection drug user. The pregnancy was uncomplicated, and the mother had a CD4+ T-cell count of over 1,000 cells/mm^3 at the time of delivery. The infant was normal at birth but required hospitalization for 8 days because of mild respiratory distress syndrome. Laboratory studies on the infant found a negative culture of cord blood for HIV. However, the infant's blood culture was positive at 19 and 51 days of age, and the PCR was positive at 33 days of life. Subsequently, HIV antibodies disappeared by 12 months of age. Multiple cultures of peripheral blood lymphocytes and plasma for HIV were negative between 3 months and 5 years of age. The child was asymptomatic and had no laboratory evidence of HIV infection at 5 years of age. The authors believed that the infant was infected but cleared the HIV infection by immunologic or other mechanisms. This case report was followed up by a search for similar cases of spontaneous resolution of perinatal HIV infection in infants by other investigators; however, no similar cases have been reported.

Subsequently, Clerici et al. reported that specific cytotoxic T-lymphocyte (CTL) responses to HIV peptides were common among antibody-negative individuals who had remained uninfected, despite frequent exposure to HIV.[12] They hypothesized that clearing of an HIV infection by highly exposed individuals might not be uncommon. However, alternative explanations for their findings could be that some of the CTL results lacked specificity or that the CTL responses occurred because of immunization with viral peptides or proteins, rather than true HIV infection (ie, HIV replication and nucleic acid integration).

Case Series

A second type of descriptive epidemiologic study is a case series. In this type of study, data from a cluster or series of cases are reported. No comparison is made with controls; instead, the exposures of the cases are often described. These case series may be reported in sufficient epidemiologic detail that it is possible to infer the means of transmission and the risk factors for infection. A case series of AIDS patients, which was reported early in the epidemic and prior to the identification of HIV, is described below.

AIDS Cluster

A cluster of homosexual men with Kaposi's sarcoma (KS) and/or *Pneumocystis carinii* pneumonia (PCP) was reported in 1984, prior to the identification of the HIV.[13] The investigators enumerated the sexual contacts of the first 19 homosexual male AIDS patients reported from Southern California. One of the men had sexual contacts with 12 of the AIDS patients within 5 years of the onset of their symptoms. Four of the patients from Southern California had contact with a non-California AIDS patient, who was also the sex partner of four AIDS patients from New York City. Ultimately, 40 AIDS patients in 10 cities were linked by sexual contact in this extensive sexual network (Figure 3–2). This remarkable study led the investigators to conclude that AIDS was caused by a sexually transmitted agent. The sexual network linking these patients with the new disease (AIDS) was remarkably similar to the networks of patients with syphilis that were described four decades earlier. At the epicenter of this cluster was "patient 0," who estimated that he had had about 250 different male sexual partners each year from 1979 through 1981 and was able to name 72 of his 750 partners

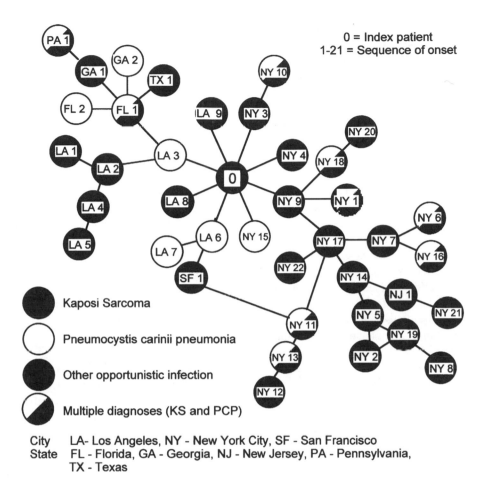

0 = Index patient
1-21 = Sequence of onset

● Kaposi Sarcoma

○ Pneumocystis carinii pneumonia

● Other opportunistic infection

◐ Multiple diagnoses (KS and PCP)

City   LA- Los Angeles, NY - New York City, SF - San Francisco
State   FL - Florida, GA - Georgia, NJ - New Jersey, PA - Pennsylvania,
        TX - Texas

Figure 3–2 Sexual contacts among homosexual men with AIDS. Each circle represents an AIDS patient. Lines connecting the circles represent sexual exposures. Indicated city or state is place of residence of a patient at the time of diagnosis. "0" indicates Patient 0 (described in text). *Source:* Reprinted from *American Journal of Medicine*, Vol. 76, D. Auerbach et al., Cluster of Cases of the Acquired Immune Deficiency Syndrome, Patients Linked by Sexual Contact, pp. 487–492, Copyright 1984, with permission from Excerpta Medica Inc.

during this 3-year period; 8 of these partners had developed AIDS.

Ecologic Studies

Ecologic studies are another type of epidemiologic study. Ecologic studies measure the exposure and rates of disease at a population level, rather than at an individual level. Thus, they compare the rates of exposure to risk factor(s) in different populations and the association with the rates of disease in the same populations. In an ecologic study, whether an individual member of a population is exposed and has disease or whether there is an association between a risk factor and a disease at the individual level is unknown. Furthermore, it is not possible to assess whether there are confounding factors at the individual level in the relationship between the exposure and disease. This may lead to biased or erroneous conclusions. Despite these caveats, ecologic studies may be useful to explore hypothesized associations and to test hypotheses that may not be easily tested by other types of studies. Ecologic studies also may be conducted with relatively less financial or other resources than other epidemiologic studies. Data may be available from national or community-wide surveys of exposures and disease rates, which can be accessed inexpensively. Ecologic studies also allow for comparisons between populations that are too geographically dispersed for individual-based study designs. In some populations, the range of exposure may be too narrow to allow easy analysis of the association with a disease outcome at an individual level within that population. Studies of host nutrition status, such as vitamin A, on the outcome of an infection might best be evaluated in a population containing vitamin A–deficient individuals or by comparing infection outcome in several populations with different vitamin A levels. Similarly, studies of the relationship between infectious agents and unusual outcomes, such as the liver fluke *Ophisthorcus viverini* and bile duct cancer or *Helicobacter pylori* and stomach cancer, can be strengthened by ecologic data from populations with widely varying rates of infections and cancer. In addition, the concept of "herd immunity" to infectious diseases is a concept that developed based on ecologic considerations. The proportion of a population that is immune to an infectious disease can influence the risk of infection in an individual in the population. Ecologic studies are also extremely important for assessing the population impact of intervention programs. For example, the efficacy of measles vaccination is well established from randomized clinical studies, but population effectiveness of a vaccination program can be assessed only by surveillance, using an ecologic

design. Two ecologic studies, one of rheumatic fever and one of HIV infection are described below.

Crowding and Rheumatic Fever

Early studies led to the hypothesis that household crowding was an important environmental factor in the transmission of Group A streptococci and high rates of acute rheumatic fever. Conversely, it has been hypothesized that the reduction in household crowding may be one of the factors in the decreased rates of acute rheumatic fever in the last half of the twentieth century in comparison with earlier periods.[14] The data in Figure 3–3 show the association between the incidence of rheumatic heart disease per 100,000 and the number of persons per room in various districts in the city of Bristol, England in 1927–1930.

Circumcision and HIV Transmission

Because of the physical differences in the penile epithelium between circumcised and uncircumcised males, it has been hypothesized that uncircumcised males might be at higher risk for HIV infection. Circumcised men have been found to have lower rates of other sexually transmitted diseases (STDs).[15] An ecologic study of circumcision rates and HIV seroprevalence was conducted in several African countries.[16] Data on circumcision practices were extracted from an ethnographic database, the Human Relations Area File in New Haven, Connecticut, and combined with HIV seroprevalence data from a variety of published scientific literature sources and governmental data. These data were mapped to demonstrate geographical overlap between cultures that do not practice male circumcision and a high seroprevalence rate of HIV infection among males (Figure 3–4). This study raises the possibility that lack of male circumcision increases the risk of HIV transmission. However, there are obvious behavioral, cultural, and religious differences between ethnic groups that are correlated with circumcision frequency and sexual behavior, which could influence the risk of HIV transmission. Because an ecologic study

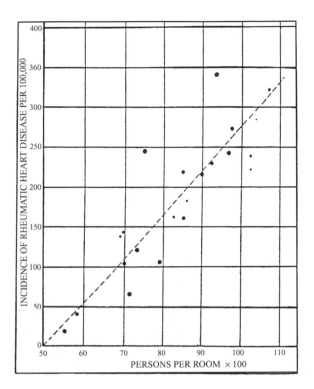

Figure 3–3 The correlation between the incidence of rheumatic heart disease per 100,000 and the number of persons per room (× 100), as found by Perry and Roberts in various districts of the city of Bristol, England, in 1927–1930. (The size of the dots indicates roughly the comparative population size of the districts.) *Source:* Reprinted with permission from E. Kass, Infectious Diseases and Social Change, *Journal of Infectious Diseases,* Vol. 23, No. 1, p. 113, © 1971, University of Chicago Press.

design does not collect individual-level data, it cannot control for these confounding factors. However, an increased risk of HIV infection in uncircumcised men is biologically plausible and has been found for other STDs. Furthermore, a randomized clinical trial of circumcision would be very difficult. Therefore, although these ecologic data are not as scientifically rigorous as are data studied in a clinical trial, they provide useful information on this association.

Analytic Studies in General

Several different types of analytic studies have been used to study the natural history or risk factors for an infection. Among these are

cross-sectional, cohort, case-control and nested-case-control studies, and clinical trials. In these types of studies, the epidemiologist measures exposures and disease status in individuals to evaluate associations (Table 3–1). These study designs differ in

- their temporal nature, whether they are conducted at a given point in time or are conducted over an interval of time
- the characterization of subjects, whether they define individuals according to their risk factors for disease or according to their disease status
- the measures of association between risk factors and disease

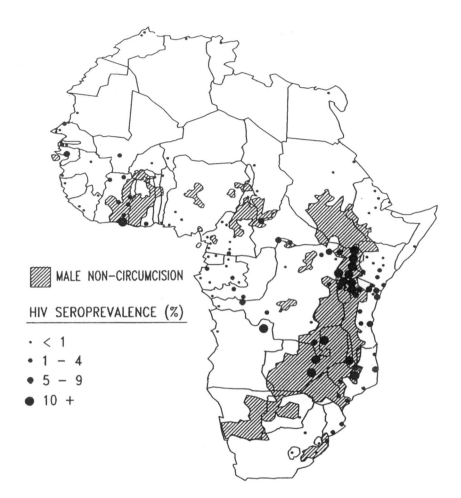

Figure 3–4 Map of Africa showing political boundaries and usual male circumcision practice, with point estimates of general adult population HIV seroprevalence superimposed. *Source:* Reprinted with permission from S. Moses et al., Geographical Patterns of Male Circumcision Practices in Africa: Association with HIV Seroprevalence, *International Journal of Epidemiology*, Vol. 19, p. 693–697, © 1990, Oxford University Press.

Temporal Differences in Study Designs

Epidemiologists may be able to measure the occurrence of disease and other characteristics in a population at a given point in time—a cross-sectional study. A cross-sectional study can measure the prevalence of disease in a population. Cross-sectional and case-control studies measure the association between a dis-

ease and possible risk factors. Although correlates of disease are not always causes of the disease, a causal association is more likely if the association is strong, consistent in several studies, and biologically plausible. These study designs may collect exposure data at the time that cases and controls are selected or they may use previously collected data to add temporal depth to their study. Later in the chapter, case-control

Table 3-1 Summary of the Basic Analytic Study Designs

Study Design	Temporal Nature	Characterization of Subjects at Enrollment	Measures of Association
Cross-sectional	Point in time May collect retrospective data	Exposure and disease status measured simultaneously	$\text{Prevalence of disease} = \dfrac{\text{N with disease}}{\text{Total population}}$
Case-control	Point in time May collect retrospective data	Diseased and nondiseased	$\text{Relative Risk} = \dfrac{\frac{\text{N exposed with disease}}{\text{Total N exposed}}}{\frac{\text{N unexposed with disease}}{\text{Total N unexposed}}}$ $\text{Odds Ratio} = \dfrac{\frac{\text{N exposed with disease}}{\text{N exposed without disease}}}{\frac{\text{N unexposed with disease}}{\text{N unexposed without disease}}}$
Cohort	Follow participants over time	Exposed and nonexposed	$\text{Prevalence} = \dfrac{\text{N with disease}}{\text{N total cohort}}$
Clinical trial	Follow participants over time	Similar with respect to disease status, randomly assigned an exposure status (treatment)	$\text{Relative Risk} = \dfrac{\frac{\text{N treated with disease}}{\text{N treated}}}{\frac{\text{N untreated with disease}}{\text{N untreated}}}$ $\text{Incidence of disease} = \dfrac{\text{N with disease}}{\frac{\text{N persons}}{\text{Unit of time}}}$ $\text{Odds Ratio} = \dfrac{\frac{\text{N treated with disease}}{\text{N treated without disease}}}{\frac{\text{N untreated with disease}}{\text{N untreated without disease}}}$

studies that are "nested" in cohort studies are discussed.

In contrast, cohort studies are often but not always longitudinal studies, and participants are followed over time. In cohort studies, a researcher identifies and enrolls a population (cohort) that does not have the disease at baseline and measures various factors to identify those that precede the development of disease and those that may be causal factors. When such associations are confirmed in multiple studies and if the factors can be shown to have a biologic association with disease, it can fulfill the epidemiologic criteria to be considered a cause or cofactor in the disease.

Exposure Status versus Disease Status

All of the study designs measure the strength of the association between disease and a characteristic or exposure of a population. However, the approaches are based on different definitions of the study population. The study population can be defined according to disease or exposure status, or both (Figure 3–5). In a cross-sectional design, the study population is defined simultaneously by exposure characteristics and disease status. Patients with the disease are compared to nondiseased controls, and risk factors, or exposures, are measured in the two groups.

Prospective cohort studies enroll persons who are at risk of developing a disease but who are disease free at baseline. Possible risk factors, or exposures, (ie, interview data and/or biologic specimens) are measured, as is the incidence of new cases of the disease. Multiple biologic specimens, eg, serum, cells, tissues, etc., can be collected and stored in a repository for subsequent testing when new hypotheses are developed.

Disease status is used for enrollment in case-control and cross-sectional studies. In a case-control study, the researcher determines eligibility using a specific definition of disease status and compares the prevalence of exposure between those with and without disease. In a case-control study, it is usually possible to specify multiple rigorous criteria for the enrollment of a case, so that the case definition is not arguable. However, this may make selection of a suitable control population more difficult.

Measures of Association

Regardless of the study design, the goal is to measure the association between exposure to a risk factor and the occurrence of a disease. Both cross-sectional and prospective studies can express the data obtained in a 2×2 table or a $2 \times X$ (several categories) table. In these tables, the number of study participants who are exposed are stratified according to their disease status. In a $2 \times X$ table, there may be multiple levels of exposure (Exhibit 3–2).

The calculation of the association between exposure and disease differs, based on the de-

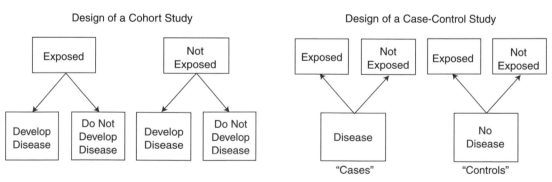

Figure 3–5 Cohort and case-control study designs. *Source:* Reprinted with permission from L. Gordis, *Epidemiology*, p. 163, © 1996, W.B. Saunders Company.

Exhibit 3–2 Epidemiologic Data Presentation

Epidemiologic data can be presented according to the disease and exposure status of the study participants. In the simplest case, the data may be presented as a 2 × 2 table. In instances where there are multiple
exposures, the 2 × 2 table may be generalized to include as many exposure categories as necessary.

2 × 2 Table				*2 ×X Table*		
		Disease Status			Disease Status	
		+	−		+	−
Exposure	Yes	A	B	High	A	B
Status	No	C	D	Medium	C	D
				Low	E	F
				None	G	H

In the 2×X table, the "Exposure Status" label appears at left with rows High, Medium, Low, None.

sign of the study. In a cross-sectional study, in which the proportion of diseased individuals from a defined reference population is not fixed by the study design, the association between exposure and disease is termed the *relative risk* (RR) and is expressed as follows:

$$RR = \frac{\dfrac{A}{(A+B)}}{\dfrac{C}{(C+D)}} = \frac{\text{Prevalence of disease in exposed}}{\text{Prevalence of disease in nonexposed}}$$

The above equation shows that if the prevalence of disease among those exposed is greater than the prevalence in the unexposed, the RR will be greater than 1, and if the difference is large (ie, statistically significant) the exposure is a risk factor for the disease. Conversely, if the prevalence in the exposed is significantly less than the prevalence in the unexposed, the RR will be less than 1, and the exposure is protective. Less commonly, data from a cross-sectional study may be analyzed to determine the ratio of odds of exposure in cases and controls, the odds ratio (OR), as described below.

In a prospective cohort study, the incidence rate, usually expressed as the number of cases of disease per unit of time or per person-years of observation is used instead of the prevalence.

$$RR = \frac{\text{Incidence/person-years in exposed}}{\text{Incidence/person-years in non-exposed}}$$

Statistical Significance

To determine whether the association is statistically significant, the epidemiologist must be able to demonstrate that the results are unlikely to be explained by chance alone. Epidemiologists commonly use the 95% confidence interval to illustrate the possible range of values that the RR could take, given the distribution of the data. In other words, the researcher is confident that, 95% of the time, the measured RR will be between the upper and lower limits of the confidence interval if the experiment were repeated. If the confidence interval does not include one, then the researcher can report that there is a statistically significant association, within the 95% confidence limits, between the exposure and the disease. The use of the 95% confidence limits as indicating "statistical significance," though standard, is arbitrary. Other confidence limits could be used in some circumstances and sometimes are. One could also calculate the "p-value," or the probability of a chance association, instead of the 95% confidence limits. The p-value, in contrast to the 95% confidence limits, gives only the probability of a chance association and not the strength, or importance, of the association. Weak associations can have a significant p-value if the sample size is very large. Therefore, the 95% confidence limit is preferable, because it more clearly depicts the strength of the association, as well as demonstrating its statistical significance.

The method usually used to calculate the 95% confidence limit of the RR is shown below.[17]

$$\text{Variance of natural log (RR)} = \frac{\frac{B}{A}}{(A+B)} + \frac{\frac{D}{C}}{(C+D)}$$

Standard error of the natural log(RR) = (Variance lnRR)$^{1/2}$

95% Confidence Interval lnRR = lnRR $\pm z_{\alpha=0.05}$ * SE (lnRR)

upper limit lnRR = lnRR + 1.96 * SE (lnRR)

lower limit lnRR = lnRR − 1.96 * SE (lnRR)

upper limit RR = $e^{\text{upper limit lnRR}}$

lower limit RR = $e^{\text{lower limit lnRR}}$

In contrast, case-control studies, which have a predetermined proportion of diseased and disease-free participants (ie, a given number of controls are chosen per case), compare the RR of exposure among those with and without disease. The formula is shown below:

$$\text{RR of exposure} = \frac{A/A+C}{B/B+D}$$

However, although the RR of exposure can evaluate the strength of the association between a risk factor and disease, it is not an intuitively easy measurement to evaluate. Instead, the odds of disease among exposed, or OR, is more commonly calculated from case control data.

$$\text{Odds Ratio} = \frac{AD}{BC}$$

The 95% confidence interval for the OR is calculated in a similar manner to the method used for calculating the confidence interval of RR in a cohort study[17]:

$$\text{Variance of lnOR} = \frac{1}{A} + \frac{1}{B} + \frac{1}{C} + \frac{1}{D}$$

Standard error of the lnOR = (Variance lnOR)$^{1/2}$

95% Confidence Interval lnOR = lnOR $\pm z_{\alpha} = 0.05$ * SE (lnOR)

upper limit lnOR = lnOR + 1.96 * SE (lnOR)

lower limit lnOR = lnOR − 1.96 * SE (lnOR)

upper limit OR = $e^{\text{upper limit lnOR}}$

lower limit OR = $e^{\text{lower limit lnOR}}$

In a case-control study, the OR of disease may be a close approximation of the RR of disease when the prevalence of the disease in the population is low. As a rule of thumb, when the prevalence of disease is less than 5%, the RR and OR are considered equal.

$$\text{RR} = \frac{A/A+B}{C/C+D} = \frac{AD}{BC} = OR$$

When the disease is rare, A and C are very small, A + B is approximately equal to B, and C + D is approximately equal to D.

$$\frac{A/B}{C/D} = \frac{AD}{BC}$$

In addition to these simple measures of exposure and disease associations, a variety of other statistical methods is available to the infectious disease epidemiologist. Powerful computer programs for exploratory analysis, graphing, and statistical software for simultaneous control of the effect of multiple variables in disease outcome are now available to epidemiologists. A clear understanding of the statistical tools used in analysis is vital to achieving accurate results in the analysis of data, because these computer programs will give results even when inappropriately applied. A description of these methods is beyond the scope of this chapter. The reader is advised to consult other references for a detailed description of these methods: Breslow and Day,[18] Rothman and Greenland,[2] Diggle, Liang, and Zeger,[3] and Brookmeyer and Gail.[19]

Analytic Study Designs, Some Specific Details

Cross-Sectional Studies

Cross-sectional studies measure the occurrence of disease in a population at a single point in time; this measurement is called the *prevalence*. Case-control studies collect data on participants that are used to evaluate the prevalence of disease with respect to exposures of interest. The prevalence is a measure that is very useful to public health professionals in assessing the current burden of disease in a community. This "snapshot" of a disease is inherently static, but if multiple cross-sectional studies are conducted in a population, changes over time may be evaluated. However, incidence data are often more useful in making future projections. Cross-sectional studies suffer some limitations in their ability to draw conclusions about cause and effect. Because measurements of disease are being made concurrently with the measurements of related characteristics, it is often not possible to determine for certain whether the exposure preceded the disease. However, this is sometimes possible. Cross-sectional studies also can be done at several times within a defined cohort. Some examples are described below.

Cross-Sectional Studies of HIV Prevalence in Young Men in Northern Thailand

Multiple cross-sectional studies of HIV prevalence in male military conscripts in Thailand have been used to evaluate the national HIV control program. Serial cross-sectional studies of HIV prevalence and behavioral risk factors among 21-year-old men conscripted into the Royal Thai Army (RTA) were conducted between 1991 and 1998.[20] The HIV/AIDS epidemic began in Thailand in 1988 and spread rapidly among urban and rural populations, especially in Northern Thailand. The predominant means of spread was by heterosexual sex, although transmission by injecting drug use, homosexual sex, and perinatal transmission also occurred.

The government responded to this widespread, rapidly evolving epidemic with a program called the *100% condom program*. This program included intensive health education about the risk of HIV transmission, especially during commercial sex, the provision of free condoms, and the promotion of their use wherever commercial sex occurred.

The serial cross-sectional studies were used to document temporal trends in HIV prevalence, changes in the frequency of commercial sex, condom use, and the prevalence of STDs in these young men. These data were an unbiased estimate of the prevalence of HIV and associated risk factors because selection of the conscripts was by a random lottery system. Approximately 9% of all eligible 21-year-old men were conscripted by lottery each year. Men were not excluded based on their HIV status, a history of male-to-male sexual behavior, or injecting drug use. Furthermore, because the average age of sexual debut was 17 years, HIV prevalence in 21-year-old males represented recently acquired infection and could be used to evaluate the success of the Thai control program.

The prevalence of HIV declined from 11.9% in 1991–1993 to 4.7% in 1997, whereas the lifetime history of an STD declined from 42% to 4.2% during this period. The use of sex workers in the past year declined from 60% in 1991 to 18% in 1997, and condom use during commercial sex increased from 67% in 1991 to 95% in 1997 (Figure 3–6). These cross-sectional data documented the effectiveness of the HIV prevention program in Thailand.

HIV Cross-Sectional Studies within a Cohort

Multicenter AIDS Cohort Study. Any particular visit of the individuals enrolled in a cohort study is an opportunity to conduct a cross-sectional analysis. In many cohort studies, the study population is characterized initially at baseline. Such cross-sectional studies allow for description of the cohort being followed and a preliminary assessment of the association of risk factors with disease outcome. The Multicenter AIDS Cohort Study (MACS) enrolled about 5,000 homosexual men in 1984 from four urban areas (Los Angeles, Chicago, Baltimore-Washington, and Pittsburgh) in a prospective study to evaluate the risk factors and natural history of HIV/AIDS. Enrollment criteria included participants who were homosexual, over 18 years of age, and willing to be followed with repeated interviews and physical exams (Table 3–2). After the HIV antibody test became available, the MACS study was able to measure the HIV seroprevalence among study participants at the baseline visit, even though they had been enrolled prior to the availability of an HIV antibody test (Table 3–3).[21] HIV seroprevalence rates were reported according to the participants' demographic characteristics, including

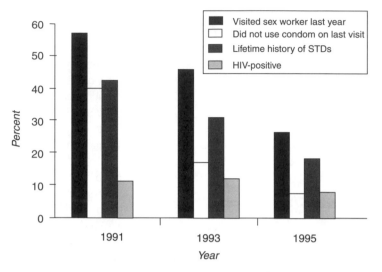

Figure 3–6 Sexual behavior, STDs, and HIV in 21-year-old men in Northern Thailand, 1991–1995. *Source:* Data from Nelson et al., *The New England Journal of Medicine*, Vol. 335, pp. 297–303, © 1996, the Massachusetts Medical Society.

city of residence, age, race, educational level, and occupational group. These data give a "snapshot" of the HIV prevalence and risk factors for HIV infection in the MACS population. They demonstrated that men who were 25–34 years old, nonwhite, with no more than a high school education, and who were service or craft/repair workers had a higher prevalence of HIV infection early in the study. The HIV prevalence at baseline varied in the men from the participating cities; HIV prevalence was 11% in subjects from Pittsburgh, 29% in Baltimore-Washington, 30% in Chicago, and 42% in Los Angeles. The number of partners and sexual practices were similar in men from the different sites. However, men from Los Angeles were more likely to have had sex with a partner who developed AIDS, reflecting the fact that the epidemic was older in Los Angeles. Prevalence of HIV infection at baseline was also associated with having had receptive anal intercourse with a larger number of partners and reporting a history of an STD.

Women's Interagency HIV Study. Another cohort study is the Women's Interagency HIV Study (WIHS), which was initiated to study the effect of HIV-related immune suppression on gynecologic pathology and the natural history of HIV in women (Table 3–2).[22] A cross-sectional study was done in this cohort to evaluate the association between HIV and human papilloma virus (HPV) infection among over 2,500 subjects, comprised of both HIV-negative and HIV-positive women who were enrolled at six clinical sites throughout the United States. Data collected included physical exams, medical history, behavioral and demographic factors, as well as $CD4^+$ cell count and quantitative RT-PCR measurement of HIV RNA and prevalence of HPV infection using hybrid capture and PCR amplification. This allowed the investigators to examine the association between HIV and HPV prevalence.[23]

In this study, HIV-positive women with a $CD4^+$ T-cell count of less than 200 cells/mm³ were at the highest risk of HPV infection, regardless of HIV RNA load (OR = 10.13; 95% confidence interval [CI] = 7.32, 10.34). A lower risk was seen among women with a $CD4^+$ T-cell count greater than 200 cells/mm³ but who had a high viral load, HIV RNA greater than 20,000 copies/ml (OR = 5.78, 95% CI: 4.17–8.08). The

Table 3–2 Enrollment Criteria for the Multicenter AIDS Clinical Study, the AIDS Link to the Intravenous Experience (ALIVE), and the Women's Interagency HIV Study (WIHS)

Characteristics	MACS (N = 4,955)	ALIVE (N = 2,960)	WIHS (N = 2,058)
Risk group	Men who have sex with men	Injected drugs at least once after 1978	Women with and without HIV infection
Age group	18–70 years	Over 18 years	Over 13 years
Gender	Males	Males and females	Females
Recruitment method	Existing HBV study, word of mouth referrals, community outreach, media outreach, clinic referral	Street recruitment, word of mouth, clinic/hospital/ treatment center referral	Community outreach, hospital-based and research programs, women's support groups, drug treatment, word of mouth, HIV testing sites, clinic referral
HIV serostatus	Unknown	Tested at first visit	Tested at first visit
AIDS	AIDS-free	AIDS-free	AIDS and AIDS-free
Study visit schedule	6-month visits	6-month visits	6-month visits
Physical exam	All	All HIV-seropositives, subset HIV-seronegatives	All
Routine specimens	Serum, plasma, lymphocytes, throat washings/saliva, urine, feces, semen	Serum, plasma, lymphocytes	Serum, plasma, lymphocytes, cervical lavage, urine, throat washings/saliva
Risk exposure data	1-hour interviewer-administered questionnaire	1-hour interviewer-administered questionnaire	1-hour interviewer-administered questionnaire

lowest risk was for women with a CD4$^+$ T-cell count greater than 200 cells/mm^3 and a low viral load, less than 20,000 HIV-RNA copies/ml. This study suggested there was a correlation between HIV-related immune suppression and HPV infection. The next step would be to evaluate the association in a prospective study design so that a causal link could be evaluated.

Case-Control and Nested Case-Control Studies

Case-control studies are the natural extension of a descriptive case series study. They are also related to a cohort study when the cases and controls are drawn from or can be related back to a defined or similar population, ie, a population

Table 3–3 Cross-Sectional Analysis of Data from the Multicenter AIDS Cohort Study (MACS)

	% Seropositive*			
	Baltimore/ Washington DC	Chicago	Los Angeles	Pittsburgh/ Tristate Area
Age (years)				
18–24	29	30	42	11
25–34	35	49	53	26
35–44	31	42	52	19
45+	18	33	38	11
Race				
White	30	42	51	20
Black	47	60	52	35
Other	46	50	41	27
Educational level				
≤12th grade	35	60	65	26
Some college	34	46	51	21
Some graduate work	27	33	46	17
Occupation				
Management/professional	29	39	47	21
Technical/sales	32	39	51	18
Service	36	57	62	23
Craft/repair	38	71	52	21
Operator/laborer	30	41	50	24

*Prevalence of ELISA antibody to human immunodeficiency virus and relationship to demographic features among homosexual men, by center of the MACS, at entry, April 1984–April 1985.

Source: Reprinted with permission from R. Kaslow et al., The Multicenter AIDS Cohort Study: Rationale, Organization, and Selected Characteristics of the Participants, *American Journal of Epidemiology*, Vol. 126, p. 317, © 1987, Oxford University Press.

"set." In a case-control study, a group of persons with a disease—the cases—is compared with a group of persons without the disease—the controls. Because the proportion of those with disease in the study is fixed by the study design, the analysis is based on comparing the rate of exposure in those with and without the disease. In a case-control study, the researcher concentrates on assembling a group of persons with and without disease. This fundamental characteristic of the study design has several advantages. The

study of rare diseases is possible because resources can be efficiently used in evaluating the known or readily available cases of a disease. More than one exposure can be evaluated because the original study population was not restricted with respect to exposure. Typically, case-control studies have smaller sample sizes than do cohort studies, allowing for greater resources to be expended per participant and for lower costs to the study overall. Resources can be used to define disease status and the absence of disease with certainty, reducing the risk of misclassification bias.

Case-control studies are especially useful for evaluating potential risk factors in an outbreak of an infectious disease, because they can be done quickly and efficiently. However, the determination of exposure data may be difficult. Sometimes, the exposure may have occurred many years prior to the onset of the disease, so recall bias may be a problem. However, in acute outbreaks of infectious diseases, such as the toxic shock syndrome or food-borne outbreaks, the exposures are recent, so recall bias may be less important than when the time from exposure to disease is long. Recall often can be differential; persons who have developed a disease that is putatively linked to an exposure may recall exposure more readily than will those in whom

no disease occurred. Also, case-control studies of chronic infectious diseases may be affected by survival bias, ie, the cases enrolled are the survivors. Case-control studies are sensitive to biases because the study population is highly selected (Exhibit 3–3). However, it would be incorrect to assume that other study designs are not also susceptible to some of these same biases.

In analytical case-control studies, the researcher attempts to determine the exposures among the cases and controls. Because the analysis is based on comparisons within the study sample, generalizability of the results to the overall population is less important than the appropriate selection of the control population. The overriding consideration in the selection of controls is to select them in such a way that they

Exhibit 3–3 Biases of Epidemiologic Studies

Response-bias occurs when persons who have a disease or their medical care providers examine their past behaviors and exposures so carefully that they are more likely to report behaviors or risk that they feel are associated with a disease. Conversely, they may also be more likely to suppress information that they feel would incriminate them as the cause of their own illness.

Ibrahim-Spitzer bias is when the selection of cases and controls results in a distorted measure of association between the exposure and disease.

Prevalence-incidence bias, Neyman bias, may occur if the duration of disease is affected by exposure. Prevalence incidence bias can raise or lower the observed association between an exposure and a disease. If persons who are exposed to a factor have a more rapid course of disease, they may die before they can be identified by researchers. This will spuriously reduce the relative risk. Conversely, if exposure increases survival, the relative risk measured by the study will be higher than the true association.

Latency bias occurs if the analysis is begun prior to the development of disease among exposed cases. For example, liver cancer cases would not be manifested if a study of the role of Hepatitis C infection in cancer was initiated only a few months after exposure.

Berksonian bias occurs if there is referral bias of exposed persons to study personnel.

Detection bias occurs when persons who are known to be exposed to a hypothesized etiologic exposure undergo more rigorous screening. Thus, exposed persons are more likely to be cases because the sensitivity of screening is higher among exposed than unexposed.

Nonresponse bias cases may be either too sick to participate or have died prior to the study. Researchers may have to rely on exposure ascertainment data from surrogate respondents. Thus, data may be collected differently from cases and controls.

are representative of the same population from which the cases arose. Studies have sought controls from other patients in hospitals or clinics, friends of the cases, family members of cases, neighborhood or geographic controls, or other accessible populations. Whereas the risk of disease may differ between cases and controls, controls must be at risk of developing disease. For example, HIV seronegative persons are not suitable controls for a study of KS in AIDS patients. Researchers must also decide whether controls should be chosen from populations with other diseases or from nondiseased persons. Frequently, data are available on persons diagnosed with another disease as a result of treatment for the other disease that can be of use in comparing risk factor exposures between cases and controls. When controls with other diseases are selected, it is important to ensure that the exposure being evaluated is not also related to the control's disease. Sometimes, it may be difficult to rule out the presence of disease in persons who have not received certain diagnostic procedures. However, a study may compromise generalizability or external validity when it increases the level of diagnostic information required for controls.

Generally, researchers choose to minimize differences between cases and controls with respect to other known risk factors for the development of disease. Controls may be matched with cases to varying degrees. Controls may be simply drawn from homogenous populations, such as clinics that serve only specific types of patients. More closely matched controls may be chosen from subpopulations that closely conform to the demographic characteristics of the cases. Individual matching may also be used. Individual matching can reduce the variability between the cases and controls with respect to confounding factors, known and unknown, but there are several potential drawbacks. The inability to find a matched control for a particular case could result in exclusion of the case. This would be a particular problem if cases were rare. Matching increases the complexity of enrollment of par-

ticipants, and this complexity could result in errors in enrollment. Because cases and controls have been chosen so that they are similar with respect to the matching variables, analysis of these characteristics with respect to disease is no longer possible. The data may be expressed in a 2×2 table. Instead of each study participant being counted in the table, data are entered by pairs. For example, a pair where both the case and control are exposed would be recorded as one data point in the A cell of the table. When a matched design is used in a case-control study, the OR is expressed as the ratio of the discordant pairs.

		Controls	
		Exposed	Not exposed
Case	Exposed	A	B
	Not exposed	C	D

$$\text{Odds ratio (matched pair)} = \frac{B}{C}$$

One of the major problems with case-control studies is the reliability and validity of the measurement of the exposure. Also, it may not be possible to determine whether the exposure occurred prior to the onset of disease. One type of study design that can be used to avoid these issues is a *nested case-control* study. Cases are selected from a cohort after the onset of illness, and they are matched with controls from the same cohort on whom similar exposure information is available and who have had the same opportunity to be diagnosed with disease. Controls should have been followed for a similar length of time as the cases, and they should have received the same diagnostic procedures. Many of the biases that can arise in reconstructing retrospective exposure data are reduced or eliminated when previously collected data from a cohort study are used. Furthermore, nested case-control study designs have the advantage that the researcher can be certain that exposure proceeded the onset of disease. Analysis of stored specimens from the cohort study also ensures that changes in laboratory methods or artifacts due to specimen storage do not affect the study results differentially between cases and controls.

There are two commonly used methods for selecting controls in the nested case-control study. When controls are matched to cases by selecting participants from the cohort who are disease free at the time the case becomes ill, the procedure is referred to as *incidence density sampling*. A second method is to select controls from the cohort at baseline—a case-cohort design. In the case-cohort study, all or some known proportion of the original cohort is sampled for the analysis. When the case-cohort design is used, it is possible to estimate the prevalence of disease in the cohort and to calculate the population-attributable risk.[24]

Examples of case-control and nested case-control study designs are given below. The first two studies are case-control studies. First is a study of the association of KS and PCP and risk behaviors among homosexual men. The second is a study that evaluated the association between Reye's syndrome and aspirin use. Following these are examples of nested case-control studies. These studies evaluated the association of Epstein-Barr virus (EBV) infection and Hodgkin's disease (HD), and the association of KS and human herpes virus type 8 (HHV-8) infection. The third is a case-cohort study that evaluated the risk of HIV transmission due to needlestick exposures in health care workers (HCWs).

Case-Control Studies, Examples

Kaposi's Sarcoma and Pneumocystis carinii *Pneumonia in Homosexual Men*

After the recognition of the cluster of homosexual/bisexual men with KS and PCP in 1981, the Centers for Disease Control and Prevention (CDC) did a case-control study to determine the factors that placed these men at increased risk of AIDS.[25] For this study, 50 men with KS or PCP were matched by age and geographic area with 120 controls, who were homosexual men without AIDS. The rates of different exposures were compared between the cases and controls. The variable most strongly associated with illness was a greater number of male sex partners per year. Compared with controls, cases were also more likely to have been exposed to feces during sex, have had syphilis or hepatitis B virus infection, have been treated for enteric parasites, and had a higher reported lifetime use of various illicit substances, especially amylnitrite (Table 3–4). These results led the investigators to hypothesize that the illness was spread sexually and was associated with certain aspects of the homosexual lifestyle. When a similar disease appeared in injection drug users, transfusion recipients, and hemophiliacs, the hypothesis was strengthened that AIDS was caused by a specific infection.[26] The hypothesis that the agent was sexually transmitted was strengthened further when studies of the wives of men with hemophilia and AIDS or lymphadenopathy found that the wives also had low CD4+ lymphocyte counts.[27]

Reye's Syndrome and Aspirin Exposure

Another postinfectious syndrome, Reye's syndrome, was studied using a case-control design. The first case-control study of Reye's syndrome was conducted in Phoenix, Arizona, in 1976. This study showed a significant association between the use of aspirin during influenza illness and Reye's syndrome.[28] Subsequently, the incidence of Reye's syndrome in the United States increased significantly between 1972 and 1983. A number of case-control studies was done, and all of them showed a significant association with a similar OR.[29–31] Because of some lingering concerns about the representativeness of controls in these studies, the CDC did a case-control study in which controls were selected from four different populations for each case.[31] This case-control study agreed with the results of the other studies and showed a significant association between aspirin use for influenza and Reye's syndrome. Because of these findings, the

Table 3–4 Rates of Risk Behaviors Measured in a Case-Control Study

	Patients	Controls	
	Cases (N = 50)	Clinic (N = 78)	Private Practice (N = 42)
Median male sexual partners per year	61	27	25
Mean feces exposure scale	2.3	1.9	1.9
History of syphilis (%)	68	36	36
History of non-B hepatitis (%)	48	30	33
History of drugs for enteric parasites (%)	44	19	50
Use of ethyl chloride (%)	50	35	38
Lifetime nitrite use (days)	336	168	264

Source: Data from H. Jaffe et al., National Case-Control Study of Kaposi's Sarcoma and Pneumocystic Carinii Pneumonia in Homosexual Men, *Annals of Internal Medicine*, Vol. 99, pp. 145–151, © 1983 American College of Physicians-American Society of Internal Medicine.

CDC[32] and the American Academy of Pediatrics recommended that physicians warn parents of the risk of aspirin use for influenza, and the U.S. Food and Drug Administration mandated warning labels about this hazard on aspirin bottles. In the last decade, Reye's syndrome has virtually disappeared as aspirin use during influenza has declined (Figure 3–7).[33]

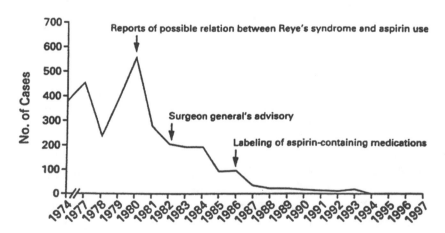

Figure 3–7 Number of reported cases of Reye's syndrome in relation to the timing of public announcements of the epidemiologic association of Reye's syndrome with aspirin ingestion and the labeling of aspirin-containing medications. *Source:* Reprinted with permission from Belay et al., Reye's Syndrome in the United States from 1981 through 1997, *The New England Journal of Medicine*, Vol. 340, pp. 1377–1382. Copyright © 1989 Massachusetts Medical Society. All rights reserved.

Nested Case-Control Studies

Epstein-Barr Virus Infection and Hodgkin's Disease

For several years, epidemiologists have questioned whether HD might be caused by an infectious agent, especially in those with onset at an earlier age. Some investigators have found evidence of an increased prevalence of EBV antibodies in patients with HD. Also, EBV is known to cause other tumors, especially nasopharyngeal carcinoma, and to persist after the initial infection. However, EBV infection is not uncommon. To show a causal association, it was necessary to demonstrate that EBV infection preceded the development of HD.

A community-based public health epidemiologic study in Washington County, Maryland, afforded the opportunity to test the hypothesis that EBV might be etiologically related to HD.[34] In this study, a sera repository was collected in 1963. Over two decades later, specimens from persons who had developed HD in the interim were selected, matched with controls, and tested for serologic evidence of EBV. The data showed a significant association between EBV antibodies prior to the onset of HD in cases, compared with matched controls (RR = 2.6–4.0 for various serologic markers of infection). This evidence strengthened the argument that EBV infection might be in the causal pathway for the development of HD because EBV infections preceded the onset of HD by years in many cases.

Kaposi's Sarcoma and HHV-8 (KSHV)

The presence of nucleic acid sequences of a new herpes virus (HHV-8) were detected in the lesions of AIDS patients with KS by Chang et al.[35] It then became important to determine whether infection with HHV-8 preceded the occurrence of KS in patients with HIV-1 infection. The availability of specimen repositories from several large cohorts of homosexual men allowed investigators to perform nested case-control studies. The sera were examined at baseline for antibodies to HHV-8 to estimate the RR of subsequent KS in men with and without HHV-8

antibodies. Also, Kaplan-Meier survival analysis was done to estimate the time-dependent risk of KS in HIV-positive men after HHV-8 infection. Nested case-control studies showing an association between HHV-8 infection and KS have been published from several cohorts, including a Danish Homosexual Cohort, an Australian Cohort, and the Multicenter AIDS Cohort Study (MACS).[36-38]

Case-Cohort Study of HIV Seroconversion among Health Care Workers

A nested case-cohort study of the risk of HIV seroconversion among HCWs in France, the United Kingdom, and the United States was published in 1995.[39] This study was done to determine whether treatment with zidovudine (or other antiretroviral drugs) after parenteral exposure in HCWs reduced the rate of HIV transmission. Several animal studies suggested that postexposure prophylaxis conferred protection after challenge with Simian immunodeficiency virus (SIV). Furthermore, at the time of the study, zidovudine had been shown to be effective in preventing vertical transmission of HIV. Prospective studies suggested that the risk of HIV transmission after parenteral exposure was only 0.35%.[40] Therefore, a prospective study, or clinical trial, would need to be extraordinarily large to have sufficient statistical power to evaluate the benefit of therapy. Also, recruitment of participants for a randomized clinical trial would be difficult because the unproven antiretroviral therapy was generally felt to be effective in preventing HIV transmission.

Accordingly, a case-cohort study using the available data from the United States and France was analyzed in which the exposure and treatment history of all known cases of HIV transmission to HCWs (N = 31 cases) was compared with that of all reported uninfected exposed HCWs (N = 679, cohort). Exposure was defined as those who had a documented penetrating injury with an instrument contaminated by blood from an HIV-positive patient. Cases and cohort members had received either zidovudine or no antiretroviral prophylaxis and had been followed at least 6 months, as of August 1994. The risk factors for HIV infection and protective effect of zidovudine are shown in Table 3–5.

Based on this study, it was recommended by the CDC that all HCWs receive zidovudine after percutaneous exposure to HIV-infected blood. However, it is clear that there are some potential biases in this study. For example, if there was significant underreporting of HCWs in whom transmission failed to occur and who had not received prophylaxis, the transmission rate in the control group could be inflated. This referral (or enrollment) bias would decrease the measured OR and increase the apparent protective efficacy of zidovudine postexposure prophylaxis above the actual efficacy. Certainly, data from a randomized controlled clinical trial could provide more valid data. However, clinical trials are not always feasible or ethical to conduct, and other study designs must often be used to answer important policy questions.

Cohort Studies

Enrollment

The word *cohort* was originally used to describe a unit of 300–600 men in the ancient Roman army. In epidemiology, a cohort is a group of persons with similar characteristics who are followed over time. The characteristic used to define the cohort may be an exposure, an occupation, a genetic trait, a geographic location, or another population characteristic determined by the epidemiologist. To conduct a prospective cohort study, participants who are disease free at baseline but at risk for disease are enrolled and followed over time to measure the occurrence of disease.

A cohort study is best suited for diseases with high incidence rates among exposed persons and frequent exposures to the variable of interest. The study needs to have adequate numbers of individuals who are exposed and develop disease after enrollment for the statistical analysis to have sufficient power to detect associations. If a disease were rare, even among exposed people, an unrealistically large cohort would have to be assembled. If exposures were uncommon, this could also affect the size of the population needed in the cohort. Cohorts can be assembled for which there are special resources available for follow-up. For example, members of HMOs or occupational groups with employment records can be selected. Occupational cohorts may also represent persons with high exposure to an agent. For example, HCWs were an ideal group from which to draw a cohort to study the risk of HBV, CMV, and HIV transmission.[40] Unfortunately, although the high levels of exposure and

---

Table 3–5 Risk Factors for HIV Infection among HCWs after Percutaneous Exposure to HIV-Infected Blood

Risk Factors	Adjusted OR	(95% CI)
Deep injury	16.1	(6.1–44.6)
Visible blood on device	5.2	(1.8–17.7)
Procedure involving needle placed directly in vein or artery	5.1	(1.9–14.8)
Terminal illness in source patient	6.4	(2.2–18.9)
Postexposure use of zidovudine	0.2	(0.1–0.6)

OR, odds ratio; CI, confidence interval.

Source: Reprinted from *Morbidity and Mortality Weekly Report*, Vol. 44, pp. 929–931, Centers for Disease Control and Prevention.

the ensuing high numbers of cases may make demonstrating a link between an exposure and an outcome easier, the unusual exposure levels may make results of such cohorts more difficult to generalize to the population. Nevertheless, internal validity, ie, whether an exposure and disease are truly related in the study population, is more important than generalizability to populations outside the study. Cohort studies can be very expensive and often require a large staff and great motivation on the part of the study subjects to remain in follow-up. Cohort studies with large losses to follow-up may not yield data that are interpretable, because the risks for disease may be different in those lost to follow-up than in the subjects who were successfully followed. The enrollment criteria for three HIV/AIDS cohorts—the Multicenter AIDS Cohort Study (MACS), the AIDS Link to the Intravenous Experience (ALIVE), and the Women's Interagency IIIV Study (WIIIS) arc shown in Table 3–2.

Although most cohort studies enroll and follow subjects prospectively, cohorts may also be assembled retrospectively, after disease has occurred. Such a study could look at only previously collected medical or exposure records or incorporate previously collected data with current and future assessment of disease among those exposed.

A retrospective cohort, or historical cohort design, takes advantage of records and specimens collected in the past and can generate results more rapidly than can a prospective design, which must wait for the development of disease. Within existing cohorts, subgroups that have been followed for a shorter duration that enroll all or some of the original cohort members can be studied. These studies can be referred to as *nested cohort studies*. Nested cohorts are able to study participants enrolled in the initial cohort and data collected by the original cohort, either concurrent with the nested cohort or collected previously. This allows researchers to test hypotheses prospectively that were not proposed at the outset of the original cohort.

Data Collection

Cohort studies collect information on exposure and on the development of disease. Simplistically, a cohort is assembled from a group of exposed individuals, and the study measures the incidence of disease in the group. Practically, however, cohorts assemble persons with a range of risk behaviors and measure the incidence of disease across a range of behaviors. Often, it is possible in cohort studies to measure a dose-response effect of increasing disease incidence (because of higher attack rates or shorter incubation periods) with higher levels of exposure. Furthermore, in cohort studies, the subjects can develop infection or disease of varying severity. Thus, defining the appropriate endpoint is critical. In some cohort studies, several endpoints may be measured. For example, a study of influenza could measure serologically or virologically confirmed infection, clinical illness, illness with a physician visit or with work loss, hospitalization, or death. In addition, some studies of influenza vaccine in the elderly have found the vaccine to be more efficacious in preventing death than it is in preventing infection.[41]

An interviewer-administered questionnaire can collect more detailed and complex information, can allow for more flexibility in collecting information, and often results in more complete and standardized information being collected. Interviewer-administered questionnaires can also create a stronger bond with the study participants, so they are more likely to share information and are more likely to continue their participation in the study. In some populations, literacy levels may be low, necessitating an interviewer-administered design. Other cohort studies have relied on less expensive data collection techniques, such as mail or telephone interviews. These data collection techniques commonly have lower response rates than do interviewer-administered questionnaires but are significantly less expensive. Repeated interviews of ongoing cohorts may encounter problems with "socially desirable responding" to questions in a behavioral interview. In this situation, participants respond to questions according to what they believe the interviewer might view as desirable behavior. This is not always intentional misreporting or "lying" about behavior by the subject. Sometimes, the subject's memory is influenced by the social situation of the interview. Care must be taken to ensure that interviewers are well trained and that the questionnaire is carefully conducted to minimize these potential biases. One recent technique that has been evaluated as a technique to reduce socially desirable responses uses an audio-adapted computer assisted interview (ACASI). The use of ACASI to measure risk behavior has resulted in higher levels of study participants reporting unprotected sex and injection drug use in a cohort of adolescents.[42]

Analysis

Unlike other epidemiologic study designs, cohort studies are able to measure the rate at which participants develop disease per unit of time— the incidence rate. The incidence rate is the number of people who develop disease divided by the cumulative time in the study for all participants up until the time that they develop disease.

To measure associations, cohort studies compare the incidence rate of disease among persons with different exposures or other characteristics at baseline or during the follow-up period. The ratio of the incidence rates according to exposures is expressed as the relative risk, risk ratio, or relative hazard of disease (Table 3–1). Analysis may be extended to include Kaplan-Meier types of survival curves and Cox Proportional Hazard analysis, in which data are stratified according to exposure characteristics and survival curves are compared. Cohort studies can also use data obtained by testing multiple biologic specimens collected from subjects during the course of the study.

In addition to methods that define exposure at an arbitrary baseline time point, there are analytical methods that take into account changes in exposure among individuals over time. Because cohort studies follow participants over time, the level of exposure to different risk factors may fluctuate for an individual over time. For example, an individual who uses illicit drugs may have times of abstinence and episodes of heavy drug use. Exposures that fluctuate over time, either qualitatively (eg, present/absent) or quantitatively (eg, heavy/light), are termed *time-dependent covariates*. Those covariates that don't change, eg, sex, histocompatibility locus antigen (HLA) type, ethnicity, age at baseline, are termed *fixed covariates*. It may be useful to think of cohort studies as a study of the group, not of the individual. Although participants contribute data to the study at each visit, how those data are distributed in the analysis depends on their risk behaviors at that point in time. A single individual may contribute data to both the exposed and the unexposed categories over the course of the cohort study. The fluctuation in personal behaviors is accounted for in the person time analysis and gives cohort analysis considerable statistical power, as each data point from each participant is used.

The ability to assess time-dependent covariates is useful when assessing the effects of long-term therapy on chronic disease outcomes. The patients may have periods when they go off treatment (eg, due to side effects) or may even change therapy, so that a baseline assessment of exposure would lead to misclassification of such patients. In studies of HIV therapies, for example, therapies can start, stop, and change several times over a year.

The analysis of longitudinal data requires attention to some of the assumptions of the statistical models. Longitudinal data contain repeated measurements on risk behaviors for a single individual over time. The distribution of these risk behaviors is not normal, nor is it independent. For example, a person who injects illicit drugs frequently will probably continue to inject at a high frequency. A plot of a hundred measurements of injection frequency on a single participant would differ from single measurements on a hundred participants. The variation in data from the single person would be much less than the variability in data from a hundred individuals. Many statistical programs assume that the

those participating in NNIS and others, in the investigation and control of nosocomial outbreaks.

Nosocomial infections are a very important health problem in the United States, and antibiotic-resident organisms often may be selected for and transmitted in this setting. It has been estimated that over 2 million patients develop a nosocomial infection in the United States each year, at a cost of approximately $3.5 billion. The NNIS is the only ongoing surveillance program of nosocomial infections in acute care hospitals in the United States. Data from the NNIS program are described in detail in Chapter 13.

EMERGING INFECTIONS

Recently, considerable attention has been directed at emerging and reemerging infections. This topic is covered in detail in Chapter 2 of this book. A sensitive system of surveillance for the early detection of emerging infections is a critically important component of the public health response to this problem.

The Institute of Medicine of the National Academy of Sciences reviewed the problem of emerging infectious diseases in 1991.[32] This expert committee recommended that the CDC develop a strategy for improved early detection and response to the threat of emerging infections. The CDC established an Emerging Infections Program (EIP) in seven states—California, Connecticut, Georgia, New York, Maryland, Minnesota, and Oregon. The goals of the EIP are to improve national surveillance for new and emerging infectious diseases, conduct applied epidemiologic and laboratory research, develop prevention and control measures, and strengthen the national public health infrastructure.

FoodNet and PulseNet

The Food-Borne Diseases Active Surveillance Network (FoodNet) is the food-borne disease component of CDC's EIP. FoodNet is a collaborative project among CDC, the seven EIP sites, the U.S. Department of Agriculture, and the U.S. Food and Drug Administration (FDA). It consists of active surveillance for food-borne diseases and related epidemiologic studies designed to help improve public health officials' understanding of the epidemiology of food-borne disease in the United States. The total population included in the special surveillance efforts of the FoodNet catchment areas is 20.3 million people, or 8% of the population of the United States. FoodNet provides a network for responding to new and emerging food-borne diseases of national importance, monitoring the burden of food-borne diseases, and identifying the source of specific food-borne diseases.

The program includes surveillance of several populations, including the following:

- active laboratory-based surveillance
- survey of clinical laboratories
- survey of physicians
- survey of the population
- case-control studies

Closely linked to FoodNet is another laboratory-based program called PulseNet. PulseNet is a national network of public health laboratories that performs DNA fingerprinting of bacteria that might be the cause of food-borne illnesses. The network permits rapid comparison of the DNA fingerprint patterns through an electronic database at the CDC. The DNA fingerprinting method used is pulsed-field gel electrophoresis (PFGE). The PFGE methods are described in some detail in Chapter 8. The data from FoodNet and PulseNet allow a better understanding of the epidemiology of food-borne diseases of national significance.

Tuberculosis Surveillance

Enhanced tuberculosis surveillance was established as part of the CDC's EIP in response to the reemergence of tuberculosis in the United States, related in part to the HIV/AIDS epidemic and in part to the reduced public health funding and attention toward tuberculosis in the decades prior to the AIDS epidemic. The increased attention that tuberculosis has received recently has included increased funding to health departments for more active case detection, directly observed therapy of active cases with effective drug combinations (termed DOTS), and molecular characterization of all isolates from patients in the seven EIP states. These molecular epidemiologic studies of isolates from patients with recent tuberculosis has led to a reassessment of the proportion of cases in adults that are due to reactivation versus recent tuberculosis. Studies from several locations have suggested that recent infections in adults are more common than had been previously believed; recent infections have accounted for about 35% of active cases in some areas.[33] Also, several clusters of tuberculosis cases acquired by casual contact and unusual exposures, such as bronchoscopy, have been documented.[34] These issues are reviewed in greater detail in Chapter 14.

Influenza Surveillance

Influenza has probably received more systematic global surveillance than any other disease in the last several decades. Active surveillance of influenza is necessary to monitor the emergence of new influenza viruses that arise by genetic drift or reassortment (genetic shift). The detection of new influenza viruses on a global basis is required to have sufficient lead time to produce and distribute new influenza vaccines. Because of the great genetic variability of influenza viruses, the vaccine must be reformulated on an annual basis. Therefore, the World Health Organization (WHO) has established a global network of influenza surveillance laboratories, where isolates from infected persons are characterized serologically and genetically. Each year, a panel of experts meets and makes a prediction as to which of the circulating viruses is most likely to be responsible for an epidemic during the ensuing influenza season. Vaccine preparation for the next year is based on the advice of these experts (see Chapter 16).

In addition to this program of global influenza surveillance, the CDC maintains an influenza surveillance program in the United States. This program, which is described in more detail in Chapter 16, monitors influenza and pneumonia deaths in adults in 121 U.S. cities. Also, special influenza surveillance programs include monitoring visits to sentinel physicians and hospital emergency rooms, as well as obtaining data concerning hospital admissions and school absenteeism in selected populations. For several years, Baylor University in Houston, Texas, has maintained comprehensive community-wide surveillance of influenza in Harris County, Texas, with funding from the National Institutes of Health (NIH) to evaluate the influenza morbidity and mortality at the population level.[35]

Hepatitis

The hepatitis program at CDC has established the Sentinel County Study, a collaborative network of county health departments for the purpose of monitoring the epidemiology of viral hepatitis. This program has been in operation since 1982. The counties involved in this surveillance program are provided with personnel to do active surveillance of hepatitis occurring in residents of these sentinel counties. This surveillance includes maintaining regular active contact with physicians, other health care providers, and laboratories to detect all cases of hepatitis. Each hepatitis case is interviewed to determine their epidemiologic risk factors, and laboratory evaluation is done to establish the type of hepatitis virus responsible for the infection. The data from the Sentinel County study have been of considerable value in monitoring the incidence, temporal trends, and risk factors for infection with the different hepatitis viruses in the United States. Although viral hepatitis is one of the reportable diseases in the United States, the reporting is incomplete, and the passively reported data do not provide reliable estimates of the type of hepatitis or the risk factors for infection. The epidemiology of viral hepatitis and the data from the Sentinel County study are reviewed in more detail in the chapter on hepatitis (Chapter 19).

VACCINE ADVERSE EVENT REPORTING SYSTEM

The National Childhood Vaccine Injury Act of 1986 mandated the reporting of certain adverse events following vaccination to help ensure the safety of vaccines distributed in the United States. This Act led to the establishment of the Vaccine Adverse Event Reporting System (VAERS) in November 1990. The program is operated jointly by the CDC and FDA. VAERS receives about 800–1,000 reports each month from health care providers, vaccine manufacturers, and vaccine recipients or their parents or guardians. One of the dilemmas in public health is the imbalance between the tremendous benefits from vaccines during the twentieth century in reducing morbidity and mortality and the high degree of suspicion that the public has about the dangers of new vaccines or vaccines in general. This has led to reluctance to develop, test, and license new vaccines among some pharmaceutical firms, due to concerns about litigation, and even vaccines given to healthy persons are blamed for a health event that is entirely coincidental or fortuitous. This situation, which is inimical to further advances in public health, has been addressed in part by the VAERS surveillance program. Although VAERS is a passive reporting system and does not include denominator data, it has identified a complication of intussusception among recipients of a recently licensed recombinant rotavirus vaccine that has been shown to be attributable to the vaccine only in about 1 in 5,000–10,000 recipients of the vaccine on further study.[36] This passive reporting system has already proved to be quite valuable.

In 1991, the Centers for Disease Control and Prevention, in collaboration with several large health maintenance organizations (HMOs), established another surveillance system to monitor adverse reaction to vaccines. This program is called the Vaccine Safety Datalink Project (VSD).[37] The VSD program contains a large database of vaccinated children and adults where adverse events can be linked to denominator data on the number of vaccines administered.

Because the HMO populations included in VSD are relatively stable and receive all of their health care through the HMO, these data are less subject to bias than passive reporting systems.

OTHER SURVEILLANCE DATA

There are several surveillance systems in the United States that have been established to obtain data for other purposes that could be utilized to evaluate infectious diseases issues. Among these are the Surveillance, Epidemiology, and End Results (SEER) project of the National Cancer Institute and the National Health and Nutrition Assessment Study (NHANES) of the National Center for Health Statistics.

SEER Study

The SEER project of the National Cancer Institute of NIH includes cancer registries in eleven geographic areas, including six states, one territory, and four metropolitan areas. Through contacts with hospitals and pathologists, the occurrence of incident cases of cancer are monitored, and ascertainment is believed to be very complete. Data collected on cancer patients include demographic characteristics; exposures, such as industrial or occupational histories; characteristics of the cancer (site, morphology, stage); treatment; and outcomes. These patients have been enrolled in a number of studies. They are a useful population for the study of infectious causes of cancer, such as hepatitis B virus (HBV), hepatitis C virus (HCV), *Helicobacter pylori*, human papillomavirus (HPV), Epstein-Barr virus, and other infections.

National Health and Nutrition Survey

The NHANES involves a random sample of the U.S. population, which is done about every 10 years to evaluate the prevalence of health conditions and the nutritional status of the U.S. population. Randomly selected subjects are asked to participate in a survey that includes a detailed assessment of health conditions and disabilities, a physical examination, and collection of blood specimens. The blood specimens are evaluated for several biochemical and nutritional components, and a repository is created. Several studies of infectious diseases have been evaluated using the repository and questionnaire data, including the prevalence of infection with HBV, HCV, and herpes simples viruses types 1 and 2. These data are discussed in Chapters 19 and 20.

The Behavioral Risk Factor Surveillance System

The Behavioral Risk Factor Surveillance System is an ongoing telephone survey that is conducted by over 40 state health departments in the United States. The survey includes standardized questions on various behavioral risk factors for disease, including cigarette smoking, alcohol use, seat belt use, and exercise. These data are analyzed and published by the CDC and are very useful in evaluating temporal trends in health risk behaviors. Additional questions are added periodically.

Drug Abuse Warning Network

The Drug Abuse Warning Network (DAWN) collects data on morbidity and mortality related to illicit drug use from hospital emergency departments and medical examiners or coroners' offices in 27 metropolitan areas. It is a useful source of data on the types of illicit drugs in common use in a geographic area and the associated health problems associated with their use. The DAWN data have been useful in detecting changing types of drug use that have adverse health consequences. The DAWN study is especially useful for detecting changes in the rates of drug overdose.

International Surveillance Systems

In addition to the numerous sources of data on health events in the United States listed above,

there are various sources of international surveillance data. Most national governments have established surveillance programs on cancer and infectious diseases. Some of those data are published in the *Weekly Epidemiologic Record* of the WHO. Also, the International Union Against Tuberculosis and the International Cancer Control Organization in Lyon, France, collect and publish data on tuberculosis and cancer, respectively.

OTHER SURVEILLANCE ISSUES

Types of Surveillance

As noted above, for various diseases, it is important to focus on laboratory surveillance, health provider surveillance, pathology surveillance, or patient surveillance, or to use randomly selected populations to be surveyed by telephone or interviews.

Confidentiality of Data

For many diseases, it is of critical importance to maintain the confidentiality of surveillance data. For some conditions, such as HIV/AIDS, the issues of confidentiality are critical and must be considered in order to obtain valid data and to prevent harm to the persons surveyed. The issue of confidentiality arose over a plan to test sera from NHANES participants for HIV antibodies. After the plan was proposed initially, it was dropped because of fears that testing the sera for HIV would substantially reduce the participation rate and the representativeness of the sampled population if counseling and informed consent were required of the subjects studied. If only persons at low risk to HIV participated in NHANES, it would not only compromise the validity of the HIV prevalence estimate but of other health conditions measured in NHANES, as well. Eventually an anonymous, random survey of HIV prevalence in the general population was done by the NCHS.[38]

One method of dealing with this ethical and scientific dilemma is to use blinded, anonymous serologic surveys to estimate the prevalence of HIV in critical populations. This method was used, originally in Massachusetts, to determine the prevalence of HIV in pregnant women.[39] In this type of surveillance, the heel stick samples of blood from newborn infants, which are mandated by law for screening infants for phenylketonuria (PKU), hypothyroidism, and glucose-6-phosphate deficiency, are blinded (ie, names are removed), and the same specimens are tested for HIV antibodies. This blinded screening avoids selection bias (and the need for informed consent), because all infants are screened, and it gives valid data on the prevalence of HIV in pregnant women. Because maternal antibodies are passively transferred to the infant, the prevalence of HIV antibodies in a newborn reflects the infection status of the mother, not the infant. Whenever this type of blinded screening is done, it is important that the mother be provided with access to screening that is not blinded, so that she can elect to be screened, receive the results, and be counseled, and the HIV-positive women can be provided therapy to prevent transmission to the infant. Nevertheless, the results from blinded screening can provide valid and valuable public health data on the prevalence of HIV (or another infection) in all pregnant women in a geographic area. This method of blinded anonymous surveillance of HIV seroprevalence has been extended to include other populations, such as aliquots of sera from hospital or clinic patients from populations that were not selected because of HIV-related conditions. These blinded serosurveys often provide useful data on HIV prevalence in selected populations.[40]

COMMUNICATION AND PRESENTATION OF DATA

The primary purposes of a surveillance system are to collect data on the health status and/or risk factors for disease in a population and to analyze and interpret the data in a manner that will lead to prevention and control of disease. Therefore, a critical component of this activity is the interpretation and communication of the data

in an ongoing fashion, so that health care providers or officials can take appropriate action when necessary. Investigations of epidemics of infectious diseases and reporting the results of the investigation and control measures instituted in a widely available publication, such as the *MMWR*, with interpretive comments to put the epidemic in context, and wide distribution of these reports to health officials, news organizations, and the general public often have implemented changes in policies or procedures and prevented future epidemics.

Presentations of data on endemic infectious diseases are also important to assess progress or lack of progress toward a healthier society. The CDC issues annual reports on the epidemiology of several diseases, where longer-term trends are analyzed. Also, CDC regularly presents the weekly reports of infectious diseases in a graphic form, in which the number or rates of reported cases of several infectious diseases are compared with the number reported in recent weeks or in a comparable period in a previous year (Figure 4–4). Another method of data presentation is to show the temporal trends of disease incidence in reference to a targeted rate of the disease in years 2000 or 2010. This type of graph allows the reader to determine whether a predetermined goal is likely to be met. These PHS goals were specified and published in the PHS publication, *Healthy People, 2000* (Figure 4–5).

GUIDELINES FOR EVALUATING A SURVEILLANCE SYSTEM

The CDC has published a set of attributes and criteria by which to evaluate a surveillance system. These criteria can be used to evaluate an existing surveillance system or to establish a new system. The judgment of which criteria are most important depends on the primary purposes for which the surveillance data will be used. Some surveillance systems that are designed to eradicate a disease or to control an epidemic of a serious disease need to be comprehensive, rapid, and sensitive. Therefore, the efforts and funding allocated to such a system will need to be much

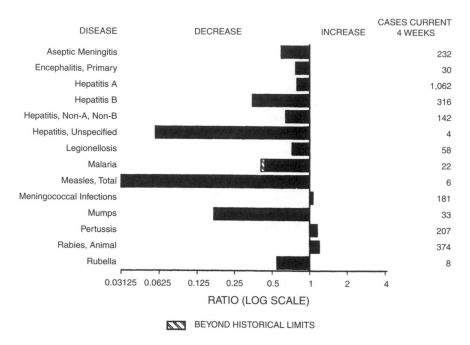

DISEASE	DECREASE	INCREASE	CASES CURRENT 4 WEEKS
Aseptic Meningitis			232
Encephalitis, Primary			30
Hepatitis A			1,062
Hepatitis B			316
Hepatitis, Non-A, Non-B			142
Hepatitis, Unspecified			4
Legionellosis			58
Malaria			22
Measles, Total			6
Meningococcal Infections			181
Mumps			33
Pertussis			207
Rabies, Animal			374
Rubella			8

0.03125   0.0625   0.125   0.25   0.5   1   2   4

RATIO (LOG SCALE)

▨ BEYOND HISTORICAL LIMITS

Figure 4–4 Notifiable disease reports, comparison of 4-week totals ending February 4, 1995, with historical data—United States. *Source:* Reprinted from Centers for Disease Control and Prevention, National Center for Infectious Diseases.

greater than an ongoing system of surveillance of an endemic disease, where the immediate and eventual health costs are less. In the latter situation, a passive reporting system, where the criteria for a case are quite specific but less sensitive, may be sufficient to detect major fluctuations in incidence, even when many cases go undetected and/or unreported.

The attributes of a surveillance system reviewed by CDC were as follows:

- *Sensitivity*: To what extent does the system identify all or most cases in a target population? As described above, good sensitivity may be more important for a surveillance system designed to control an outbreak or to evaluate an intervention than for monitoring disease trends.
- *Timeliness*: This refers to how rapidly reports are received, evaluated, and analyzed

and the information provided to those in a position to intervene. This may be critical to control an outbreak of an acute disease.
- *Representativeness*: This refers to whether the likelihood of reporting a disease is the same within subgroups of the population or in different populations. If surveillance reports are not representative, this could affect the application of control efforts.
- *Predictive Value Positive*: This refers to the specificity of the case report. To what extent are the reported cases really cases? This is an important attribute of surveillance systems in most situations.
- *Simplicity*: This refers to both the system's structure and ease of operation. Surveillance systems should be as simple as possible, while still meeting their objectives. It is not wise to collect data that will not be used.

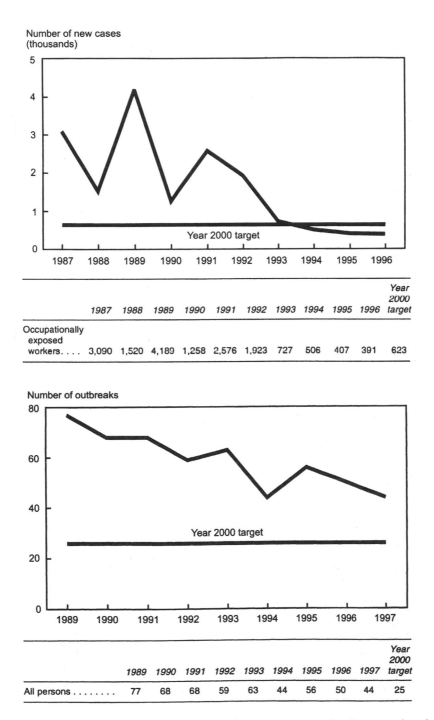

	1987	1988	1989	1990	1991	1992	1993	1994	1995	1996	Year 2000 target
Occupationally exposed workers....	3,090	1,520	4,189	1,258	2,576	1,923	727	506	407	391	623

	1989	1990	1991	1992	1993	1994	1995	1996	1997	Year 2000 target
All persons........	77	68	68	59	63	44	56	50	44	25

Figure 4–5 Top, Number of new cases of hepatitis B infections among occupationally exposed workers: United States, 1987–96, and year 2000 target for objective 10.5. Bottom, Outbreaks of infections due to *Salmonella enteriditis*: United States, 1989–97, and year 2000 target for objective 12.2. *Source:* Reprinted from the Centers for Disease Control and Prevention, National Center for Infectious Diseases, Salmonella Surveillance System.

• *Acceptability*: This refers to the willingness of individuals and organizations to participate in the surveillance system. Obviously, this is a critical characteristic of all surveillance systems.

• *Flexibility*: This refers to a system's ability to adapt to changing information needs or operating conditions with little additional costs in time, personnel, or funding. Some disease-reporting systems are quite flexible and can accommodate the need to monitor new diseases. Generally, simple systems are more flexible. The system that reports the 52 diseases that are officially reported by all the states to the CDC is generally quite flexible. A newly recognized or emerging infectious disease usually can be added to the list. The decisions as to what diseases are to be reported are made regularly by the Council of State and Territorial Epidemiologists, and the definitions to be used to report cases are developed in consultation with the CDC.

CONCLUSION

Surveillance is a critical epidemiologic and public health tool for the control and prevention of infections and other diseases. The type of surveillance system needed and the details of its operation must be considered in the light of how the data will be used. In other words, what are the purposes of surveillance of a specific disease? Perhaps the best example of the successful and creative use of a surveillance system has been the central role of specific surveillance in the eradication of smallpox and the current application to the global effort to eradicate poliomyelitis. The details of the structure and operation of surveillance systems to control a number of infectious diseases are given in other chapters of this book.

REFERENCES

1. Centers for Disease Control and Prevention (CDC). Comprehensive plan for epidemiologic surveillance. Atlanta, GA: CDC; 1986.

2. Thacker SD, Berkelman RL. Public Health surveillance in the United States. *Epidemiol Rev.* 1988;10:164–190.

3. Hartgerink MJ. Health surveillance and planning for healthcare in the Netherlands. *Int J Epidemiol.* 1976; 5:87–91.

4. Wilcox WF, ed. *Natural and Political Observation Made upon the Bills of Mortality.* John Graunt (reprint of first edition, 1662). Baltimore: Johns Hopkins University Press, 1937.

5. Frank JP; Sigerist H, trans. The people's misery: Mother of disease. An address delivered in 1790. *Bull History Med.* 1941;9:81–100.

6. Langmuir AD. William Farr: Founder of modern concepts of surveillance. *Int J Epidemiol.* 1976;5:13–18.

7. Chapin CV. State health organization. *JAMA.* 1916;66: 699–703.

8. Francis T Jr, Korus RF, Voight RB, et al. An evaluation of the 1954 poliomyelitis vaccine trials. Summary report. *Am J Public Health.* 1955;45(5, 2).

9. Nathanson N, Langmuir AD. The Cutter incident: Poliomyelitis following formaldehyde inactivated poliovirus vaccine in the United States in the spring of 1955. *Am J Hyg.* 1963;78:16–28.

10. Langmuir AD. The surveillance of communicable diseases of national importance. *N Engl J Med.* 1963;268: 182–192.

11. Luik J, Kendal AP. Impact of influenza epidemics on mortality in the United States from October 1972 to May 1985. *Am J Public Health.* 1987;77:712–716.

12. Serfling RE. Methods for the current statistical analysis of excess pneumonia: Influenza deaths. *Public Health Rep.* 1963;78:494–566.

13. Centers for Disease Control and Prevention. Case definitions for surveillance purposes. *MMWR.* 1997; 46(RR19)1–15.

14. Centers for Disease Control and Prevention. Revision of the surveillance case definition for acquired immunodeficiency syndrome. *MMWR.* 1987;36:35–55.

15. Centers for Disease Control and Prevention. 1993 revised classification system for HIV infection and expanded surveillance case definition for AIDS for adolescents and adults. *MMWR.* 1992;41:1–19.

16. CDC guidelines for evaluating surveillance systems. *MMWR.* 1988;37:1–18.

17. Minkoff HL, McCalla S, Delike, et al. The relationship

of cocaine use to syphilis and human immunodeficiency virus infection among inner city parturient women. *Am J Obstet Gynecol.* 1990;163:521–526.

18. Centers for Disease Control and Prevention. Gonorrhea among men who have sex with men—selected sexually transmitted disease clinics, 1993–1996. *MMWR.* 1997; 46:889–892.

19. Centers for Disease Control and Prevention. Summary of notifiable diseases, United States, 1990. *MMWR.* 1991;39:30.

20. Shasby DM, Shope TC, Dowas K, et al. Epidemic measles in a highly vaccinated population. *N Engl J Med.* 1977;296:585–589.

21. The National Vaccine Advisory Committee. The measles epidemic: The problems, barriers and recommendation. *JAMA.* 1991;266:1547–1552.

22. Marks JS, Hayden GF, Orenstein WA. Measles vaccine efficacy in children previously vaccinated at 12 months of age. *Pediatrics.* 1978;62:955–960.

23. Orenstein WA, Markowitz L, Preblod SR, et al. Appropriate age for measles vaccination in the United States. *Dew Biol Stand.* 1985;65:13–21.

24. Patriarca PA, Laender F, Palmeira E, et al. A randomized trial of alternative formulations of oral polio vaccine in Brazil. *Lancet.* 1988;1:429–433.

25. Ukena T, Esher H, Bessette R, et al. Site of injection and response to hepatitis B virus vaccine. *N Engl J Med.* 1985;313:579–580.

26. Pappaioanou M, Fishbein DR, Dreesen DW, et al. Antibody response to pre-exposure human diploid-cell rabies vaccine given concurrently with chloroquine. *N Engl J Med.* 1986;314:280–284.

27. Foege W. The eradication of vaccine-preventable diseases. In: Levine MM, Woodrow GC, Kapes JB, Cobon GS, eds. *New Generation Vaccines.* New York: Marcel Dekker; 1997.

28. Fenner F, Henderson DA, Arita C, et al. *Smallpox and Its Eradication,* 1st ed. Geneva: World Health Organization; 1988.

29. Mukinda VBK, Mwema G, Kilanda M, et al. Reemer-

gence of human, monkey pox in Zaire. *Lancet.* 1997; 349:1449–1450.

30. Pan American Health Organization. Director announces campaign to eradicate poliomyelitis from the Americas by 1990. *Bull Pan Am Health Org.* 1985;19:213–215.

31. Robbins FL, de Quadros LA. Certification of the eradication of indigenous transmission of wild poliovirus in the Americas. *J Infect Dis.* 1997;175(suppl. 1):S281–S285.

32. Lederberg J, Shope RE, Oaks SC Jr., eds. *Institute of Medicine, Committee on Emerging Microbial Threats to Health: Emerging Infections.* Washington, DC: National Academy Press; 1992.

33. Small P, Hopewell P, Singh S, et al. The epidemiology of tuberculosis in San Francisco. *N Engl J Med.* 1994; 330:1703–1709.

34. Michele T, Cronin W, Graham NMH, et al. Transmission of mycobacterium tuberculosis by a fiberoptic bronchoscope. *JAMA.* 1997;278:1093–1095.

35. Perrotta DM, Decker M, Glezen WP. Acute respiratory disease hospital patterns as a measure of impact of epidemic influenza. *Am J Epidemiol.* 1985;122:468–476.

36. Centers for Disease Control and Prevention. Intussusception among recipients of rotavirus vaccine, United States, 1998–1999. *MMWR.* 1999;48:577–581.

37. Chen RT, Glasser JW, Rhodes PH, et al. Vaccine safety datalink project: a new tool for improving vaccine safety monitoring in the United States. *Pediatrics.* 1997; 99:765–773.

38. McQuillan GM, Ezzati-Rice TM, Siller DB, Visschev N, Morley P. Risk behavior and correlates of risk for HIV infection in the Dallas County Household Survey. *Am J Public Health.* 1994;84:747–753.

39. Gwinn M, Pappaianou M, George JR, et al. Prevalence of HIV infection in childbearing women in the United States: surveillance using newborn blood samples. *JAMA.* 1991;265:1704–1708.

40. Centers for Disease Control and Prevention. *National HIV Serosurveillance Summary: Results through 1992.* Atlanta: U.S. Department of Health and Human Services; 1994.

CHAPTER 5

Outbreak Epidemiology

Diane M. Dwyer and Carmela Groves

Outbreak epidemiology is the study of a disease cluster or epidemic in order to control or prevent further spread of disease in a population. The word *epidemic*, defined as an increase in the number of cases of a disease above what is expected, is derived from the Greek, meaning "that which is upon the people." This meaning enriches our understanding of epidemics by emphasizing the burdensome toll they have on a population or "a people." This definition also allows us to realize that epidemics are not always caused by infectious agents. Many other hazards, such as chemicals or physical conditions, can cause unusually high numbers of cases of disease in a given population. Nevertheless, the techniques used to investigate and control outbreaks are generally similar, regardless of the etiology of the disease.

Accounts of outbreaks have been recorded throughout the centuries. Cholera, influenza, malaria, smallpox, and the plague are extensively documented as causes of epidemics and pandemics that have altered the outcome of wars, disrupted political structures, killed millions of people, and affected the lives of countless others.[1] The prevention of disease through improved sanitation was recognized even before the causes of these diseases had been identified.

Today, there are new challenges in the control of infectious diseases. Public health officials and health care providers face the emergence of new diseases and the re-emergence of diseases that were no longer thought to be a threat to the public's health.[2] The intentional use of biologic agents or their toxins (eg, anthrax, plague, botulism, and smallpox) as weapons of bioterrorism has recently gained increasing attention. Changes in the environment; in industrial practices; in agriculture and food processing; in international transportation of people, foods, and goods; and changes in human behaviors have increased the risk of disease and the speed at which communicable disease can spread. Concurrently, the number of people at high risk and the density of human populations have increased. People with immunosuppression (eg, those infected with human immunodeficiency virus), the elderly, or people with medical therapy for cancer, kidney failure, etc are more susceptible to infectious diseases, including ones that may not have been medical concerns in the past. These compromised individuals may present with unusual symptoms that complicate the diagnosis, and their infections may be more difficult to treat. Immunosuppression may also increase the infectiousness of the individual, either by increasing the number of infectious organisms that the individual sheds or by increasing the length of time that the individual is infectious. The increasing density of the human population, especially in some developing nations, creates situations that foster the spread of new and old infectious diseases. However, the advantage is not all to the microbes. Advances in laboratory techniques and medical interventions, such as antibiotics, sanitation, and epidemiology, have increased our ability to identify and control infectious diseases.

In recent years, the news media have enhanced outbreak awareness. The names of organisms such as *Escherichia coli* O157:H7, Ebola virus, *Cryptosporidium*, Group A *Streptococcus* ("the flesh-eating bacteria"), and antibiotic-resistant *Streptococcus pneumoniae* conjure up reports of outbreaks that have been sensationalized in the press. Although some may take issue with the manner in which these reports have been presented, the reports have brought the results of outbreak investigations to the attention of the public. That *E. coli* O157:H7 can cause fatal hemolytic uremic syndrome, especially in children, was demonstrated in the U.S. outbreaks caused by contaminated ground beef and in the Japanese outbreak caused by contaminated radish sprouts.[3,4] The speed at which international diseases could become threats to U.S. citizens was underscored by the reports of Ebola virus isolated in monkeys in Reston, Virginia.[5] Reports of outbreaks of strains of *Mycobacterium tuberculosis* and *S. pneumoniae* that are resistant to antibiotics have raised the public awareness of the danger of inappropriate or excessive antibiotic use. Investigation of outbreaks such as these allows epidemiologists to identify risk factors and to determine preventive measures that will limit and control the spread of disease. This chapter will review the methods used to investigate and control outbreaks of infectious disease.

SURVEILLANCE AND OUTBREAK DETECTION

Outbreaks may come to the attention of health professionals through a report from a doctor's office, a hospital, a nursing home, a laboratory, or even a patient's call to the health department. Alternatively, outbreaks may be recognized through analysis of reports of individual cases of disease.

In the United States, individual cases of certain diseases are "nationally notifiable" (Table 5–1), ie, the Council of State and Territorial Epi-

demiologists (CSTE) and the federal Centers for Disease Control and Prevention (CDC) recommend that 52 notifiable diseases be included in national surveillance.[6] States have individual laws, regulations, or both that govern which diseases and conditions are reportable and the method and timing of reporting. Reporting of outbreaks is generally included in a state's disease reporting system.

In routine passive surveillance in public health, reporting occurs from multiple sources. Physicians, laboratories, hospitals, prisons, schools, child care centers, other facilities, and vital records departments (eg, using death records) may generate reports (Figure 5–1). Cases are generally reported to state or local health departments with information such as diagnosis, name, age, gender, address, and date of onset. Reports may also include additional information, such as laboratory results, treatment, occupation, setting of occurrence, and risk factors (Figure 5–2 and Figure 5–3). Case reports usually without personal identifiers are then transmitted weekly from states to the CDC for inclusion in national summary data published in the *Morbidity and Mortality Weekly Report*.

Information collected as part of the disease reporting system is compiled and evaluated at the local, state, and federal level. The information collected as part of the surveillance network is available for additional epidemiologic evaluation. These data represent years of continuous data collection that can be used to examine disease trends in a community. However, these data are not collected for the conduct of epidemiologic studies. Rather, surveillance data are collected to detect disease and to describe cases found in a community. Epidemiologic *research* data ideally would be collected to address specific hypotheses. Surveillance data are collected according to those procedures that maximize consistency and minimize the barriers to reporting. Surveillance databases often include data collected by passive reporting and have only minimal information on cases. Research data may, instead, require more detailed data collection to examine specific hypotheses and may re-

Table 5–1 The 52 Infectious Diseases Designated as Notifiable at the National Level during 1997

Acquired immunodeficiency
   syndrome
Anthrax
Botulism*
Brucellosis
Chancroid*
Chlamydia trachomatis genital
   infection
Cholera
Coccidioidomycosis*
Congenital rubella syndrome
Congenital syphilis
Cryptosporidiosis
Diphtheria
Encephalitis, California
Encephalitis, eastern equine
Encephalitis, St. Louis
Encephalitis, western equine
Escherichia coli O157:H7
Gonorrhea

Hemophilus influenzae
   (Invasive Disease)
Hansen disease (leprosy)
Hantavirus pulmonary
   syndrome
Hemolytic uremic syndrome
   post-diarrheal
Hepatitis A
Hepatitis B
Hepatitis C/non-A, non-B
HIV infection, pediatric
Legionelldosis
Lyme disease
Malaria
Measles (Rubeola)
Meningococcal disease
Mumps
Pertussis
Plague
Poliomyelitis, paralytic

Psittacosis
Rabies, animal
Rabies, human
Rocky Mountain spotted fever
Rubella
Salmonellosis*
Shigellosis*
Streptococcal disease,
   invasive, group A
Streptococcus pneumoniae,
   drug-resistant*
Streptococcal toxic-shock
   syndrome
Syphilis
Tetanus
Toxic-shock syndrome
Trichinosis
Tuberculosis
Typhoid fever
Yellow fever

Note: Although varicella is not a nationally notifiable disease, the Council of State and Territorial Epidemiologists recommends reporting of cases of this disease to CDC.
  * Not ourrently published in the *MMWR* weekly tables.

Source: Reprinted from the Centers for Disease Control and Prevention.

---

quire employees dedicated to managing complex data collection systems. Because of these differences, surveillance data may be inadequate to answer some epidemiologic questions. However, surveillance data are an excellent source of information to establish baseline rates and detect outbreaks, to identify new problems or trends in a community, to evaluate programs, to assist health professionals in estimating the magnitude of a health problem, and to identify possible hypotheses that can be explored by enhancing surveillance or by a research study.

Because outbreak epidemiology is concerned primarily with the control of disease, the sensitivity of the surveillance or reporting network is of paramount importance. If cases of disease are not reported, an outbreak may not be detected or may continue unabated.

Most commonly, outbreak investigations are conducted by facilities (eg, hospitals, nursing homes) or at the local or state public health level. Generally, the CDC is consulted in multistate outbreaks or in outbreaks of diseases that require resources or skills that state and local agencies are unable to provide. The laboratory and epidemiologic capabilities of the CDC are used to assist with domestic and international disease outbreaks of unusual etiology or of major public health significance.

Local and state health departments make the decision to conduct an outbreak investigation based on health regulations and on their professional judgment regarding the outbreak and its public health impact or implications. Regardless of the etiologic agent, the setting in which the disease may have been transmitted, or the popu-

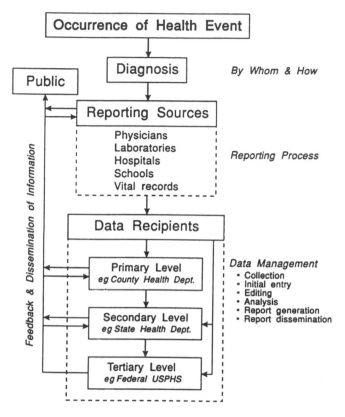

Figure 5–1 The flow of surveillance information. *Source: Public Health Surveillance*, W. Halperin and E. Baker, eds., p. 30, Copyright © 1992, Van Nostrand Reinhold. Reprinted by permission of John Wiley & Sons, Inc.

lation at risk, it is possible to summarize the basic steps and goals of the investigation. The primary motivation of any outbreak investigation is to control the spread of disease within the initial population at risk or to prevent the spread to additional populations. Many outbreaks occur in confined populations, groups, or settings, such as a food-borne outbreak at a wedding banquet or a pot luck dinner. Fortunately, these outbreaks generally have a single exposure, where the contaminated vehicle may have been consumed or eliminated before the first cases are apparent. In other outbreaks, where transmission is ongoing, such as legionellosis among hospitalized patients, the epidemiologic investigation must be initiated quickly and control measures imple-

mented to halt transmission. Regardless of the current transmission status, prevention of disease requires that the investigation seek to identify the etiologic agent, its source, the mode of transmission, and the vehicle. Information learned is important in preventing and controlling outbreaks of the same disease in the future and may be useful in linking sporadic cases to the same source.

OUTBREAK INVESTIGATION

Based on experience with outbreak investigations, there is a series of steps that can be used to guide any epidemiologic field investigation.[7–10] The outbreak epidemiologist is the "Sherlock

MARYLAND CONFIDENTIAL MORBIDITY REPORT
SEND TO LOCAL HEALTH DEPARTMENT

NAME OF PATIENT — LAST	FIRST	M	DATE OF BIRTH OR AGE MO DAY YR	M☐	W☐. B☐. Asian☐. Am.Ind.☐. Unk ☐
				F☐	Hispanic: Yes ☐. No☐. Unk.☐

ADDRESS	CITY OR TOWN	ZIP CODE	COUNTY

TELEPHONE NO.	OCCUPATION	WORKPLACE, SCHOOL, CHILD CARE FACILITY, ETC (NAME, ADDRESS)

DISEASE OR CONDITION (IF STD OR TB COMPLETE REVERSE SIDE ALSO)	DATE OF ONSET MO DAY YR	ADMITTED NO ☐ YES ☐	DATE ADMITTED MO DAY YR	HOSPITAL

PERTINENT CLINICAL INFORMATION:

LABORATORY TEST(S) IF VIRAL HEPATITIS
pos neg date

	pos	neg	date
HAV IgM	☐	☐	_____
HBsAg	☐	☐	_____
HBcAb	☐	☐	_____
HBcIgM	☐	☐	_____
HBsAb	☐	☐	_____
HCV AB	☐	☐	_____

(SPECIMEN, TEST, RESULT, DATE)

SURVIVED ☐
DIED ☐
DATE _____

IMPORTED
INTERSTATE ☐
YES INTERNATIONAL ☐
NO ☐
UNK ☐

SUSPECTED SOURCE

ACQUIRED IMMUNODEFICIENCY SYNDROME (AIDS) AND SYMPTOMATIC HIV INFECTION   LABORATORY TEST(S)

FEVER, WEIGHT LOSS, OR DIARRHEA ☐	SECONDARY CANCERS (KS, etc.) ☐	CD4 + T-cells < 200/µL ☐	
MYELOPATHY, OR PERIPHERAL NEUROPATHY ☐	OTHER CONDITIONS ATTRIBUTED TO	ELISA ☐	
SECONDARY INFECTIONS (PCP, etc.) ☐	HIV INFECTION ☐	WESTERN BLOT ☐	
		OTHER _____ ☐	

REPORTED BY:	ADDRESS	TELEPHONE NO.	DATE OF REPORT MO DAY YR

☐ CHECK HERE IF YOU NEED ADDITIONAL MORBIDITY REPORT CARDS   DHMH-1140   5/94

SEXUALLY TRANSMITTED DISEASE (STD) (SEE INSTRUCTIONS)
STAGE OF SYPHILIS

PRIMARY ☐   SECONDARY ☐   EARLY LATENT (LESS THAN 1 YR) ☐   CONGENITAL ☐   OTHER STAGES ☐ SPECIFY _____

GONORRHEA   OTHER STD (SPECIFY)

UNCOMPLICATED ☐   PID ☐   RECTAL ☐   PHARYNGEAL ☐   OPHTHALMIA NEONATORUM ☐   OTHER ☐ (SPECIFY) _____

Specify Lab Test (RPR or VDRL, FTA - ABS, FTA - IgM, Darkfield, Smear, Culture, Other)   TREATMENT GIVEN

DATE	TEST	RESULTS	DATE	DRUG	DOSAGE

TUBERCULOSIS DISEASE (SEE INSTRUCTIONS)
MAJOR SITE OF DISEASE

FOREIGN BORN: YES ☐

Pulmonary ☐ Pleural ☐ Lymphatic ☐ G/U ☐ Military ☐ Bone Joint ☐ Meningeal ☐ Peritoneal ☐ Other ☐ _____

COUNTRY _____

Additional Sites: _____

DATE ENTERED USA _____ NO ☐ UNK ☐

SUPPORTING BACT./HISTOLOGICAL EVIDENCE   CHEMOTHERAPY

SPUTUM SPECIMEN: DATE _____

	POS	NEG	PENDING	NOT DONE
SMEAR	☐	☐	☐	☐
CULTURE	☐	☐	☐	☐

CURRENT RX, DATE STARTED _____
INH ☐, RIF ☐, PZA ☐, EMB ☐
SM ☐, OTHER ☐ _____
NONE ☐

TUBERCULIN TEST
PPD _____ mm
DATE _____
NOT DONE ☐

OTHER SPECIMEN: TYPE _____ DATE _____

	POS	NEG	PENDING	NOT DONE
SMEAR	☐	☐	☐	☐
CULTURE	☐	☐	☐	☐
HISTOLOGY	☐	☐	☐	☐

DATE _____

DIRECTLY OBSERVED THERAPY
YES ☐   NO ☐.   UNK ☐

PREVIOUS RX FOR TB DISEASE
YES ☐ YEAR _____, NO ☐. UNK ☐

PREVIOUS INH PROPHYLAXIS
YES ☐ YEAR _____, NO ☐. UNK ☐

X-RAY
NORMAL ☐
ABNORMAL
NON-CAVITARY ☐
CAVITARY ☐
NOT DONE ☐

5/94

Figure 5–2 Morbidity Case Report Form for transmission to the state or local health department. *Source:* Reprinted from Maryland Department of Health and Mental Hygiene.

Source of Case Report _____

Date of Case Report _____

Gastroenteritis Case Report Form
Maryland Department of Health & Mental Hygiene
Epidemiology & Disease Control Program

Disease	☐ Campylobacteriosis ☐ Shigellosis ☐ Unknown
	☐ Salmonellosis ☐ Other _____

Status	☐ Sporadic Case ☐ Outbreak

Patient Data

Name _____ Last _____ First

Telephone _____ Home _____ Work

Address _____ Street

_____ County _____ City _____ State _____ Zip

Age _____ | Date of Birth _____ / _____ / _____

Race   ☐ White   ☐ Hispanic   ☐ Other
        ☐ Black   ☐ Asian   ☐ Unknown

Occupation, Student, or Situation _____

Name of Employer, School or Day Care _____

Clinical and Lab Data

Date of Onset _____ / _____ / _____   Time _____ am or pm

☐ Diarrhea   ☐ Bloody Stool   ☐ Cramps

☐ Fever   ☐ Vomiting   ☐ Other _____

Duration of Symptoms _____ days

Outcome   ☐ Survived   ☐ Died

Hospitalized   ☐ Yes   ☐ No

Name of Hospital

Date Admitted _____ / _____ / _____   Date Discharged _____ / _____ / _____

Date of Death _____ / _____ / _____

Name of Lab confirming diagnosis

Was the culture of specimen sent to the State Lab for
serotyping or confirmation?   ☐ Yes   ☐ No   ☐ Unknown

Agent (Check one)

☐ Campylobacter   Serotype _____

☐ Giardia

☐ Salmonella Group _____ Serotype _____

☐ Shigella   Serotype _____

☐ Other _____

Type of Specimen
☐ Bacterial   ☐ Viral   ☐ Ova and Parasite   ☐ Serological

Source of Specimen
☐ Stool   ☐ Urine
☐ Blood   ☐ Other _____

Travel

Did patient travel to another state or country in the 2 weeks
prior to symptom's onset?   ☐ Yes   ☐ No

Where _____ When _____

Animal Contact

Did patient have contact with the following animals [   ] hours/
days* prior to symptom's onset?

☐ Dogs   ☐ Parakeets   ☐ Cows

☐ Cats   ☐ Chickens   ☐ Turtles

☐ Ducks   ☐ Other _____

Food History

Did patient eat any of the following within [   ] hours/days*
prior to onset of illness?

	Yes	No	Unknown
1. Eggs			
a. Cooked eggs: scrambled, hard fried, other _____	☐	☐	☐
b. Undercooked eggs: poached, soft, scrambled, sunny side up, other _____	☐	☐	☐
c. Raw eggs: egg nog, Caesar salad, hollandaise sauce, meringue, bearnaise, other _____	☐	☐	☐
2. Raw or undercooked poultry (chicken, turkey)	☐	☐	☐
3. Raw or undercooked red meat	☐	☐	☐
4. Raw (unpasteurized) milk	☐	☐	☐
5. Homemade/unpasteurized cheese	☐	☐	☐
6. Raw or undercooked fish/shellfish	☐	☐	☐

Other Exposure

Within [   ] hours/days* prior to onset of symptom(s) did
patient:

	Yes	No	Unknown
1. Handle raw poultry?	☐	☐	☐
2. Have exposure to a day care or nursery?	☐	☐	☐
3. Have household member or sexual partner with similar symptoms?	☐	☐	☐
4. Hike, camp, fish, swim?	☐	☐	☐
5. Drink from a spring, stream or lake?	☐	☐	☐
6. Take antibiotics in month prior to onset of illness?	☐	☐	☐

Disposition

Work or school restrictions?   ☐ Yes   ☐ No

Is yes, specify _____

Was patient advised of appropriate precautions?   ☐ Yes   ☐ No

If yes, how?

☐ Telephone   ☐ Fact Sheet   ☐ In Person   ☐ In Writing

DHMH 4458 (June 1992)

continues

Figure 5–3 continued

Food History for Foodborne Diseases. List the foods eaten within [   ] hours/days* prior to onset:

[12 hours]   [24 hours]   [48 hours]   [72 hours]

Breakfast _____

_____

_____

Lunch _____

_____

_____

Dinner _____

_____

_____

_____

Household Members. List all household contacts, even if asymptomatic; give onset if symptomatic:

Name	Age	Relationship to Case	Symptoms Y/N?	Onset of Symptoms	Lab Testing (Date Collected, Result)	Occupation/Employer School/Grade, Day Care

---

Summary of Investigation - action taken on patients and contacts - outcome:

_____

_____

_____

_____

_____

_____

_____

_____

Name of person completing form   Date of Interview

* Use the incubation period which applies to the agent/disease under investigation: e.g., Bacillus cereus (1-24 hours), Campylobacter (1-10 days), Clostridium (6-24 hours), E. coli (9-60 hours), Giardia (5-25 days), Listeria (3-70 days), Salmonella (6-72 hours), Shigella (12-96 hours), Staphylococcus (30 min.-7 hours), Typhoid fever (1-3 weeks), Vibrio (4-96 hours), Viral agent (24-72 hours).

Figure 5–3 Maryland Gastroenteritis Case Report Form. *Source:* Reprinted from Maryland Department of Health and Mental Hygiene.

Holmes" or disease detective of public health. Outbreak investigation is a systematic process of evaluating data to form hypotheses, then collecting additional data to test the hypotheses. An understanding of the basic steps of outbreak epidemiology can guide the type of data to collect and how to collect them; however, each outbreak is unique, and it is equally important to be aware of how the current outbreak differs from previous outbreaks.

The steps for conducting an outbreak investigation are outlined in Exhibit 5–1. A hallmark of outbreak epidemiology is that these steps do not necessarily proceed in a specified sequence. In actuality, several steps in the investigation usually occur simultaneously. These steps are tailored to the situation and depend on factors such as the urgency to implement control measures; the availability of staff, resources, and time; and the difficulty in obtaining the data. Activities may be performed concurrently by multiple persons. Action and reaction proceed, based on new and cumulative information. Most obviously, implementation of control measures is central to the goal of any outbreak investigation. Measures to control the spread of disease must be imple-

mented early in the investigation and may be altered as data are collected and analyzed.

Prepare for Field Work

Preparing for the outbreak investigation and planning the investigation are critical to a successful outcome. It is imperative to identify the investigation team members, to assign responsibilities, to begin the investigation as soon as possible, and to conduct progress meetings at regular intervals. The multidisciplinary investigative team may be composed of epidemiologists, health care professionals, laboratorians, sanitarians, etc. Often, the personnel who initiate an outbreak investigation are predetermined: health departments, hospitals, schools, or nursing homes commonly have personnel responsible for disease control who are dedicated to outbreak activities when the need arises. For many small scale epidemiologic investigations, the initial outbreak "team" will be a single epidemiologist or other professional who will assess the situation and determine what needs to be done. As the investigation proceeds, personnel may need to be added or reassigned to carry out the investigation.

Successful investigations require effective communication at all levels of authority. Summaries or specific findings need to be shared on an ongoing basis (as appropriate and as allowed by confidentiality laws) with critical individuals and parties, such as facilities or businesses where the outbreak occurred, colleagues, health care providers, other regulatory agencies, the media, or the public. In the United States, communication among the local health department, state health department, and federal agencies such as the CDC, the Food and Drug Administration (FDA), and the U.S. Department of Agriculture (USDA) is routine.

Confirm the Existence of an Outbreak— Verify the Diagnosis

An early step of any outbreak investigation is to confirm the existence of an outbreak. Impor-

---

Exhibit 5–1 Steps in an Outbreak Investigation

Prepare for field work
Confirm the existence of an outbreak—verify the diagnosis
Identify and count cases and exposed persons
  Select a case definition
  Identify cases, population at risk, and controls
Choose a study design
Collect risk information
Tabulate the data in terms of time, place, and person
Collect specimens for laboratory analysis
Conduct an environmental investigation
Institute control measures
Formulate and test hypotheses
Conduct additional systematic studies
Communicate the findings

tant questions to ask are: Are there cases in excess of the expected baseline rate for that disease and setting? Is the reported case actually a case of the disease or a misdiagnosis? Do all (or most) of the "suspect cases" have the same infection or similar manifestations? For some diseases, a single case is sufficient to warrant an outbreak investigation. For example, anthrax, human rabies, food-borne botulism, polio, or bubonic plague are so rare in the United States and so serious that an investigation would be initiated with a single suspected case. Those investigating an epidemic must be aware of the background level of disease in a population under surveillance. For example, malaria infection *acquired* in the United States would be treated quite differently than a case of malaria acquired in Sub-Saharan Africa. A review of existing state, local, or facility baseline rates of disease can be compared with the current case number. It is important to take into account the population in which the cases are occurring. Cases of diarrhea in a nursing home may be a common occurrence, whereas the same number would represent an outbreak if they occurred clustered in time among healthy adults after a picnic. It is also important to consider seasonal variations in disease rates. Influenza outbreaks can be expected to occur in the winter; whereas, bacterial enteric diseases are more common in the summer.

As an outbreak investigation is initiated, it is important that the diagnosis be confirmed—and that the specificity of the case definition be good. This involves a review of available clinical and laboratory findings that support the diagnosis and often involves obtaining more clinical or laboratory information than is initially reported. For example, before deciding that *Neisseria meningitidis* is the organism causing disease, the investigator must confirm that the specimen was taken from a sterile body site (eg, blood or cerebrospinal fluid), rather than from a body site where the organism may be a part of the normal flora (eg, throat). Several cases of rash illness in a school may signal a scabies outbreak if the diagnosis is confirmed, or they may simply represent a cluster in time of rashes of different etiologies and, therefore, not an outbreak.

Identify and Count Cases and Exposed Persons

Select a Case Definition

A case definition is needed to identify and count cases in order to determine who may be affected by the outbreak. Components of the case definition may include information about time and place of exposure, laboratory findings, and clinical symptoms. For example, an early definition in a food-borne outbreak may read: "A case of illness is defined as any diarrhea, vomiting, abdominal cramps, headache, or fever that developed after attending the implicated event." This broad definition neither assumes that all cases will have the same symptoms, nor does it make any assumptions about the risk factors for illness (eg, those who ate a particular food or had contact with specific people). This initial case definition has greater emphasis on sensitivity than on specificity. As additional information is gathered about the cases, the nature of exposure, and the symptoms, the case definition can be refined as appropriate to improve the specificity. A subsequent case definition may state that "A case of illness is defined as diarrhea or vomiting with onset within 96 hours of consuming food served at the implicated meal." This refined definition is more specific and will serve to exclude unrelated cases of gastroenteritis or other illnesses.

In outbreak investigations, as in routine surveillance, cases of disease are commonly separated into those that are *confirmed* and those that are *probable* cases. Confirmed cases are generally those with laboratory findings (such as a positive culture or antigen test, antibody titer rise, or a positive polymerase chain reaction [PCR]) for the organism, and probable cases are those who have certain symptoms meeting a clinical case definition but without laboratory confirmation.[11] For some diseases (eg, pertussis), a case can be confirmed if there is a compatible clinical illness and the case is epidemiologically linked to a laboratory-confirmed case. Frequently, laboratory confirmation is complicated by a number of factors: People may test positive for the organism for a short time around the acute phase of illness; some pathogens produce toxins for which there is no laboratory test; the organism may be shed only transiently or intermittently; antibody tests may be difficult to interpret if individuals had been exposed to the pathogen in the past; persons with mild disease may not seek medical attention and, thus, will not have laboratory tests completed; and persons may be treated at different medical facilities with different laboratory procedures. If laboratory confirmation is important and the outbreak is identified rapidly enough, the outbreak investigation team may want to collect samples promptly or obtain multiple specimens to confirm the initial cases in order to establish the agent responsible for the outbreak. However, this commitment of resources may not be necessary to confirm every case during the investigation. If the case definition can be made sufficiently specific without the use of laboratory tests, collecting and testing specimens may only represent an additional burden and expense to the exposed population and the research team.

Identify Cases, Population at Risk, and Controls

During the outbreak investigation, the investigator should seek to identify additional cases not known or reported at the time of the initial report. Case finding techniques used to enhance surveillance for additional cases include reviewing existing surveillance data (eg, morbidity reports received by a health department or monthly summaries of illness); reviewing outbreak/complaint logs kept by the local health department; reviewing past laboratory data; and surveying hospitals, emergency rooms, or physicians. In certain outbreaks, such as those occurring in a restaurant where there is no list of attendees, a useful technique for finding additional cases and controls is questioning known cases to identify others who were in attendance (see section on case control studies).

The investigator should identify the population at risk or the exposed group in which to conduct expanded surveillance for cases. The exposed group or cohort will vary, depending on the setting, and it may not always be possible to identify or enumerate the entire population at risk. Examples of exposed groups include a group of persons who attended a wedding banquet; all people who dined in a food establishment on one particular day; children who attend a day care center, their household members, and the employees of the center; or all persons who were exposed to an implicated manufactured lot or shipment of a commercial product. The exposed population, therefore, can range from as few as one person to as many as thousands of individuals in multiple locations. Identification of persons at risk can be facilitated by records maintained by the establishments involved. Wedding invitation lists, guest books, credit card receipts, and customer lists are often available and are very helpful to investigators. However, individuals located by use of their credit card receipt may be concerned about how the investigators got their names. Explaining the purpose of the investigation and how information will be handled may be vital to securing their cooperation in the investigation. State and federal public information laws vary in what information is to be held confidential in outbreak situations.

Choose a Study Design

During an outbreak investigation, the study design is chosen based on factors such as the size and availability of the exposed population, the speed with which results are needed, and the available resources. The characteristics of the exposed population are generally determined after interviewing a few of the initial cases. Exposed populations fall into four broad categories: small enumerable exposed groups, large enumerable exposed groups, large or small groups where the exposure situation can be pin-pointed but where the exposed population can-not be enumerated, and finally, cases of disease where the exposed population is not known or identifiable. The study design that is chosen will then dictate the appropriate analysis and hypoth-esis testing as discussed below.

Cohort Studies

Cohort studies, which include persons based on their exposure status, are appropriate when it is possible to enumerate or assemble a list of per-sons potentially exposed and to contact the people in a timely manner. Outbreaks that are suspected to have occurred at a specific event, such as a party, or in a specific place, such as a worksite or cruise ship, are often suited to cohort investigations. If the group is small enough, a study can be designed to include all of the people in the exposed cohort. Alternatively, a selection (using a random number table or selecting a ran-dom starting point and then choosing, eg, every fourth name) can be made from a large enumer-ated exposed population. The demographic sta-tistics, attack rates, and relative risks are calcu-lated when data are collected on the cohort or on a randomly selected fraction of the cohort. (See section on formulating and testing hypotheses.)

Case Control Studies

For outbreaks associated with large events (such as a convention or a state fair), or for community-wide outbreaks or uncommon dis-eases reported from a population, especially where the potential exposure is unknown, it may not be possible or economically feasible to ob-tain or assemble a list of all those exposed or to interview all people in the cohort or exposed population. These outbreak investigations lend themselves to studies that include all or a se-lected group of cases, and a selected group of not-ill individuals for comparison. A full de-scription of the types of case control studies, their nomenclature, and their analyses can be found in several references. [12–14]

When a list of a large cohort of potentially ex-posed people is available (ie, the cohort can be enumerated) but a cohort study is not desirable or feasible, information on identified cases can be included and compared with information from a random sample of not-ill persons chosen from the baseline cohort, eg, the list of those ex-posed (called a case control study within a spe-cific cohort, a case cohort study,[14] or a cumula-tive ["epidemic"] case control study[13]). The number of not-ill people for comparison, and the manner in which the not-ill participants are cho-sen, differentiates these studies from traditional case control studies. These studies maximize the number of cases included, and include a man-ageable number of not-ill people for compari-son. The analysis of data is based on odds ratios, but attack rates and relative risks can also be cal-culated if the study group is a known fraction of the total cases and not-ill people.

Another common outbreak situation arises when cases are occurring within a known ex-posed population (eg, attendees at a state fair or a specific restaurant) but the exposed population cannot be enumerated and there is no list of at-tendees from which to identify cases and con-trols. In this situation, it is important to secure data on a representative sample of people who were potentially exposed. Cases can be identi-fied from reports of illness. Both cases and con-trols can be identified from the exposed group through friends of cases or through media re-ports, credit card receipts, lists of hospital pa-tients, etc. Publicizing through a press release in local print or on television and radio may be nec-essary to secure a sufficient number of not-ill participants. People who know someone who became ill are more likely to know about the out-break investigation and volunteer to participate. The volunteers, however, may share characteris-tics with those who are cases and may not repre-sent all of those who attended the event. Small groups may be identified who attended a larger event, eg, a church group who attended a na-tional convention or a state fair, and the group members may serve as a source of investigation participants. The use of such identified groups can aid recruitment because they may have a list of participants for inclusion. For outbreaks such as these, analysis of the data would necessarily proceed using odds ratios as in a case control study because data are neither available on the entire cohort nor from a known fraction of the group of exposed persons.

For situations in which an exposed cohort or population is not known or identifiable, a case control study design is appropriate to determine risk factors for disease. Examples of this situation include increases in the number of community-wide cases of an unusual *Salmonella* serotype, or the need to identify risk factors for sporadic cases of *Campylobacter* infection. In these situations, cases are selected based on their disease status rather than their exposure status. All known cases are included in the study along with a group of controls, selected, for example, by random digit dialing, or from friends or neighbors of cases. For increased statistical power, up to four controls per case are selected. A further refinement of the case control study is the matched case control design. In these studies, controls are matched to cases with respect to potentially confounding variables. In matched case control studies the effect of these matched variables is removed from the analysis so that the effect of other factors can be more readily observed. For example, to determine the risk factors for a cluster of cases of a rare *Salmonella* serotype, all known cases would be interviewed. Controls may be identified by randomly calling homes with incrementally higher or lower telephone numbers from the case's telephone number. If a household is found in which a member matches the case within a certain age grouping, that person is included as a control in the study and is interviewed.

Because outbreak investigations are primarily concerned with the prevention of the spread of disease, the speed at which case control studies can be assembled makes them an attractive alternative to cohort studies. The case control design is also efficient with respect to collection of data and the expense of conducting the study. The toxic shock syndrome epidemic of 1980 was alarming for the speed at which cases occurred and the severity of the illness.[15,16] Investigation was needed as rapidly as possible. Using a case control study design, investigators assembled study populations using cases and selecting as controls their friends of the same sex. Controls were matched to cases within 3 years of age. Lives were saved because of the speed at which these investigations were completed and the subsequent speed at which health interventions were initiated (see Box).

Collect Risk Information

As the case investigation continues, the investigator assimilates information regarding the affected population to answer questions regarding person, place, and time (also referred to as Who? What? When? and Where?). As part of the investigation, the investigator may use a questionnaire or survey instrument to collect pertinent data (Exhibit 5–2). Questionnaires should be administered as soon as possible. The ability to recall one-time exposures after an event is poor, even in the best of circumstances, and will diminish rapidly with time. Initially, questionnaires may need to be broad and encompassing to capture as much information regarding suspected exposures, such as in widely distributed or geographically clustered outbreaks like the large crytosporidiosis outbreak in Milwaukee.[17]

The questionnaire instrument collects pertinent information about the exposed population or the cases and controls, and about the situation under investigation. Questionnaires usually include variables sufficient to define cases and to identify exposures. Each survey must be tailored to the outbreak and the possible routes of exposure for the agent involved. Demographic information allows the investigator to answer the Who? question and usually includes personal identifiers, such as the person's name, home address, telephone number, age, gender, race/ethnicity, occupation/school, and work address.

Investigation of Toxic-Shock Syndrome

Identified as a severe systemic illness in children, toxic-shock syndrome (TSS) burst on the national scene when cases suddenly appeared, first in Wisconsin and Minnesota and then nationwide, among young adult women during their menstrual periods. The disease was serious and caused substantial mortality. Recovery was complete among survivors; however, recurrences were common during a subsequent menses unless the *S. aureus* vaginal infection was effectively treated with antibiotics. Eventually, 941 cases were reported from every state in the United States. However, 247 (26%) of the cases occurred in Minnesota and Wisconsin.

In the interest of speed and because the number of cases was small, a case control study design was chosen. To control for unknown confounders and to assemble a study population rapidly, the investigators chose to use friends of cases for the initial investigation. Controls were the same gender as the cases (female) and matched to cases within 3 years of age. In the initial investigations, conducted June 13–19, 1980, one control was matched to each case. These studies implicated tampons and hormonal contraception as risk factors for TSS during menstruation. However, women had been using tampons and hormonal contraception for years. Why an outbreak now? And why were the cases concentrated in Wisconsin and Minnesota? The epidemiologic team was aware that a new brand of tampons had been marketed in these states, and they suspected that these super-absorbent tampons might be associated with the outbreak. Although a few brands of tampons were common among women with TSS, these tampon brands were found to be popular with women in general (as measured by market share). A third case control outbreak investigation was conducted September 5–8, 1980. In this study, cases were matched to three age- and gender-matched controls. To reduce misclassification bias, participants were asked to get any boxes of tampons they had in the house and to read the brand information to the telephone interviewer. In this investigation, one brand of super-absorbent tampons was identified and subsequently recalled September 22, 1980. The incidence of TSS declined dramatically and fell even further when polyacrylate tampons (super-absorbent tampons) were withdrawn altogether, although some cases are still reported.

These variables are used to characterize both the ill and well populations. Clinical information helps the investigator with the What? and When? questions and includes symptoms of illness, date and time of onset and length of symptoms, specimen collection dates and results, severity of illness, medical care sought, and outcome information, such as hospitalization or death. These variables allow the characterization of identified cases and assist with hypothesis generation. Exposure information helps the investigator to answer the Where? and When? questions and helps detail the suspected event or situation that put the individuals at risk. The questionnaire should consider exposures other than the most obvious exposure. For example, if ill individuals all at-

Exhibit 5–2 Sample Questionnaire for a Food-Borne Disease Outbreak

---

Food-Borne Illness Questionnaire—(Date)

The Health Department is investigating some reports of illness that occurred after the _____ (event) _____ on __ day, _____.
It is important that **anyone who attended** fill out a questionnaire, even if you did not get sick.

Last name _____ First name _____ Age _____

Home phone number: (__ __ __) __ __ __ -__ __ __ __   Sex: M F (circle one)

Did you eat at this event?   Yes   No

Please circle YES for any food item you ate at the event and circle NO for each item that you did not eat.
All items should be marked.

	Ate item?				Ate item?	
Food 1	Yes	No		Food 7	Yes	No
Food 2	Yes	No		Food 8	Yes	No
Food 3	Yes	No		Food 9	Yes	No
Food 4	Yes	No		Food 10	Yes	No
Food 5	Yes	No		Food 11	Yes	No
Food 6	Yes	No		Food 12	Yes	No

Did you have any drinks on ice?	Yes	No	
Did you have any soft drinks on ice?	Yes	No	
Did you have any alcoholic drinks on ice?	Yes	No	(Number_____)
Did you have any noniced alcoholic drinks?	Yes	No	(Number_____)

Was anyone in your household ill with diarrhea or vomiting in the week preceding the event?
Yes   No   (If yes, Who? & When?_____)

Have you become ill **since** attending the event?   Yes   No

    If yes, please circle YES or NO for **each** of the following symptoms:

Diarrhea	Yes No	If yes, total number of stools on worst day _____
		Was there any blood in your stool? Yes No
Stomach cramps	Yes No	
Nausea	Yes No	
Vomiting	Yes No	
Fever	Yes No	If yes, what was your highest temperature?_____
Headache	Yes No	
Body aches	Yes No	
Chills	Yes No	

Date illness began: _____   Time illness began: ___:___ AM? or PM? (circle answer)

Still having symptoms? Yes   No   (If no, symptoms ended: Date: ___ Time: ___:___ AM? or PM?)
Did you take any medicines for this illness? Yes   No   If yes, what medicines? _____
Did you go to your doctor or an emergency room for this illness?   Yes   No
  If yes, did they collect specimens? Yes   No   If yes, name of doctor: _____
Were you **admitted** to the hospital for this illness? Yes No   If yes, name of hospital: _____

---

tended a wedding, they should be asked not only about the wedding but also about events related to the wedding, such as a common hotel swimming pool exposure, or attendance at other events, such as the rehearsal dinner.

Errors in recall can result in "baseline noise" or misclassification bias. Misclassification bias occurs when persons are randomly incorrectly classified with respect to exposure or illness. Misclassification bias results in the measured risk of disease for persons exposed being lower than the actual risk. Thus, a study could underestimate or miss a significant exposure. Exhibit 5–3 shows an example of how a 20% misclassification of exposure among all attendees at a dinner underestimates the true relative risk by half. One technique used to aid respondents is to ask directed questions of what they "usually" would eat. Using these questions in combination with more traditional food survey questions may

help to reduce misclassification bias. Such questions might be, If given a choice between chicken salad and roast beef, which would you usually take? In addition to improving the quality of data collected, timely collection of data allows for a faster public health response, such as closure of a facility or a product recall or embargo.

The Tennessee Department of Health and Environment conducted a planned study to determine the degree of misclassification of food consumption after a luncheon.[18] By comparing video tapes of the luncheon to participants' answers on a subsequent food survey, investigators found that 32 attendees failed to report 58 food items actually selected and reported selecting 24 items not actually selected, or a total of 82 errors. Only 12.5% of participants made no errors.

The design of the survey instrument is determined by how much the investigative team al-

---

Exhibit 5–3 Example of the Effect That Misclassification Bias Has on the Relative Risk Calculation

The table below shows the *true exposures* to birthday cake and *true illness* in a cohort of 210 people who attended a banquet: 50% of those who ate cake became ill, compared with only 10% of those who did not eat the cake. The true relative risk of illness is 5.0, or "Those who ate birthday cake were five times as likely to become ill, compared with those who did not eat cake."

Ate Birthday Cake	Ill	Not Ill	Attack Rate	Relative Risk
Yes	30	30	30/60 = 50%	50%/10% = 5.0
No	15	135	15/150 = 10%	

Now, assume that, on the questionnaire, 20% of all attendees made an error in whether or not they ate birthday cake. The table below shows the resulting calculation with the relative risk underestimated at 2.5.

Ate Birthday Cake	Ill	Not Ill	Attack Rate	Relative Risk
Yes	30 − 6 + 3* = 27	30 − 6 + 27 = 51	27/78 = 34.6%	34.6%/13.6% = 2.5
No	15 − 3 + 6 = 18	135 − 27 + 6 = 114	18/132 = 13.6%	

Note: 30 people ate birthday cake, minus 20% (or 6) who make an error and say they did not eat cake, plus 20% of the 15 (or 3) people who did not eat cake but in error say that they did.

ready knows. In cases where some of the epidemiologic questions have been answered, the questionnaire can be more specific. Questions can be in a closed format with "yes" or "no" answers, or they can be quantitative (eg, maximum number of stools per day or amount of food consumed). This assures consistency in response and facilitates analysis of the data. In cases where less is known, investigators must keep an open survey instrument to collect any information that may be of use. In such instances, the initial interview or survey instrument should include open-ended questions to encourage people to recall how, where, and over what period they may have been exposed. The questionnaire must be flexible enough to take into account the variable incubation periods for different diseases. For example, two diseases that might initially be reported as diarrheal diseases, salmonellosis and giardiasis, have incubation periods of 1–3 days and 7–10 days, respectively. Until the agent is known through laboratory results, the questionnaire would need to be broad enough to cover exposures during both periods of risk. The epidemiologist must evaluate all the questionnaires to see whether any common links can be found. This sort of evaluation will require knowledge about the clinical syndrome, incubation period, duration, possible etiologies, and possible routes of transmission. This detailed initial process may be conducted even verbally, with as few participants as necessary to define the outbreak better. Once the questionnaire can be simplified, a new, more specific questionnaire without open-ended questions can be administered to a larger group of participants to complete the investigation.

More than one questionnaire can be used during an investigation to capture the necessary information. The initial questionnaire may not be specific enough to answer all of the epidemiologic questions of interest, such as the qualitative and quantitative details of exposure. Furthermore, different populations affected by the epidemic may have different roles in its transmission. For example, a survey of patrons of a food establishment might be administered to the exposed group to find cases and to record clinical and risk information. A different questionnaire would be administered to food service workers that would collect information on illnesses prior to the event, food preparation and handling, hygiene practices, food intake at the event, and any illnesses after the event. Similarly, in a hospital nursery outbreak, the questionnaires completed on newborn cases and controls would be very different from the questionnaires for hospital personnel.

Tabulate and Orient the Data in Terms of Time, Place, and Person

The organization of data is critical to the timely and successful analysis of the outbreak data. A useful tool to organize data is the *line listing*. An example of a line listing is provided in Figure 5–4. Using a spreadsheet-style format, key variables on each ill person are listed, either on paper or computerized. Information on well persons can also be included. A line listing allows the investigator to visualize and summarize pertinent variables quickly, including the total number of cases, the number of individuals with specific symptoms, their ages, gender, hospitalization, date and time of onset, exposures, and rates of illness. Another traditional method for organizing outbreak data is to use cards, where each person's characteristics are recorded on a single index card. Sorting the cards in different ways allows investigators to determine risk factors for cases. Obviously, card and paper methods were devised prior to the use of computers, and any of the spreadsheet or database programs available today can be used for data management and analysis. The CDC has developed the EpiInfo computer software program, in which questionnaires can be created, data entered and analyzed, and line listings produced. This program is currently in worldwide use because it is free, easy to use, has modest computer requirements, is designed specifically for surveillance systems and outbreak epidemiology, and is sufficiently powerful for most investigations. Information on EpiInfo can be obtained from the CDC home page on the Internet (www.cdc.gov).

List for Residents _____ Employees _____ (check one)

Name of Facility: _____   Address: _____
Contact Person: _____   Telephone: _____

Name	Age	Sex	Room No. or Shift & Unit*	Date of Onset	Shift of Onset	Duration of Illness	Fever (Record Highest Temp.)	Cough	Sore Throat	Runny Nose	Congestion—Nasal	Congestion—Chest	Muscle Aches	Vomiting or Diarrhea	Pneumonia	X-Ray Results (if taken)	Influenza Vaccine This Season Y/N	Hospitalized Y/N	Death (Date)	Viral Throat Culture (Date)	Bacterial Throat Culture (Date)	Rapid Antigen Detection (Date)	Serology—Acute (Date)	Serology—Convalescent (Date)	Treatment (List)

Signs and Symptoms (columns: Fever through Pneumonia)

Laboratory Results (if applicable) (columns: Viral Throat Culture through Treatment)

*List shift and unit (or ward) for employee cases.

Figure 5–4 Line listing for respiratory illness outbreaks

Visual representations of data can be helpful in understanding an epidemic. Spot maps of cases by residence, site of care, or location in a facility can help explain the occurrence of cases. More complex methods of combining outbreak data with other sources of data are explained in the chapter on Geographical Information Systems (GIS). Graphs, such as an epidemic curve, or *epi-curve*, provide a visual summary of data (Figure 5–5). The epidemic curve depicts the frequency of cases over time by plotting the number of cases by date or time of onset. This provides information regarding the nature and time course of the outbreak. The epi-curve can allow an estimate of the incubation time of the infection, which may help in the identification of the organism. The time from the presumed exposure to the peak of the epidemic curve is the hypothesized median incubation time. The epi-curve can also give an indication of whether transmission is continuing or has ended. This information is vital to knowing whether control

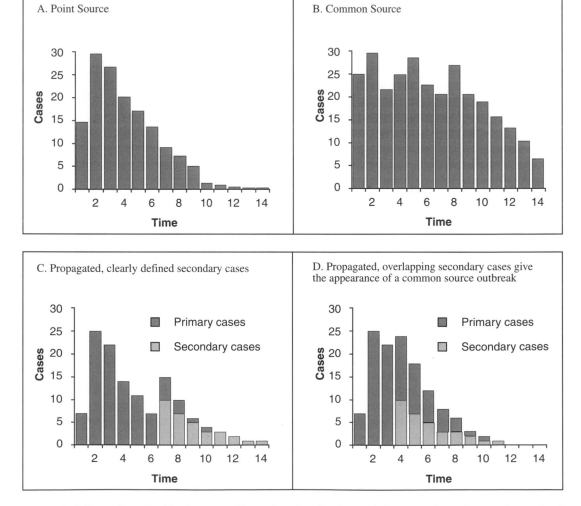

Figure 5–5 Examples of epidemic curves illustrating that the shape of the curve gives clues to the mode of transmission and incubation period

measures may be needed because the current outbreak is continuing and whether control measures are containing the outbreak. Epidemics in which the number of cases rises abruptly and falls again in a log linear fashion are possible *point source* epidemics: The population at risk was exposed at one point in time. Cases occur suddenly after the minimum incubation time and continue for a brief period of time related to the variability in the incubation time in infected individuals. Unless there is secondary spread of the pathogen to others not exposed originally, the epidemic ends. In cases where there is continued exposure of individuals, a *common source* epidemic, cases rise suddenly after the minimum incubation time but do not disappear completely because more individuals continue to be exposed to the source. Third, a *propagated* outbreak will show an increase in cases after exposure, then a fall in the number of cases after the epidemic has exhausted those susceptible from the initial exposure. Later, there is a second increase in cases one incubation period after the peak of the first cases, due to secondary cases infected by person-to-person spread. Because an incubation period may be shorter than the rate at which case rates decline after the initial exposure, propagated outbreaks and common source outbreaks can be difficult to distinguish on the basis of their epi-curves alone.

Perform Laboratory Analysis

The laboratory investigation consists of collecting and testing appropriate specimens. To identify the etiologic agent, the collection of laboratory specimens needs to be appropriately timed. Examples of specimens include food and water samples, other environmental samples (eg, air settling plates), and clinical specimens (eg, stool, blood, sputum, or wound specimens) from cases and controls. Hypotheses about the suspected agent and source should guide the laboratory tests that are performed. Further description of organisms through speciation and other specialized laboratory testing, such as pulsed field gel electrophoresis (PFGE),[19] plas-

mid analysis,[20] PCR,[21-23] or DNA fingerprinting (restriction fragment length polymorphism [RFLP]),[24] is useful to link cases with each other and with the hypothesized source(s). For example, to confirm the source in a legionellosis investigation, it is important to obtain an isolate of *Legionella* from the patient and from the epidemiologically implicated water source to determine whether the isolates are identical. Chapter 8 covers the methods and use of laboratory techniques in more detail.

Conduct an Environmental Investigation

An assessment of the environment where the exposure occurred should be performed when appropriate. The environmental investigation assists in answering How? and Why? questions. This includes an inspection of the facility, a review of practices and procedures for the operation, and an assessment of employee illness. Staff members (including paid employees and volunteers) at facilities such as day care centers, restaurants, and health care facilities may play a key role in outbreaks and may be either the source of the problem or cases in the outbreak. Their evaluation as potential sources and cases, as well as the information they provide in the environmental investigation, may be critical.

The facility assessment may include an inspection by an environmental specialist or other investigator to review procedures and compliance with existing regulations and to identify breakdown of preventive measures. Timely inspection of facilities is of utmost importance to the control of an outbreak. When violations are noted, corrective actions are recommended and compliance monitored. In a food-borne outbreak, an inspection should focus on the kitchen and food preparation areas, whereas in a legionellosis outbreak, inspection should focus on water sources, such as the cooling tower, heating and ventilation systems, potable hot water and plumbing systems, and other areas of water aerosolization, such as showers, decorative fountains, and respiratory equipment. In a nursing home outbreak with person-to-person spread, inspection and interviews should focus on adherence to appropriate infection control procedures, including hand washing and exclusion of ill employees.

While conducting the physical inspection of the facility, the investigator must pay careful attention to the details of the suspected procedure, eg, food preparation, administration of medications, hand washing, or endoscope cleaning. Investigating each step in a procedure with observations of their use and open-ended questions enables the epidemiologist to identify potential problem areas or violations. A review of existing standard operating procedure manuals or materials is helpful in the process. In the United States, food providers are recommended (or, in some states required) to have a hazard analysis, critical control point (HACCP) procedure outlined for each food product they serve.[25] The HACCP plan outlines the ingredients, food preparation techniques, storage until serving, serving conditions, and handling of leftover food (Figure 5–6). However, the investigator must assess how the procedure was done at the time of the outbreak, instead of how the procedure should be done or how it is usually done. For example, in an outbreak of egg-associated *Salmonella* serotype Enteritidis in Maryland, pasteurized eggs were always used in the preparation of crab cakes, and the crab cakes were reportedly cooked to an adequate internal temperature according to their procedure. On one occasion when no pasteurized eggs were available and the facility was exceptionally busy, the facility used fresh shell eggs in the mixture and the crab cakes were not cooked to an internal temperature necessary to kill *Salmonella*. Thus, *Salmonella* in the raw shell eggs and breaks in the usual operating procedures were responsible for the outbreak.[26]

The investigator may need to replicate the process described to determine where the break in food handling procedures occurred. A Maryland outbreak of cholera was found to be associated with a coconut dessert prepared in an individual's home.[27] The cook explained that the commercial, fresh-frozen coconut milk had been brought to a boil. After replicating the recipe and cooking procedures, investigators found that coconut milk brought to a low boil reached only 160° F. After "boiling," the coconut milk had been allowed to sit on the counter for several hours at room temperature in the summer before being eaten, offering an excellent opportunity for the *Vibrio cholerae* organisms to multiply.

Implement Control Measures

As soon as preliminary data indicate the magnitude and severity of the outbreak, a hypothesis should be made regarding the time, place, and person; the suspected etiologic agent(s); and the mode of transmission. Steps should be taken to contain the outbreak. Additional recommendations for control may be developed as the investigation progresses and new information is gathered. Appropriate control measures depend on knowledge of the etiologic agent, the mode of transmission, and other contributing factors. Public health law gives health officials substantial authority to take action to prevent the spread of disease to others. Some examples of control measures include:

- recalling or destroying remaining contaminated food products[27,28]
- restricting infected workers from high-risk occupations[29]
- closing affected facilities to prevent continued exposure
- correcting procedural practices identified as inadequate or improper (such as food handling in a salmonellosis outbreak,[30] or patient care practices in a methicillin-resistant *Staphylococcus aureus* outbreak[31])
- recommending a prophylactic therapeutic agent and/or vaccine (eg, use of rifampin in an outbreak of meningococcal disease)[32]
- enforcing hand washing (eg, in an outbreak of nosocomial gastroenteritis)
- educating the public about risk and prevention (eg, recall of beef contaminated with *E. coli* O157:H7, coupled with the message to cook hamburger to greater than or equal to 160° F)[28]

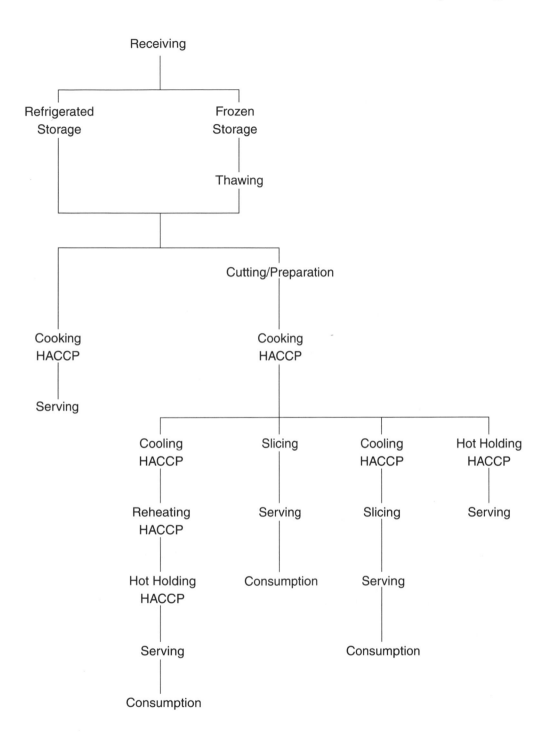

Figure 5–6 Sample hazard analysis, critical control point chart that follows an item (eg, raw meat) from the point of receiving the raw product through storage and cooking to the point of consumption. *Source:* Reprinted from Maryland Department of Health and Mental Hygiene.

Surveillance for additional cases will allow the investigator to evaluate how the control measures are working. Depending on the disease and the incubation period, additional reports of cases may be expected, even after control measures have been implemented and control achieved. For example, successful control of an outbreak of hepatitis A (with an incubation period of 2–6 weeks) does not prevent additional cases from occurring that were exposed in the past and incubating at the time that control measures were implemented.

Recommendations or control measures from an outbreak investigation may lead to the development of procedural changes, guidelines, regulations, or laws that will be applied more broadly as public health policy and are intended to prevent additional cases or outbreaks in similar settings in the future.

Formulate and Test Hypotheses

As the outbreak is investigated, data are assessed informally so that control measures can be implemented and hypotheses can be developed that may lead to further data collection or data analysis. Data are also assessed formally, using standard descriptive and analytic epidemiologic techniques to determine the specific cause(s) of the epidemic.

A primary goal of data analysis is to determine means of transmission and the source and the vehicle of the agent, so that the most effective preventive measures can be initiated. Laboratory data can be conclusive but may not be available, especially at the beginning of an outbreak. An evaluation of symptoms, including their description, frequency, and severity, is a first step in determining the probability of the causal agent. Also, the mean, median, mode, and range of the incubation period can be determined from the epi-curve or by direct calculation. As mentioned above, it is important to separate primary and secondary cases of disease, when possible, to avoid errors in estimating the incubation period. The epi-curve and interviews can be used to determine whether the epidemic is most likely a point source, a common source, or a propagated epidemic.

Another goal of data analysis is to determine the risk factors for disease. As has been done throughout the investigation, analysis starts by answering global questions and works toward answering more specific questions—nesting more specific questions within the context of having answered the broader ones. Initially, analysis will be directed toward determining what population is at risk for disease. Initial hypotheses will be questions such as, Are people who attended the wedding at greater risk of disease than the general public (was there an outbreak)? Subsequently, the question will be, Among those who participated in the wedding party events are people who ate at the wedding buffet, or swam in the pool, or attended the rehearsal dinner at greater risk of disease than those without these exposures? More specifically, the hypotheses will be in the form, Among those who ate at the buffet, are people who ate the Caesar salad (or other specific food item) at greater risk than those who did not? To answer these questions, measures of risk will be calculated.

The measure of risk used in outbreaks investigated using cohort design is the *risk-specific attack rate* (eg, food-specific attack rate for foodborne outbreaks), which is the number of persons who became ill who reported the risk behavior divided by the total number of people who reported that risk behavior. Commonly, the risk-specific attack rate is expressed as a percentage. Exhibits 5–4, 5–5, and 5–6 illustrate the nested hypothesis testing in a typical outbreak of diarrheal disease associated with a picnic. In Exhibit 5–4, 42.9% (30 of 70) of attendees who ate hors d'oeuvres were ill (that is, the risk-specific attack rate for hors d'oeuvres was 42.9%, higher than the attack rates for other risk factors examined).

The second step of analysis is to compare the attack rates for different groups. In this way, it can be determined whether persons reporting a particular behavior are at higher risk of illness than those who do not report the risk behavior. The *relative risk* (RR) is the attack rate among

Number of new cases (thousands)

Exhibit 5–4 Example of the Attack Rate and Relative Risk Calculations in a Typical Outbreak

An outbreak at a company picnic outing has investigators looking at several aspects of the event. Using a cohort study design, questionnaires were administered to all picnic attendees.

Risk Factor Present	Cases N = 35	Not Cases N = 100	Risk-Specific Attack Rate (AR)
Swimming	15	39	$\frac{15}{54} = 27.7\%$
Volleyball	5	20	$\frac{5}{25} = 20.0\%$
Ate box lunch	20	95	$\frac{20}{115} = 17.3\%$
Ate evening hors d'oeuvres	30	40	$\frac{30}{70} = 42.9\%$

To determine which risk factors were associated with an increased risk of disease, the investigators made a two-by-two table and calculated the relative risk of disease.

		Case	Not Case	AR	
Swimming	Yes	15	39	$\frac{15}{54} = 27.7\%$	Relative Risk $= \frac{27.7\%}{24.7\%} = 1.1$
	No	20	61	$\frac{20}{81} = 24.7\%$	

		Case	Not Case	AR	
Ate hors d'oeuvres	Yes	30	40	$\frac{30}{70} = 42.9\%$	Relative Risk $= \frac{42.9\%}{7.7\%} = 5.6$
	No	5	60	$\frac{5}{65} = 7.7\%$	

those exposed to the risk factor divided by the attack rate in those who were not exposed. If those who ate hors d'oeuvres were no more likely to become ill than those who did not, the attack rates would be equal, and the RR would be one. If those who ate hors d'oeuvres were *more* likely to become ill than those who did not, this ratio would be *greater than one,* and hors d'oeuvres would be a *risk factor* for illness. Conversely, if the ratio is less than one, having that factor would have been protective against illness. In Exhibit 5–4, the attack rate in those who ate hors d'oeuvres is divided by the attack rate in those who did not, or 42.9% divided by 7.7%, for an RR of 5.6. In this example, the statement could be made that those who ate hors d'oeuvres were more than five times as likely to become ill than those who did not eat hors d'oeuvres. Usually, additional statistical calculations are made, including the *confidence interval* around this

Exhibit 5–5 Follow-up Analysis Using a Case Control Study To Determine the Odds of Disease According to Consumption of Specific Hors d'Oeuvres

These findings raised the investigators' interest in the specific hors d'oeuvres. Fifteen of the cases answered additional questions. Twice as many controls were selected as were cases.

	Ate Stuffed Mushrooms				*Ate Nachos*	
	Yes	No			Yes	No
Case	9	6	Case		8	7
Control	6	24	Control		20	10

$$\text{Odds Ratio} = \frac{9 \times 24}{6 \times 6} = 6.0$$

$$\text{Odds Ratio} = \frac{8 \times 10}{7 \times 20} = 0.6$$

point estimate of risk and the *probability* that this result occurred by chance (see below).

In a case control study, the total population exposed to the risk factor is not available; the ratio of cases to controls is determined by the investigator. Therefore, in the case control study design (or, frequently, in the case cohort design, unless the cases and not-ill individuals are a known fraction of the cohort of ill and not-ill individuals), it is not possible to measure the risk-specific attack rates. However, it is possible to measure the number of cases who reported the risk behavior and compare this to the number of controls who report the same risk behavior. In the example in Exhibit 5–5, a small case control study was done within the picnic cohort in order to determine which hors d'oeuvre was the culprit. Fifteen cases and 30 controls were asked additional questions. In this case control study, the question was, How many cases ate stuffed mushrooms? rather than, How many of those who ate stuffed mushrooms became cases? as would be asked in a cohort study. The odds ratio (OR) is used to compare the odds of risk behaviors between cases and controls. The odds of eating stuffed mushrooms in cases (9/6, or 3:2) is divided by the odds in controls (6/24, or 1:4). Thus the OR or relative odds is 6.0. The OR is interpreted in the same manner as the relative risk: Values greater than one indicate that the risk behavior is associated

with being a case (a risk factor), values less than one indicate that the risk behavior is associated with being a control (a protective factor). An OR greater than one would be stated as "the relative odds of eating stuffed mushrooms among cases compared to controls was 6.0." Confidence intervals and probabilities can be calculated for the OR as well.

In an outbreak investigation, it is important to consider the possibility that there may be relationships between the variables that influence their association with the risk of disease. Three commonly seen relationships are: *interaction*, *effect modification*, and *confounding* of the data. Variables are said to interact if the presence of one changes the risk of disease for another. In an additive model, the effect of a variable increases the risk of the other as though the risks were being added. If the risk of disease in those people exposed to both risk factors *exceeds* the sum of the two individual risks, the two factors are said to show positive additive interaction or synergism. Similarly, the presence of a multiplicative interaction is evaluated against a multiplicative model for disease risk where the baseline risk is multiplied in the presence of one or more factors.[12]

In the example provided in Exhibit 5–6, a third analysis of the picnic data was conducted to examine additive interactions. All of the guests who had eaten the evening hors d'oeuvres were

Exhibit 5–6 Additional Analysis To Determine Whether There Was Interaction between Foodstuffs Consumed at the Picnic

The investigators were concerned that one of the ingredients used in the preparation of the stuffed mushrooms was also used in a dipping sauce for chips. In particular, they were concerned about a prepared meat product used to stuff the mushrooms and to flavor the dipping sauce. To determine whether the two hors d'oeuvres were independent risk factors for illness, the investigators first reviewed the risk of disease for participants who ate the mushrooms and for those who ate the dipping sauce. They then conducted a cohort study because they were using data from the entire cohort who ate the evening hors d'oeuvres (N = 70), and they were able to calculate relative risks.

		Case	*Not Case*	*AR*	
Ate	Yes	15	9	$\frac{15}{24}=62.5\%$	
Stuffed					Relative Risk = 1.9
Mushrooms	No	15	31	$\frac{15}{46}=32.6\%$	

		Case	*Not Case*	*AR*	
Ate	Yes	16	14	$\frac{16}{30}=53.3\%$	
Dipping					Relative Risk = 1.5
Sauce	No	14	26	$\frac{14}{40}=35.0\%$	

Next, they conducted a stratified analysis to determine the risk-specific attack rates of people who ate both of the hors d'oeurves, dipping sauce only, stuffed mushrooms only, and neither item.

Ate Dipping Sauce

			Yes						No		
		Case	*Not Case*	*AR*				*Case*	*Not Case*	*AR*	
Ate	Yes	4	1	$\frac{4}{5}=80.0\%$		*Ate*	Yes	11	8	$\frac{11}{19}=57.9\%$	
Stuffed						*Stuffed*					
Mushrooms	No	12	13	$\frac{12}{25}=48.0\%$		*Mushrooms*	No	3	18	$\frac{3}{21}=14.3\%$	

Based on these results, investigators concluded that both stuffed mushrooms and dipping sauce were each risk factors for illness, without evidence of additive interaction between them. An investigation was initiated into the common ingredient—prepared meat. Further laboratory tests confirmed that packages of prepared meat were contaminated, and appropriate control measures instituted.

further queried about whether they had eaten specific items including stuffed mushrooms and dipping sauce. First, a two-by-two table was constructed for each item and it was found that the relative risk of disease was 1.9 for those who had eaten the stuffed mushrooms and 1.5 for those who had eaten the dipping sauce. Second, a stratified analysis was performed, where the risk of disease after eating stuffed mushrooms was stratified according to whether or not the guest also ate the dipping sauce. In this analysis, it was found that those who ate *both* the mushrooms and the dipping sauce were over five times more likely to be cases than those who ate neither (80% vs 14.3%; the risk attributable to consuming both items above the baseline rate of disease is 80% minus 14.3% or 65.7%). The risk of disease after consuming both is slightly lower than the sum of the risks of only eating stuffed mushrooms and the risk of only eating the dipping sauce, ie, 65.7% is slightly lower than 77.3%, the sum of the individual risks (57.9% – 14.3%) + (48.0% – 14.3%). An additive risk model makes biological sense in this example: If both items were equally contaminated and people ate equal amounts of both items, then those who ate both items would get twice the dose of the pathogenic agent. Although the number of people in the example is small, the combined risk is approximately the sum of the risk of the two items alone—or no evidence of additive interaction.

Another type of relationship is effect modification. Effect modification is when the value of one variable affects the relative risk or odds ratio of another variable. For example, age is often an effect modifier: The risk of disease is higher among infants and the elderly who consume a particular food. Confounding occurs when the causal effect of one variable is modified by the value of another variable. For example, it may initially appear that gender is a risk factor for a particular disease until it is determined that a second factor is differentially distributed by gender. A preliminary review of the data might show that male participants at an event were more likely to be cases than were female participants. After additional investigation, it was found that the water fountain near the men's restrooms was contaminated; thus, more men were exposed than were women. The variable gender was confounded by whether the participant drank from a contaminated water fountain. When investigating an outbreak, it is important to consider the possibility of interaction or confounding and to continue to explore the relationships between variables to ensure that any of these effects in the data have been evaluated.

The OR and RR are similar measures of risk that can be used and interpreted interchangeably when the attack rate in the population being studied is less than 5%. This is done because many find it simpler to describe or to conceptualize the risk and relative *rate* of disease than are the *odds* and relative odds of disease. The assumption that the OR approximates the RR is known as the *rare disease assumption*; mathematically, the OR estimates the RR at low attack rates. Although the rare disease assumption is usually valid in epidemiologic research on diseases of low prevalence, it is commonly *not* valid in outbreak investigations. Attack rates of 30% or more are common in outbreak studies—clearly much higher than the 5% cutoff used by convention. It is important to realize that the OR and RR are both valid measures of the association between disease and the risk factor at any level of attack rate. However, when the disease is common, the investigator may often not be able to use the OR to estimate the RR. For example, the OR in Exhibit 5–5 for stuffed mushrooms is 6.0; whereas the RR in Exhibit 5–6 is 1.9. Both measures point to an association between the mushrooms and illness.

It is possible for associations to be found that are due to chance, rather than because of any true association between the risk factor and disease. Statistical tests (eg, *p*-value and confidence interval) are used to evaluate the possibility that the findings are due to chance alone. These statistical tests assess the possibility that the distribution of cases by risk group could have happened by chance alone. In other words, How likely is it that, by chance alone, 30 of the 70 people who ate hors d'oeuvres became ill, versus 5 of the 65 who did not eat them? If the possibility that this distribution of data would occur by chance is less than 5% ($p < .05$), the distribution of the data is attributed to an association between the factors, ie, exposure is associated with disease. In outbreak studies, it is common for multiple comparisons to be made, eg, the risk of disease is compared for exposure to 20 different foods. If the cutoff value for statistical significance is set at 5% ($p < .05$), it would be expected that one of 20 comparisons would appear to be a significant association by chance alone. To correct for multiple comparisons, the most conservative approach is to lower the *p* value, according to the number of comparisons being made. To assess the possibility that the distribution is by chance alone, the statistical test will make some assumptions about the distribution of data. For instance, the test will commonly assume that the data are "normally distributed." This means that the test is comparing the distribution of data found in the study to a hypothetical data set, where the distribution of data would fit a normal curve. If there are very few people (less than 40) in the study, the assumption of normally distributed data may be false. Some corrections have been devised to overcome the assumption of normality, such as Cornfield or Fisher's exact test. These alterations to the basic statistical equations are available in most software packages, including EpiInfo.

In some outbreak investigations, the data are sufficiently complex that analysis using two-by-two tables is difficult or insufficient. Stratifying the data may be necessary to remove confounding factors. Logistic regression may also be used to control for certain variables. However, the basic goal remains the same: to determine the important risk factors for disease and to prevent its spread or recurrence.

Outbreak investigations should look beyond the current circumstances to determine how to prevent future outbreaks. In food-borne outbreaks, determination that a particular food was responsible for the disease is only the first step. It may be possible to follow the flow diagram of the food production to determine how the food became contaminated with the pathogen or how the food was improperly handled so that a pathogen could persist or multiply. Corrections to the handling of the food should be made to prevent problems in the future. This step may take the investigation across state or national boundaries. In Exhibit 5–6, once the prepared meat in the stuffed mushrooms is determined as the most likely cause of illness, the investigators can further query the food handlers who prepared the item by developing an HACCP chart, detailing food preparation, storage, and serving. Laboratory data, if available, will be used to support the epidemiology.

In the case of the cholera outbreak in Maryland, epidemiology and laboratory results pointed to the coconut milk as the vehicle for *Vibrio cholera*.[27] It was determined that raw coconut was washed in stream water in the country of origin. Subsequently, the coconut milk was not pasteurized but, instead, frozen and shipped to the United States. The contamination from the stream water exposed U.S. residents to pathogens from thousands of miles away. Changes in U.S. import laws may be required to reduce the risk of future outbreaks.

Plan Additional Studies

The data derived from the outbreak investigation may lead to questions that can be answered only with further planned studies, including epidemiologic research or laboratory investigation at academic, private, or governmental agencies. Outbreaks of *E. coli* O157:H7 have identified undercooked hamburger and apple cider as vehicles. In follow-up, institutional review board-approved case control studies of sporadic cases of diarrhea in numerous states caused by this pathogen are under way to determine additional specific risk factors. Similarly, nationwide outbreaks of *Salmonella* serotype enteritidis linked to grade A shell eggs led to studies of chickens, the hen house environment, the heat lability of the pathogen, the transport and storage requirements of eggs, etc, with the goal of preventing future cases.

Communicate Findings

Investigators communicate interim findings and recommendations verbally and in writing during the investigation to those needing to know, such as the facility or public health agencies. At the conclusion of the investigation, the investigators should write a summary report to document the investigation, the actions taken, and the outcome. If the investigation was conducted by a local, state, or federal health agency, the report becomes a document that will provide feedback to the personnel at the facility or site where the outbreak occurred. Final reports may,

in some instances, lead to recommendations, publications, or regulatory changes that will prevent disease and improve outbreak response in the future (see Box).[33]

CONCLUSION

Outbreaks afford opportunities to gain information about diseases, pathogens, and changing risk factors for disease. Epidemiologic field investigations or outbreak investigations involve a series of methodical, well-planned steps for the collection and analysis of data. Armed with the knowledge of how to investigate an outbreak, the

---

An Outbreak of Oyster-Related Norwalk-Like Virus Gastroenteritis Traced to Fecal Contamination from Fishing Boats

Background: In November 1993, we investigated an outbreak of gastroenteritis associated with eating raw oysters.

Methods: We interviewed 14 groups of two or more ill persons who had eaten raw oysters together. Source beds for oysters were identified using oyster sack tags and dealer records. Oyster harvesters were interviewed. Stool samples from ill persons were tested by electron microscopy (EM) and reverse transcription-polymerase chain reaction (RT-PCR) for Norwalk-like virus (NLV); viral genome was also sequenced.

Results: Of 78 raw oyster eaters, 65 (83%) became ill, compared with 2 (5%) of 41 associated persons who did not eat raw oysters (Risk Ratio [RR] = 17.1, 95% Confidence Interval [CI] 4.4–66.3). The 67 persons had vomiting (71%) or diarrhea (92%) 5–60 hours after eating (median 31 hours). Nine stool samples from persons in three of the groups were

tested for NLV; six were positive by EM, and nine were positive by RT-PCR. Viruses sequenced to date are identical. In the 13 outbreaks where tracing information was available, implicated oysters were harvested November 9–13 from a single area of beds remote from sewage contamination and ship traffic. Four harvesters who did not eat oysters were ill with vomiting and diarrhea while working in the implicated beds on November 7–9 and disposed of their feces and vomitus overboard.

Conclusions: Because the infectious dose for NLV is small (1–10 virus particles) and because oysters concentrate enteric pathogens, virus-containing stool from four ill harvesters may have contaminated a sufficient number of oysters to cause this outbreak. Enforcement of regulations governing waste disposal by fishing boats might prevent similar outbreaks from occurring.

Source: Reprinted from M.A. Kohn et al., An Outbreak of Oyster-Related Norwalk-Like Virus Gastroenteritis Traced to Fecal Contamination from Fishing Boats, presented at the Epidemic Intelligence Service 43rd Annual Conference, 1994, Centers for Disease Control and Prevention.

epidemiologist is able to execute a timely and thorough study of the cause and contributing factors of an outbreak while quickly taking measures to control the outbreak. Cooperation and communication are key elements in the smooth operation of this process. Issues of confidentiality and the release of information should be taken into account, with the operating procedure of the jurisdiction guiding the action to release information. Public health officials in local, state, and federal agencies can provide expert advice and assistance in the investigation of outbreaks.

REFERENCES

1. Zinsser, H. Lice and History—The Biography of a Bacillus: A Bacteriologist's Classic Study of a World Scourge. Boston: Atlantic, Little, Brown; 1963.

2. Lederberg J, Shope RE, Oaks SC Jr, eds. *Institute of Medicine—Emerging Infections: Microbial Threats to Health in the United States.* Washington, DC: National Academy Press; 1992.

3. Bell BP, Goldoft M, Griffin PM, et al. A multistate outbreak of *Escherichia coli* O157:H7-associated bloody diarrhea and hemolytic uremic syndrome from hamburgers: the Washington experience. *JAMA.* 1994; 272(17):1349–1353.

4. Yukioka HK. *Escherichia coli* O157 infection disaster in Japan 1996. *S Eur J Emerg Med.* 1997;4(3):165.

5. Centers for Disease Control. Ebola virus infection in imported primates—Virginia, 1989. *MMWR.* 1989; 48(38):831–838.

6. Centers for Disease Control and Prevention. Summary of notifiable diseases, United States, 1997. *MMWR.* 1998;54(46):iii–iv.

7. Goodman RA, Buehler JW, Koplan JP. The epidemiologic field investigation: science and judgment in public health practice. *Am J Epidemiol.* 1990;132:9–16.

8. Dwyer DM, Strickler H, Goodman RA, Armenian HK. Use of case-control studies in outbreak investigations. *Epidemiol Rev.* 1994;16:109–123.

9. Reingold AL. Outbreak investigations—a perspective. *Emerg Infect Dis.* 1998;4:21–27.

10. El-Gazzar RE, Marth EH. Foodborne disease: investigative procedures and economic assessment. *Environ Health.* 1992;55:24–26.

11. Centers for Disease Control and Prevention. Case definitions for infectious conditions under public health surveillance. *MMWR.* 1997;46(RR-10):1–5.

12. Schlesselman JJ. *Case-Control Studies: Design, Conduct, Analysis.* New York: Oxford University Press; 1982.

13. Rothman KS, Greenland S. *Modern Epidemiology.* 2nd ed. Philadelphia: Lippincott-Williams & Wilkins; 1998:108–111.

14. Szklo M, Nieto FJ. *Epidemiology: Beyond the Basics.* Gaithersburg, MD: Aspen Publishers; 1999:1–51.

15. Langmuir AD. Toxic-shock syndrome—an epidemiologist's view. *J Infect Dis.* 1982;145(4):588–591.

16. Centers for Disease Control. Toxic-shock syndrome, United States, 1970–1982. *MMWR.* 1982;31(16):201–204.

17. MacKenzie WR, Hoxie NJ, Proctor ME, et al. A massive outbreak in Milwaukee of cryptosporidium infection transmitted through the public water supply. *N Engl J Med.* 1994;331:161–167.

18. Decker MD, Booth AS, Dewey MJ, et al. Validity of food consumption histories in a foodborne outbreak investigation. *Am J Epidemiol.* 1986;124(5):859–863.

19. Centers for Disease Control and Prevention. Multistate outbreak of *Salmonella* serotype Agona infections linked to toasted oats cereal—United States, April-May 1998. *MMWR.* 1998;47(22):462–464.

20. Morris JG Jr, Dwyer DM, Hoge CW, et al. Changing clonal patterns of *Salmonella enteritidis* in Maryland: evaluation of strains isolated between 1985 and 1990. *J Clin Microbiol.* 1992;30:1301–1303.

21. Kohn MA, Farley TA, Ando T, et al. An outbreak of Norwalk virus gastroenteritis associated with eating raw oysters: implications for maintaining safe oyster beds. *JAMA.* 1995;273:466–471.

22. Dowell SF, Groves C, Kirkland KB, et al. A multistate outbreak of oyster-associated gastroenteritis: implications for interstate tracing of contaminated shellfish. *J Infect Dis.* 1995;171:497–503.

23. Moe CL, Gentsch J, Ando T, et al. Application of PCR to detect Norwalk virus in fecal specimens from outbreaks of gastroenteritis. *Clin Microbiol.* 1994;32:642–648.

24. Braden CR, Templeton GL, Cave MD, et al. Interpretation of restriction fragment length polymorphism analysis of *Mycobacterium tuberculosis* isolates from a state with a large rural population. *J Infect Dis.* 1997;175:1446–1452.

25. US Public Health Service. Food Code, 1998 Recom-

mendations of the United States Public Health Service, Food and Drug Administration. National Technical Information Service Publication.

26. Maryland Department of Health and Mental Hygiene, Epidemiology and Disease Control Program, Division of Outbreak Investigation. Unpublished data.

27. Taylor JL, Tuttle J, Pramukul T, et al. An outbreak of cholera in Maryland associated with imported commercial frozen fresh coconut milk. *J Infect Dis*. 1993;167: 1330–1335.

28. Centers for Disease Control and Prevention. *Escherichia coli* O157:H7 infections associated with eating a nationally distributed commercial brand of frozen ground beef patties and burgers—Colorado. *MMWR*. 1997;46(33):777–778.

29. Rodriguez E, Parrott C, Rolka H, et al. An outbreak of viral gastroenteritis in a nursing home: importance of excluding ill employees. *Infect Control Hosp Epidemiol*. 1996;17:587–592.

30. Meehan PJ, Atkeson T, Kepner DE, Melton M. A foodborne outbreak of gastroenteritis involving two different pathogens. *Am J Epidemiol*. 1992;136:611–616.

31. Boyce JM, Jackson MM, Pugliese G, et al; the AHA Technical Panel on Infections within Hospitals. Methicillin-resistant *Staphylococcus aureus* (MRSA): a briefing for acute care hospitals and nursing facilities. *Infect Control Hosp Epidemiol*. 1994;15:105–115.

32. Jackson LA, Schuchat A, Reeves MW, Wenger JD. Serogroup C meningococcal outbreaks in the United States: an emerging threat. *JAMA*. 1995;273:383–389.

33. Kohn MA, Farley T, Curtis M, et al. An outbreak of oyster-related Norwalk-like virus gastroenteritis traced to fecal contamination from fishing boats. Abstract presented at: Epidemic Intelligence Service 43rd Annual Conference; April 18–22, 1994.

CHAPTER 6

Mathematical Modeling: The Dynamics of Infection

Joan L. Aron

INTRODUCTION

Mathematical models are important for understanding the population dynamics of the transmission of infectious agents and the potential impact of infectious disease control programs. As an example, consider the information available for a decision to introduce an immunization program to control an infectious agent circulating in a population of 50 million people. Studies of the biology of the agent could identify its basic biochemical and genetic characteristics and possibly even its entire genome. Studies of the clinical effects of the agent could describe the natural history of disease, including the likelihood of permanent damage or death. Studies of the epidemiology of the agent could estimate its prevalence and incidence in various demographic subgroups and identify likely modes of transmission and various risk factors. Studies of the vaccine itself could determine its level of efficacy in protecting an individual from infection or disease. Nevertheless, an enormous extrapolation is required to contemplate the effect of an immunization program on 50 million people and the populations of the infectious agent they harbor. Therein lies the role of the mathematical model.

Still, personal common sense, a so-called mental model, might seem to be more reliable than extensive computer calculations based on a mathematical model whose details are comprehended fully by only a few individuals. After all,

the quality of a mathematical model of complex phenomena depends on the accuracy of its underlying assumptions, which cannot always be verified. However, mental models for making decisions are often ambiguous, difficult for others to comprehend, and just plain wrong.[1] The way out of this quandary is an approach to analyze and understand the differences between mental models and mathematical models, where the term *mathematical model* is used here interchangeably with *computer model* because computer software is often used to construct mathematical models. Insights about the role of mathematical models in evaluating social and economic policies also apply to infectious disease control policies:

> Computer modeling is thus an essential part of the educational process rather than a technology for producing answers. The success of this dialectic depends on our ability to create and learn from shared understandings of our models, both mental and computer. Properly used, computer models can improve the mental models upon which decisions are actually based and contribute to the solution of the pressing problems we face.[1(p228)]

Public health professionals can gain a better understanding of infectious disease epidemiology by becoming intelligent "consumers" of the literature on mathematical models. Furthermore, public health professionals frame the questions to be addressed, thereby playing a major role in guiding the development of applications of mathematical models.

As a first step in introducing mathematical models to public health professionals, it is necessary to define what a mathematical model is (and, by implication, what it is not). A mathematical model is an explicit mathematical description of the simplified dynamics of a system. The use of the word *simplified* is essential because the art and science of modeling require the appropriate selection of information in order to achieve a specific purpose. A model is therefore always "wrong," but may be a useful approximation, permitting conceptual experiments that would otherwise be difficult or impossible. The results of mathematical models can help determine the plausibility of epidemiologic explanations, improve understanding by a demonstration of unexpected interrelationships among empirical observations, and predict the impact of changes on the dynamics of a system. An extensive literature on mathematical models of the epidemiology of infectious diseases is closely linked to the field of population biology, which incorporates aspects of ecology, demography, and genetics, as well as mathematics and statistics.[2-8]

The transition from a clinical and biologic understanding of the course of an infectious disease to a mathematical model of the dynamics of transmission requires selection of features of the disease to represent in the model. For example, the population size of an infectious agent that replicates inside a host may grow from a small inoculum and later decline and disappear altogether (Figure 6–1). It is common to represent this process as a series of stages of infection, starting with a susceptible host who becomes infected. The level of infection must grow for the infected host to be able to transmit the infection to others, that is, to become infective. The latent period refers to the period of time that elapses before an infected host becomes infective. When the host is no longer able to transmit infection, the host is removed from the cycle of transmission in the population. Removal might involve death caused by the infection or the acquisition of natural immunity that clears infection and prevents reinfection. (Mortality unrelated to the infection may occur at any stage and is not part of the natural history of infection per se.) Removal might also involve curative treatment that leaves the host free of infection and disease, and prevents the host from reinfection. For some diseases, removal does not occur because a host becomes susceptible to reinfection after recovery. The relative length and importance of different stages vary with the host population and the agent.

The distinction between infection and disease is essential. Figure 6–1 shows stages of infection relevant to the dynamics of transmission. In general, symptoms of disease might occur before or after the host becomes infective. The period of time from infection until the onset of symptoms is the incubation period, which is not to be confused with the latent period. Hypothetical incubation and symptomatic periods appear in italics in Figure 6–1. In cases of asymptomatic infection, symptoms never appear. In some situations, acute symptoms that occur close in time to the period of infectivity could be followed by damage that persists long after the infection is cleared from the body. The appearance of symptoms is important for case diagnosis and treatment, case definition in a disease surveillance program, and estimation of the harm caused by disease as the justification for a disease control program. However, the fundamental process represented in mathematical models of the epidemiology of infectious diseases is the transmission of infectious agents.

Transmission occurs when a susceptible host contacts an infective host and the infectious agent initiates an infection in the susceptible host. Contact is defined according to the appropriate mode of transmission for a specified agent, such as direct person-to-person transmission of measles via coughs or indirect vector-borne transmission of malaria via mosquito bites. The ability of the agent to infect people is dependent on inherent characteristics of the agent; some infectious agents are more readily

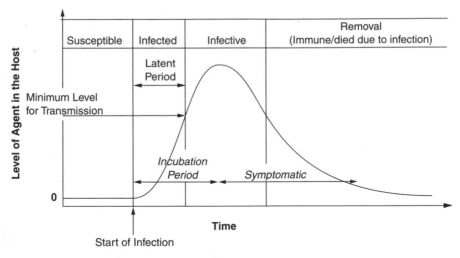

Figure 6–1 Population size of an infectious agent replicating inside a host and classification of stages of infection

transmitted than are other infectious agents under similar conditions. Mathematical models characterize transmission in terms of infection rates related to the frequency of contact between individuals and the likelihood of transmission given a contact between a susceptible host and an infective host.

If the chain of transmission from infective host to susceptible host is maintained in a population, the infection is considered to be endemic. In other words, one would expect to find the infectious agent somewhere in the population at any time. However, the chain of transmission may be interrupted for many reasons. Environmental and social conditions may no longer support transmission of the infectious agent (in effect, reducing contact), treatment may interfere with the infectious stage, or most of the host population may be immune. The last situation is called *herd immunity*, to suggest the analogy between the immune status of a population preventing spread of infection, and the immune status of an individual host preventing internal replication of an infectious agent. The term *herd* is used instead of *population* because of a history of related work on infections in large herds of animals. Mathematical models provide a

theoretical framework for understanding how transmission is maintained and can be interrupted.

This chapter will focus on infections that are directly transmitted and confer life-long immunity. The prototypical example of this class of infections is the measles virus, which causes a respiratory infection transmitted from person to person. If a person survives a case of measles, that person cannot be infected again. The basic model structure also provides a framework for adding structural details to address other epidemiologic problems. An important theme is that different models, characterized by type and degree of complexity, are appropriate for different kinds of questions.

The class of infections represented by the measles virus has several advantages that make it especially useful as an introduction to mathematical models of the epidemiology of infectious disease. The model needs to account for relatively simple characteristics of transmission. The infectious agent is transmitted from one human host to another without a disease vector. An individual who is not infected can be clearly defined as either susceptible or immune without intermediate stages of immunity. Immunity is acquired after a single infection. Although these model assumptions may seem restrictive, several childhood immunizable diseases have these characteristics.

The application of mathematical models to childhood immunizable diseases has contributed to the development of important concepts that are used widely in the field of public health. These concepts illustrate basic features of the epidemiology and control of infectious disease that might not be readily understood in personal mental models. Analysis according to the age of the host is particularly critical. Immunization of a percentage of the population does not necessarily result in a proportionate drop in incidence across all age groups and, indeed, may even increase incidence in some age groups. Further, even if the only laws affecting immunization apply to school entry, it does matter whether children are immunized at school entry or well before school entry. Another problem is that extrapolating the conditions for interrupting transmission from one population to another is often invalid. If a small town is able to interrupt transmission of a respiratory infectious disease by immunizing 70% of its population, the same target is unlikely to have the same effect in a metropolitan area. It is also risky to assume that immunization can be delivered as a single time-limited campaign, even if such a campaign is followed in one instance by a few years free of infection and disease. Careful comparison of the results of mathematical modeling with erroneous ideas demonstrates the utility of modeling.

BASIC THEORY FOR SIR MODEL

The basic theory for the dynamics of transmission of directly transmitted infections that confer life-long immunity describes a population divided into three classes or states. The classes are taken from the depiction of the natural history of infection in Figure 6–1. The first class is susceptibles (S) who can acquire infection. The second class is infectives (I) who can transmit infection to susceptibles. The third class is re-

movals (R) who are immune or dead as a consequence of infection. Because many conclusions from the basic model are not affected by the class of individuals shown in Figure 6–1 with latent infection, that is, those who are infected but not yet infective, discussion of this class is deferred until later in this chapter. The initial letters of the names of the three classes (S, I, R) are used to name the SIR model. Throughout this chapter, the last class always refers to immune individuals. The immune individuals are often called *recovered*, and the process of removal from infective to immune is often called *recovery*.

The development of the basic theory is structured around three important concepts—endemicity, age at infection, and mass immunization/herd immunity. *Endemicity* refers to an endemic infection, that is, an infection that is always present in a population. *Age at infection* refers to the age of a susceptible host when infection occurs. The distribution of ages at which infection occurs is characteristic of a particular infection that is endemic in a particular population. The average age at infection is an indirect indicator of the underlying dynamics of transmission whose components may be difficult to measure directly. Mass immunization is a strategy to control disease by administering a vaccine to a large segment of a population. It may even be possible to create herd immunity so that transmission is completely interrupted because of a high percentage of immune individuals. The theory of mass immunization and herd immunity is based on the concepts of endemicity and age at infection.

Endemicity

Empirical Example

Infectious agents can have very different patterns of endemicity in populations. An epidemiologic comparison of poliovirus and hepatitis B virus demonstrates how differences in natural history affect endemicity. Both kinds of viruses have been studied in seroprevalence surveys that use the presence of antibodies as an indicator of prior exposure to virus. A prevaccine poliovirus study in an isolated Eskimo village in Greenland examined the prevalence of antibodies to the three different types of poliovirus according to age of the host (Figure 6–2a).[9] For each type of poliovirus, there appeared to be an age cutoff that split the population into an older group previously exposed to the poliovirus and a younger group who had not been previously exposed. This pattern is consistent with the introduction and extensive spread of the virus in the population, followed by rapid disappearance of the virus from the population in a short period of time. Poliovirus disappears in an isolated population because those infected with poliovirus develop immunity to the infection, and too few susceptibles remain to maintain transmission. In contrast, another study of Eskimos in Greenland showed that the prevalence of antibodies to hepatitis B virus rose slowly with age (Figure 6–2b).[9] This pattern is consistent with some risk of exposure present all of the time. The key to understanding the difference between hepatitis B and polio is the hepatitis B carrier state, which is a chronic infection in an individual host, indicated by the presence of the hepatitis B surface antigen. In the hepatitis B study population, the prevalence of the hepatitis B surface antigen rose with age of the host (see Figure 6–2b). The establishment of the hepatitis B carrier state in some individuals allows hepatitis B virus to remain endemic in a population where poliovirus transmission cannot be maintained.

The dynamics of poliovirus display the characteristics of an infection obeying the basic assumptions of the SIR model. The presence of the carrier state in hepatitis B infection is not part of the assumptions of the SIR model. Analysis of the SIR model helps to develop a deeper understanding of the phenomenon of epidemic spread and disappearance.

Assumptions in the Threshold Theorem

The formulation of the SIR model is based on the Kermack-McKendrick Threshold Theorem.[6] The Kermack-McKendrick Threshold Theorem considers population size in relation to area, that is, population density. The variables X, Y, and Z denote the population densities of the three classes in a SIR model (Figure 6–3). The population is closed, which means that no one enters or leaves the population. Although the assumption that the population is closed appears to ignore births, deaths, and migrations that happen in every human population, a population can be effectively closed during an epidemic if the epidemic moves quickly through the population before the processes of demographic change have a significant effect. (For other applications in which the removals are not immunes but, rather, deaths from the disease, the removals are counted as part of the population during the course of the epidemic.) Short-term travel movements in and out of the defined population may also violate the assumption of a closed population. However, in many settings, travel may not contribute very much to transmission during the time scale of an epidemic, especially for children, who typically travel less than do adults. Under the assumption of a closed population, the three classes add up to a fixed total population density, N.

Transmission of the infectious agent is characterized by a mass-action term (βXY) for the rate of transfer of individuals from the susceptible class X to the infective class Y. The contact parameter β incorporates an area of movement per person per day and a probability that a contact between an infective and a susceptible results in transmission of the infectious agent. The multiplication of X and Y corresponds to mass-action mixing, the simplest assumption for random mixing. The removal of infectives is characterized by a term (γY) for the rate of transfer of individuals from the infective class Y to the immune class Z. The recovery parameter γ is a rate, but it is easier to think about the transition from the infective state to the immune state in terms of $1/\gamma$, the average duration of infectivity. A rapid rate of recovery results in a short duration of infectivity. The model is written as a system of differential equations showing the rates of change of the population densities of X, Y, and Z with time t (see also Figure 6–3).

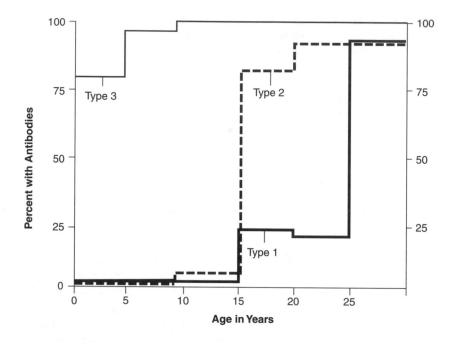

a

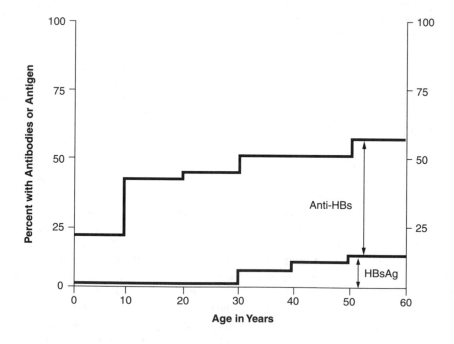

b

Figure 6–2 (a) Age distribution of poliomyelitis antibodies in an isolated Eskimo village, Narrsak, Greenland; and **(b)** age distribution of hepatitis B surface antigen (HbsAg) and antibody to HbsAg (anti-HBs) in Eskimos of southwest Greenland. *Source:* Reprinted with permission from J.A. Yorke et al., *American Journal of Epidemiology*, Vol. 109, p. 106, © 1979, The Johns Hopkins University School of Hygiene and Public Health.

Susceptibles ⟶ Infectives ⟶ Removals

$$X \xrightarrow{\quad\beta XY\quad} Y \xrightarrow{\quad\gamma Y\quad} Z$$

$$\frac{dX}{dt} = -\beta XY \qquad \frac{dY}{dt} = \beta XY - \gamma Y \qquad \frac{dZ}{dt} = \gamma Y$$

Figure 6–3 SIR model for a closed population

$$\frac{dX}{dt} = -\beta XY$$

$$\frac{dY}{dt} = \beta XY - \gamma Y$$

$$\frac{dZ}{dt} = \gamma Y \qquad\qquad (1)$$

$$X + Y + Z = N$$

Results from the Threshold Theorem

The conditions for transmission in an epidemic model are usually analyzed in terms of a scenario in which a single infective is introduced into an otherwise susceptible population. For the Kermack-McKendrick Threshold Theorem using population density, the introduction of an infective corresponds to a very small density of infectives. In the system described in Equation (1), an epidemic will start only if the density of susceptibles X exceeds a threshold γ/β.

The threshold condition is derived from an analysis of the growth in the density (or number) of infectives, Y, at $t = 0$, which is the conventional starting time. An epidemic means that the number of infections grows beyond the number initially introduced.

$$\text{At } t = 0, \frac{dY}{dt} = (\beta X - \gamma)Y > 0 \text{ if } X > \frac{\gamma}{\beta} \qquad (2)$$

If the density of susceptibles exceeds the threshold γ/β, the rate at which susceptibles become

infectives (βXY) exceeds the rate at which infectives are removed (γY). That is, the net rate of growth of the population density of infectives is positive. Because it is assumed that almost everyone is susceptible at the outset ($X \cong N$), the statements about the density of susceptibles, in effect, refer to the population as a whole. In other words, the initiation of an epidemic requires that the population density exceed the threshold γ/β. If there is an epidemic, it eventually terminates. At the end of the epidemic, the population consists of susceptibles below the threshold density and removals (immunes). A more detailed mathematical analysis of the system in Equation (1) may be found elsewhere.[10]

Hypothetical SIR Epidemic in Baltimore City

A hypothetical infection in Baltimore City provides an example to demonstrate calculations of the variables and the parameters of the SIR model, as well as the progress of the epidemic. The threshold condition is stated in terms of the density of susceptibles required for an epidemic to spread and an alternative formulation of secondary cases per introduced case. Evidence of the great power and generality of this restatement of the threshold condition will be seen later in this chapter.

Baltimore City has a population density, N, of 8,700 people per square mile. The epidemic is assumed to start with $X = 8,699$, $Y = 1$, and $Z = 0$. The contact term β incorporates an area of movement per person per day of .001 square miles. Thus, a typical infective would encounter an average of 8.7 (8,700 × .001) people per day, virtually all of whom are susceptible at the start of the epidemic. The parameter β is reduced from .001 to .0004 because it is further assumed that only 40% of contacts between susceptibles and infectives result in transmission. So the number of people infected per day by a single infective at the start of the epidemic would be only 3.48 (βN). The recovery parameter γ of .5 per day means that a person is infective, on average, for 2 days before becoming immune. Under these assumptions, the threshold condition in Equation (2) for the density of susceptibles becomes 1,250 people per square mile (.5/.0004). In this example, the population density of 8,700 people per square mile clearly exceeds the threshold, so the epidemic spreads. The SIR epidemic for the system in Equation (1) demonstrates the classic rise and fall in the population density of infectives, Y, over time as the epidemic progresses (Figure 6–4).

The assumptions about the contact parameter β can be subtle. The key assumption is that everyone in the population has a typical pattern of contact, characterized by the population density and a typical area of movement. However, it is sometimes erroneously stated that everyone in the population must have an equal chance of contacting everyone else in the population. Because this pattern of contact is obviously impossible for large populations in cities or countries, it would be easy to reject the model for failure to meet this assumption. This misinterpretation is encouraged when population size is used to define population density. For example, one could achieve the same numerical results for Baltimore City by constructing a new unit of area to be 80.8 square miles and using the total city population of 702,979 instead of 8,700 people per square mile.

An alternative expression of the threshold condition is in terms of secondary cases per introduced case instead of population density. Simply put, the epidemic will spread if a single case introduced into a susceptible population generates more than one new case. Therefore, the threshold density of 1,250 people per square mile becomes a threshold of one secondary case. The number of secondary cases generated by a single introduced case is the product of the number of new cases generated per day and the num-

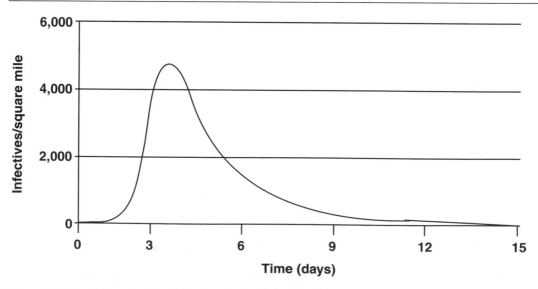

Figure 6–4 Population density of infectives during SIR epidemic

ber of days of infectivity. As discussed earlier, the values for the Baltimore City example are 3.48/day (βN) and 2 days ($1/\gamma$), respectively. Because there are, on average, 6.96 secondary cases per introduced case, the epidemic will spread.

There are other ways of describing the progress of an epidemic. The ratio of the population density of infectives, Y, to the total population density, N, yields the prevalence, that is, the proportion of the population that is infective. For example, the value in Figure 6–4 of 5,000 infectives per square mile corresponds to roughly 57% of the population. In addition, the ratios of population density and proportion of infectives to the average duration of infectivity provide approximate measures of incidence (see relationships among prevalence, incidence, and the duration of infectivity in Chapter 2). For example, the value in Figure 6–4 of 5,000 infectives per square mile corresponds to an incidence of 2,500 people per square mile per day, or roughly 29% of the population per day at that point in the progress of the epidemic. These numbers translate to about 202,000 cases per day for the city as a whole. The true incidence of infection may actually be shifted in time because, technically, this approximation estimates the rate at which infective cases become immune rather than the rate at which susceptible individuals become infective. Epidemic statistics are often cited in terms of incident cases for entire populations in political jurisdictions. Although such reporting is useful for public health services, it may generate confusion among population density, population size, and assumed patterns of contact in the underlying model of transmission. It should be noted that the shape of the epidemic curve remains the same for all of these alternative measurements, except that the delays in appearance of symptoms and reporting may shift the observed timing.

Epidemiologic Insights from the Threshold Theorem

The development of the SIR epidemic theory and the Kermack-McKendrick Threshold Theo-

rem have led to important epidemiologic insights about endemicity for directly transmitted infections that confer life-long immunity. The central result has been a better understanding of the dynamics of the susceptible population.

Epidemics cannot spread in a population of susceptibles whose density is very low. If the density of susceptibles is sufficient for the initial spread of epidemics, infection in the population cannot be sustained (ie, become endemic) without an influx of susceptibles. If new susceptibles do not arrive quickly enough, the population is effectively "closed," and the infection dies out. The episodic appearances and disappearances of poliovirus in remote Eskimo villages demonstrate the consequences of an inadequate supply of susceptibles (Figure 6–2a). Endemicity of infection generated by a steady influx of susceptibles is discussed in the section on age at infection.

Epidemics can wax and wane as a function of the supply of susceptibles. Although the role of the susceptible population may seem obvious in retrospect, the study of the causation of epidemics has been characterized by vigorous debate. An old epidemic theory postulated the need for increases and decreases in the transmissibility of the agent.[11]

Finally, the eradication of an infection by mass immunization can be understood in terms of reducing the density of susceptibles below a threshold required for the spread of infection. Thus, herd immunity is theoretically possible because eradication can, in principle, be achieved with less than 100% effective immunization. The section on mass immunization and herd immunity provides more details.

Age at Infection

Empirical Example

Infections that obey the basic assumptions of the SIR model remain endemic in open populations with a steady influx of susceptibles. For these endemic infections, the distribution of age of the susceptible host at time of infection may vary by disease and location. For example, the average ages of measles and whooping cough (pertussis) cases reported in Maryland from 1908 to 1917 demonstrate differences between urban and rural areas and differences between the two diseases (Table 6–1). The average age of measles cases is lower in urban areas (6.9 years) than in rural areas (10 years). Similarly, the average age of pertussis cases is lower in urban areas (4.9 years) than in rural areas (6.5 years). A comparison within urban and rural areas shows that pertussis tends to strike at younger ages than does measles. Analysis of the SIR theory of endemic infection helps to develop a deeper understanding of the underlying population dynamics of infection reflected in the relationships observed in Table 6–1.

SIR Model of Endemic Infection

An influx of susceptibles is required to maintain transmission of an infection characterized by the basic assumptions of the SIR model. An influx of susceptible hosts changes a closed population to an open population (see Figure 6–5). The simplest formulation of a SIR model of an endemic infection permits the derivation of new concepts about endemicity. Three basic elements characterize the turnover of population. First, the steady influx of susceptibles is assumed to be the births in the host population. The short period of passive immunity provided by maternal antibodies is ignored. Second, mor-

tality unrelated to the infection acts equally on all epidemiologic classes in the model. Third, the total population size remains fixed because the influx of births exactly balances the loss due to mortality. The influx of births is represented by B, and the deaths are represented by $\mu X + \mu Y + \mu Z$, where μ is the mortality rate. When the parameters for birth and death are added to the system in Equation (1), the result is the system in Equation (3).

$$\frac{dX}{dt} = -\beta XY + B - \mu X$$
$$\frac{dY}{dt} = \beta XY - \gamma Y - \mu Y$$
$$\frac{dZ}{dt} = \gamma Y - \mu Z \qquad (3)$$
$$B = \mu N, \; X + Y + Z = N$$

Basic Reproduction Ratio

The basic reproduction ratio, R, is the number of secondary cases generated from a single infective case introduced into a susceptible population. (R is sometimes called R_0, and the basic reproduction ratio is sometimes called the *basic reproductive rate*.) If R is greater than 1 and there is a steady influx of births of susceptibles, as shown in Equation (3), an infection obeying the basic assumptions of the SIR model becomes endemic. The threshold condition for the basic reproduction ratio is the generalization of the alternative formulation of the threshold condition in terms of secondary cases per introduced case. R is the product of an effective contact rate and the average duration of infectivity. In terms of the notation for the hypothetical Baltimore City example, these values are 3.48/day (βN) and 2 days ($1/\gamma$). (Technically, the effect of mortality can alter the duration of infectivity because of the chance of dying during the period of infectivity. This effect can be ignored for practical purposes if this chance of dying is small.) It may be useful to re-express the effective contact rate

Table 6–1 Average Age at Infection in Maryland, 1908–1917

	Age at Infection (yrs)	
Disease	*Urban*	*Rural*
Measles	6.9	10.0
Whooping Cough	4.9	6.5

Note: Age at infection is measured as age of the cases.
Source: Data from C.V. Broome et al., Epidemiology of Pertussis, *Journal of Pediatrics*, Vol. 98, pp. 362–367, © 1981.

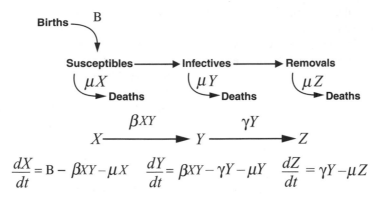

Figure 6–5 SIR model for a population with births and deaths

in terms of new parameters for contact rate c and the probability of transmission per contact q.

$$R \cong (\beta N)(1 / \gamma) = cq(1 / \gamma) \qquad (4)$$

With c of 8.7 people per day, q of .4, and $(1/\gamma)$ of 2 days, the basic reproduction ratio has a value of 6.96 that exceeds the threshold of a single secondary case. By focusing on the contacts instead of just population density, attention is directed to the underlying social and biologic determinants of transmission. For example, if regional schools in rural districts bring children together from large areas, the contact rate is not as small as would be expected on the basis of residential population density alone.

Equation (4) shows that larger R is associated with greater contact rate, greater duration of infectivity, and greater probability of transmission per contact. In turn, greater contact rate is often associated with greater population density, especially for respiratory infections. Therefore, R would be expected to be higher in urban areas than in rural areas in regional comparisons of a particular infection. (As noted above, social mixing patterns may make the differences less pronounced than the differences in residential population density.) Also, greater duration of infectivity and greater probability of transmission per contact are associated with greater infectiv-

ity of infectious agents and reflect intrinsic differences between different infectious agents. In comparisons of different infections within the same population, one would expect R to be consistently higher for some infections.

The great contribution of the SIR theory is that the value of R can be used to analyze the dynamics of transmission, both when infection has just been introduced into a population and when infection has long been endemic. When R is greater than 1, the dynamics of infection in the system of equations in (3) tend toward an equilibrium with infection present, ie, an endemic equilibrium. At the equilibrium (denoted with the bar over the variable), the fraction susceptible, $\overline{X}/N$, is equal to the inverse of the basic reproduction ratio:

$$\frac{\overline{X}}{N} = \frac{1}{R} \qquad (5)$$

The intuitive explanation is that a single case will generate, on average, R new cases if everyone else is susceptible but only a single new case at the endemic equilibrium. (If the number of cases is growing, the dynamics of infection cannot be at an equilibrium.) That means that only a fraction, $1/R$, of the possible contacts is susceptible at the endemic equilibrium. From Equation

(5), it is clear that the susceptible fraction at equilibrium decreases with larger R.

The susceptible fraction is also related to the mean life expectancy L and the average age at infection A:

$$\frac{\overline{X}}{N} \cong \frac{A}{L} \qquad (6)$$

A more detailed explanation of the reasoning based on following the experience of a birth cohort may be found elsewhere.[13] However, an intuitive explanation is that the earlier a birth cohort experiences infection (smaller A), the fewer will be the people remaining susceptible at equilibrium (smaller $\overline{X}$). Combining Equation (5) and Equation (6) yields a relationship between the basic reproduction ratio and the average age at infection:

$$R \cong \frac{L}{A} \qquad (7)$$

The larger basic reproduction ratio R is associated with lower average age at infection A. [A variation on the formula in Equation (7) shows the value 1 added to the right-hand side. This variation is related to technical differences in the definition of the average age at infection,[13] but the effects are minor in most situations.]

The relationship in Equation (7) provides a basic understanding of the average ages of measles and pertussis cases in Maryland shown in Table 6–1. Urban areas have higher population density, which is associated with greater contact rates for respiratory infections. Therefore, measles and pertussis should have higher basic reproduction ratios in urban areas. In turn, these higher basic reproduction ratios in urban areas are associated with lower average ages at infection reflected in the average age of reported cases. It is important to focus on the contact pattern and not on urban living per se. For example, a study of hepatitis A found lower ages at infection in rural areas, a reversal of the urban–rural

pattern described for measles and pertussis.[14] Apparently, poor sanitation is more important than population density in determining contact rates for hepatitis A, whose mode of transmission is fecal-oral.

Equation (7) also helps elucidate the differences between measles and pertussis. If pertussis tends to occur at younger ages than measles in the same populations, pertussis should have a larger basic reproduction ratio than measles. Pertussis could be more infective than measles because of a longer duration of infectivity or a greater probability of transmission per contact, or both.

Admittedly, this reasoning about infectivity of different infectious agents is indirect. However, this indirect reasoning was bolstered by empirical evidence of an inverse relationship between infectivity and the average age at infection. A study of measles, varicella, and mumps in England compared the (infection) attack rates of susceptibles within households[15] of an index case with the average age of cases in the community (Table 6–2). The attack rate is an indicator of infectivity because it measures the percentage of susceptible people in the household who become ill from an initial case in the household. In the English study, the attack rate was highest for measles and lowest for mumps, whereas the average age of the reported cases was lowest for measles and highest for mumps. Such studies are more difficult to perform after diseases are controlled by immunization programs. However, a study of pertussis[16] in unvaccinated household contacts demonstrated a very high attack rate that is consistent with an infection even more contagious than measles (Table 6–3).

Mass Immunization and Herd Immunity

Immunization and the Basic Reproduction Ratio

Immunization, when effective, transfers an individual directly from the susceptible class to the immune class without experiencing disease. Mass immunization is a program to control dis-

Table 6–2 Empirical Evidence for Inverse Relationship between Infectivity of Agent and Average Age at Infection

| | Disease | | |
Factor	Measles	Varicella	Mumps
Exposures	266	282	264
Transmissions	201	172	82
Exposure Attack Rate	75.6%	61.0%	31.1%
Average age at Infection (yrs)	5.6	6.7	11.5

Note: Medical records were used to determine which household members were susceptible to the infection. All susceptibles in the household of an index case were considered as possible exposures.

Source: Data from R.E. Hope Simpson, Infectiousness of Communicable Diseases in the Household (Measles, Chickenpox and Mumps), *Lancet*, pp. 549–554, © 1952.

ease by vaccinating large segments of the population; mass immunization policy often aims for universal coverage. When many people are immunized, the dynamics of transmission are altered. Potentially infectious contacts that would have been made with susceptible individuals are made instead with immune individuals. From the perspective of an infectious agent that requires a steady supply of susceptible hosts to maintain propagation, mass immunization transforms a high-density population into a low-density population.

Table 6–3 Pertussis Secondary Attack Rates in Unvaccinated Household Contacts

Statistic	<1 Year Old	1–5 Years Old
Total Contacts	9	5
Illnesses	8	5
Attack Rate	89%	100%

Source: Data from C.V. Broome et al., Epidemiology of Pertussis, *Journal of Pediatrics*, Vol. 98, pp. 362–367, © 1981.

The effect of mass immunization is to reduce the basic reproduction ratio. A change in the basic reproduction ratio refers to permanent changes in the conditions of transmission as a result of an ongoing immunization program. If, for any reason, the immunization program does not continue, the original conditions for transmission will eventually return as new susceptibles enter the population. Defining R′ to be the basic reproduction ratio after immunization and *v* to be the proportion vaccinated and effectively immunized,

$$R' = R(1-v) \tag{8}$$

A higher proportion immunized means a lower basic reproduction ratio after immunization. The theoretical proportion immunized does not include the administration of vaccine to individuals who are already immune as a result of natural infection. Consequently, because older individuals are more likely to have been exposed to infection, careful assessment of the effectiveness of immunization programs should consider the age of the recipient of vaccine. If, for example, substantial transmission occurs before the typical age at which a child enters school, immunization at time of school entry is less likely to reach susceptible individuals than is immunization at younger ages.

Eradication

When the basic reproduction ratio is reduced below 1, transmission is, in theory, eradicated, and herd immunity is achieved.

$$R' < 1 \tag{9}$$

The magnitude of the basic reproduction ratio before the start of an immunization program is an indicator of the difficulty of disease eradication because the proportion that should be immunized to achieve eradication increases with the magnitude of the basic reproduction ratio. Figure 6–6 illustrates how the target immunization level for eradication increases if the

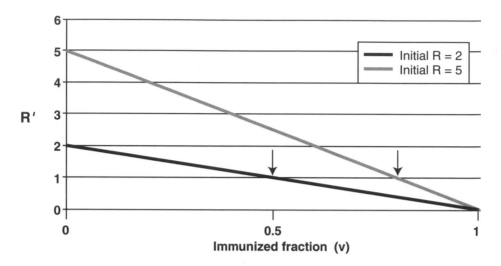

Figure 6–6 Basic reproduction ratio after immunization

---

preimmunization basic reproduction ratio increases from 2 to 5. More generally, the target level of immunization to achieve herd immunity may be expressed by combining Equation (8) and Equation (9):

$$v > 1 - \frac{1}{R} \qquad (10)$$

Selected values of the target level of immunization are shown in Table 6–4. It should be noted that many estimates of the basic reproduction ratio for SIR-type diseases are at least 10, meaning that at least 90% of the population must be effectively immunized. Eradication by mass immunization still requires a large effort, even with the help of the herd immunity principles.[17]

The theory also demonstrates that it is generally invalid to use a target level of immunization simply because it was effective in another location. If there are important differences in the dynamics of transmission, as reflected in the value of the basic reproduction ratio, the target levels must differ also. For example, one would expect the target levels for eradication of a respiratory

infection to be higher in an urban setting than in an otherwise comparable rural setting because the basic reproduction ratio is probably higher.

Increased Average Age at Infection

If mass immunization reduces transmission without interrupting it, then $1 < R' < R$. Total incidence is reduced but, because a lower basic reproduction ratio is associated with a higher average age at infection, the average age at infection is increased. That is, the population that remains unimmunized indirectly experiences the effect of mass immunization by a delay in the age at

---

Table 6–4 Immunization Percentage To Achieve Herd Immunity

Preimmunization Basic Reproduction Ratio	Target Immunization Percentage
2	50%
5	80%
10	90%
20	95%

which infection occurs. Despite the drop in the total number of cases, older age groups may actually experience an increase in the number of cases.

The impact of measles immunization provides an excellent example of this phenomenon. After the measles immunization program was introduced in the United States in 1963, the overall risk of measles infection was dramatically reduced. During the program, however, measles became a new risk on college campuses as measles cases appeared at ages older than was typical before the immunization program began.[18] The risk of measles on college campuses has subsequently been reduced through the introduction of a second dose of vaccine in 1989 to compensate for primary vaccine failure, in combination with campus policies to require proof of immunization.

DEVELOPING APPLICATIONS

Extensions of the SIR Model

The basic SIR model provides useful insights about the persistence of infection in populations, factors determining the average age at infection, the response to mass immunizations, and the possibilities of interrupting transmission. However, the development of applications usually requires the incorporation of considerably more epidemiologic detail than shown earlier. The challenge is identifying specific questions and the level of information needed to address them. Several examples of extensions of the SIR model will be used to illustrate the issues.[13]

Age Differences in Contact Rates

The simple SIR model makes a strong general prediction that mass immunization raises the average age at infection. However, the simple SIR model assumes that everyone in the population has the same contact rate, regardless of age. The limitations of the simple SIR model can be seen in an explicit description of how the average age at infection should change in response to immunization. If A is the average age before immunization, A_I is the average age after immunization, and v is the fraction effectively immunized,

$$A_I(1 - v) = A \qquad (11)$$

For example, if $v = .5$, then the average age of the cases should double after the immunization program is in place. However, a study of the impact of immunization in Britain shows that the results of the simple SIR model do not make reliable quantitative predictions about the magnitude of the increase in the average age of measles cases.[19,20] During the period from 1970 to 1980, when measles vaccine uptake in children was around 50%, the effect of immunization was to raise the average age of the cases from 4.5 to 5.5 years, much smaller than the doubling predicted by the simple model. The reason for the discrepancy is thought to be the enhanced contact rates among school-aged children that accelerated the rate of exposure at around the age of 5 years. Therefore, the results of the simple SIR model applied to the study of the average age at infection are only semi-quantitative, in that the model can reliably identify the direction of change but not the magnitude of change.

Other models of the impact of immunization in Britain have estimated the percentage of the population that needed to be effectively immunized in order to eradicate measles.[21–23] Three different models yielded 96%, 89%, and 76%. The differences among the three predictions correspond to different assumptions about disease contact rates for adults—low for 76%, intermediate for 89%, and high for 96%. The adult contact rates are important because the average age at infection increases as an immunization program is implemented. The degree of difficulty of eradication is related to transmission patterns among adults. Projections of the eradication of disease based on studies of children may be misleading when extrapolated to adults.

Latent Period

Infectious diseases typically have a latent period between the time that a host becomes infected and a host is able to transmit infection to others. For an analysis of latency, an exposed but latent class E transforms the model from SIR to SEIR. The importance of the latent period depends on the epidemiologic problem under investigation. For example, the values of the immunization thresholds needed to eradicate infection and the reservoirs of infection when systems are at an endemic equilibrium depend on the basic reproduction ratio but not usually on latency. Latency does not affect the basic reproduction ratio unless there is a probability of dying during the period of latency. For the diseases presented in this chapter, the probability of dying during the period of latency is usually small enough to have a negligible effect on the basic reproduction ratio. However, latency always affects time-dependent phenomena, such as the speed of the epidemiologic response to changes in immunization or the speed of an epidemic. For example, in following a chain of measles transmission, the generation time from case to case is approximately 14 days. Because the latent period accounts for the majority of the generation time, the elimination of the latent period would significantly accelerate the spread of disease.

Demographic Effects

Epidemiologic models usually assume a fixed population size for diseases affecting human populations. This simplifying assumption is justified on the basis that the dynamics of infectious agents operate on a much faster time scale than do changes affecting human populations. However, the difference between crude birth rates and crude death rates in many developing countries is large enough to affect the population dynamics of infection and, in particular, contribute to the reduction of the average age at infection.[2]

Spatial Effects

The fact that populations are geographically dispersed has important implications for the spread of disease and the design of disease control programs. Measles is one of many diseases whose geographic aspects have been studied in detail.[24] Explicit representation of a collection of populations (a metapopulation) permits joint analysis of characteristics for individual populations, such as birth rate and population size, and contacts between populations in a region (geographic coupling).[25] Before a measles immunization program was introduced in England and Wales, the pattern of maintenance or interruption of transmission at a local level was strongly influenced by geographic coupling. New technologies for geographic information systems have expanded opportunities for studying spatial characteristics of disease (see Chapter 9).

Stochastic Effects

Deterministic models, which are the focus of this chapter, have fixed rules for change. Given the same initial conditions, a deterministic model will produce the same result. However, there is also an extensive literature on stochastic, or probabilistic, models in which chance plays a role. Deterministic models tend to be more appropriate when many infectives are circulating and immunization levels are moderate. Stochastic effects tend to be more important when few infectives are circulating, immunization levels are high, and cases tend to occur in clusters. In some settings, the differences between deterministic formulations and stochastic formulations may be quite substantial.[2,26,27]

Other Epidemiologic Models

Modes of Transmission

Vector-borne transmission is indirect transmission, in that one person can infect another person only by transmitting the infectious agent through an invertebrate animal, ie, the disease vector, which is typically an insect, tick, or snail (see discussion of vector-borne disease in Chapter 22). The specific details of transmission cycles are as varied as the diseases and vectors involved, but the example of malaria can be used to demonstrate the basic concepts. The cycle of transmission starts when a person harboring the infectious stage of malaria in the blood is bitten by an anopheline mosquito that ingests the infectious stage. The malaria parasite develops and migrates to the salivary glands of the mosquito vector, and the cycle of transmission continues when the mosquito transfers the parasite while biting another human host. A standard model for this process counts both the human and the mosquito population, dividing each population into those who are susceptible and those who are infected.[28] The only contacts are mosquito bites that transmit infections from people to mosquitoes and from mosquitoes to people. As with infections that are transmitted directly from person to person, the basic reproduction ratio of the number of new human cases generated from an initial human case in a susceptible population is a fundamental concept. However, the basic reproduction ratio must be generalized as the product of two quantities:

1. the number of mosquitoes that become infective by biting an infective person
2. the number of people who become infective due to the bites of an infective mosquito

Models of transmission of infection by sexual contact share some features with both direct transmission and vector-borne transmission. Homosexual contact is structured as direct transmission, and heterosexual contact is structured as vector-borne transmission, in which females and males are counted as separate populations. That is, the basic reproduction ratio of transmission considers how many new cases among females are generated from a single infected female (or how many new cases among males are generated from a single infected male). It may also be useful to construct separate subpopulations within a homosexual population (ie, use the structure of a heterosexual transmission model) if specific sexual practices result in asymmetric patterns of risk between partners. The sharing of needles for injecting drugs, resulting in the spread of blood-borne diseases,

can be considered a form of direct transmission. Although all contact patterns display some heterogeneity within populations, the effects are perhaps the most extreme for sexual contacts. The existence of a subset of the population with very high contact rates, called *superspreaders* or the *core population*, is central to models of sexually transmitted infections.[2,29] Such social heterogeneity renders population averages very misleading; an understanding of the spread of sexually transmitted disease in a population depends on detailed studies of personal sexual behavior.

In zoonotic diseases, the reservoir of infection is maintained in a vertebrate animal population, and humans are infected only occasionally.[30] The model structures that have been applied to the human population are used for the animal host population; the framework may be applied to animal infections whether or not they present a problem to humans.[31]

Another mode of transmission is vertical transmission, in which a parent transmits infection to unborn offspring. This may be of importance in maintaining transmission in the reservoir of infection in some circumstances, such as transovarial transmission by ticks[32] and hepatitis B transmission in humans.[2] For populations of ticks, a full ecologic model of the growth of the affected population is required. A model of hepatitis B transmission can incorporate population turnover of births and deaths in a manner similar to that shown in Figure 6–5, except that there are two types of births—infected and uninfected. In contrast, the transmission of HIV from mother to fetus is a tragic consequence of other modes of transmission, but it is not a major contributor to the reservoir of infection.

Natural Histories

The most fundamental distinction in the natural history of infection is whether or not immunity is acquired after infection. For epidemiologic purposes, the key consideration is whether a person is subject to repeated infection and not whether there is some evidence of an immunologic response. (For some diseases, an immunologic response may not be effective, at least not at first.) Hethcote[10] provides a comparative analysis of the SIR model in which a person acquires immunity and the SIS model in which a person reverts to the susceptible state after infection. For either natural history, an infection will spread initially if the basic reproduction ratio exceeds 1. However, in a closed population, infection will become endemic in the SIS model and will disappear in the SIR model. The maintenance of transmission in a SIR model with births and deaths is also discussed.

An elaboration of the SIS model of infection and reinfection counts the number of parasites in a host. This structure has been used extensively for diseases caused by worms, such as schistosomiasis, and is considered a model for macroparasites.[2] In contrast, the models used in this chapter are considered models for microparasites that typically are smaller and replicate inside their hosts. Analysis of the replication of macroparasites is in terms of the number of parasites generated per parasite. Persistent infection, which is characterized as SI, is also important for facilitating transmission of infection. This kind of infection is often asymptomatic and may be referred to as a *carrier state*, as with hepatitis B virus.[2]

Host Genetic Factors

Genetic factors of the host that affect susceptibility to infection can be incorporated into models by dividing the host population into subgroups based on genotypes. Although this type of heterogeneity has played a relatively small role in epidemiologic models, it has been explored for a subset of the population that develops an asymptomatic carrier state of hepatitis B infection.[2] The genetics of host–parasite interactions are being investigated in diverse ways,[33,34] and more is being learned about the importance of host genetic factors in a variety of infectious diseases, including Puumala hantavirus infection, tuberculosis, Lyme disease, and HIV/AIDS.[35] With advances in understanding the ge-

netic basis of disease, it is expected that models of the epidemiology of infectious diseases will incorporate more genetic information.

Health Impacts

An analysis of the dynamics of transmission alone is not sufficient to inform policy makers. Measures of the impact of infectious diseases and other health problems are used to identify priorities for action. Measures of the burden of disease based on estimates of mortality and disability have become more widespread,[36] although such estimates are not without controversy. Translating a disease burden into economic impacts is another step that takes into account the cost of treatment and the cost of morbidity and mortality. For example, the global AIDS epidemic has been analyzed in terms of the cost of treating an AIDS patient, the effect on the health care sector, and the effect on poverty due to the loss of adults in a household.[37] Another important area of application is planning for economic development projects in terms of an economic analysis of environmental impacts, including possible adverse health impacts.[38,39] For example, water development projects in Africa have long demonstrated the capacity to increase the incidence of malaria or schistosomiasis.[40]

CONCLUSION AND PROSPECTS

This chapter has focused primarily on mathematical models of directly transmitted infections that confer life-long immunity, such as measles and many other childhood immunizable diseases. The model and its extensions are usually referred to as *SIR*, for epidemiologic states corresponding to people who are susceptible, infective, or recovered/removed. A central concept is the basic reproduction ratio, which is the number of secondary cases generated from a single case in an otherwise susceptible population. The basic reproduction ratio affects patterns of endemicity, the age at which a host becomes infected, and the epidemiologic response to mass immunization. Mathematical analysis demonstrates how the basic reproduction ratio depends on the structure of the host population and the characteristics of the infectious agent.

This chapter has also provided a brief overview of issues in developing applications beyond the basic SIR model. Common extensions of the SIR model involve the age structure of contact patterns and latent periods, as well as demographic, spatial, and stochastic effects. An understanding of the SIR model forms the basis for understanding applications to infectious diseases with different modes of transmission, different natural histories, or a strong dependence on host genetic factors. For any disease, links between the dynamics of transmission and health impacts are needed for the analysis of policies for disease control and prevention.

Trends in research reveal two apparently contradictory directions. On the one hand, adverse effects of global environmental change on public health are a growing concern.[41] Models of the dynamics of transmission of infectious diseases should be linked to models of environmental phenomena on a global scale.[42] On the other hand, microbial change is a major cause of the emergence and re-emergence of infectious diseases.[43] Models should examine the dynamics of infection at the level of replication of the infectious agent, taking into account genetic changes[44,45] and the dynamics of the immune response,[46] for an overall evolutionary perspective.[47] Both macro and micro factors must be considered in practical applications to public health, such as the development of an immunization program to combat a large epidemic of diphtheria in the former Soviet Union.[48]

The complexity of the dynamics of transmission can easily overwhelm any attempt to develop mathematical models of multiple factors operating at radically different scales. Quantitative predictions will require highly detailed models. However, it is important to remember that the development of applications has an inherent tension between simple and complex models. As stated in the introduction, mathematical models are supposed to aid the educational process and not simply be "black boxes" that produce answers. For conceptual understanding, a limited number of assumptions are an advantage.

The tradeoff between simplicity and complexity arises again and again in different contexts. Experiences in other fields are useful in gaining insight about this issue in the epidemiology of infectious diseases. An evaluation of a global model of population and resources led to the comment below on the problem of losing conceptual understanding of a complex model:

> Although the model suppresses a great deal of detail, it is complicated enough to make understanding difficult. When you discover some new aspect of its behavior, it can be difficult to track down the mechanism responsible. Thus, adding more structure in the cause of realism would not necessarily teach us much. We might well reach a point where we could not understand the model any better than we understand the real world.[49(p516)]

A report on the use of geographic information systems emphasizes the problem of making decisions using highly detailed data:

> Realistic modeling of spatial and temporal phenomena generally demands disaggregation (ie, large detailed models and/or databases)—but in terms of decision-making, such levels of disaggregation are usually counterproductive. Decision-making demands aggregation, and therein lays the dilemma. From a scientific viewpoint, we must disaggregate "to be real"—from a decision-making viewpoint, we must aggregate "to be real."[50(p28)]

In selecting an appropriate degree of complexity during the process of model development, it is essential to focus on specific questions to be addressed.[13] Variations of a model with different levels of structure may be useful in different phases of development.

The challenge of developing and utilizing mathematical models to aid in understanding and controlling the spread of infectious diseases continues to evolve. It is hoped that researchers and practitioners in public health can use the concepts and approaches presented in this chapter as a starting point in meeting the challenge.

REFERENCES

1. Sterman JD. A skeptic's guide to computer models. In: Barney GO, Kreutzer WB, Garrett MJ, eds. *Managing a Nation: The Microcomputer Software Catalog.* Boulder, CO: Westview Press; 1991:209–229.

2. Anderson RM, May RM. *Infectious Diseases of Humans.* London: Oxford University Press; 1991.

3. Scott ME, Smith G. *Parasitic and Infectious Diseases: Epidemiology and Ecology.* San Diego, CA: Academic Press; 1994.

4. Mollison D, ed. *Epidemic Models: Their Structure and Relation to Data.* Cambridge: Cambridge University Press; 1995.

5. Grenfell BT, Dobson A, eds. *Ecology of Infectious Diseases in Natural Populations.* Cambridge, UK: Cambridge University Press; 1995.

6. Bailey NTJ. *The Mathematical Theory of Infectious Diseases and Its Applications.* New York: Oxford University Press; 1975.

7. Levin SA, Hallam TG, Gross LJ, eds. *Applied Mathematical Ecology. Biomathematics.* Vol. 18. Berlin: Springer-Verlag; 1989.

8. Hastings A. *Population Biology: Concepts and Models.* New York: Springer-Verlag; 1997.

9. Yorke JA, Nathanson N, Pianigiani G, Martin J. Seasonality and the requirements for perpetuation and eradication of viruses in populations. *Am J Epidemiol.* 1979; 109:103–123.

10. Hethcote HW. Three basic epidemiological models. In: Levin SA, Hallam TG, Gross LJ, eds. *Applied Mathematical Ecology.* Berlin: Springer-Verlag; 1989:119–144.

11. Fine PEM. John Brownlee and the measurement of infectiousness: an historical study in epidemic theory. *J R Stat Soc [A].* 1979;42:347–362.

12. Anderson RM. Directly transmitted viral and bacterial infections of man. In: Anderson RM, ed. *Population Dynamics of Infectious Diseases.* London: Chapman and Hall; 1982.

13. Aron JL. Simple versus complex epidemiological models. In: Levin SA, Hallam TG, Gross JJ, eds. *Applied Mathematical Ecology.* Berlin: Springer-Verlag; 1989: 176–192.

14. Lobel HO, McCollum RW. Some observations on the ecology of infectious hepatitis. *Bull WHO.* 1965;32: 675–682.

15. Hope Simpson RE. Infectiousness of communicable diseases in the household (measles, chickenpox, and mumps). *Lancet.* 1952;2:549–554.

16. Broome CV, Preblud SR, Bruner B, et al. Epidemiology of pertussis, Atlanta, 1977. *J Pediatr.* 1981;98:362–367.

17. Fine PEM. Herd immunity: history, theory, practice. *Epidemiol Rev.* 1993;15(2):265–302.

18. Centers for Disease Control. Current trends. Practices in college immunization—United States. *MMWR.* 1987; 36(14):209–212.

19. Fine PEM, Clarkson JA. Measles in England and Wales. I. An analysis of factors underlying seasonal patterns. *Int J Epidemiol.* 1982;11:5–14.

20. Fine PEM, Clarkson JA. Measles in England and Wales. II. The impact of the measles vaccination programme on the distribution of immunity in the population. *Int J Epidemiol.* 1982;11:15–25.

21. Anderson RM, May RM. Directly transmitted infectious diseases: control by vaccination. *Science.* 1982;215: 1053–1060.

22. Anderson RM, May RM. Age-related changes in the rate of disease transmission: implications for the design of vaccination programmes. *J Hyg (Camb).* 1985;94: 365–436.

23. Schenzle D. An age-structured model of pre- and post-vaccination measles transmission. *IMA J Math Appl Med Biol.* 1984;1:169–191.

24. Cliff A, Haggett P, Smallman-Raynor M. *Measles: An Historical Geography of a Major Human Viral Disease from Global Expansion to Local Retreat, 1840–1990.* Oxford, UK: Blackwell Reference; 1993.

25. Finkenstadt B, Grenfell B. Empirical determinants of measles metapopulation dynamics in England and Wales. *Proc R Soc Lond B Biol Sci.* 1998;265(1392): 211–220.

26. Nasell I. The threshold concept in stochastic epidemic and endemic models. In: Mollison D, ed. *Epidemic Models: Their Structure and Relation to Data.* Cambridge, UK: Cambridge University Press; 1995:71–83.

27. Diekmann O, Heesterbeek H, Metz H. The legacy of Kermack and McKendrick. In: Mollison D, ed. *Epidemic Models: Their Structure and Relation to Data.* Cambridge, UK: Cambridge University Press; 1995: 95–115.

28. Aron JL, May RM. The population dynamics of malaria. In: Anderson RM, ed. *Population Dynamics of Infectious Diseases.* London: Chapman and Hall; 1982:139–179.

29. Hethcote HW, Yorke JA. Gonorrhea: transmission dynamics and control. *Lect Notes Biomath.* 1984;56:1–105.

30. Wilson ML. Ecology and infectious disease. In: Aron JL, Patz JA, eds. *Ecosystem Change and Public Health.* Baltimore, MD: Johns Hopkins University Press. In press.

31. Barlow ND. Critical evaluation of wildlife disease models. In: Grenfell BT, Dobson AP, eds. *Ecology of Infectious Diseases in Natural Populations.* Cambridge, UK: Cambridge University Press; 1995:230–259.

32. Smith G, Basanez M-G, Dietz K, et al. Macroparasite group report: problems in modelling the dynamics of macroparasitic systems. In: Grenfell BT, Dobson AP, eds. *Ecology of Infectious Diseases in Natural Populations.* Cambridge, UK: Cambridge University Press; 1995:209–229.

33. Wakelin D. Host populations: genetics and immunity. In: Scott ME, Smith G, eds. *Parasitic and Infectious Diseases: Epidemiology and Ecology.* San Diego, CA: Academic Press; 1994:83–100.

34. Lively CM, Apanius V. Genetic diversity in host-parasite interactions. In: Grenfell BT, Dobson AP, eds. *Ecology of Infectious Diseases in Natural Populations.* Cambridge, UK: Cambridge University Press; 1995: 421–449.

35. McNicholl J. Host genes and infectious diseases. *Emerg Infect Dis.* 1998;4(3):423–426.

36. Murray CJL, Lopez AD. *The Global Burden of Disease: A Comprehensive Assessment of Mortality and Disability from Diseases, Injuries and Risk Factors in 1990 and Projected to 2020.* Cambridge, MA: Harvard University Press; 1996.

37. World Bank. *Confronting AIDS: Public Priorities in a Global Epidemic.* New York: Oxford University Press; 1997.

38. World Bank. *Economic Analysis and Environmental Assessment. Environmental Assessment Sourcebook Update*, no. 23, Environment Department. Washington, DC: World Bank; 1998.

39. World Bank. *Health Aspects of Environmental Assessment. Environmental Assessment Sourcebook Update*, no. 18, Environment Department. Washington, DC: World Bank; 1997.

40. Hunter JM, Rey L, Scott D. Man-made lakes and man-made diseases: towards a policy resolution. *Soc Sci Med.* 1982;16:1127–1145.

41. WRI/UNEP/UNDP/World Bank. *World Resources 1998–99.* New York: Oxford University Press; 1998.

42. Aron JL, Patz JA, eds. *Ecosystem Change and Public Health.* Baltimore, MD: Johns Hopkins University Press. In press.

43. Lederberg J. Emerging infections: an evolutionary perspective. *Emerg Infect Dis.* 1998;4(3):366–371.

44. Burke DS. Evolvability of emerging viruses. In: Nelson AM, Horsburgh CR, eds. *Pathology of Emerging Infections.* Washington, DC: American Society of Microbiology Press; 1998.

45. Burke DS, Grefenstette JJ, Ramsey CL, De Jong KA, Wu AS. Putting more genetics into genetic algorithms. *Evolutionary Computation.* 1998;6(4):387–410.

46. Perelson AS, Nelson PW. Mathematical analysis of HIV-1 dynamics in vivo. *SIAM Rev.* 1999;41(1):3–44.

47. Levin BR, Lipsitch M, Bonhoeffer S. Population biology, evolution, and infectious disease: convergence and synthesis. *Science.* 1999;283(5403): 806–809.

48. Vitek CR, Wharton M. Diphtheria in the former Soviet Union: reemergence of a pandemic disease. *Emerg Infect Dis.* 1998;4(4):539–550.

49. Hayes B. Balanced on a pencil point. *Am Scientist.* 1993;81(6):510–516.

50. Glass GE, Aron JL, Ellis JH, Yoon SS. *Applications of GIS Technology to Disease Control.* Baltimore, MD: Dept. of Population Dynamics, Johns Hopkins School of Hygiene and Public Health; 1993.

CHAPTER 7

Microbiology Tools for the Epidemiologist

James Dick and Nikki M. Parrish

INTRODUCTION

Medical microbiology is the study of interactions between organisms that result in infectious disease. Despite our concentration on microorganisms that cause disease, the vast majority of microorganisms we continuously interact with do not result in disease. In fact, many are beneficial and essential for our health and well-being. Pathogenic viruses, bacteria, fungi, and parasites have cellular structures, products, or toxins that permit them to cause disease in a specific host. These are termed *virulence factors* and can be classified into those factors that permit the microorganism to:

1. colonize
2. evade host defense mechanisms
3. invade and disseminate

The resulting host response, combined with virulence factors, results in toxicity or tissue damage to the host. Alternatively, some microorganisms produce toxins that, in and of themselves, cause pathology to the host.

Of equal importance in understanding the interactive nature of infection and disease is an understanding of the host mechanisms that continually operate to prevent infection. Only a small number of microorganisms associated with man and animals causes disease, despite the vast numbers of bacteria that inhabit our mouth, teeth, gastrointestinal tract, urogenital tract, and skin. The prevention of infection and disease is in large part due to an array of defense mechanisms that we have developed to deal with these continuous intimate interactions. Mechanical barriers are typically the first line of defense. Examples include: skin and mucous membranes as a physical barrier, ciliated cells and mucus in the respiratory tract, and the washing action of tears and urine. A variety of chemicals are produced at these sites, many by resident normal flora, such as fatty acids and propionic acid, which prevent colonization by pathogens. Other compounds produced by the host that are inhibitory include lysozyme in tears, blood, urine, and sweat; acid in the stomach, vagina, and skin; basic polyamines and complement in plasma; and acute-phase proteins, such as β-antitrypsin, fibrinogen, C-reactive protein, and β_2-microglobulin. In addition to mechanical and chemical mediators, phagocytic cells such as macrophages, polymorphonuclear neutrophils, monocytes, and eosinophils are all components of nonspecific host resistance or innate immunity. Specific immunity in man and other vertebrates is the function of both the humoral immune system, involving antibody-mediated B-cell functions, and the cellular immune system, involving T-lymphocyte–mediated functions. A compromise in any of these defense mechanisms can lead to infection and disease in the host. Pathogens of low virulence or pathogenicity, as well as true pathogens, can cause infection in these situations and are termed *opportunistic pathogens.*

In this chapter, a basic broad overview of the classification, taxonomy, structure, and methods of diagnosis of infectious agents is presented. Although by no means comprehensive, it is hoped that the information will provide a basis of understanding for further in-depth study of microbiology as it relates to infectious disease epidemiology.

TAXONOMY, CLASSIFICATION, AND STRUCTURE OF INFECTIOUS AGENTS

Early biologists realized that microorganisms such as algae, protozoa, fungi, and bacteria did not readily fit into the already established plant and animal kingdoms. This led to the proposal by Haechel in 1886 of a third kingdom, the Protista. Because the observations that led to the establishment of this third kingdom were well known before the discovery and descriptions of viruses, they were not included in this classification system. Subsequent advances in the biologic sciences, specifically microscopy, led to a further subdivision of the Protista into eukaryotic cells, which included the algae, fungi, and protozoa, as well as members of the plant and animal kingdoms and prokaryotic cells that represent the bacteria. The terms *eukaryotic* and *prokaryotic* reflect only the presence of a true nucleus, eukaryotic, or the absence of a well-delineated nucleus, prokaryotic. Significant structural and other biologic differences are described in Table 7–1, although the presence of transition forms can result in a blending of some of the listed characteristics.

A variety of characteristics has been used to name and identify microorganisms. These included initially phenotypic properties and morphology, such as size and shape, staining characteristics, biochemical properties, physiology, metabolism, ecologic niche, etc. Currently, taxonomy is moving toward a genetic basis for differentiation among microorganisms. Genetic methods use DNA and RNA homology and nucleic acid base sequence similarity to evaluate relatedness. Highly conserved genes with variable regions, such as bacterial 16 and 23s ribosomal RNA genes, are commonly used to differentiate bacteria. Microorganisms are taxonomically organized into orders, families, genera, and species. The naming of microorgan-

---

Table 7–1 Comparison of Eukaryotic and Prokaryotic Cells

Characteristic	Eukaryotes	Prokaryotes
Form	Multicellular	Single cells
Nucleus	Nuclear membrane	DNA in contact with cytoplasm
Organelles	Membrane-bound organelles present	No organelles
Sterols	Always	Only in *Mycoplasma*
Ribosomes	80s = 40s + 60s	70s = 30s + 50s
Cell wall	Absent or cellulose	Peptidoglycan
Mitosis	Yes	No

isms, with the exception of the viruses, is binomial and includes the genus and species name, eg, *Staphylococcus aureus*. Microorganisms can be further subdivided on characteristics that do not warrant a separate species designation but do differentiate a specific member of a species or strain from other members or strains of a particular species. Differences or similarities used for subspecies or strain designation within a species can include a variety of parameters, such as structural or functional differences, phenotypic differences, antigenic differences in surface or subsurface structures, and genomic polymorphism. Strain differentiation is an important component of epidemiologic studies, in light of the significant diversity within species among microorganisms.

VIRUSES

Viruses are the smallest of the infectious agents, with the possible exception of prions or agents of spongiform encephalopathies, eg, scrapie and Creutzfeldt-Jakob disease. Viruses range in size from 20 to 200 nm and, as such, are not readily visible by light microscopy. They contain a single form or type of nucleic acid, either DNA or RNA, which functions as their genome. In addition to a single form of nucleic acid, viruses compositionally may contain proteins, lipids, and glycoproteins as structural components, depending on their level of complexity. Viruses are obligate intracellular parasites, and their replication is host-cell–dependent, directed by their DNA or RNA. Viral subversion of the host's cellular machinery favors the synthesis of viral nucleic acid and structural proteins. Viral infection is very host-cell–specific and depends on the presence of specific surface receptors (attachment molecules) for successful entry. There are viruses specific for almost every organism. The ultimate outcome of virus-infected cells varies for different viruses and includes a spectrum from rapid lysis (influenza) to continued growth of the cell and continued release of new virus particles (adenovirus). Some viruses are capable of integrating their

nucleic acid into the host cell genome, establishing a latent (herpes viruses) or quiescent state. Latency can continue for long periods of time before reactivation with initiation of viral replication and subsequent lysis of the host cell (herpes viruses).

Classification

Viruses are classified into families, genera, and species, as are other microorganisms, but are not named in a generally binomial classification, ie, genus and species. Commonly, viruses are referred to by their single names. The viral classification system is based on the nature of the following:

1. viral genome: DNA or RNA; single- or double-stranded, linear or circular, segmented or nonsegmented; and genome capping with a protein or polynucleotide
2. size and shape of the capsid and whether it is enveloped or nonenveloped
3. method of replication
4. pathophysiology of the virus such as host range, antigenic composition, vectors and tissue tropism
5. physical/chemical features, such as susceptibility to acid or lipid solvents

The medically important DNA viruses are shown in Table 7–2. Significant differential features include: single- or double-stranded DNA, linear or circular DNA, and the presence or absence of capsid protection, ie, enveloped or naked. Similarly, the medically important RNA viruses are categorized in Table 7–2. Although the criteria are similar to those used to categorize DNA viruses, the following criteria are used: RNA viruses that possess polycistronic RNA and use of messenger RNA (mRNA) to produce a large single protein that is subsequently cleaved to yield several smaller proteins. These include the Coronaviridae, Paramyxoviridae, Picornaviridae, Togaviridae, and Rhabdoviridae. Alternatively, viruses with segmented genomes without polycistronic RNA, requiring cleavage of nested genes, include Arenavirus,

Table 7–2 Classification of Viruses

Family	Example	Genome Size, Kilobases of Kilobase Pairs	Envelope
RNA Viruses			
Single-stranded			
Picornaviridae	Poliovirus	7.2–8.4	No
Togaviridae	Rubella virus	12	Yes
Flaviviridae	Yellow fever virus	10	Yes
Coronaviridae	Coronaviruses	16–21	Yes
Rhabdoviridae	Rabies virus	13–16	Yes
Paramyxoviridae	Measles virus	16–20	Yes
Orthomyxoviridae	Influenza viruses	14	Yes
Bunyaviridae	California encephalitis virus	13–21	Yes
Arenaviridae	Lymphocytic choriomeningitis virus	10–14	Yes
Retroviridae	HIV	3–9	Yes
Double-stranded			
Reoviridae	Rotaviruses	16–27	No
DNA Viruses			
Single-stranded			
Parvoviridae	Human parvovirus B-19	5	No
Mixed strandedness			
Hepadnaviridae	Hepatitis B	3	Yes
Double-stranded			
Papovaviridae	JC virus	8	No
Adenoviridae	Human adenoviruses	36–38	No
Herpesviridae	Herpes simplex virus	120–220	Yes
Poxviridae	Vaccinia	130–280	Yes

Bunyavirus, Orthomyxoviridae, Reovirus, Rotavirus, and the Retroviridae. The RNA viruses are further subdivided on the basis of transcription requirements for their RNA. Positive-strand viruses use their RNA as messenger RNA (mRNA) for translation for required protein. In contrast, negative-stranded RNA viruses require their own RNA-dependent RNA polymerase with production of mRNA and subsequent translation of essential proteins.

Structure

The complete infectious virus is termed a *virion*. It is composed of its specific nucleic acid, DNA or RNA, surrounded by a protein coat known as the *capsid*. The capsid is further subdivided into capsomers, repeating identical morphologic protein subunits. Each capsomer subunit is composed of one or more polypeptides. Viruses construct several different capsid shapes, according to how these proteins combine. Arrangement of capsomers in the shape of an icosahedron (polygon with 20 faces) results in cubic symmetry. In a cubically symmetrical virus, some capsomers are surrounded by five (penton) capsomers, whereas others are surrounded by six (hexon) capsomers. In helical viruses, the capsid proteins are arranged around the helical nucleic acid core. In addition to icosahedral and helical viruses, a third structural category, known as *complex viruses*, is more complicated than either icosahedral or helical viruses. The viral genome can have an associated protein complex that is referred to as the *nucleocapsid* and forms the viral core. Enveloped viruses possess a lipoprotein coat that surrounds the virion and is acquired from infected host cell membrane. Nonenveloped viruses are termed *naked viruses*. Finally, viruses may possess glycoprotein spikes, known as *peplomers*, which protrude from the envelope and function in the attachment of the virus to target host cells.

BACTERIA

Classification

The classification of bacteria has a longer history than does the classification of viruses, due to their earlier discovery. As with other organisms, prokaryotic bacteria are named using the binomial system of genus and species (Exhibit 7–1). Further subdivision can occur among species, such as subspecies, serotype, etc. Early groupings of bacteria grew and continue to be based on morphologic and biochemical characteristics that formed the basis for their taxonomic classification. More recently, genetic methods indicative of the phylogenetic or evolutionary relationships among the various genera have been applied for classification. Morphologic classification of bacteria has developed on the basis of staining characteristics, shape, and size of the microorganism when visualized by light microscopy. The gram stain reaction, which is a reflection of cell wall structure of bac-

teria, has been used extensively for classification. The gram stain procedure is a relatively simple staining method that utilizes gentian or crystal violet (purple dye) as the initial stain, followed by fixation with iodine, decolorization with 95% ethanol or acetone-alcohol, and final counterstaining with safranin (a red dye). Crystal violet and iodine form large aggregates within the cell, which, depending on the nature of the cell wall, will be retained or washed out by the action of alcohol. Cells that retain the crystal violet–iodine complex will appear blue/purple, whereas those with thinner cell wells will stain red/pink with the safranin counterstain. Bacteria that retain the dye and stain blue/purple are referred to as *gram-positive bacteria*, whereas those that do not retain the dye and stain red/pink are referred to as *gram-negative bacteria*. Another widely used stain for differentiation of bacteria is the acid-fast stain, also known as the *Ziehl-Nielsen stain*. The acid-fast stain differentiates members of the genus *Mycobacterium*, which includes *M. tuberculosis* and *M. leprae,* the etiologic agents of tuberculosis and leprosy. The differentiation is based on the ability of mycobacteria to retain a primary carbolfuchsin stain when decolorized with 95% alcohol containing 3% HCl. All other bacteria will decolorize during the acid wash. In addition to differential staining characteristics, bacteria are also morphologically classified on the basis of their shape and arrangement. Three general shapes have been identified:

1. cocci—round or spherical cells
2. bacilli—rod-shaped cells
3. curved, spiral forms

Further descriptive terms include *coccobacilli*, which are short, rod-shaped cells, and *pleomorphic cells*, which demonstrate variable morphologies. Morphologically, bacteria are also frequently described in terms of this arrangement. For example, *Streptococcus pneumoniae* is frequently described as gram-positive diplococci (pairs of cocci), whereas *Staphylococcus aureus* is most often described as gram-positive cocci in clusters. These descriptions reflect the

Exhibit 7–1 Examples of Bacteria of Medical Importance

Family Genus and Species	Disease
Gram-positive cocci	
Staphylococcus	
S. aureus	Abscess, toxic shock, food poisoning
S. epidermidis	Nosocomial infections
Streptococcus	
S. pyogenes (Group A)	Pharyngitis, rheumatic fever, glomerulonephritis, toxic shock
S. agalactiae (Group B)	Neonatal meningitis
S. pneumoniae	Lobar pneumonia, meningitis
Enterococcus	
E. faecalis	Nosocomial infections
Gram-positive bacilli	
Bacillus (spore-forms)	
B. anthracis	Anthrax
Clostridium (spore-forms)	
C. botulinum	Botulism
C. tetani	Tetanus
C. perfringens	Gas gangrene, food poisoning
C. difficile	Pseudomembranous colitis
Listeria	
L. monocytogenes	Meningitis
Corynebacterium	
C. diphtheriae	Diphtheria
Actinomyces	
A. israelii	Actinomycosis
Nocardia	
N. asteroides	Pulmonary disease, brain abscess
Gram-negative spirochetes	
Borrelia burgdorferi	Lyme disease
Treponema pallidum	Syphilis
Leptospira interrogans	Leptospirosis
Acid-fast gram-positive bacilli	
Mycobacterium	
M. tuberculosis	Tuberculosis
M. leprae	Leprosy
M. avium complex	Disseminated infection in immunocompromised hosts
Gram-negative bacilli	
Enterobacteriaceae	Urinary tract infection, diarrhea
Escherichia coli	Meningitis, bacteremia
Klebsiella pneumoniae	Pneumonia, urinary tract infection

continues

Exhibit 7–1 continued

Family Genus and Species	Disease
Enterobacteriaceae (continued)	
Salmonella typhi	Typhoid fever
Salmonella species	Diarrhea, food poisoning
Shigella species	Diarrhea, gastrointestinal disease
Yersinia enterocolitica	Gastroenteritis
Yersinia pestis	Bubonic plague
Pasteurella multocida	Cat bite infections
Hemophilus influenzae	Meningitis, pneumonia, otitis media, and epiglottiditis
Bordetella pertussis	Whooping cough
Brucella species	Brucellosis
Francisella tularensis	Tularemia
Legionella pneumophila	Legionnaires' disease
Pseudomonas aeruginosa	Opportunistic infections
Bacterioides fragilis	Anaerobic abscesses
Fusobacterium nucleatum	Abscesses, oral infections
Gram-negative curved or helical bacilli	
Campylobacter jejuni	Gastroenteritis
Helicobacter pylori	Gastritis, peptic ulcers
Vibrio cholerae	Cholera
Vibrio parahaemolyticus	Gastroenteritis
Gram-negative cocci	
Neisseria	
N. gonorrhoeae	Gonorrhea
N. meningitidis	Meningitis
Gram-negative, obligate intracellular bacteria	
Rickettsia	
R. prowazekii	Epidemic typhus
R. rickettsii	Rocky Mountain spotted fever
Coxiella burnetii	Q fever
Chlamydia	
C. trachomatis	Lymphogranuloma venereum
C. pneumoniae	Pneumonia
Trachoma	
C. psittaci	Psittacosis
Ehrlichia	
E. chaffiensis	Ehrlichiosis
Mycoplasma (lacking a cell wall)	
Mycoplasma pneumoniae	Pneumonia
Ureaplasma urealyticum	Urethritis

characteristic arrangement and shape of particular bacteria upon microscopic examination of gram-stained specimens.

The ability of most bacteria to grow in vitro has resulted in biochemical classification, as well as morphologic classification of most bacteria. These taxonomic characteristics are based on the metabolic and physiologic differences between different groups of organisms and are most commonly referred to as *phenotypic characteristics*. A variety of methods has been developed to test for the presence or absence of particular enzymes. Commonly used taxonomic classification tests by this method include determining whether a bacteria can use specific nutrients for growth or whether it metabolizes particular substrates, such as carbohydrates. Other phenotypic methodologies directly test for the presence of an enzyme, such as catalase. Catalase is an enzyme that breaks down H_2O_2 to water and oxygen and can be readily tested by applying hydrogen peroxide to a growing colony. The solution will bubble, due to the release of oxygen, if the organism possesses the catalase enzyme. The presence of particular enzyme systems is most commonly detected by colorimetric assays wherein, if the enzyme is present, there will be a pH change or production of a colored product in the culture medium. Similarly, antigen-antibody reactions have been utilized to distinguish between species, subspecies, or serotypes within a genus. In these tests, antibodies that bind to specific bacterial surface antigens can be used to identify bacteria that produce these proteins. Relatively recent advances in genetics have resulted in classification methodologies that are indicative of evolutionary and phylogenetic relationships. Application of these methods has resulted in the reclassification of many bacteria at the genus level. Genetic methods have gone through an evolution with earlier tests, utilizing the measurement of DNA homology of the *entire* chromosome as the determinant of genetic relatedness. Although still used as a tool for genetic classification, hybridization techniques using cloned or amplified *portions* of

the genome have also been developed that look for the presence of a specific DNA sequence. These methods have found extensive utilization in diagnostic microbiology. Current genetic taxonomy has evolved to the use of sequence analysis of highly conserved genes for determination of phylogenetic relationships. The most commonly used genes are the ribosomal RNA genes, which include the 16s, 23s, and 5s genes. These genes are found in all prokaryotes and contain both highly conserved and variable regions. Sequence, ie, base changes, in these genes reflect evolutionary and phylogenetic relationships among bacteria.

Bacterial Structure

Figure 7–1 illustrates the basic structure of a bacterial cell. Although all of the structures shown in Figure 7–1 are involved in the life and survival of these versatile cells, many are important virulence factors and are briefly described with emphasis on their roles in pathogenesis. Figure 7–2 shows bacterial cell structure. Moving from the outermost structures inward, the flagella are long, complex structures that are responsible for motility or movement. They are nonessential (not all bacteria have them) and are composed of protein, which is an important antigen (H antigen) for identification and classification among those bacteria that possess them. Fimbriae or pili are short, nonflexible structures that surround the surface of the cell. As with flagella, they are nonessential but function in adherence. In bacterial pathogens, these structures are responsible for adherence to host cell membranes through a very specific interaction, which frequently determines the organotropism of a particular pathogen. A type of pili known as *sex* or *F pili* permits attachment and DNA transfer between similar species through a process known as *conjugation*. This process is the most common method for acquisition of antibiotic resistance determinants by bacteria. Capsules are secreted polysaccharides and, in some cases, proteins that surround some bacterial cells. In

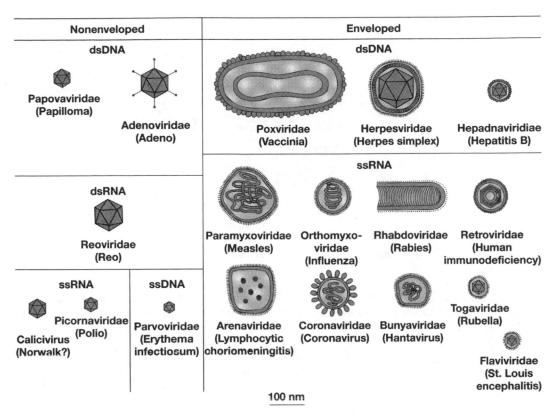

Figure 7–1 The 18 families of animal viruses pathogenic for human. *Filoviridae* is not included because human infection by this family of viruses has not been documented in the United States. *Source:* Reprinted with permission from E.J. Baron et al, *Medical Microbiology: A Short Course*, p. 606, Copyright © 1994. Reprinted by permission of Wiley-Liss, Inc., a subsidiary of John Wiley & Sons, Inc.

general, they are nonessential. In the environment, their primary function is to prevent dehydration of the cell, but in pathogens, they are a major virulence factor through interference of phagocytosis by the host. The cell wall is an essential component of all bacteria, with the exception of the mycoplasma. In addition to determining the size and shape of the cell, it serves as an exoskeleton, preventing lysis of the cell. As discussed earlier, the differences in cell wall structure form the basis for taxonomic differences or groupings of bacteria through the gram-stain reaction. As shown in Figure 7–3, an es-

sential component of both gram-positive and gram-negative cell walls is peptidoglycan. This is the essential structural component of all bacterial cell walls. Peptidoglycan is a complex polymer composed of alternating units of *N*-acetyl-glucosamine and *N*-acetyl muramic acid in a β-1, 4 linkage. The polysaccharide chains are cross-linked through peptide bonds between a pentapeptide chain (typically, four amino acids ending in D-alanine) and the muramic acid residue of *N*-acetyl muramic acid. This interlinked polymer forms the strong backbone for all other cell wall components. The gram-positive cell

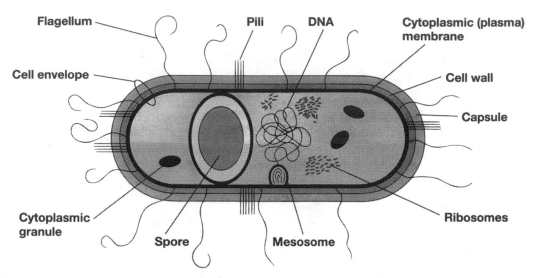

Figure 7–2 Schematic diagram illustrating bacterial cell structure. *Source:* Reprinted with permission from E.J. Baron et al., *Medical Microbiology: A Short Course*, p. 8, Copyright © 1994. Reprinted by permission of Wiley-Liss, Inc., a subsidiary of John Wiley & Sons, Inc.

wall is composed of a very thick layer of peptidoglycan. Despite its thickness, the gram-positive cell wall offers no permeability barrier to the cytoplasmic membrane. A unique component of the gram-positive cell wall is teichoic acid. This polymer is composed of either glycerol or ribitol with phosphate linkages. It is frequently attached to the cytoplasmic membrane and can activate host macrophages with the release of interleukin-1 and tumor necrosis factor alpha (TNF-α). In contrast to the gram-positive cell wall structure, gram-negative bacteria have a significantly more complex cell envelope. The outermost portion of the gram-negative cell wall is a lipid bilayer referred to as the *outer membrane*. Under the outer membrane is an area called the *periplasmic space*, which contains a variety of metabolic and transport enzymes. The peptidoglycan layer of gram-negative bacteria is significantly thinner than that of gram-positive bacteria. The outer leaflet of the outer membrane contains lipopolysaccharide (LPS) or endotoxin, a major virulence factor of gram-negative bacteria. Lipopolysaccharide is a three-component molecule. Lipid A is the toxic component of LPS and is located innermost in the lipid bilayer. Extending from lipid A is the core, an oligosaccharide composed of some unusual sugars. The composition of the core oligosaccharide is similar among all gram-negative bacteria. The outermost portion of LPS is a series of repeating oligosaccharides, the somatic antigen, which is a primary antigenic determinant of the cell. In addition to LPS, the outer membrane of gram-negative bacteria has a variety of proteins associated with it. A group of these outer membrane proteins are porins. These proteins are frequently trimers (three identical proteins bound together) and have a central channel that provides for the passage of hydrophilic compounds through the hydrophobic outer membrane. Unlike gram-positive bacteria, the cell wall of gram-negative bacteria does present a permeability barrier to the cell, due to the presence of the hydrophobic outer membrane. Hydrophilic compounds with a molecular weight greater than

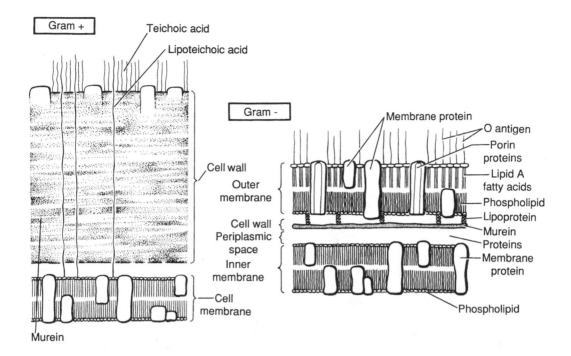

Figure 7–3 The envelope structure of a gram-positive (*left*) and a gram-negative (*right*). Capsules and append-ages are not shown, nor are surface proteins such as the M protein of streptococci indicated. Note the 20-fold greater amount of peptidoglycan in the gram-positive. The outer membrane of the gram-negative envelopes shows O antigen polysaccharide molecules covering the outer layer. *Source:* Reprinted with permission from M. Schaechter, G. Medoff and B.I. Esenstein, *Mechanisms of Microbial Disease*, p. 31, © 1993, Lippincott Williams & Wilkins.

approximately 800 cannot pass through the porin protein channels. Beneath the cell wall, all bacteria are surrounded by a cytoplasmic mem-brane, which is the primary osmotic barrier for the cell. The cytoplasmic membrane is a lipid bilayer composed of phospholipids and protein. Unlike eukaryotic cells, bacteria do not have ste-rols, such as cholesterol, in their membranes. Within the cytoplasm, ribosomes for protein synthesis and the bacterial chromosome are the essential structural components. In addition, many bacteria possess granules that can be visu-alized within the cytoplasm. These granules are most commonly storage depots for nutrients.

FUNGI

The study of pathogenic fungi and the diseases they cause is known as *medical mycology*. Fungi are eukaryotic organisms, which include a wide variety of forms, from single-cell microscopic yeasts to the multicellular and macroscopic mushrooms and toadstools. There are over 100,000 different species of fungi, which play an essential role in degrading organic waste in na-ture. Despite their ubiquitous nature, only a few fungi are of medical importance (Table 7–3). As eukaryotes, the fungi have a defined nucleus, surrounded by a nuclear membrane, a

Table 7–3 Selected Fungi of Medical Importance

Fungus	Classification	Disease
Malassezia furfur	Yeast	Superficial mycoses
Trichophyton rubrum	Filamentous	Tinea, cutaneous mycoses
Microsporum audouinii	Filamentous	Tinea, cutaneous mycoses
Epidermophyton floccosum	Filamentous	Tinea, cutaneous mycoses
Candida albicans	Yeast	Mucocutaneous and systemic mycoses
Sporothrix schenckii	Dimorphic	Subcutaneous mycoses
Histoplasma capsulatum	Dimorphic	Systemic mycoses, histoplasmosis
Blastomyces dermatitidis	Dimorphic	Systemic mycoses, blastomycosis
Coccidioides immitis	Dimorphic	Systemic mycoses, coccidioidomycosis
Paracoccidioides brasiliensis	Dimorphic	Systemic mycoses, paracoccidioidomycosis
Penicillium marneffei	Dimorphic	Systemic mycoses, penicilliosis
Cryptococcus neoformans	Yeast	Systemic mycoses, opportunistic cryptococcosis
Candida species	Yeast	Opportunistic infections
Aspergillus fumigatus	Filamentous	Opportunistic infections
Aspergillus flavus	Filamentous	Opportunistic infections
Rhizopus species	Filamentous	Opportunistic infections
Mucor species	Filamentous	Opportunistic infections
Absidia species	Filamentous	Opportunistic infections
Pneumocystis carinii	Dimorphic, cysts, and trophozoites	Opportunistic infections, pneumonia

plasma membrane that contains sterols, mitochondria, golgi apparatus, 80S ribosomes, and a cytoskeleton, as well as a cell wall or exoskeleton.

Characteristics of Pathogenic Fungi

The pathogenic fungi have two forms: yeasts, which are unicellular and reproduce by exten-sion of buds from the mother cell; and molds, which are multicellular, with a division of function among the individual cellular components. Molds grow as a filamentous, branching strand of connected cells, which form what is called a *hypha*. Hyphae may have intracellular divisions or septa, or may lack them entirely. The majority of fungi can be grown in vitro and form colonies that are either cottony or velvety in appearance. In contrast, yeast grows as moist, smooth colonies similar to bacteria. Fungi are classified by the type and method of sexual reproduction. Fungi not known to reproduce sexually have been classified together and produce spores that are called *conidia*. Spores or reproductive structures of sexual origin are referred to as *spores*, with a prefix that describes the origin of the spore. Examples include: arthrospores, which are formed within a septate hypha; chlamydospores, which also develop within a hyphal strand; blastospores, which are the sexual spores of yeasts and are the daughter buds from yeast cells; and sporangiospores, which develop within a saclike structure known as a *sporangium* (Figures 7–4 and 7–5). These terms are frequently prefixed with *micro* or *macro*, which refer to the size of the spore.

Many of the truly pathogenic fungi have two growth forms and can exist as either molds or yeasts, depending on environmental conditions. This phenomenon is known as *dimorphism*. This yeast-filamentous or filamentous-yeast transition is most commonly associated with environment or functional roles, such as free-living versus parasite or pathogen. In most cases, the infectious or pathogenic form of the dimorphic fungi is the yeast form, with the filamentous or mycelial form being found in the environment. An exception to this exists with *Candida*, in which the pathogenic form is most commonly associated with the filamentous or pseudohyphal form (aggregates of newly budded cells that remain attached and become elongated), whereas the yeast form is associated with colonization or noninvasive behavior.

Classification

Historically, the fungi have been classified on the basis of morphologic characteristics and type or lack of sexual reproduction. As a group, the fungi are included in a separate biologic kingdom called *Fungi*. Within the kingdom are five phyla: *Zygomycota, Ascomycota, Basidiomycota, Deuteromycota*, and *Mycophycophyta*. Pathogenic fungi are found in the first four phyla, with the majority belonging to the *Ascomycota* and *Deuteromycota*. Members of the various phyla, genus, and species are frequently referred to or grouped by replacing the suffix *ota* with *etes*.

Fungi of medical importance can be grouped according to the type or location of infection that they cause. These groupings include:

1. superficial mycoses or infections that involve only the outermost layers of the skin and hair
2. cutaneous mycoses that involve primarily the epidermis

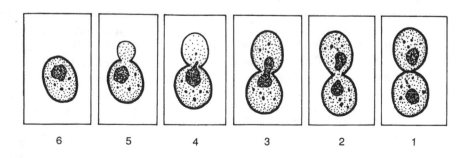

Figure 7–4 Vegetative reproduction of yeast. *Source:* Reprinted with permission from M. Schaechter, G. Medoff and B.I. Esenstein, *Mechanisms of Microbial Disease*, p. 563, © 1993, Lippincott Williams & Wilkins.

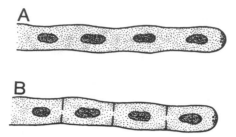

Figure 7–5 Somatic hyphae. **A.** Apical portion of nonseptate (coenocytic) hypha; the protoplasm is continuous and multinucleated. **B.** Apical portion of septate hyphae; protoplasm is interrupted by cross walls. *Source:* Reprinted with permission from M. Schaechter, G. Medoff and B.I. Esenstein, *Mechanisms of Microbial Disease*, p. 563, © 1993, Lippincott Williams & Wilkins.

3. subcutaneous mycoses that cause infections of the dermis and subcutaneous tissue
4. systemic mycoses, which are infections of internal organ systems

The systemic mycoses can be further subdivided into those caused by true or primary pathogens, which are capable of causing disease in healthy individuals, and opportunistic pathogens, which are marginally pathogenic and cause disseminated or deep-tissue infection in compromised or debilitated hosts.

There are four fungi associated with superficial mycoses. *Malassezia furfur* is a lipophilic yeast that causes a mild, asymptomatic infection of the stratum corneum known as *pityriasis* or *tinea versicolor*. *Phaeoannellomyces wenckii* is the etiologic agent of tinea negra palmaris, an asymptomatic infection, usually of the palms of the hands, which produces flat areas of pigmentation. *Piedraia hortae* and *Trichosporon beigelii* are the etiologic agents of black piedra and white piedra, respectively. The piedras are diseases of the hair shaft. Cutaneous mycoses can be caused by a variety of fungi and include such diseases as ringworm and athlete's foot, etc. Although yeasts such as *Candida* species and some other miscellaneous fungi can cause infections of the skin, the most common etiologic agents of cutaneous infections include

members of the genera *Microsporum, Trichophyton,* and *Epidermophyton*. As a group, these agents are referred to as *dermatophytes,* and the diseases they cause are termed *tineas*, which are further described by the specific area of the body infected. For example, infection of the head is termed *tinea capitis*; infection of the body is termed *tinea corporis*, etc.

Subcutaneous mycoses are caused by a variety of fungi, which are found in soil and other environmental sources. Infection occurs by direct inoculation through broken skin, with the subsequent development of a localized infection, which rarely disseminates beyond the regional lymphatics. The most common cause of subcutaneous mycoses is *Sporothrix schenckii*, a dimorphic fungus on plant surfaces and in the soil. Infection occurs through implantation of microconidia of the filamentous stage into tissue through a puncture or abrasion, with subsequent conversion to the yeast form, resulting in an ulcer and potential spread to the lymphatic system. Two other subcutaneous infections include mycetoma and chromoblastomycosis. Mycetoma is a subcutaneous infection, usually of the foot or ankle, as a result of inoculation. Mycetomas are rare in the United States and are caused by a variety of relatively unusual fungi. Similar to mycetoma, chromoblastomycosis is most commonly a disease of the tropics. The disease manifests as a warty or cauliflower-like growth on the foot or ankle as a result of subcutaneous fungal growth. There are multiple etiologic agents of chromoblastomycosis, with the majority producing dark brown, pigmented hyphae in tissue and culture.

The primary etiologic agents of systemic mycoses include *Histoplasma capsulatum*, *Blastomyces dermatitidis*, *Coccidioides immitis*, *Paracoccidioides brasiliensis*, and *Cryptococcus neoformans*. All except *Cryptococcus neoformans*, a yeast only, are dimorphic fungi, existing as yeasts in vivo during infection and in the filamentous hyphal form in the soil. The infective stage is the microconidium of the hyphal form. The route of entry for all of the primary systemic mycoses is the respiratory tract with potential dissemination, if not controlled by the host, to other organ systems. Person-to-person transmission does not occur. The epidemiology of the systemic mycoses varies geographically. *H. capsulatum* and *B. dermatitidis* are found predominantly in Mississippi, Missouri, and the Ohio River valleys and, for *B. dermatitidis*, Canada. In contrast, *C. immitis* is found primarily in the soil of North, Central and South America, as well as the Southwestern United States; *P. brasiliensis* is found only in South and Central America.

The opportunistic systemic mycoses include a spectrum of fungi, from the primary system fungi described above to the usually nonpathogenic, saprophytic *Aspergillus* or *Rhizopus* species. Opportunistic fungi cause disease in hosts that have a depressed immune system, such as infants, diabetics, the elderly, patients with AIDS, or patients receiving cytotoxic drug therapy. As a group, they are ubiquitous and are frequently found as part of the normal flora. Initial infection can progress to serious system diseases, depending on the degree and duration of immunosuppression of the host. The most common opportunistic fungi are members of the genus *Candida*, particularly *C. albicans*, *Aspergillus fumagatus*, and *A. flavus*, members of any of the three genera of the *Zygomycetes*, *Rhizopus*, *Mucor*, *Absidia*, and *Pneumocystis carinii*. Also, one species of the genus Penicillium, ie, *P.*

marheffei, is a frequent opportunistic pathogen causing disseminated mycotic infections in AIDS patients in Southeast Asia.

MEDICAL PARASITOLOGY

The study of protozoan and animal parasites that infect humans is known as *medical parasitology*. Organisms considered in this field fall into two major categories: the protozoa and the helminths, in which the adult stage is a worm. A few parasites of medical importance from each of these categories are discussed in the following section.

Protozoa

The protozoa belong to a subkingdom, Protozoa, because they are neither plant nor animal. The morphology of protozoa varies widely and includes oval, spherical, and elongated cells that can range in size from 5–10 μm to 1–2 mm. Structurally, the protozoa resemble other eukaryotic cells in possessing a cytoplasmic membrane that encloses cytoplasm containing membrane-bound nuclei, mitochondria, 80S ribosomes, and a variety of specialized organelles associated with higher life forms. The majority of protozoa are aquatic, living in soil water, rivers, oceans, etc. However, a relatively small subset is obligate parasites in animals capable of producing both acute and chronic disease (Table 7–4).

Like fungi, many protozoa are capable of both asexual and sexual reproduction. Asexual reproduction usually involves division of a cell into two daughter cells of equal size and composition through transverse (crosswise) or longitudinal (lengthwise) fission. Some species are capable of unequal fission or division through budding or multiple fission. In contrast, the method of sexual reproduction involves the fusion of two morphologically disparate cells (conjugation) with exchange of nuclear material and segregation of two daughter cells. Reproductive cycles of some protozoa are complex, in that a part of the life cycle is required in one host, such as a

Table 7–4 Major Disease-Causing Protozoa in Humans

Disease	Causative Agent	Transmission to Humans	Important Reservoir Hosts	Geographic Location
Amoebiasis	*Entamoebae histolytica*	Ingestion of cysts	Humans	More prevalent in tropical/ subtropical regions
Balantidiasis	*Balantidium coli*	Ingestion of cysts	Hogs, humans	Worldwide
Giardiasis	*Giardia lamblia*	Ingestion of cysts	Humans	Worldwide
Trichomoniasis vaginitis	*Trichomonas vaginalis*	Contact	Humans	Worldwide
West African sleeping sickness	*Trypanosoma gambiense*	Inoculation (bite of tsetse fly, *Glossina* species)	Humans, animals	West Africa
East African sleeping sickness	*Trypanosoma rhodesiense*	Inoculation (bite of tsetse fly, *Glossina* species)	Humans, animals	Eastern and Central Africa
Chagas' disease	*Trypanosoma cruzi*	Reduviid bugs (contamination from feces)	Humans, armadillos, opossums	Southern US, Central and South America
Leishmaniasis (visceral)	*Leishmania donovani*	Inoculation (bite of sandfly, *Phlebotomus* species)	Humans, dogs	Middle and Far East Africa
Leishmaniasis (cutaneous)	*Leishmania tropica*	Inoculation (bite of sandfly, *Phlebotomus* species)	Humans, dogs	Near East, Mediterranean, Africa, southern Russia, and southern Asia
Leishmaniasis (mucocutaneous)	*Leishmania braziliensis*	Inoculation (bite of sandfly, *Phlebotomus* species)	Humans, possibly dogs	South America
Malaria	*Plasmodium falciparum*	Inoculation (Anopheline mosquitoes)	Humans	Tropics
	Plasmodium vivax	Inoculation (Anopheline mosquitoes)	Humans	All areas where malaria is endemic
	Plasmodium ovale	Inoculation (Anopheline mosquitoes)	Humans	Tropics
	Plasmodium malariae	Inoculation (Anopheline mosquitoes)	Humans	Tropics, subtropics, temperate zones

human or other vertebrate, and another stage is required in an invertebrate host. In instances where two different hosts are required in the life cycle, the host in which sexual reproduction occurs is known as the *definitive host*, whereas the host in which only asexual multiplication occurs is termed the *intermediate host*. Not unlike spore-forming bacteria, some protozoa are capable of forming cysts under the influence of unfavorable environmental conditions. During conversion to the cyst form, protozoa become morphologically round or oval and secrete a protective coating around themselves that is resistant to temperature changes, toxic chemicals, and drying. Encysted protozoa are capable of survival outside of their specific host until they gain access to a new host, with resumption of growth and infection.

Classification

As with bacteria and fungi, only a limited number of the ~40,000 species of protozoa cause disease in humans. Pathogenic protozoa are found throughout the phylogeny of the subkingdom, Protozoa. In the following sections, members of three phyla are discussed: *Sarcomastigophora*, *Ciliophora*, and *Apicomplexa*.

In the phylum *Sarcomastigophora*, amoebae comprise a subphylum known as *Sarcodina*. Amoebic infections of humans are generally confined to the intestine but can occasionally involve other organs of the body, such as the liver, lungs, spleen, pericardium, and brain, if carried by the bloodstream. Amoebae do not possess complex organelles and do not undergo sexual reproduction, but rather multiply by binary fission. They are known for their ability to acquire food through the use of fingerlike projections known as *pseudopodia*, meaning "false feet." These projections are also used for motility. Under adverse conditions, many species are capable of forming cysts that can change into actively feeding trophozoites when conditions are more favorable.

Of the *Sarcodina*, *Entamoeba* is the most prevalent genus found associated with humans. In most instances, species of this genus exist as normal flora of the human intestinal tract. However, one species in particular, *Entamoebae histolytica*, is a potential pathogen in humans. Infections with *E. histolytica* are referred to as *amebiasis* and can be the cause of amebic dysentery. In such cases, actively growing organisms (trophozoites) invade the intestinal mucosa, resulting in lesions that can cause a range of symptoms from a few daily loose stools with small amounts of blood and mucus to acute cases with numerous intestinal ulcers causing severe diarrhea and substantial amounts of blood and mucus. In a small proportion of individuals, these intestinal ulcers may erode into adjoining blood vessels, allowing spread to other organs, especially the liver and lungs, and eventually leading to abscess formation.

Amebiasis is more prevalent in tropical and subtropical regions than in temperate zones and is often associated with poor sanitary conditions. In most instances, transmission is the result of ingestion of cysts from chronic carriers who shed the cyst form of the organism in their feces. Unlike acute cases, which tend to shed the trophozoite forms in feces, cysts are relatively resistant to harsh environmental conditions and, therefore, survive long enough to establish new infections.

Also in the phylum *Sarcomastigophora*, the subphylum *Mastigophora* comprise a group of flagellated protozoa commonly divided into two groups: those causing disease in the intestinal or genital tracts of humans (intestinal flagellates) and those transmitted by blood-sucking insects (hemoflagellates). Intestinal flagellates can produce a spectrum of disease, ranging from asymptomatic to severe, whereas the hemoflagellates may produce severe disease that is often fatal.

Of the intestinal flagellates, *Giardia lamblia* is the only one that produces specific intestinal disease. The actively growing form of this organism is bilaterally symmetric, with two nuclei and four pairs of flagella that provide its motility. It also produces cysts. Infections in adults range from asymptomatic to mild, including abdominal cramps and diarrhea. However, in severe cases, malabsorptive deficiencies may result in the small intestine. This organism is ubiquitous throughout the world and in the United States and may contaminate surface water. Furthermore, as it is resistant to chlorine, even treated water supplies can become contaminated if the water is not properly filtered.

Another flagellated protozoan, *Trichomonas vaginalis*, is the causative agent of trichomoniasis, a relatively common sexually transmitted disease infecting both men and women. Infection in both men and women can be asymptomatic or in women can cause a thin, watery, vaginal discharge, accompanied by burning and itching. This parasite does not form cysts and has four anterior flagella with one posterior flagellum that forms the outer edge of an undulating membrane.

Hemoflagellates are those flagellated protozoa that are transmitted to humans by the bites of infected, blood-sucking insects. Two genera are of importance in this particular category: *Trypanosoma* and *Leishmania*. In both cases, cells of each of these genera pass through similar stages in their life cycles. This involves development in both vertebrate and invertebrate hosts. Four principal stages are typically involved in the life cycles of these parasites and are characterized by the presence or absence of an undulating membrane and flagella: trypomastigotes, which characteristically possess an undulating membrane running the entire length of the organism, the outer edge of which is formed by a single flagellum that extends anterior to the cell; the epimastigotes, in which the undulating membrane originates in the central part of the cell; the promastigotes, which lack an undulating membrane but have a single anterior flagellum; and amastigotes, which are rounded, nonmotile forms. It is important to remember that for each species of parasite, some forms develop in the vertebrate host and others develop in the invertebrate host.

Trypanosomes are the causative agents of West and East African sleeping sickness. Specifically, *Trypanosoma gambiense* is the etiologic agent of West African sleeping sickness,

and *T. rhodesiense* is the etiologic agent of East African sleeping sickness (also known as *Rhodesian trypanosomiasis*). Transmission occurs as the result of a bite from an infected tsetse fly, and the organisms migrate through the blood, eventually invading the lymph nodes, which results in attacks of fever. These attacks can be intermittent and recur over a period of weeks to months, often resulting in heart damage. As the disease progresses, trypanosomes invade the central nervous system, causing a meningoencephalitis, resulting in slurred speech and difficulty walking. Later stages are characterized by convulsions, paralysis, mental deterioration, and increasing sleepiness that ultimately progresses to coma and death. This process may take several months to reach its ultimate conclusion. Although West and East African sleeping sickness are similar in clinical presentation, the East African form of the disease typically progresses much more rapidly, with death occurring well before the onset of the meningoencephalitis. Frequently, myocarditis is the cause of death.

Another disease caused by a trypanosome is American trypanosomiasis, also known as Chagas' disease. This disease is found in the southern United States and Central and South America. The causative agent of this disease is *T. cruzi*, which is transmitted to humans by the contamination of the bite of an infected reduviid bug (kissing bug). Reduviid bugs are large bugs that are common inhabitants of houses in tropical climates. They shed trypanosomes in their feces. As the bugs feed, they continually defecate, contaminating the bite site and, thus, infecting the host. This particular species of trypanosome is unable to multiply outside the cell in its vertebrate host; thus, it undergoes a morphologic change to the amastigote form and is found multiplying in virtually every cell in every organ of the body. The organ most often affected is the heart, and growth of the parasite in this organ induces an inflammatory reaction that enlarges the heart. Death usually results from disturbances in heart rhythm or congestive heart failure.

The genus *Leishmania* is another hemoflagellate that infects humans. All species of this parasite are transmitted from one animal to another by the bite of an infected sandfly of the genus *Phlebotomus*. In general, the form of the parasite introduced by the bite of the sandfly is the flagellated promastigotes (the form present in the insect's gut), which transform into nonmotile amastigotes that then proliferate in cells of the reticuloendothelial system, specifically, macrophages and endothelial cells. Three particular species of this genus are of particular medical importance in humans. *Leishmania tropica*, the causative agent of cutaneous leishmaniasis, *L. braziliensis*, the causative agent of mucocutaneous leishmaniasis, and *L. donovani*, the causative agent of visceral leishmaniasis. These diseases vary in regions of the world in which they are found and in severity of disease. Cutaneous leishmaniasis occurs primarily in the Near East, Mediterranean countries, Africa, southern Russia, and southern Asia. It is characterized by a papule that appears at the bite site and eventually develops into an ulcer. Secondary bacterial infection can be a problem but, in general, the ulcer heals within a year, leaving a depigmented scar. Mucocutaneous leishmaniasis is a variant of the cutaneous form, involving the mucous membranes of the nasopharyngeal area. If untreated, the nasal septum, lips, and the soft palate may be destroyed, resulting in asphyxiation due to airway collapse or secondary bacterial infection. This form of leishmaniasis is typically found in South America. Visceral leishmaniasis, also known as *kala-azar*, is a form of the disease in which the parasites are able to invade the reticuloendothelial system throughout the body, especially the liver and spleen. As a result, these organs become enlarged, causing abdominal swelling, and often culminate in death an average of two years after onset of initial symptoms.

In the phylum *Ciliophora*, only one of these free-living species, *Balantidium coli*, causes disease in humans. Actively growing trophozoites are covered in tiny, hairlike projections called *cilia,* which provide motility in aqueous environments. This organism has both a macronucleus that controls the metabolic activities of the cell and a micronucleus involved in sexual reproduction of the cell, which divides by transverse fission. In addition, this parasite is capable of forming cysts that provide a means of transmission upon ingestion of contaminated food or water. *B. coli* typically resides in the lumen of the intestine, obtaining food by ingesting bacteria. Occasionally, this organism can cause symptoms not unlike those seen in amebic dysentery.

The phylum *Apicomplexa* contains one class, the Sporozoa, which is of relevance to human disease. Members of this particular class are obligate parasites of animal hosts. Among the diseases caused by these organisms are malaria and toxoplasmosis, as well as intestinal infections. Because the life cycles of the Sporozoa are much more varied than those of the other protozoa, only a few of them are covered in this chapter.

Malaria is caused by one of four parasites belonging to the class Sporozoa: *Plasmodium vivax, P. ovale, P. malariae*, and *P. falciparum*. Although the clinical signs and symptoms can vary with each species of malaria, in general, these include chills and fever at intermittent, regular intervals, followed by profuse sweating. Because the life cycle of the malarial parasite is complex and varies by species, only a brief description is presented here. In general, transmission occurs when an individual is bitten by an infected female mosquito of the genus *Anopheles*. Sporozoites are released into the bloodstream of the host from the salivary glands of the mosquito as it feeds. Subsequently, the sporozoites migrate to the hepatocytes of the liver and undergo one or more rounds of asexual reproduction before returning to the bloodstream as merozoites, where they invade red blood cells. Interestingly, two species of parasite, *P. ovale* and *P. vivax,* are associated with relapsing malaria. This particular form of disease is caused by dormant parasites in the liver, which may erupt weeks, months, or years after the initial episode. Merozoites undergo several developmental stages and asexual reproduction within the red blood cells, eventually causing rupture of the cells and release to the bloodstream, where other red blood cells can then be infected and the process started again. It is during the time of red blood cell rupture and parasite release that the symptoms of the disease are present. In addition, after asexual reproduction has occurred in the red blood cells, some of the merozoites do not divide, but rather undergo a transition to male and female gametocytes. These, in turn, are ingested by a feeding mosquito, and the gametocytes are converted into male and female gametes that fuse, producing a zygote during sexual reproduction in the gut of the mosquito. The zygote undergoes several developmental transitions within the mosquito before once again reaching the sporozoite stage and repeating the infectious cycle.

In endemic areas, significant morbidity and mortality are the result of anemia, due to the high level of parasitized red blood cells. *P. falciparum*, the most dangerous of the malarial parasites, is adept at invading red blood cells and, in addition, can induce conformational changes in these cells that result in blocked capillaries, leading to hemorrhages in the brain, lungs, and kidneys. For this reason, severe infection with this species of parasite is often fatal.

Toxoplasmosis is caused by another member of the class Sporozoa, *Toxoplasma gondii*. This parasite is one of the most widespread in the world, infecting vertebrate hosts. Very often, the disease is mild to asymptomatic in humans; however, it can present a particular threat in neonates and immunocompromised individuals. This parasite is widespread throughout the animal kingdom and, thus, a common source of infection for humans is ingestion of undercooked or raw meat containing either the trophozoite or cyst forms. In particular, these parasites undergo their sexual reproduction in the intestinal cells of members of the cat family and are shed as oocysts in the feces of these animals. Infection can also result from ingestion of these oocysts, which release enclosed sporozoites that then travel to infect epithelial cells, leukocytes, the reticuloendothelial system, and the central nervous system. The parasites then multiply within these cells.

Cryptosporidium, the causative agent of cryptosporidiosis, is also included in the class Sporozoa. Both the sexual and asexual reproductive cycles occur in one host. Infectious oocysts are shed in the feces, which can then infect another susceptible host. Clinically, the disease is characterized by mild to severe diarrhea and nausea that spontaneously resolve in an average of 1–10 days. Although infection with *Cryptosporidium* produces asymptomatic to mild, self-limiting illness in most individuals, it can cause a persistent diarrhea in immunocompromised patients and may even be fatal.

Helminths

The numbers of invertebrates that parasitize humans are seemingly endless. Helminths are typically classified into two phyla: Platyhelminthes, or flatworms, and Aschelminthes, or roundworms. Generally speaking, many live only in the intestinal tract of a parasitized host, whereas others invade organs such as the liver, lungs, blood, brain, and subcutaneous tissue. Most of these parasites are large, macroscopic organisms.

The flatworms are the most primitive of the Platyhelminthes and characteristically have no digestive tract or only a rudimentary one. They are typically flat, and most contain both male and female reproductive organs (hermaphroditic). Although many require an alternation of hosts to complete their life cycles, humans are often the definitive host for the adult worms, and other animals are the hosts for the intermediate stages.

Intestinal cestodes, or tapeworms, of humans inhabit the intestinal tract. Adult tapeworms are long and ribbonlike, and are divided into segments with a head, which has either suckers or hooks that provide for attachment to the intestinal wall. In general, the animal in which the larval stage develops into an adult worm is the definitive host, and the animal in which the eggs develop into the larval stage is the intermediate host. Humans are the only definitive host for the beef and pork tapeworms, *Taenia saginata* and *T. solium*, respectively. *Taenia saginata* is acquired by ingestion of beef infected with the larval stage of the parasite. Once the larvae reach the small intestine, the worm head emerges and attaches itself to the intestinal mucosa. Mature worms can reach a length of 8–12 meters. Eggs are passed in the feces and can infect other animals, such as cattle. The eggs subsequently hatch, and the embryos disseminate throughout the body, particularly the muscles. There, they develop into the larval stage, or cysticercus, which will die in about 9 months if not ingested by the definitive host, humans. Most infections are asymptomatic, although malnutrition, anemia, and weight loss can result. The adult pork tapeworm develops similarly to that of the beef tapeworm and can attain a length of 2–3 meters. However, pigs can ingest eggs on fecally contaminated food. The larvae that develop can survive for several years in the musculature of the animal. If the larvae are ingested, very often, no symptoms are present. Unlike infection with the beef tapeworm, humans can serve as an intermediate host. This arises when an individual ingests food or water contaminated with fecal material containing eggs from another human carrier. These eggs hatch, and the resulting larvae disseminate throughout the body, forming cysticerci. The resulting condition, cysticercosis, can cause an asymptomatic infection if either the subcutaneous tissues or muscles are involved. However, more severe complications and death can occur if vital organs become infected, such as the central nervous system. Another tapeworm infection of humans is acquired by eating raw or undercooked fish infected with *Diphyllobothrium latum*, the fish tapeworm.

Other Platyhelminthes of human medical importance are the trematodes, also known as *flukes*. Adult worms are typically smaller than the cestodes, ranging in size from 1 mm to several centimeters and use suckers to attach themselves to host tissue. These parasites are found worldwide, although most human infections occur in the Far and Near East. Trematodes require snails as their intermediate host. In general, parasite eggs hatch in fresh water and undergo several larval stages, one of which involves the snail, until the infective-stage larvae are formed.

Humans become infected by ingestion of infective-stage larvae or, as in the case of the schistosomes, the larvae burrow directly through the skin of an individual standing in contaminated water. These parasites are typically classified as intestinal, liver, lung, or blood flukes. Intestinal flukes, such as *Fasciolopsis buski*, involve humans only accidentally. Liver flukes, such as *Fasciola hepatica*, mature into adult worms in the bile ducts of the liver. Lung flukes, such as *Paragonimus westermani,* cause a major disease of the lungs, paragonimiasis, and are found only in the Far East. Blood flukes of the genus *Schistosoma* cause schistosomiasis and vary by anatomic region in which the adult worms reside. For example, adult worms may reside in the inferior mesenteric veins of the large intestine (*S. mansoni)*, the superior mesenteric veins of the small intestine (*S. japonicum),* or the rectal vessels and veins surrounding the bladder (*S. haematobium*). In the latter case, ulceration of the bladder is common, thus leading to the presence of blood in the urine.

Aschelminthes

Nematodes, or roundworms, are small and possess functional digestive systems, including an anus. Human infections caused by these worms are largely divided into intestinal roundworms and blood and tissue roundworms. Of the intestinal roundworms, *Trichinella spiralis* is the cause of trichinosis in carnivorous animals. Human infection usually is the result of ingestion of the encysted larvae in undercooked or raw pork. After ingestion, the cysts reach the intestine, where the larvae are liberated and develop into adult worms. Adult female worms penetrate the intestinal mucosa, producing larvae that then migrate via the lymphatics to the muscles, etc, and become encysted. The severity of symptoms varies with the magnitude of the initial infection. Thus, infection can be asymptomatic or severe, with initial symptoms including fever, diarrhea, and malaise, due to the activities of the adult worms in the intestines. In severe cases, muscle pain throughout the entire body can also occur, due to migration of the larvae into the skeletal muscles. However, this is most commonly seen in cases of moderate to heavy infection. In addition, although encystment occurs only in muscle, larvae can infect other organs of the body, such as the lungs, heart, meninges, and brain. In particular, myocarditis, the most common cardiac lesion caused by the larvae, can lead to arrhythmias and congestive heart failure. Thus, invasion of any of these organs during the early weeks of infection can be fatal.

Ascaris lumbricoides is the largest nematode infecting humans and often attains a length of 20–30 cm. It is most frequently found in the tropics and some areas of the southern United States. Humans become infected by ingesting infectious eggs containing second-stage larvae. Once in the intestine, the larvae hatch, penetrate the intestinal mucosa, and eventually reach the lungs after the portal circulation picks them up. Once in the lung, the parasites undergo differentiation, are coughed up and swallowed, and eventually return to the small intestine, where adult worms remain attached. Only in cases of heavy infection are symptoms such as abdominal pain or complications arising from invasion of the liver, etc, seen.

Whipworm disease, caused by *Trichuris trichiura*, is found primarily in the tropics and occasionally in the southern United States. The adult worm lives in the human cecum and is attached to the intestinal mucosa. Eggs are passed in feces, and, as a result, transmission occurs via ingestion of contaminated food or water. Heavy infections are associated with chronic diarrhea, abdominal pain, vomiting, constipation, headache, and, in some cases, anemia.

Pinworms, *Enterobius vermicularis*, are strictly human parasites. Humans become infected by ingestion of fertilized eggs. As in the preceding example, adult worms live in the cecum. Female worms migrate to and lay their eggs in the perianal area, which produces an intense itching. Most infections are asymptomatic and resolve after all of the female worms have died. Human hookworm disease is caused by *Necator americanus* and *Ancylostoma duodenale*. Both species are widely distributed in tropical regions; however, *A. duodenale* is also present in Europe. The eggs of both species are passed in the feces and develop into rhabditiform, or first-stage larvae, which are generally noninfectious. These larvae feed on vegetation and bacteria in the soil and subsequently develop into infectious, filariform larvae. Filariform larvae infect a host by direct penetration of the skin, usually of the foot, and migrate to the lungs, where they are coughed up and swallowed. Adult worms reside in the small intestine, attached to the mucosa. Although the life cycles of these two species are similar, only *N. americanus* has an obligatory requirement for development in the lungs, whereas *A. duodenale* can bypass this particular stage. In addition, *A. duodenale* can also infect a host orally, as well as by direct skin penetration.

Symptoms of hookworm disease range from mild to severe and include headache, fever, nausea, and hemoptysis due to the migration of the larvae in the lungs, intestinal symptoms such as diarrhea and vomiting, and, in extreme cases, anemia, due to the feeding activity of the worms in the intestines. Creeping eruption, also known as *cutaneous larva migrans*, can also result from the migration of the larvae beneath the skin.

Blood and tissue nematodes, unlike their intestinal counterparts, are not spread by fecal-oral transmission. Most are carried from one host to another by the bite of an arthropod vector. In general, most worms in this category belong to the superfamily *Filarioidea*, and the human infection they cause is called *filariasis*.

Adult worms generally range in size from 2 to 30 cm in length, and females are ordinarily twice the size of males. Unlike other nematodes, females do not lay eggs, but rather give birth to prelarval forms known as *microfilariae*. Microfilariae are subsequently picked up by a blood-sucking vector, which then transmits the filariae from one host to another. These parasites are divided largely into two groups, based on the habitat of the adult worms: the lymphatic group

(*Wuchereria bancrofti* and *Brugia malayi)* and the cutaneous group (*Loa loa* and *Onchocerca volvulus*). *Wuchereria bancrofti* is the etiologic agent of elephantiasis. This disease is seen extensively in the Pacific Islands and Africa, and occurs sporadically in the Near and Far East and Central and South America. The disease is caused by transmission of infective larvae to humans by the bite of a mosquito. Within the human host, the larvae enter the lymphatic vessels and nodes and eventually develop into adult worms. Because the adult worms tend to prefer the lymphatics of the lower extremities, in extreme cases, especially in endemic areas, fibrous tissue can develop around the worms, leading to an obstruction of lymphatic flow and resulting in massive edema in the legs, scrotum, breasts, or female genitalia. This condition is also known as *elephantiasis*. However, this particular complication is relatively rare, and more often, light infections cause only slightly enlarged lymph nodes. *Brugia malayi,* the causative agent of Malayan filariasis, is similar in life cycle to *W. bancrofti*. It is endemic on the Malay Peninsula, although it is also present in India, Indonesia, Thailand, Ceylon, and Vietnam.

Loa loa, often referred to as the *African eye worm*, is found only in Africa. This parasite is transmitted by either mango or deer flies in which microfilariae undergo development. Unlike other filarial parasites, adult worms of this particular species migrate through the subcutaneous tissue throughout the body and, in some cases, can affect the facial area. There they can be seen as they migrate across the bridge of the nose or the subconjunctival tissue of the eye.

The disease frequently referred to as *river blindness* is caused by *Onchocerca volvulus*. This parasite is typically found in Central Africa and in some areas of Central and Northern South America. Infection is transmitted to humans by the bite of infected sandflies carrying infectious larvae. Adult worms reside in subcutaneous tissue and routinely become encased in a fibrous capsule that can often be seen beneath the skin. Microfilariae migrate from the capsules and move throughout the dermis and connective tis-

sue and can cause ocular lesions, which may ultimately result in blindness.

DIAGNOSTIC MICROBIOLOGY

Since the study of microorganisms began with their initial observation in 1683 by Antony van Leeuwenhoek, using the first microscope, continuous progress has resulted in the discovery and development of methods to detect and identify members of this previously unseen universe. Historically, this initially involved improvements in microscopy and methods to cultivate microorganisms outside of their normal hosts. The subsequent development of immunology and the sensitivity and specificity of antigen-antibody reactions led to a rapid expansion of noncultural techniques for the detection and identification of microorganisms. This has culminated in the face of molecular genetics into even more extraordinarily sensitive and specific molecular methods for detection of microbial pathogens. With the development of many of these technologies has come their application to older methods, such as microscopy and culture, which has resulted in continued improvement in specificity and accuracy. In the following section, the four major categories of microbial detection—microscopy, culture, immunology, and those utilizing molecular/nucleic acid methods—are briefly reviewed.

MICROSCOPY

Light Microscopy

The current light microscope contains a built-in light source and a compound lens system, which means that at least two separate lenses are used. Specimens are visualized by transillumination, with light being focused on the object, which is then seen against a bright background. The major components of the microscope can be divided into lens systems and mechanical parts. The purposes of microscopy include:

1. magnification of an image
2. maximization of resolution

3. optimization of the contrast between structures, organisms, cells, and background

The lens system utilized today in microscopes offers a variety of magnifications through a number of objective lenses in conjunction with a fixed (usually 10×) ocular lens. Light microscopes should be equipped with objective lenses of low-power (10×), high-dry (40×), and oil immersion (100×), which will result in final magnifications, in conjunction with the ocular lens, of 100×, 400×, and 1,000×, respectively. As important as magnification, resolving power is an essential component of microscopy. Resolving power is the ability of the lens system of the microscope to distinguish two objects as separate, rather than one. Resolving power is dependent on the wave length (L) of light used to illuminate the specimen or object and the numerical aperture of the microscopic system. Numerical aperture is a measure of the angle of the maximum cone of light that can enter the objective lens of the microscope. Resolving power of the microscope can be optimized through proper use of the condenser, which focuses light into the plane of the specimen. The most commonly used condensers can produce a numerical aperture of 1.25. Resolving power can also be increased by adjusting the medium through which the light passes between the specimen or object and the objective lens. Special oils, termed *immersion oil*, have a refractive index similar to glass, permitting more light to be incorporated in the image, thus improving resolving power. Visualization of bacteria usually requires the use of the 100× objective and immersion oil. This combination will result in resolution of approximately 0.2 microns.

Optimization of resolving power and magnification may require further adjustment of contrast and must be incorporated into microscopic systems to differentiate or distinguish various elements within a microscopic field. This is due to the similar refractive indices of many microorganisms and the matrices in which they are being observed. Although some adjustment can be made through a decrease or increase in admitted light, the majority of biologic structures cannot be visualized without the use or application of differential stains. Biologic stains are basically dyes that are used to improve contrast between structures in specimens and objects. The contrast is improved through a color differentiation, ie, attraction of a particular dye molecule, based on charge, pH, or other physiochemical interaction between a specific structural component and the dye. Due to the relative nonspecific staining characteristics of dyes, most staining techniques involve a stepwise application of chemicals for differentiation. These usually include a primary stain, which is amphoteric and can act either as an acid or a base, depending on the predominance of anionic (acidic) or cationic (basic) moieties in the dye. In general, basic dyes stain structures that are acidic, such as nuclear chromatin, whereas acid dyes react with basic structures, such as cytoplasm and cell walls. The second step involves the application of mordant, which fixes the primary stain to its target, followed by decolorization, which removes unbound dye/stain from the structure in the microorganism. Finally, a secondary or counterstain is added to provide color to nontargeted structures or microorganisms. This process is best explained by the gram-stain and acid-fast stain of bacteria, described earlier.

Variations on bright-field microscopy are employed in the diagnosis of infectious disease. Dark-field microscopy is utilized to increase apparent resolving power of light microscopy below 0.2 microns. In dark-field microscopy, the condenser, which focuses light directly onto a plane, is replaced by a special dark-field condenser, which permits entry of light only from the periphery or circumference of the object or structure. As a result, objects within the field or specimen appear to glow. Although there is no real increase in resolution, this technique does permit the visualization of microorganisms with diameters between 0.1 and 0.2 microns. This technique has been limited in application to visualization of spirochetes, such as *Treponema pallidum*, the causative agent of syphilis, in secondary syphilitic lesions; *Borrelia burgdorferi*, the agent of Lyme disease in spinal fluid; and *Leptospira* species in urine or blood.

Fluorescence Microscopy

Fluorescence is a phenomenon that occurs when a molecule is impacted by a given wavelength of light and emits light at a wavelength longer than the one to which it was exposed. In fluorescent microscopy, specimens are labeled with a fluorescent dye (molecule) and exposed to ultraviolet (UV) light of a specific wavelength, which results in emission of longer wavelength visible light. Specificity or selectivity is dependent on the nature of the fluorescent dye and the staining process. Examples of this direct fluorescence staining technique are auramine-rhodamine dye staining of mycobacteria and acridine orange staining of bacteria. The specificity of the mycobacterial fluorescent system is the staining technique, which utilizes the acid-fast nature of this group of bacteria. In contrast, acridine orange at low pH can intercalate into nucleic acid with bacterial nucleic acid fluorescing green when the appropriate UV wavelength light is utilized. Fluorescent microscopy is significantly more sensitive than light microscopy because organisms that bind and retain dye are visualized as brightly glowing objects in a dark background.

Another powerful adaptation of this technique combines the sensitivity of fluorescent microscopy with the specificity of antigen–antibody reactions. In this technique, a fluorescent dye is linked to a specific antibody that binds only to a specific antigen. Use of this method can detect the presence and cellular location of any antigen or, depending on the antigen, organism. Similarly, different antigens within a single specimen can be detected by using antibodies labeled with dyes that emit visible light of different colors. Antigen detection is termed *direct fluorescent antibody technique*. Indirect fluorescent antibody methods are utilized to determine the presence of antibody through the use of a labeled antibody, usually of another mammalian species, directed against specific classes of antibody.

Electron Microscopy

The resolving power of any microscope is directly related to the wavelength of light, which is used for visualization. The use of a beam of electrons decreases the resolution from 0.2 microns in the light microscope to 0.0005 microns in the electron microscope, which utilizes an electron beam. Although the substantial increase in resolution of electron microscopy has led to significant scientific discoveries in the ultrastructure of microorganisms, a major disadvantage is the inability to examine living cells. In addition, the preparation process can result in the creation of artifacts. Two types of electron microscopy are available that include transmission and scanning. Transmission electron microscopy uses an electron beam that travels directly through the specimen with a resulting two-dimensional image. Scanning electron microscopy produces a three-dimensional image of the specimen or object through the use of modified electron beams. In electron microscopy, contrast is achieved through differences in electron density. As a result, specimens are treated with chemicals to accentuate the electron density differential. To optimize this electron density differential, three methods of preparation have been developed: negative staining utilizes a heavy metal, such as uranium or gold, to stain the background, leaving the target structures lighter; freeze-etching involves rapid cooling of the specimen with subsequent fractures along planes of the object or specimen; and, finally, osmium tetroxide or glutaraldehyde fixation and embedding in epoxy resins with very thin, fine sectioning of the specimen and, in some cases, enhancement with heavy metal treatment.

CULTURE

Almost all medically important bacteria and fungi can be cultivated outside of the host on artificial culture media. Due to the growth characteristics of bacteria, a single cell, when placed on appropriate culture medium and environmental conditions, will reproduce to numbers sufficient to be visible to the naked eye (ie, colony) or other means of detection (Exhibit 7–2). Media utilized to cultivate microorganisms are of two general types, defined and undefined. Defined media are formulated from chemically known ingredients in known quantities. Undefined media are prepared from ingredients in which not all of the components are known but do contain adequate amounts of essential or growth-promoting ingredients. Examples of ingredients frequently used in undefined culture include partial digests of animal or vegetable protein, yeast extract, serum, or blood. The majority of diagnostic media is undefined because of their lower cost and their ability to support the growth of a broad range of pathogenic organisms. Culture media can be prepared as a fluid, broth media, or as a solid media through the addition of a gelling agent—most commonly, agar, a polysaccharide extracted from specific types of seaweed. Agar becomes liquid upon boiling and does not solidify until cooled to <50°C. The advantage of solid or agar media contained in a petri dish is the ability to isolate single cells that will form visible colonies following incubation. Isolated colonies growing on a solid surface represent pure cultures, ie, a single strain, which is required for subsequent identification and susceptibility testing, using standard methodologies.

Nutritionally, pathogenic microorganisms require a source of energy, electrons, carbon, nitrogen, oxygen, sulfur, and phosphorus. In addition, trace elements, such as potassium, calcium, magnesium, and iron, are all required for normal growth, as are very low concentrations of zinc, copper, manganese, nickel, boron, and cobalt.

Exhibit 7–2 Media Used for Growth and Isolation of Pathogenic Bacteria

Medium	Cultivation
Enrichment Media	
Brain-heart infusion broth	Most bacteria
Trypticase soy broth	
Thioglycolate broth	Anaerobes, facultative anaerobes
Blood agar	Most pathogens
Chocolate agar	Most pathogens, including *Hemophilus* and *Neisseria* species
Selective Media	
MacConkey	Nonfastidious gram-negative bacteria-differential for lactose fermentation
Colistin-nalidixic acid Blood agar	Gram-positive bacteria only
Hektoen agar	*Salmonella* and *Shigella* species
Specialized Media	
Thayer-Martin medium	Selective for *N. gonorrhoeae* and *N. meningitidis*
Thiosulfate-citrate-bile-sucrose agar	Selective for *Vibrio* species
Bordet-Gengou agar	Selective for *Bordetella pertussis*
Lowenstein-Jensen medium	Mycobacteria

Similarly, many of the more fastidious microorganisms require vitamins, which function as coenzymes or precursors for coenzymes. The use of complex media components, such as yeast extract, in media formulations for the routine growth and recovery of microbial pathogens obviates the need to add trace minerals and vitamins. Bacteriologic media are usually categorized into three groupings: enrichment, selective, and differential media.

Enrichment Media

Enrichment media are formulated to encourage the growth of a wide variety of bacteria, although a single medium that will support the growth of all bacteria has not been found. Examples of enrichment media used for the recovery of pathogenic bacteria include blood agar, chocolate agar, trypticase soy broth, and brainheart infusion broth. Selective media are used when specific pathogens are sought from specimens or sites that contain normal flora. In these instances, the pathogen of interest may be overgrown, due to a slower growth rate or smaller numbers being present at the site. Selective media usually contain chemicals, dyes, or antibiotics that are inhibitory to contaminating bacteria but not the specific pathogen of interest. Differential media contain indicator systems that permit the differentiation of groups of organisms, based on a selective metabolic or physiologic characteristic. Commonly, this includes the addition of a specific carbohydrate and a pH indicator to the base media. Fermentation of the carbohydrate results in a reduction of pH and a color change in the colony. Erythrocytes added to base media can also be differential in indicating hemolysin and the presence or absence of a hemolysis, a common virulence factor. Frequently, the properties of enrichment, selective, and differential media are combined in the same medium. Culture media commonly used in the clinical laboratory are listed in Exhibit 7–2.

In addition to the rational requirements for in vitro growth of microorganisms, the optimum physical conditions for successful cultivation must be considered. Most human pathogens are mesophiles, growing at temperatures from 25° to 40°C, with the optimum being 37°C. Similarly, the ideal pH range for most bacteria lies between 6.5 and 7.5. The principal gases that effect bacterial growth are oxygen and carbon dioxide. Aerobic organisms require oxygen for growth and can be cultivated in an air atmosphere. In contrast, anaerobic bacteria cannot use oxygen as a terminal electron acceptor; oxygen is toxic and they cannot be cultivated in an air atmosphere. Facultatively anaerobic bacteria do not require oxygen for growth, although if it is available, they are capable of using it as a terminal electron acceptor. Facultative anaerobes are capable of growth in the presence or absence of air. Microaerophilic organisms require low levels of oxygen but cannot tolerate the level of oxygen present in atmospheric air. Microaerophilic organisms are cultured in an atmosphere of 5–10% carbon dioxide.

In addition to visualization of growth through colony formation on agar media or turbidity in broth media, several methods have been developed that do not depend on visual changes for detection of growth. The techniques include detection of carbon dioxide as a result of bacterial metabolism, bioluminescence, changes in electric impedance, and chromatographic detection of metabolic end products. All of these methods require growth or metabolism by the microorganism for successful detection.

Viruses and some other microorganisms are obligate intracellular pathogens and, as such, cannot be cultivated using the techniques described above. Because growth and replication of these pathogens require living cells, three techniques have been used: inoculation of tissue or cell culture, embryonated hens' eggs, and experimental animals. Tissue culture is the most common method of viral culture. Cells are grown as monolayers, one cell in thickness, in flasks, and in the presence of nutrient media until a confluent layer of cells is achieved. Cell culture monolayers are of three basic types: primary cell culture, transformed haploid or heteroploid cell lines, and diploid cell lines or stains. In primary cell culture, the cells have a normal chromosome count (diploid) and are derived from initial cell cultivation from a tissue source such as monkey and human embryonic kidney cells. Continued subculture and regrowth of primary cell lines usually result in one of two events: the cells will eventually die or they will undergo spontaneous transformation. Transformed cell lines have altered growth characteristics; the chromosome count varies (haploid or heteroploid); and their susceptibility to viral infection can be altered. In addition, transformed cell lines are immortal, in that they can be subcultured or regrown through serial passage many times without dying. Transformed cells can also be obtained from malignant cells or tissue, or through mutagenesis in vitro. A common transformed cell line used diagnostically is Hep-2, derived from a human epithelial carcinoma. The third type of tissue culture or cell strain is composed of diploid cells, usually of fibroblast origin that can be subcultured or regrown through 30–40 passages, prior to dying out or transforming. The ability to cultivate virus in vitro is highly dependent on the specific cell line in which it is placed. As a result, successful cultivation of human viral pathogens requires the use of a number of cell lines for diagnosis unless a specific viral pathogen is being sought.

Microbial growth in cell culture can be visualized or detected through a variety of methods. Most commonly, growth can be detected through cytopathic effect. Lytic or cytopathic viruses produce alterations in cell morphology during replication in susceptible cell lines, which can be observed directly by light microscopy. The morphologic changes observed are usually characteristic of a particular virus growing in a specific cell line. For example, respiratory syncytial viruses cause fusion of cells to produce multinucleated giant cells, termed *syncytia*.

Viruses that produce proteins expressed on the membrane of infected cells that bind to erythrocytes can be detected by hemadsorption and hemagglutination. Addition of susceptible erythrocytes to an infected cell culture, followed by incubation, will result in hemadsorption—ad-

herence of the red blood cells to the cell surfaces. Sufficient release of completed virions of virus processing a hemagglutinin into the fluid culture media can be detected through addition of erythrocytes into the media, with the observation of subsequent clumping. Detection and visualization of viruses that produce little or any cytopathic effect (CPE) do not possess hemagglutinins or do not completely replicate in cell culture can be achieved through immunologic or nucleic acid probes. For immunologic detection, antibody directed at a specific viral antigen is added to the cell culture, with detection being visualized by fluorescence through a direct or indirect immunologic technique. Another commonly utilized immunologic method for viral identification is neutralization. In this technique, viral infectivity is neutralized through mixing of subcultured virus with specific individual antibodies against different viruses and inoculation of cell lines with treated and untreated aliquots of the unknown viral agent. The identity of the virus is indicated by an inability of the virus to grow in the presence of specific antibodies compared to untreated controls. Finally, animal inoculation is used in the recovery of some viruses. Suckling mice in the first 48 hours of life are very susceptible to viral infection. Depending on the virus, the mice can be inoculated intracerebrally, subcutaneously, or intraperitoneally. Evidence of viral replication/infection is manifested by clinical disease.

Confirmation and identification of the infecting virus can be achieved through histology, immunofluorescent staining, or detection of specific antibody response. Arboviruses and rabies virus are detected using this system.

DIAGNOSTIC IMMUNOLOGY

Previously used techniques for the investigation of infectious diseases included culture, serologic tests, and biochemical assays. Initially, serodiagnosis was achieved through a variety of techniques, including antigen antibody, agglutination, and complement fixation. However, these techniques were labor intensive and lacked specificity and sensitivity. These drawbacks improved significantly with the development of immunofluorescence, radioimmunoassays, and enzyme immunoassays.

In general, the use of immunoassays for the diagnosis of infectious diseases involves one of two main principles: testing for specific microbial antigens or testing for specific microbial-antigen antibodies. These assays may involve the detection of a microbial antigen directly from a clinical specimen or the detection of a specific antigen, once an organism is cultured in vitro.

Tests for antibodies may be designed to detect any antibody isotype or a particular isotype, such as IgM or IgG. Precautions must be taken in using IgM or IgG, due to markers for infection as a result of the temporal expression of each of these isotypes. For example, IgM appears rapidly following infection, peaks within 7–10 days, and wanes after several weeks. In contrast, detectable IgG requires 4–6 weeks to develop and persists longer than IgM. In general, the presence of IgM antibodies is indicative of recent infection. However, because IgM appears on second exposure to most agents and may persist in some individuals for long periods of time, interpretation of results must be carefully evaluated for each infectious agent. Therefore, in most cases, paired sera are required for the measurement of total antibody. This includes both an early sample taken the first week to 10 days after onset of symptoms and a subsequent sample taken during convalescence (3–4 weeks). In general, a fourfold rise or greater in antibody titer indicates a positive test. Other antibody isotypes, such as IgA and IgE, are not routinely used in immunodiagnosis. This is largely due to the amount of variability present in IgA levels and persistence, and the fact that IgE plays little role in dealing with infectious agents other than parasites.

In terms of sensitivity and specificity in immunodiagnostics, several important terms and how they are applied should be remembered. In addition to the traditional meaning of the term, *sensitivity,* in reference to immunodiagnostics,

may also refer to the minimum level of antigen or antibody, which can be detected by a given test. *Specificity* may also refer to the ability of a particular assay to distinguish one antigen from another. The following sections contain a brief summary and outline of several of the most commonly used immunodiagnostic methods.

Complement Fixation

Complement refers to series of serum proteins that become activated by a variety of biologic mechanisms. One of the functions of complement includes lysis of red blood cells (RBCs) in the presence of RBC-specific antibody, which has become the basis for the complement fixation test. This assay involves incubation of test serum in the presence of a particular microbial antigen. If antibodies to that antigen are present, ie, indicating infection, complement is activated and depleted from the sample. As a result, reaction mixtures containing RBCs as an indicator of complement activity will not be lysed, due to the depleted complement in the sample. In the event that the test sample does not contain antigen-specific antibody, complement is not depleted, and the RBCs are lysed. This particular type of diagnostic assay has some inherent problems associated with it, including the fact that it is relatively labor intensive and can lack sensitivity. In addition, other factors in the serum can activate complement nonspecifically, producing false-positive results.

Agglutination Assays

Agglutination assays involve the immobilization of a particular antigen or antigen-specific antibody on polystyrene beads or latex particles that are then mixed with a test specimen. This specimen is then examined for evidence of clumping. These reactions are typically performed in a tube or on a slide and often are measured photometrically. In addition, agglutination assays can usually be completed within 30 minutes and the antigen- or antibody-coated beads are relatively stable for long periods of time.

This particular type of assay has been especially useful in the detection of soluble antigens from sterile body fluids, such as cerebrospinal fluid, urine, and serum, especially in the case of infections due to *Haemophilus influenzae*, *Streptococcus pneumoniae*, *Neisseria meningitidis*, *Cryptococcus neoformans*, and both Groups A and B streptococci. However, they have not been developed for rapid diagnosis of viral infections because this method lacks sensitivity for this particular type of agent.

Neutralization and Hemagglutination Inhibition Assays

Both of these assay types are used primarily for viral identification. Hemagglutination inhibition is used to detect viruses containing hemaglutinin, such as the influenza virus. This assay requires a mixture of viral hemaglutinin, RBCs, and a test sample. If virus-specific antibodies are present, they react with the viral hemaglutinin, thus preventing agglutination of the RBCs. The neutralization assay is one of the most important standard techniques for the detection of cultivable viruses. Test samples are mixed with virus and subsequently incubated in the presence of a susceptible cell type. If antibodies to the particular virus are present, adsorption to the cells or another stage of viral replication will usually be blocked, resulting in a decrease in infectivity, which can then be measured.

Enzyme Immunoassay

The discovery that antibodies could be labeled with enzymes that could subsequently be used in histochemical staining procedures led to the development of enzyme immunoassays (EIAs), also known as *enzyme-linked immunoabsorbent assays* (ELISAs). A detailed discussion of the variety of formats possible for EIAs is beyond the scope of this text; therefore, only a brief outline of the general principles involved will be presented here. In general, several types of EIAs are currently in use and can be divided into two broad categories: assays that detect microbial antigens and assays that detect antigen-specific antibodies (Figure 7–6). Antigen detection methods are either direct or indirect, whereas antibody detection methods are either competitive or noncompetitive. Both types of EIAs typically involve the use of a solid-phase (eg, microtiter plates, tubes, beads, or nitrocellulose membranes) to which an antigen or antibody is immobilized by passive adsorption. In the direct EIA, an antigen-specific antibody is attached to a solid-phase support and mixed with a test sample. Subsequently, an enzyme-labeled detector antibody is added, followed by a chromogenic enzyme substrate. The amount of color generated is directly proportional to the amount of antigen present in the test specimen. The indirect EIA utilizes the same two initial steps as the direct method; however, once the test specimen has been added, a specific, unlabeled detector antibody is added, followed by an enzyme-labeled antiglobulin (against the detector antibody). Once the chromogenic enzyme substrate is added, a color change will occur if the antigen in question is present in the test sample. Results are determined as mentioned above for the direct EIA. Antibody detection is achieved largely through the use of competitive or noncompetitive EIAs. The noncompetitive EIA requires the attachment of a specific antigen to a solid support, which is then mixed with a particular test specimen containing specific antibody. Subsequently, an enzyme-labeled antiglobulin specific for the test specimen antibody is added, along with a chromogenic enzyme substrate. The amount of color produced is directly proportional to the amount of specific antibody present in the test specimen. The competitive version of this assay differs slightly, in that the test specimen is added simultaneously with an enzyme-labeled antibody specific for the antigen bound to the solid support. This is followed by the addition of a chromogenic enzyme substrate, and the amount of color produced is inversely proportional to the amount of antigen-specific antibody present in the test sample.

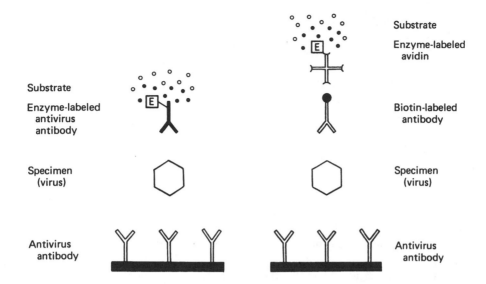

Figure 7–6 Enzyme immunoassays (EIA or ELISA) for detection of virus and/or viral antigen. *Left:* Direct. *Right:* Avidin–biotin. *Source:* Reprinted with permission from D.O. White and F.J. Fenner, *Medical Virology*, 4th edition, p. 197, © 1994, Academic Press, Inc.

Radioimmunoassay

Radioimmunoassay, or RIA, is a technique similar to EIA. However, a radioactive rather than an enzyme label is used, and specific binding is determined using a gamma- or beta-ray counter, depending on the isotope. Therein lie the disadvantages of RIA—adherence to radiation safety protocols and the restrictions that accompany working with radioactive substances. In addition, the immunoreagents used for RIAs are typically not stable for as long a period of time as those used in EIAs.

Fluorescent Antibody Techniques

Fluorescent antibody (FA) techniques have been widely used in the past for the detection of both microbial antigens and antigen-specific antibodies, and still have many applications today. Tests can be either direct or indirect and typically involve fixation of microbial antigens to glass slides, followed by testing of a patient's serum. In the direct method, a fluorescein-labeled antibody specific for a particular antigen is incubated with a test specimen fixed on a glass microscope slide. If the antigen is present in the specimen, a bright yellow-green fluorescence will be observable when viewed under a fluorescent microscope. The indirect method involves the use of a primary, unlabeled, antigen-specific antibody and a fluorescein-labeled anti-immunoglobulin specific for the primary antibody. Both are incubated with the test specimen, and results are interpreted the same as for the direct FA. This particular technique allows for the differentiation of IgM and IgG and is more sensitive and specific in identifying viruses, as compared with traditional cell culture. Unfortunately, this type of assay requires cells containing viral antigen and, therefore, cannot be used for detection of virus in samples such as serum or feces. However, FA is commonly used for the detection of antibodies to *Legionella pneumophila* and serodiagnosis of several parasitic diseases, including malaria, leishmaniasis, African trypanosomiasis, pneumocystosis, toxoplasmosis, and schistosomiasis. It can also be used for the direct detection of antigen in clinical samples and is used in the diagnosis of respiratory syncytial virus, influenza virus type A, and parainfluenza viruses types 1 through 3.

MOLECULAR DIAGNOSTICS

Over the past 10 years, advances in molecular biology have resulted in the application of these techniques in diagnostic microbiology. Although microscopy, culture, and phenotypic characterization remain the mainstay for microbial diagnosis, application of molecular techniques can potentially enhance the speed, sensitivity, and sometimes the specificity of diagnosis and identification of etiologic agents. A variety of molecular techniques has evolved from initial hybridization and nucleic probes, including signal amplification, target amplification, and postamplification technologies.

The underlying principle of nucleic acid probe technology is the selection of unique genomic sequences for a particular group of etiologic agents or specific genes with subsequent cloning, synthesis, and utilization. Probes can hybridize with either DNA or RNA with high specificity to complementary sequences of the target nucleic acid. Hybridization is detected by labeling the probe with radioisotopes, enzymes, antigens, or chemoluminescent compounds that can be measured through instrumentation specific for the label. Three nucleic acid probe hybridization methods have evolved: liquid-phase, solid-phase, and in situ hybridization; for liquid-phase hybridization, a single-stranded probe that does not hybridize to itself is utilized. The most common method used in diagnostics is the hybridization protection assay. A labeled probe is mixed with the potential target and subjected to alkaline hydrolysis. The signal molecule is protected from hydrolysis, if hybridized, and is detected directly in the liquid specimens. In solid-phase hybridization, nucleic acid-bound nylon membranes or nitrocellulose are hybridized with the nucleic acid probe. Unbound probe is washed off, and hybridization can be detected using any of the signal systems mentioned earlier. In situ hybridization utilizes tissue or whole cells fixed to microscope slides. Probes are hybridized targets in the cells, using the same principles employed in solid-phase hybridization. The sensitivity of this method is limited by penetration of the probe into the cell, but does have the advantage of visualization by microscopy of the location and cell type in which hybridization is occurring. Nucleic acid probes have been used successfully for the detection of fastidious, slow-growing, or nonculturable, organisms and antibiotic resistance genes, as well as for identification of phenotypically difficult microorganisms.

Signal amplification methods are designed to increase the signaling capacity of the hybridization reaction of a probe to its target through an increase in the concentration of the label. Signal amplification methods increase the amount of signal generated by a fixed amount of probe/target hybrid. These methods do not increase the amount of target, as do amplification methods. These methods offer the potential advantage of being less susceptible to contamination, an inherent problem with target amplification, but are comparatively limited in sensitivity. Two examples of signal amplification techniques are a solution hybridization antibody capture assay that uses chemiluminescent detection and the branched DNA (bDNA) probe assay. The former utilizes RNA probes that hybridize with DNA target sequences to form an RNA-DNA hybrid. These hybrids are captured on a solid surface by attached antibodies specific for RNA-DNA hybrids. The immobilized hybrids are then reacted with another enzyme-conjugated antibody specific for the hybrids. Signal amplification occurs through multiple antibody binding to the hybrid, with detection through the addition of a chemiluminescent substrate. The branched DNA probe technique uses a branched multiple probe–enzyme complex. This system utilizes three probes for detection of a primary probe (target-specific), a branched secondary probe, and a short enzyme-labeled tertiary probe. The primary probes are used to capture target on a solid surface. Branched oligonucleotide probes (bDNA amplifiers) specific for the hybridized primary probe are added, followed by the short enzyme-labeled tertiary probes. Chemiluminescent substrate is then added, and the signal can be quantitated.

The polymerase chain reaction (PCR) has in many ways revolutionized diagnostic microbiology. Because it was the first amplification technology, it has to date had the widest application. Other target amplification systems that have been developed but have not received as wide an application as PCR include: transcription-mediated amplification (TMA) and similar methodologies, and strand displacement amplification (SDA). As a target amplification method, PCR is based on the ability of DNA polymerase to copy a strand of DNA when two primers (oligonucleotides) bind to complementary strands of target DNA. The enzyme initiates elongation at the 3′ end of a primer bound to the target strand of DNA. The sequence between the two specific primers is amplified exponentially with each cycle of PCR. A cycle consists of three steps:

1. a DNA denaturation step, in which the double-stranded target DNA is separated into single strands
2. primers anneal or bind to their complementary target sequences at a lowered temperature
3. DNA polymerase synthesizes or extends the target sequences between the primers

With each cycle, the PCR product or target sequences are doubled. The reaction is performed in a programmable thermal cycler, usually with 30–50 cycles, resulting in amplification of <100 copies of target sequence to a detectable level. There has been a variety of adaptations to PCR, which include:

- RT-PCR, developed to amplify RNA targets through the initial use of the enzyme reverse transcriptase for conversion of the RNA target to cDNA
- nested PCR, designed primarily to increase sensitivity through the use of two primer sets directed at the same target, one set within the other
- multiplex PCR, in which two or more sets of primers specific for different targets are utilized in the same reaction

Other technologies for target amplification include transcription-mediated amplification systems and strand displacement amplification. In addition to target amplification, two systems, QB replicase (QBR) and the DNA ligase reaction, are based on amplification of a probe.

The application of molecular technology to the diagnosis of infectious disease has enhanced the speed, sensitivity, and specificity of microbial diagnosis. Although improving the ability of the clinical laboratory to make some diagnoses, before developing and implementing this technology in the laboratory for a particular microorganism, a definite need should be established. In general, molecular techniques are warranted in situations where currently available culture techniques are unable to recover or grow the organism in vitro, or instances where current methods are too insensitive, too costly, or too time consuming.

The application of molecular technology in the diagnostic laboratory has also revealed a variety of limitations. Perhaps the most serious of these limitations is the potential for contamination of true negative specimens from carryover or cross-contamination from positive controls or true positive specimens. Due to the amplification inherent in PCR, minute contamination of a specimen can result in a false-positive result. In contrast, a number of factors can result in false-negative results. Most commonly, this is the result of the inhibitors of the enzymes utilized in the amplification reaction mixture. An additional limitation of the majority of molecular tests is their narrow detection scope. Each test can detect only one pathogen. For the detection of more than one pathogen, additional tests have to be performed. This is a disadvantage when compared with culture systems that are capable of detecting multiple pathogens simultaneously from the same specimen. The final disadvantage of currently utilized molecular technology is cost. This includes reagent, equipment, space, and labor costs, which significantly exceed the cost incurred by conventional microbiologic methods.

SUGGESTED READING

Ajello L, Hay RJ. Medical mycology, Vol. 4. In: Collier L, Balows A, Sussman M, eds. *Topley and Wilson's Microbiology and Microbial Infections*, 9th ed. New York: Oxford University Press; 1998.

Baron EJ, Chang RS, Howard DH, Miller JN, Turner JA. *Medical Microbiology: A Short Course*. New York: Wiley-Liss; 1994.

Barrett JT. *Microbiology and Immunology Concepts*. Philadelphia: Lippincott-Raven Publishers; 1998.

Flint SJ, Enquist LW, Krug RM, Racaniello VR, Skalka AM. *Virology, Molecular Biology, Pathogenesis, and Control*. Washington, DC: American Society of Microbiology (ASM) Press; 2000.

Garcia LS, Bruckner DA. *Diagnostic Medical Parasitology*, 3rd ed. Washington, DC: ASM Press; 1997.

Mandell GL, Bennett JE, Dolin R. *Principles and Practice of Infectious Diseases*, 5th ed. Philadelphia: Churchill Livingstone; 2000.

Murray PR, Baron EJ, Pfaller MA, Tenover FC, Yolken RH. *Manual of Clinical Microbiology*, 7th ed. Washington, DC: ASM Press; 1999.

Mims CA. *The Pathogenesis of Infectious Disease*, 3rd ed. Orlando, Fla: Academic Press; 1987.

Nelson KE, Kaufman L, Cooper CR, Merz WG. *Penicillium mannettei*: biology and infections with this emerging fungal pathogen. *Infect Med*. 1999;16:118–121.

Salyers AA, Whitt DD. *Bacterial Pathogenesis: A Molecular Approach*. Washington, DC: ASM Press; 1994.

Schaechter M, Medoff G, Esenstein BI. *Mechanisms of Microbial Disease*, 2nd ed. Baltimore: Williams & Wilkins; 1993.

Volk WA, Gebhardt BM, Hammarskjold M-L, Kadner RJ. *Essentials of Medical Microbiology*, 5th ed. Philadelphia: Lippincott-Raven Publishers; 1996.

CHAPTER 8

Molecular Epidemiology and Infectious Diseases

Susan M. Harrington and William R. Bishai

The last 20 years have seen significant advances in the ability of the clinical microbiologist to identify substrains of bacterial pathogens and use this information to track infectious diseases. Most strain typing has focused on bacteria, but fungi and viruses can also be typed. Pathogens are identified in the clinical microbiology laboratory according to their species. Speciation is part of a medical diagnostic evaluation for a particular infectious disease. However, most routine clinical evaluations do not include identification to the substrain level of a particular pathogen. For example, strains of *Staphylococcus aureus*, implicated in many nosocomial hospital infections, are identified to the species level, but are not routinely evaluated for evidence of belonging to a particular type. Similarly, *Haemophilus influenzae* isolates can be identified by serotype, as well as by species. However, the subtyping is not part of a routine microbiology culture result. Serotyping is generally only performed to rule out serotype b infection in children.

Strain typing is used to determine how close isolates of the same species are relative to one another. When one finds isolates that have originated from different patients are related or identical to one another, it suggests a common source of the infection. This information is useful to epidemiologists who are responsible for tracking communicable diseases within a health care institution or a community. Such information helps them to identify point sources and transmission patterns of infections so that appropriate interventions can be applied.

Likewise, when isolates are found to differ, it suggests a different origin of infection. Hence, if two people are diagnosed with tuberculosis in the same community at the same time, the determination that the substrain analysis shows differences indicates that the individuals are highly unlikely to have passed the infection between them.

In short, the goal of strain typing is to distinguish epidemiologically related isolates from those that are unrelated based on the premise that related isolates will share detectable characteristics that will distinguish them from others. As with other kinds of epidemiologic investigations, control strains known to be unlinked epidemiologically must be included in a subtyping analysis. A typing system must be able to delineate control strains from those thought to be part of an outbreak or cluster. The ability of a typing method to distinguish epidemiologically related isolates from epidemiologically unrelated isolates is termed "discriminatory power." It is important to mention that, although strain typing is a powerful tool for the epidemiologist, it should be done with clear goals in mind and should be used to enhance a sound epidemiologic investigation.

EXAMPLE APPLICATIONS

Strain typing systems are widely used to characterize bacteria, fungi, and, more rarely, viruses. Often the laboratory is asked to subtype isolates when an epidemiologist notices increased isolation of a microbe on routine surveillance of microbiology culture results. For example, an increase in *S. aureus* in a hospital intensive care unit (ICU) or long-term care facility may indicate a possible outbreak. Sometimes a relatively rare organism recovered over a short period of time from patients not obviously linked epidemiologically may be an indication of disease transmission. Three cases of *Listeria monocytogenes* bacteremia, noted in two departments in the same hospital within a 2-week time period, led investigators to suspect a common source of contamination. Molecular typing quickly determined the isolates to be distinct and no further investigation was indicated.[1] As part of a prospective study of tuberculosis transmission in Baltimore, two patients whose only link was the hospital wherein they were treated were found to have the same *Mycobacterium tuberculosis* subtype. On further examination, the second patient was thought to have acquired tuberculosis from a contaminated bronchoscope that had been used on the other patient 2 days earlier.[2]

Reports of unusual pathogens (e.g., those with rare antimicrobial resistance patterns or unexpected isolates from environmental sources) alert microbiologists and epidemiologists to potential outbreaks. Molecular analysis of plasmid DNA has been found useful in demonstrating the clonality of a relatively rare strain of chloramphenicol resistant *Salmonella* in California. The Los Angeles County Health Department Laboratory noticed a 4.9 times increase in this species, of which 87% were chloramphenical resistant. A case-control study showed the illness to be associated with consumption of ground beef derived from feedlots using antibiotics in cattle. The strain was further linked to contaminated beef, slaughterhouses, and dairy farms.[3]

Strain typing techniques are now used for other clinical applications as well. To determine if isolates of the same genus and species cultured from a patient weeks or months apart represent re-infection with a new strain or recrudescence of a previous infection, they might be typed by molecular methods. In one report, an immunocompromised child had episodes of bacteremia 4 months apart with the same uncommon gram-negative bacterium, *Flavobacterium meningosepticum*. Molecular analysis by pulsed-field gel electrophoresis showed the isolates to be indistinguishable. The two episodes of sepsis likely resulted from an indwelling central catheter that harbored small numbers of organisms.[4] In another example, 1 year after having been adequately treated for a *M. tuberculosis* infection, a patient with human immunodeficiency virus (HIV) was again found to have active disease. Was the therapy inadequate or had the patient been re-infected? Molecular studies showed the second strain recovered to be the same as the first, except for a mutation rendering it resistant to rifampin. The strain was presumed to have become resistant *in vivo* during rifabutin prophylaxis to prevent infection with *Mycobacterium avium*. Hence, molecular analysis proved reactivation of disease with a new antibiotic resistance in the patient's original strain.[5]

Additionally, molecular techniques may be used to determine if multiple blood cultures drawn over 1 or more days yielding coagulase-negative *Staphylococci* or other skin flora represent a true bacteremia or culture contamination. Multiple strains isolated from a true bacteremia generally have the same molecular type, whereas skin contamination will likely produce heterogeneous strains.[6,7]

Finally, as important pathogens such as *S. aureus* and *Streptococcus pneumoniae* evolve, acquiring new antimicrobial resistance genes, or as new microbial pathogens emerge, molecular typing techniques can be used to investigate these strains within the health care environment and community at large.

DEFINITIONS AND BACKGROUND

Throughout this chapter, vocabulary known to the microbiologist and molecular biologist will be used. To create a framework for the reader, some basic concepts with respect to strain relatedness will be defined. Strain typing methods that preceded molecular techniques will be discussed. An overview of microbial nucleic acids and ways in which the genetic content of a microbe can vary will be given. The laboratory techniques used to detect genetic change will also be explained in this section before specific molecular typing methods are presented.

Relevant Concepts and Conventional Strain Typing Methods

An isolate refers to the bacterium or other microbe recovered from a primary microbiology culture. Typically, an isolate is characterized only by its source and its genus and species. The word "strain" is applied after some further testing is performed. Isolates can be grouped as a single strain based on characteristics they have in common. They can be considered unique strains if the "test" distinguishes them from other strain types tested. Clones are isolates that have been derived from the same parent strain. Strains are considered clones if they are indistinguishable from one another. Although progeny strains are produced from indistinguishable isolates, normally occurring genetic mutations will cause them to diverge gradually. Therefore, after multiple generations, daughter strains may no longer be identical, but will likely be clonally related.

Relationships among strains are to some extent relative. They may depend on which test is used for characterization. Different techniques provide information about different aspects of the organism. Also, isolates may be related to varying degrees depending on the amount of mutation within a species and the number of generations between the isolates.[8]

Before the advances in molecular biology of the last 10 or 20 years, the techniques used to characterize microorganisms were based on their phenotypic characteristics. The phenotype of an organism is derived from the expression of the genetic material. Biotyping, antimicrobial susceptibility patterns, serotyping, bacteriocin typing, phage typing, and protein-based methods are all examples of phenotypic tests. Each of these measures varies within a species and each has observable properties. Although more discriminatory molecular methods have replaced these for accurate strain typing, the information provided by phenotypic results should not be minimized.

As part of the speciation of bacteria and yeasts, organisms are tested for the expression of various metabolic functions such as biochemical reactions and growth under selected environmental conditions. The results produced in these tests provide characteristic patterns for identification, and they are referred to as the "biotype." Sometimes isolates of a particular species will be observed with an unusual biochemical marker distinguishing them from other strains of that species. However, biotyping is usually not a sensitive indicator of strain differences.

As bacteria are speciated, the clinical laboratory almost always performs susceptibility testing of that microbe to a panel of antibiotics appropriate for therapy. The susceptibility results are reported as susceptible, intermediate, or resistant to each antibiotic. A numeric minimum inhibitory concentration (MIC) value is also often reported as an indicator of the degree of susceptibility. The susceptibility of the organism to the panel of antibiotics is termed the "antibiogram." Two isolates found to have the same antibiogram may be an early indicator that clonal dissemination is occurring. For highly resistant species, such as vancomycin resistant enterococci or methicillin resistant *S. aureus,* antibiograms are of limited use because few changes will be seen in the susceptibility profile between isolates. Isolates with vastly different antibiograms are most likely unrelated. Sometimes two antibiograms will differ by only one or a few antibiotic susceptibilities. Strains producing such patterns may be clonally related. Bacteria can become antibiotic resistant depending on the selective pressure of antibiotics in the environment or the presence of other resistant species that can transfer resistance genes. Conversely, organisms can also lose antibiotic resistance genes carried on extrachromosomal plasmids. Overall, antibiograms provide highly standardized, prospective data and are an excellent place to start in making strain comparisons.

Some bacteria can be differentiated by serotype. Antigenic determinants (e.g., cell surface carbohydrates, membrane proteins, and lipopolysaccharides) are variable and can be detected with specific antibody. Serotyping continues to be a useful method for species such as *H. influenzae, S. pneumoniae, Neisseria meningitidis, Salmonella* and *Shigella* species, *Escherichia coli,* and some viruses. Not only can serotyping differentiate stains, but certain serotypes are markers of virulence. For example, *H. influenzae* type b causes severe invasive disease and *E. coli* O157:H7 can cause hemolytic uremic syndrome. Influenza viruses can be typed to determine which serotypes are circulating, and this information used for vaccine development. Serotyping, however, is limited as an epidemiologic typing method, because the discriminatory power is less than other, molecular methods. Additionally, serotyping can be expensive, and it is useful for only a limited number of organisms for which antisera have been developed.[9]

Bacteriophage typing had long been the standard typing method for *S. aureus*. A bacteriophage is a viral particle that is capable of infecting bacterial cells and causing cell lysis. The isolates to be typed can be tested for susceptibility to a panel of different bacteriophage to produce a pattern known as the "phage type." This method, however, is technically demanding and requires stock strains of bacteriophage which are generally available only in reference laboratories. Bacteriocin testing is similar to phage typing. A bacteriocin is a toxin to which a bacterium may be susceptible. Strains to be typed are tested with a set of bacteriocins to achieve a bacteriocin profile. As with phage typing, this method is expensive and technically difficult.[9]

The presence, size, and function of proteins can be used to distinguish strains of bacteria. Proteins can be isolated from whole cell preparations or from cell wall fractions. Sodium dodecyl sulfate–polyacrylamide gel electrophoresis (SDS-PAGE) is then used to separate the protein extracts based on molecular mass. Protein bands can be visualized with radioactive labels, by stain, or by the Western blot technique. For the latter method, the proteins in the gel are transferred to a nitrocellulose membrane. Antibody is added, which will bind to specific proteins of interest on the membrane. The first antibody is detected with a second conjugated antibody that gives a signal with an enzyme-substrate system.[10] A drawback of this method is the numerous bands that are often detected, making interpretation difficult. Electrophoretic protein typing is rarely used for outbreak investigations today.

A second protein based method is multilocus enzyme electrophoresis (MLEE). Extracts containing metabolic enzymes from the bacteria are separated by electrophoresis in starch gels. The location for each enzyme in the gel is detected with a colorimetric substrate specific to that enzyme. Because the electrophoretic mobility of the enzymes depends on their exact amino acid content, it is strain specific. Evaluated as a profile, the electrophoretic mobilities or isoenzyme patterns are referred to as an "electrophoretic type." Moderately discriminatory, this technique is not in widespread use because it is technically demanding.[10]

As with all living forms, bacteria are composed of four classes of biochemicals: nucleic acid, protein, lipid, and carbohydrate. Methods exist for identifying intraspecies differences for each of these four categories, some of which have already been discussed. However, in the last two decades, methods based on the presence, size, and sequence of nucleic acids have come to predominate in the field of molecular epidemiology. These methods are referred to as "genotypic" because they are based on the genetic content of the microbe.

The Basics of Microbial Nucleic Acids and Mutational Change

The primary location of the genetic content of a microorganism is its chromosome. Most bacteria contain a single, circular chromosome composed of double-stranded DNA (dsDNA). Fungi are eukaryotes and carry multiple linear chromosomes. An understanding of the components of DNA is essential to the basic theory of molecular epidemiology. All dsDNA have two complementary strands, which pair by hydrogen bonding. A sugar-phosphate backbone and the nucleotide bases adenine (A), guanine (G), thymidine (T), and cytosine (C) comprise each strand. Adenine pairs with thymidine and guanine with cytosine. It is the order or sequence of these base pairings that determines the genetic content. Molecular biologists measure chromosomes, specific genes, or other DNA fragments by their length in base pairs (bp). In fact, some genome sequencing projects have been completed, and the number of base pairs in the chromosome and the complete DNA sequence for these species have been determined. On average, bacterial chromosomes range in size from 800 kilobases (kb) to 10,000 kb. In addition to the chromosome, there may be ancillary segments of DNA known as episomes or plasmids. Such extrachromosomal DNA elements usually range in size from 1 to 200 kb. The organism's total genetic content (i.e., chromosomal and episomal DNA together) is referred to as the genome. Molecular epidemiologists determine strain relatedness by detecting changes in the genome. Several ways exist in which variations in the genetic content of a bacterium can occur (Exhibit 8–1).

Mutational Changes

Mutations are mistakes in copying the DNA of a parent bacterial strain during the replication process of binary fission. The basal mutation rate for most bacterial species is about one error in 10^8 base pairs per generation. Hence, in an organism that has a genome size of 10^7 DNA base pairs, a base pair replication error will be made once every 10 generations. Two general types of mutations are seen: (1) the substitution of one base for another is a point mutation; and (2) fragments of DNA inserted into or deleted from the chromosome result in a chromosomal rearrangement. Most mutations are inconsequential or si-

Exhibit 8–1 Types of Alterations in DNA That Can Be Detected by Molecular Epidemiology

Mutations in chromosomal DNA
- DNA point mutations
- DNA insertions
- DNA deletions
- DNA rearrangements

Mobile genetic elements
- Insertion sequences
- Transposons
- Conjugative plasmids
- Lysogenic phages

Excessory genetic material
- Multicopy plasmids
- Single copy plasmids
- Accessory chromosomes

lent (i.e., they do not lead to physiologic or functional changes in the mutated progeny cell). In organisms that replicate quickly and are present in large environmental reservoirs, significant genetic drift is observed. If the basal rate of genetic replication errors is assumed to be constant, then the more genetic differences between two isolates of the same species, the more time has passed since the two originated from a common ancestor. Hence, it is possible to identify numerous changes of subspecies of most bacterial organisms, and to estimate the distance in evolutionary time between isolates.

Mobile Genetic Elements

Most bacterial species contain mobile genetic elements that create variability in the genome. These are pieces of DNA capable of moving themselves around the chromosome. A common type of mobile genetic element is the transposon. Duplicative transposons can copy themselves and can insert a second copy at another site within the bacterial chromosome. Mobile genetic elements, such as transposons, lead to more easily detectable changes in the bacterial chromosome than point mutations resulting from the basal rate of mutation. Later in this chapter we will see how transposable elements can be used as part of a strain typing system.

Plasmids

Finally, accessory genetic elements can be used to identify differences between species. In addition to the chromosome, many species contain small, circular pieces of self-replicating DNA known as plasmids, which are present in single or multiple copies in the cytoplasm of the bacterial cell. Often these plasmids are nonessential and may come and go over time within a particular bacterial subpopulation. Some plasmids, however, carry elements that code for functional genes (e.g., metabolic enzymes, virulence factors, or antibiotic resistance). Antibiotic use can create selective pressure to maintain a plasmid. Likewise, absence of antibiotic can lead to loss of plasmids. Plasmids carried by a species (and their type and size) may be useful in identifying subspecies of the same strain.

Molecular Biology Tools Available to the Molecular Epidemiologist

Some understanding of basic molecular biology laboratory techniques will be useful before the discussion of specific typing methods is presented. The next section is a brief overview of selected "tools." The reader is referred to *Molecular Cloning: A Laboratory Manual*[11] or *Diagnostic Molecular Microbiology Procedures and Applications*[12] for more detail on specific procedures.

Restriction Endonucleases

Restriction endonucleases or restriction enzymes are "work horses" for strain identification techniques. These are enzymes that scan double-stranded DNA searching for specific sequences. When a specific recognition sequence innate to the restriction enzyme is found, the enzyme cleaves the double-stranded DNA. Table 8–1 shows several restriction enzymes and the sequences at which they cut.

In addition to having different recognition site sequence specificities, restriction endonucleases

also have different restriction site length specificities. This information is illustrated in Table 8–1, which shows restriction enzyme *Hae*III and *Sau*3AI. Both of these are four base pair recognition endonucleases, which are sometimes called four-base cutters. Table 8–1 also shows six-base cutters, *Eco*RI and *Hin*dIII, as well as two eight-base cutters, *Pac*I and *Not*I .

As also shown in Table 8–1, four-base cutters will cleave DNA much more frequently than do six- or eight-base cutters. In DNA that is evenly distributed in its AT and GC content (50:50), a four-base cutter will be expected to cleave every 256 bp on average, whereas a six-base cutter does so every 4,096 and an eight-base cutter every 65,530 bp. Hence, four-base cutters or "frequent cutters" cleave chromosomal DNA into many small pieces distributed around 250 bp, whereas 6-base cutters cleave DNA into a moderate number of intermediate size fragments of approximately 4,000 bp, and finally eight-base cutters or "infrequent cutters" create very large fragments of approximately 65,000 bp in size.

In addition, the frequency of cutting is not only dependent on the number of bases in the recognition site but is also dependent on the percent GC and percent AT of the organism. If a bacterial species is GC rich, a restriction endonuclease whose recognition site is biased toward AT will be an infrequent cutter and a restriction endonuclease whose recognition site has a heavy GC content will be much more common than expected. A good example of this occurs in *M. tuberculosis,* which is 67% GC and 33% AT in its DNA content. The eight-base cutter *Pac*I, which recognizes the AT-rich sequence TTAATTAA, is expected to cut DNA, containing equal amounts of AT and GC base pairs about every 65,530 bp. However, because of the heavy GC content of *M. tuberculosis* DNA, *Pac*I fails to cut even once within its 4.7 million base pairs.

If a mutation has occurred at a restriction endonuclease site, the alteration of bases will prevent the enzyme from cutting. This is illustrated in Exhibit 8–2, where a change from an AT base pair to a CG base pair in an *Eco*RI endonuclease restriction site destroys the recognition sequence

Table 8–1 Some Common Restriction Endonucleases and Their Recognition Site Specificities

Restriction Enzyme	Recognition Sequence	Base Pairs Recognized (N)	Approximate Frequency of Cutting (bp)
*Hae*III	5'—GG↓CC—3' 3'—CC↑GG—5'	4	256
*Sau*3AI	5'—↓GATC—3' 3'—CTAG↑—5'	4	256
*Eco*RI	5'—G↓AATTC—3' 3'—CTTAA↑G—5'	6	4096
*Hind*III	5'—A↓AGCTT—3' 3'—TTCGA↑A—5'	6	4096
*Pac*I	5'—TTAAT↓TAA—3' 3'—AAT↑TAATT—5'	8	65,530
*Not*I	5'—GC↓GGCCGC—3' 3'—CGCCGG↑CG—5'	8	65,530

Note: **Arrows** indicate the place in the DNA sequence where cutting occurs.

and prevents *Eco*RI cleavage. Likewise, insertion or deletion of DNA may lead to the creation or elimination of a restriction site. The use of restriction enzymes is fundamental to many molecular typing tests. Isolates that are clones will have the same DNA base sequence and, therefore, share the same spacing of restriction sites.

When the chromosome of a microbe is cut with a restriction enzyme, many DNA fragments of a variety of lengths are produced according to the spacing of the restriction enzyme recognition sites for that restriction endonuclease. Base mutations (insertions, deletions, or point mutations) that alter restriction enzyme recognition sites

Exhibit 8–2 Sequence Recognized by Restriction Enzyme *Eco*RI

5'—G↓AATTC—3' 3'—CTTAA↑G-5'	Recognition sequence for *Eco*RI. **Arrows** indicate site of enzyme cleavage.
5'—**GCATTC**—3' 3'—**CGTAAG**—5'	A point mutation occurs. AT base pair changed to CG. Restriction site specificity is lost.
5'—**GAAGC**AATTC—3' 3'—**CTTCG**TTAAG—5'	A DNA insertion occurs. Addition of four base pairs. Restriction site specificity is lost.

Note: Point mutations or DNA insertions or deletions cause loss of restriction specificity as shown.

will change the number and size of some of the restriction fragments. Also, nucleotides inserted or deleted between restriction sites will alter the length of restriction fragments.

Changes in the genome sequence (which may be detected by altered patterns of restriction enzyme cleavage) are called "polymorphisms." Restriction fragment length polymorphism (RFLP) refers to variations in the lengths of restriction fragments; different RFLP patterns indicate genetic differences between strains and suggest that the strains are not clonal. Figure 8–1 is a schematic diagram of the bacterial chromosome illustrating this principle. Organisms 1 and 2 are clones and, therefore, have an identical restriction site distribution as depicted by the lines cutting the circular chromosome. Organism 3 is unrelated and has a different restriction site pattern. The differences between organisms may be visualized by separating the fragments resulting

from restriction enzyme digestion by gel electrophoresis. Nucleic acid probes and Southern hybridization may also be used to identify specific restriction fragment differences. Only restriction fragments with specificity for the probe are detected (highlighted bands on Figure 8–1). Southern hybridization using a DNA probe to a region known to be highly variable is an efficient, sensitive way of detecting RFLPs.

Gel Electrophoresis

A technique known as gel electrophoresis is used to separate DNA molecules. Agarose gels are formed with wells into which small amounts of solutions containing DNA are placed. Agarose is a polysaccharide derived from seaweed, which forms a large matrix through which DNA fragments must migrate. DNA is negatively charged and, when a positive electrode is placed

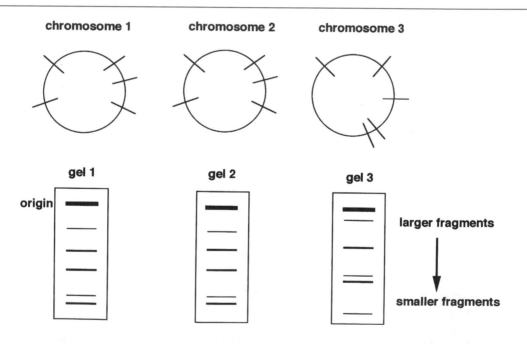

Figure 8–1 Restriction fragment length polymorphism of three bacterial chromosomes. Lines on circles indicate sites for cutting with a restriction enzyme. Organisms 1 and 2 share restriction endonuclease sites and, therefore, have identical banding patterns on gel electrophoresis as depicted. Bacterium 3 has different restriction sites. The fingerprint for organism 3 is different from the other two.

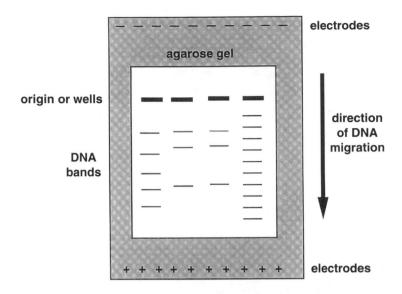

Figure 8–2 Conventional agarose gel electrophoresis. Fourth lane from left indicates molecular weight marker. *Source:* Copyright © 2000, Susan M. Harrington.

at the distal end of the gel and a negative electrode at the proximal end, the DNA migrates in a lane toward the positive charge (Figure 8–2). Usually, this migration occurs on the basis of size; small fragments run more rapidly than large fragments. After the separation under an electric charge, the gel is removed from the electrophoresis running box and stained using a variety of intercalating fluorescent chemicals such as ethidium bromide, which enables visualization of the DNA bands. A molecular weight marker or size standard is always run on the same gel to determine DNA band size.

Standard agarose gel electrophoresis enables the separation of fragments of DNA ranging from 50 bp to about 15,000 bp. Beyond 15,000 bp, the DNA molecules are too large to fit easily through the agarose gel matrix and the fragments fail to migrate proportionally to their size. Thus, segments greater than 15,000 bp tend to accumulate at the origin of the agarose gel.

A modification of standard agarose gel electrophoresis is pulsed-field gel electrophoresis (PFGE). PFGE is an adaptation that enables large fragments of DNA ranging from 10,000 bp

to 5 million base pairs to be separated on the basis of size. This technique uses standard agarose gels; however, the electric field in which the DNA migrates is not applied in only one direction as in conventional electrophoresis. PFGE uses alternating electric fields, in which the current is applied for varying lengths of time in each direction, depending on the size of fragments to be separated. Several electrode configurations have been used by investigators. The most popular system is the contour-clamped homogeneous electric field (CHEF). The CHEF apparatus consists of a hexagonal array of electrodes producing two electric fields at 120° angles to one another (Figure 8–3). The length of time that the current is applied in each direction is referred to as the "switch time" or "pulse time." Larger DNA molecules require longer pulse times and smaller fragments are separated adequately with shorter pulse times. PFGE can be used to separate the fragments created by restriction endonuclease digestion of bacterial or fungal genomic DNA. Such digestion generally yields about 10 to 20 bands that have a range of fragment sizes. The array of small, medium, and large size frag-

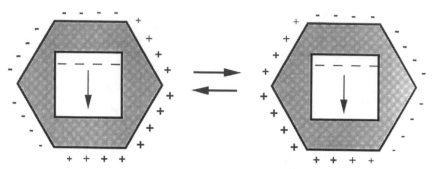

Figure 8–3 Schematic diagram of pulsed-field gel electrophoresis (PFGE) by the contour-clamped homogeneous electric fields (CHEF) technique. Alternation of current is shown. The figure on the left indicates current from northwest to southeast. The figure on the right shows the current from northeast to southwest. **Vertical arrows** indicate net migration of DNA fragments in the gel. *Source:* Copyright © 2000, Susan M. Harrington.

ments is separated by "ramping" the pulse time. With ramping, the pulse time is increased incrementally from just a few seconds up to several minutes over the course of the run.[13] Most users of PFGE purchase CHEF equipment, which can perform these intricate electrical switches with little programming by the operator. However, such CHEF equipment can be expensive.

Handling pieces of DNA that are large requires great care because such DNA fragments are fragile. For PFGE, DNA is extracted from cells that have been immobilized in agarose so that the DNA is not broken by agitation, vibration, or excessive pipetting.

Hybridization and Nucleic Acid Probes

Hybridization refers to the pairing or annealing of nucleic acid, both RNA and DNA, to complementary nucleic acid strands. Because of the rules of base pairing (that A pairs with T and C pairs with G), single strands of nucleic acid will anneal or hybridize to complementary strands that have the correct sequence of matching base pairs to form a complete set of Watson-Crick pairs. Nucleic acid probe technology is based on the principle of hybridization. Sequences derived from specific genes or other DNA sequences can be used as probes to find places in the genome—the target—where these

same sequences (or their complements) occur. The probe anneals to the target creating new, hybrid dsDNA.

In the process of Southern hybridization, target DNA, which has been digested with a restriction enzyme, is separated by size with agarose gel electrophoresis. The DNA bands are transferred by capillary action or "blotted" onto a nylon or nitrocellulose membrane and immobilized so that they will not come off even in liquid solutions (Figure 8–4A). The target DNA, now on the membrane, is chemically treated to permit access to probe DNA. At this point, probe DNA is added and hybridization is allowed to occur at the appropriate temperature. In this process, the double-stranded probe is first separated by boiling and then quickly added to the solution containing the membrane. The probe DNA seeks out sequences that are complementary to it and anneals to the target DNA bands immobilized on the membrane. Probe DNA is typically labeled with a radioisotope, or a fluorescent or chemiluminescent substrate. Following hybridization, the membrane is used to expose X-ray film (for radioisotope labeled DNA) or treated with appropriate reagents (for fluorescent or chemiluminescent labeled DNA) to develop the indicator on the probe. This permits visualization of the target bands among all the bands on the membrane (Figure 8–4).

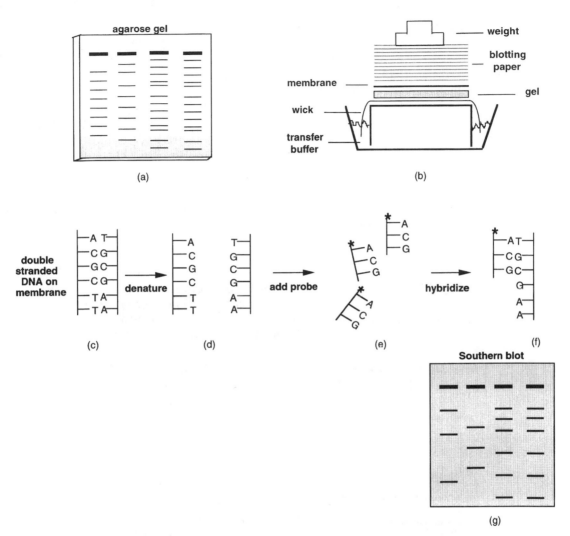

Figure 8–4 (a) Agarose gel electrophoresis. (b) Southern transfer of DNA from agarose gel to nylon membrane, steps involved in hybridization of probe DNA to target DNA on nylon membrane. Double-stranded DNA (c) is separated to the single-stranded form (d). Labeled probe (*) is added (e). Probe hybridizes to complementary DNA to form labeled dsDNA (f). Only bands from the agarose gel (a) with DNA sequence complementary to probe will hybridize. The hybridized Southern blot (g) shows target bands detected by labeled probe. *Source:* Copyright © 2000, Susan M. Harrington.

Polymerase Chain Reaction

Adapted successfully as a tool for the molecular epidemiologist, polymerase chain reaction (PCR) is a tool used to amplify short sequences from among a diverse DNA pool such as a bacterial chromosome. The limits of PCR are 5 to 10,000 bp sequences; beyond this amplification methods fail and other techniques are necessary to obtain large quantities of longer pieces of DNA. In a standard PCR reaction, two specific oligonucleotide primers are mixed with template

DNA. Oligonucleotides are very short segments of DNA, typically 15 to 30 bp in length. The template is the DNA that contains the sequences to be amplified. Template DNA is generated by lysing bacterial, fungal, or viral cells to release the genome. The oligonucleotides are chosen based on the target sequence to be amplified within the template DNA. One oligonucleotide primer is complementary to the top strand at one end of the target sequence and the second oligonucleotide is complementary to the bottom strand at the opposite end of the target sequence (Figure 8–5).

Polymerases are enzymes that facilitate DNA replication. Because PCR requires high and low temperatures, thermostable polymerases (e.g., the DNA polymerase enzyme from *Thermus aquaticus* [*Taq*]) are used to amplify the target

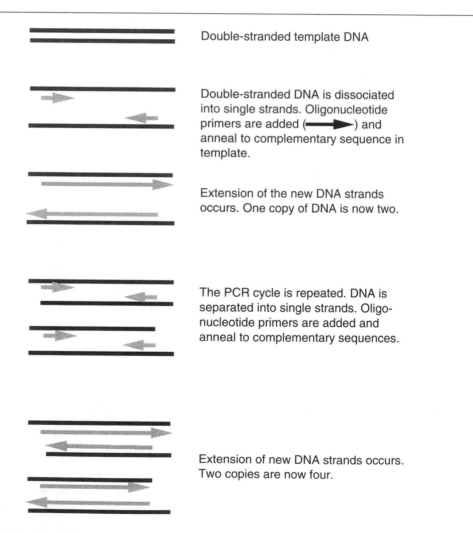

Double-stranded template DNA

Double-stranded DNA is dissociated into single strands. Oligonucleotide primers are added (━━►) and anneal to complementary sequence in template.

Extension of the new DNA strands occurs. One copy of DNA is now two.

The PCR cycle is repeated. DNA is separated into single strands. Oligonucleotide primers are added and anneal to complementary sequences.

Extension of new DNA strands occurs. Two copies are now four.

Figure 8–5 Polymerase chain reaction (PCR) amplification of template DNA. Two cycles of PCR are shown. Double-stranded DNA is separated into single strands. Primers anneal. New DNA strands are created through extension. Typical PCR reactions are 30 to 40 cycles long, creating millions of copies of double-stranded DNA.

sequence. A typical PCR reaction mix contains template DNA, oligonucleotide primers, *Taq* polymerase, Mg^{++}, deoxyribonucleotide triphosphate bases, and a suitable buffer. Approximately 30 cycles are usually conducted in which first the template DNA is dissociated by heating to 94°C. Annealing occurs by cooling to 55°C; at this stage, the oligonucleotides have an advantage because of their high concentration and they bind to the target more quickly than the original complementary strand. Finally, an extension phase occurs at 72°C where the *Taq* polymerase adds the correct nucleotides to the short primer oligonucleotide strand to create a new complementary strand. The result after 30 cycles of dissociation, annealing, and extension is a large amplification of the target sequence, namely, the sequence between the two oligonucleotide primers called the PCR product from the diverse and low concentration template DNA (Figure 8–5). The amplified PCR product DNA can then be analyzed by gel electrophoresis, restriction endonuclease analysis, or Southern hybridization.

A common application of PCR is the detection of microbial DNA in clinical specimens. PCR is particularly useful when the microbe of interest either grows slowly or cannot be cultivated by conventional techniques. PCR has the power to turn one copy of dsDNA into more than a billion copies. This power brings with it an important drawback. DNA from other samples or DNA from previous PCR reactions can contaminate the test, causing false-positive results. In recent years, a number of advancements in PCR methodologies have helped investigators minimize contamination. Most important among these is the physical separation of the steps involved. Processing, PCR reaction setup, and analysis of postamplification products are performed in different rooms. Protocols also exist that call for the addition of chemicals, photochemicals, and enzymes, which inactivate contaminating nucleic acids. Finally, laboratory technicians take particular care with technique, including working in biologic safety hoods, wearing gloves and gowns, cleaning surfaces, and using specialized equipment. With apprecia-

tion of the intricacies of the method, PCR is a robust and indispensable tool.

As typing methods are the focus of this chapter, the next section will examine how these techniques use frequent and infrequent cutting enzymes, PFGE, hybridization, and PCR to detect strain differences based on DNA sequence and restriction site specificities.

SPECIFIC TECHNIQUES OF MOLECULAR EPIDEMIOLOGY

In this section the methodologies of the most commonly used nucleic acid molecular methods are described. Strengths and weakness of each method and some examples are included. With the exception of DNA sequencing, all of these methods rely on visualization of DNA bands, whether they are from plasmids, restriction digests, hybridization, or PCR products. These banding patterns are the "DNA fingerprints" used to compare one isolate with another.[14]

Evaluation of Typing Systems

It is important to keep in mind that typing systems measure different biologic properties and perform with varying degrees of success depending on the organism and technical requirements. No one system is best for all species, although several newer methods can be applied to almost all bacterial species, especially those causing the majority of nosocomial outbreaks. As with other clinical laboratory methods, strain typing techniques must be carefully evaluated before they are used to answer epidemiologic questions. The specific question that needs to be answered may lead to the selection of one method over another.

To be widely useful, a typing system must give an interpretable result for every isolate of a given species. This is referred to as typeability. Plasmid analysis, one of the earliest typing methods, detects the extrachromosomal DNA of bacteria. However, not all strains within a species will contain plasmids, rendering them nontypeable by this method.

Additionally, reproducibility is a critical factor. An assay cannot be considered reliable if the same results are not obtained when an isolate is tested multiple times in the system. Some molecular methods are highly technique dependent in this sense. For example, the reaction conditions, reagents, and template DNA used in the arbitrary primed PCR reaction must be carefully standardized or a different result could be obtained with each run. Standardization is another important component. Interpretation of results is much more reliable when methods are performed in the same way from batch to batch.[9]

Discriminatory power is the ability of the typing technique to distinguish unrelated isolates from epidemiologically related strains. It is critical to include epidemiologically unrelated strains in the evaluation of new typing systems. Many methods are able to link closely clustered isolates; however, the more difficult aspect is to exclude unassociated strains. Often some isolates are found with a molecular link for which no epidemiologic link exists. The key is to minimize this phenomenon with the most powerful typing tool available.[9] It must also be understood that to some degree the ability to discriminate related from unrelated isolates is species dependent. For example, the number of different clones of methicillin resistant *S. aureus* is much more limited than for methicillin susceptible strains. This is a result of the way the methicillin resistance gene was acquired by some strains of the species.[15] The limited number of clones could cause one to falsely link strains that are truly unrelated. For methicillin resistant *S. aureus* it is important to compare isolates over a short time frame and to combine laboratory results with careful epidemiologic analysis.

The ease of interpretation or readability of DNA fingerprints varies. Some methods such as chromosomal restriction endonuclease analysis produce many bands that are difficult to distinguish because they are so close together. Faint or very bold bands can be equally difficult to discern. Interpretability can vary between methods or even between applications of a single method.

For example, in Southern hybridization methods one probe may yield a much more readable RFLP than another.

Issues of cost-effectiveness, ease of use, ease of interpretation, and turn-around time must also be considered. As molecular methods have become more discriminatory, they have required more expensive and sophisticated machinery, including PCR thermocyclers, PFGE equipment, DNA sequencers, and computer software for archiving data and comparing run-to-run results. The time to results for these powerful techniques may be from 1 or 2 days for PCR to a week for pulsed-field gel electrophoresis. The technical expertise needed to perform molecular techniques also varies from simple DNA extraction to lengthy hybridization procedures. Finally, interpretation of banding patterns and results is method dependent as well.

The choice of a typing method is dependent on all of these parameters; it will vary with the needs and capabilities of individual laboratories. As each method is presented, it will be evaluated based on these criteria.

Plasmid Analysis

As described, some bacterial strains harbor extrachromosomal DNA called plasmids. Plasmids are frequently found in the *Enterobacteriaceae* and in gram-positive organisms responsible for many nosocomial hospital infections such as *Staphylococci* and *Enterococci*. Analysis of plasmid DNA is one of the oldest of the nucleic acid–based methods for strain typing and has been used in the evaluation of many outbreaks.[16] Plasmids are easily extracted from bacterial cells in a process that takes only several hours. The plasmid preparation can then be evaluated by agarose gel electrophoresis to analyze the number and size of the plasmid(s) from each strain. Because plasmids are frequently present in bacterial cells and easily extracted for analysis with inexpensive electrophoresis equipment found in many laboratories, this method can easily be applied in many investigations.

Practically, some difficulties may be encountered when plasmid gel electrophoresis is performed. Plasmid DNA can range in size from just a few kilobases to almost 200 kb. The larger DNAs separate poorly, tending to bunch together at the top of the gel. Moreover, different plasmids of the same size could have different sequences, a characteristic unappreciated if size alone is evaluated. During extraction, the covalently closed, circular nature of plasmids is often disturbed, yielding nicked circular and linear forms. A single plasmid could appear as three bands by gel analysis, because these forms migrate differently in the gel. Hence, plasmid gels can have poor reproducibility and can be difficult to interpret. These problems can be overcome by cutting the plasmid DNA with a restriction enzyme. Often referred to as plasmid restriction enzyme analysis (REA), this method creates smaller, linear fragments that migrate faithfully according to size, and they are more easily interpreted. Restriction enzyme cutting is dependent on DNA sequence; therefore, REA can distinguish if single, large plasmids are the same in both DNA content and size. The number of REA bands will increase proportionately with the number of plasmids. However, as band number increases, interpretation becomes more difficult.

When applying this method, the variable nature of plasmids must be appreciated. Depending on the environment and the antibiotic resistance genes or virulence factors encoded by the plasmids that a bacterium harbors, plasmids can be gained or lost because of selective pressures. Hence, depending on what antibiotic therapy is in use, strains involved in an outbreak can evolve through changes in plasmid content even as the outbreak is being evaluated.[17] Movement of plasmids (or the transposable elements that they carry) between strains of the same species and even between species has been observed.[18,19] Thus, a plasmid epidemic could be observed.[20] Plasmid results must be evaluated carefully in comparison to the susceptibility profiles of the organisms isolated at the time of an outbreak.

Two other factors should be considered when using plasmid analysis. First, all strains will not give a result because some do not carry plasmids. Second, plasmid analysis focuses on only a small part of the genome, two bacterial strains can have the same plasmid content, but unique chromosomes. With all of this in mind, it is probably best to apply this typing technique to studies that are relatively limited in time span and to combine plasmid analysis with another method.

Restriction Endonuclease Analysis of Chromosomal DNA

Analysis of chromosomal DNA is an alternative to plasmid typing methods. The chromosome is the more stable genetic element, not subject to gain and loss as is the plasmid. A RFLP is produced by extracting the DNA and cutting with a restriction enzyme. Hundreds of fragments approximately 0.5 to 50 kb in length are produced, which are separated by gel electrophoresis. To produce these relatively small fragments "frequent cutting" restriction enzymes such as *Bam*HI, *Hind*III, and *Eco*RI are used. As with plasmid analysis, this method does not require specialized equipment. DNA can be extracted and restriction digested in just a few hours with minimal technical expertise. Gels are usually run overnight to achieve the best possible separation of bands. The major advantage to chromosomal REA is that with the correct selection of restriction enzyme all bacterial species are typeable. However, the large number of bands produced makes interpretation difficult. Multiple fragments can migrate together and very large bands can group together at the top of the gel.[10] Some investigators preferentially analyze the high molecular weight (top) portion of the gel, which is usually most interpretable.[21]

The extraction procedures used do not separate plasmid from chromosomal DNA. Two isolates with the same chromosome, but distinct plasmids, could have slightly different patterns. Although largely replaced by newer methods, chromosomal REA has continued to be of value especially for nosocomial outbreaks of *Clostridium difficile*.[10,21]

RFLP Analysis Using REA with Southern Hybridization

The interpretability of chromosomal REA has been improved with the addition of nucleic acid probes targeted to specific multicopy genes, insertion sequences, or mobile genetic elements such as transposons. First, DNA cut with a frequent cutting restriction enzyme is separated in agarose as described above. The DNA fragments are transferred from agarose to a membrane by the Southern blot technique. The DNA fragments immobilized on the membrane can then be hybridized with a nucleic acid probe. Only a small portion (ideally 10 to 20) of the thousands of restriction fragments will have specificity for the probe and will be detected. This is the technique referred to as restriction fragment length polymorphism. RFLP detects the number of copies of sequence homologous to the probe and reflects the size of the restriction fragments containing those sequences. The number of bands will be proportional to the number of copies of the target as long as the target does not contain a restriction site. When a single restriction site is present within the target sequence, the probe will hybridize along both sides of the restriction site and two bands will be produced for each copy of target. Several probes are most commonly used for RFLP typing; however, theoretically, any repetitive sequence with species specificity can work. For example, the *mec* gene, which encodes methicillin resistance, and Tn554, a transposon, have both been used as probes of chromosomal digests for *S. aureus*.[15,22] Other types of probes have included insertion sequences, toxin production genes, and even random chromosomal sequences.[12] However, most of these probes are specific to only a single species and sometimes only to strains within a species carrying the gene of interest.

Ribotyping is a popular approach, almost universally applicable to all bacterial species. Ribo-

somal RNA or DNA homologous to the ribosomal operon is used as the probe. The ribosomal operon, which encodes the rRNA transcripts essential to make a ribosome, is highly conserved within bacterial species and is usually present in multiple copies in the chromosome. Organisms such as *E. coli* and *Klebsiella* and *Staphylococcus* species have from five to seven copies of this element, producing easily interpreted, ribotype patterns with 10 to 15 bands.[23] In a study comparing 12 typing methods for *S. aureus*, ribotyping was highly sensitive, identifying all outbreak-associated strains. However, as demonstrated in this study, unrelated isolates are sometimes grouped with an outbreak strain.[22]

Although ribotyping uses a commercially available standardized probe, the choice of restriction enzyme is not standardized. In fact, the most discriminatory enzyme varies between species. An increase in discrimination can be obtained by combining the results with two or more enzymes.[22] Although ribotyping results are easily interpreted and very reproducible, other more discriminatory methods are now available for many organisms.[24,25]

Ribotyping is not of value for strain delineation of *M. tuberculosis* because only one copy of the ribosomal operon is present. Several repetitive elements have been studied as probes for RFLP.[26,27] Currently, the method of choice proposed by van Embden et al. uses IS6110, an insertion sequence present in 1 to approximately 20 copies in *M. tuberculosis* complex organisms, to probe *Pvu*II digested genomic DNA.[28] This method has been applied in many studies, including transmission in large cities and HIV infected populations, epidemiology between nations, laboratory contamination, and outbreaks.[29–33] Figure 8–6 is an example of an IS6110-probed Southern blot *of M. tuberculosis*. Matched pairs are found in lanes 6 and 7, as well as in lanes 8 and 9. Lanes 1 and 10 contain a well-characterized *M. tuberculosis* strain that is included as a molecular weight marker. Inclusion of a bacterium as a marker instead of purchasing one commercially is highly desirable. Not only does using a live organism serve as a

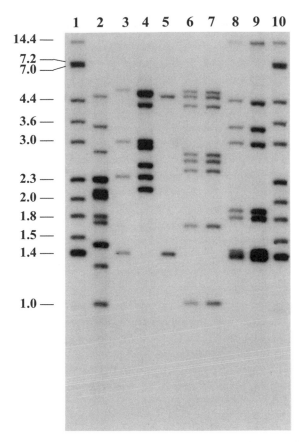

Figure 8–6 Restriction fragment length polymorphism of *Mycobacterium tuberculosis* with IS6110 probe. **Lanes 2 to 9** contain clinical isolates. **Lanes 1 and 10** are the molecular weight marker Mt 14323. Molecular weights are shown in kilobase pairs.

determiner of molecular size, it is also a useful extraction control. To be confident of the extraction process in the laboratory, every time this strain is extracted and cut with the indicated restriction enzyme, the same number and size of bands must be obtained.

Rarely, *M. tuberculosis* or related organisms will lack IS6110. Most of these strains have come from cases in Southeast Asia. Additionally, up to 25% of isolates have less than six IS6110 bands.[34] Isolates with low band numbers are shown in lanes 3 and 5 of Figure 8–6. It follows that the fewer bands, the less reliable is

the discrimination. For IS6110 typing or for other methods, isolates with few bands should be repeated with a second probe or by another procedure.

Ribotyping and other RFLP techniques generally produce interpretable banding patterns that are highly reproducible. An advantage of these tests is that they do not require a lot of expensive equipment. However, they may take up to a week to perform and require considerable technical expertise. An automated ribotyping instrument, The Riboprinter (Qualicon), is now available. Up to 32 organisms can be typed in a single day.

However, the cost of the instrument and associated reagents is prohibitive for most laboratories.

Pulsed-Field Gel Electrophoresis

First described in 1984 by Schwartz and Cantor, pulsed-field gel electrophoresis is one of the most widely used and discriminatory typing techniques.[13] Developed to separate large DNA molecules, PFGE is ideal for electrophoresis of the fragments created by digestion of a genomic DNA extract with infrequent cutting restriction enzymes. Optimally, 10 to 20 bands are produced. A major strength of PFGE is that probes and Southern blotting usually are not needed. The low number of bands can be visualized by staining followed by Polaroid photography.

With the appropriate restriction enzyme, PFGE can be used to type most bacteria and a number of fungal species. Rarely, DNA from isolates will be degraded and an uninterpretable pattern will result. This has been observed for *C. difficile*.[21] As with all strain typing methods, no one restriction enzyme is considered standard. Choice of restriction enzyme depends on the percent GC content of the organism, as previously described. Some enzymes inherently work better than others do. A review of the literature is helpful before spending time in trial-and-error choosing a restriction enzyme for a particular species. Lists of organisms and restriction enzymes used for PFGE have been published.[8,12]

Fungi have multiple individual chromosomes that vary in size. These can be extracted for separation as whole chromosomes or cut with restriction enzymes. Both the number and size of chromosomes can also vary within a particular fungal species. Separation of such intact chromosomes generates a type of fingerprint referred to as an electrophoretic karyotype. Interpreting karyotypes can be difficult if the chromosomes migrate closely to one another. Some investigators digest these DNAs with restriction enzymes, yielding smaller, more distinguishable bands.[35,36]

Probably, PFGE is the method most frequently used for outbreak investigations involv-

ing common nosocomial pathogens. It has been shown to be highly discriminatory in outbreaks caused by many organisms such as *Staphylococcus, Candida, E. coli, Enterococcus,* and *Enterobacter*.[37–40] Figure 8–7 shows some examples of vancomycin resistant *Enterococcus faecium* (VRE) from a hospital ICU outbreak. A total of 13 VRE were isolated from patient cultures over a 5-week period. Seven of these were characterized as belonging to the outbreak cluster. Lanes 2 to 4 in Figure 8–7 are indistinguishable outbreak isolates. The VRE isolate in lane 5 was considered a clonally related strain within the outbreak because it has only two bands different from the main outbreak strain. Lane 6 contains an environmental strain isolated from the surface of an intravenous machine. Because it shares many bands with the outbreak strain, this strain is also possibly related to the outbreak cluster. The strains in lane 7 and 8 are from patients unrelated to the outbreak. It was believed that these two patients were colonized before admission. The isolate in lane 9 was recovered 4 months after the outbreak; its banding pattern suggests that it is a progeny isolate that has diverged from the outbreak strain. The end lanes contain *Not*I-digested *E. faecalis* (ATCC 47077) as a molecular weight marker.[8]

Because PFGE fingerprints are highly reproducible, interpretation is fairly straightforward. However, interpretation can become time consuming when several isolates, which differ by only a few bands, are compared as illustrated in Figure 8–7. When many isolates are compared, it is often necessary to run those with similar fingerprint patterns side-by-side on the same gel. Some investigators are using computer databases and analysis software to compare large numbers of strains run on multiple gels. It should be kept in mind, however, that no software can substitute for visual comparison of isolates run in adjacent lanes.

In addition to the expense of the PFGE apparatus, the total time required to perform the test is a disadvantage of this method. DNA extraction procedures take approximately 2 to 3 days, although more rapid methods have been devel-

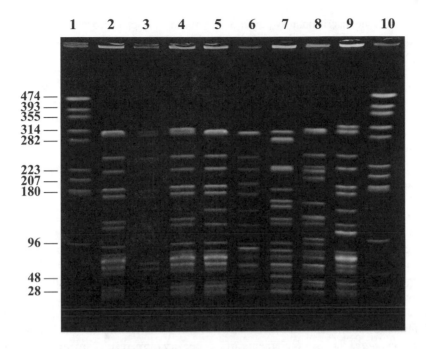

Figure 8–7 Pulsed-field gel electrophoresis of vancomycin resistant *Enterococcus faecium*. **Lanes 2 to 5, 7, and 8** are patient isolates recovered during an outbreak in an ICU. **Lane 6** contains an isolate cultured from the surface of an IV machine. **Lane 9** is a strain isolated 4 months later. The molecular weight marker, *Not*I-digested *E. faecalis* ATCC 47077, is in lanes **1 and 10**. Molecular weights are in kilobase pairs.

oped.[41] The electrophoresis time is also lengthy; 24 hours is a typical running time, and a fair amount of technical expertise is necessary. To prevent mechanical breakage of chromosomal DNA, all extraction steps must be carefully performed with preparations embedded in agarose.

PCR-Based Methods

All of the methods presented to this point need a fairly large amount of DNA for gel electrophoresis. PCR-based strain typing techniques require only a small amount of DNA from the clinical isolate. In addition, DNA from organisms that cannot be grown by conventional culture methods can be amplified and used to delineate strain differences. Compared with RFLP and PFGE, PCR fingerprinting is rapid with results available within a day.

Three basic variations of PCR fingerprinting have been described. The first, PCR-RFLP, uses PCR to amplify known variable regions of the genome. A restriction endonuclease is then used to digest these PCR products, yielding several smaller DNA fragments. For example, in a method called Vir typing, the gene for the antiphagocytic M protein in *Streptococcus pyogenes* is amplified and digested with *Hae*III, producing an RFLP.[42] The DNA fragments are visualized by conventional gel electrophoresis. No hybridization or PFGE equipment is needed. Species-specific virulence genes such as the M protein gene of *S. pyogenes*, the coagulase gene of *S. aureus*,[43] or genes coding for rRNA have been useful for this method. However, the requirement for a known variable genetic region limits applicability. Only well-characterized regions specific to a given species will be discriminatory. Hence, the discriminatory power of PCR-RFLP varies, depending on the organism and the gene being amplified. This method does, however, generate easily interpreted, reproducible fingerprints.[9]

The second method, repetitive element PCR or rep-PCR, uses PCR to amplify regions between known sequences. Oligonucleotide primers homologous to the ends of sequences that are present in multiple copies prime PCR reactions to amplify the sequences between repeats. Repetitive sequences may be spaced somewhat randomly throughout the chromosome. It follows that the DNA fragment lengths between the repetitive elements are also variable. Amplification of the sequences between the repeats, therefore, produces a range of fragment lengths or a DNA fingerprint. The repetitive extrapalindromic sequences of *E. coli* (rep), the enterobacterial repetitive intergenic consensus (ERIC) elements of *Enterobacteriaceae*, the BOX elements of gram-positive bacteria and regions between ribosomal RNA genes are some of the repetitive elements used for this technique.[12,44] Applicable to many bacterial species, rep-PCR is a discriminatory method. Discriminatory power can be enhanced with multiple primer sets.[45]

Arbitrary primed PCR (AP-PCR) or random amplified polymorphic DNA (RAPD) is the third PCR fingerprinting technique. A single, short oligonucleotide primer (8 to 10 bp) is designed with random sequences. The number of recognition sites for this primer in the template DNA is not generally known. PCR is performed at a low annealing temperature to facilitate binding of oligonucleotide to the template in the regions that may lack perfect sequence homology. When primers anneal sufficiently close to each other (within ~1 kb), in the correct orientation and on opposite DNA strands, amplification of the region between the arbitrary primers takes place. These primers will anneal at random locations throughout the template. As with rep-PCR, products of various sizes will result. The PCR products can be separated by gel electrophoresis yielding a fingerprint pattern.[46] An advantage of this method is that no sequence infor-

mation about the organism is required. Many bacterial species, fungi, and some parasites have been typed successfully with AP-PCR.[45] An example of a RAPD fingerprint pattern is given in Figure 8–8.

Whereas typeability is excellent for this method, batch-to-batch reproducibility is sometimes poor. Alteration in concentration of primers, template DNA, *Taq*, or Mg[++] will influence results. Different lots of *Taq* or primer, or use of a different thermocycler, can affect fingerprints, as can contamination with a product from a previous run. Frequently, nonspecific bands will be produced when any of these variables are changed. To show if nonspecific bands are present, inclusion of a control tube that lacks template DNA is recommended. This sample should not have any visualized bands. Although a strength of AP-PCR is its ability to type strains with a small amount of nucleic acid that may not be very pure, results are much more reproducible if DNA is used at a standardized quantity and of fairly high quality.[44] Unfortunately, quantification and DNA purification increase the technical difficulty and time required to perform this test.

In general, AP-PCR is a more rapid method and is less technically demanding than RFLP or PFGE because fewer steps are involved. However, AP-PCR can be more difficult to interpret than either RFLP or PFGE. The bands seen on AP-PCR gels generally vary in intensity, depending on reaction conditions, the ability of the arbitrary primers to anneal to template, and the efficiency of the elongation step. AP-PCR is probably best used with relatively small numbers of isolates compared within the same run on the same day.[9,19] A number of studies have demonstrated AP-PCR to have discriminatory power similar to PFGE and better than some other methods. Multiple primer sets have been used to increase discrimination.[47]

None of the PCR-based methods are standardized. Various primers, whether for arbitrary or intergenic amplification, and different restriction enzymes have been used for strain typing. However, because of so much run-to-run variability, interlaboratory comparisons are not ad-

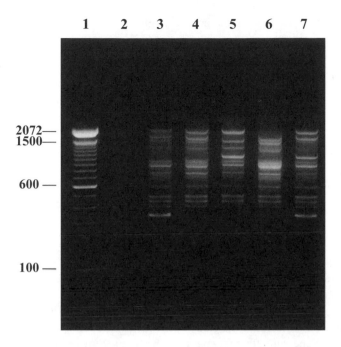

Figure 8–8 Arbitrary primed polymerase chain reaction of *Penicillium marnefii*. **Lanes 3 to 7** contain isolates showing different banding patterns. **Lane 2** is a control which lacked template DNA. **Lane 1** is the 100 base pair DNA ladder (Gibco BRL). Molecular weights are given in base pairs. Courtesy of Sharon Howat.

vised. Therefore, standardized methods for comparison are less important than with other applications.[44]

DNA Sequencing

DNA sequencing is an emerging strain typing method. Well-characterized genes or DNA sequences, which are relatively variable, are PCR amplified. Following amplification, the nucleotide sequences (i.e., the order of the A, T, C, G bases) are determined by gel electrophoresis with an automated sequencing instrument. The nucleotide sequences can then be aligned to find base differences between isolates. DNA sequence typing has been described for some bacteria and for HIV-1.[9] For example, the protein A gene of *S. aureus* contains a variable number of 24 bp repeats that can be determined by DNA sequencing. Haefnagels-Schuermans et al.

evaluated strain difference based on protein A variability. However, the discriminatory power was low.[48] Future application of this method depends on identification of appropriate variable regions for sequencing and availability of expensive automated sequencers. The role of DNA sequencing in molecular epidemiology remains to be seen.[9]

Interpretation of Results

As molecular typing methods have been described, the interpretability or readability of the fingerprint has also been discussed. This is not the same as the interpretation of results. With the exception of DNA sequencing, all of these methods produce a DNA fingerprint, or banding pattern, for each isolate. As the fingerprints are compared, the similarity or differences between them must be evaluated. All of the bands from an isolate are compared with those in the other lanes on the gel.

The simplest comparison is that of two isolates having the same DNA fingerprint. These are more accurately described as "indistinguishable" rather than identical. Each of the molecular typing methods evaluates only a portion of the genome (i.e., restriction endonuclease sites, a specific gene, or amplified sequence). It is impossible to say that two microorganisms are exact clones based on these types of tests. Clearly, mutations in the genome will occur that will not be detected by these methods. At the opposite end of the spectrum, it is fairly easy to decide that two isolates having vastly different fingerprints are not clonally related. The difficult interpretations are those in which isolates vary by just a few bands. Such strains may be related to each other, but how closely?

The relative relatedness of organisms can be expressed in terms of the number of genetic events or changes to the chromosome that occur from one generation to the next. For example, two organisms that demonstrate changes in the chromosome produced by one genetic event may be categorized as "probably related." Strains that differ by two genetic events are characterized as "possibly related." Isolates differing by three or more genetic events are most likely "unrelated." It seems reasonable to categorize strains based on these definitions of relative relatedness.[8] However, it is much more difficult to decide the number of fingerprint band differences that place strains into these categories. Tenover et al. present a detailed discussion of molecular typing methods and the way in which mutations affect banding patterns.[19] Additionally, the way in which changes in fingerprint patterns are evaluated varies widely between laboratories.

Some interpretive criteria used by investigators in molecular epidemiology can be found in the literature. The guidelines for PFGE have probably been those most widely applied. One genetic change would cause up to a three-band difference between two isolates. Hence, isolates with one- to three-band differences are probably related. Two genetic events would alter the PFGE pattern by anywhere from four to six bands. Strains with four- to six-band differences are possibly related. Unrelated strains differ by more than six bands. Most investigators evaluating strain typing data in an outbreak will designate the most common type by a letter or number, i.e., strain A. Isolates which differ from A by one to three bands are subtypes of A. Isolates with more than three band differences are given new letter designations. In practice, as many fingerprints are compared, categorizing strains which "may be related" becomes complex. For example, two isolates may each be subtypes of strain A and vary from one another by more than four bands. These subtype strains would represent new type strains B and C if evaluated apart from the type A strain. This emphasizes the importance of evaluating strain types over a limited time period relative to an outbreak. Differences between epidemiologically unrelated strains will occur randomly. Two such strains could, therefore, have only minor molecular differences and be grouped as subtypes if no epidemiologic information is considered. Hence, interpretive guidelines can give misleading information if applied in a larger context without epidemiologic data.[8]

These interpretive criteria are valid for PFGE because the whole chromosome is assessed. For other typing systems, interpretation is less easily defined. Many genetic events can occur which will not be detected. For example, substitution mutations of DNA that do not alter restriction sites or target areas for probes will not be detected by RFLP methods.[19] Although no standard approach to RFLP interpretation has been proposed, some investigators have designated isolates with one-band differences subtypes of one another. Isolates with two or more band differences represent new strain types.[22]

For rep-PCR and AP-PCR, no standard approach is found for analyzing minor differences in band patterns such as changes in intensity or a one-band size shift. Frequently, a second set of PCR primers is used to see if similar results are consistently obtained. Any mutational event may be responsible for the alterations seen in PCR fingerprints if that mutation occurs at a primer binding site. Additionally, insertions or deletions of DNA between primer binding sites will alter the banding pattern. However, all mutations will not be detected by this method. In a manner similar to interpretation of RFLP, isolates having a one-band difference by PCR fingerprinting may be considered subtypes of each other. PCR patterns having two or more bands different are generally categorized as different strains.[19,49]

Plasmid analysis strains with three or more plasmids that are the same by gel electrophoresis are considered indistinguishable. Confidence in the discriminatory ability of this method declines if fewer than three plasmids are present. Although strains containing only one identical plasmid have been helpful in elucidating outbreaks, better discrimination can also be achieved with plasmid REA.[19]

Computer-Assisted Analysis

Sometimes the epidemiologist needs to compare isolates in large populations or over a lengthy period of time. This circumstance requires between-gel comparisons, which cannot be done without strict standardization of the method (i.e., the same DNA extraction procedure, electrophoresis conditions, molecular weight standards, and so on). Computer system assistance is also very helpful. Such systems allow gels, photographs, or autoradiographic images to be scanned and stored as digitized files. A molecular size standard with a well-characterized pattern is included in the two end lanes and often in the middle of every gel. The bands in the other lanes are then "normalized" to the standard to account for variability between gels. Depending on the computer program, either band sizes or band positions relative to the standard are stored for subsequent comparisons. Analysis software finds bands automatically, but allows the user the flexibility to add, delete, or move bands after visual inspection. Within-gel and between-gel band matching can then be accom-

plished as desired. The user can also set deviation or percent tolerance for matching around each band, which further minimizes within-gel and between-gel differences and enhances strain matching. The microprocessors use various numerical indices (e.g., Dice coefficients) to assign percent similarities to selected isolates. Finally, graphical representation of strain relatedness can be accomplished in the form of dendrograms based on several grouping methods (e.g., UPGMA, neighbor joining). A dendrogram links isolates according to percent similarity in a manner similar to a phylogenetic tree. Currently, three popular computer fingerprinting systems are available: Dendron (Solltech, Inc., Oakdale, IA), Whole Band Analysis (BioImage, Ann Arbor, MI), and GelCompar or Molecular Analyst Fingerprinting Plus (Biorad Laboratories, Hercules, CA). Each of these systems is unique but each performs the basic functions outlined.[50]

When done in a rigorously standardized fashion, fingerprinting software allows the user to accomplish many comparisons that would otherwise be very time consuming. Computerized analysis does have limitations, however. Although these systems can correct for differences that arise between gels, they do so imperfectly. They are unable to correct for great variability. The degree of matching is determined by the percent deviation around the bands selected by the operator. Overmatching or undermatching can occur, depending on this setting. Because the systems use mathematical methods to match strains, isolate 1 may match perfectly to isolate 2 and isolate 3, but isolates 2 and 3 may not match each other at 100% similarity. However, all three of these may be grouped together in a mathematical cluster. Such cluster analysis must be carefully interpreted. It is best to allow the computer program to find strains that are closely related and then run these strains on the same gel in adjacent lanes. Visual inspection of banding patterns is often better to determine relatedness than computer software. Finally, dendrograms must also be interpreted with caution. The tree structure is highly dependent on the grouping method chosen and can lead to false conclusions. Some grouping methods give different tree structures, depending on the order in which strains are added to the tree. Distance between strains on the tree may be relative, not absolute. It is probably best to use dendrograms only as graphical representations of large groupings of strains. The distance between individual isolates or small clusters should not be interpreted as representative of genetic distance.

In summary, computer software is very helpful in archiving fingerprint data from a large number of strains. Although computer systems can be good at finding similar or matching indistinguishable isolates in the database, closer comparison should be done by testing related isolates on the same gel.

CONCLUSION

Before strain typing is initiated, epidemiologic investigations should always start with simple questions based on current case findings and microbiology. Controls known to be epidemiologically unrelated to cases should be included to ensure adequate discrimination and the most appropriate strain typing method for that species applied. The method chosen will also depend on the epidemiologic question to be answered and practical issues such as cost, ease-of-use, equipment availability, and time to results. By definition, different typing methods measure different biological properties, and they sometimes group isolates differently, which is to be expected. For this reason, a combination of molecular tests is sometimes utilized. This can be in the form of two different primers for RAPDs, two different restriction enzymes for PFGE, two RFLP probes, or two different methods altogether.

Currently, PFGE- and PCR-based tests have the highest discriminatory power for strain de-

lineation of most common nosocomial pathogens and many fungal species. They have largely replaced plasmid fingerprinting, chromosomal REA, and even ribotyping. Exceptions exist, however, such as for *M. tuberculosis* where IS6110 RFLP is the recommended method. Unfortunately, high equipment costs and the need for technical expertise render the most discriminatory methods unsuitable for small laboratories. However, a number of larger hospitals and academic centers are offering fingerprinting services on a per isolate basis.

Molecular strain typing has truly advanced the field of infectious disease epidemiology. As part of a classic epidemiologic investigation, molecular epidemiology has been used to determine the source of an outbreak and distinguish cases from noncases. Potential sources of infection (e.g., fomites or the environment) can be surveyed during an outbreak. Pathogens recovered can then be analyzed with these methods to determine any links to patient infections. Molecular methods are now considered standard to ongoing infectious disease outbreak investigations. Additionally, strain typing has been used to answer clinical questions such as if therapy should be altered because of relapse of an infection or if a new strain or resistance gene was acquired. Whether multiple isolates of the same species are indistinguishable or represent various contaminants has also been a recent application of these methods.

The future of DNA fingerprinting is exciting. Many genome sequencing projects are under way. As detailed DNA sequence information is published, the structure and function of many more genetic elements may be determined. This information will likely be useful for the rapid assessment of strain differences, which should have even more impact on intervention and outcomes.

REFERENCES

1. La Scola B, Fournier P, Musso D, et al. Pseudo-outbreak of listeriosis elucidated by pulsed-field gel electrophoresis. *Eur J Clin Microbiol Infect Dis.* 1997:756–760.

2. Michele T, Cronin W, Graham N, et al. Transmission of *Mycobacterium tuberculosis* by a fiberoptic bronchoscope. *JAMA.* 1997; 278:1093–1095.

3. Spika J, Waterman S, Soo Hoo G, et al. Chloramphenicol-resistant *Salmonella newport* traced through hamburger to dairy farms. *New Engl J Med.* 1987; 316:565–570.

4. Sader H, Jones R, Pfaller M. Relapse of catheter-related *Flavobacterium meningosepticum* bacteremia demonstrated by DNA macrorestriction analysis. *Clin Infect Dis.* 1995; 21:997–1000.

5. Bishai W, Graham N, Harrington S, et al. Rifampin-resistant tuberculosis in a patient receiving rifabutin prophylaxis. *N Engl J Med.* 1996; 334:1573–1576.

6. Zaidi A, Harrell L, Rost J, et al. Assessment of similarity among coagulase-negative staphylococci from sequential blood cultures of neonates and children by pulsed-field gel electrophoresis. *J Infect Dis.* 1996; 174:1010–1014.

7. Hartstein A, Valvano M, Morthland V, et al. Antimicrobic susceptibility and plasmid profile analysis as identity tests for multiple blood isolates of coagulase-negative staphylococci. *J Clin Microbiol.* 1987; 25:589–593.

8. Tenover F, Arbeit R, Goering R, et al. Interpreting chromosomal DNA restriction patterns produced by pulsed field gel electrophoresis: criteria for bacterial strain typing. *J Clin Microbiol.* 1995; 33:2233–2239.

9. Arbeit R. Laboratory procedures for the epidemiologic analysis of microorganisms. In: Murray P, Jo Baron E, Pfaller M, et al., eds. *Manual of Clinical Microbiology.* 6th ed. Washington, DC: ASM Press; 1995:190–208.

10. Maslow J, Mulligan M, Arbeit R. Molecular epidemiology: application of contemporary techniques to the typing microorganisms. *Clin Infect Dis.* 1993; 17:153–164.

11. Maniatis T. *Molecular Cloning: A Laboratory Manual.* Sambrook J, Fritsch E, Maniatis T, eds. Cold Spring Harbor: Cold Spring Harbor Laboratory Press; 1989.

12. Persing D. *Diagnostic Molecular Microbiology Procedures and Applications.* Persing D, Smith T, Tenover F, et al., eds. Rochester, MN: Mayo Foundation; 1993.

13. Schwartz D, Cantor C. Separation of yeast chromosome-sized DNAs by pulsed field gradient gel electrophoresis. *Cell.* 1984; 37:67–75.

14. Pfaller M, Herwaldt L. The clinical microbiology laboratory and infection control: emerging pathogens, antimicrobial resistance, and new technology. *Clin Infect Dis.* 1997; 25:858–870.

15. Kreiswirth B, Kornblum J, Arbeit R, et al. Evidence for a clonal origin of methicillin resistance in *Staphylococcus aureus. Science.* 1993; 259:227 230.

16. Mayer L. Use of plasmid profiles in epidemiologic surveillance of disease outbreaks and in tracing the transmission of antibiotic resistance. *Clin Microbiol Rev.* 1988; 1:228–243.

17. Locksley R, Cohen M, Quinn T, et al. Multiply antibiotic-resistant *Staphylococcus aureus*: introduction, transmission, and evolution of nosocomial infection. *Ann Intern Med.* 1982; 97:317–324.

18. Rubens C, Farrar W, McGee Z, et al. Evolution of a plasmid mediating resistance to multiple antimicrobial agents during a prolonged epidemic of nosocomial infections. *J Infect Dis.* 1981; 143:170–181.

19. Tenover F, Arbeit R, Goering R. How to select and interpret molecular strain typing methods for epidemiological studies of bacterial infections: a review for healthcare epidemiologists. Molecular Typing Working Group of the Society for Healthcare Epidemiology of America. *Infect Control Hosp Epidemiol.* 1997; 18:426–439.

20. Tompkins L, Plorde J, Falkow S. Molecular analysis of R-factors from multiresistant nosocomial isolates. *J Infect Dis.* 1980; 141:625–636.

21. Kristjansson M, Samore M, Gerding D, et al. Comparison of restriction endonuclease analysis, ribotyping, and pulsed-field gel electrophoresis for molecular differentiation of *Clostridium difficile* strains. *J Clin Microbiol.* 1994; 32:1963–1969.

22. Tenover F, Arbeit R, Archer R, et al. Comparison of traditional and molecular methods of typing isolates of *Staphylococcus aureus. J Clin Microbiol.* 1994; 32:407–415.

23. Hinojosa-Ahumada M, Swaminathan B, Hunter S, et al. Restriction fragment length polymorphisms in rRNA operons for subtyping *Shigella sonnei. J Clin Microbiol.* 1991; 29:2380–2384.

24. Gordillo M, Singh K, Murray B. Comparison of ribotyping and pulsed-field gel electrophoresis for subspecies differentiation of strains of *Enterococcus faecalis. J Clin Microbiol.* 1993; 31:1570–1574.

25. Martin I, Tyler S, Tyler K, et al. Evaluation of ribotyping as epidemiologic tool for typing *Escherichia coli* serogroup O157 isolates. *J Clin Microbiol.* 1996; 34:720–723.

26. van Soolingen D, Hermans P, de Haas P, et al. Occurrence and stability of insertion sequences in *Mycobacterium tuberculosis* complex strains: evaluation of an insertion sequence-dependent DNA polymorphism as a tool in the epidemiology of tuberculosis. *J Clin Microbiol.* 1991; 29:2578–2586.

27. van Soolingen D, de Haas W, Petra E, et al. Comparison of various repetitive DNA elements as genetic markers for strain differentiation and epidemiology of *Mycobacterium tuberculosis. J Clin Microbiol.* 1993; 31:1987–1995.

28. van Embden J, Cave M, Crawford J, et al. Strain identification of *Mycobacterium tuberculosis* by DNA fingerprinting: recommendations for a standardized methodology. *J Clin Microbiol.* 1993; 31:406–409.

29. Small P, Hopewell P, Singh S, et al. The epidemiology

of tuberculosis in San Francisco. *N Engl J Med.* 1994; 330:1703–1709.

30. Alland D, Kalkut G, Moss A, et al. Transmission of tuberculosis in New York City. *N Engl J Med.* 1994:1710–1716.

31. Yang Z, Mtoni I, Chonde M, et al. DNA fingerprinting and phenotyping of *Mycobacterium tuberculosis* isolate from human immunodeficiency virus (HIV)-seropositive and HIV-seronegative patients in Tanzania. *J Clin Microbiol.* 1995; 33:1064–1069.

32. Yang Z, de Haas P, van Soolingen D, et al. Restriction fragment length polymorphism of *Mycobacterium tuberculosis* strains isolated from Greenland during 1992: evidence of tuberculosis transmission between Greenland and Denmark. *J Clin Microbiol.* 1994; 32:3018–3025.

33. Small P, McClenny N, Singh S, et al. Molecular strain typing of *Mycobacterium tuberculosis* to confirm cross-contamination in the mycobacteriology laboratory and modification of procedures to minimize occurrence of false-positive cultures. *J Clin Microbiol.* 1993; 31: 1677–1682.

34. Burman W, Reves R, Hawkes A, et al. DNA fingerprinting with two probes decreases clustering of *Mycobacterium tuberculosis. Am J Respir Crit Care Med.* 1997; 155:1140–1146.

35. King D, Rhine-Chalberg J, Pfaller M, et al. Comparison of four DNA-based methods for strain delineation of *Candida lusitaniae. J Clin Microbiol.* 1995; 33:1467–1470.

36. Merz W. *Candida albicans* strain delineation. *Clin Microbiol Rev.* 1990; 3:321–334.

37. Roman R, Smith J, Walker M, et al. Rapid geographic spread of a methicillin-resistant *Staphylococcus aureus* strain. *Clin Infect Dis.* 1997; 25:698–705.

38. Diekema D, Messer S, Hollis R, et al. An outbreak of *Candida parapsilosis* prosthetic valve endocarditis. *Diagn Microbiol Infect Dis.* 1997; 29:147–153.

39. Keene W, Sazie E, Kok J, et al. An outbreak of *Escherichia coli* O157:H7 infections traced to jerky made from deer meat. *JAMA.* 1997; 277:1229–1231.

40. Shi Z, Liu P, Lau Y, et al. Epidemiological typing of isolates from an outbreak of infection with multidrug-resistant *Enterobacter cloacae* by repetitive extragenic palindromic unit b1-primed PCR and pulsed-field gel electrophoresis. *J Clin Microbiol.* 1996; 34:2784–2790.

41. Matushek M, Bonten M, Hayden M. Rapid preparation of bacterial DNA for pulsed-field gel electrophoresis. *J Clin Microbiol.* 1996; 34:2598–2600.

42. Hartas J, Hibble M, Sriprakash K. Simplification of a locus-specific DNA typing method (vir typing) for *Streptococcus pyogenes. J Clin Microbiol.* 1998; 36: 1428–1429.

43. Goh S, Byrne S, Zhang J, et al. Molecular typing of *Staphylococcus aureus* on the basis of coagulase gene polymorphisms. *J Clin Microbiol.* 1992; 30:1642–1645.

44. Tyler K, Wang G, Tyler S, et al. Factors affecting reliability and reproducibility of amplification-based DNA fingerprinting of representative bacterial pathogens. *J Clin Microbiol.* 1997; 35:339–346.

45. van Belkum A. DNA fingerprinting of medically important microorganisms by use of PCR. *Clin Microbiol Rev.* 1994; 7:174–184.

46. Welsh J, McClelland M. Fingerprinting genomes using PCR with arbitrary primers. *Nucleic Acids Res.* 1990; 18:7213–7218.

47. van Belkum A, Kluytmans J, van Leeuwen W, et al. Multicenter evaluation of arbitrarily primed PCR for typing of *Staphylococcus aureus* strains. *J Clin Microbiol.* 1995; 33:1537–1547.

48. Haefnagels-Schuermans A, Peetermans W, Struelens M, et al. Clonal analysis and identification of epidemic strains of methicillin-resistant *Staphylococcus aureus* by antibiotyping and determination of protein A gene and coagulase gene polymorphisms. *J Clin Microbiol.* 1997; 35:2514–2520.

49. Woods C Jr, Versalovic J, Koeuth T, et al. Analysis of relationships among isolates of *Citrobacter diversus* by using DNA fingerprinting generated by repetitive sequence-based primers in the polymerase chain reaction. *J Clin Microbiol.* 1992; 30:2921–2929.

50. Gerner-Smidt P, Graves L, Hunter S, et al. Computerized analysis of restriction fragment length polymorphism patterns: comparative evaluation of two commercial software packages. *J Clin Microbiol.* 1998; 36: 1318–1323.

CHAPTER 9

Geographic Information Systems

Gregory E. Glass

A common definition of geographic information systems (GIS) is that they are procedures to input, store, retrieve, manipulate, analyze, and output data that have spatial attributes associated with them.[1] Typically, the results are presented as maps or images that summarize the data or analyses performed on the data. Infectious disease epidemiology, almost by the very nature of the interaction of hosts and the pathogens within the environment (as well as vector and reservoir populations with vector-borne and zoonotic diseases), lends itself to GIS, at least as a way to summarize the sometimes complex relationships associated with disease transmission.

Snow's classic study of cholera transmission around Broad Street in London in the mid-1850s is often summarized by the map of deaths he plotted in relation to the Broad Street pump, as well as the pump's spatial relationship to other features such as workhouses, residences, and factories (Figure 9–1). As such, the manual construction of a map to present these data conforms to the definition of a GIS. Despite the convincing nature of the data when presented in this way, it is critical to keep in mind an important feature of Snow's analysis that generally characterizes the limited application of GIS in epidemiology: The map that he created did not lead him to conclude that (1) cholera was a water-borne illness and (2) the pump was the source of contagion (contrary to popular lore), rather, the map was a method that he used to summarize his data to his audience and a tool he used to try to convince others of his conclusions. As Vandenbroucke[2] recently noted, "As an historical example, it remains important to remember that Snow's theory on the communication of cholera was not derived from his epidemiologic observations, but preceded them." Although Snow applied GIS well, it was a relatively restricted application. The restriction has been due, historically, to technical limitations rather than to conceptual ones.

Although the spatial distribution of cases is recognized as important in understanding infectious disease transmission, the statistical and geographic tools have not been generally available to make the examination of spatial distributions of infectious diseases an important analytical method for epidemiologic investigations. The increased development of GIS as an analytical approach in epidemiology results from improved access to automated computer systems and their associated software. To date, most of the progress in spatial epidemiology has been made where point exposures to a single factor (e.g., a pollutant or radiation) is responsible for human disease. An analogous situation occurs during outbreak investigations from a single source of infection. Although the graphical presentation of these data is little removed from Snow's early representations, demonstrating the spatial consequences of epidemiologic processes deduced from more traditional means can be compelling. For example, in 1979 an outbreak of anthrax was reported from the Sverdlovsk region in Russia involving deaths of both

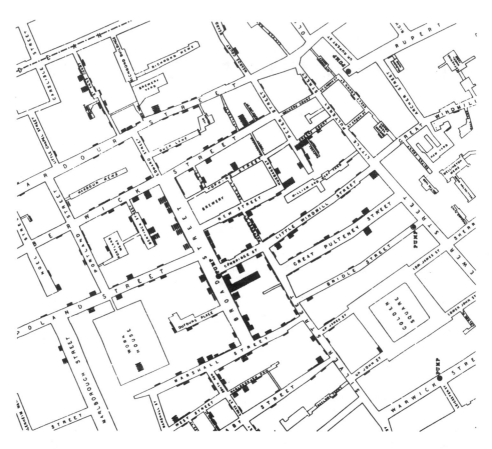

Figure 9–1 Map of the cholera outbreak in London around Golden Square and the Broad Street pump, indicating deaths, the pumps in the vicinity, and various land use features as drafted by John Snow. *Source:* Historical Collection, Institute of the History of Medicine, The Johns Hopkins University.

humans and domestic animals. Occasional anthrax outbreaks had been known from that region since at least the early 1900s. Anthrax is a disease caused by infection with *Bacillus anthracis*, and the severity of the disease caused by infection varies with the route of exposure. Cutaneous infection is least likely to cause mortality, whereas ingesting contaminated meat has a higher rate of mortality and inhalation of the agent is commonly fatal. Official reports of the investigation indicated the outbreak was associated with contact with naturally infected animals. However, rumors persisted that the outbreak was related to an accidental release of bacteria from a military facility. Subsequent

epidemiologic investigations, summarized by Meselson et al.[3] with the mapping of human and animal cases, indicated both the locations and timing (based on meterologic conditions) were immediately downwind of the military facility (see Chapter 2). Examination of autopsy materials confirmed the human cases resulted from inhalation rather than ingestion of the bacteria.

Probably one of the most striking early examples that moved beyond simple graphic representation and demonstrated the power of examining spatial patterns in infectious diseases was Maxcy's[4] implication of rodent arthropod vectors in the transmission of murine typhus. Comparison of the spatial distributions of typhus cases in Montgomery, Alabama, from 1922–1925, by places of residence and places of occupation, showed substantial aggregation by place of occupation, rather than residence. Thus, the differences in the spatial distributions of cases by alternate, possible places of exposure provided a means to evaluate different epidemiologic hypotheses. Maxcy hypothesized that if human lice served as vectors of typhus (as was assumed by many at that time), then multiple cases should occur in and around the same household because of close human contact. However, spatial clustering of cases was more evident when place of occupation was examined (Figure 9–2); typhus was especially common among workers associated with food services, leading Maxcy to propose that an arthropod vector associated with food services was responsible. Subsequent work[5] showed the vector of murine typhus to be the rat flea, whose hosts infested many of the food facilities at that time.

Clearly, one factor limiting the use of spatial data was the methodological difficulties associated with manipulating spatial data. The problem with manually plotting information, such as Maxcy's, multiplies significantly with each environmental factor examined, the spatial (and temporal) relationships of these factors, and the epidemiologic associations to be evaluated. These difficulties have been greatly reduced by the accessibility of relatively powerful computing systems in epidemiologic research and the development of dedicated GIS software that is designed to perform functions associated with mapping spatial data. When coupled with spatial analytic methods that have developed during the past two decades, it seems that we may be able to use the spatial patterns of infectious diseases in an analytical fashion, rather than intuitively, to provide important clues to the epidemiology of infectious diseases. This is true even when multiple environmental factors interact to influence disease rates. The most intriguing possibility of these systems is that they will allow us to develop and test hypotheses about infectious disease epidemiology in ways that have previously been impossible.

This chapter provides an overview of GIS with its structure discussed in functional terms. The influence of computer systems on the field means that many software systems have been developed to apply to spatial data, each with its own limitations. The field of GIS is rapidly growing and various textbooks exist as introductions to the methods and approaches of the technology.[6,7] Thus, after the brief overview of GIS, the rest of the chapter contains discussion of each of the major applications of GIS as they apply to infectious disease epidemiology. A series of case studies, from simple situations involving data storage through analysis and decision making, is provided. These examples represent studies that will provide some ideas of the broad scope of the technology's application.

OVERVIEW

Geographic information systems can be used for a variety of purposes in infectious disease epidemiology and these functions are fairly general to any field using spatial data. GIS can be used to help collect and store data, manage data, query data, model the processes generating the data, and make programmatic decisions. It is important to realize that these latter tasks, especially modeling and decision making, are not independent of the earlier functions; the quality of modeling, for example, is critically influenced by how well data have been collected and managed.

An excellent recent synopsis of GIS can be found in Vine et al.[8] Briefly, a major feature that distinguishes GIS from other computer-based systems is that a GIS contains within the stored data information concerning the spatial relationships among geographic features, and provides methods to study the relationships among selected, relevant features. Two major formats are used to represent these features. Software systems tend to be predominantly one or the other, but more recent versions usually provide algorithms for alternating between formats. GIS tend to present data in either vector or raster formats.

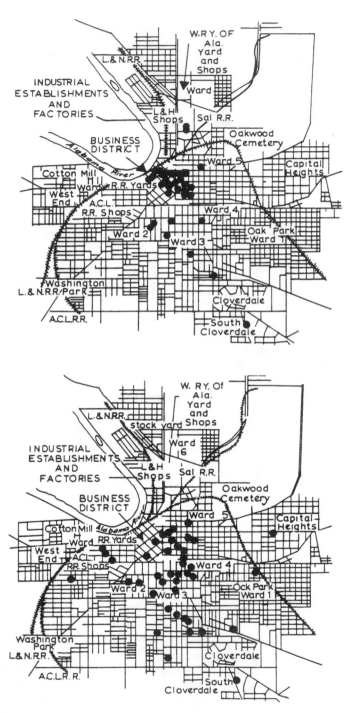

Figure 9–2 The distribution of cases of typhus fever in Montgomery, Alabama, plotted by K.F. Maxcy in 1926. **Top** shows distribution of cases by place of work (or residence if unemployed); **bottom** by place of residence. The more focal distribution of cases by place of work (**top**) was used by Maxcy to infer that endemic typhus was not transmitted by lice.

Vector Format

Vector format GIS represent features in two-dimensional space as points, lines, or polygons. Raster format GIS represent features in two-dimensional space in (usually) a uniform grid. Other data formats, such as quadtrees, which are something of a hybrid format, also exist but they are generally less common in their current usage. The major conceptual difference between vector- and raster-based systems is in how the data are represented. In vector format, points are located by specific x,y coordinates that typically represent a specific place on the earth's surface. Lines are interconnected points, linked one to another, whereas polygons represent features with areas and are joined line segments in which the first and last point have the same coordinates. These three types of features are used to represent objects on a map. For example, points might be used to indicate the location of health care facilities, lines might be used to represent transportation networks (e.g., roads), and polygons may be used to indicate the geographic extent of a service area for the clinics. In vector formats, the points, lines, and polygons are usually thought of as being fairly precisely located and, in the case of polygons, the area to the inside of the polygon's boundary is assumed to be homogeneous. This is only approximately true for most environmental features and this raises an issue of data quality that must be assessed in any analysis.

How objects are represented in vector format depends on the scale at which the data are gathered. For example, a clinic might be presented as a point at one scale but as one moves to a larger scale (zoom in), such as floor plans, the outside walls of the buildings making up the clinic may be best represented by polygons. Issues related to choice of scale for GIS application are critical to the study design and outcome. The choice of scale, to some extent, is often determined by the initial resolution of the epidemiologic data. Consider, for example, that Lyme disease, a tickborne bacterial infection, is a nationally reportable disease in the United States. However, the summary data may only be available at state or, at best, county level. Consequently, the scale for the GIS applications of the problem may be no better than county resolution, with cases known to occur somewhere within the county boundary. This indicates that a fairly small scale is most appropriate for presentation of these data and this scale places limits on the types of questions that can be addressed. In properly maintained databases, the minimal mapping unit (or the extent of smallest feature identified) is indicated, which is an important consideration in the selection of databases for study.

Raster Format

By contrast, raster formats are typically represented as grids of a study area, and locations are determined by the row and column locations much like a Cartesian coordinate system so that each x,y coordinate represents the location of a cell. Probably the most obvious example of raster-based data is satellite imagery in which reflected light from the earth is recorded by sensors on the satellite. The brightness of the reflected light is recorded for an area of the earth's surface. This area represents the spatial resolution of the image. No points and lines are used in raster formats, as all features have some minimal area assigned to them. Additionally, polygons, as used in vector formats, do not exist but are represented by large numbers of adjacent cells with the same data value. This data format has two consequences in GIS. First, the locations of points, lines, and boundaries of areas are approximate in that they are located somewhere within the specified cells, although their precise locations are not specified. This means that the locations of features are somewhat "fuzzy"—which may be more realistic for natural features, such as habitat edges. Spatial accuracy of raster features is determined by the spatial resolution of the grid. The raster format sometimes provides a more detailed characterization of features in the inside of regions than vector formats, which assume features are uniform within a polygon. Second, because the spatial resolution is determined by the interval distances between the rows and columns, the shorter the intervals, the finer the resolution. This produces a computational trade-off between improved spatial resolution, made by increasing the numbers of rows and columns and the size of the database. This is because, unlike vector formats, the data value for each cell has to be recorded. To minimize the size of files and the time needed to process data, various methods of data encoding have been developed to try to reduce the computational loads associated with raster formats.

Data Structure

The development of relational databases in which different databases can be linked by a common, key field was a major contribution for integrating GIS within infectious disease epidemiology. Relational database structures make it possible to use GIS as a tool within a larger, investigative analysis rather than forcing studies within specified data frameworks. Data for GIS can be derived from a variety of sources, both specifically for study (e.g., survey data) and as part of the regular duties of agencies (administrative data). As long as at least one of the variables in the gathered data can be linked to a geographic location (e.g., postal codes, addresses, census tracts, states, provinces, countries), the information can be incorporated in a GIS.

More typically, studies derive information from both administrative and specific study design sources. Information on environmental conditions (e.g., land use/land cover patterns, property ownership patterns, soils, watersheds) can all be accessed from appropriate governmental agencies that gather the data as part of their administrative responsibilities. These data can form a portion of the analysis, whereas specific survey data to study disease incidence, morbidity patterns, and so forth can be gathered as part of a specific study by investigators who then attempt to link observed disease patterns with the spatial distribution of environmental covariates.

Remotely sensed information is a source of accurate, updated information for environmental data. Such information can be gathered from various sources, such as airplanes, for survey studies, but most current sources that have a nearly administrative purpose are remotely sensed data recorded from satellites. Various satellite platforms are actively gathering data and vary in their spatial resolution, temporal resolution, duration of data gathering, and the portions of the electromagnetic spectrum that are scanned. For example, the current Landsat Thematic Mapper platform surveys each region of the earth every 16 days. It scans in seven regions (bands) of the electromagnetic spectrum—three in the visible portion and four in the infra-red region, with a spatial resolution of approximately 30 m. By contrast, the Advanced Very High Resolution Radiometer (AVHRR) system surveys each region twice daily, scanning in five bands of the electromagnetic spectrum, with a spatial resolution of 1.1 km. Analysis of archived satellite imagery is a useful method to examine changes in environmental conditions over time or to review environmental conditions at the times of previous disease outbreaks. The choice of satellite data is influenced then by both the time when the epidemiologic data were gathered and the spatial and temporal resolution needed for the environmental data. Interpretation of the satellite imagery, or any remotely sensed data, can be a difficult task and requires substantial training. Thus, in GIS, the remotely sensed data serve as an updated data source on environmental conditions, but the quality of the interpretation involves skills and techniques outside of GIS.[9]

Data quality, especially when not gathered by the investigators, is a substantial, often ignored, issue. Epidemiologists are often used to considering misclassification errors associated with attribution (false-positive and false-negative findings); however, four additional sources of error can be overlooked in GIS analyses: spatial, resolution, interpretive, and temporal errors.

Spatial errors involve misplacement of mapped features to their locations in the coordinate system. These errors can occur from simple data entry mistakes or from the methods used to locate the mapped features. An example of spatial errors introduced by methodologies concerns address-matching algorithms using digitized street maps. Digitized street map databases in vector formats often use an "arc-node" design to code information where street intersections are nodes and the streets are the arcs. The numbering of the buildings is not done by actually locating each property boundary. Rather, the "even" and "odd" sides of the streets are indicated in the file and the possible range of addresses are given. The geographic location of a residence is then determined by the linear interpolation of the building number relative to the range of numbers for the street.

Introduced errors by this coding method can be striking in some areas where block numbers have specific local meaning. In Baltimore, Maryland, blocks north and south of Baltimore Street are numbered in 100s north or south (e.g., 600 block of North Wolfe Street). At the intersection the block changes in units of 100. Even if only 10 buildings, numbered 600 through 618 occupy one side of a block, on the next block the first building is numbered 700. Thus, with the arc-node format all the buildings will be mapped within the lower one fifth of each block even though they cover its entire length. If the spatial resolution of the study is not too fine, this error can be relatively insignificant; however, if exposures need to be specified with a high degree of spatial accuracy, the error could be substantial. Regardless, such errors need to be identified and empirically evaluated for each study.

Resolution errors can occur because the databases that make up the GIS inherently have some level of spatial resolution, or detail. This is sometimes known as a minimal mapping unit. That is, because of limitations of resources or space, the databases are abstractions of the real world they represent. For example, a database of forest boundaries rarely, if ever, shows the exact location of each tree in the forest. Rather, the edge of the forest is approximated to some level of resolution. In addition, open spaces in the forest that support small meadows or grasslands may not be shown if these open spaces are too

small (i.e., they are smaller than the minimal mapping unit). This abstraction is necessary but can limit the usefulness of a particular database for a specific study. Even if every environmental feature, such as each tree, could be located, epidemiologic investigations of infectious diseases rarely have sufficient accuracy themselves to make such detail meaningful. An example of this is Lyme disease, a bacterial infection transmitted by small, hard-bodied ticks. Clearly, an epidemiologic investigation that attempts to identify environmental risk factors of the disease requires identifying places of exposures for cases. However, the ticks associated with most disease transmission in the eastern United States are so small that only a few individuals can accurately identify where or when exposure occurred to any useful level of accuracy. Many people do not even recall getting tick bites.

The epidemiologic issue related to place of exposure is often a critical one with the application of GIS. Placing a "case" on a map has significant implications for any viewer of the data, but such conclusions may be incorrect. This is especially true when the place of exposure is unknown. The example of Maxcy's study[4] of murine typhus is a classic example of such a phenomenon. Recently, for example, Kitron et al. examined the risk of LaCrosse encephalitis (LAC) in Illinois.[10] This California group encephalitis virus is transmitted by mosquitoes and can produce severe disease, primarily in children. However, most cases are clinically not apparent and the symptoms vary widely, making diagnosis difficult. Consequently, it is difficult to identify where and when cases of LAC are likely to occur. Kitron et al. combined a GIS with spatial analyses to identify clusters of LAC cases, specifically to determine if regions existed where cases occurred at higher than expected frequencies. Their results showed significant spatial clustering in the state within three counties surrounding Peoria. Demonstration of this clustering then allowed them to investigate what environmental factors occurred within the regions around these sites. Identifying these conditions would permit targeted interventions that would minimize environmental impacts associated with controlling mosquito vectors and to reduce most cases of LAC in the region.

Another condition in which the place of exposure is subject to significant error is when the time between exposure and onset of disease is relatively long, such as with human immunodeficiency virus (HIV), acquired immune deficiency syndrome (AIDS), or tuberculosis. Under this condition, use of current place of residence or place of work, for example, could give misleading results. This is especially critical during the occurrence of syndromes whose causes are unknown. Thus, workers using a GIS need to take special care in selecting what data are to be presented and how they are to be shown.

Interpretive errors are misclassification errors in the databases. In many cases when databases are obtained from other sources such errors are difficult to estimate unless "ground truthing," in the case of environmental data, is conducted. Epidemiologists often fail to appreciate the level of error in these databases, especially when they are presented as maps. For example, remotely sensed data (e.g., those collected by satellites) can be used to interpret land cover patterns. Land cover is classified based on the reflectance patterns from regions of the electromagnetic spectrum using various classification algorithms. However, when sites are "ground truthed" and compared with their predicted land cover, error rates of 15% to 20% are common, especially in complex environments, such as residential or rural environments.[11]

Improvements in the classification algorithms remain a major research focus. For example, Gong[12] demonstrated that the use of evidential reasoning and artificial neural networks substantially improved classification rates of environmental data from multiple sources compared with the more traditional approaches.

All of the developed databases have a temporal aspect associated with their collection. This is evident for epidemiologic data gathered during an outbreak investigation, for example. However, it is easy to forget that spatial databases gathered for a GIS also have temporal components that can change rather dramatically over various time scales. For example, soil databases may be relatively time invariant, whereas land cover, especially in rapidly developing areas, can change within a few years and precipitation patterns can vary in a matter of hours. Consequently, using databases in GIS as part of infectious disease studies can produce classification errors if the environmental conditions during the time of the study differ substantially from those when the database was created. In many areas of the world recently updated databases simply do not exist, hence the interest and application of remote sensing in these GIS.

APPLICATION EXAMPLES

Data Collection and Storage

A major feature of computerized systems is their capacity to input and store large quantities of data with relative ease. When data are being collected to answer a specific focused research question, the data gathered are often limited to those variables needed to test the hypotheses associated with the question. In these cases, the data collection and storage needs may be relatively small and a GIS primarily serves to present the data visually.

By contrast, some agencies are required to gather certain data as part of their administrative responsibilities. These data files can be extensive, both in the numbers of records included and in the number of data fields incorporated into each record. If spatial attributes are associated with these data, especially if they are combined from multiple sources, a GIS can prove a useful system for organizing and updating the data.

Schistosomiasis is a disease caused by infection with various species of parasitic worms of the genus *Schistosoma*. The disease causes substantial morbidity worldwide and is often associated with large-scale agro-ecosystem developments. Infection in humans requires contamination of water sources by infectious individuals, subsequent development in snail hosts, and then infection of susceptible people who contact contaminated water.

This complex interplay of hosts and environmental variables creates significant data storage issues when detailed epidemiologic studies of transmission patterns are undertaken. However, GIS can be exceptionally useful for such storage. For example, the Schistosomiasis Research Program (SRP), a joint effort of the Egyptian Ministry of Health and the U.S. AID, undertook as part of its research program a detailed ecological study of environmental factors associated with schistosome transmission at six sites in Egypt. Irrigation canals at these sites represented the primary source of environmental exposure. The sites were sampled once a month for more than a year. The issues related to data storage involved the large number of environmental variables being recorded at a very fine spatial scale over the extended period of the project. Every 50 m 84 variables were recorded including factors related to the type of canal, the abundance and size of host snails, whether the snails were infectious, the abundance of other species of snails, water chemistry, aquatic vegetation, and temperature. Because irrigation systems in these villages typically were 50 to 70 km long, it was usual to have 1,400 collecting locations at each of the six sites. This resulted in the production of large volumes of data. Nearly 50,000 sheets of data were generated for each study site. This longitudinal sampling of many data variables at many collecting locations for multiple sites presented a substantial data storage problem. Because collections were performed repeatedly at fixed collecting locations along the canals, a GIS represented a simple way of storing and organizing the data (Figure 9–3). Each collection location served as a key field in the data record and those places were geocoded to their locations along the canals. Figure 9–3, a simple schematic of the study area, shows major features of one site, such as roads, canals, and collecting sites. The primary difference from many such hand-drawn schematics is that the locations of all the features are spatially accurate and are referenced to particular locations on the earth's surface. As

a result, querying the data (see below) to identify where snail hosts were located and when transmission could occur became a simple process.

Data Management

Once data are entered, validated, and stored in the GIS, managing, updating, and editing them can be much more straightforward. GIS, in this sense, serves as a system to integrate data from various sources (e.g., paper maps, reports, administrative and test data) into a coherent system. Thus, GIS can be especially helpful in quality control issues, both those related to geographic locations and those used in evaluating consistency among different data sources.

In Baltimore, Maryland, the Baltimore City Health Department (BCIID) has as one of its responsibilities monitoring the number of cases of several reportable sexually transmitted diseases (STDs). The city has an area of approximately 240 km^2 and a population of approximately 700,000 people; however, even in this small region, substantial ethnic, racial, and socioeconomic diversity exists. The administrative data are derived from several sources, including several public health care clinics where patients can be treated and offices of private physicians who diagnose their patients and take samples for laboratory workups; a network of public and private health care systems conduct laboratory diagnoses and report the results to either the city or state health departments (depending on the source of the specimen). The data include a required array of demographic and personal information. To coordinate all the information obtained from these various sources, the BCHD developed a data management scheme[13] that allows the information from laboratory tests and clinic records to be integrated and merged into a single large database (Figure 9–4). A GIS was incorporated into the data management scheme using place of residence as the geographic identifier.

The GIS provided an additional level of quality control for the database and health care delivery. For example, examination of the data

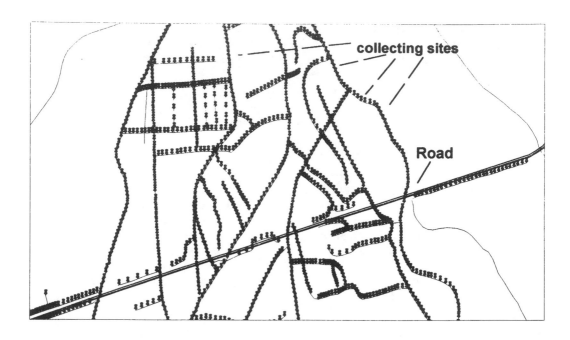

Collection Site	Date	Depth of Canal (Meters)	Site	Sampling Technique N = Canal Bed S = Surface	Non-Vector Snail Species			Schistosomiasis Vector Snail Species		
					Paspal	Phrag	Planor	Biomm9	Biom+	Bioml 13
321.0000	6/29/93	0.10	1	N		1	0	0	0	0
321.0000	6/29/93	0.10	1	S		1	0	0	0	0
322.0000	6/29/93	0.10	2	N		1	0	0	0	0
322.0000	6/29/93	0.10	2	S		1	0	0	0	0
323.0000	6/29/93	0.10	3	N		2	0	0	0	0
323.0000	6/29/93	0.10	3	S		2	0	0	0	0
324.0000	6/29/93	0.10	4	N	2		0	0	0	0
324.0000	6/29/93	0.10	4	S	2		0	1	1	2
325.0000	6/29/93	0.10	5	N	1	1	0	0	0	2
325.0000	6/29/93	0.10	5	S	1	1	0	0	0	0
326.0000	6/29/93	0.10	6	N		1	0	1	0	0
326.0000	6/29/93	0.10	6	S		1	0	0	0	1
327.0000	6/29/93	0.10	7	N	1	1	0	0	0	0
327.0000	6/29/93	0.10	7	S	1	1	0	0	0	1
328.0000	6/29/93	0.20	8	N		1	0	0	0	1
328.0000	6/29/93	0.10	8	S		1	0	0	0	0
329.0000	6/29/93	0.10	9	N	1		0	0	0	0
329.0000	6/29/93	0.10	9	S	1		0	0	0	0
330.0000	6/29/93	0.10	10	N	1		0	0	0	0
330.0000	6/29/93	0.10	10	S	1		0	0	0	0
331.0000	6/29/93	0.10	11	N	1		0	0	0	0
331.0000	6/29/93	0.10	11	S			0	0	0	0

Figure 9–3 Collecting locations and selected features at one site in Egypt used to sample for snails that serve as host for schistosome parasites. Collecting sites are densely located along canals (*thin lines*). A major road (*thick line*) bisected the region. More than 1,400 collecting locations were sampled each month during the study but the same collecting locations were revisited each time, making data storage within a geographic information system feasible.

showed substantial differences in the quality of data reporting by public and private providers for several important demographic variables. Public clinics reported racial data for 99% of cases compared with 72% of cases for private providers. It is thought that STDs occur at substantially different rates in different portions of the population, but the extent to which reporting bias affects these results is uncertain. In general, if such administrative data were used to make programmatic decisions such conclusions could be significantly in error.

Management of the data files using GIS also showed several places in the actual implementa-tion of both services and the data management where problems had arisen. For example, a small subsample of patients with a STD were seen at private health care systems and the public clinics for the same disease within a single day. This was not identified in the previously used system because private and public clinics used different identification numbers for the same individuals. However, the GIS identified cases with identical demographic information at the same locality. Subsequent examination of confidential infor-mation by appropriate staff identified individu-als who had been sent from the private facilities to the public clinics for treatment.

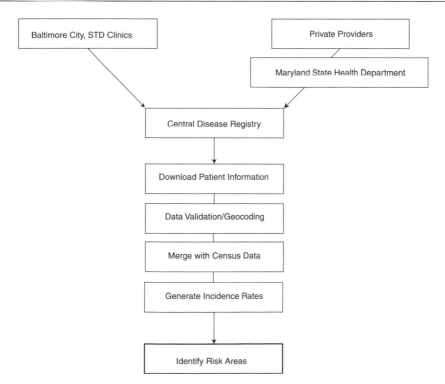

Figure 9-4 Data management of clinical information with the Baltimore City Health Department (BCHD) for sexually transmitted diseases. Cases could be seen initially at clinics run by BCHD or at private providers such as hospitals. If patients were seen by private providers, the information first was reported to the Maryland State Health Department before integration in the Central Disease Registry. The information then was downloaded to the geographic information system for validation, cleaning, and geocoding. Subsequently, the information could be merged with census information, as shown here, to generate rate maps of selected sexually transmitted dis-eases (STDs) and identify high-risk areas.

Querying

Once data management is ongoing within a GIS, its application in identifying disease patterns becomes of interest. Data querying in GIS, which represents an approach to examine past or current infectious disease patterns, is probably the most frequent use of a GIS. Querying uses many of the features specific to GIS, especially the spatial relationships of features to one another (topology). These include issues such as how close cases of disease are from a potential site of transmission, or how close they are to one another. This is often referred to as a "problem of adjacency." Querying often relies on taking survey and administrative data that are collected and using the GIS to summarize and categorize the data. Such questions usually involve determining the numbers and geographic distributions of cases of disease within a region and their relationship to various features of interest.

Adjacency problems can be addressed by several methods in GIS. Typically, fairly "low-end" GIS technology can deal with many querying tasks; when fairly sophisticated relational aspects are investigated, more powerful systems are needed.

Consider the example of schistosomiasis discussed above (Figure 9–3). An obvious question arises: Where are the snails found that serve as hosts for the schistosomes? Remembering how large the database was and how many sites were sampled, the utility of GIS queries is immediately obvious. When the database is queried for a simple tally of captures of *Biomphalaria*, the genus of snail host, throughout the year (Figure 9–5) and this is compared with all the collecting sites (Figure 9–3), it is evident that the snails are very restricted in their distribution within the canals. If only sites with large numbers of snails (e.g., 14–42 snails) are considered, these sites are extremely limited. This raises several questions that then can be further queried. What is there about these nine sites (out of 1,450 sampled) that differs from the remaining? Is it related to vegetation cover, water chemistry, other species of snails, where people conduct

certain activities? From a programmatic perspective, it also suggests that focused snail control in a very limited number of locations could have a substantial impact on the total abundance of the host snail population.

Other querying functions include extracting information from the databases for specific geographic regions. This process of overlaying features is an often-used feature of GIS that has benefited from the development of relational database formats. The value of relational databases is that they permit the linking of data from multiple sources to obtain information that is not uniquely available in any one source. The STD data obtained by the city of Baltimore provide a useful example. An important concern is whether the rates of selected STDs differ substantially within the city. Estimation of rates requires a denominator of the estimated population at risk. The STD database (Figure 9–4), however, does not include such information. It is possible to acquire from the U.S. census bureau data on the census information gathered in the city of Baltimore (Figure 9–6). A portion of the database is shown, along with a map of the census tracts in the city. Note that one of the data fields is the census tract number.

The distribution of gonorrhea cases for 1994 in Baltimore can be mapped on a similar base map to Figure 9–6 using place of residence (Figure 9–7). The geographic locations of these residencies were determined by geocoding the addresses to another database of street addresses for the city. Rates of gonorrhea were estimated by overlaying the census tract data on the locations of gonorrhea cases. The GIS was used first to count the numbers of cases in specific age-ethnicity-gender categories contained in the STD database, and then the appropriate categories from the census data were used as denominators to estimate rates. A large-scale portion of the data (Figure 9–7) shows that even in an area of intense transmission, substantial local variation in rates of disease is seen.[13] These data then might be used to identify and target regions where rates of disease are above some threshold for action.

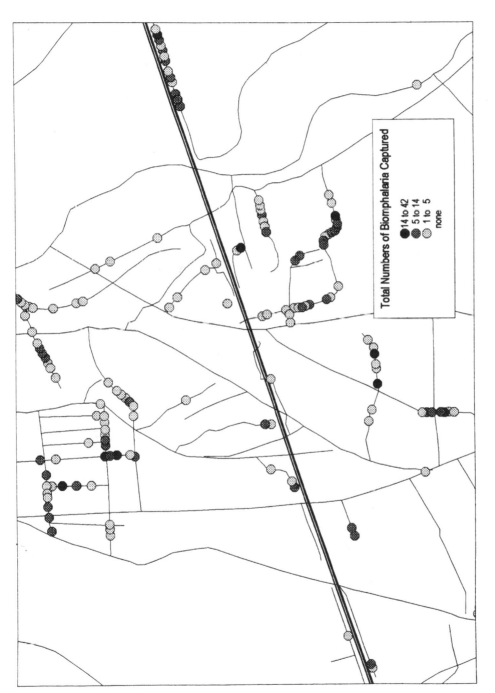

Figure 9–5 A data query of the schistosomiasis database for the map shown in Figure 9–3. This query involved locating all sites that captured *Biomphalaria*, one of the genera of snail that serves as a host for schistosoma in the region, for the entire collecting interval. Intensity of captures is shown by increasing darkness of the circles. Collecting localities that captured no snails are not indicated. Comparison with Figure 9–3 shows very few sites had any snails captured and only a few of these had significant numbers.

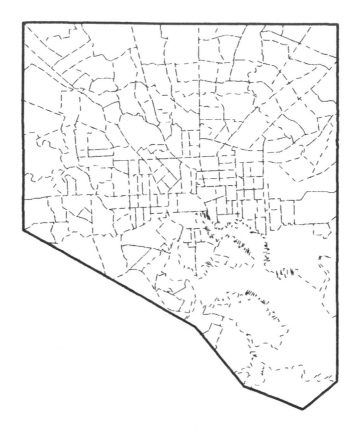

Tract90	Totalper__	Perusamp__	Per100____	Pctinsam__	Males____	Females__
010100	3,508	477	3,508	13.6	1,646	1,862
010200	3,435	494	3,431	14.4	1,613	1,822
010300	2,414	344	2,418	14.2	1,135	1,279
010400	2,244	292	2,218	13.2	1,158	1,086
010500	1,942	285	1,968	14.5	962	980
020100	2,078	260	2,148	12.1	1,012	1,066
020200	1,863	264	1,916	13.8	987	876
020300	2,088	240	1,965	12.2	1,154	934
030100	1,685	225	1,660	13.6	748	937
030200	2,763	326	2,714	12.0	1,461	1,302
040100	1,632	163	1,683	9.7	938	694
040200	1,474	159	1,497	10.6	744	730
050100	3,828	439	3,828	11.5	1,568	2,260
060100	3,246	430	3,246	13.2	1,530	1,716
060200	4,094	559	4,094	13.7	1,910	2,184

Figure 9–6 One database of census data for the city of Baltimore showing the geographic boundaries of census tracts within the city. Shown below the map is the database linked to the map indicating census tract number and population data.

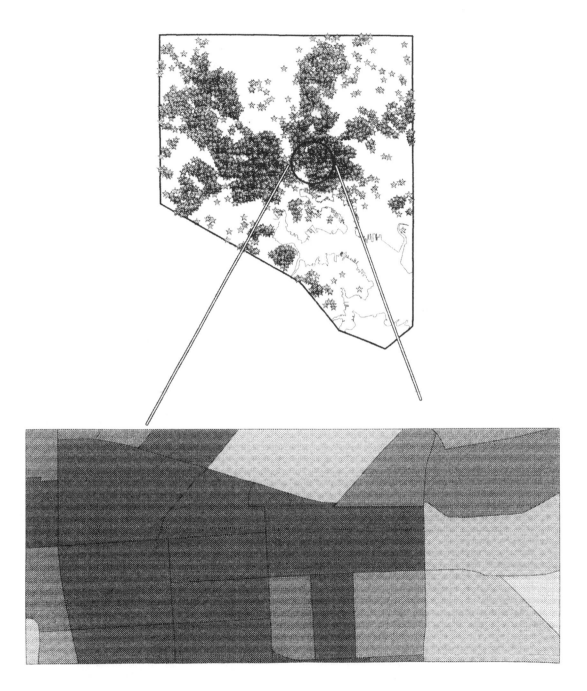

Figure 9–7 The geographic distribution of cases of gonorrhea for the city of Baltimore (*top figure*; cases have been randomly shifted to protect confidentiality). Using overlay procedures and census data (Figure 9–6), it is possible to link two unrelated databases to estimate disease rates for any portion of the city. An enlarged area is shown below. Rates of disease increase are shown with darker shading.

Another important feature of GIS that involves data querying is the ability of the system to measure distances from one feature of interest to another feature. If only two points are involved, this can be done manually. However, in the situation of multiple cases or irregular features this task becomes quite difficult, if not impossible. For example, Lyme disease is transmitted by hard-bodied ticks (genus *Ixodes*) that live in forests (see Chapter 21). To assess the importance of peridomestic exposure, it would be of interest to know how far the residences of cases of human Lyme disease are from the edge of the nearest forest (Figure 9–8). Forests have irregular boundaries, multiple cases of Lyme disease occur, and, practically, it would be impossible to measure the distance from the site of each Lyme disease case to the nearest forest edge. With aerial photographs and knowledge of where cases of disease occurred, it would be possible to estimate the distances with a ruler and a conversion method. This supposes that a procedure exists for identifying which forest edge is nearest to the site of each case. However, GIS can be used to measure the distances from the edges of all forests to each case by overlaying one data layer, the distribution of forests, with the distribution of Lyme disease cases in another layer, and calculating the distances between each case and the nearest forest edge. In the county of Baltimore, the distribution of the residences of Lyme disease cases appears to be clustered along the edge of forested areas (Figure 9–8), an observation confirmed by the histogram of cases relative to the distance from the edge of the forest. None of the persons infected resided more than 2,000 m from the edge of the forest and most lived within 100 m of the forest edge. Before confirming such a relationship, however, the distribution of all residences from the forest edges would need to be determined, as residence in or near forests can be a culturally preferred behavior.

Modeling

One obvious feature of GIS database development is that a large number of potential environmental risk factors for a selected infectious disease can be evaluated. Any feature that can be given a geographic location can be considered in the epidemiologic investigation. Consequently, the investigator is faced with the task of selecting from among these features the most appropriate ones to examine and analyze.

In some cases of infectious diseases this can be straightforward. The basic epidemiology is well understood and the environmental factors, both proximate and ultimate, are fairly clear. For many vector-borne diseases, for example, only one or a few vectors transmit the pathogen and the environmental conditions that favor the vector have been characterized. These conditions are so well defined that all that needs to be done is to overlay the distributions of the appropriate conditions to identify the predicted distribution of disease. For example, Beck et al.[14] used information on the breeding, feeding, and flight habits of *Anopheles albimanus*, a major vector of malaria in the Americas, and the locations of villages to model the predicted risk of malaria in a region of coastal Mexico using satellite imagery to identify key environmental features. It is not often appreciated, however, that the variables selected in the analysis and the way the biological information is used by the researcher represent a model of the disease process. The model is developed outside the GIS and the GIS then is used to identify where the stated conditions exist. With such models, the GIS simply serves its query function. For many infectious diseases with alternate hosts or vectors, however, such simple models cannot be developed. In addition, for many infectious diseases the conditions that cause disease outbreaks are not clearly understood, in which case the GIS can be used as an exploratory data analysis tool to develop and test hypotheses about the potential importance of environmental factors. In this situation, statistical methods are used to identify "important" factors associated with disease. The GIS can be used to query the environmental data (Figure 9–8) associated with disease. This information can be exported and analyzed by various statistical procedures. Then, the GIS can graphically represent the results.

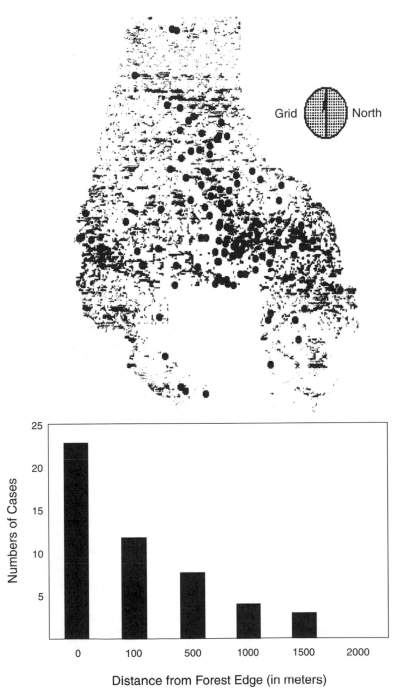

Figure 9–8 Geographic distribution of the residences (*dots*) of Lyme disease in Baltimore County in relationship to forested areas (*gray areas*). (Places of residences have been randomly shifted to protect confidentiality.) Using a buffer procedure it is possible to determine distances between the nearest forest edges and the residences of Lyme disease cases and summarize the results (*graph below map*). Results suggest nearness to forest edge may be a risk factor for disease.

Many infectious diseases with arthropod vectors are influenced by environmental conditions affecting the survival of the vector and any other hosts or reservoirs of the pathogen. Lyme disease (see Chapter 21) is common along the coastal regions of northern and central North America (as well as elsewhere). It is the most common vector-borne disease in the United States, and it is associated with substantial morbidity. In some areas, Lyme disease has a dramatic impact on outdoor activities of residents. Although exposure can be associated with recreational activities, a significant problem with Lyme disease in the northeastern United States is that much of the exposure appears to occur as part of daily activities around the place of residence.

Baltimore County, Maryland, is located along the western shore of the Chesapeake Bay, and surrounds Baltimore City on three sides. The county is a mixture of industrial, fairly high-density residential and rural environments. Since Lyme disease was recognized in Maryland, it has had the largest number of cases reported annually; its population in 1990 was approximately 700,000. In 1991, 38 cases of Lyme disease were reported.

To better understand the epidemiology of the disease, the areas within the county at high risk for the disease need to be identified. A number of environmental factors have been thought to influence the survival of the tick vector, the rodent reservoir of the Lyme disease spirochete and the white-tailed deer, the host for the adult tick. Presumably how these factors interacted were thought to influence where and how intense Lyme disease transmission would occur.

To model Lyme disease risk, a case-control design was developed using confirmed cases of Lyme disease. Place of residence was selected as the likely site of exposure. This was based on interviews conducted with patients, few of whom indicated any other likely site. Because residential site was used for exposure, control sites were a randomly selected sample of all residential addresses within the county. A GIS was used to extract environmental variables (e.g., land use characteristics, soil types, distance to forests, elevation, aquatic drainage systems) that were thought to influence Lyme disease risk from the areas around case residences, as well as randomly selected residential sites.[15] These data were analyzed by logistic regression analysis. The environmental variables, weighted by their appropriate regression coefficients, then were mapped throughout the region (Figure 9–9) as a measure of Lyme disease risk. The results of the risk map were evaluated on follow-up by comparing the numbers of cases of Lyme disease the following year, relative to a new set of randomly selected control sites. Cases were 16 times more likely to occur in high-risk than in low-risk areas the following year.

A significant risk of modeling with GIS once the databases are developed is that in many situations the number of potential environmental variables is as great or greater than the numbers of cases of disease. As such, the potential exists for the model to be unstable and dependent on idiosyncrasies of the data. This is not unique to GIS modeling and is always a risk in exploratory data analysis; however, because it is relatively easy to incorporate many variables once the databases are constructed, it is an important aspect to remember with GIS. Another potential problem with statistical modeling of spatial data exists that is rarely explicitly considered in traditional epidemiologic analyses. In general, most traditional statistical methods assume that observations are independent of one another. However, this is unlikely to be true, especially when considering the spatial distribution of infectious diseases. This is fairly obvious for contagious diseases. However, even when diseases, such as Lyme disease, are not contagious, significant spatial structure is generated by the underlying spatial correlation of environmental factors that influence the risk of disease. The major consequence for statistical models appears to be that the spatial structure creates a false sense of precision in the statistics.[16] A basic introduction to the measures and effects of spatial autocorrelation on data can be found in Griffith.[17]

Methods of analyzing spatially autocorrelated data have received special attention in geogra-

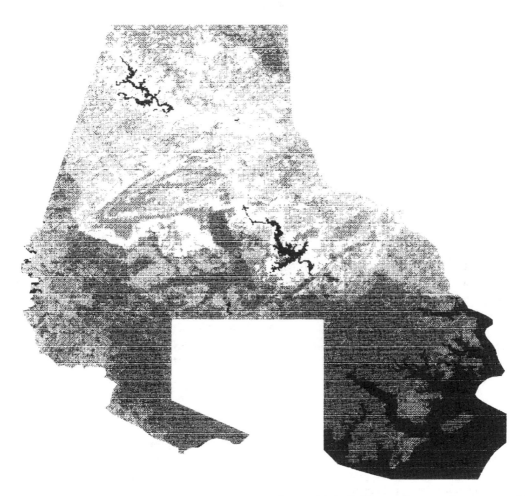

Figure 9–9 Geographic distribution of predicted Lyme disease risk in Baltimore County using a geographic information system to create an environmental database of potential risk factors for a case-control study design. Risk is mapped as four quartiles using the results of logistic regression analysis. Risk increases with increasing lightness. *Source:* Reprinted with permission from G.E. Glass et al., Environmental Risk Factors of Lyme Disease Identified with Geographic Information Systems, *American Journal of Public Health*, Vol. 85, No. 7, p. 946, © 1995, American Public Health Association.

phy. As such, many methods have been developed to estimate features that are spatially autocorrelated but have not been measured. For example, estimating the elevation of a particular point given the elevation at other points is a typical problem of spatial autocorrelation that is analogous to the problem of estimating the risk of disease at a particular location from which there is no data. Various methods have been

developed to answer this problem, such as "kriging," which attempts to use information about the internal spatial structure of the data to interpolate a "best" answer. A major practical problem with these approaches for public health is that these methods "smooth" the data. The consequence is that sites that are at very low or very high risk are regressed toward the mean. As a result, very high-risk sites are predicted to have a lower risk, whereas very low-risk sites are predicted to have a higher risk than they actually do. Such tendencies are not desirable for practical public health problems. Additionally, simple spatial techniques (e.g., ordinary kriging) exclude information on the spatial distribution of other factors, such as environmental covariates, that may influence the distribution of the outcome in question.

An alternative approach is the explicit incorporation of spatial aspects of the data, as well as the other environmental data, and any information of the known biological processes. For example, Das et al.[18] used hierarchical linear modeling to develop a spatially explicit model of tick vector abundance for adult *Ixodes* found on its principal host, white-tailed deer, that incorporated both spatial correlation of the data and overdispersion in the outcome variable, tick abundance. This hierarchical model had the advantage in both identifying environmental covariates of vector abundance, as well as factors influencing the overdispersion of the tick vectors.

Decision Making

A major application of GIS technology that has been recognized, but little used in infectious disease epidemiology, is in decision making and targeted public health interventions. Throughout this chapter the policy implications of the data collected for the various examples, such as targeting schistosomiasis control programs or developing STD interventions, have been mentioned. In principle, this use of a GIS would allow policy makers a better method of identifying areas at risk for the outcome of an infectious disease process and then direct resources toward preventing disease or targeting the at-risk population for screening and treatment while minimizing collateral (and potentially undesirable) impacts. In fact, development of accurate spatial models that incorporated the dynamics of infectious diseases might allow the testing of alternative strategies to identify the best strategy or

combination of strategies for disease control. As noted, however, this goal requires substantial, accurate databases that have been incorporated into a GIS, as well as a detailed understanding of disease processes. Given the lack of development of GIS in infectious disease epidemiology, it is not too surprising that few examples of this application exist. However, GIS should be extremely useful in targeting such interventions. The example discussed below demonstrates its application in evaluation of vaccine trials by identifying target populations at risk for Lyme disease.

Until recently, public health interventions for Lyme disease primarily involved education and encouraging individuals to take appropriate personal protective measures to reduce exposure to vectors. However, recently several recombinant vaccines have been developed and tested. Although Lyme disease represents the most common vector-borne disease in North America and may be locally common, the numbers of individuals infected often represent a very small portion of the entire population. For example, although the state of Maryland ranks fifth nationally in numbers of cases, the crude incidence in 1995 was approximately 9 per 100,000. A major problem in conducting population-based vaccine trials for diseases, such as Lyme disease, which lack a well-defined at-risk group is the large number of individuals who would need to be recruited to demonstrate efficacy of a vaccine if individuals were recruited at random. Given the tremendous costs associated with recruiting patients for vaccine trials, testing them, and following up the population for evaluation, it would be nearly impossible to conduct vaccine trials by such a population-based recruitment strategy.

Maryland was included as a site for the evaluation of a double-blind trial for one candidate vaccine. Power estimates indicated that, assuming a vaccine efficacy of 80% and 4,000 people in each of two arms of the study, it would be necessary to recruit from areas where the seasonal incidence was 500 per 100,000.[19] To identify an

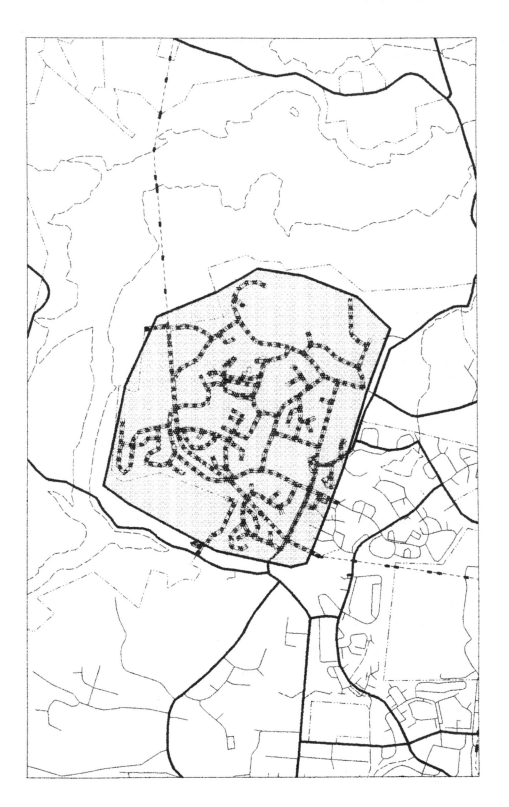

Figure 9–10 Application of geographic information system to decision making showing an overlay of high-risk area for Lyme disease shown in outlined region overlaid on street map. Street addresses falling in high-risk areas were selected to recruit individuals for vaccine trial based on the assumption that peridomestic risk was an indicator of individuals likely to be at high risk of disease.

appropriate population, therefore, the GIS and the model of Lyme disease risk described above were used to recruit individuals into the study. The map of Lyme disease risk (Figure 9–9) was overlaid with street maps of the region. Streets that overlaid high-risk areas were identified, and individuals who lived in these high-risk areas were contacted and asked to participate in the trial until 200 individuals were enrolled, the population size needed for the Maryland portion of the study (Figure 9–10). This approach reiterates the points made earlier that each use of GIS relies on the earlier ones: using databases that have been developed and checked, linking them with epidemiologic data, modeling the factors associated with disease, and then querying the results for specific conditions (residence in high risk areas).

If this strategy was successful, we would expect to see a significant increase of Lyme disease cases, compared with the crude population rate, making it possible to conduct the trial with substantially fewer participants and more power than would be possible otherwise. If the vaccine were successful, the cases should be (nearly) confined to the control group. As part of the 2-year surveillance, Lyme disease diagnostics were performed twice a year. By the end of the study Lyme disease incidence in the control group was 2% per year. This was substantially above both the crude population level and the targeted incidence rate, and was sufficient to demonstrate the effectiveness of the vaccine with a limited sample size.

CONCLUSION

The applications of GIS to infectious disease epidemiology are extremely diverse, ranging from data storage and management to modeling and programmatic decision making. As a tool for the field, GIS remains highly underutilized but this is beginning to change. The opportunities to apply the technology are only limited by the users' abilities to apply the technology. For much of the practical infectious disease epidemiology, low-end data querying systems are perfectly adequate. These systems are fairly easily mastered in a short period of time. Most important, many services are being developed in which critical data layers are professionally constructed, which minimizes the time and resources needed to create and update needed data layers. Along with this, however, will be the risk that data are used inappropriately or beyond the level of their quality. Unlike many other investigative tools in epidemiology, because GIS produces derivative products, such as maps, these errors will be more difficult to detect. Despite this concern, the opportunities for a better understanding of infectious diseases using GIS outweigh the risks.

REFERENCES

1. Aronoff S. *Geographic Information Systems: A Management Perspective.* Ottawa: WDL Publications; 1989.

2. Vandenbroucke JP. Re: "A new perspective on John Snow's communicable disease theory." *Am J Epidemiol.* 1997;146:363–364.

3. Meselson M, Guillemin J, Hugh-Jones M, et al. The Sverdlovsk anthrax outbreak of 1979. *Science.* 1994; 266:1202–1208.

4. Maxcy KF. An epidemiological study of endemic typhus (Brill's disease) in the southeastern United States with special reference to its mode of transmission. *Public Health Rep.* 1926;41:2967–2995.

5. Woodward TE. President's address: typhus verdict in American history. *Trans Am Clin Climatology Assoc.* 1970;82:1–8.

6. Ripple WJ. GIS for resource management: a compendium. *Am Soc Photo Remote Sens.* 1987.

7. Antenucci JC, Brown K, Croswell PL, Kevany MJ. *Geographic Information Systems: A Guide to the Technology.* New York: Van Nostrand Reinhold; 1991.

8. Vine MF, Degnan D, Hanchette C. Geographic information systems: their use in environmental epidemiologic research. *Environ Health Perspect.* 1997;105:598–605.

9. Sabins FF. *Remote Sensing: Principles and Interpretation.* 3rd ed. New York: WH Freeman and Company; 1997.

10. Kitron U, Michael J, Swanson J, Haramis L. Spatial analysis of LaCrosse encephalitis in Illinois. *Am J Trop Med Hyg.* 1997;57:469–475.

11. Harris R. *Satellite Remote Sensing: An Introduction.* London: Routledge and Kegan Paul; 1987.

12. Gong P. Integrated analysis of spatial data from multiple sources: using evidential reasoning and artificial neural network techniques for geological mapping. *Photo Eng Remote Sens.* 1996;62:513–523.

13. Becker KM, Glass GE, Brathwaite W, Zenilman JM. Geographic epidemiology of gonorrhea in Baltimore, Maryland, using a geographic information system. *Am J Epidemiol.* 1998;147:709–716.

14. Beck LR, Rodriguez MH, Dister SW, et al. Assessment of a remote sensing–based model for predicting malaria transmission risk in villages of Chiapas, Mexico. *Am J Trop Med Hgy.* 1997;56:99–106.

15. Glass GE, Schwartz BS, Morgan JM, Johnson DT, Noy PM, Israel E. Environmental risk factors for Lyme disease identified with geographic information systems. *Am J Public Health.* 1995;85:944–948.

16. Breslow NE. Extra-poisson variation in log-linear models. *Applied Statistics.* 1984;33:38–44.

17. Griffith DA. *Spatial Autocorrelation: A Primer.* Washington, DC: Association of American Geographers; 1987.

18. Das A, Lele SR, Glass GE, Shields T, Patz JA. Spatial modeling of vector abundance using generalized linear mixed models: application to Lyme disease. *Biometrics.* 1999;(in press).

19. Steere AC, Sikand VK, Meurice F, et al. Vaccination against Lyme disease with recombinant *Borrelia burgdorferi* outer-surface lipoprotein A with adjuvant. *N Engl J Med.* 1998;339:209–215.

CHAPTER 10

Vaccines—Past, Present, and Future

Steffanie A. Strathdee and Anita M. Loughlin

INTRODUCTION

A vaccine is any biologically derived substance that elicits a protective immune response when administered to a susceptible host. The first documented account of vaccination is attributed to a Buddhist nun who described how smallpox scabs were dried, ground, and blown into the nostrils of susceptible persons in approximately A.D. 1000 to protect them from disease.[1] The first scientific attempt at vaccination occurred in 1796, when Edward Jenner proved that persons inoculated with cowpox were resistant to challenge with Variola virus, the etiologic agent responsible for smallpox.

Worldwide improvements in sanitation and vaccination have led to impressive declines in the incidence and mortality of many infectious diseases throughout the twentieth century. Perhaps the greatest public health achievements of this era were the global eradication of smallpox in 1977 and the near elimination of polio. Despite these achievements, a significant proportion of the estimated 17.3 million deaths attributed to infectious and parasitic diseases in 1997 could have been prevented by existing vaccines (Table 10–1). Despite the existence of highly effective measles vaccines, about one million children die from measles each year, 50% of whom live in Africa. Although a tuberculosis vaccine has been available since 1927, this disease remains uncontrolled in many parts of the world (see Chapter 14 on Tuberculosis).

In this chapter, we describe various types of traditional and experimental vaccines, the role of vaccines in the eradication of specific infectious diseases (eg, smallpox, polio), and recent technological advances in vaccine development. We also summarize fundamental concepts relating to vaccine efficacy and effectiveness and barriers to achieving adequate vaccine coverage.

ACTIVE VERSUS PASSIVE IMMUNIZATION

Protection from many infectious diseases can be conferred by either passive or active immunization. *Passive immunity* refers to protection conferred to a susceptible host through the transfer of animal or human products (eg, immunoglobulin), usually by injection. Passive antibody transfer from mother to child in utero or through breastfeeding plays an important role in preventing disease in newborns. Although maternal antibodies do not necessarily provide full protection from infection, immunization of pregnant women against tetanus has led to dramatic reductions in the incidence of neonatal tetanus.[2] A disadvantage of passive immunity is that it is typically short-lived. Protection conferred by immunoglobulin lasts only a few weeks; maternal antibodies can protect newborns for up to six months.

Active immunity refers to protection produced by the host's own immune system and relies on the ability of the host to generate an immune re-

Table 10–1 Leading Causes of Death World-wide from Infectious Diseases in 1997

Type of Disease	Estimated Deaths (millions)
Acute lower respiratory infections	3.7
Tuberculosis*	2.9
Diarrhea†	2.5
HIV/AIDS‡	2.3
Malaria‡	1.5–2.7
Total	~17.3

* BCG vaccine first licensed in 1927.

† Vaccines currently available for cholera and typhoid; shigella and rotavirus vaccines under development.

‡ No licenced vaccine available.

Source: World Health Organization, World Health Report 1998.

munization. The extent of the host's immune response has an important bearing on vaccine efficacy, which is discussed in detail later.

TYPES OF VACCINES

Traditionally, vaccines have been considered to fall into two main groups. The antigenic agent used in active immunization can be: (1) a live organism that has been attenuated (ie, weakened) or (2) an inactivated form that is either whole or fractionated (eg, protein or polysaccharide component). Recombinant vaccines are developed through genetic manipulation, and these can be either live or inactivated. Below, we describe characteristics of the various types of vaccines, as well as a newer experimental approach involving vaccination with naked DNA. A summary of characteristics for specific vaccine-pre-

sponse following exposure to specific antigen(s). Antigens are foreign bodies—usually proteins—that are recognized by the immune system as non-self. The goal of immunization is to elicit a protective immune response that mimics natural infection with a wild-type (ie, pathogenic) microorganism without causing serious clinical illness. Features of an ideal vaccine are tabulated in Exhibit 10–1.

Factors that affect the host immune response include the type and dose of antigen, the route of administration (eg, intramuscular, subcutaneous, oral), the presence or absence of maternal antibody, host factors (eg, age, immunosuppression, genetic predisposition), and specific characteristics of the vaccine (Exhibit 10–1). Timing is also an important consideration. For most vaccines, immunization must take place before natural infection occurs, allowing for several weeks to generate an adequate immune response. During some outbreaks (eg, hepatitis A, measles), passive immunization offers effective short-term protection, especially when there is insufficient time for susceptibles to mount an adequate immune response following active im-

Exhibit 10–1 Characteristics of an Ideal Vaccine

1. Produces a good humoral, cell-mediated, and local immune response, similar to natural infection, in a single dose.
2. Elicits protection against clinical disease and reinfection.
3. Provides protection for several years, preferably a lifetime.
4. Results in minimal immediate adverse effects or mild disease with no delayed effects that predispose to other diseases.
5. Induced immunity confers protection to multiple strains of the organism.
6. Can be administered simply in a form that is practically, culturally, and ethically acceptable to the target population(s).
7. Vaccine preparations do not require special handling (eg, cold chain).
8. Does not interfere significantly with the immune response to other vaccines given simultaneously.
9. Costs and benefits associated with receiving the vaccine clearly outweigh the costs and risks associated with natural infection.

ventable diseases and the types of vaccines used in most immunization programs is found in Table 10–2.

Whereas traditional vaccines are designed to prevent infection, some vaccines prevent or minimize the consequences of infection. Toxoid vaccines prevent tissue damage from bacterial toxins (eg, tetanus or diphtheria toxin). Inactivated poliovirus vaccine does not prevent wild-type polio virus from multiplying in the intestinal tract, but immune barriers induced by this vaccine prevent the virus from causing central nervous system disease. A new recombinant rotavirus vaccine does not prevent infection but reduces the severe consequences of disease caused by dehydration.

The public health burden of specific cancers may be also considerably reduced through the introduction of preventive or therapeutic vaccines. The inclusion of hepatitis B (HBV) vaccine in several national immunization programs is hoped to reduce the incidence of liver cancer; however, barriers to achieving adequate coverage persist (discussed in more detail later). Preventive vaccines are under development for human papillomavirus (HPV) infection, which accounts for approximately 95% of all cervical cancers. In the future, it is hoped that antitumor vaccines can be used to boost host immune responses to promote tumor destruction.[3]

Live Attenuated Vaccines

Bacteria and viruses are referred to as being attenuated if they have been rendered nonpathogenic. Bacteria can be attenuated through laboratory culture, and viruses through serial passaging. Both bacteria and viruses can be attenuated through genetic manipulation. The potential role of attenuated organisms in vaccination was identified soon after Jenner's landmark smallpox vaccination study in 1796. In the 1870s, Louis Pasteur recognized that inoculating a weakened form of chicken cholera protected chickens against challenge with the wild-type virus. Pasteur then developed an attenuated anthrax bacilli vaccine that was first administered to livestock

in 1881, and an attenuated live rabies vaccine that was used to immunize two human volunteers in 1885.[4] In 1909, the Bacille Calmette-Guerin (BCG) tuberculosis vaccine was the first live attenuated bacterial vaccine developed for humans.

Live attenuated organisms must replicate, or multiply, in the host to induce an adequate immune response. Live vaccines typically generate a stronger immune response than do inactivated vaccines, and immunity is often life-long, due to immunologic memory. Live vaccines have the advantage of inducing both humoral and cell-mediated immunity. In simplistic terms, *humoral immunity* refers to immunoglobulin (Ig) production. Antigen recognition by lymphocytes (T cells and B cells) leads to clonal expansion of specific antibodies that are directed against a particular antigen and a generation of memory cells. The primary humoral immune response to a new antigen involves short-term production of IgM antibodies, which is superceded by longer-lasting, higher-affinity IgG antibodies. If the host is re-exposed to the same antigen, a rapid expansion of memory cells results in a secondary immune response involving IgG but not IgM antibodies. Cell-mediated immunity includes nonspecific responses that are often the first-line attack directed against invading organisms. This includes phagocytes, natural killer cells, cytotoxic T cells, and complement. For a detailed account of the humoral and cell-mediated response to infectious agents, the reader is referred elsewhere.[5-8]

Another potential advantage of live vaccines is the possibility of horizontal transmission, which refers to the transmission of vaccine virus to susceptible persons. Horizontal transmission of vaccine virus has been described for live oral polio vaccine[9] and a newly developed rotavirus vaccine.[10] Although horizontal transmission may serve to enhance vaccine coverage, this feature is not necessarily beneficial because there is potential for live attenuated viruses to revert to virulence. For this reason, horizontal transmission of vaccine strains requires careful monitoring and surveillance, should it be known to occur.

Table 10-2 Summary of Selected Vaccine-Preventable Diseases and Estimated Vaccine Efficacy

Organism	Disease	Primary Route(s) of Exposure	Preferable Vaccine in Current Use	Estimated Vaccine Efficacy
Corynebacterium diphtheriae	Diphtheria	Respiratory	Inactivated diphtheria toxoid	97%
Clostridium tetani	Tetanus	Wound	Tetanus toxoid	100%
Bordetella pertussis	Pertussis (whooping cough)	Respiratory	Acellular component vaccine	71–84%
Hemophilus influenzae type B	Meningitis, Epiglottitis, Pneumonia, Arthritis, Cellulitis	Respiratory	Polysaccharide-protein conjugate	95–100%
Paramyxoviridae	Mumps, Orchitis	Respiratory	Live attenuated (MMR)	95%
Rubella virus	Measles	Respiratory	Live attenuated (MMR)	95%
Polio virus	Polio	Oral-fecal	Oral Polio Vaccine (OPV), Inactivated Polio Vaccine (IPV)	95% 99%
Hepatitis B virus	Hepatitis, Liver cancer	Parenteral, Mucosal	Recombinant	95%
Varicella virus	Chicken pox, Shingles	Respiratory	Live attenuated	95%
Yellow fever virus	Yellow fever	Vector (*Aedes aegypti*)	Live attenuated	85–95%
Mycobacterium tuberculosis	Tuberculosis	Respiratory	Live attenuated *M. bovis* (BCG)	Estimates vary widely
Streptococcus pneumoniae	Pneumonia, Bacteremia, Meningitis	Respiratory	Polysaccharide	60–70%
Influenza virus (type A)	Influenza	Respiratory	Inactivated	90%

Because the host does not differentiate between natural infection with a wild-type organism and an attenuated form of the same virus, live vaccines can cause severe adverse effects, especially among persons with incompetent immune systems (eg, immunosuppressed persons, infants, persons with HIV/AIDS). In most cases, adverse effects caused by live vaccines are less severe than is natural infection but, nevertheless, all unintended consequences of vaccination must be carefully assessed during clinical trials of vaccine safety, efficacy, and effectiveness, and through surveillance.

Antibodies induced by live attenuated vaccines can sometimes be rendered inactive by circulating antibodies that cross-react with the attenuated organism. Interference can be caused by antibody produced during intercurrent natural infections, immune globulin administered during recent passive immunization, or maternal antibodies. Measles vaccine is particularly sensitive to circulating maternal antibodies, which has complicated immunization schedules in preschool children.[11] In rare cases, antibodies induced by one vaccine can inhibit the immune response to another, a situation that bears consideration when several vaccines are administered simultaneously. Previous concerns that administering yellow fever and cholera vaccines simultaneously could reduce the long-term immune response to both vaccines have not been borne out by recent studies[12]; however, the Centers for Disease Control and Prevention (CDC) recommends that these vaccines be administered at least three weeks apart. In addition, some antimalarial drugs (eg, chloroquine) interfere with live cholera vaccine.[12]

Immunization programs that incorporate live vaccines also need to take appropriate measures to protect the vaccine from environmental conditions (eg, heat, light). The system of storage and transport of vaccine from manufacturer to client is called the *cold chain*. Although stabilizing agents (eg, magnesium chloride) can be used to safeguard the viability of live vaccines, failure to maintain the cold chain can compromise efficacy. This is particularly a problem in developing countries. When appropriate, simultaneous administration of several live vaccines (eg, measles, mumps, rubella [MMR]) reduces cost and minimizes cumbersome handling, shipping, and storage requirements.[13]

Inactivated Vaccines

Inactivated vaccines refer to either whole viruses or bacteria that are "killed," using heat or chemicals (eg, formalin), or fractional components of the organism that are extracted and purified. These components include toxoid, polysaccharide, conjugate, and multiple subunit vaccines. As early as 1888, it was discovered that the diphtheria bacillus (*Corynebacterium diphtheriae*) produced a powerful toxin.[14] In the early twentieth century, chemical inactivation of bacterial toxins led to the first toxoids for diphtheria and tetanus. Another type of inactivated vaccine is based on polysaccharides that are typically derived from bacterial cell walls (eg, pneumococcus, meningococcus, *Hemophilus influenzae* type b [HiB]). These vaccines primarily induce short-lived nonspecific IgM but no immunologic memory. Polysaccharide-based vaccines are not consistently immunogenic for the elderly, immunocompromised persons or infants, and are not recommended for children under two years of age.[2] In some cases, polysaccharides can be chemically linked, or conjugated, to a protein carrier that can boost the immune response. This approach has been successfully used to maximize the immune response to HiB, which was the first conjugate vaccine licensed for use in humans.

By definition, inactivated vaccines are not alive, and, therefore, they cannot replicate in the host or revert to virulence. They are not rendered ineffective by circulating antibody and require less stringent handling procedures. Inactivated vaccines are associated with fewer adverse effects, which are usually localized to the injection site. Although these properties are favorable, the immune response associated with inactivated vaccines is typically restricted to humoral immunity. Several doses are usually required to boost the specific antibody level, or *titre*; otherwise, immunity usually wanes over time.

In cases where the antigenic component of the organism has not easily been isolated, whole inactivated viruses and bacteria have formed the basis of vaccine preparations. These vaccines are more likely to induce adverse effects, in which case, they are referred to as *reactogenic*. This was a common problem with whole cell pertussis vaccine, which led to the development of an acellular form that is associated with fewer side effects.

Recombinant Vaccines

In the last two decades, much attention has focused on genetic manipulation of organisms to generate either live attenuated or inactivated vaccines. Several different approaches have been used. Hepatitis B vaccine was the first recombinant DNA vaccine and was licensed in 1986. Development of this vaccine relied on clonal expansion of the primary immunogen, hepatitis B surface antigen (HBsAg), which was expressed in *Saccaromyces cerevisiae* yeast cells. This technique has evolved rapidly to generate many new vaccines. For example, *Escherichia coli* has been used to express lipoprotein from *Borrelia burgdorferi*, the bacteria responsible for Lyme disease.[15] The first human vaccine for Lyme disease was licensed in 1998.

Another approach to developing a recombinant vaccine involves deletion or modification of genes that are known to confer pathogenicity. This method has been used to construct an oral typhoid vaccine and numerous others. Recently, genetic manipulation of rhesus monkey and human rotavirus genomes enabled the development of vaccines for rotavirus, the major etiologic agent responsible for diarrheal deaths in children. Development of rotavirus vaccines took advantage of the fact that human and animal (ie, bovine, rhesus) strains of the virus readily underwent reassortment. The resultant multivalent vaccine increases the potential to provide protection against multiple serotypes.[16] First-generation rhesus rotavirus vaccines have

been associated with a high level of protection in clinical trials in Venezuela, the United States, and Finland.[10]

A third approach to recombinant vaccine development involves insertion of a gene from one organism to another, usually a live virus. The modified virus subsequently acts as a carrier, or vector, that expresses the foreign gene. Using this innovative approach, canarypox virus has been used to express HIV glycoproteins. This modified canarypox virus is currently being evaluated in clinical trials as a candidate HIV vaccine.[17] Vaccinia virus and adenovirus have been used to express rabies G protein.[18,19] The former vaccine vector has been used to immunize wildlife against rabies.[18]

DNA Vaccines

DNA vaccines differ from traditional vaccines, in that the naked DNA coding for a specific component of a disease-causing organism is injected directly into the body. The delivery system is either a saline solution injected through a hypodermic needle or DNA-coated gold beads propelled into the body, using "gene guns." Although no DNA vaccine is currently licensed, DNA vaccination represents a considerable technological advance that may revolutionize immunization. Developed extensively throughout the 1990s, this approach offers the possibility of safer and cheaper vaccines, even for diseases where there has been only limited success with traditional vaccines. DNA vaccines are currently under development for malaria, rotavirus, influenza virus, and HIV, among other pathogens.

There are several potential advantages associated with DNA vaccines. First, the actual production of the immunizing protein takes place in the cells of the vaccinated host. This theoretically eliminates the risk of the vaccine causing the infection that it is intended to prevent, which is a concern with traditional live attenuated vaccines. Second, like live vaccines, DNA vaccines have the ability to elicit wide-range humoral and cell-mediated immune responses that are potentially long term. Third, DNA vaccines are very stable and can be stored under a vast array of conditions, which eliminates the need for a cold chain. For this reason, they may be particularly suitable in developing countries. Finally, DNA vaccines may lend themselves to generic production methods that will simplify and standardize vaccine production.

An important shortcoming of DNA vaccines is that they are limited to developing immune responses against protein components. Therefore, they cannot substitute for traditional polysaccharide-based vaccines (eg, pneumococcal vaccine). There are also new safety concerns posed by these vaccines. If DNA from the vaccine were incorporated into host chromosomes, for example, foreign DNA theoretically could turn on oncogenes or turn off tumor suppressor genes, which could conceivably predispose vaccinees to cancer. Therefore, the safety and efficacy of DNA vaccines will need to be carefully evaluated to ensure that the benefits outweigh the short-term and long-term risks.

IMMUNIZATION SCHEDULES

The goal of an effective immunization program is to vaccinate a high proportion of susceptible persons early in life (ie, before they are potentially exposed to the infectious agent). In the United States, infants and children are immunized against hepatitis B; diphtheria; tetanus; pertussis; HiB; polio; measles, mumps, and rubella (MMR); and Varicella virus (Table 10–3). Rotavirus vaccines are likely to be recommended for routine childhood immunizations in the near future.[20] Alternative immunization schedules are available from other sources for children who have missed primary immunization series or who were inadequately immunized.[21]

Immunization schedules differ from country to country, depending on the burden of disease in the population, the availability of an efficacious and effective vaccine, economic factors, and the level of priority that is placed on vaccine-preventable diseases. In addition to the routine vaccinations listed in Table 10–4, the World Health Organization (WHO) also recommends vaccination against tuberculosis (ie, BCG) and yellow fever in countries where these diseases are endemic.

Target Populations

In the United States, identifiable high-risk populations have specific immunization recommendations (Table 10–3). Missed opportunities to vaccinate are major causes of outbreaks in school-aged children. Assessment of adolescents at routine health care visits is warranted to ensure completion of primary vaccine series for newer vaccines (eg, varicella, hepatitis B vaccine) and to provide boosters for MMR and tetanus toxoid.[7]

Adult vaccination is an important part of preventive medical care. Routine adult vaccines include pneumococcal vaccine and influenza and tetanus toxoid. In higher-risk individuals, MMR, hepatitis B, hepatitis A, and varicella vaccines are recommended. The U.S. Public Health Service and the CDC also provide immunization recommendations for international travelers, depending on the country of destination.[22] Travelers should be immunized against infections that are endemic in specific regions (eg, measles, hepatitis A and B, yellow fever, meningococcus, typhoid, polio, rabies, plague, Japanese encephalitis). HiB, pnuemococcal, and meningococcal vaccinations are recommended for immunosuppressed persons who are at high risk of invasive bacterial infections. However, depending on the level of immune suppression, vaccine-induced immune responses may not be optimal, and some persons may remain susceptible.

Conditions That Contraindicate Vaccination

Immunization schedules are modified when an individual has a contraindication to a particular vaccine (Exhibit 10–2). Mild illnesses (eg, low-grade fever, upper respiratory infection, otitis media, mild diarrhea) or breastfeeding are not contraindications for immunization. Previous or

Table 10–3 Recommended Childhood Immunizations Schedule, United States, January–December 1998

Recommended Age or Age Range*	Hepatitis B†	Diphtheria, Tetanus, Pertussis	H. influenzae type B	Polio	Measles, Mumps, Rubella	Varicella
Birth	Hep B-1					
1 mo						
2 mos	Hep B-2	DTaP-1	Hib-1	IPV		
4 mos		DTaP-2	Hib-2	IPV		
6 mos	Hep B-3	DTaP-3	Hib-3			
12 mos			Hib	Polio		
15–18 mos		DTaP			MMR	VAR
4–6 yrs		DTaP		Polio	MMR	
11–12 yrs	Hep B‡	Td			MMR‡	VAR‡
14–16 yrs						

* Box indicates acceptable age range for vaccination.

† For infants born to HBsAg negative mothers, the second dose of hepatitis B vaccine should be administered at least one month after the first dose. The third dose should be administered at least 4 months after the first dose and at least 2 months after the second dose, but not before 6 months of age.

‡ Children are assessed to assure receipt of complete vaccine series. Vaccine is given if indicated.

Source: Reprinted from the Centers for Disease Control and Prevention.

Table 10–4 The Immunization Schedule for Infants Recommended by the WHO Expanded Program on Immunizations

| Age | Vaccines | *Hepatitis B Vaccine (alternative schemes)* | |
		For Countries Where Perinatal Transmission of HBV Is Frequent (eg, SE Asia)	*For Countries Where HBV Perinatal Transmission Is Less Frequent (eg, Sub-Saharan Africa)*
Birth	BCG, OPV-0	HBV-1	
6 wks	DTP-1, OPV-1	HBV-2	HBV-1
10 wks	DPT-2, OPV-2		HBV-2
14 wks	DPT-3, OPV-3	HBV-3	HBV-3
9 mos	Measles (MMR) Yellow fever*		

*In countries where yellow fever poses a risk.

Source: Reprinted from http://www.who.int/gpv-dvacc/service/immschedule.htm.

suspected anaphylactic reaction to a vaccine component is the strictest contraindication to immunization. When it is considered that a concurrent moderate or severe illness might be exacerbated by a vaccine-induced immune response, immunization may be delayed. Contraindications are specific to live attenuated vaccines, which pose a threat to immunosuppressed persons and to the fetus. Because measles can be a severe illness in an HIV-infected person, MMR immunization is recommended for HIV-infected persons before they become severely immunosuppressed. Among blood product recipients, circulating antibody present in transfused blood components can interfere with the replication of live vaccine virus. Therefore, it is recommended that MMR and varicella vaccinations be postponed for a period following blood or blood product transfusions.

VACCINE DEVELOPMENT

Vaccine innovation includes identification and characterization of antigens that induce neu-

tralizing antibody, identification of genetic clones that produce these antigens, vaccine biochemical formulation, numerous animal studies, and extensive manufacturing to mass-produce vaccine. Vaccine science, innovation, and manufacturing are critical components in the development of safe and efficacious vaccines for national immunization programs.

Licensure of any new vaccine requires that efficacy be demonstrated from preclinical studies. The vaccine manufacturer begins this process upon filing an Investigational New Drug (IND) application with U.S. Food and Drug Administration (FDA). All information concerning vaccine formulation, vaccine manufacturing, stability and sterility testing, and results of animal testing is submitted to the FDA prior to conducting human trials. The FDA approves the implementation of human studies only if the new vaccine demonstrates preliminary potency, safety, and effectiveness in animal studies.

The following section outlines the objectives of preclinical and clinical trials involving candidate vaccines. The following series should be

Exhibit 10–2 Contraindications for Vaccinations

Severe allergy to vaccine component
Severe illness
Immunosuppression (live vaccines only)
HIV infection (live virus vaccines except measles vaccine)
Pregnancy (especially live vaccines)
Encephalopathy (pertussis vaccine only)
Recent receipt of blood products (MMR and varicella)

considered hierarchical in nature; that is, the decision to progress to the next phase is based on promising results from the previous set of studies. Table 10–5 provides an overview of the progression of human vaccine studies.

Preclinical Studies

Animal testing is used to develop assays that assess the humoral and cellular immune response to candidate vaccines. Through a series of studies, appropriate animal models are used to determine the dose–response relationship and to identify optimal routes of administration and dosing schedule necessary to achieve the maximum beneficial dose (ie, the dose that maximizes the protective immune response and minimizes serious adverse events). Animal studies represent the first step in evaluating vaccine safety. A list of vaccine-induced toxicities is established, which may include severe systemic effects, organ systems damage, carcinogenicity, and teratogenicity. Provided that potential benefit is deemed to outweigh potential harm, results from these animal models proceed to subsequent testing in human studies.

Phase I: Dose Finding and Safety

Following FDA review and approval by a local institutional review board (IRB), early vaccine studies in humans are conducted to evaluate vaccine dose and safety and to assess whether the vaccine is biologically active. Specific toxicities (eg, local and systemic reactions, hematologic abnormalities) are evaluated in both phase I and phase II safety and immunogenicity studies, which usually take the form of randomized controlled trials. Rules for stopping an immunization series are established from the onset and are adapted as more data are collected.

Most preventive vaccine clinical trials begin with trials in healthy, adult volunteers. Childhood vaccines are first tested in healthy adults and older children, prior to testing in infants. For some vaccines (ie, HIV vaccines), initial clinical trials may be conducted in previously infected persons and subsequently among uninfected healthy adults. Adult studies typically begin with a single fixed dose of vaccine in a small number of volunteers (eg, 5–10 subjects). Postinoculation serologic assays measure the level and duration of the immune response. Adverse events are carefully enumerated and graded for severity, duration, and the relationship to vaccination. Small sequential studies may be conducted, whereby the vaccine dose is increased until a beneficial dose is established. Additional phase I or phase I/II safety and immunogenicity studies are performed in children and infants to fine-tune the dose, define the vaccine schedule, and continue monitoring immune response and vaccine safety in these age groups.

Phase II: Safety and Immunogenicity Trials

In phase II studies, safety, immunogenicity, and preliminary estimates of probable efficacy are the primary endpoints. Safety and immunogenicity endpoints are predefined, based on preclinical and phase I studies. The vaccine is tested in healthy persons representing the population for which the vaccine is indicated. Sample size needs to be sufficiently large to measure benefit (ie, evidence of immunogenicity) without compromising the ability to estimate rates of adverse events. Studies of 50–100 persons can measure adverse events at a rate of 10 in 100 doses and estimate the beneficial effect that occurs in 10% ($\pm$ 10%) or more of the population. As in phase I

Table 10–5 Progression of Vaccine Clinical Trials

	PHASE I Dose-Finding and Safety	PHASE II Safety and Immunogenicity	PHASE III Randomized Double-Blinded Placebo-Controlled Vaccine Efficacy Trial
Purpose	These studies determine the dose response and/or beneficial dose (BD). The BD is defined as the dose that achieves immunologic response without severe adverse events (SAEs). Route of administration and dosing schedule necessary to achieve BD with lowest chance of SAEs are evaluated. Evidence of immune response (eg, rise in antivaccine antibody titer) is assessed and surrogate serologic markers for vaccine efficacy are defined.	These studies measure the proportion of side effects (general, serious, nonreversible) and assess evidence of efficacy. Immune response is assessed by determining the proportion of subjects who achieve a predetermined immunologic response (eg, two- or fourfold rise in antibody titer). In a comparative trial, the proportion of side effects and level of immune response can be compared between dose group or between vaccine and placebo groups.	These studies estimate the vaccine efficacy, by comparing the infection incidence in the vaccinated (new vaccine) with the incidence in placebo or standard vaccine group. They continue to enumerate side effects and determine the proportion of subjects with all side effects and severe side effects. Also, they may examine the feasibility of adding vaccination to ongoing immunization program.
Population	Healthy adults with no conditions that contraindicate vaccination.	Healthy adults, children (receiving booster dose), or infants (receiving primary series) with no conditions that contraindicate vaccination.	Adults, children, or infants at risk of infection, who are otherwise healthy with no conditions that contraindicate vaccination.
Study Design	Open label study in single or sequential samples.	Open label prospective cohort studies or small randomized controlled trials are used to assess fixed doses of vaccine or to compare differing doses or vaccine schedules.	Randomized double-blinded trial of new vaccine versus standard vaccine or placebo.
Sample Size	Number needed to estimate beneficial dose. Series of small studies (eg, 5–10 persons each).	Number needed to estimate proportion of persons who achieve a favorable immunologic outcome without hindering the study's ability to measure side effect levels. Samples may range from 20 to 200 persons.	Number needed to estimate the difference between intervention and control groups or to measure vaccine efficacy. Samples may range from 100 to more than 10,000 persons.

continues

Table 10–5 continued

	PHASE I	PHASE II	PHASE III
	Dose-Finding and Safety	*Safety and Immunogenicity*	*Randomized Double-Blinded Placebo-Controlled Vaccine Efficacy Trial*
Endpoints	*Dose Finding:* Dosing schedule and route of administration that are required to achieve beneficial immunologic response, ie, rise in neutralizing antibody titer. *Safety:* Number and proportion of expected or unexpected adverse events, including local reactions (pain and swelling) and systemic reactions (allergy and fever). *Biologic Effect:* Proportion of persons who achieve surrogate measure of protective immune response.	*Safety:* Expected and unexpected adverse events are enumerated, graded for severity and relationship to vaccine. Adverse events include local reactions (pain, erythema, swelling, induration); systemic reactions (allergic reaction, fever, arthralgia, myalgia, lymphadenopathy, hepatic, renal, hematologic, neurologic-irritability, fussiness, gastrointestinal, cardiac reaction); or other toxicities. *Immunogenicity:* The proportion of persons who achieve protective immune response (after 1 or multiple doses of vaccine) is used as an indicator of clinical efficacy. Markers for protective immune response include: • neutralizing antibody titer and rise in antibody titer from baseline • proliferation of specific cytotoxic T lymphocytes	*Efficacy:* The number of new infections in the vaccinated versus the control group. Vaccine efficacy is also measured in all study participants, then within strata by number of doses received. Clinical or biologic efficacy is estimated by comparing the proportion of vaccinated and controls who achieve a defined threshold of protective immune response (such as a fourfold rise in neutralizing antibody). This measure is important when determining whether new vaccine is equivalent to standard vaccine. *Safety:* Number and grade of adverse events in both groups. *Feasibility:* Large clinical trials begin to demonstrate the feasibility of adding a new vaccine to an immunization program. Feasibility indicators include: follow-up rates (completion and dropouts), tolerability and acceptability of vaccine, as well as barriers to compliance to immunization schedule.
Measures of Effect	Estimates of single means or proportions.	Estimate of single proportion (or mean) or difference between two proportions (or means) for comparative trial.	Estimate of difference between two means or proportions. Estimate of vaccine efficacy (VE).

studies, postinoculation serologic assays are performed to measure the level and duration of the immune response. Participants are closely evaluated for severity and duration of adverse events. Expected adverse events and severity grades are listed in toxicity tables used to standardize safety evaluations. Correlates of protection provide evidence of vaccine clinical efficacy. These are immunologic markers of immune response to the vaccine, such as seroconversion (ie, development of neutralizing antibodies), rise in antibody titer (ie, booster response), and development of cell-mediated immune response (eg, cytotoxic T lymphocytes).

Phase III: Comparative Efficacy Trials

Comparative efficacy trials determine the impact of vaccination on prevention of infection and begin to assess the feasibility of administering vaccinations in at-risk populations. Vaccines that are shown to be safe and immunogenic in phase I and II trials advance to phase III randomized comparative trials to assess true vaccine efficacy. Phase III trials involve large numbers of susceptible persons in "real world" settings. The definitive study design for determining vaccine efficacy is the randomized, double-blinded, placebo-controlled trial. Often, multiple clinic sites are required to recruit a large enough sample to demonstrate vaccine efficacy with adequate study power. Sample size requirements depend on the incidence of infection in an unvaccinated population (or a similar vaccinated population if a standard vaccine is already available), as well as the reduction in incidence one expects to observe in the vaccinated population. In phase III trials, vaccine efficacy is calculated as the observed reduction in incidence in the vaccinated versus the unvaccinated population, expressed as a percentage:

$$VE = \frac{I_{controls} - I_{vaccinated}}{I_{controls}} \times 100$$

Randomization strives to achieve comparability between vaccinated and unvaccinated groups with respect to demographic characteristics and risk factors for natural infection. Nevertheless, residual confounding may persist. The nature and extent of confounding depends on factors relating to the host, agent, and environment. For example, risk factors for most childhood infections include other immunizations, attendance in day-care or school, exposure to infected individuals, and general health status. In vaccine trials of HIV, HBV, and hepatitis C, risk factors that require consideration include the number of unprotected sexual acts and sharing of potentially contaminated injection equipment. For infections such as malaria that are transmitted by a vector (eg, *Aedes* sp), it is important to take into account the level of endemicity of *Plasmodium* sp and participants' use of mosquito nets and insect repellents. Appropriate adjustment for these potential confounders is crucial, because differential exposure to the infectious agent across the vaccinated and control groups can bias estimates of vaccine efficacy.

VACCINE EFFICACY AND VACCINE EFFECTIVENESS

Measures of vaccine efficacy (VE) are calculated from prelicensure, randomized, double-blind, clinical trials. Results from postlicensure observational studies associate disease outcomes with vaccine failure in fully vaccinated and inadequately vaccinated individuals, and in populations with low vaccine coverage. Whereas vaccine trials measure efficacy, the overall estimate of protective effect calculated from an observational epidemiologic study is more accurately defined as vaccine effectiveness (VE*).[23] Overall vaccine effectiveness is the result of both the vaccine's direct effect, which refers to its ability to protect individuals from infection, and its indirect effect, which is its ability to reduce the spread of the infection in a population (Figure 10–1).[24,25] For a discussion of the ways in which vaccines can indirectly decrease the duration of disease, alter susceptibility, or reduce the infective period of an organism in a given population, refer to Halloran et al.[25–27] Table 10–6 summa-

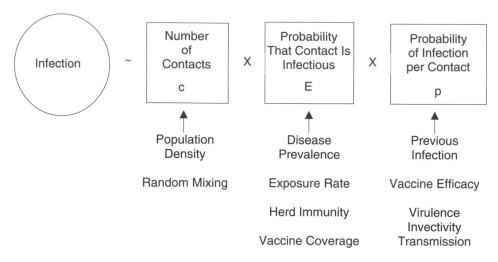

Figure 10–1 Dynamics of infection in a population

rizes equations for calculating vaccine effectiveness.

In any given population, spread of disease is a function of the rate of contact (c), the probability of exposure to an infectious agent (E), and the probability that exposure leads to infection (p). Determination of VE* generally assumes that infected, immune, and susceptible persons are randomly mixed in the population and that the population is sufficiently dense so that contact (c) will be common.[25–27] The probability of exposure is related to both the prevalence of disease and the number of immune persons in the population. *Herd immunity*, which refers to the level of immunity in a population, depends on the extent of immunity acquired from previous epidemics, as well as other factors, such as vaccine coverage. The probability that contact with an infected person will result in infection is a function of an individual's susceptibility and the virulence of the organism. Individual susceptibility can be reduced if a previous infection conferred protective immunity or if the person received an efficacious vaccine prior to exposure.

In a randomized clinical trial, vaccine efficacy is calculated, using the following equation, where VE represents vaccine efficacy, I_{unv} represents incidence in the unvaccinated, and I_{vac} represents incidence in the vaccinated:

$$VE = \frac{I_{unv} - I_{vac}}{I_{unv}}$$

The following equation is derived from dividing by the incidence in the unvaccinated:

$$VE = \frac{I_{vac}}{I_{unv}} = 1 - \frac{C_{vac} \times E_{vac} \times P_{vac}}{C_{unv} \times E_{unv} \times P_{unv}} = 1 - RR$$

As demonstrated by these equations, the ratio of incidence in the vaccinated to unvaccinated groups is a measure of relative risk (RR). The equation VE = 1 – RR is useful in epidemiologic studies, where vaccine effectiveness (VE*) can be assessed. Vaccine effectiveness (VE*) approximates vaccine efficacy (VE) under the following circumstances:

1. when exposure (E) to the infectious agent is not dependent on vaccination status and does not differ across comparison groups
2. when the vaccinated and unvaccinated persons arise from the same population, such that the rate of contact (c) is equivalent

Table 10–6 Vaccine Effectiveness Equations

Prospective Studies	*Cohort*	$VE^* = 1 - RR$
	Outbreak Investigation (Attack Rates or Cumulative Incidence)	$VE^* = 1 - AR_{vac} / AR_{unv}$
	Household Spread (Secondary Attack Rate)	$VE^* = 1 - SAR_{vac} / SAR_{unv}$
	Longitudinal Follow-up with Time to Event Data	
	Life-Table (Hazard Ratio)	$VE^* = 1 - \lambda_{vac} / \lambda_{unv}$
	Person-Time (Cumulative Incidence)	$VE^* = 1 - CI_{vac} / CI_{unv}$
Retrospective Studies	*Case Control Studies*	$VE^* = 1 - OR$

Unmatched

$VE^* = 1 - (a/c) / (b/d)$
ratio of the odds of vaccination in cases and controls

!	*Case*	*Control*
Vaccinated	a	b
Unvaccinated	c	d

Matched

$VE^* = 1 - b/c$
ratio of discordant pairs

!	*Control*	
Case	*Vaccine*	*No vaccine*
Vaccine	a	b
No vaccine	c	d

Logistic Regression Model or Proportional Hazard Model

$VE^* = 1 - e^{\beta vac}$

Source: Adapted with permission from M.E. Halloran, C.J. Struchiner, and I.M. Longini, Study Designs for Evaluating Different Efficacy and Effectiveness Aspects of Vaccines, *American Journal of Epidemiology*, Vol. 146, No. 10, pp. 789–803, © 1997, The Johns Hopkins University School of Hygiene and Public Health.

If the comparison groups are similar, vaccine effectiveness, $VE^* = 1 - p_{vac}/p_{unv}$, is a function of the ratio of individual immunity in the vaccinated and unvaccinated groups and can be estimated by $VE^* = 1 - RR$.[25–27]

EPIDEMIOLOGIC STUDIES

After licensure, vaccines are distributed among heterogeneous populations at risk of disease, who will vary in age, infirmity, access to health care, and risk of exposure. At this point, observational studies play an important role in assessing vaccine effectiveness. In contrast to randomized clinical trials evaluating vaccine efficacy, case control and cohort studies evaluate the combination of vaccine efficacy and the success of a given immunization program. A significant decline in the overall incidence of disease is one indicator that the vaccine itself and the immunization campaign have contributed to the prevention of disease. However, vaccine effectiveness can be suboptimal, due to a variety of factors. For example, the potency of an inactivated vaccine can be reduced if a specific lot of vaccine was less antigenic, whereas the potency of a live attenuated vaccine can be compromised if the cold chain was not maintained. Vaccine effectiveness can also be low, due to incomplete vaccine coverage, which is discussed further in another section.

Seldom, if ever, do vaccine efficacy and/or coverage attain 100%. Outbreaks among vaccinated populations can and do occur. Observational studies are often used to determine whether vaccine failures contribute to epidemics in the general population or within subgroups, and these lend themselves to the study of risk factors for vaccine failure. Vaccine effectiveness can be measured within a population experiencing an outbreak, special populations at risk of infection (eg, the elderly, children in day care, people in refugee camps), or as part of community-wide surveillance of vaccine-preventable diseases.

Vaccine effectiveness can be determined by comparing risk of disease among vaccinated and nonvaccinated groups. In general, an ideal study includes groups of comparable susceptibility before vaccination, equal exposure to disease before and after vaccination, and equal risk of being diagnosed with disease during the study period.[24] As in randomized trials of vaccine efficacy, it is important to ensure that these groups are comparable with respect to exposure, risk of infection, access to the vaccine, and opportunity for diagnosis. Potential bias may occur if:

1. there is unequal exposure to disease that causes individuals to self-select for vaccination
2. vaccination status systematically differs between healthy and diseased persons
3. disease is differentially diagnosed in the vaccinated versus the unvaccinated[24,28]

Essential components to any epidemiologic study include definition of a case, standardized case finding, ascertainment of vaccine status, and level of exposure.

An a priori case definition of infection or disease should be sensitive and specific. A case definition that poorly represents the disease in question may lead to imprecise estimates of vaccine effectiveness.[28,29] For invasive infections (eg, bacteremia and meningitis), the organism is isolated and cultured; such laboratory confirmation yields a sensitive and specific case definition. Although it is not essential for every observational study, laboratory confirmation of cases generally increases the point estimate of vaccine effectiveness.[24]

Vaccination may prevent clinical disease but not infection or it may reduce the severity of disease, resulting in a differential disease diagnosis in the vaccinated versus unvaccinated groups. Therefore, to avoid bias, a case definition must detect a spectrum of mild, moderate, and severe disease. The point estimate of vaccine effectiveness will be biased by the extent to which groups differ in assessment, medical care and diagnosis, validity of parental history of disease, and quality of medical records. Providers often underreport disease that they may deem to be less important to public health. Therefore, if case finding is established solely through passive surveillance, this may bias estimates of vaccine effectiveness. In any study, it is crucial to assure that case finding occurs with the same degree of rigor in both the vaccinated and unvaccinated groups.

Equal effort must be made to confirm vaccination status in diseased and nondiseased persons. Reliance on the self-reporting of vaccination status or inaccurate vaccination records (eg, school records) may result in misclassification. When possible, self-reported vaccine histories should be confirmed through provider records, which are also important in confirming vaccination dates, vaccine type, manufacturer and lot number, and expiration dates.

The definition of *vaccination* must also be clear. When multiple doses of vaccine are required to develop full protection, the appropriate comparison is between persons who receive no vaccine and those who receive a complete course. If it is assumed that one or two doses induces some immunity, inclusion of these persons into the unvaccinated group would enrich that group with "nonsusceptibles," thereby lowering the attack rates in the unvaccinated group, relative to attack rates in the vaccinated. This, in turn, lowers the estimate of vaccine effectiveness. Alternatively, if the vaccinated group includes persons receiving less than the full series, the vaccinated group would be enriched with "suceptibles," resulting in increased attack rates. This would result in decreased estimates of vaccine effectiveness.[24] Vaccine effectiveness for one, two, and three doses compared with no vaccination can be calculated from prospective cohort and case control studies.

Observational studies evaluiating vaccine effectiveness are vulnerable to selection factors that can cause rates derived from diseased and nondiseased or vaccinated and unvaccinated groups to differ systematically. Factors such as age, sex, race, socioeconomic status, place of work or residence, attendance in school, day care, and residence in jails or nursing homes may independently be related to both risk of disease and to vaccination status. Therefore, these studies must diligently control for confounding factors in the design (eg, through stratification or matching) or, alternatively, by making appropriate adjustments of vaccine effectiveness in the analysis.

In highly endemic areas and/or where there are adequate resources, surveillance is conducted among cohorts of vaccinated and unvaccinated persons. Upon establishing vaccination status at baseline, the cumulative incidence of infection in vaccinated persons (CI_{vac}) is compared with the cumulative incidence of infection in unvaccinated persons (CI_{unv}), estimating the relative risk.[27] Other types of epidemiologic study designs that are used to evaluate vaccine effectiveness are described in detail below. In-depth discussion on these field methods is found in Halloran et al.[26,27]

Seroprevalence Cross-Sectional Studies

Evidence of vaccine efficacy and effectiveness is often correlated with some protective level of antibody in serum. In a cross-sectional study, a single serum sample is drawn, and antibody levels are correlated with past records of vaccination and disease. The comparison of the proportion of subjects who have been vaccinated with protective antibody with the proportion of subjects not vaccinated with protective antibody is a prevalence ratio (PR). In this case, the calculation of vaccine effectiveness is VE* = 1 − PR. One advantage of seroprevalence studies is the ability to assess quickly the vaccine-induced immunity, measured according to the length of time since vaccination. These results should be interpreted with caution, because antibody responses wane over time, and the absence of antibody does not necessarily indicate susceptibility.

Prospective Studies

Populations at high risk of infection can be defined during an outbreak investigation, a household contact study, or in a highly endemic area. Using methods such as personal interviews and medical records review, vaccination status can be confirmed and a cohort of vaccinated and unvaccinated persons followed for the purpose of identifying new cases of disease. Prospective studies yield valid estimates of RR when the disease is common and exposure (ie, vaccination status) is rare.[30] In situations where the attack rate (AR) is expected to be high and the population is a mix of vaccinated and unvaccinated persons, a prospective study is useful for evaluating vaccine effectiveness.

In outbreak studies, vaccination status is established at baseline, and the RR is used to compare the AR in the vaccinated (AR_{vac}) and the unvaccinated (AR_{unv}). Households of primary cases represent highly exposed populations that warrant close observation. As high-risk households are identified, vaccination status is confirmed for each member, and any secondary cases are identified. To estimate vaccine effectiveness, the RR is calculated as the ratio of vaccinated secondary cases (SAR_{vac}) to unvaccinated secondary cases (SAR_{unv}) from all households. Time-to-event analyses (ie, survival analysis) are also useful for estimating RR. Using Cox proportional hazards models, the hazard ratio is an estimate of the instantaneous relative risk, which is the ratio of the probability of disease in the vaccinated group at some time point (λ_{vac}), relative to the probability of disease in the unvaccinated (λ_{unv}) at the same time point.[25–27]

In prospective studies, factors that erroneously increase the attack rate in the vaccinated, relative to the unvaccinated, will cause vaccine effectiveness to be underestimated, whereas any erroneous increase in the attack rate in the unvaccinated, relative to the vaccinated, will lead to an overestimate of vaccine effectiveness.

Case Control Studies

Case control studies can be an appropriate study design for assessing vaccine effectiveness when the disease is rare. One advantage is that data pertaining to multiple risk factors of vaccine failure can be collected and evaluated. Cases are often identified through a surveillance system, such as direct laboratory reporting or national surveillance databases. To avoid bias, controls should be selected from the same population as cases and should not significantly differ with respect to their probability of vaccination or exposure to infection. As in other case control studies, a matched or unmatched design may be used. The odds ratio (OR) is used to estimate RR or, in this case, VE*. The OR is calculated as the ratio of the odds of vaccination in the cases, relative to the odds of vaccination in the controls, or the ratio of discordant pairs for unmatched and matched designs, respectively. Vaccine effectiveness is calculated as VE* = 1 – OR. When logistic models are used to calculate the OR for disease in the vaccinated, the equation VE* = 1 – $e\beta_{vac}$ is the measure of vaccine effectiveness, where $e\beta_{vac}$ is the expotentiated log OR of disease in the vaccinated population. In case control studies, VE* is underestimated when vacci-

nation rates are erroneously overreported in the cases, relative to the controls and overestimated when controls are more likely to be misclassified as being vaccinated, relative to cases.[28]

Monitoring Adverse Events

Comparative studies continue to collect information on adverse events. Additional post-licensure monitoring is achieved through the use of surveillance systems to track vaccine-related adverse events, which is a mandate of the National Childhood Injury Act of 1986. By 1998, a nationwide vaccine adverse event reporting system (VAERS) was established by the U.S. Department of Health and Human Services.[31] VAERS is a passive reporting system designed to collect case-series data to detect rare events and identify trends in commonly reported adverse events. A strength of VAERS is its demonstrated feasibility as a cost-effective public health system for identifying potential harmful effects of mass vaccination. Health care providers and vaccine manufacturers are required to report all adverse events associated with the administration of a U.S. licensed vaccine. VAERS is especially important with newly licensed vaccines and in the assessment of new indications for vaccinations.

Like many passive reporting systems, VAERS case-series data are biased, due to under- and/or overreporting of suspected vaccine reactions.[31,32] Rates of adverse events cannot be calculated because the system does not collect denominator data (ie, number of persons vaccinated or number of doses given). However, VAERS data can be used to identify clusters of rare adverse events, such as associations between oral polio vaccine and poliomyelitis, and DTP with Sudden Infant Death Syndrome (SIDS). Following identification of adverse event clusters, clinical, epidemiologic, and laboratory investigations are required to assess causality. Studies that substantiate severe adverse disease may lead to the withdrawal of vaccine, the development of safer vaccines, or compensation for persons who experienced an adverse event.

The Vaccine Safety Datalink (VSD) Project is another effort to improve postlicensure monitoring of vaccine-related adverse events. Beginning in 1991, the CDC, in partnership with health maintenance organizations (HMOs), established large cohorts of vaccinated children.[33] Subsequently, the VSD has expanded to monitor vaccine-related adverse events in adolescents and adults. VSD data are generated during routine health care visits and contain adverse event as well as denominator data (number vaccinated and doses administered) on large stable populations. As such, the system is less subject to underreporting or other biases common to passive surveillance systems. The VSD thus provides a rapid and economic means of conducting postlicensure comparative studies of vaccine safety.[33]

DIRECT IMPACT OF VACCINATION

"The impact of vaccination on the health of the people worldwide is difficult to exaggerate. With the exception of safe water, no modality, not even antibiotics, has had such a major effect upon reducing mortality and subsequent population growth."[34] This direct impact from widespread use of vaccines can be easily understood when one examines incidence rates of specific diseases over time. Below, we highlight disease trends in poliomyelitis, measles, and invasive *Hemophilus influenzae* type b to illustrate the impact of effective vaccines and vaccine programs.

Polio

The increased incidence of paralytic poliomyelitis coincided with improvements in hygiene and societal developments in the 1930s and 1940s (Figure 10–2). Between 1940 and 1952, the incidence of paralytic polio in the United States rose from less than 12 cases per 100,000 persons to about 37 cases per 100,000 persons. Although the total number of cases declined before the first vaccine was introduced in 1955, the proportion of paralytic cases increased from a rate of 66% to 88% of all cases.[35]

The Salk inactivated polio vaccine (IPV), was the first vaccine licensed in 1955. After licensure, the United States began a mass immunization campaign, and the incidence of poliomyelitis fell dramatically as more and more children were immunized. A 90% reduction in the number of poliomyelitis cases was attained with Salk IPV alone. As a result, the death rate declined from 1.9 per 100,000 cases between 1915 and 1924 to 0.1 per 100,000 cases in 1961. The Salk IPV did not induce sufficient mucosal immunity to protect against reinfection, and outbreaks continued to occur, including a high proportion of cases that were fully vaccinated.[35,36]

The Sabin oral live attenuated vaccine (OPV) was licensed for human use in 1961–1962, after which the incidence of poliomyelitis continued to decline further; in 1964, only 59 polio cases were reported in the United States. In 1960, a total of 2,525 paralytic cases was reported, compared with 61 in 1965.[35,36] Thus, the Sabin OPV quickly became the vaccine of choice in the United States and in most other parts of the world (see section in this chapter entitled "Toward Global Eradication of Polio").

Measles

Regional elimination of measles began in 1989, when the World Health Assembly resolved to reduce measles morbidity and mortality by 90% and 95%, respectively, by 1995. The goal to eliminate indigenous measles in the United States was set in 1978. In September 1999, the CDC reported a record low number of measles cases; only 100 measles cases were confirmed in 1998, most of which were imported or associated with an imported case. Very soon, measles may no longer be an indigenous disease in the United States.[37]

Five years prior to measles vaccine licensure (1958–1962), the average annual number of reported measles cases in the United States was 503,282, with approximately 500 deaths per year.[38]

Epidemic cycles of measles occurred every 2–3 years, and the actual annual number was esti-

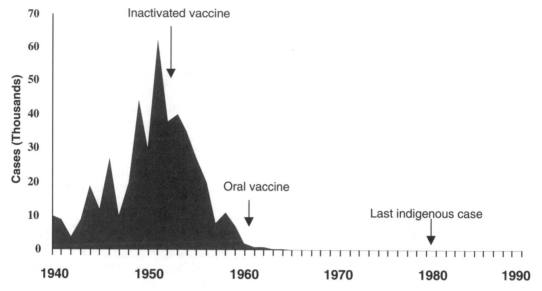

Figure 10–2 Poliomyelitis cases reported in the United States, 1940–1990. *Source:* Reprinted from the Centers for Disease Control and Prevention.

mated to be about 3–4 million. More than 50% of the population had experienced measles by age 6, and more than 90% had measles by age 15, with the highest incidence between ages 5 and 9 years.[39] The first live attenuated measles vaccine (Edmonston B strain) was licensed for use in 1963 (the currently available vaccine, the Enders-Edmonston strain, was licensed in 1968). Following initial licensure, the incidence of measles decreased by more than 98%, and the 2–3 year epidemic cycles no longer occurred (Figure 10–3).[39]

In the United States, between 1985 and 1988, 42% of measles cases occurred in children who were vaccinated on or after their first birthday, and 68% of cases were in school-aged children who had been appropriately vaccinated. However, of the latter group, only 16% had been appropriately vaccinated. The measles outbreaks in 1985 and 1986 led to a recommendation in 1989 of universal reimmunization of children against measles, either at school entry or at entry into middle school or junior high school.[39]

Once again, a resurgence of measles occurred between 1989 and 1991. There were 18,193 measles cases in 1989, 27,786 in 1990, and 9,643 in 1991. During this resurgence, the age distribution changed, and children 5 years and younger accounted for 45–48% of the new cases. The principal cause of the measles epidemic of 1989–1991 was failure to vaccinate children at the recommended age.[40,41] Pockets of low immunization coverage were observed in inner-city communities, and the highest measles incidence occurred among Hispanic and African American children. Surveys conducted in areas experiencing preschool measles outbreaks indicated that as few as 50% of children had been vaccinated for measles by their second birthday and that African American and Hispanic children were less likely to be appropriately vaccinated. Reported cases of measles declined rapidly after the 1989–1991 resurgence. This decline was due primarily to intensive efforts to vaccinate preschool children. Measles vaccination levels among 2-year-old children have increased from

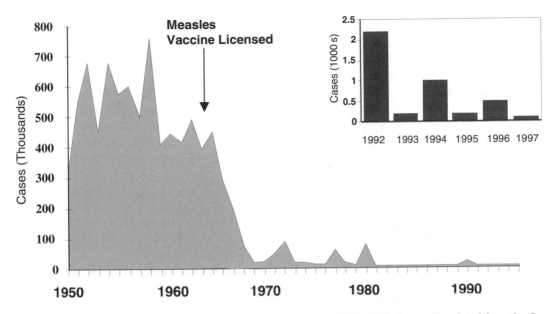

Figure 10–3 Reported measles cases by year in the United States, 1950–1997. *Source:* Reprinted from the Centers for Disease Control and Prevention.

70% in 1990 to 91% in 1996. Since 1993, fewer than 1,000 cases have been reported annually.[39]

Measles incidence increased in 1994, due primarily to several large outbreaks among communities with religious and philosophic exemptions to vaccination. Smaller outbreaks were reported in unvaccinated preschool populations, vaccinated school populations (vaccine failures), college students, and adult communities. With increased intensity of measles vaccination, the number of preschool and school-aged measles outbreaks has declined. The CDC recommends that adults born in 1957 or later receive one dose of MMR upon college entrance or entrance to other post-high-school educational institutions.

In contrast, many developing countries have not yet achieved high rates of measles immunization coverage. The 1990 World Summit for Children adopted a goal of vaccinating 90% of children worldwide against measles by the year 2000.[42]

Hemophilus Influenzae Type B

Prior to the advent of an effective vaccine, it was estimated that 1 in every 200 children would develop an invasive *Hemophilus influenzae* type b (Hib) infection before the age of 5 years.[43] Subsequently, 60% of infected children developed bacterial meningitis, and 10% of these children died while many more suffered permanent impairments, ranging from hearing loss to mental retardation.

Since 1993, invasive Hib disease has decreased by 95%, and elimination in the United States is imminent (Figure 10–4). This decline began with the introduction of capsular polysaccharide Hib vaccine in 1985. This vaccine induced antibody in the majority of children aged 18 months and older but was less immunogenic in younger children. This vaccine was recommended for children at least 2 years of age, but most of the invasive disease occurred in children less than 1 year of age.[43] To overcome poor im-

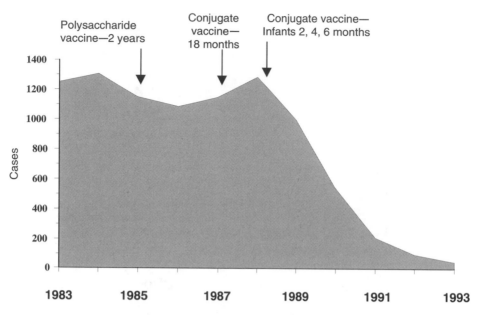

Figure 10–4 Hemophilus influenzae type B cases per year, United States, 1983–1993. *Source:* Reprinted from the National Institutes of Health.

munogenicity of polysaccharide-only vaccine, particularly in young infants, Hib polysaccharide-protein conjugates were developed. The first Hib conjugate vaccine was licensed in 1987 for children aged 18 months and older. In 1988, similar vaccines were licensed for children as young as 2 months of age, based on clinical trials showing over 90% efficacy of these vaccines in fully immunized infants.[44] By 1997, 93% of all 2-year-old children in the United States completed the Hib vaccine series. From 1989 to 1997, the race-adjusted incidence of Hib invasive disease among children younger than 5 years of age decreased by 99%, from 34 cases to 0.4 cases per 100,000 children.[45] Progress toward elimination of invasive Hib continues in the United States and in Europe. The importance of the disease is only now being recognized in many developing countries.

THE ROLE OF VACCINES IN ERADICATION OF SPECIFIC DISEASES

Eradication of a given communicable disease implies total control over morbidity, disability, mortality, and subclinical disease beyond control of the etiologic agent(s) itself. As suggested by Evans, eradication is achieved when there is no risk of infection or disease in the absence of vaccination or any other control measures.[46] The need to immunize susceptibles before natural infection occurs is a formidable obstacle in the case of many childhood diseases. Factors that favor the eradication of a communicable disease are provided in Exhibit 10–3.

An immunization program need not achieve 100% coverage to provide protection against disease in a community. Herd immunity implies

Exhibit 10–3 Factors Associated with Potential for Eradication of a Communicable Disease

---

Factors Associated with the Disease
Ease of diagnosis and treatment
Low prevalence of subclinical disease
High disease burden and economic impact
Immunity is long term or life-long
Disease cannot be reactivated
Disease has predictable seasonality

Factors Associated with the Etiologic Agent
Lack of an animal reservoir or vector
Only one causative agent or serotype
Short incubation period

Factors Associated with the Host or Target Population
Correlates or protection can be demonstrated

Host cannot be reinfected with the agent
Host cannot shed the organism once infection is resolved
Public acceptance of the vaccine and other control measures is high

Factors Associated with the Vaccine
Can confer long-lasting protection in a few injections
Minimal handling and storage requirements (eg, cold chain)
Simple administration
Can be administered simultaneously with other vaccines or adapted to schedules and timing of the national childhood immunization programs
Few short- or long-term adverse effects
Low cost to produce and purchase vaccine

Source: Adapted with permission from A.S. Evans, The Eradication of Communicable Diseases: Myth or Reality?, *American Journal of Epidemiology*, Vol. 122, No. 2, p. 200, © 1985, The Johns Hopkins University of Hygiene and Public Health.

---

that some level of immunity in a community can provide protection to susceptible (nonimmunized) persons. This collective immunologic protection represents an indirect effect of a vaccine beyond the level of the individual toward the level of the population.[25] However, the concept of herd immunity assumes that susceptible persons mix randomly within the population, which is often not the case. Groups of nonimmunized persons who share common characteristics (eg, age, religion, culture) often cluster together in relatively restricted geographic settings. The degree of herd immunity required to prevent an epidemic varies according to the specific disease, the extent to which an infected individual is capable of transmitting the infection, the duration of the infectious period, the size of the population, and mixing patterns within and between other populations.

The global eradication of smallpox provides the gold standard against which other eradication programs will inevitably be judged. Systematic application of smallpox vaccine began in Mexico and in Guatemala around 1805 and elsewhere in North America and Europe.[47] Prior to the initiation of a global immunization program aimed at its eradication, smallpox vaccine was offered to all age groups, but only those at risk (eg, health care workers, travelers) were specifically targeted. As a result, incomplete coverage caused outbreaks to continue throughout the world.

The first attempt at global immunization of smallpox was in 1956, but this effort was not successful in containing the disease. In 1967, there were still 10–15 million cases of smallpox per year, causing at least 2 million deaths and 100,000 cases of blindness.[47] In 1967, a global smallpox eradication program was established that included an additional strategy of surveillance/containment. This approach emphasized extensive case-finding and tracking of the origin of the outbreak, coupled with immunization of remaining susceptibles.[47] In addition, a standardized, lyophilized ("freeze-dried") vaccine had become available, and rapid, effective administration of vaccine was made possible through the development of the bifurcated needle. These factors, combined with leadership, political will, and adequate resource allocation, ended the smallpox pandemic. The last known case was observed in Somalia in 1977. Since this time, vaccination against smallpox has been considered unnecessary. In 1980, the WHO officially declared that smallpox had indeed been eradicated, representing the most significant public health achievement of the twentieth century.

Toward Global Eradication of Polio

Although incidence and prevalence of polio-induced paralysis decreased after the introduction of the Salk (IPV) and Sabin (OPV) vaccines in the 1950s, polio continued to take its toll in developing countries. In 1988, the World Health Assembly set a target to eradicate polio from the world by the year 2000. From the outset, eradication of polio appeared more difficult, compared with smallpox. Three serotypes of polio virus exist, with no considerable cross-immunity. Polio infection is associated with a higher prevalence of subclinical infections, a longer incubation period, and multiple routes of exposure. Moreover, several doses of OPV or IPV are usually needed to induce immunity.

Despite these obstacles, progress toward eradication of polio over the last 10 years has been impressive. The virus was eradicated from the Western Hemisphere in 1991. In 1998, the WHO estimated that global routine immunization coverage with three doses of OPV was 82%. Globally, numbers of cases have decreased by 80% since 1988, suggesting that eradication of polio may soon be a reality. In 1999, however, vaccine coverage varied widely by country, with the lowest coverage rates in Africa. Regions of Africa reached immunization coverage levels over 50% for the first time only in 1994. Polio cases today are largely confined to the poorest and most densely populated developing countries, where health delivery systems are inadequate. The major remaining reservoirs of polio are South Asia and West and Central Africa.[48]

Appropriate evaluation of an immunization program is essential for establishing whether control has been attained and whether a pool of susceptibles exists that could represent the potential for new outbreaks. Evaluation should include surveys to assess vaccine coverage, coupled with clinical and/or serologic confirmation of immunity. Sentinel surveillance should be maintained to identify the persistence of wild-type, indigenous, or imported virus, as well as live vaccine virus.[49] Ideally, this should include serology, as well as measures of morbidity (eg, acute flaccid paralysis, lameness). Only with systematic application of these methods will it be possible to determine whether polio or any other agent has been successfully eradicated.

Potential for Eradication of Other Communicable Diseases

The ability to control or attempt eradication of a communicable disease varies by country, according to demographic, environmental, hygienic, and economic factors.[48] Apart from criteria that need to be taken into account when considering a specific communicable disease for eradication, such programs require political will, financial resources, and unwavering commitment to meet predefined goals. In 1974, WHO created an Expanded Programme on Immunization (EPI), which initially aimed to eliminate six diseases: tuberculosis, diphtheria, neonatal tetanus, whooping cough, poliomyelitis, and measles (Table 10–7). Prior to this initiative, less than 5% of children in developing countries were being immunized against these preventable childhood diseases. In more recent years, new vaccines have been added to EPI (eg, TB, HBV,

Vaccines—Past, Present, and Future 279

Table 10–7 Year of Introduction of Selected First-Generation Vaccines for Use in Humans and Year of First National and Expanded Programme on Immunization (EPI)

Vaccine*	Year First Introduced	Year of First National Immunization Program	Year Beginning EPI
Smallpox	1798	1804	1956
Plague	1897	–	–
Diphtheria	1923	mid-1940s†	1974
Pertussis	1926	mid-1940s†	1974
Tuberculosis (BCG)	1921	1949	1974
Tetanus	1927	mid-1940s†	1974
Yellow Fever	1935	1989	1989 (endemic countries)
Oral Polio Vaccine	1962	1974	1974
Measles	1964	1974	1985
Mumps	1967	1977	–
Rubella	1969	1970	–
Hepatitis B	1981	1990	1995
Hemophilus influenzae Type B	1985	1985	pending
Varicella-Zoster	1984	1989	–

* Not necessarily the vaccine currently in use.
† Approximate time period of wide use in the United States.

Notes:
- 1974 EPI established with six targeted diseases: diphtheria, pertussis, tetanus, measles, polio, and tuberculosis (BCG).
- Rubella and mumps vaccines were never adapted into the EPI as single-antigen vaccines.

yellow fever), although the number of countries participating in the various programs varies considerably. Since the establishment of EPI, major progress has been made toward the elimination of other communicable diseases in various parts of the world. For example, routine administration of tetanus toxoid has virtually eliminated neonatal tetanus.

In a response to poor vaccine coverage in preschool children, the United States launched the Childhood Immunization Initiative in 1993. Its five strategies include improving the quality and quantity of immunization services; reducing vaccine costs; increasing community participation, education, and partnerships; improving systems for monitoring diseases and vaccinations; and improving vaccines and vaccine use.

Following establishment of this program, measles, diphtheria, mumps, pertussis, tetanus, HiB, and congenital rubella have been virtually eliminated from the United States. However, there are known subpopulations of nonimmunized persons that represent the potential for new outbreaks.

Despite the successes described above, many infectious diseases are unlikely to be eradicated. Global eradication of measles has proven to be a difficult task, due to the narrow window of opportunity available to vaccinate after loss of protective maternal antibodies and exposure to natural infection. Control of influenza is hampered by the multiplicity of antigenic types, high contagiousness of the disease, and the persistence of multiple reservoirs (ie, swine, fowl) for the origin of new recombinant viruses. Eradication of urban yellow fever proves difficult because jungle fever persists in endemic areas. Whereas vaccines against several herpes viruses (eg, Epstein-Barr virus, herpes simplex, cytomegalovirus, HHV-8) are under development and a vaccine against varicella is commercially available, herpes virus infections are characterized by widespread subclinical infections, multiple routes of exposure, and heterogeneity of serologic subtypes that can become reactivated. Apart from biologic considerations, it must be recognized that some vaccines that have been proven both efficacious and effective have not been licensed, due to high cost, low public health priority, or lack of endorsement from pharmaceutical companies.

BARRIERS TO VACCINE IMPLEMENTATION AND COVERAGE

Seemingly insurmountable barriers are encountered in the attempt to deliver proven vaccines to those who need them the most. Because most vaccines are developed and manufactured in developed countries, steps must be taken to ensure that live vaccine can be transported and stored in a developing country in a viable form, maintaining the cold chain where

appropriate. Staff must be trained in vaccine administration, safe injection techniques, and program management. To increase vaccine acceptability, public education campaigns are required, using materials that are sensitive to local language and culture.

Even in developed countries, proven vaccines do not necessarily reach those individuals who are at highest risk of infection. Although hepatitis B has been added to childhood immunization schedules in many developed countries, immunization levels are low among injection drug users and homosexual/bisexual men, who remain at high risk of infection (Exhibit 10–4).

Pockets of low coverage in most, if not all, countries are capable of perpetuating disease transmission. Even when adequate coverage has been achieved, births, in-migration, waning immunity, and requirements for multiple doses indicate that diligence is required to maintain herd immunity. Threats to achieving and maintaining coverage include wars, civil unrest, and natural disasters that can destroy the health infrastructure supporting immunization programs. The possibility of changes in the natural history of some diseases (eg, new route of infection, new reservoir or host, reactivation of latent disease) underscores the need for continued sentinel surveillance in national and global immunization programs. The high cost of many proven vac-

---

Exhibit 10–4 Barriers to Achieving High Coverage with Recombinant Hepatitis B Vaccine in the United States

1. One quarter of HBV-infected persons deny known risk factors for HBV infection.
2. Access to high-risk populations (eg, homosexual/bisexual men, injection drug users, illegal aliens from endemic countries) is difficult because populations are "hidden"; high-risk behaviors are highly stigmatized.
3. Low awareness of HBV infection and consequences of disease (ie, hepatitis, liver cancer).
4. Low acceptability of vaccine schedule.
5. Lack of third-party reimbursement to cover vaccine costs.
6. Rapid acquisition of HBV infection among high-risk populations.
7. Age-specific decline in immunogenicity of vaccine.
8. Waning of induced immunity over time (ie, protection estimated to last 13 years).

cines also prevents many countries from adding them to their national immunization programs. If global eradication of major vaccine-preventable diseases is to be upheld as a realistic goal, devel-

oped countries, nongovernmental organizations, and pharmaceutical companies must fulfill their obligation to support immunization programs in resource-poor countries.

REFERENCES

1. Hume EH. *Vaccines*. Baltimore: W.B. Saunders Company; 1940.

2. Rappouli R. New and improved vaccines against diphtheria and tetanus. In: *New Generation Vaccines*. 2nd ed. New York: Marcel Dekker; 1997:417–436.

3. Hellstrom KE, Hellstrom I, Chen L. Antitumor vaccines. In: *New Generation Vaccines*. 2nd ed. New York: Marcel Dekker, Inc; 1997:1095–1116.

4. Pasteur L. *Vaccines*. Paris: W.B. Saunders Company; 1885.

5. Abbas A, Lichtman A, Pober J. *Cellular and Molecular Immunology*. 3rd ed. Philadelphia: W.B. Sanders Company; 1997.

6. Janeway C, Travers P. *Immunobiology*. 3rd ed. New York: Garland Publishers; 1997.

7. Huston DP. The biology of the immune system. *JAMA*. 1997;22:1804–1814.

8. McDonnell WM, Askari FK. Immunization. *JAMA*. 1998;22:2000–2007.

9. Levine MM, Tacket CO, Galen JE, et al. Progress in development of new attenuated strains of *Salmonella typhi* as live oral vaccine against typhoid fever. In: *New Generation Vaccines*. 2nd ed. New York: Marcel Dekker; 1997:437–446.

10. Perez-Schael I, Guntinas MJ, Perez M, et al. Efficacy of the rhesus rotavirus based quadrivalent vaccine in infants and young children in Venezuela. *N Engl J Med*. 1997;337:1181–1187.

11. Black F. Measles in acute viral infections. In: Evans AS, ed. *Viral Infections of Humans: Epidemiology and Control*. 2nd ed. New York: Plenum Medical Co; 1989:521–522.

12. Kollaritsch H, Que JU, Kunz C, Wiedermann G, Herzog C, Cryz SJ. Safety and immunogenicity of live oral cholera and typhoid vaccines administered alone or in combination with antimalarial drugs, oral polio vaccine, or yellow fever vaccine. *J Infect Dis*. 1997;175(4):871–875.

13. Guess HA. Combination vaccines: issues in evaluation of effectiveness and safety. *Epidemiol Rev*. 1999;2(41): 89–95.

14. Roux E, Yersin A. Contribution a l'etude de la diptherie. *Ann Inst Pasteur*. 1888;2:629–661.

15. Steere AC, Sikand VK, Meurice F, et al, and the Lyme Disease Vaccine Study Group. Vaccination against Lyme disease with recombinant *Borrelia aburgdorferi* outer-surface lipoprotein A with adjuvant. *N Engl J Med*. 1998;339(4):209–215.

16. Kapikian AZ, et al. Efficacy of a quadrivalent rhesus rotavirus based human rotavirus vaccine aimed at preventing severe rotavirus diarrhoea in infants and young children. *J Infect Dis*. 1996;174:S65–72.

17. Clements-Mann ML, Weinhold K, Matthews TJ, et al. Immune responses to human immunodeficiency virus (HIV) type 1 induced by canarypox expressing HIV-1MN gp120, HIV-1SF2 recombinant gp120, or both vaccines in seronegative adults. *J Infect Dis*. 1998; 177(5):1230–1246.

18. Brochier B, Kieny MP, Costy F, et al. Large-scale eradication of rabies using recombinant vaccinia-rabies vaccine. *Nature*. 1991;354:520–522.

19. Prevec L, Campbell JB, Christie BS, Belbeck L, Graham FL. A recombinant human adenovirus vaccine against rabies. *J Infect Dis*. 1990;161:27–30.

20. Clemens J, Kechich N, Naficy A, Glass R, Rao M. Public health consideration of new rotavirus vaccines for infants: a case study of tetravalent rhesus rotavirus-based reassortant vaccine. *Epidemiol Rev*. 1999;2(41): 24–42.

21. Watson JC, LeBaron CW, Hutchins MD, Hadler SC, Williams WW. General recommendations on immunization recommendations of the Advisory Committee on Immunization Practices (ACIP). *MMWR*. 1994;43(RR-01):10.

22. National Center of Infectious Disease. *Travelers' Health*. http://www.cdc.gov/travel (7 September 1999). Accessed 12 November 1999.

23. Comstock GW. Vaccine evaluation by case-control or prospective studies. *Am J Epidemiol*. 1990;131(2):205–207.

24. Ornestein WA, Bernier RH, Hinman AR. Assessing vaccine efficacy in the field: further observations. *Epidemiol Rev*. 1988;10:212–241.

25. Halloran ME, Haber M, Longini IM, Struchiner CJ. Direct and indirect effects in vaccine efficacy and effectiveness. *Am J Epidemiol*. 1991;133(4):323–331.

26. Halloran ME, Struchiner CJ, Longini IM. Study designs for evaluating different efficacy and effectiveness as-

pects of vaccines. *Am J Epidemiol.* 1997;146(10):789–803.

27. Halloran ME, Longini IM, Struchiner CJ. Design and interpretation of vaccine field studies. *Epidemiol Rev.* 1999;21(1):73–88.

28. Rodrigues LC, Smith PG. Use of the case control approach in vaccine evaluation: efficacy and adverse effects. *Epidemiol Rev.* 1999;21(1):56–72.

29. Basch PF. *Vaccine and World Health: Science, Policy and Practice.* New York: Oxford University Press; 1994.

30. Kelsey JL, Thompson WD, Evans AS. *Methods in Observational Epidemiology.* New York: Oxford University Press; 1986.

31. Chen RT, Rastogi SC, Mullen JR, et al. The Vaccine Adverse Event Reporting System (VAERS). *Vaccine.* 1994;5(6):542–549.

32. Braun MM, Ellenberg SS. Descriptive epidemiology of adverse events after immunization: reports of the Vaccine Adverse Event Reporting System (VAERS) 1991–1994. *J Pediatr.* 1997;131(4):529–535.

33. Chen RT, Glasser JW, Rhodes PH, et al; the Vaccine Datalink Team. Vaccine Safety Datalink Project: a new tool for improving vaccine safety monitoring in the United States. *Pediatrics.* 1997;99:765–773.

34. Plotkin SL, Plotkin SA. A short history of vaccination. In: Plotkin SA, Mortimer EA, eds. *Vaccines.* Philadelphia: W.B. Saunders Company; 1998.

35. Ogra PL. Poliomyelitis as a paradigm for investment in and success of vaccination programs. *Pediatr Infect Dis J.* 1999;18:10–15.

36. Atkinson W, et al, eds. Poliomyelitis. In: *Epidemiology and Prevention of Vaccine Preventable Diseases.* Atlanta, GA: Centers for Disease Control and Prevention, Department of Health and Human Services; 1997:81–99.

37. Centers for Disease Control and Prevention. Epidemiology of Measles—United States, 1998. *MMWR.* 1999;48(34):749–753.

38. Atkinson W, et al, eds. Measles. In: *Epidemiology and Prevention of Vaccine Preventable Diseases.* Atlanta, GA: Centers for Disease Control and Prevention, Department of Health and Human Services; 1997:117–137.

39. Centers for Disease Control and Prevention. *Impact of Vaccine Universally Recommended for Children, 1999.* Available at: http://www.cdc.gov/od/oc/media/fact/impvacc.htm. Accessed 12 November 1999.

40. The National Vaccine Advisory Committee. The measles epidemic: the problems, barriers, and recommendation. *JAMA.* 1991;266:1547–1552.

41. Georges P. Childhood immunizations. *N Engl J Med.* 1992;327[25]:1794–1800.

42. Center for Disease Control. Progress toward global measles control and regional elimination, 1990–1997. *MMWR.* 1998;47(48):1049–1054.

43. Cochi SL, Broome CV. Vaccine prevention of *Haemophilus influenzae* type b disease, past, present and future. *Pediatr Infect Dis.* 1985;5:12–19.

44. Santosham M, Wolff M, Reid R, et al. The efficacy in Navajo infants of a conjugate vaccine consisting of *Haemophilus influenzae* type b polysaccharide and *Neisseria meningitides* outer membrane protein complex. *N Engl J Med.* 1991;324:1767–1772.

45. McCollough M. Update on emerging infections from the Centers for Disease Control and Prevention. *Ann Emerg Med.* 1999;334:109–111.

46. Evans AS. The eradication of communicable diseases: myth or reality? *Am J Epidemiol.* 1985;122(2):199–207.

47. Fenner F, Henderson DA, Arita I, Jezek Z, Ladnyi ID. *Vaccines.* Philadelphia: W.B. Saunders Company; 1994.

48. World Health Organization. Measles, acute respiratory virus, and poliomyelitis vaccines. http://www.who.int/gpv-dvacc/research/virus1.htm. Accessed 12 November 1999.

49. Evans AS. Criteria for control of infectious diseases with poliomyelitis as an example. *Prog Med Virol.* 1984;29:141–165.

CHAPTER 11

Nutrition and Infectious Diseases

Richard D. Semba

INTRODUCTION

This chapter provides a practical introduction to the relationship of nutrition to infectious diseases. The main focus is on developing countries where the problems of malnutrition and infection are more common, although the prevalence of malnutrition in some situations in industrialized countries may be high as well.[1] Micronutrients play essential roles in growth, development, and function of the immune system. The main cause of immunodeficiency worldwide is nutritionally acquired immunodeficiency syndrome (NAIDS), which affects more than 100 million children and several million women.[2,3] The close association between malnutrition and infection has been likened to a vicious cycle in which malnutrition, immunodeficiency, and infection are closely linked (Figure 11–1). Within this cycle is found increased morbidity and mortality associated with malnutrition.

IMPACT OF NUTRITION ON HEALTH

Malnutrition is defined as compromised biological function due to the inadequate intake, absorption, metabolism, storage, and utilization of nutrients, including protein energy and micronutrients. Infection can be an underlying cause of malnutrition,[3] given that infection can influence intake, absorption, and others aspects of nutrient metabolism. Undernutrition is another term used for malnutrition. Agreement is not always found regarding the level at which malnutrition will compromise biological function, which biological functions are most affected, and how to measure such function. Because malnutrition is manifested most often as alterations in growth, weight, and lean body mass, epidemiologic studies typically rely on anthropometric indicators for the assessment of malnutrition in populations.[4] Anthropometric indicators are usually compared with reference populations.[5]

In children, malnutrition has been defined as mildly underweight, or weight-for-age less than two standard deviations below the National Center for Health Statistics (NCHS) reference population mean.[6] Z-scores for weight-for-age, height-for-age, and weight-for-height are also used to classify malnutrition in children; however, a wide variety of classification systems and cut-offs for malnutrition exists.[7] Mid-upper arm circumference can be used to screen for malnutrition when weight and height are difficult to obtain and the exact age of the child is unknown (Figure 11–2).[7]

Weight-to-height ratios or body mass indices (BMIs) are usually used to define nutritional status in adults. Quetelet's index (weight/height^2) is considered the best body mass index for most adult population groups.[7] A body mass index less than 19.0 is considered to be underweight for adults.[8] Other means of nutritional assessment that can be incorporated in epidemiologic studies of infectious diseases include additional anthropometry, dietary assessment, biochemical

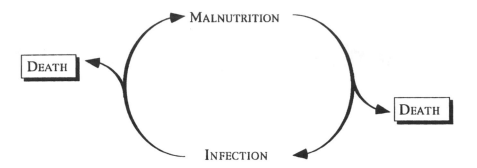

Figure 11–1 Vicious cycle of malnutrition and infection

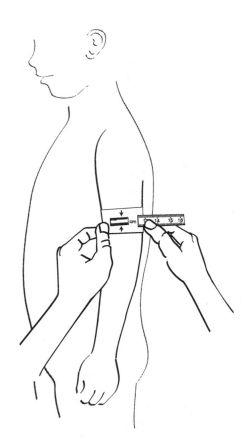

Figure 11–2 Measurement of mid-upper arm circumference using a Zerfas tape. *Source:* Copyright © 2000, Richard Semba.

measures, clinical assessment, immunologic studies, and body composition analysis. These methods are discussed in detail elsewhere.[7,9]

Nutrition can have a major influence on many basic indicators of health of populations, especially in developing countries. Infectious diseases contribute a large part to these indicators, and malnutrition is often an underlying cause of infectious disease. These health indicators include the under-five mortality rate, incidence of low birthweight, and the maternal mortality rate, all of which are discussed below.

Child Mortality

Worldwide, 98% of all deaths in children younger than 15 years occur in developing countries.[10] Among these children, the leading causes of death are perinatal causes, acute respiratory infections, diarrhea, measles, and malaria (Figure 11–3).[3] Malnutrition was estimated to be an underlying cause of 55% of these deaths.[11] Child mortality rates are usually expressed as under-five mortality rate (U5MR), which is the probability of dying between birth and exactly age 5 years expressed per 1,000 live births. The range and magnitude of these rates vary considerably around the world, from 211 to 320 per 1,000 live births in countries such as Niger, Angola, Sierra Leone, Afghanistan, Liberia, Guinea-Bissau, Mali, Malawi, Mozambique, and Somalia to 4 to 8 per 1,000 live births in Finland, the United States, and the United Kingdom. Thus, the U5MR is often 50 to 80 times greater in some developing countries compared with industrialized countries.

Micronutrient deficiencies clearly affect child survival. Studies suggest that perhaps up to one half of the mortality rate due to infectious diseases in children in developing countries could be prevented by improving micronutrient intake. Clinical trials suggest that improving vitamin

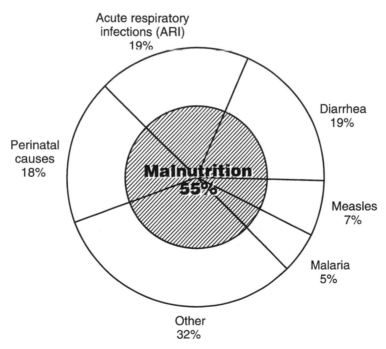

Figure 11–3 Malnutrition and the leading causes of death in children

A[12,13] and iodine status[14,15] could reduce child mortality from infectious diseases in various populations in developing countries by one third to one half. Improvement of zinc status can have an impact on reducing child morbidity from infectious diseases.[16–19] Some micronutrient clinical trials are highlighted in Table 11–1.

Low Birthweight

Low birthweight, defined as birthweight less than 2,500 g, is a major risk factor for neonatal morbidity and mortality in both developed and developing countries. Low birthweight infants have a perinatal mortality rate (mortality rate in the first 7 days of life), which is 5 to 35 times greater than infants with normal weight.[20] The extent to which infectious diseases contribute to this perinatal mortality is incompletely characterized. Prematurity (gestational age <37 weeks) and intrauterine growth retardation (IUGR) are two major determinants of low birthweight.[21] Factors that appear to contribute to low birthweight include genetic and constitutional factors (infant sex, race, maternal height), demographic factors (maternal age, socioeconomic status), obstetric factors (parity, birth interval), nutritional status, and maternal morbidity during pregnancy (malaria).[22] The highest prevalence of low birthweight is found in south Asia, accounting for 25%, 33%, and 50% of births in Pakistan, India, and Bangladesh, respectively.[3] In contrast, 7% of infants born in the United States, Japan, and the United Kingdom are of low birthweight.

Micronutrient status during pregnancy can influence the incidence of low birthweight infants in some populations. Folic acid supplementation during pregnancy has been shown to increase birthweight of infants in South Africa and India,[23,24] and to reduce the incidence of neural tube defects. A low zinc intake is associated with increased risk of low birthweight infants,[25] and zinc supplementation during pregnancy has been shown to reduce low birthweight in pregnant African-American women in Alabama,[26] although this effect has not been observed else-

where.[27] During human immunodeficiency virus (HIV) infection, pregnant women with low serum vitamin A levels had lower birthweight infants,[28] and a recent clinical trial shows that vitamin A supplementation for HIV-infected pregnant women reduces the incidence of low birthweight by one third (Semba et al., unpublished data).

Maternal Mortality

An estimated 600,000 maternal deaths occur per year worldwide,[3] and most of these deaths occur in developing countries. Maternal mortality is defined as the death of a woman while pregnant or within 42 days of termination of pregnancy, irrespective of the duration or site of the pregnancy, from any cause related to or aggravated by the pregnancy or its management, but not from accidental causes.[29] Maternal mortality rates are expressed as the annual number of maternal deaths per 100,000 live births. Major causes of maternal mortality include severe anemia, hemorrhage, eclampsia, induced abortion, infections, dystocia, and postpartum sepsis.[30–32] Maternal mortality rates as high as 1,500 to1,800 maternal deaths per 100,000 live births have been reported in Afghanistan, Bhutan, Chad, Guinea, Mozambique, Nepal, Sierra Leone, and Somalia,[3] compared with rates of 9 to15 maternal deaths per 100,000 live births in the United States, France, and the United Kingdom. The maternal mortality rates in some developing countries seem to be 100 to 200 times higher than in many industrialized countries; however, the accuracy of maternal mortality data from many developing countries may be problematic.

Programs advocating safe motherhood aim at reducing the high maternal mortality in developing countries, and these programs have typically promoted the improvement of medical treatment for obstetrical emergencies.[30,32] Some evidence suggests that improving maternal iron status can influence maternal mortality,[33,34] although well-designed studies are needed to confirm these observations.[35] Low serum vitamin A levels during pregnancy are associated with increased

Table 11–1 Some Clinical Trials Examining Effects of Micronutrients on Infections

Micronutrient	Population	Dose	Outcome	Reference
Vitamin A	Preschool children in Nepal, Indonesia, India, Africa	60 mg retinol equivalent (RE) q 4–6 mo*	Overall one third reduction in child mortality	12, 13
Vitamin A	Children with measles, Tanzania, South Africa	60 mg RE ×2	>50% reduction in mortality	12
Vitamin A	Preschool children in malaria region, Papua New Guinea	60 mg RE q 3 mo	One third reduction in malaria morbidity	53
Iodine	Six-week-old infants, Indonesia	100 mg once	72% reduction in mortality	14
Zinc	Preschool children, India	10 mg q day	Reduction in incidence of diarrhea	19
	Children with diarrhea, India	20 mg q day	Reduction of persistent diarrhea and dysentery	16
	Preschool children, Mexico	20 mg q day	Reduction in infectious disease morbidity	18

*Other studies used weekly dosing or vitamin A fortification.

mortality in HIV-infected pregnant women in Malawi.[36] A study from Nepal suggests that either vitamin A or beta-carotene supplementation throughout the reproductive years, including pregnancy, can reduce maternal mortality by 30% to 50%.[37] This study supports the idea that adequate nutrition can effectively complement obstetric care in reducing maternal mortality.

RELATIONSHIP OF NUTRITION WITH INFECTIOUS DISEASES

Malnutrition is a major determinant of morbidity and mortality for many major infectious diseases, and the role of micronutrients in the immunity to different infections is a rapidly growing and promising area of investigation.

Diarrheal Disease

Diarrheal disease causes an estimated 19% of all child deaths worldwide.[3] Malnutrition and associated immunodeficiency are important risk factors for diarrheal disease among infants and young children in developing countries.[38] Children who are malnourished (low weight-for-age, low mid-upper arm circumference) have an increased prevalence of diarrhea and a higher mortality rate.[39] Micronutrient deficiencies described during diarrheal disease include that of vitamins A, D, and B$_{12}$, folate, copper, iron, magnesium, selenium, and zinc.[12,39] Recent clinical trials show that supplementation with vitamin A[12,13,40] or zinc[16–19] can reduce the morbidity and mortality of diarrheal disease in children.

Lower Respiratory Infections

Worldwide, lower respiratory infections account for 19% of all child deaths.[3] Vitamin A deficiency causes pathologic alterations in the mucosal epithelium of the respiratory tract, including keratinization and loss of ciliated cells, mucus, and goblet cells. Epidemiologic studies demonstrate that vitamin A deficiency is associated with lower respiratory infections[12]; how-

ever, vitamin A supplementation appears to have little effect on reducing lower respiratory infections in children[41] and respiratory syncytial virus infection.[42,43] Vitamin D or calcium deficiency may be important risk factors for lower respiratory infections in children.[44] Zinc supplementation appears to reduce the morbidity of respiratory infections in infants in Guatemala.[45]

Measles

Measles causes an estimated 2 million deaths per year, and despite measles immunization, periodic and serious outbreaks occur because of lapses in immunization programs, vaccine failure, and problems related to optimal timing of immunization. Case fatality rates during acute, complicated measles infection are often 10% to 30%, depending on age and nutritional status of the children. Low serum vitamin A levels are associated with greater mortality in acute, complicated measles infection.[46] Randomized, placebo-controlled clinical trials show that vitamin A supplementation can reduce the mortality of measles by 50% or more, and high-dose vitamin A supplementation is now recommended as standard therapy for measles, both in developing countries and in selected circumstances in the United States.[12] Vitamin A supplementation for measles is one of the most important examples of the use of micronutrients as disease-targeted therapy.

Tuberculosis

Approximately 1.8 billion individuals, or about one third of the world's population, are infected with *Mycobacterium tuberculosis*, and most of these individuals have latent infection. Malnutrition is a major risk factor for the progression of tuberculosis[47]; however, tuberculosis control programs tend to focus on chemoprophylaxis and chemotherapy alone, rather than on improvement of host nutritional status. Cod-liver oil, a rich source of vitamins A and D, was used as treatment for tuberculosis for more than

100 years, prior to the development of antibiotics.[48] The role of nutrition and tuberculosis remains a major area of neglect, despite the promise that micronutrients have shown as therapy for other types of infections and the long record of the use of vitamins A and D for treatment of pulmonary and miliary tuberculosis in both Europe and the United States.

Malaria

Malaria affects about 400 million individuals each year, resulting in 1 to 2 million deaths worldwide,[49] and malaria is reemerging worldwide.[50] Vector control and antimalarial drugs have been the traditional strategy against malaria, and, until recently, little attention has been paid to improving host nutritional status. Low serum or plasma vitamin A levels have been described during *Plasmodium falciparum* infection,[51] and low zinc status has been observed in areas where malaria is endemic.[52] Recently, two separate, randomized, placebo-controlled clinical trials conducted in Papua, New Guinea, demonstrate that vitamin A or zinc supplementation can reduce malarial morbidity in preschool children by 30% to 50%.[53]

Human Immunodeficiency Virus Infection

Human immunodeficiency virus infection is associated with a microenteropathy, malabsorption, steatorrhea, and anorexia. Low circulating micronutrient levels have been described in all stages of HIV infection and in many different risk groups.[54,55] Plasma or serum levels or intake of vitamins A, E, and B$_6$, selenium, and zinc have been associated with increased disease progression and mortality.[56–59] HIV wasting syndrome is an important part of the clinical spectrum of the infection.[60] Micronutrient and oral nutritional supplementation for HIV infection has been explored in a few clinical trials,[54,61] and a recent important study demonstrates that multivitamin supplementation to HIV-infected women reduces fetal mortality and low birthweight by approximately 40%.[62]

MICRONUTRIENTS AND IMMUNITY TO INFECTIOUS DISEASES

Micronutrients can influence immunity to infectious diseases through their roles in immune function.[63] Micronutrient deficiencies, such as that of vitamin A and zinc, can have a major impact on T- and B-cell function, generation of antibody responses, and function of other immune effector cells (Table 11–2). Micronutrients, such as vitamin E, vitamin C, zinc, and selenium, can play a role as strong antioxidants and influence the clinical course of infections. Oxidative stress, which occurs during infections, refers to the condition when the balance between pro-oxidants and anti-oxidants is upset and overproduction of free radicals and resulting pathology occurs.[64] Activated macrophages and neutrophils have important roles in the killing of microorganisms through the generation of free radicals. Free radicals can damage host bystander cells, causing oxidation of nucleic acids, chromosomal breaks, peroxidation of lipids in cell membranes, and damage to collagen, proteins, and enzymes.

The study of the relationship between nutrition and immunity is a rapidly growing field known as "nutritional immunology."[65] Investigators who wish to study the relationship between micronutrients and infectious diseases must often focus on one or two micronutrients for practical reasons. Considerable cost and complexity are involved in providing a comprehensive study of micronutrient status during infection, although a comprehensive approach would be ideal because micronutrient deficiencies often occur simultaneously. A brief overview of the relationship of specific micronutrients in immunity to infection follows.

Vitamin A

Vitamin A, or all-*trans* retinol, is an essential micronutrient for immunity, growth, cellular differentiation, maintenance of mucosal surfaces, reproduction, and vision.[12] Two main di-

Table 11–2 Selected Micronutrients and Immunity

Micronutrient	Sources	Functions	Relative Importance to Immune Function	Assessment
Vitamin A	Dairy products, carrots, dark green leafy vegetables, cod-liver oil	Growth, vision, reproduction	++++	Serum or plasma levels, relative dose response, dark adaptation
Vitamin D	Sunlight exposure, egg yolks, fish liver oils	Calcium and phosphorus metabolism, bone mineralization	++(?)	Serum or plasma 25-hydroxyvitamin D
Vitamin E	Seeds, nuts, margarine	Antioxidant	+++	Serum or plasma levels
Iron	Red meat, poultry, fish, beans	Oxygen transport, enzymes	++	Hemoglobin, transferrin receptor, ferritin
Iodine	Seafood, iodized salt	Growth, development, metabolism	++(?)	Urinary iodine, goiter prevalence, serum T4 or thyrotropin
Zinc	Shellfish, beef, chicken, beans	Growth, reproduction	++++	Serum or plasma levels, hair zinc

etary forms of vitamin A exist, either pre-formed vitamin A, found in foods such as butter, egg yolks, and cod-liver oil, and provitamin A carotenoids, found in foods such as spinach, carrots, mangoes, and papayas. Approximately 90% of the vitamin A in the body is stored in the liver, and the adult liver can contain sufficient vitamin A to last more than 1 year. Vitamin A acts as a regulator of more than 300 genes through its active metabolites, all-*trans* and 9-*cis* retinoic acid, and specific nuclear receptors that are in the steroid and thyroid hormone receptor superfamily.[66]

Vitamin A exerts a wide ranging effect on different compartments of the immune system, including the growth, maturation, and function of T and B lymphocytes, the expression of certain cytokines, and the maintenance of mucosal surfaces of the respiratory, gastrointestinal, and genitourinary tracts.[67,68] A hallmark of vitamin A deficiency is an impaired ability to mount an antibody response to protein antigens.[68] Traditionally, it has been considered that the main clinical manifestations of vitamin A deficiency are nightblindness and xerophthalmia (changes in the conjunctiva and cornea of the eye),[12] although it is becoming apparent that increased incidence and severity of infections are part of the spectrum of vitamin A deficiency. Infants, preschool children, pregnant women, and lactating women are at the highest risk of developing vitamin A deficiency.[12] Abnormal urinary losses of vitamin A can occur during infections, which can then accelerate the depletion of the body's vitamin A stores.[69] Because vitamin A is a fat-soluble vitamin, steatorrhea can interfere with intestinal absorption of it.

Methods used to assess vitamin A status include serum or plasma vitamin A levels by high performance liquid chromatography (HPLC), the relative dose response and modified relative dose response tests (which indirectly measure liver reserves of vitamin A), measurement of breast milk vitamin A, dark adaptometry, pupillary responses, and conjunctival impression cytology.[70]

Vitamin D

Vitamin D includes steroids with the biological activity of vitamin D_3. Vitamin D is produced in the skin on exposure to sunlight; it is also available from dietary sources such as egg yolks and fish liver oils. Vitamin D regulates calcium and phosphorus metabolism and bone mineralization. The clinical syndrome of vitamin D deficiency is rickets in children and osteomalacia in adults.[71] Vitamin D acts to regulate genes via specific nuclear receptors, and its receptor may interact with nuclear retinoic acid receptors, which provides some basis for the interaction between vitamins A and D.[66] Vitamin D plays a role in monocyte function, and this has been studied most extensively in tuberculosis.[72] A recent epidemiologic study in Ethiopia suggests a link between pneumonia and vitamin D deficiency.[44] Methods for the assessment of vitamin D status include measurements of serum vitamin D levels (25-hydroxyvitamin D) by HPLC.[7]

Vitamin E

Vitamin E refers to tocopherol and tocotrienol compounds, of which α-tocopherol is the most active and abundant isomer. Rich dietary sources of vitamin E include seeds, nuts, margarine, and vegetable oils. Vitamin E is a strong antioxidant that protects against cellular damage by inhibiting peroxidation of polyunsaturated fatty acids in cell membranes. A clear-cut deficiency syndrome of vitamin E has not been described in humans.[73] Vitamin E may protect immune effector cells against free radical reactions.[74–76] Methods of assessing vitamin E status include measurements of serum vitamin E levels by HPLC.[7]

B Complex Vitamins

The B complex vitamins include thiamin, riboflavin, niacin, vitamin B_6, vitamin B_{12}, and folate. These vitamins participate in the metabolism of carbohydrates, fats, and proteins, and in hematopoiesis and synthesis of DNA. Some evidence suggests that vitamin B_6, vitamin B_{12}, and folate may play a role in immune function.[77,78] The possible role of these micronutrients in the pathogenesis of infectious disease needs further clarification.

Vitamin C

Vitamin C, or ascorbic acid, is involved in a variety of biological reactions, including conversion of dopamine to norepinephrine, carnitine synthesis, iron absorption, and folate metabolism. Citrus fruits, peppers, green vegetables, potatoes, and berries contain high levels of vitamin C. Deficiency of vitamin C results in scurvy, a syndrome characterized by skin lesions, hemorrhages, joint effusions, and weakness. The therapeutic efficacy of vitamin C as treatment for symptoms of the common cold remains controversial,[79] and evidence is limited that vitamin C is involved in immune function.[80] Most current investigation of vitamin C in infectious diseases is concerned with the role of vitamin C as a potent antioxidant.

Iron

Iron plays an important role in oxygen transport, as an electron carrier in cytochromes, and in certain iron metalloenzymes.[81] Iron deficiency is associated with anemia,[82] impaired psychomotor development,[83,84] lower work capacity,[85] prematurity,[86] and higher maternal mortality.[33,34] An estimated 2 billion people suffer from iron deficiency anemia worldwide.[82] Pregnant women, women of childbearing age, infants, and children are at higher risk of developing iron deficiency anemia. A high cereal diet (which can interfere with iron absorption), chronic diarrhea, malabsorption, and blood loss from pregnancy, menstruation, and intestinal parasites[87] can contribute to iron deficiency. Although iron deficiency can adversely affect neutrophil and lymphocyte function, the relationship between iron deficiency and infection is unclear.[88] Some early studies suggested that iron

supplementation could increase susceptibility to malaria; however, recent studies show that iron deficiency should be corrected in children with malaria.[89] Oral iron therapy does not appear to exacerbate infections in most areas of the world,[88] and reducing iron deficiency still remains a formidable challenge worldwide.

Selenium

Selenium, an essential trace element contained in the enzyme glutathione peroxidase, protects cells against oxidative damage.[90] Selenium is found in seafoods, some meats, and grain products, depending on the selenium content of the soil. Keshan's disease, a cardiomyopathy, and Kashin-Beck disease, an osteoarticular disorder, occur in areas where the soil is low in selenium. Selenium appears to influence the function of T lymphocytes.[91] Recent studies with a murine model for coxsackie B–induced myocarditis suggest that selenium deficiency can increase virulence of the coxsackie B virus.[92] The biological importance of selenium is being established, and whether selenium status is important during infections in humans needs further clarification.

Iodine

Iodine deficiency can result in goiter and a wide spectrum of mental, psychomotor, and growth abnormalities.[93] Iodine functions as a component of thyroxine (T_4), and 3,5,3'-triiodothyronine (T_3), two hormones required for normal growth, development, and metabolism. Nuclear thyroid hormone receptors can bind with retinoic acid receptors, suggesting that an interaction occurs between vitamin A and thyroid status.[66] Rich sources of iodine include seafood and iodized salt. An estimated 1.6 billion people worldwide may not consume adequate amounts of iodine.[94] Increased rates of stillbirths, abortions, and infant mortality have been noted in areas with endemic iodine deficiency, and a recent clinical trial suggests that iodine supplementation can reduce infant mortality.[14]

Iodination of irrigation water in a severely io-dine-deficient area of China resulted in a large decrease in infant mortality.[15] The role of iodine deficiency in immune function is not well-estab-lished[14] and further studies of the relationship between iodine deficiency and infections are needed.

Zinc

Zinc is an important trace element needed for the function of more than 300 metalloenzymes, including those involved in proteins, fats, and carbohydrates; regulation of RNA synthesis through zinc fingers; synaptic transmission; and the function of protein kinase C.[95] Rich dietary sources of zinc include shellfish, beef, chicken, fish, nuts, and beans. Zinc deficiency is charac-terized by growth retardation, reproductive ab-normalities, increased infections, and skin and neurologic disorders. Zinc deficiency usually arises because of inadequate dietary intake of zinc, and pregnant and lactating women, infants, and preschool children are at the highest risk of zinc deficiency.

Zinc plays an important role in the growth, development, and function of neutrophils, mac-rophages, natural killer cells, and T and B lym-phocytes.[96] A large series of randomized, pla-cebo-controlled clinical trials suggests that zinc supplementation can reduce the morbidity of di-arrheal disease, respiratory disease, and ma-laria.[16–19,45] These studies suggest that the impor-tance of zinc status in resistance to infections is only just being realized. The measurement of zinc status remains somewhat problematic, and plasma or serum zinc levels can be measured us-ing atomic absorption spectroscopy and special-ized trace element handling techniques.[7]

COST-EFFECTIVENESS OF NUTRITIONAL INTERVENTIONS

Malnutrition has been ranked first as the lead-ing risk factor to the burden of disease, account-ing for 15.9% of disability-adjusted life years (DALYs) worldwide.[97,98] DALYs are the sum of life years lost from premature mortality and years lived with disability adjusted for severity.[97,98] For developing countries, interventions that consist of micronutrient supplementation or fortification are attractive, because supplementation and forti-fication are extremely inexpensive compared with other types of interventions. In a World Bank analysis of the world's major medical interven-tions, vitamin A supplementation was the most cost-effective health intervention known.[99]

CONCLUSION

Nutrition is a major determinant of morbidity and mortality from infectious diseases. Some micronutrients play essential roles in the growth, development, and function of the immune system and influence oxidative stress. Epidemiologic studies of infectious diseases should include characterization of nutritional status. At a mini-mum, basic anthropometric indices such as weight and height should be a basic part of any epidemiologic investigation of infectious dis-eases. Nutritional assessment can be expanded to more sophisticated measures of specific micro-nutrients, dietary intake, and body composition. Major indicators of health (e.g., child mortality, birthweight, and maternal mortality) are influ-enced by host nutritional status. Micronutrients have been shown to influence the clinical course of diarrheal and lower respiratory disease, measles, and malaria. The potential role of mi-cronutrients in the clinical course of tuberculosis, a major reemerging disease, remains unknown.

Micronutrient interventions such as that of vi-tamin A and zinc have been a major subject of investigation in the last two decades because of their programmatic applicability and extremely high cost-effectiveness. Improvement of agri-cultural practices, food fortification, and modifi-cation of dietary behavior are part of an inte-grated approach to nutrition. The potential use of micronutrients such as vitamin A, vitamin D, vi-tamin E, zinc, iodine, and selenium as disease-targeted therapy shows promise and needs fur-ther study. Future studies will undoubtedly focus on the use of multiple micronutrient combinations in supplements. Micronutrients such as vitamins A, C, and E and zinc may enhance immune function or other biological functions even in the absence of a specific micronutrient deficiency; thus, micronutrient supplementation can be used to correct a deficiency or in other cases to provide a megadose type of supplementation.

REFERENCES

1. Naber THJ, Schermer T, de Bree A, et al. Prevalence of malnutrition in nonsurgical hospitalized patients and its association with disease complications. *Am J Clin Nutr.* 1997;232–1239.

2. Beisel WR. Nutrition and immune function: overview. *J Nutr.* 1996;126(Suppl.10):2611S–2615S.

3. UNICEF. *The State of the World's Children 1998.* Oxford and New York: Oxford University Press; 1998.

4. Shorr IJ. *How to Weigh and Measure Children: Assessing the Nutritional Status of Young Children in Household Surveys.* New York: United Nations Department of Technical Co-operation for Development and Statistical Office; 1986.

5. World Health Organization. *Measuring Change in Nutritional Status. Guidelines for Assessing the Nutritional Impact of Supplementary Feeding Programmes for Vulnerable Groups.* Geneva: World Health Organization; 1983.

6. Mason JB, Musgrove P, Watson F, Habicht JP. Undernutrition. In: Murray CJL, Lopez AD, eds. *Quantifying Global Burden Health Risks: The Burden of Disease Attributable to Selected Risk Factor.* Cambridge: Harvard University Press; 1996.

7. Gibson RS. *Principles of Nutritional Assessment.* New York: Oxford University Press; 1990.

8. Bray GA. Definition, measurement, and classification of the syndromes of obesity. *Int J Obes Relat Metab Dis.* 1978;2:99–112.

9. Jelliffe DB, Jelliffe EFP. *Community Nutritional Assessment: With Special Reference to Less Technologically Developed Countries.* Oxford: Oxford University Press; 1990.

10. Murray CJL, Lopez AD. Mortality by cause for eight regions of the world: Global Burden of Disease Study. *Lancet.* 1997;349:1269–1276.

11. Pelletier DL, Frongillo EA Jr, Schroeder DG, Habicht JP. The effects of malnutrition on child mortality in developing countries. *Bull World Health Organ.* 1995; 73:443–448.

12. Sommer A, West KP Jr. *Vitamin A Deficiency: Health, Survival, and Vision.* New York: Oxford University Press; 1996.

13. Beaton GH, Martorell R, L'Abbe KA, Edmonston B, McCabe G, Ross AC, Harvey B. *Effectiveness of Vitamin A Supplementation in the Control of Young Child Morbidity and Morality in Developing Countries.* Administrative Committee on Coordination/Subcommittee on Nutrition, State-of-the-Art Nutrition Policy Discussion Paper No. 13, United Nations; 1993.

14. Cobra C, Muhilal, Rusmil K, et al. Infant survival is improved by oral iodine supplementation. *J Nutr.* 1997; 127:574–578.

15. DeLong GR, Leslie PW, Wang SH, et al. Effect on infant mortality of iodination of irrigation water in a severely iodine-deficient area of China. *Lancet.* 1997; 350:771–773.

16. Sazawal S, Black RE, Bhan MK, et al. Zinc supplementation reduces the incidence of persistent diarrhea and dysentery among low socioeconomic children in India. *J Nutr.* 1996;126:443–450.

17. Ninh NX, Thissen JP, Collette L, Gerard G, Khoi HH, Ketelslegers JM. Zinc supplementation increases growth and circulating insulin-like growth factors (IGF-1) in growth-retarded Vietnamese children. *Am J Clin Nutr.* 1996;63:514–519.

18. Rosado JL, López P, Muñoz E, Martinez H, Allen LH. Zinc supplementation reduced morbidity, but neither zinc nor iron supplementation affected growth or body composition of Mexican preschoolers. *Am J Clin Nutr.* 1997;65:13–19.

19. Sazawal S, Black RE, Bhan MK, Jalla S, Sinha A, Bhandari N. Efficacy of zinc supplementation in reducing the incidence and prevalence of acute diarrhea—a community-based, double-blind, controlled trial. *Am J Clin Nutr.* 1997;66:413–418.

20. Tinker A, Koblinsky MA. *Making Motherhood Safe.* World Bank Discussion Papers No. 202. Washington, DC: The World Bank; 1993.

21. Kramer MS. Determinants of low birthweight: a methodological assessment and meta-analysis. *Bull World Health Organ.* 1987;65:663–737.

22. Kramer MS. The etiology and prevention of low birthweight: current knowledge and priorities for future research. In: Berendes H, Kessel S, Yaffe S, eds. *Advances in the Prevention of Low Birthweight: An International Symposium.* Washington, DC: National Center for Education in Maternal and Child Health; 1991.

23. Baumslag N, Edelstein T, Metz J. Reduction of the incidence of prematurity by folic acid supplementation in pregnancy. *Br Med J.* 1970;1:16–17.

24. Iyengar L, Rajalakshmi K. Effect of folic acid supplement on birth weights of infants. *Am J Obstet Gynecol.* 1975;122:332–336.

25. Scholl TO, Hediger ML, Schall JI, Fischer RL, Khoo CS. Low zinc intake during pregnancy: its association with preterm and very preterm delivery. *Am J Epidemiol.* 1993;137:1115–1124.

26. Goldenberg RL, Tamura T, Neggers Y, et al. The effect of zinc supplementation on pregnancy outcome. *JAMA.* 1995;274:463–468.

27. Caulfield LE, Zavaleta N, Shankar AH, Merialdi M. Potential contribution of maternal zinc supplementation during pregnancy to maternal and child survival. *Am J Clin Nutr.* 1998;68:499S–508S.

28. Semba RD, Miotti PG, Chiphangwi JD, et al. Infant mortality and maternal vitamin A deficiency during human immunodeficiency virus infection. *Clin Infect Dis.* 1995;21:966–972.

29. World Health Organization. *Manual of the International Statistical Classification of Disease, Injuries, and Causes of Death.* Vol. 1. Geneva: World Health Organization; 1977.

30. World Health Organization. *Essential Elements of Obstetric Care at First Referral Level.* Geneva: World Health Organization; 1991.

31. Ronsmans C, Vanneste AM, Chakraborty J, van Ginneken J. Decline in maternal mortality in Matlab, Bangladesh: a cautionary tale. *Lancet.* 1997;350:1810–1814.

32. Maine D. *Safe Motherhood Programs: Options and Issues.* New York: Columbia University, Center for Population and Family Health; 1991.

33. Alauddin M. Maternal mortality in Bangladesh: the Tangail district. *Stud Fam Plann.* 1986;17:13–21.

34. Harrison KA. Tropical obstetrics and gynecology. 2. Maternal mortality. *Trans R Soc Trop Med Hyg.* 1989; 83:449–453.

35. Allen LH. Pregnancy and iron deficiency: unresolved issues. *Nutr Rev.* 1997;55:91–101.

36. Semba RD. Overview of the potential role of vitamin A in mother-to-child transmission of HIV-1. *Acta Paediatr.* 1997;421(Suppl.):107–112.

37. West KP Jr, Katz J, Khatry SK, et al. Double blind, cluster randomised trial of low dose supplementation with vitamin A or beta carotene on mortality related to pregnancy in Nepal. The NNIPS-2 Study Group. *Br Med J.* 1999;318:570–575.

38. Baqui AH, Sack RB, Black RE, Chowdhury HR, Yunus M, Siddique AK. Cell-mediated immuno-deficiency and malnutrition are independent risk factors for persistent diarrhea in Bangladeshi children. *Am J Clin Nutr.* 1993;58:543–548.

39. Tomkins A, Behrens R, Roy S. The role of zinc and vitamin A deficiency in diarrhoeal syndromes in developing countries. *Proc Nutr Soc.* 1993;52:131–142.

40. Bhandari N, Bahl R, Sazawal S, Bhan MK. Breast-feeding status alters the effect of vitamin A treatment during acute diarrhea in children. *J Nutr.* 1997;127:59–63.

41. The Vitamin A and Pneumonia Working Group. Potential interventions for the prevention of childhood pneumonia in developing countries: a meta-analysis of data from field trials to assess the impact of vitamin A supplementation on pneumonia morbidity and mortality. *Bull World Health Organ.* 1995;73:609–619.

42. Dowell SF, Papic Z, Bresee JS, et al. Treatment of respiratory syncytial virus infection with vitamin A: a randomized, placebo-controlled trial in Santiago, Chile. *Pediatr Infect Dis.* 1996;15:782–786.

43. Bresee JS, Fischer M, Dowell SF, et al. Vitamin A therapy for children with respiratory syncytial virus infection: a multicenter trial in the United States. *Pediatr Infect Dis J.* 1996;15:777–782.

44. Muhe L, Lulseged S, Mason KE, Simoes EAF. Case-control study of the role of nutritional rickets in the risk of developing pneumonia in Ethiopian children. *Lancet.* 1997;349:1801–1804.

45. Ruel MT, Rivera JA, Santizo MC, Lonnerdal B, Brown KH. Impact of zinc supplementation on morbidity from diarrhea and respiratory infections among Guatemalan children. *Pediatrics.* 1997;99:808–813.

46. Markowitz L, Nzilambi N, Driskell WJ, et al. Vitamin A levels and mortality among hospitalized measles patients, Kinshasa, Zaire. *J Trop Pediatr.* 1989;35:109–112.

47. Hudelson P. Gender differentials in tuberculosis: the role of socio-economic and cultural factors. *Tuber Lung Dis.* 1996;77:391–400.

48. Williams CJB, Williams CT. *Pulmonary Consumption, Its Etiology, Pathology, and Treatment.* 2nd ed. London: Longmans, Green, and Company; 1989.

49. Murphy GS, Oldfield EC III. Falciparum malaria. *Infect Dis Clinics North Am.* 1996;10:747–775.

50. Krogstad DJ. Malaria as a reemerging disease. *Epidemiol Rev.* 1996;18:77–89.

51. Friis H, Mwaniki D, Omondi B, et al. Serum retinol concentrations and *Schistosoma mansoni* intestinal helminths, and malarial parasitemia: a cross-sectional study in Kenyan preschool and primary school children. *Am J Clin Nutr.* 1997;66:665–671.

52. Gibson RS, Heywood A, Yaman C, Sohlstrom A, Thompson LU, Heywood P. Growth in children from the Wosera subdistrict, Papua New Guinea, in relation to energy and protein intakes and zinc status. *Am J Clin Nutr.* 1991;53:782–789.

53. Shankar AH, Genton B, Semba RD, et al. Effect of vitamin A supplementation on morbidity due to *Plasmo-*

dium falciparum in young children in Papua New Guinea: a randomised trial. *Lancet.* 1999;354:203–209.

54. Semba RD. Micronutrients and micronutrient replacement therapy. In: Miller TL, Gorbach SL, eds. *Nutritional Aspects of HIV Infection.* New York: Chapman and Hall; 1999:54–62.

55. Semba RD. Micronutrients and the pathogenesis of human immunodeficiency virus infection. In: *Proceedings of the 16th International Congress of Nutrition.* Montreal, Canada; 1998.

56. Graham NMH, Sorensen D, Odaka N, et al. Relationship of serum copper and zinc levels to HIV-1 seropositivity and progression to AIDS. *J Acquired Immune Defic Syndr.* 1991;4:976–980.

57. Baum MK, Shor-Posner G, Lu Y, et al. Micronutrients and HIV-1 disease progression. *AIDS.* 1995;9:1051–1056.

58. Tang AM, Graham NMH, Saah AJ. Effects of micronutrient intake on survival in human immunodeficiency virus type 1 infection. *Am J Epidemiol.* 1997;143:1244–1256.

59. Tang AM, Graham NMH, Semba RD, Saah AJ. Association between serum vitamin A and E levels and HIV-1 disease progression. *AIDS.* 1997;11:613–620.

60. Kotler DP, Grunfeld C. Pathophysiology and treatment of the AIDS wasting syndrome. In: Volberding P, Jacobson MA, eds. *AIDS Clinical Review 1995/1996.* New York: Marcel Dekker; 1996:229–275.

61. Pichard C, Sudre P, Karsegard V, et al., and the Swiss HIV Cohort Study. A randomized double-blind controlled study of 6 months of oral nutritional supplementation with arginine and omega-3 fatty acids in HIV-infected patients. *AIDS.* 1998;2:53–63.

62. Fawzi WW, Msamanga GI, Spiegelman, et al., and Tanzania Vitamin and HIV Infection Trial Team. Randomised trial of effects of vitamin supplements on pregnancy outcomes and T cell counts in HIV-1-infected women in Tanzania. *Lancet.* 1998;351:1477–1482.

63. Beisel WR. Single nutrients and immunity. *Am J Clin Nutr.* 1982;35:417–468.

64. Baruchel S, Wainberg MA. The role of oxidative stress in disease progression in individuals infected by the human immunodeficiency virus. *J Leukocyte Biol.* 1992;52:111–114.

65. Beisel WR. History of nutritional immunology: introduction and overview. *J Nutr.* 1992;122(Suppl. 3):591–596.

66. Chambon P. A decade of molecular biology of retinoic acid receptors. *FASEB J.* 10:940–954.

67. Semba RD. Vitamin A, immunity, and infection. *Clin Infect Dis.* 1994;19:489–499.

68. Semba RD. The role of vitamin A and related retinoids in immune function. *Nutr Rev.* 1998;56:S38–S48.

69. Alvarez JO, Salazar-Lindo E, Kohatsu J, Miranda P, Stephensen CB. Urinary excretion of retinol in children with acute diarrhea. *Am J Clin Nutr.* 1995;61:1273–1276.

70. International Vitamin A Consultative Group. *A Brief Guide to Current Methods of Assessing Vitamin A Status.* Washington, DC: The Nutrition Foundation; 1993.

71. Fraser DR. Vitamin D. *Lancet.* 1995;345:104–107.

72. Crowle AJ, Ross EJ. Comparative abilities of various metabolites of vitamin D to protect cultured human macrophages against tubercle bacilli. *J Leukocyte Biol.* 1990;47:545–550.

73. Meydani M. Vitamin E. *Lancet.* 1995;345:170–175.

74. Meydani SN, Barklund PM, Liu S, et al. Vitamin E supplementation enhances cell-mediated immunity in healthy elderly subjects. *Am J Clin Nutr.* 1990;52:557–563.

75. Meydani M, Meydani SN, Leka L, Gong J, Blumberg JB. Effect of long-term vitamin E supplementation on lipid peroxidation and immune responses of young and old subjects. *FASEB J.* 1993;7:A415.

76. Meydani SM. Vitamin E enhancement of T cell-mediated function in healthy elderly: mechanisms of action. *Nutr Rev.* 1995;53:S52–S58.

77. Rall LC, Meydani SN. Vitamin B6 and immune competence. *Nutr Rev.* 1993;51:217–225.

78. Dhur A, Galan P, Hercberg S. Folate status and the immune system. *Prog Food Nutr Sci.* 1991;15:543–560.

79. Hemilä H. Vitamin C supplementation and common cold symptoms: problems with inaccurate reviews. *Nutrition.* 1996;12:804–809.

80. Weber P, Bendich A, Schalch W. Vitamin C and human health—a review of recent data relevant to human requirements. *Int J Vitam Res.* 1996;66:19–30.

81. Beard JL, Dawson H, Piñero DJ. Iron metabolism: a comprehensive review. *Nutr Rev.* 1996;54:295–317.

82. Viteri FE. Iron supplementation for the control of iron deficiency in populations at risk. *Nutr Rev.* 1997;55:195–209.

83. Lozoff B, Brittenham GM, Wolf AB, et al. Iron deficiency anemia and iron therapy effects on infant developmental test performance. *Pediatrics.* 1987;79:981–985.

84. Walter T, de Andraca I, Chadud P, Perales CG. Iron deficiency anemia: adverse effects on infant psychomotor development. *Pediatrics.* 1989;84:7–17.

85. Basta SS, Soekirman MS, Karyadi D, Scrimshaw NS. Iron deficiency anemia and the productivity of adult males in Indonesia. *Am J Clin Nutr.* 1979;32:916–925.

86. Scholl TO, Hediger ML, Fischer RL, Shearer JW. Anemia vs iron deficiency: increased risk of preterm delivery in a prospective study. *Am J Clin Nutr.* 1992;55:985–988.

87. Stoltzfus RJ, Dreyfuss ML, Chwaya HM, Albonico M. Hookworm control as a strategy to prevent iron deficiency. *Nutr Rev.* 1997;55:223–232.

88. Walter T, Olivares M, Pizarro F, Muñoz C. Iron, anemia, and infection. *Nutr Rev.* 1997;55:111–124.

89. Menendez C, Kahigwa E, Hirt R, et al. Randomised placebo-controlled trial of iron supplementation and malaria chemoprophylaxis for prevention of severe anaemia and malaria in Tanzanian infants. *Lancet.* 1997;350:844–850.

90. Foster LH, Sumar S. Selenium in health and disease: a review. *Crit Rev Food Sci Nutr.* 1997;37:211–218.

91. Roy M, Kiremidjian-Schumacher L, Wishe HI, Cohen MW, Stotzky G. Supplementation with selenium restores age-related decline in immune cell function. *Proc Soc Exp Biol Med.* 1995;209:369–375.

92. Levander OA, Beck MA. Interacting nutritional and infectious etiologies of Keshan disease. Insights from coxsackie virus B–induced myocarditis in mice deficiency in selenium or vitamin E. *Biol Trace Elem Res.* 1997;56:5–21.

93. Delange F. The disorders induced by iodine deficiency. *Thyroid.* 1994;4:107–128.

94. Hetzel BS, Pandav CS. *S.O.S. for a Billion: The Conquest of Iodine Deficiency Disorders.* New York: Oxford University Press; 1994.

95. Walsh CT, Sanstead HH, Prasad AS, Newberne PM, Fraker PJ. Zinc: health effects and research priorities for the 1990s. *Environ Health Perspect.* 1994;102(Suppl. 2):5–46.

96. Shankar AH, Prasad AS. Zinc and immune function: the biological basis of altered resistance to infection. *Am J Clin Nutr.* 1998;68(Suppl):447S–463S.

97. Murray CJL, Lopez AD. Global mortality, disability, and the contribution of risk factors: Global Burden of Disease Study. *Lancet.* 1997;349:1436–1442.

98. Mason JB, Musgrove P, Watson F, Habicht JP. Undernutrition. In: Murray CJL, Lopez AD, eds. *Quantifying Global Burden Health Risks: The Burden of Disease Attributable to Selected Risk Factors.* Cambridge: Harvard University Press; 1996.

99. World Bank. *World Bank Development Report 1993: Investing in Health.* New York: Oxford University Press; 1993.

PART II

Emerging and Nosocomial Infections

CHAPTER 12

Emerging and New Infectious Diseases

Kenrad E. Nelson

However secure and well-regulated civilized life may become, bacteria, protozoa, viruses, infected fleas, lice, ticks, mosquitoes and bedbugs will always lurk in the shadows ready to pounce when neglect, poverty, famine, or war lets down the defenses. And even in normal times they prey on the weak, the very young and the very old, living along with us, in mysterious obscurity waiting their opportunities. About the only genuine sporting proposition that remains unimpaired by the relentless domestication of a once free-living human species is the war against these ferocious little creatures, which lurk in the dark corners and stalk us in the bodies of rats, mice, and all kinds of domestic animals; which fly and crawl with the insects, and waylay us in our food and drink and even in our love. *Hans Zinsser; Rats, Lice and History, 1934.*

Despite the optimistic forecasts often made in the 1960s and 1970s about the eventual control or even elimination of most of the major infectious diseases of developed Western countries, the outlook has changed in the 1980s and 1990s. Most dramatic has been the appearance of the acquired immune deficiency syndrome (AIDS) pandemic, which most likely arose from human contact with a modified or recombinant primate retrovirus from an infected chimpanzee in central Africa before infections with this new human virus spread around the world within a decade.[1] The targeting of critical cells of the immune system by human immunodeficiency virus (HIV), i.e., CD4+ T lymphocytes, macrophages, and Langerhans-dendritic cells has led to the emergence of a large number of important secondary pathogens, or opportunistic infections, which could no longer be controlled by the damaged immune system of infected individuals. The HIV-1 pandemic has allowed the dramatic explosion of infections with several pathogens that had been rare or were under good control prior to the AIDS epidemic.

SOME IMPORTANT HIV/AIDS-RELATED INFECTIONS

Tuberculosis

Worldwide, the most important opportunistic infection associated with the HIV/AIDS epidemic is tuberculosis.[2] In a matter of a few years after the report of the first cases of AIDS in the United States, the downward trend in new cases of tuberculosis that had been uninterrupted since the licensure of INH in 1952 was reversed. Between 1989 and 1995, 75,000 cases in excess of the number that had been estimated to occur in the absence of the AIDS epidemic were reported in the United States. However, the global impact of the HIV pandemic has been even more striking. Tuberculosis is the most important opportunistic infection associated with AIDS and is second only to AIDS as a cause of infectious disease mortality worldwide.[2]

The increase in tuberculosis cases has commonly involved young adults who are HIV infected. Many of these cases of tuberculosis represented reactivation disease but some were progressive primary infections. Patients who are HIV-positive more often develop disseminated tuberculosis. It has been estimated that persons who are immunosuppressed have a 20% to 30% risk of developing active tuberculosis in the first year after they are infected and a 40% to 50% lifetime risk, in contrast with an estimated 5% risk in the year after infection and an overall lifetime risk of 10% among HIV-negative persons who are not seriously immunosuppressed.[3] This is evidence that an HIV infection converts many otherwise asymptomatic infections with the tubercle bacillus into clinically active and often contagious tuberculosis.

Cryptococcosis and Other Systemic Fungal Infections

One of the early hallmarks of the HIV/AIDS epidemic in Africa was a dramatic increase in the incidence of cryptococcal meningitis.[4] Because tuberculosis had been a common infection in African and Asian populations even prior to the AIDS epidemic, an increase in cryptococcosis was more noticeable to clinicians and public health officials. As with many other AIDS-associated opportunistic infections, it was possible to treat cryptococcal meningitis in AIDS patients with amphotericin-B (ambisome), even though the acute mortality remained at a rate of about 20%.[5] However, in contrast to cryptococcal meningitis in patients who were immunosuppressed from diseases other than AIDS or who were not obviously immunosuppressed, patients with AIDS were highly likely to relapse in the months following effective therapy.[6] It soon became apparent that chronic suppressive therapy with antifungal drugs would be necessary in AIDS patients to prevent the frequent relapses. Several other systemic fungal infections, including histoplasmosis, coccidiodomycosis, and disseminated *Penicillium marneffei* infections in Southeast Asia were found to be common in patient with AIDS.[7] Curiously, the rates of blastomycosis and paracoccidiodomycosis, a fungal infection endemic in Colombia, South America, seem not to be increased in patients with AIDS.[8]

Kaposi's Sarcoma

One of the early hallmarks of the AIDS epidemic was a dramatic increase in the number of patients with Kaposi's sarcoma (KS). The epidemic of AIDS in homosexual men was first recognized as an outbreak of KS with/or without *Pneumocystis carinii* pneumonia (PCP) in homosexual men in Los Angeles, San Francisco, and New York.[9] The intensive investigation of these KS and PCP cases led first to the discovery that these men were immunosuppressed and later that HIV was the viral infection causing the underlying immunosuppression in AIDS patients.[10,11] Subsequently, studies of the epidemiology of KS provided data suggesting that the disease might be due to a sexually transmitted infection other than (or in addition to) HIV. This hypothesis arose from studies of the distribution of KS, which was seen primarily in populations whose HIV infection was acquired sexually, rather than those with drug use, transfusion, or perinatal transmission as risk factors. Also, women in the United States who developed AIDS because of heterosexual contact with a male partner had significantly higher rates of KS than did women who were injection drug users.[12] Recently, studies of Chang, Moore, and colleagues have identified the sequences of a new human herpes virus (HHV-8) in the tissues of patients with KS.[13,14] Further studies of HHV-8 have shown it to be associated with KS, even among patients who are not HIV infected.[14] Data indicating that infection with HHV-8 usually precedes the occurrence of KS by months to years have been obtained by several investigators.[15,16] It is now accepted by most experts that the association between HHV-8 and KS is causal, although immunosuppression and various hormonal factors appear to modify whether or not KS will result from an HHV-8 infection and when it will occur after an infection with HHV-8.

Pneumocystis carinii Pneumonia

The other opportunistic infection that was originally identified as the hallmark of AIDS before the identification of HIV was PCP occurring in a person without a malignancy or congenital immunodeficiency syndrome. Prior to the use of active antiretroviral therapy and specific prophylaxis for PCP, the disease occurred in nearly 75% of AIDS patients.[17] The fact that AIDS patients often had both PCP and KS led to the original hypothesis that AIDS was due to generalized immunosuppression, especially involving cell-mediated immune function. Although PCP has been reported from all risk groups of AIDS patients, it has been reported rarely among patients in Africa.[18] The reasons for this are unclear. However, some investigators have carefully studied African AIDS patients with bronchoscopy and autopsy, and have found the organism to be uncommon among these patients.[19]

Mycobacterium avium and other Nontuberculous Mycobacteria

Mycobacterium avium infections are especially common in patients with severe immunosuppression from AIDS. Typically, *M. avium* complex (MAC) infections occur in patients with CD4+ cell counts below 50/mL. Recently, clinical trials have shown that prophylaxis with clarithromycin or rifabutin is effective in preventing MAC infections in AIDS patients with severe immunosuppression. In addition to preventing clinical symptoms from MAC infections, the use of these drugs appears to prolong the survival of AIDS patients when prophylaxis is successful.[20] Infection with several other nontuberculous mycobacterial species, especially

M. kansasii, also has been reported in AIDS patients.

Cytomegalovirus, Herpes Simplex Virus Type 2, and Varicella-Zoster Virus

Persistent and recurrent infections with many herpes viruses are quite common in AIDS patients. Typically, cytomegalovirus (CMV) infections occur and present as CMV retinitis in patients with CD4+ cell counts below 50 cells/mL. If immunosuppression cannot be reversed with effective antiretroviral therapy, prophylactic therapy is necessary to prevent relapse and further retinal damage from occurring after successful treatment. Recent studies indicate that the risk of primary or recurrent CMV retinitis has been greatly reduced by treatment with combination antiretroviral drugs that include protease inhibitors and that continuation of CMV prophylaxis may not always be necessary to prevent relapses in patients with good immune recovery. Infections with CMV can also manifest as gastrointestinal or central nervous system infections. Herpes simplex virus type 2 (HSV-2) infections are commonly seen in patients with HIV infection and often occur in patients prior to severe immunosuppression. Genital ulcerations from HSV-2 infections in AIDS patients can be difficult to treat effectively and are very prone to recurrence. Similarly, dermatomal or disseminated herpes zoster VZV infections often occur in patients with HIV infection who have only moderately decreased CD4+ counts in the range of 200 to 400 cells/mL.

Other Infections

Patients with AIDS are at risk of developing a number of different opportunistic infections in addition to those described above. Infections with pneumococci are especially common. Increases in the rates of invasive pneumococcal infections (pneumonia, sepsis, and meningitis) have been proposed as a sentinel marker for the spread of HIV in a population.[21] It is characteristic of HIV infections and AIDS that clinically significant infections with an endemic pathogen increases in frequency if it is normally controlled by cellular immune mechanisms in persons exposed to the organisms. For example, in several countries in southern Europe, visceral leishmaniasis is a common manifestation of AIDS.[22] AIDS often presents as disseminated histoplasmosis among patients in the histoplasmosis belt in the Midwestern United States.[8] In Southeast Asia, especially in Northern Thailand and Southern China, disseminated *P. marneffei* infections (a fungal organism) are common clinical presentations in patients with AIDS.[7] Toxoplasmosis, cryptosporidiosis, and microsporidiosis are quite common parasitic infections in patients with AIDS.

AIDS-Associated Malignancies

In addition to a large number of opportunistic infections, AIDS patients also are at high risk of developing several malignancies. Kaposi's sarcoma is one of the most frequent AIDS-associated conditions and has been reviewed above. In addition, AIDS patients are at increased risk of non-Hodgkin's lymphoma (NHL), Hodgkin's disease, squamous cell carcinoma of the anus or penis, and cervical cancer.[23] Studies of the natural history of oncogenic human papilloma virus (HPV) in AIDS patients are under way. Chronic carriage of oncogenic HPV strains, especially HPV types 16, 18, and 31, appear to be more common in AIDS patients.[24] Typically, NHL occurs in severely immunosuppressed AIDS patients and is disseminated, commonly involving the central nervous system at the time of diagnosis.[25]

Other Conditions

Some patients with AIDS present with chronic diarrhea and severe weight loss, with or without chronic diarrhea, termed *slim disease* in Africa.[26] Such patients may or may not be infected with specific intestinal pathogens that cause chronic diarrheal disease. A number of other opportunistic pathogens, in addition to those discussed above, are relatively common in patients with HIV/AIDS.

FACTORS IN THE EMERGENCE OF INFECTIOUS DISEASES

Although there has been a marked decline in the morbidity and mortality from infectious diseases during the twentieth century related to the development and use of effective vaccines and antibiotics and a more hygienic environment, new infectious diseases have emerged, and old ones, such as tuberculosis, have re-emerged. Some of the important factors favoring the emergence and growing importance of infectious diseases, in addition to the HIV/AIDS pandemic, will be reviewed here briefly (Exhibit 12–1).

Population Growth

Perhaps the most important factor globally in the emergence of infectious diseases has been the growth of the human population, which started in the latter half of the nineteenth century. The human population had been stable for several centuries, then increased gradually with the urbanization and concentration of the labor force required for industrialization.

However, in the last several decades of the twentieth century, there has been an accelerated increase in the population of the planet. Along with this increase in population, there has been a dramatic growth in large urban populations. Some large urban centers have inadequate sanitary infrastructure, such as sewage disposal, water supply, and food distribution and storage. Nearly all large cities in both the developed and developing world have substantial populations living in crowded slums. The resultant crowding and marginal sanitary conditions have been associated with increases in infectious diseases. Most experts predict that the population increase will continue, as will the growth of megacities, in the twenty-first century. Some experts predict that the global population will grow from 6 billion currently to reach 12 to 15 billion or more persons by the mid–twenty-first century, i.e., 2.5

Exhibit 12–1 Emerging Infectious Diseases and Changes in Environment, Host, or Organism That Have Promoted Their Emergence

Infectious Disease or Organism	Factor

Arenaviruses
  Junin virus (Argentine HF)
  Machupo virus (Bolivian HF)
  Guanarito virus (Venezuelan HF)
	Changes in agriculture allowing closer contact with infected rodents

Hantavirus Sin Nombre virus (HPS)	Climatic changes allowing mice expansion
Rift Valley fever	Dams, irrigation, climate change
Filoviridae species Ebola-Marburg virus	Increased contact between infected primates and man; nosocomial spread, importation of animals
Dengue	Increased global travel, urbanization, increase in mosquito reservoir
Influenza	Integrated pig-duck agriculture, increase in global travel
HIV/(AIDS) HTLV	Changes in sexual behavior, urbanization, increase in illicit drug use, global shipment of blood products
Raccoon rabies	Trans-shipment of infected raccoons
Cyclospora cayetanensis	International shipment of raspberries
Cholera	El Niño climate change, international travel, shipment of foods
Borrelia burgdorferi (Lyme disease)	Increased deer population, increased human contact with ticks in nature
Malaria	Growth and movement of human populations, declining use and effectiveness of insecticides, crowding
Escherichia coli O157:H7 (enterohemorrhagic *E. coli*)	Growth-centralized agriculture promoting cross-contamination, global distribution of foods
Pfisteria pisticida	Changes in agricultural practices leading to pollution of rivers and estuaries, overgrowth of dinoflagellates
Quinolone-resistant *Campylobacter*	Overuse and misuse of antibiotics in agriculture and in clinical settings
Multidrug-resistant *Mycobacterium tuberculosis*	Misuse of antibiotics, crowding in prisons, slums, hospitals, etc., allowing transmission
Cryptosporidium parvum	Contamination of municipal water supplies, increases in immunocompromised populations

times the current population. Population growth to these levels could severely test our ability to control the emergence and spread of infectious diseases. More optimistic projections predict a global population of about 10 billion. Wherever the current population growth settles, the public health problems will be more severe than they are today. Limiting population growth is a critical public health issue that underlies our ability to control infectious diseases and other health and social problems.

Speed and Ease of Travel

Dramatic changes in the ability and ease of travel have occurred in the twentieth century. In the last several decades, with modern airplane travel, it is quite possible to get from a tropical rain forest in Africa or South America to a suburban or rural area in the United States during the incubation period of a disease such as Lassa fever, dengue, malaria, West Nile virus (WNV) encephalitis, or most infectious diseases.[27] This has facilitated the introduction and spread of diseases from one area to another. In fact, autochthonous transmission of malaria has occurred occasionally in the temperate zone of the United States, secondary to the introduction of malaria by a visitor from an endemic area and subsequent focal transmission by local anopheline mosquitoes.[28]

In addition to the movement of people, the food supply of the United States and most developed countries has become very international. The repeated introduction of *Cyclospora* on raspberries imported in the United States or Canada from Guatemala,[29,30] the importation of *Escherichia coli* O157:H7 into Japan on radish sprouts from the United States,[31] and the importation to the United States of chickens contaminated with quinolone-resistant *Campylobacter* from Mexico[32,33] are recent examples of the global transport of infectious pathogens.

Dam Building

The construction of large dams to provide hydroelectric power to growing populations and irrigation for rural crops has had adverse consequences in the emergence of infectious diseases. The number of large dams that have been constructed in the United States, Asia, Africa, and elsewhere in the twentieth century has increased in parallel with the population growth (Figure 12–1).

The construction of dams often has displaced rural and semirural populations and has provided a propitious environment for the growth of mosquitoes and other vector species. The construction of the Aswan high dam in upper Egypt was accompanied by a large expansion of the snail population and hundreds of thousands of *Schistosoma haematobium* infections in the populations that were exposed to the water supply.

Expansion of Human Populations into Previously Uninhabited Forested and Suburban Areas

The redistribution of the human population into areas that were previously uninhabited has had a major impact on the emergence of infectious diseases in both developed and developing countries.

The emergence of Lyme disease, human granulocytic ehrlichiosis (HGE), human monocytic ehrlichiosis (HME), babesiosis, and Rocky Mountain spotted fever (RMSF) in various areas of the United States is directly linked to the growth of suburbia and recreation in tick-infested areas. In tropical Africa, the emergence of Ebola virus, Lassa fever, monkey pox, and HIV-1 and HIV-2 infections were related to the expansion of the human population into wilderness areas and increased close exposures of humans to nonhuman primate populations.

Relocation of Animals

In addition to international travel and shipment of food, some infectious diseases have emerged because of shipment and relocation of animals. An epidemic of raccoon rabies was recognized in the Northeastern United States, which was initiated by the intentional transpor-

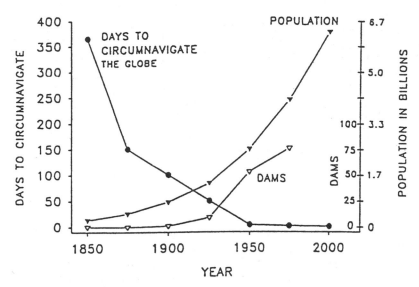

Figure 12–1 Over the last 150 years, there have been many global changes that have enhanced the probability of the emergence of new infectious diseases of humans and animals. This chart depicts three examples of such trends: The increase in the human population, the increased construction of large dams (over 75 meters high) built in the United States, 1890–1975, and the decrease in time needed to circle the globe. *Source:* Reprinted with permission from F.A. Murphy and N. Nathanson, *Seminars in Virology*, Vol. 5, p. 88, © 1994, Academic Press, Inc.

tation of raccoons from the South, especially Georgia, Alabama, Florida, and the Carolinas, to Virginia and West Virginia for hunting by sportsmen.[34] Unfortunately, the raccoons were obtained from a population of animals in which an epizootic of rabies was occurring. Subsequently, raccoon rabies has spread widely to many states in the Northeastern United States; currently, most human postexposure rabies vaccine prophylaxis in this area is given because of exposures to rabid or possibly rabid raccoons. For reasons that are unclear, there has been no transmission of rabies to humans from rabid raccoons, despite over 1,000 instances of human exposures annually in New York state and similar extensive use of vaccine after raccoon exposure in other Atlantic coastal states.

The epidemic of Ebola virus infections in rhesus macaques (*Macaca fascicularis*) monkeys imported from the Philippines to the U.S. Army primate facility in Reston, Virginia, is an-

other example of transportation of a new infectious disease with infected animals.[35] An outbreak of Marburg virus infection in laboratory workers occurred in Germany from exposure to infected monkeys imported from Africa.[36]

Global Climate Change

A major environmental factor that potentially could lead to the emergence of infectious diseases is global climate change. The changes in climate that have occurred during the past 100 years or so and are predicted to continue in the future are often termed *global warming*. Although this term is accurate, it doesn't completely capture the total complexity of global climate change. Some areas of the Earth are becoming warmer; others are not. Nevertheless, there has been an overall measured increase in average surface temperatures of the Earth during the last century. Three research programs have analyzed available data from over 7,000 stations that have recorded surface temperature around the globe. These data have been compiled and plotted by three different research groups: the National Oceanic and Atmospheric Administration (NOAA), the National Aeronautic and Space Administration (NASA), and the Climate Research Unit (CRU) of the University of East Anglia, Norwich, in the United Kingdom. Overall, these data have measured a warming of about 1°F (0.4°C) since the late nineteenth century (Figure 12–2). Although global warming during the past century seems to have been well documented, not all areas of the Earth's surface have been equally affected, and the causes of the warming and predictions for the future have been debated. However, most climatologic researchers believe that human activities that have increased greenhouse gases, such as carbon dioxide, methane, and nitrous oxide, have played a major role in the climate change of the Earth during recent decades. Data collected by Oak Ridge National Laboratory have shown dramatic increases in carbon dioxide emissions during the twentieth century from burning of fossil fuels (Figure 12–3).

Although it is difficult to predict with certainty how global climate change will affect the emergence of new infectious diseases, several recent epidemics have occurred because climate change was believed to have been important. A recent example is the infectious diseases consequent to the recent El Niño event, with warming of surface sea water temperatures in the South Pacific Ocean in 1993. This severe El Niño is believed to have led to an algal boom in the surface waters along the Pacific coast of South America. The subsequent zooplankton expansion was believed to have spread the ocean reservoir of *Vibrio cholera* along coastal South America.[37] The consequence was a new emergence of cholera, which had not been epidemic in South America during the previous century.

In the Four Corners area of New Mexico, Colorado, Arizona, and Utah, the increased rainfall associated with El Niño climate conditions is believed to have led to an expansion of the deer mouse population because of the availability of a markedly increased food supply of pinon nuts. The mice that were chronically infected with Sin Nombre hantavirus infected the human population when they invaded their homes. The outbreak of hantavirus pulmonary syndrome is believed to have been the first outbreak of infections with this virus in a human population. Serologic surveys of populations in New Mexico who might have been exposed previously did not yield evidence of previous unrecognized epidemics. The unique environmental conditions that occurred at this time allowed this virus to emerge as a significant human pathogen (Table 12–1).

An epidemic of Rift Valley fever (RVF) occurred in Tanzania and countries in East Africa between December 1997 and April 1998, which was believed to be due to an unusually large rainfall and expansion of the mosquito vector population. At least 478 deaths occurred, and an estimated 89,000 persons were estimated to have been infected in this epidemic.[38] Analysis of previous RVF virus epidemics in East Africa has determined that they have nearly always been associated with unusually high rainfall, leading to the expansion of an infected mosquito population.[39]

Many climatologists and epidemiologists are concerned that global warming associated with an increase in environmental pollution from greenhouse gases could lead to an expanded range of anopheline mosquitoes with epidemics of malaria in previously uninfected populations. Also, the expansion of the range of *Aedes aegypti* and *Aedes albopictus* could occur with modest increases in mean temperatures. This could lead to epidemics of dengue, yellow fever, and viral encephalitis (such as eastern encephalitis [EE]). Another effect of global warming is that the extrinsic incubation period of dengue virus in the mosquito vector is shortened by elevated temperatures, which increase the size of dengue epidemics.[40]

Significant global climate change could have major effects on the epidemiology of infectious diseases. One concern of climatologists is that

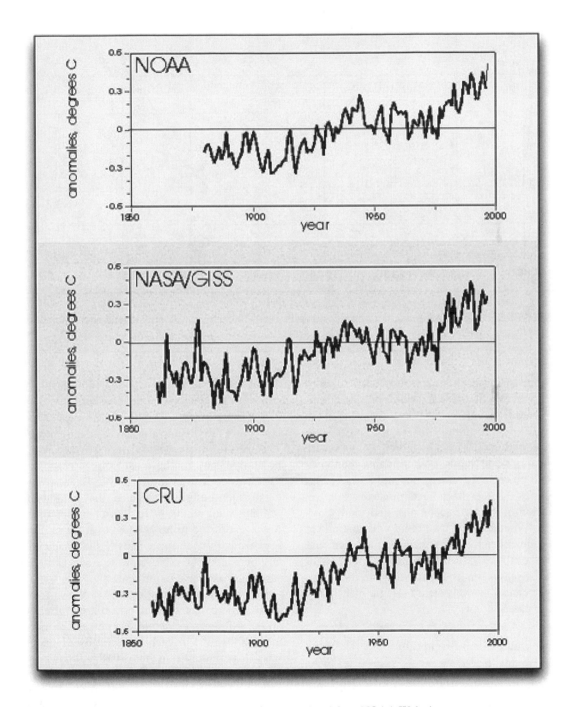

Figure 12–2 Global temperature anomalies. *Source:* Reprinted from NOAA Web site.

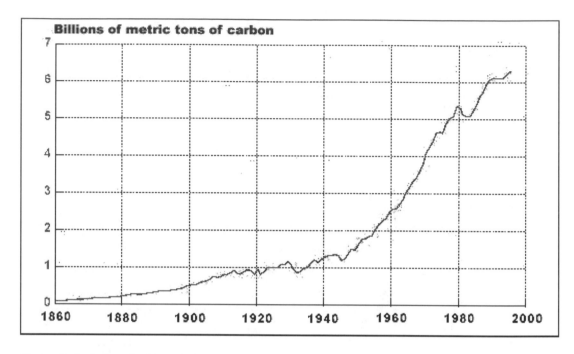

Figure 12–3 Carbon dioxide emissions from fossil fuels, 1860–2000. *Source:* Reprinted with permission from World Resources Institute.

global climate change might lead to both droughts in some areas and major increased rainfall with flooding in other areas. Warming of the Earth's surface could affect the hydrologic cycle, with increases in both drought and severe rainstorms and floods. Both droughts and floods could promote the emergence and spread of infectious diseases from contaminated water, expansion of vector populations, and food shortages. Whether global warming will continue at an accelerated rate, as some have predicted, and whether this will lead to an expansion of infectious diseases is not certain. However, the evolving scenario has sufficient biologic plausibility to be taken seriously.

War and Societal Disruption

Nearly every major war has been accompanied by significant epidemics of infectious disease that involve both the military combatants and the civilian populations. Often, the epidem-

ics of infectious disease overshadow military factors in the outcome of the conflict.[41]

There are many examples of this interaction. However, the "swine influenza" pandemic of 1918–1919, which occurred during World War I in Europe may be the most graphic example. This epidemic was unlike any influenza epidemic seen before or since, in that it targeted healthy young adults, often with a fatal outcome. It was estimated to have killed over 20 million persons worldwide and at least 43,000 U.S. military personnel. Over 80% of the American war casualties were due to influenza.[41]

Germany's General Erich Von Rudendroff blamed the defeat of the German army directly on the influenza epidemic. He noted that more than 2,000 men in each of his army divisions were ill with the flu in June 1918.[41] It has been estimated that 20% of the world's population and one of every four persons in the United States were infected during this epidemic. The virus is now believed to have arisen as a recom-

Table 12–1 Ecologic Features of Different Virus Complexes within the Genus *Hantavirus**

Virus Complex	Wildlife Host (rodent subfamily)	Geographic Distribution	Human Disease (severity)
Hantaan	*Apodemus agrarius*, striped field mouse (Murinae)	Eastern Asia, Eastern Europe	Hemorrhagic fever (severe)
Seoul	*Rattus* species, wild/laboratory rat (Murinae)	Eastern Asia, seaports worldwide	Hemorrhagic fever (moderate/mild)
Puumala	*Clethrionomys glareolus*, bank vole (Arvicolinae)	Europe, European Russia	Nephropathia epidemica (mild)
Prospect Hill	*Microtus pennsylvanicus*, meadow vole (Arvicolinae)	United States	Unknown
Sin Nombre	*Peromyscus maniculatus*, deer mouse (Sigmodontinae)	Western United States	Hantavirus pulmonary syndrome (HPS) (severe)

*Hemorrhagic fever is also known as hemorrhagic fever with renal syndrome (HFRS). In the United States, two other hantaviruses have been associated with a few cases of HPS (Black Creek Canyon virus, carried by *S. hispidus*, and Bayou virus, carried by *O. palustris*), and other new hantaviruses will probably be defined (Nichol et al., 1996).

Source: Reprinted with permission from Fields, Knipe and Hally, *Virology*, p. 1485, © 1996, Lippincott-Raven Publishers.

binant virus in swine in Kansas and transported to the European War theater by infected U.S. troops.[42]

During World War II, a major common source outbreak of hepatitis B infection occurred, due to immunization of troops with a contaminated yellow fever vaccine. The source of the contamination was human serum, which had been added to the vaccine as a stabilizer. It had been prepared from an HBV carrier, unfortunately. Also, malaria, diarrheal disease, and other infections were common in the troops during World Ward II. After the war, malaria was introduced into the United States.

During the Korean conflict, Korean hemorrhagic fever, due to a Hantaan virus, became a significant health problem among U.S. Army troops. Many U.S. soldiers serving near the de-

militarized zone developed fever, hemorrhagic phenomenon, and renal failure. The cause of the disease was not discovered for another decade. In the Gulf War of 1993, visceral leishmaniasis due to *Leishmania tropica* occurred in U.S. troops.

Civilian refugees who are displaced when fleeing political crisis in their homeland often are even more vulnerable than are military populations. Malnutrition, accompanied by outbreaks of cholera, shigellosis, and malaria is frequent among refugees in tropical areas in Africa and Asia. The United Nations High Commission on Refugees estimates that there are currently over 16 million refugees and 5.4 million internally displaced persons throughout the world.[43] Many of these refugees are highly vulnerable to epidemics of infectious diseases.

Growth of Day Care for Infants and Children Outside the Home

In the last 30 years, an increasing proportion of women with dependent infants and children has been employed full time outside the home. This includes single parents and families where both parents work. Currently, over two thirds of women with children under 18 years of age are in the work force.[44] This has necessitated a dramatic growth in the use of day-care facilities to care for preschool children. Clustering of children in day-care centers has facilitated the transmission of a number of infectious agents from one child to another, day-care staff, and, eventually, to others living in the households of children attending day-care. Because many day-care centers have substantial populations of children in diapers, the transmission of pathogenic organisms by the fecal-oral route is facilitated. Infections from organisms such as rotavirus, *Giardia lamblia, Campylobacter jejuni, Shigella* species, and hepatitis A virus (HAV) have been transmitted in the day-care setting. In fact, a substantial change in the epidemiology of hepatitis A virus infections was reported in the late 1970s in Maricopa County (Phoenix), Arizona. A significant increase in patients with jaundice due to HAV infection was related to HAV transmission in day-care settings between children and spread to household contacts.[45] Outbreaks of HAV infections in day-care centers average 12 cases in size and last 3 months in duration.[46] Typically, young children are asymptomatic or have mild infections; adults in the household or the day-care center have more severe clinical illnesses. Outbreaks are more often associated with larger centers that accept children in diapers.

Infections spread by the respiratory route and by direct contact are also common among children attending day-care centers. It has been estimated that about 10 respiratory infections per year occur among children at the peak age for respiratory infections, i.e., the second 6 months of life.[47] Most respiratory infections are viral but day care facilitates the transmission of some bacterial infections, as well.[47]

Recently, increased attention has been directed toward reducing the transmission of infections in day care by improved handwashing and disinfection of fomites, such as toys. Also, the development and licensure of new vaccines, including HAV, varicella, *Haemophilus influenzae* B, acellular pertussis, and *Streptococcus pneumoniae* have allowed improved strategies for the prevention of some day-care infections. However, public health strategies of excluding infants and children with active infections have been difficult to implement successfully, due to economic pressures on parents to work.

Increase in Nursing Home Population

The increase in the elderly population in nursing homes has been another factor promoting the transmission of infectious agents. Not uncommonly, residents of nursing homes may be given antibiotics or admitted to a hospital where they become infected or colonized with a nosocomial pathogen, such as staphylococci, enterococci, or gram-negative organisms that are resistant to multiple antibiotics. The population in nursing homes may be an important reservoir in the community for these nosocomial pathogens. Clearly, they are at increased risk of infectious diseases due to declining immunity, limited mobility, and crowding in extended-care facilities.

Antibiotic Use and Abuse

An important selective force in the emergence of pathogenic microorganisms is the widespread use of antibiotics in both the human and animal populations. Antibiotics are used for the therapy and prophylaxis of infections in humans and animals and for growth promotion in domestic animals. A recent study of *C. jejuni* infections in Minnesota between 1992 and 1998 linked many human infections with quinolone-resistant organisms to the use of these effective antibiotics as a growth factor in chickens by the poultry industry.[32] This widespread practice, which began in the United States in 1995 and earlier in Mexico, led to the emergence of these difficult-to-treat infections in humans in only a few years.[33] This illustrates the need for ecologic and public health–based decision making in agricultural industries to avoid promoting the emergence of new antibiotic-resistant human pathogens. Some studies suggest that restriction of the use of antibiotics in clinical settings might sometimes favor the re-emergence of an antibiotic-sensitive flora.[48] However, such strategies often are not entirely successful. This important topic is covered more completely in Chapter 13.

Bioterrorism

Another potential infectious disease problem that has received increased attention and publicity recently is the threat of the intentional attack of a population with infectious pathogens. Clearly, this has happened in the past. The idea of the use of infectious agents in warfare dates back to the English wars with Native American populations, where blankets impregnated with scabs from patients with smallpox were traded to Native Americans in the hopes of causing disease in the recipients.[49] Although less well documented, it is likely that some form of small-scale biologic warfare was practiced by ancient civilizations. Recently, a large community outbreak of salmonellosis in Oregon was found to be due to the intentional contamination of salad bars in multiple restaurants by followers of Bhagwan Shree Rajnesh.[50]

However, at present, the potential of biologic agents as weapons has grown with modern techniques of molecular biology to the point that an effective attack could be carried out by a group of dissidents or terrorists, as well as by a national government. Such an attack could be managed with modest financial and technologic resources. A flask of virulent *Bacillus anthracis* (Anthrax) spores deposited in a crowded area with a recirculating air supply, such as a subway in a large city, could infect thousands or tens of thousands of persons under certain conditions.

Most experts believe that the number of biologic agents that are good candidates for use as effective biologic weapons and presently available for use is limited, even though the number of organisms that could cause fatal human disease is extensive. The U.S. Department of Defense has focused attention on a few bacteria, viruses, and toxins, which are listed in Exhibit 12–2. Of these, anthrax is the leading candidate. This organism has several characteristics that make it a potentially attractive candidate for a bioterrorism attack:

1. It exists as a spore, which could remain viable under a variety of environmental conditions and could be widely dispersed and remain suspended in the air for extended distances.
2. When inhaled, the infectious dose is low, and the resultant pneumonia in suscep-

---

Exhibit 12–2 Possible Bioterrorism Agents

A. Bacteria
  1. *Bacillus anthracis* (anthrax)
  2. *Vibrio cholera* (cholera)
  3. *Yersinia pestis* (plague)
  4. *Francisella tularensis* (tularemia)
  5. *Coxiella burnetii* (Q fever)
B. Viruses
  1. Variola (small pox)
  2. Venezuelan equine encephalomyelitis
  3. Hemorrhagic fever viruses (e.g., Ebola, Sin Nombre, Hantaan, etc.)
C. Toxins
  1. Botulinum
  2. Staphylococcal enterotoxin B
  3. Ricin
  4. T-2 mycotoxins

Source: Reprinted from Walter Reed Army Institute of Research, Addressing Emerging Infectious Disease Threats: A Strategic Plan for the Department of Defense, WRAIR, DOD, Washington, DC, 1998.

tible individuals is highly fatal, especially with delayed treatment.

3. Very few civilian physicians have experience enough to recognize or treat inhalation anthrax.

4. Although a protective vaccine exists, very few persons have received this vaccine.

Furthermore, the vaccine requires multiple doses (i.e., six doses over a 2-year period), and available stores of the vaccine are limited. In addition, the efficacy of the vaccine in the prevention of anthrax in persons exposed to aerosolized spores is not certain; however, workers having occupational aerosol exposure from contaminated animal hides have been protected in the past with this vaccine.[51,52] Because of the publicity surrounding the potential of anthrax as a biologic agent, hoaxes and threats of the use of this agent have become common in the United States recently.[53] Fortunately, no attack has been carried out to date, but the potential for success is a chilling reminder of the possible risk. Other agents that have been considered by experts to be possibly useful as biologic weapons are listed in Exhibit 12–2, which was compiled and published by the U.S. Department of Defense.[54]

OTHER EMERGING INFECTIOUS DISEASES

In addition to the infectious diseases that have emerged as opportunistic pathogens in patients with HIV-related immunosuppression and AIDS, other infections have emerged in recent years because of factors favoring the increased exposure or susceptibility of human populations to infectious agents, which have been reviewed above. Several examples of recent experiences with specific emerging infectious diseases and some of the factors promoting their emergence will be reviewed.

Lyme Disease

Lyme disease was first recognized by Steere and colleagues in 1975, following the identifica-

tion of a group of children living in Old Lyme, Connecticut, who were diagnosed with juvenile rheumatoid arthritis.[55] The geographic clustering of cases, the seasonal distribution with onset of illness in the summer, and a history of a prior distinctive skin lesion, erythema chronica migrans (ECM), eventually led to the hypothesis that Lyme disease was due to an infectious agent that was transmitted by ticks.[56] Subsequently, the causative spirochete organism was identified in the salivary glands of the tick *Ixodes scapularis* by Willy Burgdorfer in studies of ticks on Shelter Island, New York. When the patients with classic Lyme disease showed evidence of specific immunofluorescent antibodies to this new organism, the conclusion was reached that Lyme Disease was caused by infection with this new organism, which was subsequently named *Borrelia burgdorferi.*[57]

In the 20 years since the recognition of Lyme disease, the number of reported cases has increased progressively, and the geographic areas of endemnicity of the disease have expanded to include the coastal Northeastern and mid-Atlantic states, several states in the Midwest (especially Minnesota, Wisconsin, and Michigan), and coastal California.[58,59] Although the clinical suspicion that a patient may have Lyme disease has increased among physicians because of the potential for chronic sequelae, there has clearly been an increase in the incidence of the disease.[59] Factors promoting the emergence of Lyme disease include the encroachment of human populations into areas infected with tick vectors and the growth of the deer populations, allowing for an increased survival and density of *Ixodes scapularis* ticks.[60] The epidemiology of Lyme disease is reviewed in more detail in Chapter 21.

Other Tick-Borne Infections

Other tick-borne infections that are endemic in the United States have been described in recent years, and these diseases may have increased in frequency as well. However, the data on temporal trends of their incidence is less clear because the only reportable tick-borne infection in the United States is RMSF. The number of reported patients with RMSF increased from about 200 to 400 cases in the 1950s and 1960s to over 1,000 cases in the late 1970s and 1980s.[61] Increased opportunities for human exposure to the vectors, primarily the Rocky Mountain wood tick (*Dermocenter andersonii*) in the Western United States and the American dog tick (*Dermocenter variabilis*) in the Eastern United States, occurred because of the expansion of suburban housing into wooded, tick-infested areas and the increased opportunities for exposure associated with recreational activities.

Two forms of human ehrlichiosis, HME due to infection with *Ehrlichia chaffeeinsis* and HGE due to infection with *Ehrlichia ewingii*, have also been recognized with increased frequency in the past few years.[62–65] These diseases are also transmitted by ticks, HME by the dog tick and HGE by the deer tick.

Another tick-borne disease, babesiosis, an infection of red blood cells with *Babesia microti*, can be transmitted to humans by tick bites in the endemic areas in the coastal Northeastern United States.[66] It is not unusual for a patient to be seen who has both Lyme disease and ehrlichiosis after exposure to tick habitats in an endemic area. It seems likely that these other tick-borne diseases have increased in frequency, similar to increases documented with Lyme disease. However, the documentation of this increased incidence has been difficult, because these diseases have not been routinely reported to health authorities.

Dengue and Other Mosquito-Borne Infections

Although dengue has been known as a human disease for over 200 years, in the last 20 years, dengue fever, dengue hemorrhagic fever (DHF), and dengue shock syndrome (DSS) have emerged as the most important arthropod-borne viral disease of humans worldwide.[67] It is now estimated that up to 100 million cases of dengue fever occur annually globally. Approximately 250,000 cases of DHF are officially reported each year, and the number probably is several times higher. The syndrome of DHF/DSS was first reported as an epidemic disease in the Philippines in 1954, and it gradually spread to other areas in Southeast Asia.[68] This more severe form of dengue carries a mortality of 5% to 15% and is believed to be related most often to an infection with a second dengue serotype in a person previously infected with another dengue virus.[69] The second dengue virus infection is believed to lead to vascular damage by immune mechanisms—associated with the formation of immune complexes—and binding to FC receptors on vascular endothelial cells in a previously sensitized host.

Several factors have promoted the emergence of dengue and its spread to new geographic areas. Increases in the use of nonbiodegradable containers and their storage in peridomestic locations have provided more breeding places for the mosquito vector, *Aedes aegypti*, in proximity to humans. A program to eradicate *A. aegypti* from the Americas was initiated by the Pan American Health Organization (PAHO) in 1947 to control yellow fever, which is also spread by the same mosquito. Efforts were successful in a number of countries. By 1972, *A. aegypti* had been eliminated from 19 countries in the Americas, representing 73% of the area originally infected (Figure 12–4). However, the campaign gradually lost steam, and funding was withdrawn. This occurred in part due to the identification of a jungle cycle of yellow fever and the recognition that, even with the elimination of *A. aegypti* from urban areas, a focus of yellow fever would persist. Hence, the disease was no longer felt to be eradicable.[70] Within about 10 years, *A. aegypti* had reestablished itself in virtually all of South and Central America (Figure 12–5). In 1981, a severe epidemic of dengue type 2 infection with the first cases of DHF/DSS in the Western Hemisphere occurred in Cuba.[71] In 1986, an explosive outbreak of dengue type 1, involving over 1 million cases, occurred in Rio de Janeiro. Subsequently, dengue epidemics have occurred in Paraguay, Bolivia, Peru, Ecuador, Colombia, and Venezuela. Recently, dengue outbreaks have been re-

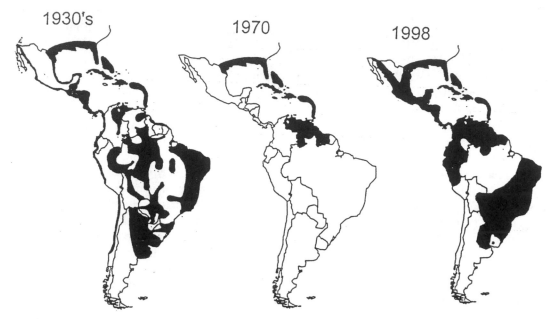

Figure 12–4 *Aedes aegypti* distribution in the Americas during the 1930s and in 1970 and 1998. *Source:* Reprinted with permission from D. Gubler, Dengue and Dengue Hemorrhagic Fever, *Clinical Microbiological Reviews*, Vol. 11, pp. 480–496, © 1998, American Society for Microbiology.

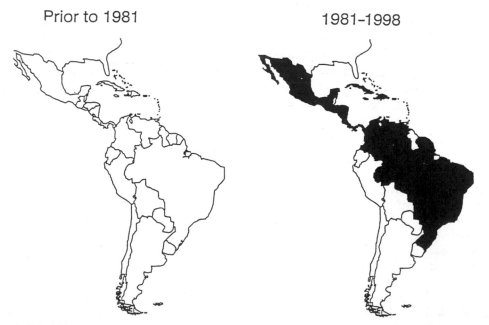

Figure 12–5 DHF in the Americas before 1981 and from 1981 to 1998. *Source:* Reprinted with permission from D. Gubler, Dengue and Dengue Hemorrhagic Fever, *Clinical Microbiological Reviews*, Vol. 11, pp. 480–496, © 1998, American Society for Microbiology.

ported for the first time in Argentina. Three of the four dengue serotypes are currently endemic in Latin America. In 1997, a second large epidemic of dengue due to dengue type 2 virus, with cases of DHF, occurred in Cuba.[72]

Reports of dengue in Africa were unusual in the 1960s and 1970s or prior to that time. In the mid-1980s, however, dengue appeared along the coast of Kenya, then in the Ivory Coast and Burkina Fasa. Dengue has spread to other African countries in recent years. Also, dengue has spread westward in Asia, into India, Pakistan, and the Middle East in the last decade.[70]

Another factor that has raised considerable concern about the potential for further spread of mosquito-borne viruses in the Americas was the introduction of *Aedes albopictus* into Houston in used truck tires imported from Southeast Asia for recapping in 1985.[73] These spare tires collected rainwater and were excellent breeding sites for these mosquitoes, which could transmit dengue and yellow fever, as well as other arthropod-borne viruses, such as eastern equine encephalitis. *Aedes albopictus* mosquitoes have also been introduced into Brazil in a similar manner; these effective vector mosquitoes are now widely distributed in 19 states of the United States (Figure 12–6). Each year, over 100 cases of dengue are reported in persons in the United States who have acquired their infections in the

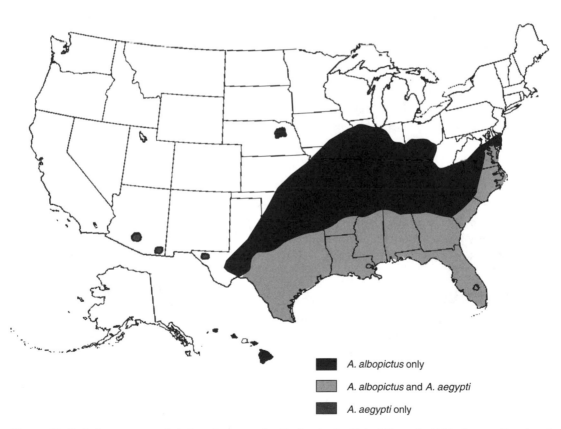

A. albopictus only

A. albopictus and A. aegypti

A. aegypti only

Figure 12–6 *Aedes aegypti* and *Aedes albopictus* distribution in the United States in 1998. *Source:* Reprinted with permission from D. Gubler, Dengue and Dengue Hemorrhagic Fever, *Clinical Microbiological Reviews*, Vol. 11, pp. 480–496, © 1998, American Society for Microbiology.

endemic areas of Asia, Latin America, or Africa.[74] It is quite possible that these viremic individuals might eventually provide a sufficient reservoir to reestablish dengue as an endemic disease in the United States, with either *A. aegypti* or *A. albopictus* as the vector.

Factors Affecting Transmission of Arthropod-Borne Viruses (Arboviruses)

Transmission of arboviruses is related to the characteristics of the virus, the distribution and biology of the vector mosquitoes, and the availability of reservoir hosts. Because of the complex interactions between man, mosquitoes, and the reservoir hosts, the prediction and the control of epidemics often can be difficult. There have been several instances of the emergence or re-emergence of arboviruses as epidemic diseases with such changes as

- building of dams and water projects, resulting in altered water distribution patterns
- deforestation and changed land use associated with the development of new communities
- introduction of new virus-amplifying hosts or the expansion of new vectors

Also, climatic changes may amplify endemic transmission by altering mosquito breeding sites and potentially by decreasing the extrinsic incubation period of the virus in the vector.[40]

Rift Valley Fever

Rift Valley fever is a phlebovirus that has been recognized for many years as a cause of disease in domestic ruminants and man in African countries south of the Sahara. In 1978, a major epidemic of RVF occurred in Egypt. This was followed by an outbreak in 1987 in Senegal after the opening of a new dam. The 1997 epidemic of RVF associated with the increased rainfall associated with El Niño weather conditions has already been discussed.[38]

Malaria

Many countries in Africa, Asia, and Latin America have experienced a major resurgence of malaria in the last 20 years. During the 1950s and early 1960s, there was great optimism that malaria could be eliminated with an aggressive program focusing on spraying of homes and other buildings with DDT.[75] However, because residual insecticide spraying was followed by resistance to DDT among anopheline mosquitoes and transmission of infection by mosquitoes that rested outdoors after biting humans emerged as new vectors, budgets for malaria control programs were cut, and the disease has reappeared in many areas. Malaria was nearly eliminated on the island of Sri Lanka but the disease has made a major comeback in the decades after the malaria control program was abandoned. Malaria has also expanded in India; resistance to chloroquine and other antimalarials among strains of *Plasmodium falciparum* has also spread worldwide in the last two decades. Currently, the malaria prevention program in many countries is focused on personal protection to avoid exposure with use of insecticides and insecticide-containing bed nets and treatment of severe cases.[76] The public health emphasis has shifted from elimination to control and treatment of malaria.

West Nile-Like Viral Encephalitis Outbreak in New York, 1999

An infectious disease physician notified the New York City Department of Health of two patients with encephalitis on August 23, 1999. The health department investigation identified a cluster of six patients with encephalitis in the same neighborhood as the two index cases. Serologic testing of these cases were positive by IgM-capture enzyme-linked immunoabsorbent assay (ELISA) for antibodies to St. Louis encephalitis (SLE) virus, a flavivirus native to North America that had not been reported previously in the New York City area. Subsequently, a total of 37 cases were identified in New York City and surrounding counties by September 28,

1999. However, officials at the Bronx Zoo noted the deaths of several birds between September 7 and 9; included were a cormorant, two captive-bred Chilean flamingoes, and an Asian pheasant. In addition, other local birds, especially crows, appeared to have increased mortality. Autopsies of these avian species revealed pathologic evidence of encephalitis. Testing of the bird tissues and human autopsy material by polymerase chain reaction (PCR) and viral isolation revealed viruses that closely resembled WNV. West Nile virus had never previously been reported in the Western Hemisphere. This virus was first isolated in the West Nile province of Uganda in 1937.[77] Subsequent outbreaks have been reported in Israel in 1950–1954 and 1957, in France in 1962, South Africa in 1974, and Romania in 1996.

Although it is not known when and how a West Nile–like virus was introduced into North America, international travel of viremic persons from endemic areas to New York or transport of virus by infected birds could have played a role. This epidemic may be a good example of the international transport of an infectious disease into a nonendemic area.

Arthropod-Borne Virus Infections

Arboviruses are important causes of encephalitis in many parts of the world. Transmission of these viruses is restricted to specific species of mosquitoes or ticks that are present in specific ecologic systems. These diseases are seasonal in temperate climates, because they depend on transmission by the arthropod host. The virus must replicate in the vector and travel from the stomach to the salivary glands before transmission can occur. The interval between infection of the vector by ingesting blood from a viremic host until the virus appears in the salivary gland of the arthropod is referred to as the *extrinsic incubation period*. This period is shorter at higher temperature.

Arboviruses are classified into four families, ie, *Togaviridae, Flaviviridae, Bunyaviridae,* and *Reoviridae.* The vectors, animal reservoir, and geographic distribution of some important representatives of these four viral families are shown in Table 12–2. The viruses are not cytopathic to the infected mosquitoes. However, some arboviruses are neurotropic in the mosquito, as well as in humans. This is especially true for Japanese encephalitis (JE) virus and may affect transmission by enhancing biting of CO_2-emitting targets, i.e., humans and other animals.

The transmission of these viruses may occur throughout the year in tropical areas. However, in temperate climates, the mechanism of survival of arboviruses over the winter is of considerable epidemiologic interest. Although it is possible that a female mosquito could hibernate after a blood meal and re-emerge the following season, this is believed to be rare. Generally, only nulliparous mosquitoes hibernate. The virus could also be reintroduced by migrating birds. Another mechanism for over wintering is the vertical transmission of the viral genome to the eggs of an infected female mosquito. This has been shown to occur for most of the viruses in the *Bunyavirus* and *Phlebovirus* groups. However, there is no good evidence of vertical transmission of other arboviruses. Ticks do survive for several years and can spread infection during subsequent seasons after they are infected.

The most widespread arboviral encephalitis in humans is JE. Infections with this virus occur as epidemics and endemic disease in Japan, Korea, Taiwan, China, Thailand, and other countries in Southeast Asia. Infection has recently spread into Nepal, India, and Pakistan. The natural cycle of the virus is between herons and other water birds and culicine mosquitoes; especially *Culex tritaeniorhynchus*, that breed in rice fields. Pigs are amplifying hosts. Infected culicine mosquitoes also spread the infection to humans (Figure 12–7). In endemic areas, most adults are immune, and clinical encephalitis is seen in children. The ratio of inapparent to apparent infection is between 50:1 and 1000:1, depending on the age of the individual. However, 20% to 30% of clinical infections are fatal, and neurologic sequelae are common in survivors. An inactivated JE vaccine is now widely used in

Table 12–2 Arboviruses That Cause Encephalitis

Family Genus Complex Virus Species	Vector	Animal Reservoir	Geographical Location	Importance in Encephalitis[a]
Togaviridae[b]				
Alphavirus[b]				
Eastern encephalitis	Mosquitoes (*Culiseta, Aedes*)	Birds	Eastern and gulf coasts of U.S., Caribbean, and South America	++
Western encephalitis	Mosquitoes (*Culex*)	Birds	Widespread; but disease in western U.S. and Canada	++
Venezuelan equine encephalitis	Mosquitoes (*Aedes, Culex, Mansonia,* etc.)	Horses and small mammals	South and Central America, Florida, and southwest U.S.	+
Flaviviridae[c]				
St. Louis complex				
St. Louis	Mosquitoes (*Culex*)	Birds	Widespread in U.S.	+++
Japanese	Mosquitoes (*Culex*)	Birds	Japan, China, southeast Asia, and India	++++
Murray Valley	Mosquitoes (*Culex*)	Birds	Australia and New Guinea	++
West Nile	Mosquitoes (*Culex*)	Birds	Africa, Middle East, and southern Europe	++
Ilheus	Mosquitoes (*Psorphora*)	Birds	South and Central America	+
Rocio	Mosquitoes (?)	Birds	Brazil	++
Tick-borne complex				
Far eastern tick-borne encephalitis[d]	Ticks (*Ixodes*)	Small mammals and birds	Siberia	+++
Central European tick-borne encephalitis	Ticks (*Ixodes*)	Small mammals and birds	Central Europe	+++
Kyasanur Forest	Ticks (*Haemophysalis*)	Small mammals and birds	India	++
Louping Ill	Ticks (*Ixodes*)	Small mammals and birds	North England, Scotland, and Ireland	+
Powassan	Ticks (*Ixodes*)	Small mammals and birds	Canada and northern U.S.	+

continues

Table 12–2 continued

Family Genus Complex Virus Species	Vector	Animal Reservoir	Geographical Location	Importance in Encephalitis[a]
Negishi	Ticks (?)	Small mammals and birds	Japan	+
Bunyaviridae[e]				
Bunyavirus				
California group				
California encephalitis	Mosquitoes (*Aedes*)	Small mammals	Western U.S.	+
La Crosse	Mosquitoes (*Aedes*)	Squirrels, chipmunks	Midwestern and eastern U.S.	+++
Jamestown Canyon	Mosquitoes (*Culiseta*)	Whitetailed deer	U.S. and Alaska	+
Cache Valley	Mosquitoes (*Culiseta*)	Livestock and large mammals	North and South America	+
Snowshoe hare	Mosquitoes (*Culiseta*)	Snowshoe hare	Canada, Alaska, northern U.S., and Russia	+
Tahnya	Mosquitoes (*Aedes, Culiseta*)	Small mammals	Central Europe	+
Inkoo	Mosquitoes (?)	Reindeer, moose	Finland and Russia	+
Phlebovirus				
Rift Valley	Mosquitoes (*Culex, Aedes*)	Sheep, cattle, camels	East Africa	+
Reoviridae				
Coltivirus				
Colorado tick fever	Ticks (*Dermacentor*)	Small mammals	Rocky Mountain area	+

[a]++++, over 10,000 cases/year; +++, common outbreaks of > 100 cases/year; ++, irregular outbreaks; +, rare occurrences.

[b]Formerly group A arboviruses.

[c]Formerly group B arboviruses.

[d]Formerly Russian spring–summer encephalitis.

[e]Several other *Bunyaviridae* (Arbia and Toseana viruses of genus *Phlebovirus*; Erve virus of genus *Nairovirus*), and *Reoviridae* (Lipovnik and Tribec viruses of genus *Orbivirus*; Eyach of genus *Coltivirus*) and single tick-borne members of *Bunyaviridae* (Bhyanjavirus) and *Orthomyxoviridae* (Thogotovirus) have been tentatively associated with CNS disease in Europe, Asia, and Africa (Dobler, 1996).

Source: Reprinted with permission from R.T. Johnson, Viral Infections of the Nervous System, 2nd Edition, © 1998, Lippincott Williams & Wilkins.

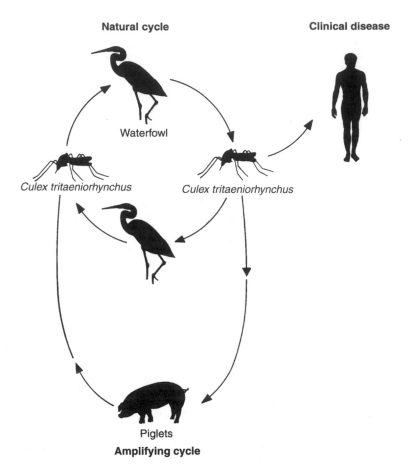

Figure 12–7 The cycle of Japanese encephalitis virus. The natural cycle is between water birds and mosquitoes, predominantly *Culex tritaeniorhynchus*. Amplification occurs in piglets and juvenile water buffalo, but older buffalo are blocking hosts. Humans are dead-end hosts. *Source:* Reprinted with permission from R.T. Johnson, *Viral Infections of the Nervous System*, 2nd Edition, p. 119, © 1998, Lippincott Williams & Wilkins.

some countries in Asia, especially Japan, Korea, and Thailand.[78] This vaccine has significantly decreased the incidence of encephalitis in these countries.

In the United States, the most widespread arboviral encephalitis is caused by SLE virus (see Chapter 2). This virus is also spread by culicine mosquitoes, primarily *Culex tarsalis*, and the natural cycle is between mosquitoes and wild birds. The SLE virus can replicate in mosquitoes at cooler temperatures, so the infection occurs even at northern latitudes.

In 1960, the La Crosse virus, a member of the California group of bunyaviruses, was first recovered from a child with fatal encephalitis in Wisconsin.[79] Since that time, the virus has been identified in states throughout the Midwestern and Eastern United States (Figure 12–8). The natural cycle of La Crosse virus involves transmission between *Aedes triseriatus* mosquitoes and small mammals, especially chipmunks and tree squirrels (Figure 12–9). The mosquito has a limited flight range and lives in tree holes in wooded areas. Persons living in suburban areas

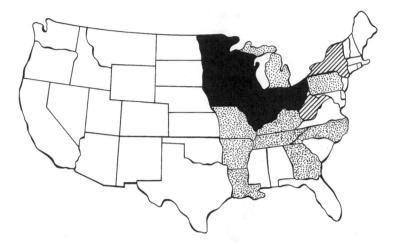

Figure 12–8 The geographic distribution of California encephalitis due to the La Crosse strain of virus. The states that reported more than 100 cases between 1964 and 1991 are *heavily shaded*, the *lined* states reported 50 to 99 cases, the *stippled* states reported 5 to 49 cases, and the *clear* states reported 4 or fewer cases. *Source:* Data from the Centers for Disease Control and Prevention.

with trees on or near their property are at highest risk of infection. A prevention strategy is to fill tree holes with concrete, tar, or other filler to eliminate breeding areas for vector mosquitoes and to dispose of used containers that could serve as "artificial tree holes."

La Crosse virus and other related viruses can be maintained in nature by transovarial transmission by an infected female mosquito. Virus survival over winter by transovarial transmission has allowed some arboviruses in the *Bunyavirus* family to become endemic in far northern latitudes. For example, the Snowshoe hare virus lives in subarctic areas that have very short summers in which mosquitoes can hatch and develop. Unless the eggs were infected when they hatched, it might not be possible for mosquitoes to acquire infection from Snowshoe hares at a rate sufficient to maintain the endemic cycle from year to year.

West Nile virus was introduced into the New York/New Jersey area in the summer of 1999. It is likely that this virus will become endemic in the United States. Other arboviruses that are endemic in the United States at present are West-

ern encephalitis (WE), SLE, California and La Crosse viruses, EE virus, and Venezuelan encephalitis (VE) virus. However, the area of endemicity is restricted to rural areas in the United States for WE and to Southern Florida for VE. Eastern encephalitis virus is found in the eastern half of the United States, primarily in the freshwater marshes of the Atlantic and Gulf Coast states. The natural cycle begins with a swamp marsh mosquito, *Culisetta melanura*, that does not bite large birds or mammals. Human infection results when *Aedes* species mosquitoes feed on infected small birds and transmit infection to man. Human infections with EE are rare because of the ecologic habitat and feeding habits of the primary vector mosquito. The possibility that human infections with EE might become more frequent because of the wide distribution of *A. albopictus* in the United States is of concern, because humans infected with this virus have high clinical attack rates and higher acute mortality than has been reported with any other arbovirus. This concern was heightened by the recovery of EE from an *A. albopictus* mosquito in Florida recently.[80]

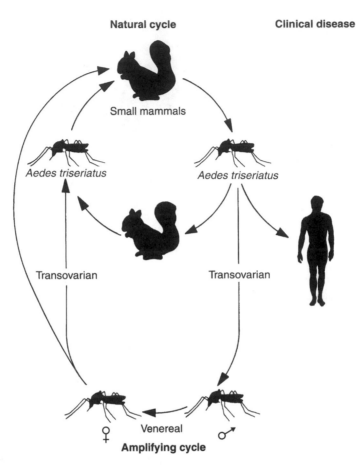

Figure 12–9 The cycle of La Crosse encephalitis virus. The inapparent cycle of the La Crosse virus is between *Aedes triseriatus*, a woodland mosquito, and chipmunks and tree squirrels. The virus is maintained over winters by transovarian transmission and is amplified by venereal transmission between the infected male nonbiting mosquito and the uninfected female, which can in turn transmit either by biting or by transovarian transmission to the next generation. Humans are the only known hosts to develop clinical disease and are dead-end hosts for the virus. *Source:* Reprinted with permission from R.T. Johnson, *Viral Infections of the Nervous System*, 2nd Ed., p. 123, © 1998, Lippincott Williams & Wilkins.

Cholera

Cholera has re-emerged as an epidemic disease in the 1990s. In 1991, cholera occurred in Latin America after an absence of over 100 years.[81] Within 2 years, cholera spread from Peru to Mexico. In 1992, a new epidemic strain, *Vibrio cholerae* 0139, appeared for the first time in India and Bangladesh.[82] There is lack of cross-immunity between classic or El Tor *V. cholerae*

01 strains and the newly recognized *V. cholerae* 0139 strain. Therefore, major outbreaks of cholera, estimated at more than 200,000 cases, occurred in India, Bangladesh, and several other countries in Southeast Asia. Travel-associated, imported cases were reported in the United States, Europe, and Japan.[81]

In addition, a massive outbreak of El Tor cholera occurred among Rwandan refugees in Goma, Zaire, during the war in Rwanda, resulting in

20,000 cases and 12,000 deaths in July 1994.[83] This outbreak, once again, demonstrated the potential for cholera to cause severe mortality in a situation of extreme civil disruption. In contrast, the cholera mortality was under 1% in Latin American countries, where good diagnostic and medical services and oral dehydration therapy were readily available. These cholera epidemics demonstrate the potential for modern societies to disseminate a potent epidemic pathogen globally. Also, *Shigella* dysentery spread in epidemic fashion in the refugee camps in Zaire.

One theory of how cholera was introduced into Latin America reported that a ship from the Orient released contaminated bilge water into a Peruvian harbor, which contaminated local shell fish and established an epidemic focus.[84] However, more recently, Colwell has reported studies indicating that the effects of global warming associated with recent El Niño conditions may have been critical in the resurgence of cholera.[37] These intriguing studies indicate that warmer sea water temperatures could expand the environmental reservoir of the organism. Warming of sea water temperatures promotes a phytoplankton expansion, followed by a zooplankton bloom. These zooplankton copepods can carry *V. cholerae* on their surfaces and in their guts in high concentration, up to 10^4 organisms per copepod. The warming of sea water temperatures and spread of the environmental reservoir of *V. cholerae* by copepods could explain the rapid widespread dissemination of cholera along coastal areas of Latin America soon after its reintroduction.[37] Because of the rapid spread of cholera recently among coastal populations of South America, copepods may have played a major role in the emergence of cholera in this area.

Escherichia coli O157:H7

E. coli O157:H7 is a recently emerged pathogen that was first incriminated as causing infections in humans in 1982.[85] This organism is now recognized as a major cause of large-scale epidemics and sporadic cases of gastrointestinal illness in North America, Europe, and Japan.[86–88]

Infections with this organism are estimated to cause about 20,000 illnesses and 250 deaths each year in the United States.[86] In contrast, infections with the organism have not been recognized to be a significant problem in most developing countries. Infections with *E. coli* O157:H7 produce a clinically distinct illness with bloody diarrhea and, in some patients, hemolysis and acute renal failure, called the *hemolytic-uremia syndrome*. This organism evolved from the ordinary intestinal flora of cattle. It emerged as a human pathogen after acquiring genetic material that would allow increased intestinal adherence, a large plasmid coding for a hemolysin, and a gene coding for severe cytotoxicity, the Shiga toxin. Also, the organism acquired the ability to withstand an acid environment.[89] This trait allowed the organism to survive the normally protective action of stomach acid and to survive in the environment in the presence of acid rain. Due to the increased resistance to acid, the infectious dose is very small, e.g., 50 to 100 organisms.

These genetic changes in the organism, acid stability, and the ability to produce the potent Shiga toxin allowed this organism to emerge as a new "super-bug." The organism is usually not pathogenic to cattle, which carry the organism in their intestinal tract without having symptoms. It has been isolated from 1% to 10% of healthy cattle and from sheep in the United States.[89] The organism can be transmitted by food, raw milk, water, and by direct person-to-person spread. Large outbreaks have occurred in the United States from improperly cooked hamburgers. These outbreaks occurred because beef was commonly contaminated with these organisms, acquired during the slaughtering process, and thorough cooking was required to disinfect the food from an organism that is highly pathogenic with small numbers of organisms. Rare or incompletely cooked hamburgers could contain an infectious inoculum of *E. coli* O157:H7 in the center of the sandwich. The modern food processing and distribution networks, i.e., corporate agribusiness, promote the cross-contamination of cattle in the slaughtering process and disseminate meat widely. Now the only defense is thorough cooking of the meat. The cultural preference for rare beef, translated into poorly cooked hamburger, increased the risk of exposure. The organism has also been transmitted by other foods, including vegetables such as alfalfa sprouts that have been contaminated with cow manure used as fertilizer or with fruit juices, such as apple cider. Often, apples used to produce cider may be harvested from the fruit that has fallen from the tree. Contamination with a small inoculum of organisms on the surface of the apples from cow manure on the ground can survive the acid environments of apple juice and the stomach. This has led to several outbreaks and recommendations are that apple juice be pasteurized to avoid this risk.[90]

Water-Borne Parasitic and Viral Infections

Cryptosporidium *Species*

The resurgence of cholera has involved primarily populations in developing countries in Asia, Latin American, and Africa. However, it has been appreciated recently that water-borne infections from newly recognized parasitic agents are a significant and increasing problem in the United States. The risk of water-borne infections was appreciated when a massive outbreak of diarrhea occurred in the spring of 1993 in Milwaukee.[91] This outbreak involved an estimated 403,000 people who received water from one of two municipal water treatment plants in the city where the water had been treated with chlorination and filtration. Between March 23 and April 9, the water treated at the city's southern treatment plant had shown marked increases in turbidity. In early April, the Wisconsin Department of Health received reports of large numbers of persons who were experiencing diarrhea that resulted in widespread absenteeism among hospital employees, students, and school teachers. At this time, little information was available about the organism involved in the outbreak. However, two laboratories identified *Cryptosporidium* oocysts in stool samples from a number of adults with typical illnesses. A sur-

vey of laboratories in the area showed no reported increased isolation of *Salmonella, Shigella, Campylobacter, E. coli* O157:H7, or other common bacterial causes of diarrhea. The epidemiologists investigating this outbreak were able subsequently to isolate *Cryptosporidium parvum* from ice that had been frozen during the period of the contamination of the water supply. A subsequent analysis of the data from the Milwaukee water system and clinical occurrences of diarrhea in the population suggests that endemic contamination of the water supply with *C. parvum* oocysts may have occurred prior to the large outbreak in April 1993.[92] This large outbreak was followed by prospective surveillance of several municipal water supplies in the United States to evaluate the risks of water-borne cryptrosporidiosis. These studies have shown that contamination of domestic water supplies with *C. parvum* oocysts is not uncommon.[93–95] Several large municipal water supplies in the United States do not filter the water to remove *C. parvum* oocysts.[94] Although chlorination of municipal water supplies is routinely practiced by most municipal water systems in the United States, *C. parvum* oocysts are resistant to chlorination. The potential for water-borne disease is increased by the fact that the infectious dose necessary to cause human disease is quite low, probably in the range of 10 to 100 oocysts per liter of water.[92,93] Furthermore, clinical laboratories do not routinely screen stool samples from diarrhea patients for *C. parvum* unless the clinician requests this evaluation. The detection of *C. parvum* in stools requires staining the stool with an acid fast stain and examining the sample microscopically for *C. parvum* oocysts. Consequently, in the Milwaukee epidemic, which involved an estimated 403,000 persons, only about 12 cases were confirmed in the laboratory.[91] This has led epidemiologists to question whether water-borne outbreaks of cryptosporidiosis might be much more common than appreciated.[92–95]

Another issue raised by this outbreak is the risk to the subset of the population who are immunosuppressed, such as persons with AIDS, those on chemotherapy, and those with malignancies. Cryptosporidia is known to be a significant pathogen in AIDS patients. The infection is not effectively treatable in this population.[93] Contamination of a municipal water supply, even at a fairly low level, could cause significant morbidity and even mortality at the population level. Other parasitic pathogens that are resistant to chlorine and could cause disease in humans with exposure to a few organisms include *Microsporidia* species, *Cyclospora*, and *Giardia lamblia*.[95] Studies are beginning to estimate the risk of water-borne infections from these pathogens in the United States and to evaluate various strategies to prevent these infections.

Cyclosporiasis

Another parasitic organism that has emerged recently as an important human pathogen in the United States is *Cyclospora cayetanensis*. Before 1996, most documented cases of cyclosporiasis in North America occurred in travelers returning from overseas, and only three small U.S. outbreaks had been reported.[96] However, in 1998, several health departments reported cases of cyclosporiasis to the Centers for Disease Control and Prevention (CDC). Ultimately, 978 laboratory-confirmed cases occurring in the spring and summer of 1996 were reported to the CDC and the Canadian Health Department. A total of 1,465 cases was eventually reported. Extensive investigation of multiple outbreaks in the United States and Canada eventually implicated raspberries imported from Guatemala as the source of these outbreaks.[29] Raspberries were first cultivated in Guatemala as a commercial crop in 1987. They were first exported in 1988, and exports have markedly increased in the mid-1990s. Another outbreak of cyclosporiasis related to Guatemalan raspberries occurred in 1997 (Figure 12–10).[30] Although the exact mode of contamination of the raspberries is unclear, it is likely that rinsing of the implicated raspberries with contaminated water prior to their export had occurred. These outbreaks emphasize the potential infection problems associated with importation of a food product that is eaten uncooked and is not easily monitored or disin-

fected before it is consumed. With the expansion of international commerce and importation of foods from many countries, this type of problem is certain to become even more frequent in the future.

Hantaviruses

A new viral infection first came to the attention of Western medicine during the Korean War in 1951, when U.S. troops stationed in Korea developed a new disease that was subsequently named *Korean hemorrhagic fever*. The disease was manifested by a febrile course with influenza-like symptoms. In about a third of the cases, hemorrhagic symptoms and hypertension, followed by severe renal failure, occurred. Over 3,000 troops were infected, and the mortality rate was about 5%.[97] The etiologic agent was not identified until 1976, after Lee et al., working in Seoul, Korea, identified the etiologic agent as a virus when it was isolated in vero cell cultures.[98] The virus was named Hantaan virus after the Hantaan River, which transects the epidemic area at the demilitarized zone separating North and South Korea. The virus was isolated from the lungs of the striped field mouse, *Apodermus agrarius*. This common animal is now recognized as the major rodent host of the Hantaan virus in rural Korea. These rodents commonly acquire the infection early in life and continuously excrete the virus in their urine for the rest of their lives. Persons who may be exposed to infected urine, such as a soldier in a foxhole, are at risk of infection. There was no evidence of person-to-person spread of infection or of water- or food-borne transmission of Hantaan virus in Korea.

Subsequently, another rodent-associated virus with some similarities to Hantaan virus was isolated from urban rats (*Rattus norwegicus* and *Rattus rattus*). Isolated cases of hemorrhagic fever were identified in urban residents and in laboratory workers who were exposed to these rats; the virus was named *Seoul virus*. It has now spread worldwide with infected rodents as passengers on commercial ships. This virus has been identified in Baltimore and has been shown

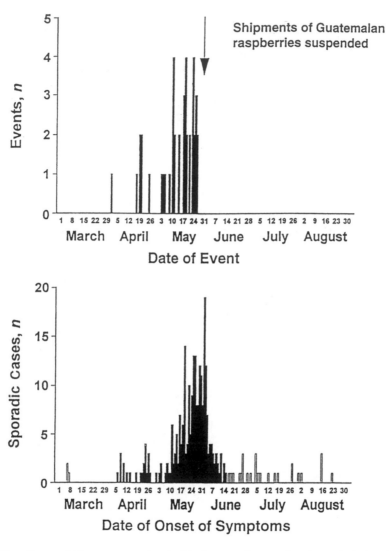

Figure 12–10 Top. Dates of 41 events associated with clusters of cases of cyclosporiasis (*n* = 762 cases) in the United States and Canada in April and May 1997. For multiday events, the date of the first day of the event is shown. The last shipment of Guatemalan raspberries in the spring of 1997 was on 28 May. **Bottom**. Dates of symptom onset for laboratory-confirmed sporadic cases of cyclosporiasis in the United States and Canada in 1997. The white bars represent 31 case-patients who became ill during the period from March through August but not during the outbreak period of April through 15 June. The black bars represent 250 case-patients whose cases were classified as having occurred during the outbreak period. The median date of symptom onset for the 250 case-patients was 26 May (range, 6 April to 15 June). Only 22 persons (8.8%) became ill in April, and most (225 [90.0%]) became ill by 4 June. The date selected as the last date of the outbreak period was 15 June because Guatemalan raspberries exported in late May could still have been available for consumption in early June and because infected persons would have become symptomatic an average of 1 week after exposure. Not all of the sporadic cases of cyclosporiasis were necessarily due to consumption of raspberries. *Source:* Reprinted with permission from B.L. Herwaldt, M.J. Beach, and the Cyclospora Working Group, The Return of Cyclospora in 1997: Another Outbreak of Cyclosporiasis in North America Associated with Imported Raspberries, *Annals of Internal Medicine*, Vol. 130, No. 3, Figure 1, pp. 210–220, © 1999, American College of Physicians.

in a preliminary case-control study to have an association with hypertension and chronic renal disease[99]; however, these data are awaiting further confirmation.

Another related virus, Puumala virus, was isolated from patients in Sweden and voles in Finland. This virus caused a syndrome, termed *Nephropathica epidemica*, which is an acute febrile disease with renal involvement.[100] Subsequently, the World Health Organization grouped the syndromes caused by these three related viruses together under the rubric *hemorrhagic fever with renal syndrome* (HFRS).

In May 1993 an apparently new disease was recognized among previously healthy young native Americans and Caucasians in New Mexico. This new disease consisted of an abrupt onset of fever, myalgia, headache, and cough, followed by the rapid development of acute pulmonary

edema and acute respiratory distress syndrome. The overall mortality in this outbreak was about 5%.[101] Eventually, 100 cases occurred among persons living in New Mexico, Arizona, and Colorado (Figure 12–11). Most patients were previously healthy young adults; the median age was 32 years, 33% were Native Americans, and 66% were Caucasians.[102] Pathologically, the disease was characterized by interstitial pneumonitis with a mononuclear cell infiltrate and focal hyaline membranes. Testing of acute and convalescent sera from these patients demonstrated seroreactivity to various hantaviruses, with the strongest reaction to Puumala virus. This finding was unexpected because, at that time, hantaviruses had not been seen in the United States, and the clinical syndrome associated with infection with other hantaviruses had included renal disease, rather than pulmonary failure. Follow-

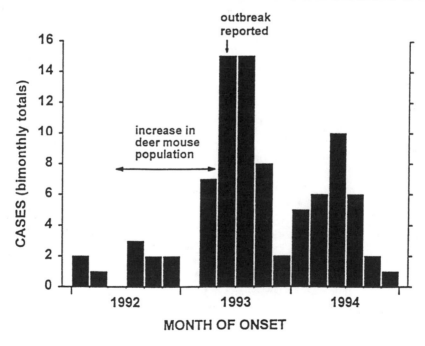

Figure 12–11 Cases of hantavirus pulmonary syndrome by month of onset, United States, 1992–1994, omitting 16 cases with onsets prior to 1992. *Source:* Reprinted with permission from N. Nathanson and S. Nichol, Korean and Hemorrhagic Fever and Hanta Virus Pulmonary Syndrome: Two Examples of Emerging Pathoviral Diseases, in *Emerging Infections*, p. 370, R.M. Krause, ed., © 1998.

ing the serologic evidence, reverse transcriptase PCR studies of hantaviruses revealed a DNA sequence similar but 30% different from Prospect Hill virus (another hantavirus).[103] The virus was eventually grown in tissue culture, using Vero E-6 cells and named Sin Nombre virus.

The rodent reservoir was eventually identified as the deer mouse, *Peromyscus maniculatus*, which had expanded 10-fold because of extraordinary climatic conditions with large amounts of precipitation in the preceding winter and spring, which provided an abundant supply of pinon nuts used as food by the mice.[104] Satellite photos of vegetation accurately identified hot spots where cases occurred and where high concentrations of deer mice were located. Apparently, this "new" infectious disease arose because of a dramatic expansion of the deer mouse population, often chronically infected with Sin Nombre virus, and invasion into the homes in the area, allowing human contact with infected aerosolized urine. Interestingly, there was no evidence of person-to-person transmission of the agent among household or hospital contacts. Population-based serologic surveys found very few asymptomatic cases. Nearly all infected cases were ill and had classic hantavirus pulmonary syndrome.

Ebola Virus

The virus that probably has raised the greatest fear and generated the most publicity about the potential of new emerging infectious agents to endanger human populations is Ebola virus, a virus in the *Filoviridae* family (Table 12–3). The first recognition of filoviruses was in 1967, when an epidemic of 31 cases and 7 deaths from viral hemorrhagic fever occurred in Marburg, Germany, among persons having contact with vervet or African green monkeys or their tissues that had been imported from Uganda.[105,106] The virus, named *Marburg virus*, was cultivated from the blood of sick humans who had become ill after exposure to the monkeys. The very unusual morphology of the Marburg virus and the

Table 12–3 Filovirus Hemorrhagic Fever Outbreaks in Humans

Virus	Contact	Location
Marburg virus	Imported African green monkeys (23% mortality)	Marburg, Germany 1967
Ebola, Zaire strain (EBO-2)	Unknown origin, close contact, and needles, 318 cases (88% mortality)	Zaire 1976
Ebola, Sudan strain (EBO-5)	Unknown origin, nosocomial transmission, 284 cases (53% mortality)	Sudan 1976 & 1979
Ebola, Reston strain (EBO-R)	Infected monkeys imported from Philippines, 4 asymptomatic human cases	Reston, Virginia, USA 1989
Ebola, Zaire strain	Contacts with chimpanzees, monkeys, other primates, and nosocomial spread, multiple outbreaks	Gabon, Zaire, Cote d'Ivore 1994–1999. Largest in Kikwit, Zaire, 317 cases (78% mortality)

potential for human-to-human transmission of this severe infection underscored the fact that this was a serious threat to human health.

In 1976, two outbreaks of infection with Ebola virus occurred in Zaire and the Sudan; together, there were more than 550 cases and 430 deaths.[107–109] In the next 20 years, an additional 18 outbreaks of Ebola virus infections in humans have been recognized.[110] Although most of these human epidemics have been initiated by contact with monkeys or other nonhuman primates, it is felt to be unlikely that monkeys are the primary reservoir for Ebola virus, because they also have experienced high mortality from infection.[110] The disease is characterized by an abrupt onset with fever, diarrhea, dysphagia, severe weakness and hemorrhagic phenomena, and, in most outbreaks, high mortality.[111] In Africa, where most of these epidemics have occurred, human-to-human transmission has been common. In the large outbreak in 1995 in Kikwit, Zaire (now the Congo), health care workers and relatives of cases acquired the disease and often succumbed.[112] Among the first 283 cases, 90 (32%) occurred in health care workers, and 28 (16%) of 173 members in the first 27 households developed disease. However, the institution of routine barrier precautions (including gowns and gloves) and the discontinuation of the ritual of bathing and cleaning of the corpse after death limited contact with infectious secretions and appeared to control further transmission.

The concept that good barrier nursing practices are adequate to control nosocomial transmission of Ebola is supported by the experience in Gabon in 1996, where 32 patients were cared for without any infections in house staff or nurses caring for the patients. A survey of family members of 27 patients who developed Ebola infection in Kikwit found a secondary attack rate of 16%; however, only those household members who had direct contact with body fluids of ill patients developed infection.[113]

Another outbreak of Ebola virus infection occurred in a monkey colony in Reston, Virginia. In this outbreak, the infected cynomolgus monkeys (*M. fascicularis*) had been imported from the Philippines, an area not known to be endemic for Ebola or other filoviruses. The monkeys were co-infected with another virus, Simian hemorrhagic fever (SMF) virus. In this outbreak, in contrast with previous outbreaks of Ebola virus, there was some evidence of aerosol transmission among the monkeys.[35,114,115] Also, four laboratory workers who had used barrier precautions in handling the monkeys developed serologic evidence of infection but remained asymptomatic.[35,114] These outbreaks underscore the potential importance of differences between strains of Ebola virus in their infectivity and pathogenicity; four subtypes of Ebola virus have been identified to date.[110]

One apparent feature of persons who survive Ebola virus infections is that they appear not to develop high titers of neutralizing antibodies.[110] Therefore, an immune serum has not been developed for the therapy of persons with acute infections. A chronic carrier state of Ebola virus has not been identified in any animal species.[110] The natural interepidemic reservoir of Ebola virus has not been defined. The genetic structures of Ebola isolates from the various outbreaks have considerable diversity, suggesting that they are not directly linked with one another, for example, through continued human-to-human transmission.[116]

Arenaviruses

The arenaviruses are a group of negative-stranded, RNA viruses that are important causes of epidemic infections in tropical areas of Africa and South America. The prototype arenavirus, lymphocytic choriomeningitis virus (LCM), was discovered in 1933 and causes benign aseptic meningitis in humans in temperate areas of North America, as well as the tropics (Table 12–4). Junin virus was recovered from patients with Argentine hemorrhagic fever (AHF) in 1958, and Machupo virus, the cause of Bolivia hemorrhagic fever (BHF) was discovered in 1960. Another disease, Venezuela hemorrhagic fever (VHF), was initially isolated in 1964.[117] Recently, VHF has been recognized as a distinct

Table 12–4 Ecologic Features of Arenaviruses Pathogenic for Humans

Virus	Natural Host	Geographic Distribution	Disease
Lymphocytic choriomeningitis virus	*Mus musculus* (house mouse)	Europe, America	Aseptic meningitis
Junin virus	*Calomys musculinus*	Argentina	Argentine hemorrhagic fever
Machupo virus	*Calomys callosus*	Bolivia	Bolivia hemorrhagic fever
Guanarito virus	*Sigmodon alstoni*	Venezuela	Venezuela hemorrhagic fever
Lassa virus	*Mastomys natalensis*	West Africa	Lassa hemorrhagic fever

human disease in the largely agricultural region of Guanarito and is caused by an arenavirus carried by rodents.[118] The extent of the public health problem from infections with the Guanarito virus is not clear.

In 1969, Lassa fever virus was isolated from a missionary nurse stationed in rural northeastern Nigeria. Following her admission to the hospital, two additional cases developed in nurses who were caring for her, and two of the three original cases died.[119] In one outbreak, 13 of 17 health care workers contracted the disease and died.[119] Subsequently, outbreaks occurred in Nigeria, Liberia, and Sierra Leone, with mortality of 20% to 60% of those infected.[119] Infections have occurred among persons working with this virus in a laboratory in the United States.[120] There was great concern after Lassa fever was first described that this virus might be the "Andromeda strain" that would spread rapidly to all human contacts, with high mortality. However, subsequent investigation suggests that spread is preventable with ordinary respiratory precautions. Various rodent species are the reservoir for the arenaviruses. These include *Mus musculus* (the house mouse) for LCM, *Mastomys* species for Lassa fever, and *Calomys* species for AHF, BHF, and VHF.

These diseases have emerged because of man-made changes in the environment that favor higher density of virus-infected rodents that have close contact with humans. Junin virus emerged as an important human pathogen in Argentina when the pampas grassland that had been a grazing area for cattle was converted into cultivated farm land for the production of maize. This led to a major expansion of population of a mouse, *Calomys musculinus*, that fed on the grain. Because these mice were frequently chronically infected with Junin virus, which they shed in their urine, the harvesting of the maize allowed humans to come into contact with the virus.

In Bolivia, an epidemic of BHF occurred in 1960, caused by a related virus, Machupo virus, when an area in eastern Bolivia was converted from cattle-raising to subsistence agriculture. This ecologic change provided a suitable environment for the expansion of the population of a small mouse, *Calomys callosus*. This mouse invaded the homes and gardens of the local inhabitants and spread the virus that caused BHF. However, unlike AHF, this epidemic is now under control, due in part to the greater pathogenicity of the virus for the carrier mouse and the more limited contact of the population with the reservoir host.[117]

Zoonotic Paramyxovirus Infections

Several epidemics of human paramyxovirus infection have occurred in recent years. These epidemics have occurred in Australia and Asia from reservoirs in domestic animals.

Hendra Virus Epidemic in Australia

In September 1994, an outbreak of respiratory disease affected 18 horses, their trainer, and a stable hand in Queensland, Australia. Fourteen horses and one human died. A novel virus was isolated from the horses and humans, and originally was named *equine morbilivirus*.[121] One of the persons who had aseptic meningitis during the original outbreak recovered but became ill with encephalitis and died 13 months later.[122] During this illness, he developed seizures with distinctive changes on magnetic resonance imaging and histologic changes in the cerebral cortex. PCR of spinal fluid, brain, and serum yielded sequences identical to those obtained during the original outbreak. Subsequently, a second, unrelated outbreak was identified in Queensland, in which two horses died and one human became infected.[123] Laboratory studies have suggested that fruit bats (*Pteropus* species) in Australia and Papua, New Guinea, may be infected and serve as the natural reservoir for this newly recognized virus, which has been renamed *Hendra virus*.[124]

Nipah Virus

Between February and April 1999, a severe outbreak of viral encephalitis occurred in the Bakit Pelandok area of peninsular Malaysia that affected more than 200 individuals and a large number of pigs.[125] The outbreak was initially thought to be JE because it involved people in close contact with pigs, a known reservoir of JE virus. However, several features of this outbreak differed from the usual clinical and epidemiologic characteristics of JE. Namely, the outbreak involved only men who were in direct contact with pigs. The illness had a very high attack rate in this population. Many of the pigs also were

sick, and most of the human cases had been immunized against JE. Among the 91 patients admitted to the University of Malaya Medical Center in Kuala Lumpur, there were 28 deaths.[125] A virus was isolated from the cerebrospinal fluid (CSF) of several patients that stained positively with antibodies against Hendra virus by indirect immunofluorescence. IgM capture ELISA showed that several patients had IgM antibodies in CSF against Hendra virus antigens. There was no clinical evidence of pulmonary involvement; however, inclusion bodies of probable viral origin were present in neurons. Electron microscopy revealed viruslike structures resembling paramyxoviruses, and nucleotide sequencing indicated that the virus was related but not identical to Hendra virus.[126] All cases had been working on pig farms and had direct contact with ill pigs. Subsequently, 11 cases were reported from Singapore among workers on pig farms. These outbreaks were controlled by culling all of the pigs from farms with infected animals.

Legionnaires' Disease

An outbreak of a new infectious disease was recognized in July 1976 that affected 182 persons in Philadelphia.[127] Most had attended the American Legion Convention in Philadelphia that was held July 21–24 and had stayed at one hotel. However, 39 persons had not actually stayed at the hotel but had exposure to the air emanating from the hotel. No evidence of human-to-human transmission was found during this outbreak. Laboratory investigation eventually isolated gram-negative bacteria by inoculating hamsters with infectious material. The organism would not grow in standard media, such as blood agar, thioglycollate broth, or tryptocase soy agar. This organism was named *Legionella pneumophila*.[128] Attack rates of illness were higher in persons staying at the hotel who had underlying illnesses or were cigarette smokers. Attack rates were 4.0% among those attending the convention, and mortality was 15.9% among those who were ill.

Another outbreak of an airborne infection had occurred 8 years previously in a county health department in Pontiac, Michigan, that affected 95 of 100 persons employed in the health department and numerous visitors, including the epidemiologists from CDC who were sent to investigate the outbreak.[129] This illness, which was called *Pontiac fever*, was characterized by self-limited symptoms of fever, chills, headache, and myalgia, lasting 2 to 5 days. In contrast to the Legionnaires' disease outbreak, none of those involved in the Pontiac fever outbreak developed pneumonia.

Subsequent to the identification of *Legionella pneumophila*, methods have been developed to diagnose infections with this bacteria and related agents. The organism can be grown on charcoal yeast extract agar, and serologic methods are also available for diagnosis. A number of outbreaks have been identified that usually involved exposure to aerosols generated by cooling towers, mist machines, shower heads, and other aerosols.[130–133] Over 30 different species of *Legionella* have been identified and 19 have been found to infect humans. The organisms have been found to replicate in freshwater amoeba and protozoa.[133,134] They grow at temperatures of 40° to 50°C and survive in chlorinated water. However, they can be eliminated by hyperchlorination or heating water to higher temperatures.[134–136] Recent studies have shown that *Legionella* strains are a common cause of endemic pneumonia, both in the community and in health care settings.

Influenza Viruses

Perhaps the most important emerging virus infection of humans is influenza. This highly contagious acute respiratory illness has caused epidemics in humans since ancient times. One influenza epidemic was recorded by Hippocrates in 412 B.C., and numerous epidemics were described in the Middle Ages.[137] Epidemics of influenza that occurred between A.D. 1500 and 1800 were reviewed by Noble.[138] He noted several features of these epidemics:

- Epidemics were sudden in onset and occurred frequently but at irregular intervals.
- Epidemics varied in severity but usually caused mortality, primarily in older persons.
- Some epidemics spread worldwide from their origins in Russia or China.

Influenza is the principle infectious disease that has been severe enough to cause major increases in mortality in the total population of the developed countries of the United States and Europe in the twentieth century, prior to the advent of the epidemic of HIV/AIDS in the early 1980s. The most severe epidemic of the twentieth century was the "Spanish Influenza" pandemic of 1918–1919. An estimated 20 to 40 million persons died in this pandemic. This epidemic was believed to be caused by a new H1/N1 swine influenza virus, to which none of the human population was immune.

A limited epidemic in humans of a totally new strain of influenza, due to an H5/N1 influenza virus, occurred in Hong Kong in the winter of 1997. Infections with this virus were fatal in a high proportion (about 30%) of the humans that were infected and caused disseminated viremia in infected persons.[139] The virus was epidemic in chickens in Hong Kong at the time. However, there was no evidence of person-to-person transmission of this new human virus; all human cases had direct contact with chickens and probably acquired their infection as a zoonotic infection. Public health authorities slaughtered a large number of infected chickens to prevent further chicken-to-human transmission of this H5/N1 virus and control this epidemic. This recent epidemic raises perplexing questions about the epidemic potential of new influenza viruses.

Staphylococcal Toxic Shock Syndrome

Infections with *Staphylococcus aureus*, a gram-positive organism, are quite common. The organism is a well-known cause of food poisoning, abscesses, pneumonia, endocarditis, and the scalded skin syndrome in humans, and causes mastitis and other infections in cattle and sheep. However, in 1978, Todd et al. reported an outbreak of a new staphylococcal disease, a severe systemic illness in young children, called *toxic shock syndrome* (TSS).[140] The illness was characterized by high fever, hypotension or shock, a generalized erythematous rash that progresses to desquamation, and multiorgan system dysfunction. Toxin-producing strains of *S. aureus* were recovered from various sites in these children with TSS.

Two years later, TSS cases suddenly appeared, first in Wisconsin and Minnesota, then nationwide, among young adult women during their menstrual period.[141,142] The disease was serious and caused substantial mortality; however, recovery was complete among survivors. Recurrences were common during a subsequent menses unless the offending *S. aureus* vaginal infection was effectively treated with antibiotics. Eventually, 941 cases were reported from every state in the United States; however, 247 (26%) of the cases occurred in women in Minnesota and Wisconsin.[143]

The pathogenesis of TSS involved the use of "super-absorbent" tampons made of a blend of synthetic materials, including poly-acrylate fibers, carboxymethyl cellulose, high-absorbency rayon-cellulose, and polyester foam. Previously, tampons had been made of rayon or a blend of rayon and cotton. These "super tampons" were much more absorbent than the traditional tampons marketed previously and could be left in place for longer periods. However, they tended to cause abrasions of the vaginal mucosa, and the blood-soaked tampons were a very good culture medium for the proliferation of *S. aureus*, which produced a chromosomally encoded toxin, designated *toxic shock syndrome toxin-1* (TSST-1). Studies have shown that over 90% of *S. aureus* strains recovered from vaginal cultures of women with TSS synthesized TSST-1, whereas the toxin is found much less frequently in other *S. aureus* isolates.[144] The TSST-1 is a member of the class of structurally related molecules called *superantigens*. TSST-1 and other superantigens bind to the major histocompati-

bility complex (MHC) class II molecules of antigen-presenting cells. This results in the stimulation of production of a number of cytokines, including several interleukins, tumor necrosis factors (TNFs) alpha, beta, and interferon gamma, leading to multiple systemic symptoms.

Importantly, the public health response in removing these highly absorbent tampons from the market as soon as they were implicated in TSS effectively controlled this devastating epidemic.[145] However, occasional sporadic cases that were not related to tampon use continued to be reported (Figure 12–12).

Streptococcal Infections

Infections from group A streptococci in the nineteenth century often were quite severe, even fatal. However, the mortality from scarlet fever, a common manifestation of toxigenic group A streptococcal infections, declined dramatically in the United States, beginning in the early twentieth century. During World War II, acute rheumatic fever, a chronic complication of group A streptococcal infections, was quite common, especially among troops stationed in crowded military barracks.[146] During this time, extensive epidemiologic studies were done to define the risk factors associated with clinical or subclinical infection with group A streptococci and subsequent acute rheumatic fever.[146]

Antibiotic treatment regimens were evaluated in carefully controlled clinical trials to develop regimens that eradicated pathogenic group A streptococci from the pharynx and prevented rheumatic fever.[147,148] This was followed by a dramatic decrease in the incidence of severe streptococcal infections, acute rheumatic fever (ARF), and poststreptococcal glomerulonephritis between the 1960s and early 1980s. Although group A streptococci were still commonly cultured from the throat in persons with and without pharyngitis, severe inflammation was uncommon, and the risk of subsequent rheumatic fever seemed to be very low. Most experts believe that the attenuated severity of acute streptococcal infections and decrease in the incidence of acute

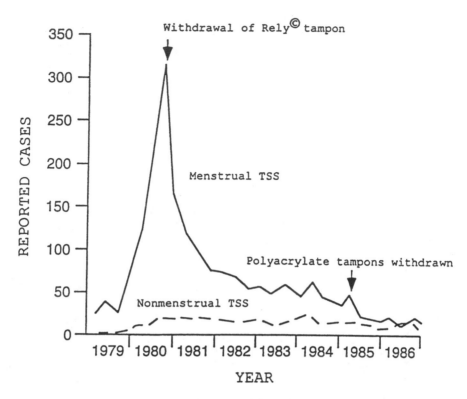

Figure 12–12 Number of reported cases of toxic shock syndrome in the United States, by year (1979–1986), based on passive surveillance. *Source:* Reprinted with permission from C.V. Broome, Epidemiology of Toxic Shock Syndrome in the United States: Overview, *Review of Infectious Disease*, Vol. 11, Suppl. 1, p. S17, © 1989, University of Chicago Press.

rheumatic fever during this period was not due to the widespread use of therapeutic antibiotics. Instead, the change in virulence was believed to be due to poorly understood changes in the epidemiology, the infectivity, or the virulence factors of streptococci causing human infections.

Suddenly, in 1985, a substantial increase in the number of cases of ARF occurred in Salt Lake City and surrounding areas; 136 cases of ARF were reported from persons living in this area in 1985 and 1986.[149] Most of the patients had typical full-blown rheumatic fever, and most were middle- or upper-class suburban or urban residents. Poor, lower-class populations from the inner cities were overrepresented in rheumatic fever patients earlier in the century.

Subsequently, Stevens and colleagues described 20 patients from the Rocky Mountain region (Utah, Idaho, Montana, and Nevada) with an unusually severe form of systemic group A streptococcal infection.[150] These patients had extensive local tissue destruction and signs and symptoms of severe systemic toxicity. Nineteen of these patients had shock, 80% had renal impairment, many had an acute respiratory distress syndrome, and six died. In some patients, necrotizing fasciitis (soft tissue and muscle necrosis) was a prominent feature. The group A streptococci that were isolated from these patients produced an exotoxin that was similar to the TSS toxin (TSST-1) produced by *S. aureus* strains isolated from patients with the staphylococcal

TSS. Subsequently, a dramatic increase in the number of patients with streptococcal TSS and necrotizing fasciitis occurred throughout the United States, Canada, several European countries, Australia, and New Zealand.[151] The organisms associated with necrotizing fasciitis were termed *flesh-eating bacteria* by the lay press.

Investigation of this resurgence of severe streptococcal disease in the past 15 years has found that most strains contain M-protein types 1 or 3 (over 80 M-protein types of streptococci have been identified). Group A streptococci are often classified on the basis of their M-protein, which is a known virulence factor. Perhaps more important, most of the organisms associated with the TSS or necrotizing fasciitis produce streptococcal exotoxin types A, B, or C. So, for unknown reasons, there appeared to be an emergence of new types of streptococci that commonly infected human populations with increased pathogenicity and virulence during the last decade of the twentieth century. The factors leading to the emergence of these more virulent streptococci are poorly understood, as was the decreased pathogenicity of Group A streptococci in the previous few decades. Possibly, host factors, such as low levels of herd immunity to these more virulent strains or genetic changes in the organisms, may have played a significant role in the emergence of these serious infections.

Transmissible Spongiform Encephalopathies

In the last 30 years, a radically new class of infectious agents, the spongiform encephalopathies, has been recognized as the cause of several diseases of man and animals (Exhibit 12–3). The infectious agents causing these diseases appear to differ from viruses, in that they do not contain nucleic acids but only proteins; they have been labeled *prions*, or *proteinaceous infectious particles* by Stanley Prusiner.[152,153] The spongiform encephalopathies are unique among the infectious diseases, in that they exhibit none of the traditional hallmarks of an infectious disease. The brain tissue of animals with these infections show spongiform changes in the cytoplasm of

Exhibit 12–3 Transmissible Spongiform Encephalopathies of Animals and Humans (Prion Diseases)

A. Animal Diseases
 Scrapie (sheep and goats)
 Transmissible mink encephalopathy
 Wasting disease of deer and elk
 Bovine spongiform encephalopathy*
 Transmissible spongiform encephalopathy
  of captive wild ruminants*
 Feline spongiform encephalopathy*
B. Human Diseases
 Kuru
 Sporadic Creutzfeldt-Jakob disease
 Familial Creutzfeldt-Jakob disease
 Gerstmann-Straussler-Scheinker disease
 Fatal familial insomnia
 New variant Creutzfeldt-Jakob disease*

*These diseases all appear to have a common source.

Source: Reprinted with permission from R.T. Johnson and C.J. Gibbs, Creutzfeldt-Jakob Disease and Selected Transmissible Spongiform Encephalopathies, *New England Journal of Medicine*, Vol. 339, pp. 1994–2004, Copyright © 1998, Massachusetts Medical Society. All rights reserved.

nerve cells without an inflammatory infiltrate; the patient or animal does not have a fever, high white cell count, or a rise in acute phase reactants or cytokines; nor is there a measurable immune response to the infectious agent.[154] Therefore, these diseases originally were felt to be degenerative, rather than infectious, and due to genetic factors, rather than infectious agents.

Scrapie

The disease of sheep called *scrapie* has been known for at least 200 years. It is widespread among sheep in Europe, Asia, and the Americas, and is also seen among goats cohabiting with affected sheep. The Scottish term *scrapie* comes from the characteristic feature of the disease, which is marked by areas of the skin denuded of fleece, due to the animals rubbing their irritated skin against fixed objects. The disease is insidious in onset but is characterized eventually by a progressive, eventually fatal, ataxia that leads to death of the affected animals in a matter of months. The affected sheep are afebrile and have normal CSF and no overt signs of infection. Pathologic lesions are limited to the central nervous system and show the characteristic noninflammatory spongiform lesions with nerve loss, cytoplasmic vacuolization of degenerating nerves, and a striking astrocytosis. The disease initially was felt to be an autosomal dominant genetic disease until two French investigators transmitted the disease to uninfected animals and found the agent to be a filterable agent.[155] Subsequently, it was demonstrated that the disease also could be transmitted to mice.[156]

The scrapie agent is unusual, in that it contains no nucleic acids and is resistant to chemicals that normally inactivate nucleic acids, such as formaldehyde, ethanol, U-V radiation, alkylating agents (such as B-propriolactone), proteases, and nucleases. However, the organism can be inactivated by autoclaving at 121°C under pressure or by exposure to extremes of pH, detergents, or phenol. The infectious agent has been felt to be an infectious protein, or prion, which is a proteinase-resistant isoform of a normal cellular protein that is characterized by abnormal folding.[152,153]

Kuru

In the 1950s, a disease was recognized among primitive Fore people living in a remote area of highland New Guinea. The disease was called *Kuru*, meaning "shivering" or "trembling" in the Fore language. The disease was characterized by an insidious onset of truncal ataxia. The ataxia progressed and became incapacitating. Eventually, ataxia occurred with every effort of voluntary movement, and death occurred uniformly 3 to 24 months after the onset of symptoms. The pathology showed spongiform changes in the brain similar to that caused by scrapie. Because of the transmission of scrapie to laboratory animals, William Hadlow, a veterinarian who had

worked with the scrapie agent, suggested that Kuru might also be due to a transmissible agent.[157] Subsequently, brain tissue from Kuru patients was inoculated into chimpanzees and transmitted the disease.[158] Epidemiologic studies indicated the likelihood that Kuru was due to ritual cannibalism of the victims after their death, usually by the Fore adult women and children (Table 12–5).[159] Consequently, the disease was more common in adult women but male and female children were affected equally, because the women fed infectious material to their children, regardless of their sex. With the suppression of cannibalism by Australian missionaries and settlers, the disease has virtually disappeared.[160]

Creutzfeldt-Jakob Disease

Creutzfeldt-Jakob disease (CJD) presents as a dementia, characterized by rapidly progressive mental deterioration, myoclonic jerking, and other neurologic signs. Classical CJD commonly begins between 55 and 70 years of age but rare cases have occurred in younger adults, even in adolescents. The disease often begins with fatigue, insomnia, and other nonspecific signs or sometimes with focal signs, such as ataxia, visual loss, or aphasia. These symptoms are followed by progressive and relentless dementia, myoclonus, and other neurologic signs. The mean duration of survival is only 5 to 6 months, and over 80% of patients die within 12 months. As in the other spongiform encephalopathies, there is no fever or other signs of infection, the spinal fluid is normal, and the brain has characteristic spongiform changes.

About 10% of patients with CJD have a family history consistent with an autosomal dominant inheritance. In most but not all of these affected families, persons with CJD have a point mutation in the gene coding for the prion protein. The majority of CJD cases (90%) have no other affected family members. CJD occurs at a rate of about 1 per million persons per year without evident clustering, aside from the 10% of familial cases, in virtually all populations.

The disease has been inadvertently transmitted by the transplantation of dural and corneal

Table 12–5 Transmission of Prion Diseases from Human to Human

Mode of Transmission	Example (no. of cases reported)	Incubation Period (years)
1. Intracranial transplantation or inoculation	a. Dural grafts (>80 cases) b. Inadequately sterilized instruments (several cases)	1.3–17 0.6–2.2 1.3–1.8
2. Extracranial transplantation	Corneal grafts (2)	1.3–1.5
3. Extracranial inoculation of neural tissue	a. Human growth hormone and gonadotropin (>100 cases) b. Arterial embolization with lyophilized dura mater (2 cases)	4–19* 3.5–7.5
4. Extracranial inoculation or oral exposure	a. Possible exposure to bovine spongiform encephalopathy prion (40 cases) b. Transmission of Kuru by ritual cannibalism (several thousand cases)	5–10* 4.40 or more

*Numbers represent minimum incubation periods since hormone was given over periods of years (time from midpoint of treatment to onset = 12 years).

Source: Reprinted with permission from R.T. Johnson and C.J. Gibbs, Creutzfeldt-Jakob Disease and Selected Transmissible Spongiform Encephalopathies, *New England Journal of Medicine*, Vol. 339, pp. 1994–2004, Copyright © 1998, Massachusetts Medical Society. All rights reserved.

grafts from infected donors. Over 80 cases have been recognized to be due to such exposures in the last 16 years.[154,161] It has also been transmitted by the intracerebral use of a sterotactic electrode to control an epileptogenic focus. This electrode had been used previously in a CJD patient and subsequently was disinfected only by soaking in alcohol; the CJD prion, like the prion causing scrapie, is resistant to disinfection by virucidal compounds. The largest number of iatrogenic cases, however, has been transmitted by the use of human growth hormone (HGH) prepared from a large pool of human pituitary tissue. The first three cases of CJD due to growth hormone were reported in 1985. Subsequently, 16 cases have occurred in the United States, 25 cases in the United Kingdom, 53 cases in France, and scattered cases elsewhere.[154,162] Fortunately, HGH is now prepared synthetically, rather than by extraction from pools of human pituitary glands, so no further patients should acquire CJD by this route. However, additional clinical cases may still appear from previous exposure, due to the long incubation period of CJD; the incubation period has ranged up to 40 years in Kuru.

Bovine Spongiform Encephalopathy and New Variant Creutzfeldt-Jakob Disease (nvCJD)

In April 1985, a dairy farmer in the south of England observed a previously healthy cow that became apprehensive, ataxic, and developed aggressive behavior. Progressive ataxia developed, and, eventually, the cow died. When tissues were sent to the central veterinary laboratory in the United Kingdom, the brain exhibited the typical features of bovine spongiform encephalopathy (BSE), a disease of cattle known to be caused by infection with a prion. Over the next few years, the number of cases of BSE in cattle in the United Kingdom grew rapidly. Sixteen cases were found in 1986, and more than 7,000 cases were found in 1989. The epidemic peaked in 1992, when 36,000 cases of BSE were reported from throughout Great Britain, Scotland, and Ireland.[154,163,164]

Eventually, over 170,000 cases of BSE were reported from more than 34,000 herds in the United Kingdom. The cattle herds with cases of BSE were scattered throughout the United Kingdom, and there was no evidence of lateral transmission of the disease between cattle in the same herd.[163] The epidemiologic pattern of disease was that of a common source outbreak. The most likely source was from contaminated bone meal that had been used for cattle feed. On investigation, it was concluded that the cause of the epidemic followed changes in the rendering process that had occurred in the 1970s. At that time, changes were introduced into the rendering process for the preparation of bone meal from animal remains, due in part to an oil crisis in the Middle East. The use of continuous heating of offal, as opposed to batch heating, was substituted to save fuel. Also, the sale of tallow became no longer profitable because of public concern about the health effects of animal fat consumption. The collapse of the tallow market resulted in more fat remaining with the offal. The added fat content probably acted to prevent the disinfection of prion proteins in the animal carcasses. Further amplification of the epidemic was probably related to the use of animal carcasses, including neural tissues from animals, such as cattle, that succumbed to BSE, for the preparation of animal feed. Bovine spongiform encephalopathy and other prion diseases have been transmitted experimentally to a number of species by the oral route; oral transmission has

been accomplished with various species of rodents and nonhuman primates.[165] These experimental data supported the hypothesis that BSE was a food-borne outbreak in the cattle.

Concern about the growing epidemic of BSE grew until the U.K. government instituted a ban against the use of carcasses from animals with possible spongiform diseases for the preparation of animal feed. In 1988, a ban on feeding ruminant-derived protein (such as cattle) to ruminants was instituted in the United Kingdom. However, as the epidemic evolved, disturbing evidence appeared suggesting cross-species infection from the BSE prion may have occurred. Domestic cats, as well as captive and exotic ruminants, died of BSE after eating animal feed containing possibly infected cattle tissues.[154] However, the public health actions that were taken had a dramatic effect on controlling the epidemic after a lag period of about 7 years, which is the median incubation period of the disease in cattle. The epidemic peaked in 1992 and has declined progressively since then.[154,163,164]

In 1989, cattle offal was banned from human food in the United Kingdom. However, because of concern about the potential transmission of BSE to humans, national surveillance of CJD was instituted in the United Kingdom in 1990. During the interval between 1990 and 1994, no unusual cases or clusters of CJD in humans were encountered.[166] However, beginning in 1994, patients with CJD with an unusual clinical presentation, course, laboratory findings, and unusual brain histopathology appeared (Figure 12–13).[166,167] Furthermore, these cases of atypical CJD were much younger than the classic cases. Because of their unusual demographic and clinical features, they were called *new variant Creutzfeldt-Jakob disease* (nvCJD).[167] Between 1994 and 1999, 39 nvCJD cases occurred in the United Kingdom and two cases in France.

New Variant Creutzfeldt-Jakob Disease

The patients with nvCJD are strikingly different from those with classic CJD. They are quite

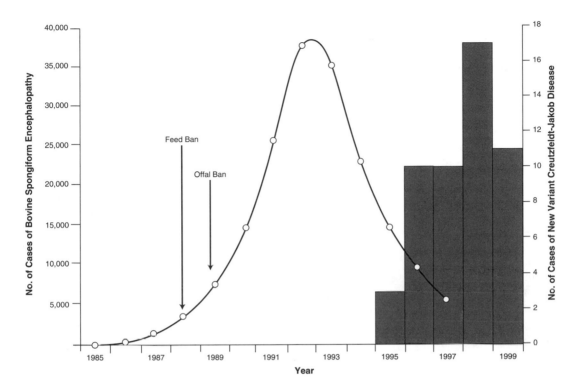

Figure 12–13 Cases of bovine spongiform encephalopathy (linear graph) and new variant Creutzfeldt-Jakob disease (bar graph) in the United Kingdom. The decline in the incidence of bovine spongiform encephalopathy began 5 years after the imposition of the ban on feeding ruminant-derived protein to ruminants. Cases of new variant Creutzfeldt-Jakob disease have been reported since February 1994. It has been postulated that these patients were exposed to contaminated meat products before the ban on cattle offal in human food was imposed in 1989. In the absence of knowledge of the duration of the incubation period in humans, this cluster of cases provides little information on the possible future incidence of the disease. Dates represent the years when cases were reported, rather than years of onset or death. *Source:* Reprinted with permission from R.T. Johnson and C.J. Gibbs, Creutzfeldt-Jakob Disease and Selected Transmissible Spongiform Encephalopathies, *New England Journal of Medicine*, Vol. 339, pp. 1994–2004, © 1998, Massachusetts Medical Society. All rights reserved.

young, with a mean age of 29 years versus 60 years for sporadic, classic CJD patients. They present with prominent psychiatric and behavioral manifestations, and have persistent painful paresthesia; the skin sensations may be similar to the sensory abnormalities leading to the scrapie lesions in sheep. Cerebellar ataxia uniformly develops, and the clinical course is prolonged, with an average survival of 14 months, compared with only 5 months in classic sporadic CJD. The electroencephalogram fails to show the typical periodic complexes of classic CJD, although some EEG abnormalities may occur. The histopathology of the brain lesions in nvCJD differs from that in classic CJD in containing diffuse amyloid plaques called *florid plaques*. When brain tissue from patients with nvCJD is inoculated into mice by the intracerebral route, the incubation period of nvCJD and BSE are identical and differ from classic CJD.[154,168]

All of the patients with nvCJD have a history of eating meat prior to their illnesses. One patient reported becoming a vegetarian within 1 year of onset of symptoms of nvCJD, but he had eaten beef previously. None reported eating cattle brains but, prior to the ban on the inclusion of cattle brain tissues in human food in 1989, these tissues were commonly included in sausages and other human foods. As a result of the epidemiologic, clinical, histopathologic, and animal inoculation data cited above, most experts currently believe that new variant Creutzfeldt-Jakob disease represents human infection with the prions of BSE, due to oral exposure to the agent in food.[168]

If this theory is correct, it raises several difficult public health issues. How many cases of nvCJD will eventually occur in the United Kingdom after the limit of the incubation period has been reached? Is it possible to transmit the disease to other humans by means other than consumption of neurologic tissues from cattle that are contaminated with BSE prions? One special concern is whether the disease is transmissible by transplantation or transfusion.[169]

Classic CJD has never been transmitted by transfusion, and no cases have been reported among patients with hemophilia or other clotting disorders who have been heavily exposed to blood and blood products, including large pools of clotting factors from many donors.[154] There is one report in the literature of the identification of CJD prions in buffy coat cells from the peripheral blood and the transmission of CJD by intracerebral inoculation of mice with infected human blood.[170] However, the higher levels of infectious prions in peripheral tissues, such as tonsillar and lymphatic tissues in patients with nvCJD, raise greater concerns about the transmission of the BSE agent than the clinical CJD prion by transfusion.[171]

Time will tell us whether this new disease, nvCJD, will persist in the human population or will disappear with the effective implementation of the public health prevention program that has been instituted in the United Kingdom to control the BSE epidemic and to prevent further human consumption of infected cattle tissues.

RESPONSES TO THE THREAT OF EMERGING INFECTIONS

Institute of Medicine

As with any public health problem, an effective plan to deal with the reality of new and emerging infections depends on the official recognition of the problem. The recognition that emerging infections constituted a substantial threat to the health of the American public and the population throughout the world was fostered by a meeting and report of the problem by a committee on emerging microbial threats to health. This committee was chaired by Nobel Laureate, Dr. Joshua Lederberg, Professor at Rockefeller University, and Dr. Robert E. Shope, Professor of Epidemiology and Director of the Arbovirus Research Unit at Yale University School of Medicine. The committee of the Institute of Medicine (IOM) met in February 1991 and convened an expert multidisciplinary committee to conduct an 18-month study of emerging microbial threats to health. The charge to the committee was "to identify significant emerging infectious disease, determine what might be done to deal with them, and recommend how similar future threats might be confronted to lessen their impact on public health."[172]

After reviewing evidence on the emergence of infectious disease presented by numerous experts, the committee made a series of recommendations, including:

1. the need for strengthened surveillance of infectious disease through CDC, National Institutes of Health (NIH), and the U.S. Department of Agriculture
2. expansion of the National Nosocomial Infection Surveillance (NNIS) system managed by the CDC
3. development by the U.S. Public Health Service of a computerized database on in-

fectious disease surveillance and vaccine and drug availability

4. increase of creative and coordinated international infectious disease surveillance through CDC, Department of Defense, NIH, and U.S. Department of Agriculture

5. increased research on agent, host, vector, and environmental factors leading to the emergence of infectious disease and expansion of the Epidemic Intelligence Service (EIS) and Field Epidemiology Training Program of CDC

6. congressional funding of a program installed in the National Health Service Corps for training in public health and related disciplines

7. development of a means for generating stockpiles of selected important vaccines

8. development of procedures to ensure availability and usefulness of critical antibiotics to maintain human health

9. development and implementation by the Environmental Protection Agency of procedures for the licensing of critical pesticides for use in infectious disease emergencies and giving of priority for funding to develop new pesticides

10. focus of attention on developing more effective ways to use education to enhance behavior change in groups at high risk of particular infectious diseases

Other National and International Agencies

Subsequent to the recommendation of the Institute of Medicine committee, several national and international health agencies have developed plans for dealing with the threat of new and emerging infections. The CDC plan focuses on more effective surveillance, improvements in the public health infrastructure, and applied research in public health prevention activities.[173] The NIH focuses on research and training. The Department of Defense plan focuses on surveillance and detection of new and emerging infectious disease, especially in international settings,

and the development of better vaccines. The World Health Organization plans to improve international surveillance and communication to detect and monitor emerging infectious diseases.

NEWLY DISCOVERED PATHOGENS

Traditionally, infectious agents have been linked to specific diseases by the isolation of an organism on artificial media, a tissue culture, recovery of the organism after inoculation of infectious material into an animal, or visualization of the organism in tissues or excretions of an infected patient. However, in the last decade or so, molecular biologists have developed methods to identify the genetic material (DNA or RNA) of infectious organisms and even sequence the genome of pathogenic organisms without ever isolating the entire intact organism *in vitro*. One of the first examples of the genetic characterization of an organism using molecular methods solely was the amplification of the nucleic acid of hepatitis C virus (HCV) and the identification of this important cause of human hepatitis in 1989.[174] Recently, additional successes have been reported in the use of molecular methods to identify the causative agents of infectious diseases. Also, epidemiologic methods have been applied to link new agents to well-studied chronic diseases. Both of these approaches have revolutionized thinking about infectious diseases and have identified "new" infectious diseases. Several examples will be reviewed briefly.

Whipples Disease

In 1907, George Whipple described a disease characterized by chronic diarrhea, with malabsorption, weight loss, polyarticular arthritis, and lymphadenopathy.[175] The intestines and lymph nodes of patients with the disease had abnormal fat deposits, and the disease was often called *intestinal lipodystrophy*. However, Whipple also noted bacilli in the walls of the intestines but repeated attempts to isolate and characterize the organisms by *in vitro* culture failed. Although steroids produced some temporary benefit, long-term antibiotic use sometimes was curative. With the advent of modern methods of molecular biology, it was possible to amplify the bacterial 16SrRNA gene and identify the causative organism as an actinomycete, which has been named *Tropheryma whippelii*.[176]

Cat Scratch Fever, Bacillary Angiomatosis, and Trench Fever

The clinical disease cat scratch fever has been known to clinicians for some time. It is characterized by fever and unilateral necrotizing lymphadenopathy involving the epitrochlear and axillary nodes that appear after a cat scratch. Recently, another syndrome, bacillary angiomatosis (BA), has been recognized in AIDS patients. This disease is characterized by nodular vascular proliferative lesions in the skin, bone, or other organs. Infection of the liver results in the formation of angiomatous lesion known as *bacillary peliosis hepatis*. Using both molecular techniques and cultures, an organism, *Bartonella henselii*, has been isolated from patients with cat scratch fever and with BA. Apparently, the organism causing the two diseases is similar, and host factors determine the clinical appearance of the resultant disease after infection. The organisms are sensitive to macrolide antibiotics, but the response is somewhat dependent on the immune competence of the infected patient. The reservoir for BA is the domestic cat, and the organisms are spread to humans by the cat flea.[177]

A related organism, *Bartonella quintana*, is the cause of trench fever, a disease that was common among soldiers serving in World War I; the disease was transmitted from one person to another by the body louse.[178] Although the disease has become very rare, cases have been described recently among homeless men.[179,180]

Helicobacter pylori: Peptic Ulcer and Gastric Cancer

Spiral bacteria have been found in the human stomach since 1906.[181] At one time, they were believed to lead to chronic inflammation and gastritis, but this theory was abandoned in favor of chronic stress, leading to acid and pepsin hypersecretion, as an explanation for the pathogenesis of chronic peptic ulcer disease. However, Warren and Marshall in Australia revived interest in the hypothesis that peptic ulcer disease might be caused by an infection when they cured a patient with chronic peptic ulcer disease by treatment with tetracycline.[182] Subsequently, they isolated the putative causative organism, which was originally called *Campylobacter pyloridis* but was later renamed *Helicobacter pylori*. The organism was linked to peptic ulcer disease and chronic gastritis, and they demonstrated that these diseases could be treated successfully with antibiotics.[182] Because some antacid regimens contain bismuth, a compound now known to be active against *H. pylori*, some of the reported successes with antacid therapy could have occurred because of the effect of bismuth on the organism. In response to skepticism about the importance of *H. pylori* as the etiologic agent of gastritis, Marshall had himself gastroscoped to prove that his stomach was normal, then ingested *H. pylori* after neutralizing his stomach acid with histamine blockers. After about 7 days, he developed epigastric discomfort and vomiting. Repeat gastroscopy showed that the organism had colonized the stomach and led to acute inflammation.[183] The organism and the pathology could be cleared with antibiotic therapy. This experiment was repeated subsequently by another investigator but the antibiotics failed to clear the *H. pylori*, and the gastritis persisted.[184] These self-experiments were followed with hundreds of studies of the association of *H. pylori* and gastric pathology. The studies have clearly and consistently shown a strong association between infections with *H. pylori* and dyspepsia, peptic ulcer disease involving both gastric and duodenal ulcers, hypertrophic gastritis, gastric cancer, and gastric lymphoma. As a result of these data, a consensus conference sponsored by the NIH in 1994 concluded that *H. pylori* infection was a major cause of peptic ulcer disease and recommended that antibiotic therapy become the mainstay of treatment.[185]

Infections with *H. pylori* are not systemic but involve only the superficial areas of the gastric mucosa. The organism secretes large amounts of urease, an enzyme that hydrolyzes urea to CO_2 and ammonia.[186] It has been hypothesized that the large amounts of ammonia produced by the urease may protect the organism from the deleterious effects of stomach acid.[187] The organism prefers to live in a neutral environment, such as is found beneath the gastric mucosa, but it can survive in an acid environment with a pH of 1.5. Infections with *H. pylori* can be detected by culture, histologic examination, or with the urease test of gastric aspirates, or it can be documented serologically by an ELISA antibody test or by using the carbon-labeled urea breath test.[188] In the breath test, the subject ingests C^{13}- or C^{14}-labeled urea, and the breakdown of the urea into C^{13} or C^{14} CO_2 by the urease-producing organisms is detected in the exhaled air.

Studies of the epidemiology of gastric cancer are also consistent with an etiologic role for *H. pylori* in this disease. Such studies have shown higher rates of *H. pylori* infection in populations living in areas with higher rates of gastric cancer. Furthermore, the prevalence of *H. pylori* is higher at early ages, especially in childhood, in countries with high gastric cancer rates. In addition, gastric cancer patients have higher rates of *H. pylori* infection than do controls.[189,190] *H. plylori* infection precedes cancer by many years.[191] The association between *H. pylori* and gastric cancer is restricted to tumors distal to the gastric cardia. Although other factors, such as smoking, may also affect the risk of gastric cancer, *H. pylori* is now believed to be of critical importance.

Gastric lymphoma is a rare disease because the stomach is not a lymphoid organ; the incidence is estimated to be about seven cases per million population per year.[192] The pathogenesis of gastric lymphoma and the association with *H. pylori* are believed to be related to the chronic inflammatory response to the infection.[193]

The theory that gastric cancer could be etiologically related to *H. pylori* infections helps to explain the epidemiology of this tumor over the last several decades in the United States.[190] Mortality from gastric cancer has shown dramatic reductions in incidence during the last several decades (Figure 12–14). This could be explained by the changes in hygiene that have occurred during the twentieth century that have afforded less opportunity for high rates of infections with *H. pylori* during childhood and gastric cancer several decades later. In contrast, in areas of the world with greater opportunities for fecal-oral transmission of *H. pylori*, the rates of gastric cancer remain high.

Chlamydia pneumoniae, CMV, *Helicobacter pylori* and Other Organisms, and Atherosclerosis

A recent hypothesis that is more controversial and uncertain than the *H. pylori*–peptic ulcer/gastric cancer association is that infections with one of several organisms may initiate or be a cofactor in coronary atherosclerosis.[194] In reality, the idea that heart attacks might be caused by a specific infection is an old idea that was popular at the end of the nineteenth century and early in the twentieth century.[195,196] However, infections have not been considered to be relevant cofactors or even evaluated systematically in the many epidemiologic studies of coronary heart disease (CHD) that have been done during the last four decades. The Framingham study of the NIH concluded that there were three primary factors in the pathogenesis of CHD, namely, elevated serum cholesterol and triglycerides, elevated blood pressure, and tobacco smoking. Some studies have found that other factors also could be important, such as stress, sedentary life style, obesity, and dietary biochemical factors other than cholesterol, e.g., homocystine. Many epidemiologic studies of CHD have identified the same risk factors. Therefore, public health programs for the prevention of CHD have emphasized reduction in animal fat in the diet and

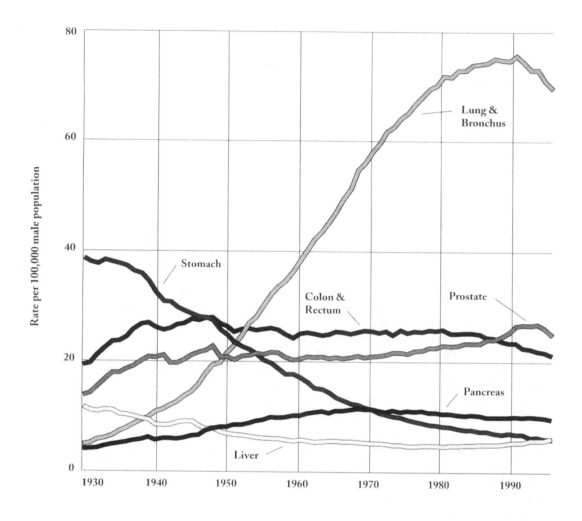

Figure 12–14 Age-adjusted cancer death rates,* males by site, U.S., 1930–1995. *Source:* American Cancer Society's Cancer Facts & Figures–1999, reprinted with permission.

reduction of serum cholesterol by diet or with the use of cholesterol-lowering drugs, blood pressure control, and prevention/cessation of cigarette smoking. The implementation of these public health programs has been accompanied by significant reduction in mortality from CHD. Nevertheless, CHD remains the number one cause of death in the United States.

Only recently has the role of infections in the etiology of CHD been suggested and studied.

Most studies have focused on one of three organisms: *H. pylori*, CMV, or *C. pneumoniae*.

H. pylori *Infection*

An association between *H. pylori* infections and CHD was first reported in 1994.[197] Since that time, a few additional studies have been reported. Most, including all of the prospective studies, have shown a modestly (and nonsignificant) elevated risk of CHD in patients with *H. pylori* infection. Many of the studies have not adequately adjusted for confounders, such as low socioeconomic status.[198] *H. pylori* leads only to a localized infection in the gastric mucosa. How, then, could it cause heart disease? It has been postulated that the pathogenetic mechanism is an autoimmune reaction between the heat shock protein 60 of *H. pylori* and a similar antigen in the endothelium of cardiac vessels.[198] Although this is an intriguing hypothesis, clearly, more data are needed on this possible association.

Cytomegalovirus

One group of investigators has reported an association between coronary stenosis, or restenosis after balloon angioplasty, and CMV antibody prevalence.[199] Another study found a significant association between carotid artery intimal narrowing and CMV antibodies.[200] Also, the CMV genome has been identified in coronary atheroma or in smooth muscle cells of coronary arteries by PCR by some investigators.[201] It is believed by some investigators that a human herpes virus might be involved in atherogenesis, because a related herpes virus causes Marek's disease, an atherosclerotic disease in chickens.

Chlamydial Pneumoniae

Chlamydial pneumoniae was first described as a distinct organism and originally named the *TWAR agent* by Grayston et al. in 1986.[202] It is now believed to be an important cause of community-acquired pneumonia in adults; it was associated with about 15% of pneumonia cases in a health maintenance organization in Seattle.[203]

Several studies have been done, and most reported a rate of *C. pneumoniae* antibodies that are twofold or more higher in patients with CHD than in matched controls. The organism is an intracellular pathogen that is capable of replication in human smooth muscle cells, endothelial cells, and macrophages.[204] It has been found in about half of the atherosclerotic lesions in the 13 pathologic studies in which it has been looked for, and it is almost never present in normal arterial walls.[198,205] However, it has also been found

in other tissues and, thus, could be merely an innocent bystander that infects already damaged tissue, in some cases. Nevertheless, because a few studies have demonstrated the organism inside the cells at the base of an atheroma, it could be the nidus that initiated atheroma formation.[205] Several randomized placebo controlled trials of prevention therapy with macrolide antibiotics have been initiated recently. A small study of roxithromycin (a macrolide antibiotic) reported lower rates of CHD in the treated patients but the differences were not statistically significant.[206,207] More evidence is needed before the role of *C. pneumoniae* in the genesis of coronary heart disease can be assessed. A recent prospective study done in physicians found no serologic evidence of an increased rate of *C. pneumoniae* antibodies prior to a first myocardial infarction.[208] However, because of the importance of CHD as a cause of morbidity and mortality, the modest elevation in risk associated with the traditional risk factors, and the intriguing preliminary data, further studies of the role of *C. pneumoniae* as an initiator or cofactor in the pathogenesis of CHD are important.

Hodgkin's Disease and Epstein-Barr Virus

Epstein-Barr virus (EBV) is known to be associated with nasopharyngeal carcinoma, a tumor that is especially common among populations living in South China. The virus has also been associated with Burkitt's lymphoma, a malignant B cell lymphoma that is highly prevalent in children living in tropical Africa. The DNA of EBV is present in multiple copies in each cell of most African Burkitt's lymphomas.

Recently, studies have been done of EBV infection in patients with Hodgkin's disease, a common tumor of unknown etiology.[209] Earlier studies had demonstrated that persons with a history of infectious mononucleosis, a common clinical manifestation of primary EBV infection in older children and young adults, had an increased risk of developing Hodgkin's disease later in life.[210] Also, patients with Hodgkin's disease commonly have elevated antibody titers to EBV viral antigens.[210] However, these antibodies might simply be due to reactivation of latent EBV after persons develop Hodgkin's disease. However, the recent report of increased antibody titers to EBV capsular antigen, nuclear antigen, and early antigen 4 or more years prior to the appearance of Hodgkin's disease, in comparison with matched controls, suggests that EBV infections may often precede the onset of the disease, which is one criterion for a causal association.[209] More data are needed on the association of EBV and Hodgkin's disease. The age distribution of Hodgkin's disease, with bimodal peaks in incidence, led to the suggestion by MacMahon that the disease might have two etiologies and that Hodgkin's disease occurring among young adults could be a sequelae of an infection, whereas disease with an older age of onset might have a different etiology.[210]

Other Chronic Diseases

An infectious etiology of a number of chronic diseases has been sought for many years. Several diseases of unknown etiology are believed likely to have an infectious etiology. Among the diseases considered most likely to be caused by infection are systemic lupus erythematosis, Kawasaki disease, multiple myeloma, multiple sclerosis, idiopathic aplastic anemia, juvenile diabetes mellitus, rheumatoid arthritis, and chronic myelogenous leukemia. Many other chronic diseases could have an infectious etiology. An enigmatic disease that spread across the globe in the 1920s was von Economo encephalitis.[160] It was followed by a form of Parkinsonism after an incubation period of 6 months to several years in about a third of the survivors. It is likely that von Economo disease was caused by an infectious agent; some have postulated that the swine influenza virus of 1918 was responsible, because nearly all cases of this type of encephalitis had previously had influenza during the 1918 epidemic. However, von Economo disease has disappeared.[160] Most current cases of Par-

kinson's disease are idiopathic, although occasionally the disease may follow acute viral encephalitis due to WE, SLE, or JE viruses or encephalitis due to Coxsackie B viruses.

CRITERIA FOR CAUSALITY

The classic criteria for establishing a causal relationship between an infectious agent and a disease was developed by Robert Koch in the 1880s, at a time when microbiology was a new science. When new organisms were being isolated from sick patients and animals, it was necessary to develop a set of standardized criteria to determine whether a given organism was causative, rather than an incidental isolate or even a contaminant. The criteria that were developed became known as the *Henle-Koch postulates*. These postulates were that:

1. A causative organism had to be consistently isolated from patients or animals with the disease.
2. It was not present in patients with other diseases or as a harmless parasite.
3. The disease could be induced in another animal or person if the organism was inoculated in pure culture after it was isolated and grown in the laboratory.
4. The organism could then be found or isolated from the experimentally infected subject.

However, new technologies are now available that often make the Henle-Koch postulates a less important criteria of causality. Modern molecular biology has required that the roles of causation be modified.[211] For example, molecular techniques such as consensus PCR allow the identification of conserved genetic sequences in the tissues of infected persons that are shared by closely related organisms. It may then be possible to demonstrate antibodies to proteins from organisms that have not been isolated. It may be possible to use such techniques to build a case for a causative relationship by establishing that the antibodies or the DNA or RNA are consistently present in persons with the disease and precede the clinical illness.[211] Another new PCR-based technique is called *representational difference analysis* (RDA). In this technique, healthy and diseased tissues are analyzed by a variant of PCR that subtracts sequences common to both specimens to find the genome of the infectious agent. The technique of RDA was utilized by Chang and colleagues to discover the human herpes virus type 8 that has been shown to cause KS.[13] HCV was discovered by scientists at CDC, NIH, and the Genetech Corporation, who created a cDNA library from the sera of HCV-infected chimpanzees and demonstrated that persons with non-A, non-B hepatitis had specific antibodies to the expressed proteins.[174,212] Subsequent PCR studies of blood from infected humans were done to characterize the sequence of the HCV genome. These new organisms were established as the cause of a human disease without isolating the agent *in vitro* and without the availability of an animal model. It was impossible to fulfill Koch's postulates to establish these organisms as the cause of a human disease.

Nevertheless, the evidence for causality is strong for each of these pathogen–disease associations. Perhaps a modification of the general criteria of causation originally developed by Bradford Hill and initially applied to assess the evidence of the etiologic association between tobacco and smoking and lung cancer should be considered in evaluating the evidence of a causal association between an organism and a disease.[213] The Bradford Hill criteria that might be used to establish the causal relationship between an organism and an infectious disease are as follows:

- Temporal association, i.e., infections with the organism, precedes the development of the disease.
- Biologic plausibility, i.e., it is biologically plausible and consistent with existing knowledge that the organism could cause the disease.
- Consistency: Evidence of infection with the organism is consistently found in patients with the disease by various investigators, using a variety of different techniques.
- Strength of the association: The relative risks of the disease are high in persons who are infected with the agent, in comparison with persons in whom no evidence of infection can be found.
- Dose–response relationship: Often, the relative risk of the disease or the length of the incubation period after infection and disease onset is related to the infectious dose.
- Removing, preventing, or decreasing the exposure is followed by a reduction in the risk of disease.

Although all of these criteria have some relevance to the determination of whether an organism is directly causative of an infectious disease, an appropriate temporal relationship, consistency of the association found by several laboratories, the specificity of the relationship, and the prevention of the disease by eliminating exposure to the putative causal organism are the most compelling. These criteria have been applied successfully to establish several new infectious diseases described in the last 20 years, including HIV/AIDS, HCV/hepatitis, and *H. pylori*/peptic ulcer.

The last two decades of the twentieth century have provided dramatically new challenges and understanding of the complex multiplicity of factors, leading to the emergence and spread of new infectious diseases. Almost certainly, the twenty-first century will bring even greater challenges to the understanding and control of infectious diseases as the population grows and our relationship with the environment becomes even more complex and better understood than it is at present.

REFERENCES

1. Gao F, Bailes E, Robertson DL, Chen Y, et al. Origin of HIV-1 in the chimpanzee, Pantroglodytes troglodytes. *Nature.* 1999;336–341.

2. Sepkowitz KA, Raffalli J, Riley C, Kiehu TE, Armstrong D. Tuberculosis in the AIDS era. *Clin Micro Rev.* 1995;8:180–199.

3. Selwyn PA, Hartell D, Lewis VA, et al. A prospective study of the risk of tuberculosis among intravenous drug users with human immunodeficiency virus infection. *N Engl J Med.* 1989;320:545–550.

4. Mitchell TG, Perfect JR. Cryptococcosis in the era of AIDS—100 years after the discovery of cryptococcus neoformans. *Clin Micro Rev.* 1995;8:515–548.

5. Dismukes WE. Cryptococcal meningitis in patients with AIDS. *J Infect Dis.* 1988;157:624–628.

6. Bozette SA, Carsen RA, Chiu J, et al. A placebo controlled trial of maintenance therapy with fluconazole after treatment of cryptococcal meningitis in the acquired immunodeficiency syndrome. *N Engl J Med.* 1991; 324:580–584.

7. Supparatpinyo K, Khamwan C, Baosoong V, Uthammachi C, Nelson KE, Sirisanthana T. Disseminated *Penicillium marneffei* infection: an emerging HIV-associated opportunistic infection in Southeast Asia. *Lancet.* 1994;344:110–113.

8. Wheat J. Endemic mycoses in AIDS: a clinical review. *Clin Micro Rev.* 1995;8:146–159.

9. Centers for Disease Control. Pneumocystis pneumonia, Los Angeles and Kaposi's sarcoma and pneumocystis pneumonia. *MMWR.* 1981;30:250–252, 305–308.

10. Barre-Sinoussi F, Chermann JC, Rey F, et al. Isolation of a T-lymphocyte retrovirus from patient at risk for acquired immunodeficiency syndrome (AIDS). *Science.* 1983;220:868–871.

11. Gallo RC, Salahudin SZ, Popovic M, et al. Frequent detection and isolation of cytopathic retroviruses (HTLV-III) from patients with AIDS and at risk for AIDS. *Science.* 1984;224:500–503.

12. Beral V, Peterman TA, Berkelman RL, et al. Kaposi's sarcoma among persons with AIDS: a sexually transmitted infection. *Lancet.* 1990;1:123.

13. Chang Y, Cesarman E, Pessin MS, et al. Identification of herpes virus-like DNA sequences in AIDS-associated Kaposi's sarcoma. *Science.* 1994;266:1864–1865.

14. Moore PS, Chang Y. Detection of herpes virus-like DNA sequences in Kaposi's sarcoma in patients with and those without AIDS. *N Engl J Med.* 1995;332: 1181–1185.

15. Melbye M, Cook PM, Hjalgram H, et al. Risk factors for Kaposi's sarcoma-associated herpes virus (KSHV/ HHV-8) seropositivity in a cohort of homosexual men, 1981–1996. *Int J Cancer.* 1998;77:543–548.

16. Grulich AE, Olsen SS, Luok. Kaposi's sarcoma-associated herpes virus: a sexually transmissible infection. *J AIDS Hum Retro.* 1999;30:387–393.

17. Phair J, Muñoz A, Detels R, et al. The risk of pneumocystis carinii pneumonia among men infected with human immunodeficiency virus type 1: multicenter AIDS Cohort Study Group. *N Engl J Med.* 1990;322: 161–165.

18. Allen S, Batongwanayo J, Kerlikowski K, et al. Two-year incidence of tuberculosis in cohorts of HIV-infected and uninfected urban Rwandan women. *Am Rev Respir Dis.* 1992;146:1439–1444.

19. Sande M, Volberding PA. Pneumocystis carinii pneumonia—current concepts. In: Saude MA, Volberding PA, eds. *The Medical Management of AIDS*, 3rd ed. Philadelphia: WB Saunders Company; 1992:261–282.

20. Pierce M, Crampton S, Henry D, et al. The effect of MAC and its prevention on survival in patients with advanced HIV infection (abstract/CB-18). *35th Interscience Conference on Antimicrobial Agents and Chemotherapy.* San Francisco, 1995.

21. Schuchat A, Broome CV, Hightower A, Costa SJ, Parkin W. Use of surveillance for invasive pneumococcal disease to estimate the size of the immuno-supressed HIV-infected population. *JAMA.* 1991;265:3275–3279.

22. Montalban C, Calleja JC, Erice A, et al. Visceral leishmaniasis in patients infected with human immunodeficiency virus. *J Infect.* 1990;21:261–270.

23. Kaplan CD, Northfelt DW. Malignancies associated with AIDS. In: Sande MA, Volberding PA. *The Medical Management of AIDS*, 6th ed. Philadelphia: WB Saunders Company; 1999:467–496.

24. Sillman FH, Sedlis A. Anogenital papilloma virus infection and neoplasia in immunodeficient women. *Obstet Gynecol Clin North Am.* 1987;14:537–558.

25. Levine AM, Sullivan-Halley J, Pike MC, et al. Human immunodeficiency virus-related lymphoma: Prognostic factors predictive of survival. *Cancer.* 1995;683:2466–2472.

26. Serwadda D, Mugerwa RD, Sewankambo NK, et al. Slim disease: a new disease in Uganda and its association with HTLV-III infection. *Lancet.* 1985;2:849–852.

27. Murphy FA, Nathanson N. The emergence of new virus diseases: an overview. *Semin Virol.* 1994;5:87–102.

28. Zucker JR. Changing pattern of autochthonous malaria transmission in the United States. *Emerg Infect Dis.* 1996;2:37–43.

29. Herwaldt B, Ackers MC, et al. An outbreak in 1996 of

cyclosporiasis associated with imported raspberries. *N Engl J Med*. 1997;336:1548.

30. Herwaldt B, Beach MJ, et al. The return of *Cyclospora* in 1997: another outbreak of cyclosporiasis in N. America associated with imported raspberries. *Ann Int Med*. 1999;130:210–220.

31. Izumiya H, Terjama J, Wada A, et al. Molecular typing of enterohemorrhagic *E. coli* O157:H7 isolates in Japan using pulse-field gel electrophoresis. *J Clin Microbiol*. 1997;35:1675–1680.

32. Smith KE, Besser JM, Hedberg CW, et al. Quinolone-resistant *Campylobacter jejuni* infections in Minnesota, 1992–1998. *N Engl J Med*. 1999;340:1525–1532.

33. Wegener HC. The consequences for food safety of the use of fluoroquinolones in food animals. *N Engl J Med*. 1999;340:1581–1582.

34. Rupprecht CE, Smith JJ. Raccoon rabies: the re-emergence of an epizootic in a densely populated area. *Semin Virol*. 1994;5:155–164.

35. Jahrling PB, Geisbert TW, Dalgard DW, et al. Preliminary report: isolation of Ebola virus from monkeys imported to the USA. *Lancet*. 1990;335:502–505.

36. Kissling RE, Robinson RQ, Murphy FA, Whitfield SG. Agent of disease contracted from green monkeys. *Science*. 1968;160:888–890.

37. Colwell RR. Global climate and infectious disease: the cholera paradigm. *Science*. 1996;274:2025–2031.

38. Centers for Disease Control. Rift Valley fever—East Africa, 1997–1998. *MMWR*. 1998;74:261–264.

39. Linthicum KJ, Anyamba A, Tucker CJ, Kelley PW, Myers MF, Peters CJ. Climate and satellite indicators to forecast Rift Valley fever epidemics in Kenya. *Science*. 1999;285:397–400.

40. Watts DM, Burke DS, Harrison BA, et al. Effect of temperature on the vector efficiency of *Aedes aegypti* for dengue 2 virus. *Am J Trop Med Hyg*. 1987;36:143–152.

41. Crosby AW. *Epidemic and Peace, 1918*. Westport, CT: Greenwood Press; 1976.

42. Taobenberger JK, Reid AH, Krafft AE, et al. Initial genetic characterizations of the 1918 "Spanish" influenza virus. *Science*. 1997;275:1793.

43. United Nations High Commission for Refugees. *The State of the World's Refugees: In Search of Solutions*. New York: Oxford University Press; 1995.

44. Aronson SS, Osterholm MT. Infectious diseases in child daycare: management and prevention, summary of the symposium and recommendation. *Rev Infect Dis*. 1986; 8:672–679.

45. Hadler SC, Webster HM, Erben JJ, Swanson JE, Maynard JE. Hepatitis A in day-care centers: a community-wide assessment. *N Engl J Med*. 1980;302:1222–1227.

46. Hadler SC, McFarland L. Hepatitis in daycare centers: epidemiology and prevention. *Rev Infect Dis*. 1986;8: 548–557.

47. Denny FW, Collier AM, Henderson FW. Acute respiratory infections in daycare. *Rev Infect Dis*. 1986;8:523–532.

48. Langlois BE, Dawson KA, Cromwell GI, Stahly TS. Antibiotic resistance in pigs following a 13 year ban. *J Anim Sci*. 1986;62:18–32.

49. Fenner F. *The History of Smallpox and Its Spread around the World*. Geneva: World Health Organization; 1988.

50. Torok TJ, Tauxe RV, Wise RP. A large community outbreak of salmonellosis carried by intentional contamination of restaurant salad bars. *JAMA*. 1997;278:389–395.

51. Brachman PS, Gold H, Plotkin SA, Fekety FR, Werrib M, Ingraham NR. Field evaluation of human anthrax vaccine. *Am J Public Health*. 1962;52:632–645.

52. Wirth JG, Green TW, Kanode RG Jr. Studies on immunity and anthrax: immunizing activity of alum-precipitated protective antigen. *J Immunol*. 1954;73:387–391.

53. Centers for Disease Control. Bioterrorism alleging use of anthrax and interim guidelines for management—United States, 1998. *MMWR*. Feb 5, 1999;4:69–74.

54. Walter Reed Army Institute of Research (WRAIR). *Addressing Emerging Infectious Disease Threats: A Strategic Plan for the Department of Defense* (DOD). Washington, DC: WRAIR, DOD; 1998.

55. Steere AC, Malawista SE, Saydman DR, et al. Lyme arthritis: an epidemic of oligoarticular arthritis in children and adults in three Connecticut communities. *Arthritis Rheum*. 1977;20:7–17.

56. Steere AC, Malawista SE, Hardin JA, Ruddy S, Askenase W, Andiman WA. Erythema chromium migrans and lyme arthritis: the enlarging clinical spectrum. *Ann Intern Med*. 1977;86:685–698.

57. Burgdorfer W, Barbour AG, Hayes SF, Benach JC, Grunwaldt G, Davis JP. Lyme disease—a tick-borne spirochetosis. *Science*. 1982;216–1317–1319.

58. Steere AC. Lyme disease. A growing threat to urban populations. *Proc Natl Acad Sci USA*. 1994;91:2378–2383.

59. Centers for Disease Control. Lyme disease—United States, 1995. *MMWR*. 1996;45:481–484.

60. Steere AC. Lyme disease. *N Engl J Med*. 1989;321:586–596.

61. Woodward TE, Dumler JS. Rocky Mountain spotted fever. In: Evans AS, Brachman PS, eds. *Bacterial Infections of Humans*, 3rd ed. New York: Plenum Press; 1998:597–612.

62. Maeda K, Markowitz N, Harley RC, Ristic M, Cox D, McDade JE. Human infection with *Ehrlichia canis*, a leukocytic rickettsia. *N Engl J Med*. 1987;310:853–856.

63. Anderson BS, Dawson JE, Jones DC, Wilson K. *Ehrlichia chaffeensis*, a new species associated with human ehrlichiosis. *J Clin Microbiol.* 1991;29:2838–2842.

64. Dumler JS, Bakken JS. Ehrlichial diseases of humans: emerging tick-borne infections. *Clin Infect Dis.* 1995; 20:1102–1110.

65. Bakken JS, Dumler JS, Chen SM, Eckman MR, Van Etta LL, Walker DH. Human granulocytic ehrlichiosis in the upper mid-west United States: a new species emerging? *JAMA.* 1994;272:212–218.

66. Ruebush TR, Juranek DD, Chisholm ES, et al. Human babesiosis on Nantucket Island: evidence for self-limited and subclinical infections. *N Engl J Med.* 1977; 297:825.

67. Gubler DJ, Clark GG. Dengue/dengue hemorrhagic fever. The emergence of a global health problem. *Emerg Infect Dis.* 1995;1:55–57.

68. Halstead SB. Dengue hemorrhagic fever—public health problem and a field for research. *Bull WHO.* 1980;58:1–21.

69. Halstead SB. Observations related to dengue hemorrhagic fever VI hypotheses and discussion. *Yale J Biol Med.* 1970;42:350–362.

70. Gubler DJ. Dengue and dengue hemorrhagic fever. *Clin Microbiol Rev.* 1998;11:480–496.

71. Guzman MG, Koori G, Bravo J, et al. Dengue hemorrhagic fever in Cuba: serological confirmation of clinical diagnosis. *Trans Roy Soc Trop Med Hyg.* 1984;78:235–238.

72. Kouri G, Guzman MG, et al. Reemergence of dengue on Cuba: a 1997 epidemic in Santiago de Cuba. *Emerg Infect Dis.* 1998;4:89–92.

73. Craven, Francy DB, Eliason DA, et al. Importation of *Aedes albopictus* and other exotic mosquito species into the United States in used tires from Asia. *J Am Mosq Contr Assoc.* 1998;4:138–142.

74. Rigau-Perez JG, Gubler DJ, Vorndam AV, Clark GC. Dengue surveillance—United States, 1986–1992, *MMWR.* 1994;43(SS-2):7–19.

75. World Health Organization. *Malaria Eradication.* From the Plenary Meeting. Geneva: World Health Organization; 1955:31–32.

76. Alonso PL, Lindsay SW, Armstrong JRM, et al. The effect of insecticide-treated bed nets on mortality of Gambian children. *Lancet.* 1991;337:1499–1502.

77. Centers for Disease Control. Outbreak of West Nile-like viral encephalitis—New York, 1999. *MMWR.* 1999;48:845–849.

78. Hoke CH, Vaughan DW, Nisalak, et al. Protection against Japanese encephalitis by inactivated vaccines. *N Engl J Med.* 1988;319:608–614.

79. Thompson WH, Kalfayan B, Anslow RO. Isolation of California encephalitis virus from a fatal human illness. *Am J Epidemiol.* 1965;81:245–253.

80. Mitchell CJ, Nichylski ML, Smith GC, et al. Isolation of eastern equine encephalitis virus from *Aedes albopictus* mosquitoes in Florida. *Science.* 1992;257:526–527.

81. Sanchez JL, Taylor DN. Cholera. *Lancet.* 1997;349:1825–1830.

82. Cholera Working Group, International Center for Diarrheal Disease Research, Bangladesh. Large epidemic of cholera-disease in Bangladesh caused by Vibrio cholera 0139. *Lancet.* 1993;342:387–390.

83. Siddigue AK, Salam A, Islam MS, et al. Why treatment centers failed to prevent cholera deaths among Rwanda refugees in Goma, Zaire. *Lancet.* 1995;345:359–361.

84. Anderson C. Cholera epidemic traced to risk miscalculation. *Nature.* 1991;354:255.

85. Riley LW, Remis RS, Helgerson SD, et al. Hemorrhagic colitis associated with a rare *Escherichia coli* serotype. *N Engl J Med.* 1983;308:681–685.

86. Armstrong GL, Hollingsworth J, Morris JG Jr. Emerging food-borne pathogens: *Escherichia coli* O157:H7 as a model of entry of a new pathogen into the food supply of the developed world. *Epidemiol Rev.* 1996;18:29–51.

87. Griffin PM, Tauxe RV. The epidemiology of infections caused by *Escherichia coli* O157:H7, other enterohemorrhagic *E. coli* and the associated hemolytic uremic syndrome. *Epidemiol Rev.* 1991;13:60–98.

88. Feng P. *Escherichia coli* O157:H7: novel vehicles of infection and emergence of phenotypic variants. *Emerg Infect Dis.* 1995;1:47–52.

89. Whittam TS, McGraw EA, Reid SD. Pathogenic *Escherichia coli* O157:H7: a model for emerging infectious diseases. In: Krause RM, ed. *Emerging Infections.* New York: Academic Press; 1998.

90. Steele BT, Murphy N, Rance CP. An outbreak of homolytic uremic syndrome associated with ingestion of fresh apple juice. *J Pediatr.* 1982;101:963–965.

91. Mackenzie WR, Hoxie NJ, Proctor ME, et al. A massive outbreak in Milwaukee of *Cryptosporidium* infection transmitted through the public water supply. *N Engl J Med.* 1994;331:161–167.

92. Morris RD, Naumora EN, Griffiths JK. Did Milwaukee experience water-borne cryptosporidiosis before the large outbreak in 1993? *Epidemiology.* 1998;9:264–270.

93. Current WL, Garcia LS. Cryptosporidiosis (review). *Clin Microbiol Rev.* 1991;4:325–358.

94. Griffiths JK. Human cryptosporidiosis. Epidemiology, transmission, clinical disease, treatment and diagnosis. *Adv Parasitol.* 1998;40:37–85.

95. Morris RD, Levin R. Estimating the incidence of waterborne infectious diseases related to drinking water in the United States. In: Reichard EG, Zappeni G, eds. *Assess-*

ing and Managing Health Risks from Drinking Water Contamination: Approaches and Applications. Great Britain: International Association of Hydrological Sciences Press; 1995.

96. Huang P, Weber JJ, Sosin DM, et al. The first reported outbreak of diarrheal illness associated with *Cyclospora* in the United States. *Ann Intern Med.* 1995;123:409–414.

97. Earle D. Symposium on epidemic hemorrhagic fever. *Am J Med.* 1954;16:619–709.

98. Lee H, Lee PW, Johnson KJ. Isolation of the etiologic agent of Korean hemorrhagic fever. *J Infect Dis.* 1978; 137:298–308.

99. Glass GE, Watson AJ, Leduc J, Kelen GD, Quinn TC, Childs J. Infection with a rat-borne hantavirus in U.S. residents is consistently associated with hypertensive renal disease. *J Infect Dis.* 1993;167:614–620.

100. Niklasson B, Leuc J. Epidemiology of nephropathica epidemica in Sweden. *J Infect Dis.* 1987;155:269–276.

101. Hughes JM, Peters LJ, Cohen MC, et al. Hantavirus pulmonary syndrome: An emerging infectious disease. *Science.* 1993;262:850–851.

102. Khan AS, Khabbaz RF, Armstrong CR, et al. Hantavirus pulmonary syndrome: the first 100 cases. *J Infect Dis.* 1996;173:1297–1303.

103. Nichol ST, Spiropoulou CF, Morzuno SP, et al. Genetic identification of a hantavirus associated with an outbreak of acute respiratory illness. *Science.* 1993; 262:914–917.

104. Stone R. The mouse-pinon nut connection. *Science.* 1993;262:833.

105. Smith CEG, Simpson DIH, Bowen ETW. Fatal human disease from vervet monkeys. *Lancet.* 1967;2:1119–1121.

106. Kissling RE, Robinson RQ, Murphy FA, Whitfield SG. Agent of disease contracted from green monkeys. *Science.* 1968;160:888–890.

107. Bowen ETN, Lloyd G, Harris WJ, Platt GS, Baskerville A, Vella EE. Viral hemorrhagic fever in southern Sudan and northern Zaire. *Lancet.* 1977;1:571–573.

108. World Health Organization. Ebola haemorrhagic fever in Sudan 1976. Report of World Health Organization International Study Team. *Bull WHO.* 1978;56:247–270.

109. World Health Organization. Ebola haemorrhagic fever in Zaire, 1976. Report of an international commission. *Bull WHO.* 1978;56:271–293.

110. Murphy FA, Peters CJ. Ebola virus: where does it come from and where is it going? In: Krause RM, ed. *Emerging Infections.* New York: Academic Press; 1998:375–410.

111. Bwaka MA, Bonnet MJ, Calain P, et al. Ebola hemorrhagic fever in Kikwit, Democratic Republic of Congo: clinical observations in 103 patients. *J Infect Dis.* 1999;179(Suppl 1):S1–S7.

112. Roels TH, Bloom AS, Buffington J, et al. Ebola hemorrhagic fever, Kikwit, Democratic Republic of the Congo, 1995: risk factors for patients without a reported exposure. *J Infect Dis.* 1999;179(Suppl 1):S92–S97.

113. Dowell SE, Mukunu R, Ksiazek TG, Khan AS, Rollin PE, Peters CJ. Transmission of Ebola hemorrhagic fever: a study of risk factors in family members, Kikwit, Democratic Republic of the Congo, 1995. *J Infect Dis.* 1999;(Suppl 1):S87–S91.

114. Preston R. *The Hot Zone.* New York: Random House; 1994.

115. Le Guenno B, Formenty P, Wyers M, Govnon P, Walker F, Boesch C. Isolation and partial characterization of a new strain of Ebola virus. *Lancet.* 1996;345: 1271–1274.

116. Jezek Z, Szczeniowski MY, Mayembe-Tamfom JJ, McCormick JB, Heymann D. Ebola between outbreaks: intensified Ebola hemorrhagic fever surveillance in the Democratic Republic of the Congo, 1981–1985. *J Infect Dis.* 1999;(Suppl 1):S60–S64.

117. Johnson KM, Halstead SB, Cohen SN. Hemorrhagic fevers of Southeast Asia and South America: a comparative appraisal. *Prog Med Virol.* 1967;9:105–158.

118. Salas R, Manziona N, Tesh RB, et al. Venezuelan hemorrhagic fever. *Lancet.* 1991;338:1033–1036.

119. World Health Organization. International symposium on arena viral infections of public health importance. *Bull WHO.* 1975;52:318–766.

120. Buckley SM, Casals J. Lassa fever, a new disease of man from West Africa III: isolation and characterization of the virus. *Am J Trop Hyg Med.* 1970;19:680-691.

121. Selrey LA, Wells RM, McCormick JG, et al. Infection of humans and horses by a newly described morbillivirus virus. *Med J Aust.* 1995;162:642–645.

122. O'Sullivan JD, Allworth AM, Paterson DL, et al. Fatal encephalitis due to novel paramyxovirus transmitted from horses. *Lancet.* 1997;349:93–95.

123. Rodger RJ, Douglas IC, Baldock FC, et al. Investigation of a second focus of equine morbillivirus infection in a coastal Queensland. *Aust Vet J.* 1996;24:243–345.

124. Williamson MM, Hooper PT, Selleck PW, et al. Transmission studies of Hendravirus (equine morbillivirus) in fruit bats, horses and cats. *Aust Vet J.* 1996;76:813–818.

125. Chua KB, Gohk J, Wong KT, et al. Fatal encephalitis due to Nipah virus among pig farmers in Malaysia. *Lancet.* 1999;354:1257–1259.

126. Centers for Disease Control. Outbreak of Hendra-like virus—Malaysia and Singapore, 1998–1999. *MMWR.* 1999;48:265–269.

127. Fraser DW, Tsai TR, Orenston W, et al. Legionnaires' disease: description of an epidemic of pneumonia. *N Engl J Med.* 1977;297:1189–1197.

128. McDade JE, Shepard CC, Fraser DW, Tsai TR, Redus MA, Dowdle WR. Legionnaires' disease: isolation of a bacterium and demonstration of its role in other respiratory disease. *N Engl J Med.* 1977;297:1197–1203.

129. Glick TH, Gregg MB, Berman B, Mallison G, Rhodes WW Jr, Kassanoff I. Pontiac fever: an epidemic of unknown etiology in a health department: 1. Clinical and epidemiologic aspects. *Am J Epidemiol.* 1978;107:149–160.

130. Dondero TJ Jr, Rendtorff RC, Mallison GF, et al. An outbreak of Legionnaires' disease associated with a contaminated air-conditioning cooling tower. *N Engl J Med.* 1980;302:365–370.

131. Myerowitz RL, Pasculla AW, Dowling JW, et al. Opportunistic lung infection due to Pittsburgh pneumonia agent. *N Engl J Med.* 1979;301:958–958.

132. Beatty HN, Miller AA, Broome CV, Goings S, Phillips CA. Legionnaires' disease in Vermont, May to October 1977. *JAMA.* 1978;240:127–137.

133. Breiman RF, Fields BS, Sanden GN, Volmer CJ, Meier A, Spika JS. Association of shower use with Legionnaires' disease, possible role of amoebae. *JAMA.* 1990; 263:2924–2926.

134. Muder RR, Yu VC, Woo AH. Mode of transmission of *Legionella pneumophila*: a critical review. *Arch Intern Med.* 1986;146:1607–1612.

135. Aibeiro CD, Burge S, Palmer S, et al. *Legionella pneumophila* in a hospital water system following a nosocomial outbreak: prevalence, monoclonal antibody subgrouping and effect of control measures. *Epidemiol Infect.* 1987;98:253–259.

136. Plouffe JF, Webster CR, Hackman B. Relationship between colonization of hospital buildings with *Legionella pneumophila* and hot water temperatures. *Appl Environ Microbiol.* 1983;46:769–790.

137. Webster RG. Influenza: an emerging viral pathogen. In: Krause RM, ed. *Emerging Infections.* New York: Academic Press; 1998:275–300.

138. Noble GR. Epidemiological and clinical aspects of influenza. In: Beare AS, ed. *Basic and Applied Influenza Research.* Boca Raton, FL: RCC Press; 1982:18–50.

139. Centers for Disease Control. Isolation of avian influenza A (H5N1) viruses from humans—Hong Kong, May–December, 1997. *MMWR.* 1997;46:1204–1207.

140. Todd J, Fishart M, Kapral F, Welch T. Toxic shock syndrome associated with phase-group 1 staphylococci. *Lancet.* 1978;2:1116–1118.

141. Davis JP, Chesney PJ, Ward PJ, et al. Toxic-shock syndrome: epidemiologic features, recurrence, risk factors and prevention. *N Engl J Med.* 1980;303:149–135.

142. Osterholm MT, Forfang JC. Toxic-shock syndrome in Minnesota: results of an active-passive surveillance system. *J Infect Dis.* 1982;145:458–464.

143. Broome CV. Epidemiology of TSS in the United States: overview. *Rev Infect Dis.* 1989;2(Suppl S1): S14–S21.

144. Musser JM, Schlievert PM, Chow AW et al. A single clone of *Staphylococcus aureus* causes the majority of cases of toxic shock syndrome. *Proc Natl Acad Sci USA.* 1990;87:225–299.

145. Centers for Disease Control. Reduced incidence of menstrual toxic-shock syndrome—United States, 1980–1990. *MMWR.* 1990;39:421–423.

146. Rammelkamp CH, Denny FW, Wannamaker LW. Studies on the epidemiology of rheumatic fever in the armed services. In: Thomas C, ed. *Rheumatic Fever.* Minneapolis, MN: University of Minnesota Press; 1952:72–89.

147. Stollerman GH, Rusoff H, Hirshfield I. Prophylaxis against group A streptococci in rheumatic fever. The use of single monthly injections of benzathine penicillin G. *N Engl J Med.* 1955;252:787–791.

148. Wood HF, Stollerman GH, Feinstein AR, et al. A controlled study of three methods of prophylaxis against streptococcal infection in a population of rheumatic children. *N Engl J Med.* 1957;257:394–399.

149. Reasy CG, Wiedmeier SE, Osmond GS, et al. Resurgence of acute rheumatic fever in the inter-mountain area of the United States. *N Engl J Med.* 1987;316:421–427.

150. Stevens DL, Tanner MH, Winship J, et al. Severe group A streptococcal infections associated with a toxic shock-like syndrome and scarlet fever toxin A. *N Engl J Med.* 1989;321:1–7.

151. Musser JM, Krause RM. The revival of group A streptococcal diseases, with a commentary on staphylococcal toxic shock syndrome. In: Krause, RM, ed. *Emerging Infections.* New York: Academic Press; 1998: 185–281.

152. Prusiner SB. Novel proteinaceous infectious particles cause scrapie. *Science.* 1982;216:136–144.

153. Prusiner SB. Prions and neurodegenerative diseases. *N Engl J Med.* 1987;317:1571–1581.

154. Johnson RT, Gibbs CJ. Creutzfeldt-Jakob disease and related transmissible spongiform encephalopathies. *N Engl J Med.* 1998;339:1994–2004.

155. Cuille J, Chelle PL. La maladic die "tremblante du mouton" est-elle inoculable. *CR Acad Sci (Paris).* 1936;203:1552–1554.

156. Chandler RC. Encephalopathy in mice produced by inoculation with scrapie brain material. *Lancet.* 1961;1: 378–379.

157. Hadlow WJ. Scrapie and kuru. *Lancet.* 1959;2:289–290.

158. Gajdusck DC, Gibbs CJ, Alpers M. Experimental transmission of a kuru-like syndrome to chimpanzees. *Nature.* 1966;209:794–796.

159. Glasse R. Cannibalism in the kuru region of New Guinea. *Trans NY Acad Sci.* 1967;29:748–754.

160. Johnson RT. *Viral Infections of the Nervous System,* 2nd ed. Philadelphia: Lippincott-Raven Press; 1998: 356.

161. Brown P. Environmental causes of human spongiform encephalopathy. In: Baker HF, Ridley RM, eds. *Prion Diseases.* Totowa, NJ: Humana Press; 1996:139–154.

162. Brown P, Gajdusek DC, Gibbs C, Asher DM. Potential epidemic of Creutzfeldt-Jakob disease from human growth hormone therapy. *N Engl J Med.* 1985;313: 728–731.

163. Nathanson N, Wilesmith J, Griot C. Bovine spongiform encephalopathy (BSE): causes and consequences of a common source epidemic. *Am J Epidemiol.* 1997; 45:959–969.

164. Collee JG, Bradley R. BSE: a decade on: part 1. *Lancet.* 1997;349:636–641.

165. Gibbs CJ, Amyx HL, Bacute A, Masters CC, Gjadusek DC. Oral transmission of Kuru Creutzfeldt-Jakob disease and scrapie to nonhuman primates. *J Infect Dis.* 1980;142:205–208.

166. Cousens SN, Zeidler M, Esmonde TF, et al. Sporadic Creutzfeldt-Jakob disease in the United Kingdom: Analysis of epidemiological surveillance data for 1970–96. *Br Med J.* 1997;315:389–396.

167. Will RG, Ironside JW, Ziedler M, et al. A new variant of Creutzfeldt-Jakob disease in the UK. *Lancet.* 1996; 347:921–925.

168. Prusiner SB. Prion disease and the BSE crisis. *Science.* 1997;278:245–251.

169. Esmonde TFG, Will RG, Slattery JM, et al. Creutzfeldt-Jakob disease and blood transfusion. *Lancet.* 1993;341:205–207.

170. Manuelidis EE, Kim JH, Mericangas JR, Manuelidis L. Transmission to animals of Creutzfeldt-Jakob disease from human blood. *Lancet.* 1985;341:896–897.

171. Hill AF, Butterworth RJ, Joiner S, et al. Investigation of variant Creutzfeldt-Jakob disease and other human prion diseases with tonsil biopsy samples. *Lancet.* 1999;353:183–189.

172. Institute of Medicine. *Emerging Infectious: Microbial Threats to Health in the United States.* Washington, DC: National Academy Press; 1992.

173. Centers for Disease Control. Preventing emerging infectious diseases: a strategy for the 21st century. *MMWR.* Sept 11, 1998.

174. Choo QL, Kuo G, Weiner AJ, et al. Isolation of a cDNA clone derived from a blood-borne non-A non-B hepatitis genome. *Science.* 1989;244:359–362.

175. Whipple GH. A hitherto undescribed disease characterized anatomically by deposits of fat and fatty acids in the intestinal and mesenteric lymphatic tissues. *Johns Hopkins Hosp Bull.* 1907;18:382–391.

176. Relman DA, Schmidt TM, MacDermott RP, Falkow S. Identification of the uncultured bacillus of Whipples disease. *N Engl J Med.* 1992;327:293–301.

177. Koehler JE, Glaser CA, Tappero JW. *Rochalimaea henselae* infection: a new zoonosis with the domestic cat as reservoir. *JAMA.* 1994;271:531–535.

178. Strong RP, ed. *Trench Fever: Report of Commission, Medical Research Committee American Red Cross.* Oxford, England: Oxford University Press; 1918:40–60.

179. Drancourt M, Mainard JC, Brouqui P, et al. *Bartonella (Rochalimaea) quintana* endocarditis in three homeless men. *N Engl J Med.* 1995;332:419–423.

180. Spach DH, Kanter AS, Dougherty MJ, et al. *Bartonella (Rochalimaea) quintana* bacteremia in inner-city patients with chronic alcoholism. *N Engl J Med.* 1995; 332:424–428.

181. Kreinitz W. Uber das Auftreten von Spirochaeten verschiedener form in Mageninhatl bei carcinoma ventricul. *Dtsch Med Wochenschr.* 1906;38:872.

182. Marshall BJ. History of the discovery of *C. pylori.* In: Campylobacter pylori *in Gastritis and Peptic Ulcer Disease.* New York: Igaku-Shoin; 1989.

183. Marshall BJ, Armstrong JA, McGeche DB, Glany RJ. Attempt to fulfill Koch's postulates for pyloric *Campylobacter. Med J Aust.* 1985;142:436–439.

184. Morris A, Nicholson G. Ingestion of *Campylobacter pyloridis* causes gastritis and raises fasting gastric pH. *Gastroenterology.* 1987;82:192–194.

185. NIH Consensus Development Panel on *Helicobacter pylori* in Peptic Ulcer Disease. *JAMA.* 1994;272:65–69.

186. Torbett GR, Hoj PB, Horne R, Mee BJ. Purification and characterization of the urease enzymes of *Helicobacter* species from humans and animals. *Infect Immunol.* 1992;60:5259–5266.

187. Marshall BJ, Barrett LJ, Prakash C, McCallum RW, Guerrant RL. Urea protects *Helicobacter* (*Campylobacter*) from the bactericidal effect of acid. *Gastroenterology.* 1990;99:697–702.

188. Brown KE, Perra DA. Diagnosis of *Helicobacter pylori* infection. *Gastroenterol Clin North Am.* 9193;22: 106–118.

189. Taylor DN, Blaser MJ. The epidemiology of *Helicobacter pylori* infection. *Epidemiol Rev.* 1991; 13:42–59.

190. Howson C, Hiyama T, Wynder E. The decline in gastric cancer: epidemiology of an unplanned triumph. *Epidemiol Rev*. 1986;8:1–27.

191. Parsonnet J, Friedman GD, Vandersteen DP, et al. *Helicobacter pylori* infection and the risk of gastric cancer. *N Engl J Med*. 1991;325:1127–1131.

192. Severson RK, Davis S. Increasing incidence of primary gastric lymphoma. *Cancer*. 1990;66:1283–1287.

193. Parsonnet J, Hansen S, Rodriguez L, et al. *Helicobacter pylori* infection and gastric lymphoma. *N Engl J Med*. 1994;330:1267–1271.

194. Ross R. Atherosclerosis: an inflammatory disease. *N Engl J Med*. 1999;340:115–126.

195. Frothingham C. The relation between acute infectious diseases and arterial lesions. *Arch Intern Med*. 1911; 8:153–162.

196. Nieto JF. Infections and atherosclerosis: new clues from an old hypothesis? *Am J Epidemiol*. 1998;148: 937–940.

197. Murry LJ, Bamford KB, O'Reilly DPJ, McCrum EE, Evans AE. *Helicobacter pylori* infection: relation with cardiovascular risk factors, ischemic heart disease, and social class. *Br Heart J*. 1995;74:497–501.

198. Danesh J, Collins R, Peto R. Chronic infections and coronary heart disease: is there a link? *Lancet*. 1997; 350:430–436.

199. Carlson J, Miketic S, Mueller KH, et al. Previous cytomegalovirus or *Chlamydia pneumonia* infection and risk of re-stenosis after transluminal coronary angioplasty. *Lancet*. 1998;350;1225.

200. Nieto FJ, Adam E, Sorlie P, et al. A cohort study of cytomegalovirus infection as a risk factor for carotid intimal-media thickening, a measure of subclinical atherosclerosis. *Circulation*. 1996;94:922–927.

201. Melnick JL, Hn CH, Burck J, Adam C, DeBakey ME. Cytomegalovirus DNA in arterial walls of patient with atherosclerosis. *J Med Virol*. 1994;42:396–404.

202. Grayston JT, Kuo CC, Wang SP, Altman J. A new *Chlamydia psittaci*, strain TWAR, isolated in acute respiratory infection. *N Engl J Med*. 1986;315:161–168.

203. Grayston JT, Campbell LA, Kuo CC, et al. A new respiratory pathogen: *Chlamydia pneumonia*, strain TWAR. *J Infect Dis*. 1990;161:618–625.

204. Gaydos CA, Summergill JT, Sabney NN, Ramirez JA, Quinn TC. Replication of *Chlamydia pneumonia* in vitro in human macrophages, endothelial cells, and aortic artery smooth muscle cells. *Infect Immunity*. 1996;64:1614–1620.

205. Kuo CC, Shor R, Campbell LA, et al. Demonstration of *Chlamydia pneumonia* in atheroscleretic lesions of coronary arteries. *J Infect Dis*. 1993;167:841–849.

206. Gupta S, Leatham EW, Carrington D, Mendall MA, Kaski JC, Camm AJ. Elevated *Chlamydia pneumonia* antibodies, cardiovascular events, and azithromycin in male surviving of myocardial infarction. *Circulation*. 1997;96:404–407.

207. Garfinkel E, Bozovich G, Gavoca A, Beck A, Martner B. Randomized trial of roxithromycin in non-Q-wave coronary syndromes: Roxis pilot study. Rox's Study Group. *Lancet*. 1997;350:404–407.

208. Ridkin PM, Jundsin RB, Stampfer MJ, Poulin S, Hennekens CH. Prospective study of *Chlamydia pneumonia* IgG seropositivity and risks of future myocardial infarction. *Circulation*. 1999;99:1161–1164.

209. Mueller N, Evans A, Harris NC, Comstock GW, et al. Hodgkin's disease and the EBV: altered antibody pattern before the diagnosis. *N Engl J Med*. 1989;320: 696–701.

210. MacMahon B. Epidemiologic evidence on the nature of Hodgkin's disease. *Cancer*. 1957;10:1045–1054.

211. Fredericks DN, Relman DA. Sequence-based identification of microbial pathogens: a reconsideration of Koch's postulates. *Clin Micro Rev*. 1996;9:18–33.

212. Kuo G, Choo Q-L, Alter HJ, et al. An assay for circulating antibodies to a major etiologic virus of non-A, non-B hepatitis. *Science*. 1989;244:362–364.

213. U.S. Public Health Service. *Smoking and Health: Report of the Advisory Committee to the Surgeon General of the Public Health Service*. Publication no. 1103. 1964:19–21.

CHAPTER 13

Nosocomial Infections

Rashid A. Chotani, Mary-Claire Roghmann, and Trish M. Perl

INTRODUCTION

The problems associated with nosocomial infections—hospital-acquired or health care associated infections—have undoubtedly existed since sick people were gathered in health care environments. Interest in the fate of patients at health care facilities has existed for centuries. In only recent decades has the rather new discipline of hospital (health care) epidemiology, which studies infectious and noninfectious adverse events, developed into an accepted medical science.

As modern medicine develops new cutting-edge diagnostic and therapeutic technologies for prolonging life and as the population ages or has compromised defenses, nosocomial infections will become one of the primary medical and public health problems that we will face. Currently, in the United States, approximately 2.5 million infections, which result in about 250,000 deaths, occur annually.[1] These numbers may significantly underestimate the problem's magnitude as more patients are discharged early and infections are being diagnosed and cared for in nontraditional medical settings. The Centers for Disease Control and Prevention (CDC) estimates that nosocomial infections contribute to 0.7% to 10.1% of deaths and cause 0.1% to 4.4% of all deaths occurring in hospitals.[2] In fact, following some medical procedures, such as cardiac surgery, nosocomial infections are the most

significant contributors to prolonged hospital stay and increased hospital mortality.[3]

Nosocomial infections also cause considerable morbidity and cost. In 1992, a nosocomial infection added an average of four extra hospital days and $2,100 to the patient's costs (Table 13–1).[1] In total, these infections added approximately $4.5 billion to the cost of the health care system.[4] Thus, hospitals or health care institutions witness a financial loss when a patient develops an infection associated with health care.

Nosocomial infections occur for four essential reasons:

1. Host factors: Patients may have a compromised immune system due to underlying disease(s), which increases their risk of developing infections from both high- and low-virulence organisms.
2. Environment: The hospital environment promotes the spread of microbial pathogens. The proximity to other patients, contamination of common equipment, exposure to water contaminated with microorganisms, presence of construction and renovation, and the often-unwashed hands of health care workers contribute to create the ideal conditions for transmission of infectious organisms.
3. Technology: Technologic advances in health care provide sophisticated methods of monitoring and caring for patients.

Table 13–1 Nosocomial Infection Morbidity and Cost per Patient, 1992

Type of Infection	Excess Hospitalization Days	Extra Cost ($)	Attributable Mortality
UTI	1	680	Very Low
SSI	7	3,152	Low
Pneumonia	6	5,683	10%
BSI	7	3,517	9%

Source: Reprinted with permission from S.K. Fridkin et al., The Role of Understaffing in Central Venous Catheter-Associated Bloodstream Infections, *Infection Control and Hospital Epidemiology*, Vol. 17, pp. 150–158, Copyright © 1996, Slack, Inc.

These advances provide new portals of entry, alter normal host flora, and may increase antibiotic resistance, thus increasing the risk of nosocomial infections.

4. Human factors: With tremendous cutbacks in the health care industry, the number and skill level of caregivers have decreased. Support staff now provide previously specialized nursing functions. Health care workers are busier than ever, allowing them little time to observe simple infection control practices, such as handwashing. These changes may contribute substantially to nosocomial transmission of organisms and development of infections.

In the United States, the type and number of infections are estimated by several surveillance systems; one of them is the National Nosocomial Infections Surveillance (NNIS) system, which was established in 1970.[5] Currently, 231 self-selected hospitals participate voluntarily and collect data using four standardized protocols for surveillance:

1. all patients (hospital-wide)
2. adult and pediatric intensive care unit (PICU) patients
3. high-risk nursery (HRN) patients
4. surgical procedures[6,7]

In the United States, based on NNIS data (January 1990 to March 1996), urinary tract infections (UTIs) accounted for 34.5% of nosocomial infections; surgical site infections (SSIs) for 17.4%; bloodstream infections (BSIs) for 14.2%; lower respiratory tract infections (LRIs) for 13.2%; and others for 20.8%.[5] This represents a change from the past, where SSIs represented 25% and BSIs 10% of nosocomial infections. These changes most likely reflect institutional-based surveillance strategies that do not capture changes in health care delivery patterns.

Approximately 90% of the nosocomial infections are caused by bacteria, with viral, fungal, protozoal, and other classes of microorganisms associated with the remaining infections.[8] Based on NNIS data, the most common pathogens isolated from any nosocomial infections are *Staphylococcus aureus* (13%), *Escherichia coli* (12%), coagulase-negative staphylococci (CNS, 11%), enterococcus (10%), and *Pseudomonas aeruginosa* (9%).[5] Like community-acquired infections, the most commonly isolated organism depends on the site of infection. *E. coli* most commonly causes UTI (24%), *S. aureus* most commonly causes SSI (20%), CNS most commonly causes BSI (31%), and *S. aureus* and *P. aeruginosa* cause 19% and 17% of nosocomial LRI.

Keeping these facts in mind, infection control programs should be organized to reduce nosocomial infections as well as the spread of resistant organisms and their associated morbidity and mortality. The ultimate goal of these programs is to improve patient care, reduce hospital stays, and reduce health-care–related costs. It is estimated that one third of nosocomial infections can be prevented by well-organized infection control programs; however, less than one tenth (6% to 9%) are actually prevented.[9,30] The components of these programs crucial in reducing nosocomial infections are:

1. a trained infection control physician (hospital epidemiologist)
2. at least one infection control nurse per 250 beds
3. a computerized surveillance system
4. a system of reporting infection rates of hospitalized patients to practicing physicians and surgeons[9,30]

HISTORY

The earliest advice regarding hospital hygiene was probably written in the fourth century B.C., in the *Charaka-Samhita*, a Sanskrit textbook of medicine, based on Indian "Vedic" medicine. The following extract demonstrates the early principles of hospital infection control:

> In the first place a mansion must be constructed under the supervision of an engineer well-conversant with the science of building mansions and houses. It shall be spacious and roomy. . . . One portion at least should be open to the current wind. It should not be exposed to smoke, or dust, or injurious sound or touch or taste or form or scent. . . . After this should be secured a body of attendants of good behavior, distinguished for purity and cleanliness of habits.[10,11]

In medieval and Renaissance Europe, hospitals were overcrowded. Pioneers such as Theodoric of Bologna[12] and Casper Stromayr,[13] tried to reform hospital practice by bathing their patients or shaving the site of operation, yet met with little success. Toward the end of the eighteenth century, Madam Necker[14] proposed "nursing the sick in a single bed." Prior to this time, up to eight patients were nursed in a bed amidst appalling squalor.

Simpson,[15,16] a Scottish surgeon, demonstrated that mortality following amputation was proportional to the size of the hospital and the degree of overcrowding. In the mid-nineteenth century, Florence Nightingale published a dramatic report after her Crimean War experiences at the military hospitals. Her report demonstrated that far more soldiers died of hospital-acquired infections than died from the primary effects of battle injuries.[17] Florence Nightingale,[18] with the help of John Farr, demonstrated a direct relationship between sanitary conditions at a hospital and postoperative complications. She proposed that ward sisters maintain records of hospital patients who developed infections and introduced broad hospital hygiene, thus pioneering the concept of nosocomial infection surveillance.

During the same era, Dr. Ignatz Semmelweis, the head of obstetrical service at the Royal Lying-In Hospital of Vienna, investigated the high maternal mortality rate. He probably undertook the first hospital-based epidemiologic study.[19] He recognized that puerperal fever was higher in the ward staffed by physicians. The physicians participated in autopsies of women with puerperal sepsis and would then return to the wards to care for women in labor. He linked the increased rates to a lack of handwashing. Once handwashing was instituted as a control measure, the ward-specific excess rate of puerperal sepsis and mortality declined.[19] (See Chapter 1.)

Louis Pasteur demonstrated that air is contaminated with living germs and that growth of germs leads to spoilage.[20,21,22] Hence, Lister[23] reasoned that microbes were responsible for wound suppuration and introduced antisepsis to surgery. He proposed controlling suppuration by preventing contaminated air from coming in contact with a wound, which would directly kill organisms. Similarly, in 1895, George Emerson Brewer,[24] an American surgeon, recognized the problem of infections after surgery and undertook an intensive surveillance project to estimate the frequency of SSIs. He reported that SSI rates among patients with clean surgery were not 5% or less, but actually 39%. These findings initiated a review of surgical techniques and environmental risk factors. In 1915, Brewer[25] reported in follow-up a steady decline of SSIs to 1.2% among patients undergoing clean surgical procedures.

In 1937, with the introduction of penicillin to treat serious staphylococcal and streptococcal infections, misconceptions developed that antibiotics could control and eventually eliminate all infectious diseases. Some physicians worried less about infections because nontoxic drugs could prevent serious complications and cure infections. In the 1940s, the concept of postsurgical antibiotic prophylaxis was introduced, and the widespread use of penicillin occurred. Shortly after this widespread use of penicillin began, strains of resistant staphylococci emerged. In the late 1950s, the first epidemics of nosocomial penicillinase-producing staphylococcus were reported in Europe and North America. In these outbreaks, patients, primarily neonates admitted to hospital nurseries without infections, subsequently developed staphylococcal sepsis.[26]

In the 1970s, gram-negative organisms emerged as the most frequent cause of nosocomial infections. In the 1980s, new gram-positive organisms, specifically, CNS, methicillin-resistant *Staphylococcus aureus* (MRSA) and fungi, primarily *Candida* species,[27] emerged as important nosocomial pathogens. Since then, organisms, both bacteria and fungi, that cause nosocomial infections have become increasingly resistant to antimicrobial agents.

For example, the prevalence of MRSA among nosocomial *S. aureus* isolates has increased from 2.4% in 1975 to 29% in 1991.[5] Infections caused by MRSA are similar to those caused by methicillin-sensitive *S. aureus* (MSSA), in that they are life threatening. However, the only therapeutic option is vancomycin, the only effective antibiotic against these resistant organisms. The frequent empiric use of vancomycin has contributed to the development of vancomycin resistance among other organisms, especially enterococci. In recent years, strains of *S. aureus* with intermediate susceptibility to vancomycin or other glycopeptide antibiotics have been documented. Should glycopeptide-intermediate susceptibility (GISA) emerge as a major pathogen, we would essentially re-enter the preantibiotic era with respect to their control.

In 1959, the first infection control practitioner (ICP) was appointed in England to control hospital-acquired staphylococcus infections.[28] It was not until 1963 that a full-time practitioner was hired to control hospital infections in the United States.[29] In 1964, Boston City Hospital conducted some of the first modern prevalence studies and reported that 15% of inpatients had nosocomial infections.[30,31] By 1968, the CDC was training ICPs in surveillance, prevention, and control of nosocomial infections, and in 1969, the Joint Commission for Accreditation of Healthcare Organizations mandated that all hospitals support an infection control nurse.

The NNIS system, created in 1970, is composed of nonrandomly selected hospitals. One of the first studies, the Study on Efficacy of Nosocomial Infection Control (SENIC) was to determine whether infection surveillance and control programs reduce the rate of nosocomial infections.[32] Data from this sentinel study estimated that 2.1 million nosocomial infections occurred per year, approximately four times the number of admissions for acute myocardial infarctions. The SENIC project demonstrated that 32% of all nosocomial infections (urinary tract, surgical site, lower respiratory tract, and bloodstream) could be prevented by well-organized surveillance and control efforts.[33] In fact, those hospitals without an established infection control and surveillance program had nosocomial infection rates 30% higher than hospitals with established programs. This study concluded that four factors were essential in decreasing nosocomial infections:

1. surveillance
2. adequate numbers of trained ICPs

3. reports that "feed back" infection rates to health care providers
4. an effective and trained infection control physician (hospital epidemiologist)

METHODS

Definition

Nosocomial infections develop in patients exposed to hospitals or to medical and surgical procedures that occur in a health care environment. An infection is considered nosocomial if it develops in a patient who has been hospitalized for 48 to 72 hours and was not incubating the infection at the time of admission. Nosocomial infections may also develop after surgical procedures. Nosocomial infections may be present on admission if they were acquired during a previous admission or outpatient medical/surgical procedure. Patients can also develop nosocomial infections in long-term care facilities and be subsequently transferred to an acute-care facility. Increasingly, an infection acquired in the hospital may manifest after discharge because of shorter hospital stays and more frequent outpatient surgical procedures.

Infections are defined using a set of standard criteria that have been developed over years. The CDC has assumed a primary role in developing definitions.[146] These definitions have been tested and validated in many acute-care settings. Separate definitions have been developed for long-term care facilities. Uniform definitions are critical to following trends within hospitals and to comparing infection rates between hospitals or data systems. Although the definitions are often based on positive culture results, these definitions may also use clinical criteria to distinguish between organisms that have colonized a body site versus those that are causing infections.

Measures of Occurrence

Nosocomial infections are evaluated by calculating rates, not the number of nosocomial infections. For instance, the presence of six nosocomial infections at a large institution (bed size >500) has different implications than the same number at a small institution (bed size <25).

Crude Infection Rate

The most common measure of occurrence, the crude infection rate, is the ratio of infections per 100 admissions or discharges.

Crude infection rate =

$$\frac{\text{number of infections}}{100 \text{ admissions or discharges}}$$

The crude infection rate can also be site specific. For example,

$$\text{Crude BSI} = \frac{\text{number of BSI}}{100 \text{ admission or discharges}}$$

Adjusted Infection Rate

To derive a rate that represents changes in the nosocomial infection rate from one period to another, the crude infection rate is often adjusted by patient-days or number of procedures. This corrects for a patient being admitted in one month and discharged in another. An example of an adjusted infection rate is the ratio of infections per 1,000 patient-days or 100 surgical procedures.

Adjusted infection rate =

$$\frac{\text{number of infections}}{1,000 \text{ patient-days}}$$

or

$$\frac{\text{number of infections}}{100 \text{ surgical procedures}}$$

The crude infection rate does not adjust for risk factors for nosocomial infections that vary among patients. The risk-adjusted infection rate adjusts the rate by the major risk factor for the infections by the number of days that a medical device (central venous catheter, urinary catheter, ventilator) is used. A recent study demonstrated that data collected for institutional nosocomial infection rates should be adjusted for risk factors, an initial attempt to correct for severity of illness.[34]

Risk-adjusted infection rate =

$$\frac{\text{number of infections in question}}{\text{number of days that a device is in place}}$$

Device-Associated Infection Rates

A device-associated infection rate is a specific example of a risk-adjusted infection rate. This method also allows the calculation of the device-associated, device-day rate, which is usually expressed per 1,000 device-days.

Device-associated, device-day rate =

$$\frac{\begin{array}{c}\text{number of device-associated} \\ \text{infections for specific site}\end{array}}{\text{number of device-days}} \times 1,000$$

Before calculating the risk-adjusted infection rate, certain steps should be followed:

1. Decide on the time period for the analysis (week, month, quarter, half, or year).
2. Select the patient population (ICU, HRN).
3. Choose the site of infection that is to be calculated (numerator).

The infection selected should be site specific and should occur in the selected population; the infection onset days should occur during the time period selected. Once the device days are determined, infections such as urinary catheter–associated urinary tract infections (UTIs) would be calculated using the following formulation:

$$\frac{\begin{array}{c}\text{number of urinary} \\ \text{catheter-associated UTIs}\end{array}}{\text{number of urinary catheter-days}} \times 1,000$$

How To Calculate the Number of Days That a Device Is in Place

In January 1998, 20 patients on the first day of the month had urinary catheters; 19 on day 2; 15

on day 3; 25 on day 4; 20 on day 5; 15 on day 6; and 15 on day 7. The number of patients with urinary catheters from days 1 to 7 is added (20 + 19 + 15 + 25 + 20 + 15 + 15), yielding 129 urinary catheter-days for the first week (Table 13–2). The total catheter-days for the entire month is the sum of the daily counts.

Device-Day Utilization

To determine the percentage of patient-days to device-days, the device utilization ratio can be calculated. The device utilization day is specifically useful for measuring infection risk among patients in ICUs or HRNs.

Device utilization =

$$\frac{\text{number of device-days}}{\text{number of patient-days}}$$

To calculate the number of patient-days, let us use an example: In January 1998, 20 patients were in the unit on the first day; 20 on day 2; 18 on day 3; 25 on day 4; 24 on day 5; 20 on day 6; and 18 on day 7. To calculate the patient-days, we would add the number of patients in the unit from day 1 to day 7. The total number of patient-days for the week is 145 (Table 13–2). Thus, the patient-days are the total number of days that patients are in a unit during a selected time period. We had calculated above the total urinary catheter-days to be 129. Thus:

$$\text{Device utilization} = \frac{129}{145} = 0.8897, \text{ or } 89\%$$

Eighty-nine percent of patient days were also urinary catheter-days for the first week of the month. Calculating the device-associated, device-day rate and utilization ratio helps ICPs to evaluate how their hospital compares with the mean rates, such as those reported by the NNIS system. Some caveats apply. If the denominator is small (<50 device-days or patient-days), this ratio will not be a good estimate of the "true" device utilization. Therefore, a longer time period should be chosen. Also, not all hospitals are similar to the hospitals included in the comparison group (i.e., NNIS hospitals). If huge varia-

Table 13–2 Device Utilization Days

Day	Number of Device-Days	Number of Patient-Days
1	20	20
2	19	20
3	15	18
4	25	25
5	20	24
6	15	20
7	15	18
TOTAL	129	145

tions in hospital infection rates are noted, reasons for these variations should be explored.

Risk Stratification for Surgical Procedures

To understand better the epidemiology of nosocomial transmission, stratification of measures of occurrence by patient or surgery characteristics can be used. In 1964, the National Research Council study stratified the risk of developing an SSI and devised the traditional wound classification.[35] Based on the probability of wound contamination at the time of surgery, this classification segregates all surgical procedures into four categories: clean, clean-contaminated, contaminated, and dirty. Experts believed that clean procedures (e.g., a coronary artery bypass graft) should be associated with a low risk of SSI, whereas dirty procedures (e.g., a ruptured appendicitis) are considered infected and should have a higher risk of becoming clinically infected. However, high rates from clean SSI were encountered in some institutions, where surgeons operated on sicker and older patients or where surgeons performed more complex procedures. The traditional wound classification fails to account for host intrinsic susceptibility and the differences in the complexity of a surgical procedure.

To account for these two components, the SENIC risk index was developed and predicted the risk of SSI twice as well as the traditional wound classification had (Table 13–3).[36] These higher-risk patients represented 50% of the surgical population and included 90% of the SSI. However, the SENIC risk index measured the host susceptibility to infection, with discharge diagnoses obtainable only upon discharge of the patient, thus precluding prospective surveillance from the date of surgery. Furthermore, all surgical procedures were considered equivalent, and the index did not account for the complexity of some procedures or their duration (Figure 13–1).

In 1991, the CDC modified the SENIC risk index and renamed it the *NNIS risk index*.[37] Three components were included in the NNIS risk index (Table 13–4). According to the NNIS risk index, the risk of infection varies from a low of 1.5%, if a patient has a score of 0, to a high of 13%, if a patient has a score of 3. Nonetheless, recent data have revealed that even these more detailed indices fail to predict the risk of SSI after certain procedures.[38] For example, these indices may not reflect an increase in the infection risk associated with prolonged hospital stay or increased exposure to procedures. Other limitations include the decrease in admissions due to more outpatient procedures and early hospital discharges, which may alter the true rate, due to a change in the denominator (the number of procedures may decrease if outpatient procedures are not included in routine surveillance) or a change in the numerator (the number of infections may decrease because infections after discharge are more difficult to detect).

Incidence and Prevalence

To measure the nosocomial infection frequency at an institution, i.e., the incidence and prevalence, surveillance surveys are performed. Incidence surveys determine the rate of new infections during a given time, whereas prevalence surveys determine the proportion of patients with infections at a given point in time. To cal-

Table 13–3 SENIC Risk Index

Risk Factors	Regression Coefficients	Score
Intraabdominal procedure	1.12	
Surgical procedure lasting longer than 2 hours	1.04	
Surgical procedure classified as either contaminated or dirty by the traditional wound classification	1.04	Score up to 4 (one point for each risk factor)
Patient with three or more discharge diagnoses	0.86	

Source: Data from L. Haley et al., Identifying Patients at High Risk of Surgical Wound Infections: A Simple Ultivariate Index of Patient Susceptibility and Wound Contamination, *American Journal of Epidemiology*, Vol. 121, pp. 206–215, 1985.

culate the incidence rate (I), the number of nosocomial infections (during a given month) is divided by the number of patients discharged/admitted (during the same month), or patient-days.[28,39]

$$I = \frac{\text{number of new nosocomial infections (during a month)}}{\text{number of patients discharged / admitted (during the same month), or patient-days}}$$

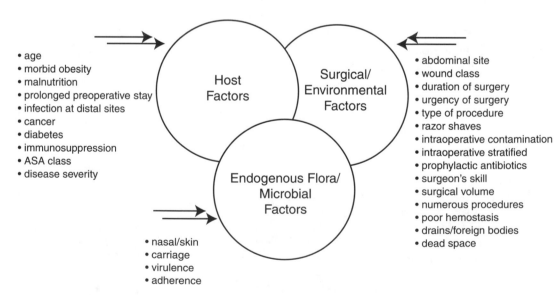

• age
• morbid obesity
• malnutrition
• prolonged preoperative stay
• infection at distal sites
• cancer
• diabetes
• immunosuppression
• ASA class
• disease severity

Host Factors

Surgical/ Environmental Factors

Endogenous Flora/ Microbial Factors

• nasal/skin
• carriage
• virulence
• adherence

• abdominal site
• wound class
• duration of surgery
• urgency of surgery
• type of procedure
• razor shaves
• intraoperative contamination
• intraoperative stratified
• prophylactic antibiotics
• surgeon's skill
• surgical volume
• numerous procedures
• poor hemostasis
• drains/foreign bodies
• dead space

Figure 13–1 Risk factors for surgical site infections. ASA, American Society of Anesthesia. *Source:* Reprinted with permission from T.M. Perl and M.C. Roy, Post-Operative Wound Infections: Risk Factors and Role of *Staphylococcus Aureus* Nasal Carriage, *Journal of Chemotherapy*, 7:Suppl. 3:29–35, © 1995.

Table 13–4 NNIS Risk Index

Risk Factors	Total Score	Risk of Infection
ASA preoperative score of 3, 4, or 5	0	1.5%
Surgical procedure lasting longer than *T* hours*	1	2.9%
Surgical procedure classified as either contaminated or	2	6.8%
dirty by the traditional wound classification	3	13.0%

Score up to 3 (1 point for each risk factor)

ASA, American Society of Anesthesia.
*T depends on the procedure being performed.

Source: Adapted with permission from C. Salemi, D. Anderson, and D. Flores, American Society of Anesthesiology Scoring Discrepancies Affecting the National Nosocomial Infection Surveillance System: Surgical-Site-Infection Risk Index Rates, *Infection Control and Hospital Epidemiology*, Vol. 18, pp. 246–247, © 1997, Slack, Inc.

In addition, incidence rates can be site or organism specific, using the number of infections at a given site in the numerator, with the denominator described above.

Prevalence surveys are designed to measure all current nosocomial infections. A prevalence survey requires planning and usually produces higher rates than do incidence surveys. This is because nosocomial infections generally are associated with longer hospitalization, so infected patients will be overrepresented in a cross-sectional survey. However, prevalence surveys are useful in large populations of high-risk patients. During a prevalence survey, infection control personnel examine all patients' medical records and interview clinical staff to identify nosocomial infections. The prevalence rate (P) is calculated by dividing the number of active (current) nosocomial infections present on a given day in hospitalized patients by the number of patients hospitalized on the same day. The prevalence rate traditionally overestimates infection rates, compared with incidence rates, but provides a picture at a single point in time.[40]

$$P = \frac{\text{number of active nosocomial infections (on a given day)}}{\text{number of patients present (on the same day)}}$$

Methods To Evaluate Risk Factors for Nosocomial Infections and the Impact of Interventions

Both observational and interventional epidemiologic studies can be used to study nosocomial infections. Observational studies, such as case control studies and cohort studies, are used to identify risk factors in outbreak investigations or epidemiologic studies and to assess outcomes. Intervention studies, such as clinical trials, are used to evaluate whether a given intervention is effective. Surveillance and outbreak investigations are routinely performed in most infection control programs. Randomized clinical trials are usually performed in infection control programs with active research programs.

Surveillance is a key component of infection control programs and is "a dynamic process for gathering, managing, analyzing and reporting data on events which occur in specific populations."[41] The building blocks of surveillance comprise:

1. collecting relevant data systematically for a specified purpose and during a defined period of time
2. managing and organizing the data
3. analyzing and interpreting the data
4. communicating the results to those empowered to make beneficial changes

This text does not permit a comprehensive discussion of surveillance. Several excellent reviews have been published recently.[1,41] Surveillance is also a method used to measure the rate of nosocomial events. The purpose of measuring the event is to determine what the baseline rate of an event is in order to compare the rate after an intervention has been instituted. Hence, surveillance may be a component of an intervention study.

The method by which cases or nosocomial infections are detected may be based on the following factors:

1. total chart review
2. selective medical record review, e.g., chart summaries—either handwritten, such as the nursing Kardex, or stored in hospital databases
3. reports of clinical symptoms from providers
4. review of microbiology reports
5. extraction of data from pharmacy records, such as antibiotic use
6. computer-based models that identify high-risk patients

Sensitivity and specificity vary for detecting nosocomial infections, when compared with the gold standard—total chart review. However, total chart review has not been shown to improve the sensitivity of detecting nosocomial infec-tions, compared with selective review of charts, based on review of microbiology reports and the nursing Kardex (74–94% vs 75–94%) and is very time intensive.[42] Case-finding methods must be applied systematically so that results are comparable over time. Most infection control practitioners choose the surveillance strategies, depending on the type of hospital, the patient population served, and the "local" epidemiology.

Outbreak investigations are the epidemiologic studies most closely identified with infection control programs, even though epidemic-related infections constitute fewer than 5% of overall nosocomial infections.[43] Outbreak investigations begin with identifying an unusual occurrence or an excessive rate of infections. Cases are defined and described in place, person, and time. Organisms should be speciated and compared for similarity, using antibiotic susceptibility and molecular technologies. If the cause of the outbreak is not overtly apparent or if a study is required to confirm the cause, a case control study is usually performed to determine risk factors.

Information on the risk factors for and the outcomes of nosocomial infection is often obtained through different types of studies. For example, knowledge of the risk factors for SSIs was obtained through a series of cohort studies in which surgical patients were followed postoperatively for SSI.[36] Information on any possible risk factors for SSI was collected on all patients in the cohort, then relative risks were calculated. The costs of nosocomial infections have been measured, using matched case control methods and cohort studies. For example, patients with nosocomial UTI were matched to controls with similar diagnoses and severity of illness, then costs and lengths of stay were compared.[44,45]

Randomized controlled trials are the best study method to prove causation; they have been used to show that sterilization/disinfection, closed urinary drainage systems, intravascular catheter care, dressing techniques, and care of respiratory therapy equipment are effective.[47] However, clinical trials have been equally important in showing what does not work. For example, a randomized clinical trial of antibiotic prophylaxis for patients with chronic urinary catheters demonstrated no difference in the rate of UTIs and febrile episodes, compared with the control group.[47]

RISK FACTORS

Hospitalized patients, in general, are at high risk for infection, due to their underlying illness (immunosuppression, diabetes); hospitalization circumstances (trauma, burns); environmental, microbiologic, and virulence factors; procedure-related interventions, such as surgery or medical care (urinary catheter, vascular catheter, ventilators); and the process of care (patient/nurse ratios, inappropriate antibiotic use). Because patient characteristics are beyond our control, reduction in nosocomial infections is best achieved by altering health care worker behaviors, procedure-related techniques and conditions, or other processes of care.

Host Factors

Host factors that contribute to hospitalized patients developing infections are extremes of age, severity of underlying illnesses, immune dysfunction (T or B cell mediated), poor nutrition, genetic factors, and loss of the body's normal protective functions (skin integrity, microbial imbalance). Extremes of age have been found to be a major significant risk factor for nosocomial infections.[34,48-51] The NNIS study indicated that 54% of the infections in adults appeared in patients aged 65 years or older.[5] Interestingly, only 23% to 24% of discharges occurred in those over 60 years of age; however, 37% to 64% of all nosocomial infections appear in this age group.[52,53]

Several studies have shown that nosocomial infections are related to underlying illness. Underlying disease, such as cancer, that causes immunosuppression can make the host highly prone to nosocomial infections. In a 2-year study[54] conducted in an oncology ICU, the over-

all infection rate was 50 per 100 patients, or 91.7 per 1,000 patient-days. Patients with granulocytopenea or acquired immune deficiency syndrome (AIDS) are immunosuppressed, exposed to many antibiotics, and hospitalized frequently for prolonged periods of time. These patients may be at a higher risk of developing nosocomial infections due to bacterial colonization and catheter placement.[55-58] Other underlying diseases put some patients at high risk for nosocomial infections. Examples are pulmonary, cutaneous, and hematologic diseases that alter host defenses by changing or modifying normal flora, breaching normal anatomic barriers, suppressing inflammatory responses, and modifying the reticuloendothelial system.[59-61]

Many different methods are currently being used to measure severity of illness; however, none is adequately validated, making nosocomial infection rates in critically ill persons difficult to use as indicators of quality of care.[62] Although one would suspect that altering the host underlying illness is important, this is rarely feasible and has not been studied. Until better measures of host factors and underlying illness can be developed, this important factor in nosocomial infections will be poorly understood.

Environment

Air, water, and the inanimate surfaces surrounding the patient are referred to as the *environment*. Contamination of the floor, walls, bed frames, chairs, water, and air of the patient's environment may lead to nosocomial infection.

Air

Malfunctioning or inadequate ventilation systems in health care facilities may not adequately filter air. *Aspergillus* species, one of the most invasive fungi, under appropriate environmental conditions can produce and disseminate several thousand spores per cubic meter of air.[63,64] These can remain suspended for long periods. Eventually, the spores settle and can contaminate surfaces. These spores remain viable for months and can become airborne when dust-generating activities are performed, such as construction or demolition. If walls or surfaces become wet and are not replaced, molds can flourish and become sources of infection.

Water

Since the etiologic agent of Legionnaires' disease was first identified in 1977,[65] numerous outbreaks of nosocomial Legionnaires' disease have been identified.[66] *Legionella* can colonize the water systems of large buildings and hospitals.[67] Hospital hot water distribution systems and water cooling towers for air conditioners have been implicated as sources of legionellosis outbreaks in patients.[68,69] Other pathogens, such as *Pseudomonas* species, *Acinetobacter* species, *Acromobacter* species, *Aeromonas hydrophila*, *Flavimonas*, certain nontuberculosis mycobacterium, and *Flavobacterium meningosepticum* have been associated with water contamination leading to infection.

Inanimate Objects

More recently, spread of resistant organisms has been linked to a contaminated environment or a fomite.[70] Both vancomycin-resistant enterococcus and MRSA have been cultured in the environment.[71–73] Also, contaminated fomites have been found to be a source of nosocomially transmitted viral respiratory infections.[74]

Microbiologic Factors

The microbiologic factors that contribute to nosocomial transmission include virulence factors, their ability to survive in the hospital environment, and antimicrobial resistance. *S. aureus* and *Pseudomonas aeruginosa* are highly virulent nosocomial pathogens; however, pathogens of low virulence can cause nosocomial infections in immunocompromised patients. Bacteria that can survive in the hospital environment can be transmitted to patients on ventilators or to those with urinary and vascular catheters. Coagulase-negative staphylococci adhere to prosthetic devices and vascular catheters; this has

become a major cause of nosocomial BSIs in patients with foreign bodies, such as prosthetic joints, valves, or permanent central venous catheters. Moreover, these pathogens live in water and soil, where they are exposed to antimicrobial substances and may develop an inherent resistance to common antibiotics. Microorganisms such as *Pseudomonas, Acinetobacter, Serratia,* and *Enterobacter* species can survive in hospital environments and can be relatively resistant to disinfectants.[75–78]

Extrinsic Factors

The extrinsic factors that contribute to nosocomial infections include medical treatment and interventions, including placement of invasive devices and operative procedures. Therapy of the patient through use of chemotherapy may cause immunosuppression and mucosal disruption and allow organisms a port of entry into the host. Equipment, such as dialysis machines or ventilators, may have complicated reservoirs, filters, or mechanisms to prevent backflow; these can malfunction and lead to organisms entering the body. Once organisms enter the body, infection may ensue. Nasogastric and endotracheal tubes have been shown to increase the risk of acquiring nosocomial pneumonia.[79] Although all of the above-mentioned extrinsic elements contribute to nosocomial infections, the most frequently implicated extrinsic factors are surgical operations and invasive devices.

In addition, the use of antibiotics can lead to imbalance in the normal symbiotic relationship of organisms in the gastrointestinal (GI) tract. As the normal state of human endogenous flora is altered, there is selective pressure in favor of antibiotic-resistant organisms. In fact, patients who received norfloxacin or fluconazole for GI tract decontamination during episodes of neutropenia[80,81] developed resistant organisms as a result of selective pressure. Organisms such as vancomycin-resistant enterococcus can proliferate when broad-spectrum antibiotics have killed the normal gastrointestinal tract gram-negative and anaerobic flora.[82]

ETIOLOGY AND TRANSMISSION

Endogenous versus Exogenous Organisms

There are four potential sources that may transmit microorganisms and lead to infections. Three of these are exogenous sources—fixed structures of the hospital, devices or instruments used at the hospital, health care personnel—and one is endogenous—the (source) patients. Exogenous infections are a direct result of pathogenic or nonpathogenic organisms directly acquired from the environment. Exogenous infections can be transmitted via the airborne route, through fomites or direct contact with carriers, by ingesting contaminated foods, or by parenteral inoculation. Endogenous source infections are divided into primary or secondary infections. Organisms that are a part of a patient's normal flora cause primary endogenous infections. Organisms that become part of the patient's flora during the hospital stay cause secondary endogenous infections.

Transmission of Microorganisms

Nosocomial transmission of organisms can be described by five routes: contact, droplet, airborne, common vehicle, and vector-borne.

Contact

The first and the most frequent route of nosocomial infections occurs by direct or indirect contact. Direct contact between body surfaces results in the transfer of microorganisms between a susceptible host and a colonized or infected individual. Direct-contact transmission usually requires personal contact. This type of transmission can occur between patient and health care provider or between two patients, with one serving as the source of the infectious microorganisms and the other as a susceptible host. Health care workers (HCWs) are important reservoirs of microorganisms. They can carry potentially infectious organisms on their hands, which can colonize their hands or nares. For example, increases in SSIs due to nasal carriage of *S. aureus* have been traced to HCWs who carry the organism.[83] Furthermore, outbreaks of *S. aureus, Candida*

albicans, and *Rhodococcus* have also occurred from colonized or infected HCWs.

Indirect-contact transmission involves contact of a susceptible host with a contaminated, usually inanimate object or with fomites (porous fungi capable of storing and transmitting infections). Fomites can be medical devices (e.g., resuscitation bags, endotracheal tubes, suction devices, ventilators, endoscopes), instruments (e.g., rectal thermometers, blood pressure cuffs, stethoscopes), dressings (especially in burn units), and toys (especially stuffed animals).[84] For example, Hughes and colleagues[85] in 1986 demonstrated that stuffed teddy bears used in a handwashing promotional campaign were heavily contaminated and colonized by organisms causing nosocomial infections.

Droplet

Infections can also be transmitted by respiratory droplets. Coughing, sneezing, and talking can produce droplets containing microorganisms. Droplets are propelled a short distance through the air and can deposit on the nasal mucosa, conjunctiva, or mouth of the host. Likewise, respiratory secretions may contain organisms that can be transmitted to HCWs or other patients while performing such tasks as suctioning or bronchoscopy. Respiratory syncitial virus and influenza are transmitted by droplets.

Airborne

Organisms are also transmitted via air (airborne), by the spread of either the evaporated airborne droplets (5 μm or smaller in size) that contain microorganisms or the dust particles with the infectious agent. These small particles can remain suspended in the air for a long period of time and can be propelled to greater distances than can droplets. Tuberculosis and viruses such as rubella and varicella are transmitted in this fashion.

Common Vehicle

Organisms can be transmitted extrinsically through common vehicles, such as food, water, medications, intravenous fluids, contaminated blood products, and medical equipment or devices.

Vector-Borne

Vector-borne transmission of microorganisms within hospitals or health care settings, is unusual in the United States. Vectors such as mosquitoes, flies, or ticks, and others can transmit microorganisms. This mode of transmission still remains a significant problem in some developing and underdeveloped countries.

TYPES OF INFECTION

Urinary Tract Infection

Definition/Impact

Nosocomial UTIs are the most common nosocomial infection in both acute and long-term health care facilities. UTIs are generally defined as bacteriuria (a single positive urine culture in patients with a urinary catheter or two positive cultures in patients without) and can be further stratified by the presence or absence of symptoms (fever, increased frequency of urination, dysuria, or suprapubic tenderness). The natural history of UTIs in patients in acute-care hospitals has been well documented.[86] The majority of bacteriuric ($>10^6$ organisms/mL of urine) patients (67%) are asymptomatic; 28% have fever or symptoms attributed to a UTI and 5% have cultured blood growing the same organism.

Risk Factors

UTIs are predominantly a device-associated infection. Five to ten percent of UTIs are associated with genitourinary manipulations, such as urologic surgery. Over 80% of UTIs are associated with indwelling urinary (Foley) catheters. The risk of UTI increases with the length of time that a urinary catheter remains in place. These catheters increase the risk for developing a UTI because they avert the normal defenses of the urologic system in multiple ways. First, bacteria can be directly inoculated into the bladder during insertion of the catheter. Second, both the inside and outside walls of the catheter serve as

conduits from the external environment to the bladder. Third, a biofilm that forms within the internal lumen of a catheter protects bacteria from antibiotics. Fourth, the catheters damage the glycosaminoglycan layer of the bladder and blunt the white blood cell immune response to infection. Finally, residual urine from the bladder that does not completely drain serves as a reservoir for bacterial growth.

Microbiology

Aerobic gram-negative rods, such as *Escherichia coli*, are the most common cause of urinary tract infection. They are usually acquired from the endogenous colonic flora of the patient. However, bacteria that are acquired after exposure to the health care environment and become part of the colonic flora, such as multiple antibiotic-resistant enterococci, can also cause UTI. The most common organisms causing urinary tract infections are shown in Table 13–5.[1,5]

Interventions

Preventing UTI in acute- and long-term care patients involves preventing bacteriuria. This can be done by:

1. avoiding indwelling urinary catheters and using alternatives, including condom catheters, suprapubic catheters, and intermittent catheterization
2. maintaining a closed drainage system for the urinary catheter
3. minimizing the duration of the catheterization

Interestingly, neither treating meatal colonization nor suppressing bacteriuria through bladder irrigation with polymyxin-neomycin or through the addition of hydrogen peroxide into the collection bag has been shown to decrease the risk of urinary infection.[88–90] In fact, antibiotic treatment of bacteriuria did not alter the rate of febrile episodes in a randomized control trial but increased the numbers of antibiotic-resistant bacteria isolated from urine cultures.[47] Therefore, the treatment of asymptomatic bacteriuria is not recommended.

Table 13–5 Most Common Organisms Causing UTIs

Setting	Microorganism(s) in Descending Order
Hospital	*Escherichia coli* Enterococci *Pseudomonas aeruginosa* *Candida* species
Intensive care unit	*Candida* species *E. coli*, enterococci *P. aeruginosa*
Long-term care facility	*E. coli* *P. aeruginosa* *Proteus mirabilis* *Providencia stuartii*

Source: Data from W.T. Hughes et al, The Nosocomial Colonization of Teddy Bears, *Infection Control*, Vol. 7, pp. 495–500, © 1986.

In summary, UTIs are the most common nosocomial infection in both acute-care and long-term care facilities. The overwhelming majority of UTIs is associated with use of a urinary catheter. Prevention should be aimed at minimizing urinary catheter use and decreasing the duration of catheterization.

Lower Respiratory Infection or Pneumonia

Impact

Approximately 300,000 cases of LRI (of the bronchi and lungs) occur each year in the United States.[91] One percent of all patients admitted to an acute-care institution developed pneumonia or bronchitis.[92,93] Nosocomial pneumonia occurs in 6 per 1,000 discharges and is the second most common nosocomial infection.[1,94,95] Of all the nosocomial infections in the United States, 18% involve the lower respiratory tract.[1,94,96,97] Up to 28.7% of patients in ICUs develop pneumonia.[98] The crude mortality rate of nosocomial pneumonia is between 20% and 50%, and the attributable mortality rate is between 30% and 33%.[93,99–106]

making it one of the most fatal nosocomial infections (Table 13–1).

Microbiology

The most common pathogens isolated from the lower respiratory tract are *S. aureus* (19%), *P. aeruginosa* (17%), and *Enterobacter* species (11%).[1,5] Trends of common pathogens isolated from 1980 to 1996 are shown in Table 13–6. Nosocomial pneumonia among immunocompromised hosts can be caused by inhalation of aerosols or droplets contaminated with *Legionella* species, *Aspergillus* species, respiratory syncytial virus (RSV), or influenza virus.[107–109] RSV and influenza A have emerged as important pathogens in recent years,[110,111] and outbreaks of nosocomial pneumonia have been documented from both of these agents.[110,112]

Risk Factors

Risk factors for developing nosocomial pneumonia include severe underlying illness, extremes of age, chronic lung disease, immunosuppression, depressed sensorium, use of histamine type 2 blockers, large volume aspiration, mechanically assisted ventilation, frequent changes of ventilator circuits (24 hours vs 48 hours), cardiopulmonary disease surgery (particularly high abdominal or thoracic incisions), presence of an intracranial pressure monitor, and fall or winter season.[93,113–120] Patients at highest risk of infection are mechanically ventilated, although they do not represent the majority of nosocomial pneumonias. Intubation increases the risk of developing nosocomial pneumonia at least fourfold[121] and increases mortality by 55%.[120] Once the first lines of host defenses are breached by intubation and placement of an endotracheal tube, patients tend to aspirate nonpathogenic bacteria that colonize the oropharynx or upper GI tract.[122]

Definition

Defining pneumonia has been a challenge because the findings are frequently nonspecific, and laboratory and radiographic findings may lag behind other physical findings or mimic

Table 13–6 Hospital-Acquired Pneumonia: Microbiology

Nosocomial Infection Surveillance (NNIS) System

Pathogen	1980–1995	1986–1990	1990–1996
Pseudomonas aeruginosa	17%	17%	17%
Staphylococcus aureus	13%	16%	19%
Enterobacter spp.	6%	11%	11%
Klebsiella spp.	12%	17%	8%

Source: Reprinted with permission from *American Journal of Infection Control*, Vol. 24, p. 380, © 1996, Mosby, Inc.

other diseases. Furthermore, colonization of the trachea with normal pathogenic organisms frequently occurs in hospitalized patients, many of whom are febrile for other reasons. Patients who develop a nosocomial pneumonia while in an acute-care hospital may develop a cough, purulent sputum with potential pathogenic bacteria in significant numbers, radiograph abnormalities, temperature of $\geq 38°$ C, and physical findings consistent with pneumonia. Any of the aforementioned criteria, including radiograph and clinical findings, are sufficient to diagnose an LRI. In neonates, radiograph findings with evidence of pneumonia alone are sufficient for the diagnosis of LRI.

Interventions

To prevent nosocomial pneumonia, the CDC recommends interventions to decrease aspiration by the patient (raising the head of bed) and prevent colonization or cross-contamination by hands of heath care workers, appropriate disinfection, appropriate sterilization of devices (especially respiratory therapy), timely vaccination, and education of patient and hospital staff.[123] The role of oral decontamination and empiric antibiotics remains controversial.

Surgical Site Infection

Impact

Each year, over 23,000,000 people undergo surgery in the United States.[124] In the United States, SSI is the third most frequent nosocomial infection, responsible for 29% of all nosocomial infections and 14% of all nosocomial adverse events.[125] SSIs cause significant morbidity and account for 55% of all the extra hospital days attributed to nosocomial infections.[126] Recent studies have demonstrated that the average SSI prolongs the hospital stay by 7.4 days.[127] These infections are estimated to cost $3,152 per infection and contribute to 42% of total extra charges attributed to nosocomial infections (Table 13–1).[128] Furthermore, SSI causes almost 2% of all deaths in the United States.[129] These numbers highlight the tremendous burden of these infections and the importance of controlling them. Because of the frequency, morbidity, mortality, and economic burden of these infections, Haley and colleagues[33] recommended that SSI should be given the highest priority for surveillance, and at least 50% of the infection control time should be directed to this activity.

Microbiology

Only 33% to 67% of infected wounds are cultured.[130] Among those, 15% to 20% of SSI are caused by *S. aureus*; whereas enterococcus and CNS species account for 15% each.[129] The remainder of SSIs are caused by gram-negative organisms and yeast. The infecting organisms vary according to the site of the surgical incision.

Risk Factors

Risk factors (Figure 13–1)[131] that increase a patient's risk of developing an SSI can be categorized as those associated with the host, those related to the surgical procedure or to the environment, and those related to the organism. The patient's risk may increase if he or she has more than one risk factor. Some mathematical models have been developed, but because they have not been validated, their widespread use in clinical medicine has not occurred.

Host Risk Factors

Patient characteristics, including the underlying medical condition(s) and the severity of the underlying disease, can increase the risk of developing an SSI. Very few controlled studies have examined the relative importance of these risk factors. Those risk factors that definitely increase the risk of developing an SSI include morbid obesity, old age, diabetes mellitus, severe underlying illness, a prolonged preoperative hospital stay, or a preoperative infection.[131,132] Several studies show that patients who are malnourished, have low albumin, have cancer, or are receiving immunosuppressive therapy are at increased risk.[134] Unfortunately, it is frequently difficult to ameliorate these risks. Occasionally, the patient's surgery is not urgent, and the health problems, such as diabetes, can be controlled or the patient surgery can be delayed until the patient's health improves. Nonetheless, studies demonstrating that reversal of these conditions reduces SSI rates have not been done.

Operative and Perioperative Risk Factors

Certain practices and procedures that occur in the operating room or during the perioperative period can increase the risk of SSI. In some cases, health care workers can alter their practices and possibly the patient's outcome. Those surgical and environmental factors that may alter the patient's risk of developing an SSI include a wound classified as contaminated or dirty, a surgical procedure involving the abdomen, a long surgical procedure, hair removal by razor (especially the night before surgery, so that preoperative colonization occurs), multiple surgical procedures, poor hemostasis during the

procedure with blood loss and the need for transfusions, presence of drains, dead space, a less-skilled or inexperienced surgeon, a low intraoperative body temperature, internal fixation of fractures, and spine fusion.[133]

Although the definition of a SSI has been debated for years, for the purposes of surveillance, a reasonable definition is used to analyze rates and to examine for trends over time. Ideally, the definition chosen should remain unchanged in order to compare data throughout the years and to see that interventions implemented reduce these rates. In 1992, a consensus group that included the Centers for Disease Control (CDC), the Society for Hospital Epidemiology of America (SHEA), and the Surgical Infection Society (SIS), modified how SSI was defined, and changed the name to surgical site infection.[135] SSIs are divided into incisional and organ-space SSIs. Incisional SSIs are further classified as involving only the skin and subcutaneous tissue (superficial incisional SSIs) or involving deep soft tissues of the incision (deep incisional SSIs). Superficial infections require that at least one of the following occur within 30 days of the operation:

- pus appears from incision
- organisms are isolated aseptically from cultured fluid or tissue
- at least one of the following: pain or tenderness, localized swelling, redness, or heat when the surgeon deliberately opens the surgical wound
- the surgeon or attending physicians diagnose the infection

SSI secondary to prosthetic devices can occur up to 1 year after the operation.

Interventions

The single most important intervention is the appropriate use and timing of perioperative antibiotic prophylaxis.[136] Pathogens that infect surgical sites during surgical procedures can be acquired from the patient, the hospital environment, or personnel. The patient's endogenous flora is responsible for most infections. In surgical procedures involving the GI, respiratory, genital, and urinary tracts, antibiotic prophylaxis has proven efficacious in reducing SSI. For most clean wound procedures, antibiotic prophylaxis is still controversial, although experts suggest giving patients prophylactic antibiotics when a foreign body implant is inserted or if an infection occurring in a "clean" procedure would be associated with severe or life-threatening consequences (e.g., valve replacement). Finally, if the perioperative antibiotic is administered after the incision, the risk of an SSI increases sixfold above the risk when it is administered 2 hours or less before the incision.[136]

Most exogenous wound contamination occurs during the operation through contact or airborne transmission of organisms; hence, events occurring after the operation (e.g., ward dressings and isolation techniques) are less likely to contribute to SSI.

Perhaps the single most important intervention to reduce nosocomial SSI is reporting surgeon-specific SSI rates. Programs that perform surveillance of wound infection rates may reduce SSI rates as much as 35% by reporting the rates associated with specific surgical teams.[135] To save resources, some programs have adopted methods that group the entire surgical population into patients who are at high or low risk of developing SSI.

One of the major challenges in infection control is deciding when to include postdischarge surveillance for detecting SSI. Recent data[37,130,137–140] show that patients are developing SSI after their discharge from the hospital (Table 13–7). Thus, surveying each patient for a defined period after their surgery should be incorporated into surveillance strategies. Telephone surveys and questionnaires sent to patients and/or physicians have been used. It is still unclear which method provides the most accurate data.[135] These studies show that SSI after either clean or clean-contaminated procedures is most likely to occur after hospital discharge, thus supporting the need for continuing surveillance after discharge.

Bloodstream Infections

Impact

Nosocomial BSIs cause about 14.2% of all nosocomial infections,[5] leading to 62,500 deaths per year[141] and accounting for $3.5 billion in cost related to excess hospital stay.[142] Between 1977 and 1981, Bryant and colleagues[143] reviewed bacteremias in over 300,000 patients discharged

Table 13–7 Percentage of SSI Detected after Discharge

Author (Year) Reference	Patient Population	% SSI Detected after Discharge
Sands (1996)[137]	Non obstetrical	84
Roy (1994)[138]	CABG*	52
Simchen (1992)[419]	Hernioraphy	51
Hulton (1992)[420]	Caesarian section	59
Weigelt (1992)[421]	General surgery	35
Law (1990)[422]	Elective procedures	59
Manian (1990)[130]	All procedures	20
Olson (1990)[423]	All procedures	30
Krukowski (1988)[424]	Appendectomy	50
Reimer (1987)[425]	All procedures	71
Brown (1987)[426]	Major procedures	46

*CABG, coronary artery bypass graft.

from four major acute-care hospitals; 51% of the bacteremias were acquired nosocomially and carried a 50% higher risk of mortality, compared with the community-acquired BSI. The crude mortality is between 25% and 50%, and the direct or attributable mortality averages about 27% to 35% in critically ill patients.[142,144] Nosocomial BSI are more common in ICUs, occurring two to seven times more often than on the ward.[144–146] Furthermore, the risk of developing nosocomial BSI increases in patients admitted to a surgical ICU (SICU), compared with those admitted to other ICUs.[106,144,146] Pittet and colleagues[144] estimated the cost attributable to a nosocomial BSI in a SICU patient to be $40,000.

The rates of nosocomial BSI vary by:

1. the type of population admitted to the hospital
2. the size of the hospital
3. the type of hospital (teaching vs nonteaching)
4. the length of hospital stay
5. the location within the hospital

NNIS data[147] from 1980 to 1989 demonstrated that BSI rates were the highest for large teaching facilities and lowest for small nonteaching facilities. During the 9-year study period, significant increases (p <0.0001) in nosocomial BSI were observed, regardless of hospital size. Although the rates were reported to be the highest in large teaching facilities, the overall increase in primary nosocomial BSI was the highest in small nonteaching hospitals (279%), followed by large nonteaching (196%), small teaching (124%), and large teaching hospitals (70%). The increase in overall nosocomial BSI could be due to a variety of factors, including host and laboratory factors and changes in health care delivery patterns. Studies[51,52,148,149] have demonstrated that elderly patients are at higher risk for nosocomial BSI. Populations are living longer, and there is an increase in older patients being admitted to hospitals who have severe underlying conditions, poor nutritional status, limited mobility, and poor host defenses, making them susceptible for developing nosocomial BSI. Another factor

accounting for the higher rates could be increased recognition of BSI through improved culture techniques in laboratories and increased frequency of blood cultures.

Definitions

Nosocomial BSI can be divided into primary and secondary types of infections. Primary BSI is caused by an unrecognized focus of infection. Bloodstream infections that are secondary to intravenous (IV) or arterial lines are considered primary bacteremias.[150] It is estimated that 50,000 to 100,000 catheter-related BSIs occur in the United States each year.[151] Two thirds of BSI are primary in origin, and 19% of them are caused by an IV or arterial line.[152] Staphylococci cause 74% of the IV or arterial line–related BSI. About 90% of intravenous catheter-related[151] BSIs are associated with central lines. Secondary sources cause 38% of nosocomial BSI. Secondary BSIs develop following a documented infection with the same organism at another anatomic site.[150] Sources for secondary BSI include LRIs, UTIs, SSIs, and infections of GI origin.[152] Nosocomial BSIs can be further subdivided as:

1. transient, that which follow manipulation of a nonsterile mucosal surface (perhaps associated with acute infection)
2. intermittent, that which clear, then recur (e.g., undrained abdominal abscess)
3. continuous, such as those due to endocarditis or suppurative thrombophlebitis

Microbiology

Coagulase-negative staphylococcus is the most common pathogen causing BSI (NNIS, January 1990–March 1996) and is isolated 31% of the time. *S. aureus* caused 16% of infections, enterococcus 9%, *Candida* species 8%, *Klebsiella pneumoniae* 5%, *Enterobacter* species 4%, and others 27%.[98] The most common nosocomial fungal cause of BSIs is *Candida* species, with an estimated overall crude mortality rate of 40% to 60%.[153] *Candida* has become the fourth most common isolate recovered from blood cultures in recent years.[153] Also, a noticeable shift toward non-*albicans Candida* species has been observed.[154–156] The attributable mortality of nosocomial BSI associated with IV catheters is between 12% and 28%.[157,158] The mortality attributable to nosocomial BSI due to particular organisms has been studied using matched case control studies. A 38% attributable mortality is reported for *Candida* species, 31% for enterococcus, and 14% for CNS.[157,159,160] All cultured blood–growing organisms should be evaluated carefully, even in the absence of clinical signs or symptoms. *Candida* species, gram-negative rods, and *S. aureus* in the blood should always be considered true pathogens. Coagulase-negative staphylococci, *Corynebacterium* species, and enterococci may represent skin contaminants. Helpful clues include cultured blood that grow organisms within 48 hours, at least 2 bottles growing the organisms and isolation of the identical organism from another sterile body fluid.

Risk Factors

Risk factors for BSI vary with underlying disease and include age greater than 65 years or less than 1 year, preexisting comorbid illness (or illness severity),[161] immunosuppression, a diagnosis of cancer, malnutrition, having multiple trauma, burns, being admitted to an ICU, long hospital stay, a surgical operation, a complicated surgery,[161] receiving antimicrobial therapy, a decreased nurse/patient ratio, and male gender.[162] One study[163] in adults at a cancer center using a multivariate analysis model showed that having a central venous catheter, poor performance status, weight loss, hematologic disease, and receiving previous antimicrobial therapy were risk factors that independently influenced outcome. Central lines have been found to be a risk factor in many settings. Among neonates in HRNs, umbilical or central IV catheters are major risk factors for BSI.[164] *Candida* species infections, for example, are more common in children with a central venous catheter placed in the femoral vein, a tunneled central venous catheter, and prolonged hyperalimentation.[165] In all patients,

predisposing factors for candidemia are similar and include acute leukemia, leukopenia, burns, GI disease, prematurity, treatment with multiple antibiotics, having a Hickman catheter, hemodialysis, and isolation of *Candida* species from anatomic sites other than the blood. A reduction in the nurse/patient ratio has been shown to be an independent risk factor for central line–associated BSIs.[166]

Interventions

Control measures for minimizing nosocomial BSI include meticulous care of intravenous catheters. Meier and colleagues[167] demonstrated that primary BSI decreased by 35% (from 1.1 to 0.7 infections per 1,000 patient-days) after the introduction of a dedicated IV therapy team. Another study[166] showed that the introduction of an IV therapy team decreased IV-related bacteremias from 4.6 to 1.5 per 1,000 patient discharges. The best approach is to use principles of basic asepsis, such as appropriate handwashing, proper disinfection of site of entry using maximum sterile barriers while inserting lines, the use of topical antimicrobials at the insertion site, timely checking and changing of dressing, and the use of subcutaneous tunnel insertion for central venous catheters. Technique has also been shown to be important in preventing catheter-related infections. Currently, central catheters are left in place unless the patient develops systemic signs and symptoms of an infection or the site becomes erythematous, tender, or purulent. Changes over guidewires of noninfected lines are permitted. However, all central catheters should be placed using maximal barrier precautions (gown, gloves, and mask).[161] In contrast, peripheral catheters are changed every 72 hours and are placed under sterile conditions but maximal barriers are not used. The CDC recommendations[161] for the prevention of vascular catheter–related infections contains pertinent information that could help reduce catheter-related infections. Finally, the procedures that ensure sterile preparation of infusates and resources that provide patient-specific equipment are also important in preventing BSIs.

In summary, nosocomial BSIs are associated with high morbidity and mortality, as well as cost. Infection control staff must perform active surveillance of patients with central venous catheters and report the rates of these infections to health care providers. Surveillance helps to identify potential infection clusters, promoting timely intervention, as well as aiding in determination of endemic rates of nosocomial BSI. Finally, and most important, clinicians must be aware of the clinical, epidemiologic, and microbiologic features of device-related BSI. These strategies might help to reduce nosocomial BSIs.

Other

Gastroenteritis and GI Infections

Nosocomial GI tract infections (unexplained diarrhea with or without an etiologic agent lasting 2 or more days in a hospitalized patient)[150,168] are a major source of morbidity and mortality, especially in children and in patients in the developing world. Hospitalized patients with diarrhea can become dehydrated, which may lead to a prolonged hospital stay. In the United States, nosocomial gastroenteritis infections occur in 10.5 per 10,000 patients discharged in the NNIS study (1985–1994 data). The infection rate varies by service and subspecialty service (Tables 13–8 and 13–9). In the underdeveloped world, the rate of this infection is substantially higher.

Definitions. As with other nosocomial infections, one must determine the incubation period of the suspected agent. Diarrhea should be defined using appropriate information about stool frequency and consistency. Other common causes of diarrhea must be ruled out, such as antacids, laxatives, cytotoxic drugs, and enteral hyperalimentation fluids.

Microbiology. Nosocomial diarrhea can be infectious or related to antibiotics. The etiologic agent can be identified in 97% of the patients who are appropriately investigated; 93% of nosocomial gastroenteritis is caused by bacterial agents, of which *Clostridium difficile* and rotavirus cause most infections. However, in pediatric hospitals or hospitals with immunocompromised patients, the role of viral agents[169–172] is underestimated unless the institution has access to laboratory methods to diagnose viral agents. Bacterial agents such as salmonella can cause severe nosocomial outbreaks and are more common outside of North America and Europe.[173,174]

Risk Factors. Risk factors for nosocomial GI tract infections include extremes of age, achlorhydria, gastrectomy and antacid use (reduction in gastric acidity helps pathogens reach the small

---

Table 13–8 Nosocomial Gastroenteritis Infection Rate by Service

Nosocomial Infection Surveillance (NNIS) System Hospitals 1985–1994

Service	Number of Infections	Rate per 10,000
Medicine	3610	15.0
Surgery	2201	12.0
Pediatric	392	10.7
Gynecology	138	5.1
Newborn	185	2.8
Obstetrics	78	1.0

Source: Adapted from S.T. Cookson, J.M. Hughes, and W.R. Jarvis, Nosocomial Gastroenteritis Infections, In *Prevention and Control of Nosocomial Infections*, 3rd edition, R.P. Wenzel, ed., © 1997, Williams & Wilkins.

Table 13–9 Nosocomial Gastroenteritis Infection Rate by Subspecialty Service

Nosocomial Infection Surveillance (NNIS) System Hospitals 1985–1994

Subspecialty Service	Number of Infections	Rate per 10,000
Burn/trauma	53	23.5
General surgery	1365	20.2
High-risk nursery	120	19.2
Oncology	365	19.1
Cardiac surgery	189	17.1
Medicine	3245	14.9
Orthopedic surgery	325	7.9
Genitourinary surgery	111	6.4
Neurosurgery	95	6.1

Source: S.T. Cookson, J.M. Hughes, and W.R. Jarvis, Nosocomial Gastroenteritis Infections, In *Prevention and Control of Nosocomial Infections*, 3rd edition, R.P.Wenzel, ed., © 1997, Williams & Wilkins.

bowel), reduced intestinal motility, alterations in the normal intestinal flora (antimicrobial therapy), and placement of a nasogastric feeding tube. The major route of transmission is fecal-oral, typically involving either spread of pathogens from person to person (direct or indirect) or in a common vehicle. Contamination of the environment has been demonstrated to be a risk factor for nosocomial transmission of agents such as *C. difficile*. In outbreaks, common-vehicle transmission has been documented, but contact spread remains the most important route for endemic disease.

Interventions. The fecal-oral route is the most important mode of transfer of enteric infections. Thus, the most important control measure is handwashing. Handwashing with soap alone can reduce enteric contaminants to a level that might not be harmful to healthy individuals. Handwashing with antiseptic soap can be used when caring for debilitated or immunocompromised patients or newborn infants, because these patients are susceptible to low doses of innoculum. Surveillance of food handling facilities must be carried out routinely by ICPs. Surveillance must include observation of food preparation, disinfection of kitchen devices, and

education of food handlers. Food handlers with active diarrhea must be removed from food handling until diarrhea resolves and stool cultures are negative. Pathogens such as enterotoxigenic *E. coli* are transmitted by food and water; thus, proper food handling techniques and chlorination of water supplies would prevent disease. *Shigella* are primarily transmitted by person-to-person contact. All persons who are culture-positive for *Shigella* should be treated with antibiotics. Salmonellosis outbreaks have been associated with contaminated colonoscopes and biopsy forceps.[175,176]

Eye Infections

Impact. Infections of the eye account for 0.5% of all nosocomial infections (0.24 per 10,000 discharges) and primarily occur in specialized hospitals.[177] Still, because they involve a sensory organ and can cause long-term debilitating effects, they are important. These infections are most frequent on pediatric units and occur at a rate of 1.8% per 10,000 discharges.

Microbiology. The most common pathogens include *S. aureus* (24%), coagulase-negative staphylococci (23%), *P. aeruginosa* (13%), *Streptococcus* species (8%), and *E. coli* (7%).

Definitions.   Ocular infections are categorized as surgical or nonsurgical. Surgical nosocomial eye infections are further classified into five categories: preseptal or orbital cellulitis, dacryocystitis, episcleritis, keratitis, and endophthalmitis. Endophthalmitis is the most devastating infectious complication of ocular surgery.[178] Nonsurgical-related nosocomial eye infections are further divided into five categories: blepharitis, conjunctivitis, keratitis, retinochoroiditis, and endophthalmitis. Conjunctivitis is the most commonly encountered nonsurgical nosocomial eye infection and most frequently occurs in the newborn.[179,180] The pathogens most commonly identified as causing nosocomial conjunctivitis include *Chlamydia trachomatis*, *Staphylococcus* species, and *Neisseria gonorrhoeae*. Outbreaks of nosocomial conjunctivitis usually have a viral etiology and are usually concurrent with community epidemics.[181] The most common causative agent is adenovirus type 8.[182]

Interventions.   A formal set of infection control policies and procedures has been shown to reduce the number of nosocomial ocular outbreaks.[183] Thus, implementation of routine infection control guidelines and appropriate disinfection of instruments can be effective control measures.

Central Nervous System Infections

Nosocomial infections involving the central nervous system are very serious, if not life threatening. These infections can arise from superficial wounds, foreign bodies (ventricular shunts), and the deep structures of the brain parenchyma. The overall incidence is 0.56 per 10,000 hospital discharges. However, the rates are higher on pediatric services (3.3 per 10,000 discharges), HRNs (2.1 per 10,000 discharges), and neurosurgical services (1.7 per 10,000 discharges). NNIS data (1975–1982) demonstrated a 15% mortality rate in patients with nosocomial central nervous system infections. Mortality related to nosocomial meningitis not associated with prosthetic devices ranges between 20% and

67%.[184–189] The most common pathogens causing central nervous system injection include coagulase-negative staphylococci (31%), gram-negative bacilli (27%) and streptococci (18%), and *S. aureus* (11%).[1]

Definitions.   Nosocomial central nervous system infections can be divided into surgical or device-related and nonsurgical-related infections. The surgical or device-related infections, i.e., SSIs, can be further categorized into three groups: organ space infections, such as meningitis/ventriculitis; superficial infections involving the skin; or deep infections involving the brain.[135] Meningitis/ventriculitis is associated with ventriculostomies; superficial and deep SSIs with subarachnoid bolts, brain abscess, subdural empyemas, and epidural abscess; and meningoencephalitis with corneal/dural implants. Nosocomial meningitis can be associated with parameningeal infections and brain abscesses that occur after head trauma, neuroinvasive procedures, sepsis, high-rish neonates, and immunosuppression.

Risk Factors.   Risk factors for nosocomial central nervous system infections are age, gender, poor physical status, underlying disease, poor nutritional status, presence of other remote infections, long preoperative stay, emergency surgical procedure, hair removal by shaving, surgeon, type of operation and skill of the surgeon, site of surgery, whether gloves were punctured, postoperative cerebrospinal fluid leak, paranasal entry, placement of a foreign body, and use of postoperative drains.[189–192]

Interventions.   Control measures include strict antiseptic preparation of skin and the use of clippers rather than shaving, meticulous surgical technique, minimization of the duration of surgery, limiting of preoperative stay, and proper use of drains. Prophylactic use of antibiotics such as cefazolin is indicated for some neurosurgical procedures and in institutions with infection rates greater than or equal to 10%.[193] Finally, adherence to infection control practices should decrease the rates of these infections.

EMERGING AND RE-EMERGING PATHOGENS

Emerging and re-emerging pathogens encompass both community-acquired and hospital-acquired microorganisms and include bacteria, fungi, and viruses. New organisms are becoming important causes of nosocomial infections, old organisms have re-emerged as nosocomial agents, and nonbacterial organisms are assuming an increasingly important role. Increased resistance or changes in resistance patterns frequently appear first in health care settings. Resistance develops under the selective pressure of antibiotics, by transfer of plasmids or chromosomal DNA, or by genetic mutation. Resistance can occur as a result of a single genetic change or can require a series of changes. Gram-positive bacteria, such as *S. aureus, Enterococcus faecium, Staphylococcus epidermidis*, and *Streptococcus pneumoniae,* have become resistant to commonly used antimicrobial agents such as oxacillin, penicillin, and vancomycin. Resistance tends to occur to multiple antibiotics. In fact, once an organism is resistant to one antibiotic in a class, it usually is resistant to all antibiotics in that class. Gram-negative bacteria, such as *Enterobacter cloacae, Klebsiella pneumoniae, P. aeruginosa*, and *E. coli,* have also become resistant to antimicrobial agents such as imipenem and ceftazidime. Fungi such as *C. albicans* are becoming resistant to some antifungal agents. The epidemiology of MRSA, vancomycin-resistant *E. faecium* (VRE), and *S. pneumoniae* are discussed, then general measures to prevent the emergence of resistant bacteria are reviewed.

Methicillin-Resistant *S. aureus*

Staphylococcus aureus is a gram-positive bacteria that colonizes the anterior nares and is a common cause of skin and soft tissue infections, BSIs, and nosocomial pneumonia. MRSA is similar to methicillin-sensitive *S. aureus* (MSSA) in its transmission and ability to cause infection, but it is resistant to oxacillin, nafcillin, and commonly cephalosporins, and erythromycin. The prevalence of MRSA continues to increase. Among *S. aureus* isolates causing nosocomial infections, MRSA increased from 2.4% in 1975 to 29% in 1991 in NNIS hospitals.[5] MRSA is more common in large hospitals with more than 500 beds, where 38% of *S. aureus* isolates are resistant to methicillin.[1] Risk factors for acquiring MRSA include prolonged hospitalization, exposure to antibiotics, and the presence of other patients with MRSA colonization or infection in the hospital.

MRSA are of interest to ICPs because they increase the overall nosocomial infection rate.[194] Infections with MRSA do not replace MSSA infections. Second, MRSA causes life-threatening infections; mortality from MRSA infections may be greater than that from MSSA infections. Third, vancomycin, a glycopeptide antibiotic, is the only drug useful to treat MRSA infections. The continued use of vancomycin may promote the growth of vancomycin-resistant organisms, such as vancomycin-resistant enterococci (VRE) and *S. aureus* with intermediate susceptibility to vancomycin or other glycopeptide antibiotics (VISA/GISA). The high prevalence of MRSA in a facility increases the use of vancomycin. Finally, a large burden of infectious MRSA represent a failure of infection control practices.

Vancomycin-Resistant Enterococcus

Vancomycin-resistant enterococci are another emerging pathogen that cause an increasing proportion of nosocomial enterococcal infections; of which two species are primary human pathogens, *E. faecalis* and *E. faecium* (most VRE are *E. faecium*). NNIS reports a 20-fold increase in VRE nosocomial infections from 1989 to 1993.[195] The overall percentage of nosocomial enterococcal isolates resistant to vancomycin increased from 0.3% to 7.3% and from 0.4% to 13.6% among ICU patients. Most nosocomial isolates resistant to vancomycin have been reported in patients in the Northeast and the Mid-Atlantic regions of the United States. Furthermore, recent data from the SCOPE hospital consortium report that 17% of nosocomial enterococcal bloodstream isolates were vancomycin resistant.[196] Although this study found the highest prevalence in the Northeast United States, it also found that 16% of enterococcal isolates from the Southwest United States, 5% from the Northwest United States, and 4% from the Southeast United States were resistant to vancomycin. Among bone marrow transplant patients, the attributable mortality of VRE bacteremia is estimated to be 38%.[197]

Enterococci are normal inhabitants of the GI tract and cause nosocomial urinary tract, bloodstream, wound, and intraabdominal infections. Although less virulent than *S. aureus*, enterococci are intrinsically resistant to multiple antibiotics. Treatment of infected patients using a penicillin and an aminoglycoside are required to kill the organism and to improve clinical outcomes.

Numerous outbreaks of VRE infection or colonization have been reported,[198–202] most commonly in patients on oncology services. Patients with serious underlying illness who have received multiple antibiotics, including vancomycin, cephalosporins, and antianaerobic drugs and who are colonized with VRE are at risk for developing a clinically significant VRE infection. Other risk factors for infection include underlying disease (AIDS, *C. difficile* diarrhea, mucositis, malignancies, immonosuppression, neutropenia), having received a bone marrow transplant, extended duration of vancomycin and antibiotic therapy, surgery, having a central line, characteristics of the patient's hospitalization (duration, ICU, transplant service, oncology, nursery), and contamination of the environment (proximity to VRE-colonized patient, equipment, electronic thermometer, ear oximeter).[200–205]

One of the primary reasons that VRE is worrisome is the potential to transfer vancomycin or glycopeptide resistance genes to other bacteria. If glycopeptide resistance spreads to MRSA, the resulting organism, glycopeptide-resistant *S. aureus*, would be a virulent organism, resistant to all available antibiotics. Transfer of glycopeptide resistance genes to *S. aureus* has occurred in the laboratory, although this phenomenon has not been documented in the clinical setting. However, *S. aureus* is already developing increased resistance to vancomycin. Six patients with infection due to *S. aureus* isolates showing intermediate susceptibility to vancomycin have been reported.[206–211] The first case was reported in Japan in 1997, when a young boy's SSI did not respond to 29 days of vancomycin treatment.[207,208] Subsequently, three other cases were reported in the United States and one in France. The sixth case was reported in February of 1999 in Hong Kong. In all cases, patients had been on long-term vancomycin or teichoplanin for MRSA infections.[206] More recent data, however, suggest these organisms evolved from MRSA.

Streptococcal Pneumonia

Streptococcus pneumoniae is a gram-positive bacteria that colonizes the naso- and oropharynx and causes respiratory infections, otitis media, sinusitis, BSI, pneumonia, and meningitis. Traditionally, pneumococci have been exquisitely susceptible to penicillin and other beta-lactams. However, penicillin-resistant pneumococcal isolates have been detected and are becoming increasingly prevalent.[212] Adults who had received a beta-lactam antibiotic during a previous hospitalization have been shown to be at increased risk for colonization or infection with penicillin-resistant *S. pneumoniae*.[213] Also, attendance in a day-care center and frequent antibiotic use are risk factors for penicillin-resistant *S. pneumoniae* colonization or infection.[214]

Control Measures

Two themes recur throughout this discussion of emerging and resistant pathogens: the control of antibiotic use and the prevention of nosocomial transmission. Controlling antibiotic use is difficult. Antibiotics are prescribed in the inpatient and outpatient settings by individual physicians, and physician behavior has been notoriously difficult to change. Clinicians tend to focus their interest on prescribing antibiotics that have maximal efficacy and safety in treating or preventing an infection in an individual patient and often are less cognizant of ecologic or epidemiologic factors of importance to infection control. There is evidence that changing antibiotic prescribing patterns can influence antibiotic resistance of specific pathogens. Reducing the use of ceftazidime has led to a reduction in ceftazidime-resistant *K. pneumoniae* infections during an outbreak, and reducing the use of cephalosporins and vancomycin have reduced VRE.[205,215]

In an era of health care reform, controlling nosocomial transmission of antibiotic-resistant pathogens has new challenges. Several recent outbreak investigations have identified a reduction in nursing staff as a risk factor associated with an increase in nosocomial infections and resistant organisms.[216,217] Infection control activities, such as handwashing and isolation, take time but are critical to reducing the transmission of these emerging pathogens.

CONTROL AND PREVENTION MEASURES

Control and prevention of nosocomial infections can occur at many levels. The SENIC study demonstrated the utility of well-developed infection control programs that include ICPs. Antibiotic control programs are of increasing importance and should now be included in infection prevention programs. Surveillance and notifying clinicians of infection rates in their patients have been shown to enhance the effectiveness of infection control. Finally, the development of policies and procedures to ensure infection prevention at all levels is necessary. Examples of such practices include handwashing among HCWs, immunization of HCWs, isolation of patients with communicable disease, antibiotic control, cleaning of the environment, and installation and maintenance of water, heating, and air-conditioning systems.

Presence of an Integrated Program

The key to controlling nosocomial infections is the presence of an integrated program, including:

- department of epidemiology and infection control
- microbiology laboratory
- occupational health services
- pharmacy
- computers/information systems

Department of Epidemiology and Infection Control

The role of this department is to measure the rates of nosocomial infections, understand their epidemiology, and devise and evaluate effective strategies for their control and prevention. The components of this program are surveillance, outbreak investigation, education, health care system employee health, antibiotic utilization, product evaluation, cost-benefit analysis, and policy and procedure guidelines. The organizational structure should include a trained hospital epidemiologist; nurse epidemiologist(s) or ICP; computer(s), microbiology, and administrative support; an infectious disease fellow; and an infection control committee. The infection control committee should be chaired by the hospital epidemiologist and should have representatives from the medical and surgical staff, hospital administration, employee health, pharmacy, microbiology, housekeeping, central supply, and engineering, as well as the ICPs.

Microbiology Laboratory

Active involvement of the microbiology laboratory is crucial for a successful infection control program. Culture reports from the microbiology laboratory are one of the most important pieces of data included in surveillance. The infection control department and the microbiology laboratory must have a close working relationship. This interaction not only provides the ICPs with timely microbiologic information, but also helps the laboratory to determine the clinical significance of isolates and to differentiate patients who are colonized from those with clinical infection. The microbiology laboratory can support the infection control department in the following ways:

- Ensure high-quality performance in the laboratory.
- Designate a person to be a consultant to the infection control department.
- Report relevant results in a timely, organized, and accessible way.
- Provide basic microbiologic training to infection control staff.
- Monitor isolates of unusual pathogens, clusters of pathogens that might indicate an outbreak, and the emergence of multidrug-resistant pathogens.
- Characterize antimicrobial susceptibility.
- Perform special procedures and molecular fingerprinting studies.
- Store isolates of epidemiologic importance.
- Conduct environmental microbiologic studies.
- Monitor commercial products, devices, or equipment that might become contaminated during manufacturing or transportation, when indicated.

Employee Health Services

Exposure events are defined when patients or hospital employees are exposed to infectious microorganisms or ectoparasites. When an individual is exposed, the goal of the infection control department is to prevent further transmission. In the event of an exposure, all patients, visitors, and staff who might have been exposed must be identified, and appropriate measures should be initiated immediately. In most institutions, an employee health department evaluates whether an employee has been exposed to or remains susceptible to a contagious disease, examines them, enforces work restrictions, and allows personnel to return to work. Infection control staff must collaborate with employee health services and develop protocols for triage, evaluation, prophylaxis, and follow-up after exposures to communicable diseases. Roles and responsi-

bilities of both departments should be identified and clear lines of communication established.

Pharmacy Service

Pharmacy is also an essential partner in infection control. This service identifies the quality, efficacy, safety, and cost-effectiveness of drugs.[218] Antimicrobials account for 15% to 30% of the overall pharmacy budget,[219] of which 25% is used in the hospital. The use and availability of antimicrobial drugs may alter the susceptibility patterns of nosocomial pathogens. Studies[220–223] have demonstrated that 23% to 37.8% of hospitalized patients receive antibiotics, of which 40% to 50% of the antibiotics are used inappropriately.[219–221] One of the easiest and the most cost-effective ways to determine the gross antibiotics utilization is based on pharmacy data. High-risk drugs, units, and patients whose antibiotic utilization rates are above those expected or that correlate with resistant organisms can be identified. Antibiotic use is the number of units, or defined daily doses, per 1,000 population in a primary health setting or per-patient days in hospital settings. This allows comparisons for trends in antibiotic use to be evaluated and to be evaluated and stratified by unit or service.

Computers

With limited resources, resulting in limited time to perform surveillance activity, computers can help ICPs manage their time more effectively. Administrative databases that contain patient demographics, clinical and pharmacy data, and microbiology and radiology reports are an important adjunct to surveillance. These data can be merged into a surveillance data system that can be stored and manipulated to facilitate surveillance. Such systems help to identify problems such as outbreaks, antibiotic susceptibility trends, nosocomial pneumonias, SSIs, UTIs, BSIs, and the emergence of important pathogens, such as MRSA and VRE. These infection control management systems need to be custom-developed with infection control and hospital informatics and the hospital information system department.

Handwashing

Handwashing is the single most important preventive strategy and remains the cornerstone of infection control.[224–228] The normal microbial flora of the skin helps to prevent colonization of hospital-acquired microorganisms. Skin flora is composed of resident and transient microorganisms. Resident microorganisms are most frequently found on the superficial skin layers, where they can survive, multiply, and be cultured. The density of normal resident microorganism populations on hands ranges between 10^2 and 10^3 colony-forming units (cfu)/cm^2.[229] They usually consist of staphylococcal species (*S. epidermidis, S. hominis*, and *S. capitis*) and micrococci. Moreover, organisms such as *S. aureus, Klebsiella-Enterobacter* group, and *Acinetobacter* species have been reported to colonize the hands of HCWs.[230–235] Larson[234] has shown that 21% of HCWs persistently carry microorganisms from the *Acinetobacter* and *Klebsiella-Enterobacter* groups. About 10% to 20% of the resident microorganisms inhabit deep epidermal layers.[236,237] In general, resident microorganisms tend not to be highly virulent but can cause infections in patients who are immunocompromised or who have implanted foreign devices. Transient microorganisms are acquired through accidental contamination and are characterized by their inability to multiply and persist. The hands of HCWs may acquire transient microorganisms from colonized or infected patients.

Many outbreaks have been reported in the ICU due to breakdowns in infection control practices.[238–242] Routine handwashing before and after contact with a patient; before and after performing invasive procedures; before and after touching wounds; and after contact with inanimate sources, such as urine-measuring devices that are potentially contaminated with microorganisms, could prevent many nosocomial infections. This simple practice substantially reduces the risk of microbial transmission from one patient to another by HCWs, as well as transmission from a contaminated site to a clean site of a patient. A brief, vigorous rubbing together of all surfaces of lathered hands, followed by rinsing under a stream of water, is adequate handwashing. Various products are available for handwashing, ranging from plain soap to detergents to antimicrobial-containing products. Microorganisms can either be removed mechanically, by washing hands with soap or detergents and rinsing; or chemically, by washing hands with antimicrobial products that can inhibit the growth or kill the microorganisms. In high-risk health care settings (such as an ICU), effective handwashing with antimicrobial agents (containing chlorhexidine), compared with washing with soap and water, was shown to reduce nosocomial infections.[243] Transient microorganisms, in contrast to resident flora, are easily removed by mechanical means. Antimicrobial soaps should be used in nurseries, neonatal units, ICUs, and when dealing with patients with immunodeficiencies or who are at risk of developing infections with resistant organisms. The handwashing facilities should be conveniently accessible—ideally, one sink per patient, located either in or immediately outside the room, with either elbow, knee, foot, or automatic temperature-adjustable taps and easy-to-use, appropriate cleansing products and dispensers. In places where sinks are not available, antimicrobial disinfectants such as foam or rinses that do not require water should be used.

Unfortunately, handwashing often is not performed as frequently as recommended. Factors that predict handwashing compliance are profession, hospital ward, time of day, patient/nurse ratio, and type of care provider.[244] Donowitz[245] examined breaks in handwashing technique among health care providers in a PICU and demonstrated that physicians did not wash their hands 79% of the time that handwashing was indicated. In this prospective study, failure to wash hands following direct patient or support equipment contact was seen 70% of the time.[245] A study examining the frequency of handwashing in an emergency department demonstrated that nurses had the highest handwashing frequency

(58.2%), which was significantly more frequent than residents (18.6%) and faculty (17.2%).[246] Compliance with handwashing rarely exceeds 40% of the times it is indicated under study conditions[247] and is particularly poor among physicians.[248–251] The handwashing compliance of different hospital professions is shown in Exhibit 13–1. Factors leading to poor handwashing compliance include lack of education, poor hygienic habits, perceived lack of importance, lack of time, dry skin, skin irritation or dermatitis, absence of suitable cleansing agent, and inadequate handwashing facilities.[246,248,252–254]

Even in today's highly technical hospital environment, adequate handwashing is still the most crucial strategy to decrease nosocomial infections. This lack of adherence and inadequate handwashing place patients at risk for acquiring nosocomial infections. Handwashing is a mundane, tedious, and repetitive task that will remain suboptimal without strict implementation of infection control practices and monitoring. The fact remains that, unless HCWs are trained to wash their hands thoroughly and without exception, the use of antimicrobial soaps and alcohol-based hand rinses, location of the sinks, and mechanism of scrubbing have little effect. Hospitals should make monitoring compliance and

---

Exhibit 13–1 Handwashing Compliance by Hospital Profession

Physicians	10–59%
Nurses	25–66%
Respiratory therapists	76%
Radiology technicians	44%
Nurses' aides	13%
Others	10–73%

Source: Data from R.K. Albert and F. Condie, Hand-Washing Patterns in Medical Intensive-Care Units, *The New England Journal of Medicine*, Vol. 304, pp. 1465–1466, © 1981, Massachusetts Medical Society and W.R. Jarvis, Handwashing—the Semmelweis Lesson Forgotten? *The Lancet*, Vol. 344, pp. 1311–1312, © 1994.

---

feedback of handwashing compliance a high priority. New and efficient techniques to improve handwashing should be evaluated because they are desperately needed.

Isolation

To transmit disease-causing organisms, a source of organisms, a susceptible host, and a mode of transmission are necessary. In a hospital setting, a source of organisms can be patients, HCWs, or visitors.

The CDC and Hospital Infection Control Practices Advisory Committee (HICPAC) have recently proposed two levels of Isolation Guidelines for Hospitalized Patients: Standard and Transmission-Based Precautions. This new system replaces the previous disease-specific systems and has integrated universal precautions and body substance isolation.

Standard Precautions are a combination of universal precautions—designed to reduce the risk of transmission of blood-borne pathogens from patients to HCW—and body substance isolation—designed to reduce transmissions of body fluid microorganisms between patients and HCWs. Standard Precautions states that blood; all patients' body fluids (except sweat), secretions, and excretions; mucous membranes; and nonintact skin be treated as potentially infectious. The components of Standard Precautions include:

- handwashing
- wearing gloves
- wearing mask, eye protection, face shield, and gowns when appropriate
- cleaning patient-care equipment
- enforcing environmental control
- cleaning linen
- enforcing occupational health and blood-borne pathogen protocols
- cohorting patients

Transmission-Based Precautions are used for infected or colonized patients (confirmed or suspected) with transmittable microorganisms. These precautions should be used in conjunction with Standard Precautions and are divided into airborne, droplet, and contact precautions (Exhibit 13–2).

Empiric isolation is crucial and based on clinical presentation and symptoms at the time of admission, before a definitive diagnosis is made. Depending on different clinical scenarios, empirical isolation, using airborne precautions (e.g., cough, fever, maculopapular, vesicular rash, tuberculosis), droplet precautions (e.g., meningitis, pertussis, influenza), and contact precautions (e.g., acute infectious diarrhea, history of previous colonization with multidrug-resistant microorganism, such as MRSA and VRE), should be implemented, pending definite diagnosis. Hospitals should have a system in place to ensure that proper empirical precautions are implemented.

Epidemic Investigation and Control

In general, nosocomial infections are endemic in nature, although approximately 5% of them occur in epidemics.[255] Wendt and Herwaldt[256] reviewed 555 published reports of outbreaks in health care institutions. Their review demonstrated that most of the outbreaks were due to bacteria (71%); however, viruses caused 12%, fungi 5%, and parasites 3%. Among bacteria, nearly half of the outbreaks were caused by gram-negative organisms. Gram-positive bacteria were associated with 36% of the outbreaks.

An increase in the incidence of nosocomial infections over the expected rates in a specified area within a time period defines an epidemic. Epidemic nosocomial infections are due either to an increase in person-to-person transmission or to a common source and are usually clustered temporally or geographically. To identify outbreaks, reliable and sensitive surveillance is crucial. Once the existence of an outbreak is established, the infection control personnel need to take certain steps, detailed in Exhibit 13–3.

Immunization

An estimated 8.8 million people work in the health care industry.[257] Health care workers are at risk for exposure to a diverse group of occupational infectious diseases, including vaccine-preventable diseases. Diseases such as diphtheria, hepatitis A and B, influenza, measles, mumps, pertussis, rubella, and varicella result in unnecessary and preventable morbidity and mortality. Nonimmune HCWs can acquire these infections from patients[258,259] or can introduce vaccine-preventable diseases into the health care environment, causing outbreaks.[259–262] A recent study demonstrated that physicians can contract measles, hepatitis B, pertussis, varicella, and influenza following patient exposure.[263] The importance of HCW vaccination and screening for vaccine-preventable diseases is briefly discussed.

Diphtheria. Although an extremely rare disease in the United States, a few cases of nosocomial transmission have been reported in the literature.[264–266] Diphtheria is re-emerging in some areas of the world where immunization rates are low. In recent years, epidemics have occurred in the new independent states of the former Soviet Union, and other areas of the world.[267–270]

Diphtheria is caused by *Corynebacterium diphtheriae* and is transmitted from infected patients by respiratory droplets or contact with skin lesions. The incubation period for diphtheria is 1 to 4 days. If diphtheria remains untreated, infected individuals are usually contagious for less than 2 weeks. Rarely, patients may shed the bacteria for 6 months or more.

Immunization with tetanus and diphtheria toxid (Td) is recommended every 10 years for adults who have received a complete immunization series. Foreign-born individuals from endemic areas without documentation of immunization should receive a primary three-dose series. Prophylaxis of unimmunized workers after contact with a patient with diphtheria with benzathine penicillin (1.2 million units intramuscular) single dose, or erythromycin (1 g/day orally) for 7 days is recommended.[271] Two weeks after the initiation of antimicrobial therapy, nasopharyngeal cultures for *C. diph-*

Exhibit 13–2 Hospital Epidemiology: New Isolation Guidelines

Transmission of Organisms

Common Mechanisms	*How?*	*Examples*
Direct and Indirect Contact	contaminated hands, contaminated equipment	MRSA
Droplet	large droplets (>5–10 μm) generated by talking	Influenza
Airborne	small droplet nuclei (1–10 μm) waft on air currents	Tuberculosis

---

Standard Precautions—used on all patients

Universal Precautions	*Body Substance Isolation*
• gloves for contact with blood or any body fluid contaminated with blood • gowns and goggles for splashes	• same as above but for any moist body substance, i.e., urine, saliva, nonintact skin

---

Transmission-Based Precautions—used for patients known or suspected to have epidemiologically important diseases

VA/CDC Name:	*Examples:*

Airborne (AFB)
• private room
• negative pressure room
• 6–12 air exchanges/hr
• respiratory protection
  1. TB-PAPR
  2. Varicella or measles—nonimmune staff should not enter
	Tuberculosis
	Disseminated Zoster
	Zoster in IC Host
	Varicella
	Measles

Droplet Precautions • private room or cohort • regular masks • do not need negative pressure	Influenza RSV, Adenovirus Mumps, Rubella Pneumonia due to *S. aureus*, DRSP during first 48 hours of treatment Invasive Meningococcus or *H. flu*
Contact Precautions (acute and nonacute) • *private room or cohort or low-risk roommate* • gloves for entry into room or *per Standard Precautions* • gowns for any contact with patient or immediate environment or *per Standard Precautions*	MRSA resistant gram-negative rods Shigella, hepA if diarrhea *C. difficile* if diarrhea Wounds that cannot be covered Scabies

Courtesy of University of Maryland, Department of Hospital Epidemiology.

Exhibit 13–3 Steps for Outbreak Investigation

---

a) determine the nature, location, and severity of the problem
b) identify cases
c) document notes regarding the outbreak in an orderly fashion
d) conduct a literature search
e) create a preliminary questionnaire
f) review medical records to establish a case definition
g) save isolates from cases, as well as suspected cases and/or source
h) summarize data into an easy-to-read line listing
i) form a hypothesis (source, mode of transmission, cause)
j) test the hypothesis by either a case control or cohort study
k) create an epidemic curve
l) demonstrate biologic plausibility
m) inform the appropriate agencies
n) institute emergency control measures

• eliminate the source, which could be environment, patient, or an HCW
• protect exposed individuals by administering chemoprophylaxis or immunization

o) evaluate the control measures
p) document and report the outbreak

---

theriae should be obtained, and, if cultures are positive, patients should receive 10 days of erythromycin. Exposed and previously immunized HCWs who have not received Td in the past 5 years should be vaccinated.[271] Exposed susceptible HCWs should be excluded from duties until completion of therapy and a negative nasopharyngeal culture.

Hepatitis A Virus.   Hepatitis A virus (HAV) is a rare cause of nosocomial infection, transmitted primarily through the fecal-oral route and, rarely, by transfusion of blood products.[272–276] Infectivity is highest 2 weeks prior to the onset of clinical symptoms or jaundice. Ninety percent of infants remain asymptomatic after HAV infection, although most adults develop jaundice (see Chapter 19).

Nosocomial outbreaks of HAV are rare but have been reported following exposure to infected neonates or children, adult patients with diarrhea or fecal incontinence, or an infected HCW. Transmission has been associated with breaks in standard hygienic practices.[241,277–280] Employees who are (a) exposed to stools of infected patients, (b) consume food prepared by infected employees, and (c) have close contact to a patient with HAV are at risk of acquiring infection. Risk factors identified for HCWs who acquired the disease were failure to comply with basic infection control practices, such as handwashing or wearing gloves and eating, drinking, or smoking in the patient care area.[241,277,279,280]

The FDA licensed hepatitis A vaccines in 1995. Two inactivated hepatitis A vaccines are available in the markets; both have efficacy greater than 94%.[281–284] Both are well tolerated and have no serious side effects. The vaccine is not routinely recommended for HCWs in the United States. Nevertheless, vaccines should be given for HCWs in high-risk areas, such as neonatal and PICUs, food service, or personnel working with HIV-infected primates or in an HIV research laboratory. In case of direct exposure to the stools of a serologically confirmed case of HIV, postexposure prophylaxis with immunoglobulin (0.02 mL/kg intramuscular) is 80% to 90% efficacious if given within 2 weeks of exposure. HCWs with suspected HAV infection should not work until jaundice or clinical symptoms subside.

Hepatitis B Virus.   Hepatitis B virus (HBV) carries a serious nosocomial transmission risk for HCWs who come in contact with blood or body fluids.[285–291] HCWs represent 2% of all reported cases of HBV infection in the United States.[292] It is estimated that approximately 1,000 HCWs became infected with HBV in 1994, which was a 90% decline from 1985.[293]

Prior to vaccine availability, it was estimated that 10% to 25% of HCWs had evidence of prior HBV infection.[294] This decline has been attributed to vaccine use and adherence to infection control practices. The virus is transmitted parenterally, sexually, and perinatally. The most important mode of occupational transmission is percutaneous exposure to infected blood or serum-derived body fluids. The infectious state is determined by the presence of hepatitis B surface antigen (HBsAg) and hepatitis Be antigen (HBeAg) in the blood. Anyone with a positive HBsAg is considered potentially infectious and is deemed to be highly infectious if HBeAg is positive. HBeAg is a marker for active viral replication, and the risk for transmission from parenteral exposure from a HBeAg-positive patient is greater than 40%.[294] The incubation period is 45 to 180 days (average 60 to 90 days).

There is clear evidence suggesting that patient-to-HCW and HCW-to-patient transmission have occurred, and many nosocomial outbreaks have been documented.[295-303] The risk of transmission depends on the infected person's HBeAg status, and level of viremia. An HCW with percutaneous, mucous membrane, or nonintact skin exposure to blood or body fluid of any patient should be considered to have been exposed to HBV until proven otherwise. A positive HBsAg in the source patient confirms exposure.

The Occupational Safety and Health Administration mandates that hepatitis B vaccine be made available to all HCWs at their employers' expense, and universal vaccination of HCWs should be the cardinal goal of occupational health services. Prevaccination serology is not necessary prior to being vaccinated, although postvaccination screening for antibody to the surface antigen (anti-HBs) is recommended. Exposed, unvaccinated HCWs should receive intramuscular hepatitis B immunoglobulin (HBIG) (0.06 mL/kg) within 24 to 48 hours[304] with the first dose of hepatitis B vaccine (1 mL intramuscular) at a different site, followed by additional doses at 1 and 6 months. Exposed, vaccinated HCWs should have their anti-HBs level measured; an antibody level of 10 mIU/mL or more indicates no need for prophylaxis. Workers whose levels have fallen below this level with a previously documented protective level should receive HBIG and a booster vaccine dose.[285,304] If an antibody response has been demonstrated after the HBV vaccine series, HBIG is not needed; these exposed HCWs can be given a booster does of HBV vaccine alone.

Influenza. Influenza is a major nosocomial pathogen, and transmission has been well documented from patients to HCW, HCW to patients, and HCW to HCW.[305-312] It has been associated with increased morbidity and mortality among patients in long-term as well as acute-care facilities. The transmission predominantly occurs through person-to-person contact with large, virus-laden droplets during close contact with infected individuals and by small-particle aerosols or droplet nuclei.[313-316] The incubation period is 1 to 2 days, and viral shedding begins approximately 1 day prior to onset of symptoms and continues up to 10 days.

Nosocomial outbreaks of influenza often occur during community epidemics and can occur in a hospital or health care setting. Numerous outbreaks have been reported in the literature, demonstrating the infectivity of influenza.[317-327] Persons at greatest risk of serious disease are: (a) people older than 65 years, (b) residents of nursing homes and chronic care facilities, (c) persons with chronic pulmonary or cardiac conditions, and (d) persons with diabetes mellitus.[328]

Influenza vaccine is recommended for HCWs each year. HCW vaccination has been shown to decrease mortality among elderly patients in long-term care facilities.[329] In the United States, influenza activity peaks between late December and early March. Thus, the ideal time to vaccinate with influenza vaccine is between October and mid-November. Vaccinating HCWs can be highly cost-effective, can reduce the risk to HCWs, and can prevent transmission from HCWs to high-risk patients.[330] During an outbreak, prophylaxis with antiviral agents (amantadine, rimantadine) for 2 weeks, in conjunction with vaccine, is recommended.[331] Recently, drugs that inhibit the enzyme neuraminidase of influenza A and B have been approved for use to treat influenza.[332–335] These agents also look promising for prophylaxis during influenza outbreaks.[336] If vaccine is not administered, antiviral agents should be given for the duration of influenza activity in the community.[328,337] By far, the best control measure in a health care setting is immunization against influenza; however, it is important that institutions have surveillance for early recognition and isolation of possibly infected individuals.[333] HCWs who are suspected to have influenza should not work until symptoms subside.

Measles. Measles is a highly contagious infection of the respiratory system. Measles is infrequent in the United States, as a result of the introduction of vaccine in 1962. However, more than 20% of young adults are seronegative.[338,339] The transmission of measles occurs by droplet and airborne transmission, especially in medical settings.[340,341] Infectious virus can survive at least several hours in the air. The incubation period is 5 to 21 days, and viral shedding begins 9 to 10 days after exposure.

Since the resurgence of measles in the United States in 1989,[259,342] many outbreaks have been documented.[259,343–349] From 1985 through 1991, 2,997 reported measles cases (4% of all reported cases) were transmitted in a medical facility,[259,350] with about half acquired in hospital inpatient units. Ninety percent of the 2,997 reported measles cases were transmitted from patients and the remaining 10% from HCWs. It has been shown that HCWs are at a 13-fold higher risk than the general population for acquiring measles.[351]

In the United States, the measles vaccine is administered in combination with mumps and rubella. It is a live-attenuated vaccine that induces 90% seroconversion with a single dose, and the second dose immunizes most of the remainder.[352,353] Documentation of immunity to measles (physician diagnosis, serologic immunity, documentation of appropriate vaccination or being born during or before 1957) should be required by the health care institution for all health care workers. Health care institutions should serologically test employees for immunity (targeted approach) and vaccinate seronegatives. This approach has shown to be cost-effective, compared with vaccination without prior screening.[354–356] However, the most important intervention to halt an outbreak is prompt administration of the vaccine. Employees with measles should not care for patients until 7 days after the appearance of rash. Exposed HCWs not immune to measles should be restricted from duty from day 5 through day 21 after exposure. People who cannot be vaccinated can be treated with IG up to 6 days after exposure. IG will not prevent measles but it does make the disease milder.

Mumps. In the United States, mumps incidence has declined steadily since 1967, when the vaccine was licensed. Between 1985 and 1987, there was resurgence of mumps, probably due to suboptimal vaccine coverage; however, since then, rates have been declining steadily. Although most cases of mumps in HCWs have been community acquired, nosocomial transmission has been documented.[357–360] Transmission occurs through droplet nuclei and direct contact with saliva of infected person. The incubation period is between 12 and 25 days (16 to 18 days average). Viral shedding may occur 6 to 9 days prior to development of parotitis and may persist 9 days after the onset of disease.[257,361]

The ideal strategy for prevention of nosocomial mumps is to have an effective vaccination program and stringent infection control practices. All HCWs should be considered susceptible unless they have documentation of immunity (physician-diagnosed mumps, serologic immunity, documentation of appropriate vaccination, or being born during or before 1957).[362] Exposed, susceptible HCW should be relieved of duty from day 5 through day 26 after exposure or until 9 days after the onset of parotitis.[363]

Pertussis. Pertussis is extremely contagious, with a greater than 80% secondary attack rate among susceptible household contacts.[364,365] Until recently, due to the widespread use of the vaccine, there had been a steady decline in the incidence of the disease. In recent years, the epidemiology of the disease has changed, and the disease now occurs more frequently among young adults and is frequently asymptomatic.[366] Recent studies indicate that HCWs often may be exposed and may develop the infection more frequently than previously appreciated.[367-370] Transmission occurs by contact with respiratory secretions or large aerosol droplets. The incubation period is between 7 and 10 days, and infectivity starts at the onset of the catarrhal stage through 3 weeks after the onset of symptoms.

Nosocomial transmission of *Bordetella pertussis* has been reported with increased frequency.[366-368,371-373] Because the clinical symptoms are less severe in adults than in children, they may go unnoticed. The failure to recognize the disease has resulted in nosocomial transmission.[367]

Although acellular pertussis vaccine has been shown to be immunogenic with lower risk of adverse events,[372,374] it has not been licensed for people older than 7 years of age. Vaccine (usually given at 4 and 6 years) immunity declines over time, with about 50% of those immunized 12 or more years earlier still immune.[375] Thus, HCWs may play an important role in disease transmission.

Prevention strategies for pertussis transmission include early diagnosis and treatment, implementation of droplet precautions, exclusion of HCWs from duties, and postexposure prophylaxis for exposed persons.[257,368,376] Postexposure prophylaxis with erythromycin (500 mg orally 4 times daily for 14 days) or trimethoprim-sulfamethazole (one tablet twice a day for 14 days) has been shown to prevent the development of clinical disease and may minimize transmission.[366,368,377,378] More recently, newer antibiotics with fewer side effects are being used. Use of the vaccine may help to prevent secondary cases.[373,379] Exposed HCWs should be excluded from duty from the onset of the catarrhal stage through the third week after the onset of paroxysms or until 5 days after initiation of effective antimicrobial therapy.[257]

Rubella. Rubella is highly contagious, but the incidence of the disease has declined steadily since 1969, when the vaccine was licensed in the United States. However, close to 20% of young adults remains susceptible to rubella.[380,381] The disease is transmitted by direct contact with infectious nasopharyngeal secretions and by aerosolized droplets. The incubation period may range from 12 to 23 days, with the rash appearing 14 to 16 days postexposure. Viral shedding may begin 1 week before through 5 to 7 days after the rash onset,[382] although infants with congenital rubella syndrome may shed virus for months. In adults, it is a mild disease, and 30% to 50% of the cases may be subclinical.

Nosocomial transmission has been well documented.[262,383-388] Outbreaks result in serious health and emotional consequences, especially if the exposure occurs during the first trimester of pregnancy. The rate of perinatal transmission is 40% to 50% overall and 90% during the first 12 weeks of pregnancy. Studies have demonstrated that medical and dental students can be the source of infection in rubella outbreaks.[262,389]

The ideal strategy for prevention of nosocomial rubella is to have an effective vaccination program and stringent infection control practices. Droplet precautions help to prevent transmission, but, for children with congenital rubella, contact precautions should be used for the first year of life unless urine and nasopharyngeal cultures are negative after 3 months of age.[390] All hospital employees, especially those working with pregnant women, should be immune to rubella and should be considered susceptible unless they have documentation of immunity (physician diagnosis, serologic immunity, documentation of appropriate vaccination). Being born during or before 1957 is acceptable evidence for immunity.[351] Also, a past history of rubella should not be accepted as criteria for immunity. Employees of child-bearing age should be checked for pregnancy and should not plan a pregnancy for 3 months after vaccine administration. Pregnant employees who are exposed should be referred for follow-up with their obstetrician, and they should be tested for anti-rubella IgM antibody.

Varicella-Zoster Virus (VZV). Varicella (chickenpox) and herpes zoster (shingles) are caused by VZV and are extremely communicable. VZV is spread through direct contact with vesicular fluid or droplets from respiratory secretions and via airborne transmission.[391-396] The incubation period is between 10 and 21 days (14 to 16 days average) but may be prolonged to 28 days after receiving postprophylaxis varicella-zoster immunoglobulin (VZIG).[397] In immunocompromised patients, the incubation period may be much shorter.[398] Viral shedding begins in the late incubation phase and can last between 4 days prior to rash development until crusting of lesions.[399]

Nosocomial transmission of VZV is well recognized, and multiple outbreaks have been reported in the literature.[393,394,400-408] Immunocompromised hosts, premature infants born to susceptible mothers, or infants born before 28-week gestation or weighing less than 1,000 g, regardless of mother's susceptibility, are at high risk for acquiring the disease.[409] In hospitals, the risk of transmission is related to air distribution patterns, and the index patient should be treated in a negative-pressure room.[394,395,410]

To reduce the risk of transmission, airborne and contact precautions are recommended, and only varicella-immune HCWs should care for patients with VZV. Studies have demonstrated that the history of varicella in adults is 97% to 99% predictive of seropositivity. Serologic testing is likely to be cost-effective in HCWs uncertain of varicella history, because between 71% and 93% will be seropositive.[351,409,411,412]

Exposure workup should include confirmation of diagnosis and extent of disease.[413,414] Ex-

posure requires either household contact or close contact with a patient with varicella or disseminated zoster. For nondisseminated zoster, exposure requires direct contact with exposed or uncovered lesion. Selected exposed individuals without measurable antibody should be considered for prophylaxis within 96 hours with VZIG (125 units/10 kg up to 625 units). All susceptible pregnant women and seronegative immunocompromised contacts should receive VZIG. VZIG does not prevent infection but modifies and attenuates the disease. Exposed HCWs should be furloughed from day 8 to day 21 after exposure and to day 28 if they receive VZIG. Post-exposure prophylaxis with VZIG does not necessarily prevent varicella and may extend the incubation period. Thus, it is not generally recommended,[415] except for immunocompromised subjects or premature infants.

In summary, health care institutions should have mandatory, comprehensive immunization programs and should bear responsibility for implementing these programs with careful planning. Success requires education of HCWs on their responsibility to seek appropriate immunization. Successful programs can be highly cost-effective and can reduce the risk of HCW infection and prevent transmission from HCW to high-risk patients, thus improving patient care and reducing HCW absenteeism.

Antimicrobial Control

In recent years, antimicrobial resistance has become a worldwide problem. Intense pressure exerted on microorganisms as a result of excessive antibiotic use in humans, animals, and agriculture has created this problem. The excessive use of antibiotics has also been linked to adverse drug reactions, adding to hospital costs. The use of antibiotics in any dosage over any period of time leads to selective pressure on the microorganism to either adapt by acquiring additional genetic resistance factors or die. In hospital formularies, antimicrobials account for the second most commonly used class of drugs. It is estimated that 23% to 40% of hospitalized patients receive systemic antimicrobial agents at any given time, and about 40% to 50% of their use is inappropriate.[220–223,416–418]

To control antimicrobial usage, hospitals need an antimicrobial utilization committee. This committee should be composed of individuals from infectious disease, pharmacy, microbiology, infection control, nursing, quality control and assurance, administration, and data management, as well as a representative physician from surgery, internal medicine, pediatrics, and obstetrics/gynecology. The chairman of infectious diseases often will head this committee. Residents should be included because they prescribe most antimicrobials. The strategies for optimizing antimicrobial use in the hospital are given in Exhibit 13–4.

In summary, antimicrobial use is the driving force behind antibiotic resistance. Bacterial pathogens that cause common illnesses are becoming increasingly resistant to the existing antibiotics. These virulent microbes will have serious implications for global epidemics. Reduction in the use of antibiotics may increase the success of treatment. Although difficult and inconvenient, antimicrobial restriction policies may control the emergence of resistant organisms and improve the outcome of treatment of nosocomial infections.

Exhibit 13-4 Strategies for Optimizing Antimicrobial Use in Hospitals

- Education of prescribers
- Clinical guidelines
- Formulary restrictions
- Pre-use approval
- Automatic stop order
- Audit of use

CONCLUSION

As we enter a new millennium, nosocomial infections are likely to increase in frequency. As our population ages, more people will be encountering the health care system and will acquire these infections, leading to further morbidity and mortality. Increases in antimicrobial resistance will complicate treatment, increasing the importance of prevention (surveillance, outbreak investigation, education, employee health, antibiotic utilization, and other processes of care). Hospital epidemiologists will need to apply creative strategies for prevention of nosocomial infections in a rapidly changing health care system. As the struggle to reduce the growth of health care costs continues, hospital epidemiology will play an important role in evaluating patients' outcomes and in improving the quality of their care.

REFERENCES

1. Emori TG, Gaynes RP. An overview of nosocomial infections, including the role of the microbiology laboratory. *Clin Microbiol Rev.* 1993;6:428–442.

2. Centers for Disease Control and Prevention. Public health focus: surveillance, prevention, and control of nosocomial infections. *MMWR.* 1992;41:783–787.

3. Kollef MH, Sharpless L, Vlasnik J, Pasque C, Murphy D, Fraser VJ. The impact of nosocomial infections on patient outcomes following cardiac surgery. *Chest.* 1997;112:666–675.

4. Perl TM, Golub JE. New approaches to reduce *Staphylococcus aureus* nosocomial infection rated: treating *S.*

aureus nasal carriage. *Ann Pharmacother.* 1998;32:7–16.

5. National Nosocomial Infections Surveillance (NNIS) report. Data summary from October 1986–April 1996, Issued May 1996. *Am J Infect Control.* 1996;24:380–388.

6. Emori TG, Culver DH, Horan TC, et al. National Nosocomial Infection Surveillance (NNIS) system: description of surveillance methodology. *Am J Infect Control.* 1991;19:19–35.

7. Gaynes RP, Horan TC. Surveillance of nosocomial infections. In: Mayhall CG, ed. *Hospital Epidemiology*

and Infection Control. Baltimore: Williams & Wilkins; 1996:1017–1031.

8. Centers for Disease Control and Prevention. National Nosocomial Infection Study report. In: *CDC Annual Summary, 1977*. U.S. Department of Health, Education and Welfare, Public Health Service; November, 1979.

9. Wenzel RP. Instituting health care reform and preserving quality: role of the hospital epidemiologist. *Clin Infect Dis*. 1993;17:831–834.

10. Anon. *Charaka-Samhita*. (Sanskrit, c. 4th century B.C.). Kavipatna AC, trans. Vol 1. Calcutta: Privately printed; 1888:168–169.

11. Selwyn, S. Hospital infection: the first 2500 years. *J Hosp Infect*. 1991;18:5–64.

12. Major RH. *A History of Medicine*. Vol 1. Oxford, England: Blackwell Publishers; 1954:294–321.

13. Stromayr C. Die handschrift des schnidt und augenarztes. Casper Stromayr [Practicia copiosa] 1559. by von Brunn W, Ed. Berlin: Idra-Verlagsanstalt; 1925.

14. Tenon JR. *Memoires sur les hopitaux de Paris*. Paris: Ph-D Pierres; 1788:138–424.

15. Simpson JY. Some propositions on hospitalism, by the late Sir JY Simpson, Bart. *Lancet*. 1870;2:698–700.

16. Simpson JY. Presidential address on public health. *Trans Natl Assoc Promotion Soc Sci*. 1867:107–123.

17. Cohen IB. Florence Nightingale. *Sci Am*. 1984;250:128–137.

18. Nightingale F. *Notes on Hospitals*. 3rd ed. London: Longman; 1863.

19. Semmelewis IP. The etiology, the concept and the prophylaxis of childbed fever. Pest, Wien, u. Leipzig. C. A. Hartleben, 1861 (reprinted in translation by FP Murphy). *Med Classics*. 5:334–773.

20. Absolon KB, Absolon MJ, Zientek R. From antisepsis to asepsis. Louis Pasteur's publication on "The germ theory and its application to medicine and surgery." *Rev Surg*. 1970;27:245–258.

21. Toledo-Pereyra LH, Toledo MM. A critical study of Lister's work on antiseptic surgery. *Am J Surg*. 1976;131:736–744.

22. Delaunay A. Centennial of the "germ theory and its applications to medicine and surgery," presented by Louis Pasteur in April of 1878. *Gac Med Mex*. 1979;115:145–149.

23. Lister J. On the effects of the antiseptic system of treatment upon the salubrity of a surgical hospital. *Lancet*. 1870;1:40,400. In: *Collected Papers*. Vol 2. Oxford, 1909. Republished, *Classics of Medicine Library*. Birmingham: 1979.

24. Brewer GE. Operative surgery at the City Hospital with preliminary report on the study of wound infection. *New York Med J*. 1896.

25. Brewer GE. Studies in aseptic technique, with a report of some recent infections at the Roosevelt Hospital. *JAMA*. 1915;64:1369–1372.

26. Wise RI, Ossman EA, Littlefield DR. Personal reflections on nosocomial staphylococcal infections and the development of hospital surveillance. *Rev Infect Dis*. 1989;11:1005–1018.

27. Schaberg DR, Culver DH, Gaynes RP. Major trends in the microbial etiology of nosocomial infections. *Am J Med*. 1991;91:72–75.

28. Centers for Disease Control. National Nosocomial Infections Surveillance system. Nosocomial infection rates for interhospital comparison: limitations and possible solutions. *Infect Control Hosp Epidemiol*. 1991;12:609–621.

29. Wenzel K. The role of the infection control nurse. *Nurs Clin North Am*. 1970;5:89–98.

30. Kislak JW, Eickhoff TC, Finland M. Hospital-acquired infections and antibiotic usage in the Boston City Hospital. *N Engl J Med*. 1964;271:834–835.

31. Barrett FF, Casey JI, Finland M. Infections and antibiotic usage among patients at Boston City Hospital. *N Engl J Med*. 1968;278:5–9.

32. Haley RW, Culver DH, Hooton TM, et al. Progress report on the evaluation of the efficacy of infection surveillance and control programs. *Am J Med*. 1981;70:971–975.

33. Haley RW, Culver DH, White JW, et al. The efficacy of infection surveillance and control programs in preventing nosocomial infections in US hospitals. *Am J Epidemiol*. 1985;121:182–205.

34. Sing-Naz N, Sprague BM, Patel KM, Pollack MM. Risk factors for nosocomial infection in critically ill children: a prospective cohort study. *Crit Care Med*. 1996;24:875–878.

35. National Academy of Sciences—National Research Council. Postoperative wound infections: the influence of ultraviolet irradiation of the operative room and various other factors. *Ann Surg*. 1964;160(Suppl. 2):1–132.

36. Haley RW, Culver DH, Morgan WM, White JW, Emori TG, Hooton TM. Identifying patients at high risk of surgical wound infection: a simple multivariate index of patient susceptibility and wound contamination. *Am J Epidemiol*. 1985;121:206–215.

37. Culver DH, Horan TC, Gaynes RP, et al. Surgical wound infection rates by wound class, operative procedure, and patient risk index. *Am J Med* 1991;91(Suppl. 3B):152S–157S.

38. Roy MC, Herwaldt A, Embrey R, Kuhns K, Wenzel RP, Perl TM. Does the Centers for Disease Control's NNIS risk index stratify patients undergoing cardiothoracic operations by their risk of surgical site infection? *Infect Control Hosp Epidemiol*. In press.

39. Freeman J, McGowan JE Jr. Day-specific incidence of nosocomial infection estimated from a prevalence survey. *Am J Epidemiol.* 1981;114:888–901.

40. Rhame FS, Sudderth WD. Incidence and prevalence as used in the analysis of the occurrence of nosocomial infections. *Am J Epidemiol.* 1981;113:1–11.

41. Pottinger JM, Herwaldt LA, Perl TM. Basics of surveillance—an overview. *Infect Control Hosp Epidemiol.* 1997;18:513–527.

42. Haley RW, Hooton TM, Schoenfelder JR, et al. Effect of an infection surveillance and control program on the accuracy of retrospective chart review. *Am J Epidemiol.* 1980;111:543–555.

43. Haley RW, Tenney JH, Lindsey JO, Garner JS, Bennett JV. How frequent are outbreaks of nosocomial infection in community hospitals? *Infect Control.* 1985;6:233–236.

44. Givens CD, Wenzel RP. Catheter-associated urinary tract infections in surgical patients: a controlled study on the excess morbidity and costs. *J Urol.* 1980; 124:646–648.

45. Coello R, Glenister H, Fereres J, et al. The cost of infection in surgical patients: a case-control study. *J Hosp Infect.* 1993;25:239–250.

46. Eickhoff TC. The Third Decennial International Conference on Nosocomial Infections. Historical perspective: the landmark conference in 1970. *Am J Med.* 1991; 91:3–5.

47. Warren JW, Anthony WC, Hoopes JM, Muncie HL Jr. Cephalexin for susceptible bacteriuria in afebrile, long-term catheterized patients. *JAMA.* 1982;248:454–458.

48. Freeman J, McGowan JE Jr. Risk factors for nosocomial infections. *J Infect Dis.* 1978;138:811–819.

49. Stamm WE, Martins SM, Bennett JV. Epidemiology of nosocomial infections due to gram-negative bacilli: aspects relevant to development and use of vaccine. *J Infect Dis.* 1977;136:151–160.

50. Ayliefe GA, Brightwell KM, Collins BJ, Lowbury EJL. Surveys of hospital infections in the Birmingham region. *J Hyg (Cambridge).* 1977;79:299–314.

51. Saviteer SM, Samsa GP, Rutala WA. Nosocomial infections in elderly: increase risk per hospital day. *Am J Med.* 1988;84:661–666.

52. Gross PA, Rapuano C, Adrignolo A, Shaw B. Nosocomial infections: decade-specific risk. *Infect Control.* 1983;4:145–147.

53. Emory TG, Banerjee SN, Culver DH, et al. Nosocomial infection in the elderly patients in the United States, 1986–1990. *Am J Med.* 1991;91:289–293.

54. Velasco E, Thuler LC, Martins CA, Dias LM, Goncalves VM. Nosocomial infections in an oncology intensive care unit. *Am J Infect Control.* 1997;25:458–462.

55. Perl T, Chotani R, Agawala R. Infection control and pre-

vention in bone marrow transplant patients. In Mayhall CG, ed. *Hospital Epidemiology and Infection Control*, 2nd ed. Baltimore: Lippincott Williams & Wilkins; 1999:803–844.

56. Craven DE, Steger KA, Hirschhorn LR. Nosocomial colonization and infection in persons infected with human immunodeficiency virus. *Infect Control Hosp Epidemiol.* 1996;17:304–318.

57. Goetz AM, Squier C, Wagener MM, Muder RR. Nosocomial infections in the human immunodeficiency virus-infected patient: a two-year survey. *Am J Infect Control.* 1994;22:334–339.

58. Stroud L, Srivastava P, Culver D, et al. Nosocomial infections in HIV-infected patients: preliminary results from a multicenter surveillance system (1989–1995). *Infect Control Hosp Epidemiol.* 1997;18:479–485.

59. Barsic B, Beus I, Marton E, Himbele J, Klinar I. Nosocomial infections in critically ill infectious disease patients: results of a 7-year focal surveillance. *Infection.* 1999;27:16–22.

60. Kampf G, Wischnewski N, Schulgen G, Schumacher M, Daschner F. Prevalence and risk factors for nosocomial lower respiratory tract infections in German hospitals. *J Clin Epidemiol.* 1998;51:495–502.

61. Berbari EF, Hanssen AD, Duffy MC, et al. Risk factors for prosthetic joint infection: case-control study. *Clin Infect Dis.* 1998;27:1247–1254.

62. Keita-Perse O, Gaynes RP. Severity of illness scoring system to adjust nosocomial infection rates: a review and commentary. *Am J Infect Control.* 1996;24:429–434.

63. Rhame FS, Streifel AJ, Kersey JH Jr, et al. Extrinsic risk factors for pneumonia in the patient at high risk of infection. *Am J Med.* 1984;76:42–52.

64. Rhame FS. Prevention of nosocomial aspergillosis. *J Hosp Infect.* 1991;18:466–472.

65. Centers for Disease Control and Prevention. Guidelines for prevention on nosocomial pneumonia. *MMWR.* 1997;46:28–34, 54–57, 74–79.

66. Joseph CA, Watson JM, Harrison TG, Bartlett CLR. Nosocomial Legionnaires' disease in England and Wales, 1980–92. *Epidemiol Infect.* 1992;112:329–345.

67. McGowan JE Jr. Environmental factors in nosocomial infection: a selective focus. *Rev Infect Dis.* 1981;3:760–769.

68. Centers for Disease Control and Prevention. Sustained transmission of nosocomial Legionnaires disease—Arizona and Ohio. *MMWR.* 1997;46:416–421.

69. Marks JS, Tasi TF, Martone WJ, et al. Nosocomial Legionnaires' disease in Columbus, Ohio. *Ann Intern Med.* 1997;90:565–569.

70. Astagneau P, Duneton P. Management of epidemics of

nosocomial infections. *Pathol Biol (Paris)*. 1998;46: 272–278.

71. Nishijima S, Sugimachi T, Higashida T, Asada Y, Okuda K, Murata K. An epidemiological study of methicillin-resistant *Staphylococcus aureus* (MRSA) isolated from medical staff, inpatients, and hospital environment in one ward at our hospital. *J Dermatol.* 1992; 19:356–361.

72. Vrankova J, Bendova E, Konigova R, Broz L. Bacteriological monitoring in the Prague Burns Center. *Acta Chir Plast.* 1998;4:105–108.

73. Warnick F. Vancomycin-resistant enterococcus. *Clin J Oncol Nurs.* 1997;1:73–77.

74. Graman PS, Hall CB. Nosocomial viral respiratory infections. *Semin Respir Infect.* 1989;4:253–260.

75. Berthelot P, Grattard F, Mahul P, et al. Ventilator temperature sensors: an unusual source of *Pseudomonas cepacia* in nosocomial infection. *J Hosp Infect.* 1993; 25:33–43.

76. Vesley D, Norlien KG, Nelson B, Ott B, Streifel AJ. Significant factors in the disinfection and sterilization of flexible endoscopes. *Am J Infect Control.* 1992;20:291–300.

77. Nosocomial infection and pseudoinfection from contaminated endoscopes and bronchoscopes—Wisconsin and Missouri. *MMWR.* 1991;40:675–678.

78. Jawad A, Heritage J, Snelling AM, Gascoyne-Binzi DM, Hawkey PM. Influence of relative humidity and suspending menstrua on survival of *Acinetobacter* spp. on dry surfaces. *J Clin Microbiol.* 1996;34:2881–2887.

79. Craven DE, Steger K. Nosocomial pneumonia in mechanically ventilated adult patients: epidemiology and prevention in 1996. *Semin Respir Infect.* March 1996; 11:32–53.

80. Carratala J, Fernandez-Sevilla A, Tubau F, Callis M, Gudiol F. Emergence of quinolone-resistant *Escherichia coli* bacteremia in neutropenia patients with cancer who received prophylactic norfloxacin. *Clin Infect Dis.* 1995;20:557–560.

81. Wingard JR, Merz WG, Rinaldi MG, Johnson TR, Karp JE, Saral R. Increase in *Candida krusei* infection among patients with bone marrow transplantation and neutropenia treated prophylactically with fluconazole. *N Engl J Med.* 1991;325:1274–1277.

82. Sherertz RJ, Reagan DR, Hampton KD, et al. A cloud adult: the *Staphylococcus aureus*–virus interaction revisited. *Annals of Intern Med.* 1996;124:539–547.

83. Perl TM. The threat of vancomycin resistance. *Am J Med.* 1999;106:26S–37S.

84. Weber DJ, Rutala WA. Role of environmental contamination in the transmission of vancomycin-resistant enterococci. *Infect Control Hosp Epidemiol.* 1997;18: 306–309.

85. Hughes WT, Williams B, Williams B, et al. The nosocomial colonization of teddy bear. *Infect Control.* 1986;7:495–500.

86. Garibaldi RA, Mooney BR, Epstein BJ, Britt MR. An evaluation of daily bacteriologic monitoring to identify preventable episodes of catheter-associated urinary tract infection. *Infect Control.* 1982;3:466–470.

87. Richards MJ, Edwards JR, Culver DH, Gaynes RP. National Nosocomial Infections Surveillance system. Nosocomial infections in coronary care units in the United States. *Am J Cardiol.* 1998;82:789–793.

88. Garibaldi RA, Burke JP, Britt MR, Miller MA, Smith CB. Meatal colonization and catheter-associated bacteriuria. *N Engl J Med.* 1980;303:316–318.

89. Warren JW, Platt R, Thomas RJ, Rosner B, Kass EH. Antibiotic irrigation and catheter-associated urinary-tract infections. *N Engl J Med.* 1978;299:570–573.

90. Thompson RL, Haley CE, Searcy MA, et al. Catheter-associated bacteriuria. Failure to reduce attack rates using periodic instillations of a disinfectant into urinary drainage systems. *JAMA.* 1984;251:747–751.

91. Gross PA. Epidemiology of hospital-acquired pneumonia. *Semin Respir Infect.* 1987;2:2–7.

92. Horan TC, White JW, Jarvis WR, et al. Nosocomial infection surveillance, 1984. *MMWR.* 1986;35:17–29.

93. Leu H-S, Kaiser DL, Mori M, et al. Hospital acquired pneumonia: attributable mortality and morbidity. *Am J Epidemiol.* 1989;129:1258–1267.

94. Centers for Disease Control and Prevention. National Nosocomial Infections Study report. Annual summary 1984. *MMWR.* 1986;35:17–29.

95. Wenzel RP. Hospital-acquired pneumonia: overview of the current state of the art for prevention and control. *Eur J Clin Microbiol Infect Dis.* 1989;70:681–685.

96. Broderic A, Mori M, Netlemann WD, et al. Nosocomial infections: validation of surveillance and computer modeling to identify patients at risk. *Am J Epidemiol.* 1990;131:734–742.

97. Boyce JM, Potter-Bynoe G, Dziobek L, et al. Nosocomial pneumonia in Medicare patients. Hospital costs and reimbursement patterns under the prospective payment system. *Arch Intern Med.* 1991;151:1109–1114.

98. National Nosocomial Infections Surveillance (NNIS) report, data summary from October 1986–April 1997, issued May 1997. A report from the NNIS system. *Am J Infect Control.* May 1997.

99. Celis R, Torres A, Gatell JM, et al. Nosocomial pneumonia: a multivariate analysis of the risk and prognosis. *Chest.* 1988;93:318–324.

100. Bartlett JG, O'Keefe P, Tally FP, et al. Bacteriology of hospital-acquired pneumonia. *Arch Intern Med.* 1986; 146:868–871.

101. Fagon JY, Chastre J, Hance AJ, Montravers P, Novara

A, Gibert C. Nosocomial pneumonia in ventilated patients: a cohort study evaluating attributable mortality and hospital stay. *Am J Med*. 1993;94:281–288.

102. Gross PA, Van Antwerpen C. Nosocomial infections and hospital deaths. *Am J Med*. 1983;75:658–662.

103. Graybill JR, Marshall LW, Charache P, Wallace CK, Melvin VB. Nosocomial pneumonia: a continuing major problem. *Am Rev Respir Dis*. 1973;108:1130–1140.

104. Stevens RM, Teres D, Skillman JJ, Feingold DS. Pneumonia in an intensive care unit: a 30-month experience. *Arch Intern Med*. 1974;134:106–111.

105. Craig CP, Connelly S. Effect of intensive care unit nosocomial pneumonia on duration of stay and mortality. *Am J Infect Control*. 1984;12:233–238.

106. Craven DE, Kunches LM, Lichtenberg DA, et al. Nosocomial infection and fatality in medical and surgical intensive care unit patients. *Arch Intern Med*. 1988;148:1161–1168.

107. Prodinger WM, Bonatti H, Allerberger F, et al. Legionella pneumonia in transplant recipients: a cluster of cases of three-year duration. *J Hosp Infect*. 1994;26:191–202.

108. Harrington RD, Hooton TM, Hackman RC, et al. An outbreak of respiratory syncytial virus in a bone marrow transplant center. *J Infect Dis*. 1992;165:987–993.

109. Pannuti C, Gingrich R, Pfaller MA, et al. Nosocomial pneumonia in patients having bone marrow transplant: attributable mortality and risk factors. *Cancer*. 1992; 69:2653–2662.

110. Hall CB, Douglas RG Jr, Geiman JM, et al. Nosocomial respiratory syncytial virus infections. *N Engl J Med*. 1975;293:1343–1346.

111. Hoffman PC, Dixon RE. Control of influenza in the hospital. *Ann Intern Med*. 1977;87:725–728.

112. Kapila R, Lintz DI, Tecson FT, et al. A nosocomial outbreak of influenza A. *Chest*. 1977;71:576–579.

113. Mosconi P, Langer M, Cigada M, et al. Epidemiology and risk factors of pneumonia in critically ill patients. *Eur J Epidemiol*. 1991;7:320–327.

114. Torres A, Azner R, Gatell J, et al. Incidence, risk, and prognosis factors of nosocomial pneumonia in mechanically ventilated patients. *Am Rev Respir Dis*. 1990;142:523–528.

115. Jimenez P, Torres A, Rodriguez-Roisin R, et al. Incidence and etiology of pneumonia acquired during mechanical ventilation. *Crit Care Med*. 1989;17:882–885.

116. Rodriguez JL, Gibbons KJ, Bitzer, et al. Pneumonia: incidence, risk factors, and outcome in injured patients. *J Trauma*. 1991;31:907–912.

117. Garibaldi RA, Britt MR, Coleman ML, et al. Risk factors for postoperative pneumonia. *Am J Med*. 1981; 70:677–680.

118. Hanson LC, Weber DJ, Rutala WA, et al. Risk factors for nosocomial pneumonia in the elderly. *Am J Med*. 1992;92:161–166.

119. Josji N, Localio AR, Hamory BH. A predictive risk index of nosocomial pneumonia in the intensive care unit. *Am J Med*. 1992;93:135–141.

120. Craven DE, Steger KA, Barber TW. Preventing nosocomial pneumonia: state of the art and perspectives for the 1990s. *Am J Med*. 1991;91:44–53.

121. Cross AS, Roup B. Role of respiratory assistance devices in endemic nosocomial pneumonia. *Am J Med*. 1981;70:681–685.

122. Torres A, el-Ebiary N, Gonzalez J, et al. Gastric and pharyngeal flora in nosocomial pneumonia acquired during mechanical ventilation. *Am Rev Respir Dis*. 1993;148:352–357.

123. Centers for Disease Control and Prevention. Guidelines for prevention of nosocomial pneumonia. *MMWR*. 1997;46:1–9.

124. Wenzel RP. Preoperative antibiotic prophylaxis. *N Engl J Med*. 1992;326:337–339.

125. Leape LL, Brennan TA, Laird N, et al. The nature of adverse events in hospitalized patients: results of the Harvard Medical Practice Study II. *N Engl J Med*. 1991;324:377–384.

126. Haley RW. Surveillance by objective: a new priority-directed approach to the control of nosocomial infections. *Am J Infect Control*. 1985;13:78–89.

127. Martone W, Jarvis W, Culver D, Haley R. Incidence and nature of endemic and epidemic nosocomial infections. In: Bennett J, Brachman P, eds. *Hospital Infections*. 3rd ed. Boston: Little, Brown and Company; 1992:577–596.

128. Public health focus: surveillance, prevalence, and control of nosocomial infections. *MMWR*. 1992;41:783–787.

129. Mayhall CG. Surgical infections including burns. In: Wenzel RP, ed. *Prevention and Control of Nosocomial Infections*. Baltimore: Williams & Wilkins; 1992:614–664.

130. Manian F, Meyer L. Comprehensive surveillance of surgical wound infection in outpatient and inpatient surgery. *Infect Control Hosp Epidemiol*. 1990;11:515–520.

131. Perl TM, Roy MC. Postoperative wound infections: risk factors and role of *Staphylococcus aureus* nasal carriage. *J Chemother*. 1995;7:29–35.

132. Society for Hospital Epidemiology of America, Association of Professionals of Infection Control, Centers for Disease Control, Surgical Infection Society. Consensus paper on the surveillance of surgical wound in-

fections. *Infect Control Hosp Epidemiol.* 1992;13: 599–605.

133. Kurz A, Sessler DI, Lenhardt R. Perioperative normothermia to reduce the incidence of surgical-wound infection and shorten hospitalization. Study of Wound Infection and Temperature Group. *N Engl J Med.* 1996;334:1209–1215.

134. Simchen E, Stein H, Sacks TG, Shapiro M, Michel J. Multivariate analysis of determinants of postoperative wound infection in orthopaedic patients. *J Hosp Infect.* 1984;5:137–146.

135. Roy MC, Perl TM. Basics of surgical-site infection surveillance. *Infect Control Hosp Epidemiol.* 1997;18: 659–668.

136. Classen DC, Evans RS, Pestotnik SL, Horn SD, Menlove RL, Burke JP. The timing of prophylactic administration of antibiotics and the risk of surgical wound infection. *N Engl J Med.* 1992;326:281–286.

137. Sands K, Vineyard G, Platt R. Surgical site infections occurring after hospital discharge. *J Infect Dis.* 1996; 173(4):963–970.

138. Roy MC, Herwaldt LA, Embrey R, Kuhns K, Perl TM. A three-year wound surveillance study in cardiothoracic (CT) surgery. Paper presented at: The 34th Interscience Conference on Antimicrobial Agents and Chemotherapy; 1994; Orlando, Florida.

139. Simchen E, Rozin R, Wax Y. The Israeli study of surgical infection of drains and the risk of wound infection in operation for hernia. *Surg Gynecol Obstet.* 1990;170:331–337.

140. Brown R, Bradley S, Opitz E, Cipriani D, Pieczarka, Sands M. Surgical wound infections documented after hospital discharge. *Am J Infect Control.* 1987;15:54–58.

141. Pittet D, Wenzel RP. Nosocomial bloodstream infections. Secular trends in rates, mortality, and contribution to total hospital stay. *Arch Intern Med.* 1995; 155:1177–1184.

142. Pittet D. Nosocomial Bloodstream Infections. In: Wenzel RP, ed. *Prevention and Control of Nosocomial Infections.* 3rd ed. Baltimore: Williams & Wilkins; 1997:711–769.

143. Bryant RE, Hood AF, Hood CE, et al. Endemic Bacteremia in Columbia, SC. *Am J Epidemiol.* 1986;123: 113–127.

144. Pittet D, Tarara D, Wenzel RP. Nosocomial bloodstream infection in critically ill patients. Excess length of stay, extra costs, and attributable mortality. *JAMA.* 1994;271:1598–1601.

145. Daschner FD, Frey P, Wolff G, Baumann PC, Suter P. Nosocomial infections in intensive care wards: a multicenter prospective study. *Intensive Care Med.* 1982;8:5–9.

146. Donowitz LG, Wenzel RP, Hoyt JW. High risk of hospital-acquired infection in the ICU patient. *Crit Care Med.* 1982;10:355–357.

147. Banerjee SN, Emory TG, Culver DH, et al. Secular trends in nosocomial primary bloodstream infections in the United States, 1980–89. National Nosocomial Infection Surveillance system. *Am J Med.* 1991;91:86–89.

148. Centers for Disease Control and Prevention. Increase in national hospital discharge survey rates for septicemia—United States. *MMWR.* 1990;39:31–34.

149. Schneider EL. Infectious diseases in the elderly. *Ann Intern Med.* 1983;98:395–400.

150. Garner J, Jarvis W, Emori G, Horan T, Hughes J. Centers for Disease Control and Prevention definitions of nosocomial infections. *Am J Infect Control.* 1988; 16:128–140.

151. Maki DG. Infections due to infusion therapy. In: Bennett JV, Brachman PS, eds. *Hospital Infections.* Boston: Little, Brown and Company; 1992:849–898.

152. Pittet D, Li N, Woolson R, Wenzel R. Microbiological factors influencing the outcome of nosocomial bloodstream infections: a 6-year validation, population based model. *Clin Infect Dis.* 1997;24:1068–1078.

153. Jarvis WR. Epidemiology of nosocomial fungal infections, with emphasis on *Candida* species. *Clin Infect Dis.* 1995;20:1526–1530.

154. Wingard JR. Importance of *Candida* species other than *C. albicans* as pathogens in oncology patients. *Clin Infect Dis.* 1995;20:115–125.

155. Rex JH, Bennett JE, Sugar AM, et al. A random trial comparing fluconazole with amphotericin B for the treatment of candidemia in patients with neutropenia. *N Engl J Med.* 1994;331:1325–1330.

156. Pfaller MA. Nosocomial candidiasis: emerging species, reservoirs, and modes of transmission. *Clin Infect Dis.* 1996;22:89–94.

157. Martin MA, Pfaller MA, Wenzel RP. Coagulase-negative staphylococcal bacteremia. Mortality and hospital stay. *Ann Intern Med.* 1989;110:9–16.

158. Smith RL, Meixler SM, Simberkoff MS. Excess mortality in critically ill patients with nosocomial bloodstream infections. *Chest.* 1991;100:164–167.

159. Miller PJ, Wenzel RP. Etiologic organisms as independent predictors of death and morbidity associated with bloodstream infections. *J Infect Dis.* 1987;156: 471–477.

160. Wey SB, Mori M, Pfaller MA, Woolson RF, Wenzel RP. Hospital-acquired candidemia: the attributable mortality and excess length of stay. *Arch Intern Med.* 1988;148:2642–2645.

161. Pearson ML. Hospital Infection Control Practices Advisory Committee. Centers for Disease Control and

Prevention. Guideline for prevention of intravascular device-related infections. *Am J Infect Control.* 1996; 24:262–293.

162. Pittet D, Davis CS, Li N, Wenzel RP. Identifying the hospitalized patient at risk for nosocomial bloodstream infections: a population-based study. *Proc Assoc Am Phys.* 1997;109:58–67.

163. Velasco E, Thuler LC, Martins CA, Dias LM, Goncalves VM. Risk factors for bloodstream infections at a cancer center. *Eur J Clin Microbiol Infect Dis.* 1998;17:587–590.

164. Gaynes RP, Edwards JR, Jarvis WR, Culver DH, Tolson JS, Martone WJ. Nosocomial infections among neonates in high-risk nurseries in the United States. National Nosocomial Infections Surveillance system. *Pediatrics.* 1996;98:357–361.

165. MacDonald L, Baker C, Chenoweth C. Risk factors for candidemia in a children's hospital. *Clin Infect Dis.* 1998;26:642–645.

166. Miller JM, Goetz AM, Squier C, Muder RR. Reduction in nosocomial intravenous device-related bacteremias after institution of an intravenous therapy team. *J Intraven Nurs.* 1996;19:103–106.

167. Meier PA, Fredrickson M, Catney M, Nettleman MD. Impact of a dedicated intravenous therapy team on nosocomial bloodstream infection rates. *Am J Infect Control.* 1998;26:388–392.

168. Wenzel RP, Osterman CA, Hunting KJ, et al. Hospital acquired infections. Surveillance in a university hospital. *Am J Epidemiol.* 1976;103:251–260.

169. Ford-Jones EL, Mindorff CM, Langley JM, et al. Epidemiologic study of 4684 hospital-acquired infections in pediatric patients. *Pediatr Infect Dis J.* 1989;8:668–675.

170. Welliver RC, McLaughlin S. Unique epidemiology of nosocomial infection in a children's hospital. *Am J Dis Child.* 1984;138:131–135.

171. Anderson LJ. Major trends in nosocomial viral infections. *Am J Med.* 1991;91:107–111.

172. Yolken RJ, Bishop CA, Townsend TR, et al. Infectious gastroenteritis in bone marrow transplant recipients. *N Engl J Med.* 1982;306:1009–1012.

173. Stamm WE, Weinstein RA, Dixon RE. Comparison of endemic and epidemic nosocomial infections. *Am J Med.* 1981;70:393–397.

174. DuPont HL. Nosocomial salmonellosis and shigellosis. *Infect Control Hosp Epidemiol.* 1991;12:707–709.

175. Lightfoot NF, Ahmad F, Cowden J. Management of institutional outbreaks of salmonella gastroenteritis. *J Antimicrob Chemother.* 1990:26;37–46.

176. Dwyer DM, Klein EG, Istre GR, Robinson MG, Neumann DA, McCoy GA. *Salmonella newport* infec-

tions transmitted by fiberoptic colonoscopy. *Gastrointest Endosc.* 1987;33:84–87.

177. Stephens JL, Peacock JE. Uncommon infections: eye and central nervous system. In: Wenzel RP, ed. *Prevention and Control of Nosocomial Infections.* 2nd ed. Baltimore: Williams & Wilkins; 1993:746–775.

178. Dhaliwal RS, Meredith TA. Endophthalmitis. In: Charlton JF, Weinstein GW, eds. *Ophthalmic Surgery Complications: Prevention and Management.* Philadelphia: JB Lippincott Co; 1995:409–430.

179. Baum JL. Current concepts in ophthalmology. Ocular infections. *N Engl J Med.* 1978;299:28–31.

180. Syed NA, Hyndiuk RA. Infectious conjunctivitis. *Infect Dis Clin North Am.* 1992;6:789–805.

181. Ford E, Nelson KE, Warren D. Epidemiology of epidemic keratoconjunctivitis. *Epidemiol Review.* 1987; 9:244–261.

182. Warren D, Nelson KE, Frorar J, et al. A large outbreak of adenovirus epidemic keratoconjunctivitis: problems in controlling nosocomial spread. *J Infect Dis.* 1989; 160:938–943.

183. Gottsch JD. Surveillance and control of epidemic keratoconjunctivitis. *Trans Am Ophthalmol Soc.* 1996;94: 539–587.

184. Buckwold FJ, Hand R, Hansebout RR. Hospital-acquired bacterial meningitis in neurosurgical patients. *J Neurosurg.* 1977;46:494–500.

185. Hodges GR, Perkins RL. Hospital associated bacterial meningitis. *Am J Med Sci.* 1976;271:335–341.

186. Durand ML, Calderwood SB, Weber DJ, et al. Acute bacterial meningitis in adults. A review of 493 episodes. *N Engl J Med.* 1993;328:21–28.

187. Mangi RJ, Quintiliani R, Anmdriole VT. Gram-negative bacillary meningitis. *Am J Med.* 1975;59:829–836.

188. Berk SL, McCabe WR. Meningitis caused by gram-negative bacilli. *Ann Intern Med.* 1980;93:253–260.

189. Mancebo J, Domingo P, Blanch L, Coll P, Net A, Nolla J. Post-neurosurgical and spontaneous gram-negative bacillary meningitis in adults. *Scand J Infect Dis.* 1986;18:533–538.

190. James HE, Bejar R, Gluck L, et al. Ventriculoperitoneal shunts in high risk newborns weighing under 2000 grams: a clinical report. *Neurosurgery.* 1984; 15:198–202.

191. Unhanand M, Mustafa MM, McCracken GH Jr, Nelson JD. Gram-negative enteric bacillary meningitis: a twenty-one-year experience. *J Pediatr.* 1993; 122:15–21.

192. Pople IK, Bayston R, Hayward RD. Infection of cerebrospinal fluid shunts in infants: a study of etiological factors. *J Neurosurg.* 1992;77:29–36.

193. Kernodle DS, Kaiser AB. Postoperative infections and

antimicrobial prophylaxis. In: Mandell D, Bennett, eds. *Principles and Practice of Infectious Diseases.* 4th ed. New York: Churchill Livingstone; 1990:2742–2753.

194. Boyce JM, White RL, Spruill EY. Impact of methicillin-resistant *Staphylococcus aureus* on the incidence of nosocomial staphylococcal infections. *J Infect Dis.* 1983;148:763.

195. Nosocomial enterococci resistant to vancomycin—United States, 1989–1993. *MMWR.* 1993;42:597–599.

196. Edmond MB, Wallace SE, McClish DK, Pfaller MA, Jones RN, Wenzel RP. Nosocomial bloodstream infections in United States hospitals: a three-year analysis. *Clin Infect Dis.* 1999;29:239–244.

197. Edmond M, Ober J, Dawson, DW, et al. Vancomycin-resistant enterococcal bacteremia: natural history and attributable mortality. *Clin Infect Dis.* 1996;23:1234–1239.

198. Edmond MB, Ober JF, Weinbaum DL, et al. Vancomycin-resistant *Enterococcus faecium* bacteremia: risk factors for infection. *Clin Infect Dis.* 1995;20:1126–1133.

199. Shay DK, Maloney SA, Montecalvo M, et al. Epidemiology and mortality risk of vancomycin-resistant enterococcal bloodstream infections. *J Infect Dis.* 1995;172:993–1000.

200. Montecalvo MA, Horowitz H, Gedris C, et al. Outbreak of vancomycin-, ampicillin-, and aminoglycoside-resistant *Enterococcus faecium* bacteremia in an adult oncology unit. *Antimicrob Agents Chemother.* 1994;38:1363–1367.

201. Livornese LL Jr, Dias S, Samel C, et al. Hospital-acquired infection with vancomycin-resistant *Enterococcus faecium* transmitted by electronic thermometers. *Ann Intern Med.* 1992;117:112–116.

202. Handwerger S, Raucher B, Altarac D, et al. Nosocomial outbreak due to *Enterococcus faecium* highly resistant to vancomycin, penicillin, and gentamicin. *Clin Infect Dis.* 1993;16:750–755.

203. Tornieporth NG, Roberts RB, John J, Hafner A, Riley LW. Risk factors associated with vancomycin-resistant *Enterococcus faecium* infection or colonization in 145 matched case patients and control patients. *Clin Infect Dis.* 1996;23:767–772.

204. Roghmann M-C, McCarter RJ, Brewrink J, Cross AS, Morris JG. *Clostridium difficile* infection is a risk factor for bacteremia due to vancomycin-resistant enterococcus (VRE) in VRE-colonized patients with acute leukemia. *Clin Infect Dis.* 1997;25:1056–1059.

205. Perl TM, DeLisle S. The emergence and control of vancomycin-resistant enterococci. In: Bartlett JG, ed. *Grand Round in Infectious Disease.* Islip, NY: Scientific Exchange, Inc; 1998:7–32.

206. Smith TL, Pearson ML, Wilcox KR, et al. Emergence of vancomycin resistance in *Staphylococcus aureus. N Engl J Med.* 1999;340:493–501.

207. Centers for Disease Control and Prevention. Update: *Staphylococcus aureus* with reduced susceptibility to vancomycin—United States, 1997. *MMWR.* 1997;46:813–815.

208. Hiramatsu K, Hanaki H, Ino T, Yabuta K, Oguri T, Tenover FC. Methicillin-resistant *Staphylococcus aureus* clinical strain with reduced vancomycin susceptibility. *J Antimicrob Chemother.* 1997;40:135–136.

209. Hiramatsu K, Aritaka N, Hanaki H, et al. Dissemination in Japanese hospitals of strains of *Staphylococcus aureus* heterogeneously resistant to vancomycin. *Lancet.* 1997;350:1670–1673.

210. Waldvogel FA. New resistance in *Staphylococcus aureus. N Engl J Med.* 1999;340:556–557.

211. Sieradzki K, Roberts RB, Haber SW, Tomasz A. The development of vancomycin resistance in a patient with methicillin-resistant *Staphylococcus aureus* infection. *N Engl J Med.* 1999;340:517–523.

212. Butler JC, Hofmann J, Cetron MS, Elliott JA, Facklam RR, Breiman RF. The continued emergence of drug-resistant *Streptococcus pneumoniae* in the United States: an update from the Centers for Disease Control and Prevention's Pneumococcal Sentinel Surveillance System. *J Infect Dis.* 1996;174:986–993.

213. Pallares R, Gudiol F, Linares J, et al. Risk factors and response to antibiotic therapy in adults with bacteremic pneumonia caused by penicillin-resistant pneumococci. *N Engl J Med.* 1987;317:18–22.

214. Reichler MR, Allphin AA, Breiman RF, et al. The spread of multiply resistant *Streptococcus pneumoniae* at a day care center in Ohio. *J Infect Dis.* 1992;166:1346–1353.

215. Meyer KS, Urban C, Eagan JA, Berger BJ, Rahal JJ. Nosocomial outbreak of *Klebsiella* infection resistant to late-generation cephalosporins. *Ann Intern Med.* 1993;119:353–358.

216. Fridkin SK, Pear SM, Williamson TH, Galgiani JN, Jarvis WR. The role of understaffing in central venous catheter-associated bloodstream infections. *Infect Control Hosp Epidemiol.* 1996;17:150–158.

217. Archibald LK, Manning ML, Bell LM, Banerjee S, Jarvis WR. Patient density, nurse-to-patient ratio and nosocomial infection risk in a pediatric cardiac intensive care unit. *Pediatr Infect Dis J.* 1997;16:1045–1048.

218. American Society of American Pharmacists. ASHP mission statement. *Am J Hosp Pharm.* 1987;44:1869.

219. Craig WA, Sarver KP. Antimicrobial usage in the USA. In: Williams JD, Geddles AM, eds. *Chemo-*

therapy. Vol 4. New York: Plenum Publishing; 1976: 293–301.

220. Jorgest GJ, Dippe SE. Antibiotic use among medical specialties in community hospitals. *JAMA.* 1981;245: 842–846.

221. Maki DG, Schuna AA. A study of antimicrobial misuse in a university hospital. *Am J Med Sci.* 1978:275; 271–282.

222. Castle M, Wilfert CM, Cate TR, Osterhout S. Antimicrobial use at a Duke University Medical Center. *JAMA.* 1977;237:2819–2822.

223. Stevens GP, Jacobson JA, Burke JP. Changing pattern of hospital infections and antibiotic use, prevalence survey in a community hospital. *Arch Intern Med.* 1981;141:587–592.

224. Ayleffe GAJ. Nosocomial infections—the irreducible minimum. *Infect Control.* 1986;7:92–95.

225. Steere AC, Mallison GF. Handwashing practices for the prevention of nosocomial infections. *Ann Intern Med.* 1975;83:683–690.

226. Lilly HA, Lowbury EJL. Transient skin flora. *J Clin Pathol.* 1978;31:919–922.

227. Bryan JL, Cohran J, Larson EL. Hand washing: a ritual revisited. *Crit Care Nurs Clin North Am.* 1995;7:617–625.

228. Garner IS, Favero MS. *Guideline for Handwashing and Hospital Environmental Control.* Atlanta: Centers for Disease Control; 1985.

229. Woodroffe RCS, Shaw DA. Natural control and etiology microbial populations on skin and hair. In: Skinner FA, Carr JG, eds. *The Normal Microbial Flora of Man.* New York: Academic Press; 1974:3–34.

230. Casewell M, Phillips I. Hands as a route of transmission of *Klebsiella* species. *Br Med J.* 1977;2:1315–1317.

231. Al-Khoja MS, Darrell JH. The skin as a source of *Acinetobacter* and *Moraxella* species occurring in blood cultures. *J Clin Pathol.* 1979;32:497–499.

232. Larson E, McGinley KJ, Grove GL, et al. Physiologic, microbiologic, and seasonal effects of handwashing of the healthcare personnel. *Am J Infect Control.* 1986; 14:51–59.

233. Pittet D, Dharan S, Touveneau S, Sauvan V, Perneger TV. Bacterial contamination of the hands of hospital staff during routine patient care. *Arch Intern Med.* 1999;159:821–826.

234. Larson EL. Persistent carriage of gram-negative bacteria on hands. *Am J Infect Control.* 1981;9:112–119.

235. Noble W. Skin as a source for hospital infection. *Infect Control.* 1986;7:111–112.

236. Price PB. New studies in surgical bacteriology and surgical technique. *JAMA.* 1938;111:1993–1996.

237. Ulrich JA. Techniques of skin sampling for microbial contaminants. *Hosp Top.* 1965;43:121–123.

238. Coovadia YM, Johnson AP, Bhana RH, et al. Multiresistant *Klebsiella aerogenes* in a neonatal nursery: the importance of infection control policies and procedures in the prevention of outbreaks. *J Hosp Infect.* 1992;22:197–205.

239. Guiguet M, Rekacewicz C, Leclercq B, et al. Effectiveness of simple measures to control an outbreak of nosocomial methicillin-resistant *Staphylococcus aureus* infections in an intensive care unit. *Infect Control Hosp Epidemiol.* 1990;11:23–26.

240. Issacs D, Dobson SR, Wilkinson AR, et al. Conservative management of echovirus 11 outbreak in a neonatal unit. *Lancet.* 1989;1:543–545.

241. Doebbeling BN, Li N, Wenzel RP. An outbreak of hepatitis A among health care workers: risk factors for transmission. *Am J Public Health.* 1993;83:1679–1684.

242. Widmer AF, Wenzel RP, Trilla A, Bale MJ, Jones RN, Doebbeling BN. Outbreak of *Pseudomonas aeruginosa* infections in a surgical intensive care unit: probable transmission via hands of a health care worker. *Clin Infect Dis.* 1993;16:372–376.

243. Doebbeling BN, Stanley GL, Sheetz CT, et al. Comparative efficacy of alternative hand-washing agents in reducing nosocomial infections in intensive care units. *N Engl J Med.* 1992;327:88–93.

244. Pittet D, Mourouga P, Perneger TV. Compliance with handwashing in a teaching hospital. Infection control program. *Annals Intern Med.* 1999;130:126–130.

245. Donowitz LG. Handwashing techniques in a pediatric intensive care unit. *AJDC.* 1987;141:683–685.

246. Meengs MR, Giles BK, Chisholm CD, Cordell WH, Nelson DR. Hand washing frequency in an emergency department. *J Emerg Nurs.* 1994;20:183–188.

247. Voss A, Widmer AF. No time for handwashing!? Handwashing versus alcoholic rub: can we afford 100% compliance? *Infect Control Hosp Epidemiol.* 1997;18:205–208.

248. Larson E, Killien M. Factors influencing handwashing behavior of patient care personnel. *Am J Infect Control.* 1982;10:93–99.

249. Larson E, Kretzer EK. Compliance with handwashing and barrier precautions. *J Hosp Infect.* 1995;30:88–106.

250. Nystrom B. Impact of handwashing on mortality in intensive care: examination of the evidence. *Infect Control Hosp Epidemiol.* 1994;15:435–436.

251. Cohen HA, Matalon A, Amir J, Paret G, Barzilai A. Handwashing patterns in primary pediatric community clinics. *Infection.* 1998;26:45–47.

252. Heenan A. Handwashing practices. *Nurs Times*. 1992; 88:70.

253. Kesavan S, Barodawala S, Mulley GP. Now wash your hands? A survey of hospital handwashing facilities. *J Hosp Infect*. 1998;40:291–293.

254. Zimakoff J, Kjelsberg AB, Larsen SO, Holstein B. A multicenter questionnaire investigation of attitudes toward hand hygiene, assessed by the staff in fifteen hospitals in Denmark and Norway. *Am J Infect Control*. 1992;20:58–64.

255. Beck-Sague C, Jarvis W, Martone W. Outbreak investigation. In: Herwaldt LA, Decker MD, eds. *A Practical Handbook for Hospital Epidemiologists*. Thorofare, NJ: SLACK Incorporated and The Society for Healthcare Epidemiology of America; 1998:135–144.

256. Wendt C, Herwaldt L. Epidemics: identification and management. In: Wenzel RP, ed. *Prevention and Control of Nosocomial Infections*. 3rd ed. Baltimore: Williams & Wilkins; 1997:175–213.

257. Bolyard EA, Tablan OC, Williams WW, Pearson ML, Shapiro CN, Deitchmann SD. Guideline for infection control in healthcare personnel, 1998. Hospital Infection Control Practices Advisory Committee. *Infect Control Hosp Epidemiol*. 1998;19:407–463.

258. Decker MD, Schaffner W. Immunization of hospital personnel and other health care workers. *Infect Dis Clin North Am*. 1990;4:211–221.

259. Atkinson WL, Markowitz LE, Adams NC, Seastrom GR. Transmission of measles in medical settings—United States, 1985–1989. *Am J Med*. 1991;91:320–324.

260. Davis RM, Orenstein WA, Frank JA Jr, et al. Transmission of measles in medical settings. 1980 through 1984. *JAMA*. 1986;255:1295–1298.

261. Poland GA, Nichol KL. Medical schools and immunization policies: missed opportunities for disease prevention. *Ann Intern Med*. 1990;113:628–631.

262. Poland GA, Nichol KL. Medical students as sources of rubella and measles outbreaks. *Arch Intern Med*. 1990; 150:44–46.

263. Lane NE, Paul RI, Bratcher DF, Stover BH. A survey of policies at children's hospitals regarding immunity of healthcare workers: are physicians protected? *Infect Control Hosp Epidemiol*. 1997;18:400–404.

264. Anderson GS, Penfold JB. An outbreak of diphtheria in a hospital for the mentally subnormal. *J Clin Pathol*. 1973;26:606–615.

265. Gray RD, James SM. Occult diphtheria infection in a hospital for the mentally subnormal. *Lancet*. 1973;1: 1105–1106.

266. Palmer SR, Balfour AH, Jephcott AE. Immunisation of adults during an outbreak of diphtheria. *Br Med J (Clin Res Educ)*. 1983;286:624–626.

267. Vitek CR, Brennan MB, Gotway CA, et al. Risk of diphtheria among schoolchildren in the Russian Federation in relation to time since last vaccination. *Lancet*. 1999;353:355–358.

268. Centers for Disease Control and Prevention. Update: diphtheria epidemic—new independent states of the former Soviet Union, January 1995–March 1996. *MMWR*. 1996;45:693–697.

269. Vitek CR, Wharton M. Diphtheria in the former Soviet Union: reemergence of a pandemic disease. *Emerg Infect Dis*. 1998;4:539–550.

270. Centers for Disease Control and Prevention. Toxigenic *Corynebacterium diphtheriae*—Northern Plains Indian Community, August–October 1996. *MMWR*. 1997;46:506–510.

271. Centers for Disease Control and Prevention. Diphtheria, tetanus, and pertussis: recommendations for vaccine use and other preventive measures. Recommendations of the Immunization Practices Advisory Committee (ACIP). *MMWR*. 1991;40:1–28.

272. Vrielink H, Reesink HW. Transfusion-transmissible infections. *Curr Opin Hematol*. 1998;5:396–405.

273. Mosley JW, Nowicki MJ, Kasper CK, et al. Hepatitis A virus transmission by blood products in the United States. Transfusion Safety Study Group. *Vox Sang*. 1994;67:24–28.

274. Lemon SM. Hepatitis A virus and blood products: virus validation studies. *Blood Coagul Fibrinolysis*. 1995;6:20–22.

275. Lemon SM. The natural history of hepatitis A: the potential for transmission by transfusion of blood or blood products. *Vox Sang*. 1994;67:19–23.

276. Noble RC, Kane MA, Reeves SA, Roeckel I. Posttransfusion hepatitis A in a neonatal intensive care unit. *JAMA*. 1984;252:2711–2715.

277. Rosenblum LS, Villarino ME, Nainan OV, et al. Hepatitis A outbreak in a neonatal intensive care unit: risk factors for transmission and evidence of prolonged viral excretion among preterm infants. *J Infect Dis*. 1991;164:476–482.

278. Ebisawa I, Kurosu Y, Hatashita T. Nursery-associated hepatitis A traced to a male nurse. *J Hyg (Lond)*. 1984;92:251–254.

279. Watson JC, Fleming DW, Borella AJ, Olcott ES, Conrad RE, Baron RC. Vertical transmission of hepatitis A resulting in an outbreak in a neonatal intensive care unit. *J Infect Dis*. 1993;167:567–571.

280. Goodman RA, Carder CC, Allen JR, Orenstein WA, Finton RJ. Nosocomial hepatitis A transmission by an adult patient with diarrhea. *Am J Med*. 1982;73:220–226.

281. Centers for Disease Control and Prevention. Prevention of hepatitis A through active or passive immunization: recommendations of the Advisory Committee on Immunization Practices. *MMWR.* 1996;45:1–30.

282. Innis BL, Snitbhan R, Kunasol P, et al. Protection against hepatitis A by an inactivated vaccine. *JAMA.* 1994;271:1328–1334.

283. Furesz J, Scheifele DW, Palkonyay L. Safety and effectiveness of the new inactivated hepatitis A virus vaccine. *CMAJ.* 1995;152:343–348.

284. Sandman L, Davidson M, Krugman S. Inactivated hepatitis A vaccine: a safety and immunogenicity study in health professionals. *J Infect Dis.* 1995;171:50–52.

285. Doebbeling BN, Wenzel RP. Nosocomial viral hepatitis and infectious transmission by blood and body products. In: Mandell GL, Bennett JE, Dolin R, eds. *Principles and Practices of Infectious Diseases.* 4th ed. New York: Churchill Livingstone, 1995:2616–2632.

286. Thomas DL, Factor SH, Kelen GD, Washington AS, Taylor E Jr, Quinn TC. Viral hepatitis in health care personnel at The Johns Hopkins Hospital. The seroprevalence of and risk factors for hepatitis B virus and hepatitis C virus infection. *Arch Intern Med.* 1993;153:1705–1712.

287. Hadler SC, Doto IL, Maynard JE, et al. Occupational risk of hepatitis B infection in hospital workers. *Infect Control.* 1985;6:24–31.

288. Levy BS, Harris JC, Smith JL, et al. Hepatitis B in ward and clinical laboratory employees of a general hospital. *Am J Epidemiol.* 1977;106:330–335.

289. Scheiermann N, Kuwert EK, Pieringer E, Dermietzel R. High risk groups for hepatitis B virus infection in a university hospital staff as determined by detection of HB antigens, antibodies, and Dane particles. *Med Microbiol Immunol (Berl).* 1978;166:241–247.

290. Shapiro CN, Tokars JI, Chamberland ME. Use of the hepatitis-B vaccine and infection with hepatitis B and C among orthopaedic surgeons. The American Academy of Orthopaedic Surgeons Serosurvey Study Committee. *J Bone Joint Surg Am.* 1996;78:1791–1800.

291. Gibas A, Blewett DR, Schoenfeld DA, Dienstag JL. Prevalence and incidence of viral hepatitis in health workers in the prehepatitis B vaccination era. *Am J Epidemiol.* 1992;136:603–610.

292. Kane M. Epidemiology of hepatitis B infection in North America. *Vaccine.* 1995;13:16–17.

293. Shapiro CN. Occupational risk of infection with hepatitis B and hepatitis C virus. *Surg Clin North Am.* 1995;75:1047–1056.

294. Diekema DJ, Bradley DN. Employee health and infection control. In: Herwaldt LA, Decker MD, eds. *A Practical Handbook for Hospital Epidemiologists.* Thorofare, NJ: SLACK Incorporated and The Society for Healthcare Epidemiology of America; 1998:291–304.

295. Snydman DR, Hindman SH, Wineland MD, Bryan JA, Maynard JE. Nosocomial viral hepatitis B. A cluster among staff with subsequent transmission to patients. *Ann Intern Med.* 1976;85:573–577.

296. Grob PJ, Bischof B, Naeff F. Cluster of hepatitis B transmitted by a physician. *Lancet.* 1981;2:1218–1220.

297. Rimland D, Parkin WE, Miller GB Jr, Schrack WD. Hepatitis B outbreak traced to an oral surgeon. *N Engl J Med.* 1977;296:953–958.

298. Ahtone J, Goodman RA. Hepatitis B and dental personnel: transmission to patients and prevention issues. *J Am Dent Assoc.* 1983;106:219–222.

299. Centers for Disease Control and Prevention. Outbreaks of hepatitis B virus infection among hemodialysis patients—California, Nebraska, and Texas, 1994. *MMWR.* 1996;45:285–289.

300. Drescher J, Wagner D, Haverich A, et al. Nosocomial hepatitis B virus infections in cardiac transplant recipients transmitted during transvenous endomyocardial biopsy. *J Hosp Infect.* 1994;26:81–92.

301. Liang TJ, Hasegawa K, Rimon N, Wands JR, Ben-Porath E. A hepatitis B virus mutant associated with an epidemic of fulminant hepatitis. *N Engl J Med.* 1991;324:1705–1709.

302. Oren I, Hershow RC, Ben-Porath E, et al. A common-source outbreak of fulminant hepatitis B in a hospital. *Ann Intern Med.* 1989;110:691–698.

303. Coutinho RA, Albrecht-van Lent P, Stoutjesdijk L, et al. Hepatitis B from doctors. *Lancet.* 1982;1:345–346.

304. Centers for Disease Control and Prevention. Protection against viral hepatitis. Recommendations of the Immunization Practices Advisory Committee (ACIP). *MMWR.* 1990;39:1–26.

305. Evans ME, Hall KL, Berry SE. Influenza control in acute care hospitals. *Am J Infect Control.* 1997;25:357–362.

306. Adal KA, Flowers RH, Anglim AM et al. Prevention of nosocomial influenza. *Infect Control Hosp Epidemiol.* 1996;17:641–648.

307. Balkovic ES, Goodman RA, Rose FB, Borel CO. Nosocomial influenza A (H1N1) infection. *Am J Med Technol.* 1980;46:318–320.

308. Serwint JR, Miller RM. Why diagnose influenza infections in hospitalized pediatric patients? *Pediatr Infect Dis J.* 1993;12:200–204.

309. Tanaka Y, Ueda K, Miyazaki C, et al. Trivalent cold recombinant influenza live vaccine in institutionalized children with bronchial asthma and patients with psy-

chomotor retardation. *Pediatr Infect Dis J.* 1993; 12:600–605.

310. Serwint JR, Miller RM, Korsch BM. Influenza type A and B infections in hospitalized pediatric patients. Who should be immunized? *Am J Dis Child.* 1991; 145:623–626.

311. Glezen WP, Falcao O, Cate TR, Mintz AA. Nosocomial influenza in a general hospital for indigent patients. *Can J Infect Control.* 1991;6:65–67.

312. Whimbey E, Elting LS, Couch RB et al. Influenza A virus infections among hospitalized adult bone marrow transplant recipients. *Bone Marrow Trans.* 1994; 13:437–440.

313. Alford RH, Kasel JA, Gerone PJ, Knight V. Human influenza resulting from aerosol inhalation. *Proc Soc Exp Biol Med.* 1966;122:800–804.

314. Moser MR, Bender TR, Margolis HS, Noble GR, Kendal AP, Ritter DG. An outbreak of influenza aboard a commercial airliner. *Am J Epidemiol.* 1979; 110:1–6.

315. Knight V. Airborne transmission and pulmonary deposition of respiratory viruses. In: Mulder J, Hers JFP, eds. *Influenza.* Groningen, Netherlands: Wolters-Noordhoff; 1972:1–9.

316. Loosli CG, Lemon HM, Robertson OH, et al. Experimental air-borne influenza infection. I. Influence of humidity on survival of virus in air. *Proc Soc Exp Biol Med.* 1943;53:205–206.

317. Nabeshima A, Ikematsu H, Yamaga S, Hayashi J, Hara H, Kashiwagi S. An outbreak of influenza A (H3N2) among hospitalized geriatric patients. *Kansenshogaku Zasshi.* 1996;70:801–807.

318. Centers for Disease Control and Prevention. Influenza A in a hospital—Illinois. *MMWR.* 1981;30:79–80.

319. Hall CB, Douglas RG Jr. Nosocomial influenza infection as a cause of intercurrent fevers in infants. *Pediatrics.* 1975;55:673–677.

320. Arden NH, Patriarca PA, Fasano MB, et al. The roles of vaccination and amantadine prophylaxis in controlling an outbreak of influenza A (H3N2) in a nursing home. *Arch Intern Med.* 1988;148:865–868.

321. Arroyo JC, Postic B, Brown A, et al. Influenza A/Philippines/2/82 outbreak in a nursing home: limitations of influenza vaccination in the elderly. *Am J Infect Control.* 1984;12:329–334.

322. Patriarca PA, Weber JA, Parker RA, et al. Efficacy of influenza vaccine in nursing homes: reduction in illness and complications during influenza A (H3N2) epidemic. *JAMA.* 1985;253:1136–1139.

323. Saah AJ, Neufeld R, Rodstein M, et al. Influenza vaccine and pneumonia mortality in a nursing home population. *Arch Intern Med.* 1986;146:2353–2357.

324. Kashiwagi S, Ikematsu H, Hayashi J, Nomura H,

Kajiyama W, Kaji M. An outbreak of influenza A (H3N2) in a hospital for the elderly with emphasis on pulmonary complications. *Jpn J Med.* May 1988; 27(2):177–182.

325. Aktas F, Ulutan F, Artuk C, Usta D, Kurtar K, Atalay S. An outbreak of influenza in hospital personnel. *Mikrobiyol Bull.* 1990;24:344–351.

326. Rivera M, Gonzalez N. An influenza outbreak in a hospital. *Am J Nurs.* 1982;82:1836–1838.

327. Malanowicz W, Tyminska K, Czarniak S, Semenicki K. Clinical picture of the 1971 influenza outbreak on the basis of hospital observation of 60 patients. *Wiad Lek.* 1974;27:1049–1054.

328. Centers for Disease Control and Prevention. Prevention and control of influenza: recommendations of the Advisory Committee on Immunization Practices (ACIP). *MMWR.* 1998;47:1–26.

329. Potter J, Stott DJ, Roberts MA, et al. Influenza vaccination of health care workers in long-term-care hospitals reduces the mortality of elderly patients. *J Infect Dis.* 1997;175:1–6.

330. Wilde JA, McMillan JA, Serwint J, Butta J, O'Riordan MA, Steinhoff MC. Effectiveness of influenza vaccine in health care professionals: a randomized trial. *JAMA.* 1999;218:908–913.

331. Mast EE, Harmon MW, Gravenstein S et al. Emergence and possible transmission of amantadine-resistant viruses during nursing home outbreaks of influenza A (H3N2). *Am J Epidemiol.* 1991;134:988–997.

332. Monto AS, Robinson DP, Herlocher ML, Hinson JM Jr, Elliott MJ, Crisp A. Zanamivir in the prevention of influenza among healthy adults: a randomized controlled trial. *JAMA.* 1999;282:31–35.

333. Monto AS, Fleming DM, Henry D, et al. Efficacy and safety of the neuraminidase inhibitor zanamivirin in the treatment of influenza A and B virus infections. *J Infect Dis.* 1999;180:254–261.

334. Calfee DP, Peng AW, Cass LM, Lobo M, Hayden FG. Safety and efficacy of intravenous zanamivir in preventing experimental human influenza A virus infection. *Antimicrob Agents Chemother.* 1999;43:1616–1620.

335. Hayden FG, Atmar RL, Schilling M, et al. Use of the selective oral neuraminidase inhibitor oseltamivir to prevent influenza. *N Engl J Med.* 1999;341:1336–1342.

336. Schilling M, Povinelli L, Krause P, et al. Efficacy of zanamivir for chemoprophylaxis of nursing home influenza outbreaks. *Vaccine.* 1998;16:1771–1774.

337. Pachucki CT, Pappas SA, Fuller GF, Krause SL, Lentino JR, Schaaff DM. Influenza A among hospital personnel and patients. Implications for recognition,

prevention, and control. *Arch Intern Med.* 1989; 149:77–80.

338. Krause PJ, Cherry JD, Deseda-Tous J, et al. Epidemic measles in young adults. Clinical, epidemiologic, and serologic studies. *Ann Intern Med.* 1979;90:873–876.

339. Crawford GE, Gremillion DH. Epidemic measles and rubella in Air Force recruits: impact of immunization. *J Infect Dis.* 1981;144:403–410.

340. Remington PL, Hall WN, Davis IH, Herald A, Gunn RA. Airborne transmission of measles in a physician's office. *JAMA.* 1985;253:1574–1577.

341. Bloch AB, Orenstein WA, Ewing WM, et al. Measles outbreak in a pediatric practice: airborne transmission in an office setting. *Pediatrics.* 1985;75:676–683.

342. Fedson DS. Adult immunization. Summary of the National Vaccine Advisory Committee Report. *JAMA.* 1994;272:1133–1137.

343. Raad II, Sherertz RJ, Rains CS, et al. The importance of nosocomial transmission of measles in the propagation of a community outbreak. *Infect Control Hosp Epidemiol.* 1989;10:161–166.

344. Rivera ME, Mason WH, Ross LA, Wright HT Jr. Nosocomial measles infection in a pediatric hospital during a community-wide epidemic. *J Pediatr.* 1991; 119:183–186.

345. Gurevich I, Barzarga RA, Cunha BA. Measles: lessons from an outbreak. *Am J Infect Control.* 1992;20:319–325.

346. Enguidanos R, Mascola L, Frederick P. A survey of hospital infection control policies and employee measles cases during Los Angeles County's measles epidemic, 1987 to 1989. *Am J Infect Control.* 1992; 20:301–304.

347. Istre GR, McKee PA, West GR, et al. Measles spread in medical settings: an important focus of disease transmission? *Pediatrics.* 1987;79:356–358.

348. Rank EL, Brettman L, Katz-Pollack H, DeHertogh D, Neville D. Chronology of a hospital-wide measles outbreak: lessons learned and shared from an extraordinary week in late March 1989. *Am J Infect Control.* 1992;20:315–318.

349. Sienko DG, Friedman C, McGee HB, et al. A measles outbreak at university medical settings involving health care providers. *Am J Public Health.* 1987;77: 1222–1224.

350. Atkinson WL. Measles and healthcare workers. *Infect Control Hosp Epidemiol.* 1994;15:5–7.

351. Centers for Disease Control and Prevention. Immunization of health-care workers: recommendations of the Advisory Committee on Immunization Practices (ACIP) and the Hospital Infection Control Practices Advisory Committee (HICPAC). *MMWR.* 1997;46:1–42.

352. Willy ME, Koziol DE, Fleisher T, et al. Measles immunity in a population of healthcare workers. *Infect Control Hosp Epidemiol.* 1994;15:12–17.

353. Cote TR, Sivertson D, Horan JM, Lindegren ML, Dwyer DM. Evaluation of a two-dose measles, mumps, and rubella vaccination schedule in a cohort of college athletes. *Public Health Rep.* 1993;108:431–435.

354. Stover BH, Adams G, Kuebler CA, Cost KM, Rabalais GP. Measles-mumps-rubella immunization of susceptible hospital employees during a community measles outbreak: cost-effectiveness and protective efficacy. *Infect Control Hosp Epidemiol.* 1994;15:18–21.

355. Subbarao EK, Amin S, Kumar ML. Prevaccination serologic screening for measles in health care workers. *J Infect Dis.* 1991;163:876–878.

356. Sellick JA Jr, Longbine D, Schifeling R, Mylotte JM. Screening hospital employees for measles immunity is more cost effective than blind immunization. *Ann Intern Med.* 1992;116:982–984.

357. Kaplan KM, Marder DC, Cochi SL, Preblud SR. Mumps in the workplace. Further evidence of the changing epidemiology of a childhood vaccine-preventable disease. *JAMA.* 1988;260:1434–1438.

358. Wharton M, Cochi SL, Hutcheson RH, Schaffner W. Mumps transmission in hospitals. *Arch Intern Med.* 1990;150:47–49.

359. Fischer PR, Brunetti C, Welch V, Christenson JC. Nosocomial mumps: report of an outbreak and its control. *Am J Infect Control.* 1996;24:13–18.

360. American Academy of Pediatrics. Summaries of infectious diseases: mumps. In: Peter G, ed. *1997 Red Book: Report of the Committee on Infectious Diseases.* 24th ed. Elk Grove Village, IL: American Academy of Pediatrics; 1997:366–369.

361. Brunell PA, Brickman A, O'Hare D, Steinberg S. Ineffectiveness of isolation of patients as a method of preventing the spread of mumps. Failure of the mumps skin-test antigen to predict immune status. *N Engl J Med.* 1968;279:1357–1361.

362. Centers for Disease Control and Prevention. Mumps prevention. *MMWR.* 1989;38:388–392, 397–400.

363. Polder JA, Tablan OC, Williams WW. Personnel health services. In: Bennett JV, Brachman PS, eds. *Hospital Infections.* 3rd ed. Boston: Little, Brown and Company; 1992:31–61.

364. Deen JL, Mink CA, Cherry JD, et al. Household contact study of *Bordetella pertussis* infections. *Clin Infect Dis.* 1995;21:1211–1219.

365. Mortimer EA Jr. Pertussis and its prevention: a family affair. *J Infect Dis.* 1990;161:473–479.

366. Weber DJ, Rutala WA. Management of healthcare

workers exposed to pertussis. *Infect Control Hosp Epidemiol.* 1994;15:411–415.

367. Valenti WM, Pincus PH, Messner MK. Nosocomial pertussis: possible spread by a hospital visitor. *Am J Dis Child.* 1980;134:520–521.

368. Christie CD, Glover AM, Willke MJ, Marx ML, Reising SF, Hutchinson NM. Containment of pertussis in the regional pediatric hospital during the Greater Cincinnati epidemic of 1993. *Infect Control Hosp Epidemiol.* 1995;16:556–563.

369. Deville JG, Cherry JD, Christenson PD, et al. Frequency of unrecognized *Bordetella pertussis* infections in adults. *Clin Infect Dis.* 1995;21:639–642.

370. Nennig ME, Shinefield HR, Edwards KM, Black SB, Fireman BH. Prevalence and incidence of adult pertussis in an urban population. *JAMA.* 1996;275:1672–1674.

371. Kurt TL, Yeager AS, Guenette S, Dunlop S. Spread of pertussis by hospital staff. *JAMA.* 1972;221:264–267.

372. Shefer A, Dales L, Nelson M, Werner B, Baron R, Jackson R. Use and safety of acellular pertussis vaccine among adult hospital staff during an outbreak of pertussis. *J Infect Dis.* 1995;171:1053–1056.

373. Linnemann CC Jr, Ramundo N, Perlstein PH, Minton SD, Englender GS. Use of pertussis vaccine in an epidemic involving hospital staff. *Lancet.* 1975;2:540–543.

374. Edwards KM, Decker MD, Graham BS, Mezzatesta J, Scott J, Hackell J. Adult immunization with acellular pertussis vaccine. *JAMA.* 1993;269:53–56.

375. Lambert HJ. Epidemiology of a small pertussis outbreak in Kent County, Mich. *Public Health Rep.* 1965; 80:365–369.

376. Garner JS. Guideline for isolation precautions in hospitals. I. Evolution of isolation practices, Hospital Infection Control Practices Advisory Committee. *Am J Infect Control.* 1996;24:24–31.

377. Management of people exposed to pertussis and control of pertussis outbreaks. *CMAJ.* 1990;143:751–753.

378. Halsey NA, Welling MA, Lehman RM. Nosocomial pertussis: a failure of erythromycin treatment and prophylaxis. *Am J Dis Child.* 1980;134:521–522.

379. Steketee RW, Wassilak SG, Adkins WN Jr et al. Evidence for a high attack rate and efficacy of erythromycin prophylaxis in a pertussis outbreak in a facility for the developmentally disabled. *J Infect Dis.* 1988;157:434–440.

380. Fliegel PE, Weinstein WM. Rubella outbreak in a prenatal clinic: management and prevention. *Am J Infect Control.* 1982;10:29–33.

381. McLaughlin MC, Gold LH. The New York rubella incident: A case for changing hospital policy regarding rubella testing and immunization. *Am J Public Health.* 1979;69:287–289.

382. American Academy of Pediatrics. Summaries of infectious diseases: rubella. In: Peter G, ed. *1997 Red Book: Report of the Committee on Infectious Diseases.* 24th ed. Elk Grove Village, IL: American Academy of Pediatrics; 1997:456–462.

383. Polk BF, White JA, DeGirolami PC, Modlin JF. An outbreak of rubella among hospital personnel. *N Engl J Med.* 1980;303:541–545.

384. Reves RR, Pickering LK. Impact of child day care on infectious diseases in adults. *Infect Dis Clin North Am.* 1992;6:239–250.

385. Greaves WL, Orenstein WA, Stetler HC, Preblud SR, Hinman AR, Bart KJ. Prevention of rubella transmission in medical facilities. *JAMA.* 1982;248:861–864.

386. Strassburg MA, Imagawa DT, Fannin SL, et al. Rubella outbreak among hospital employees. *Obstet Gynecol.* 1981;57:283–288.

387. Gladstone JL, Millian SJ. Rubella exposure in an obstetric clinic. *Obstet Gynecol.* 1981;57:182–186.

388. Centers for Disease Control and Prevention. Rubella in hospitals—California. *MMWR.* 1983;32:37–39.

389. Storch GA, Gruber C, Benz B, Beaudoin J, Hayes J. A rubella outbreak among dental students: description of the outbreak and analysis of control measures. *Infect Control.* 1985;6:150–156.

390. Recommendation of the Immunization Practices Advisory Committee (ACIP): rubella prevention. *MMWR.* 1984;33(22):301–310, 315–318.

391. Sawyer MH, Chamberlin CJ, Wu YN, Aintablian N, Wallace MR. Detection of varicella-zoster virus DNA in air samples from hospital rooms. *J Infect Dis.* 1994; 169:91–94.

392. Eickhoff TC. Airborne nosocomial infection: a contemporary perspective. *Infect Control Hosp Epidemiol.* 1994;15:663–672.

393. Josephson A, Gombert ME. Airborne transmission of nosocomial varicella from localized zoster. *J Infect Dis.* 1988;158:238–241.

394. Gustafson TL, Lavely GB, Brawner ER Jr, Hutcheson RH Jr, Wright PF, Schaffner W. An outbreak of airborne nosocomial varicella. *Pediatrics.* 1982;70:550–556.

395. Leclair JM, Zaia JA, Levin MJ, Congdon RG, Goldmann DA. Airborne transmission of chickenpox in a hospital. *N Engl J Med.* 1980;302:450–453.

396. Asano Y, Iwayama S, Miyata T, et al. Spread of varicella in hospitalized children having no direct contact with an indicator zoster case and its prevention by a live vaccine. *Biken J.* 1980;2:157–161.

397. Gordon JE, Meader FM. The period of infectivity and

serum prevention of chickenpox. *JAMA*. 1929;93: 2013–2015.

398. American Academy of Pediatrics. Summaries of infectious diseases: varicella-zoster infections. In: Peter G, ed. *1997 Red Book: Report of the Committee on Infectious Diseases*. 24th ed. Elk Grove Village, IL: American Academy of Pediatrics; 1997:573–585.

399. Brunell PA. Transmission of chickenpox in a school setting prior to the observed exanthem. *Am J Dis Child*. 1989;143:1451–1452.

400. Williams WW. CDC guidelines for the prevention and control of nosocomial infections. Guideline for infection control in hospital personnel. *Am J Infect Control*. 1984;12:34–63.

401. Hyams PJ, Stuewe MC, Heitzer V. Herpes zoster causing varicella (chickenpox) in hospital employees: cost of a casual attitude. *Am J Infect Control*. 1984;12:2–5.

402. Berlin BS, Campbell T. Hospital-acquired herpes zoster following exposure to chickenpox. *JAMA*. 1970;211:1831–1833.

403. Weintraub WH, Lilly JR, Randolph JG. A chickenpox epidemic in a pediatric burn unit. *Surgery*. 1974; 76:490–494.

404. Morens DM, Bregman DJ, West CM, et al. An outbreak of varicella-zoster virus infection among cancer patients. *Ann Intern Med*. 1980;93:414–419.

405. Meyers JD, MacQuarrie MB, Merigan TC, Jennison MH. Nosocomial varicella. Part I: outbreak in oncology patients at a children's hospital. *West J Med*. 1979;130:196–199.

406. Alter SJ, Hammond JA, McVey CJ, Myers MG. Susceptibility to varicella-zoster virus among adults at high risk for exposure. *Infect Control*. 1986;7:448–451.

407. Weber DJ, Rutala WA, Parham C. Impact and costs of varicella prevention in a university hospital. *Am J Public Health*. 1988;78:19–23.

408. Weber DJ, Rutala WA, Hamilton H. Prevention and control of varicella-zoster infections in healthcare facilities. *Infect Control Hosp Epidemiol*. 1996;17:694–705.

409. Centers for Disease Control and Prevention. Prevention of varicella: recommendations of the Advisory Committee on Immunization Practices (ACIP). *MMWR*. 1996;45:1–36.

410. Anderson JD, Bonner M, Scheifele DW, Schneider BC. Lack of nosocomial spread of varicella in a pediatric hospital with negative pressure ventilated patient rooms. *Infect Control*. 1985;6:120–121.

411. Steele RW, Coleman MA, Fiser M, Bradsher RW. Varicella zoster in hospital personnel: skin test reactivity to monitor susceptibility. *Pediatrics*. 1982;70:604–608.

412. Shehab ZM, Brunell PA. Susceptibility of hospital personnel to varicella-zoster virus. *J Infect Dis*. 1984; 150:786.

413. Haiduven DJ, Hench CP, Stevens DA. Postexposure varicella management of nonimmune personnel: an alternative approach. *Infect Control Hosp Epidemiol*. 1994;15:329–334.

414. Josephson A, Karanfil L, Gombert ME. Strategies for the management of varicella-susceptible healthcare workers after a known exposure. *Infect Control Hosp Epidemiol*. 1990;11:309–313.

415. Prevention of Varicella: recommendations of the Advisory Committee on Immunization Practices (ACIP). *MMWR*. 1996;45(RR11):1–25.

416. Buckwold FJ, Ronald AR. Antimicrobial misuse—effects and suggestions for control. *J Antimicrob Chemother*. 1979;5:129–136.

417. Kunin CM, Tupasi T, Craig WA. Use of antibiotics. A brief exposition of the problem and some tentative solutions. *Ann Intern Med*. 1973;79:555–560.

418. Pallares R, Dick R, Wenzel RP, Adams JR, Nettleman MD. Trends in antimicrobial utilization at a tertiary teaching hospital during a 15-year period (1978–1992). *Infect Control Hosp Epidemiol*. 1993;14:376–382.

419. Simchen E, Wax Y, Galai N, Israeli A. Discharge from hospital and its effect on surgical wound infections. The Israeli Study of Surgical Infections (ISSI). *J Clin Epidemiol*. 1992;45:1155–1163.

420. Hulton LJ, Olmsted RN, Treston-Aurand J, Craig CP. Effect of postdischarge surveillance on rates of infectious complications after cesarean section. *Am J Infect Control*. 1992;20:198–201.

421. Weigelt JA, Dryer D, Haley RW. The necessity and efficiency of wound surveillance after discharge. *Arch Surg*. 1992;127:77–81.

422. Law DJ, Mishriki SF, Jeffery PJ. The importance of surveillance after discharge from hospital in the diagnosis of postoperative wound infection. *Ann R Coll Surg Engl*. 1990;72:207–209.

423. Olson MM, Lee JT Jr. Continuous, 10-year wound infection surveillance. Results, advantages, and unanswered questions. *Arch Surg*. 1990;125:794–803.

424. Krukowski ZH, Irwin ST, Denholm S, Matheson NA. Preventing wound infection after appendectomy: a review. *Br J Surg*. 1988;75:1023–1033.

425. Reimer K, Gleed C, Nicolle LE. The impact of postdischarge infection on surgical wound infection rates. *Infect Control*. 1987;8:237–240.

426. Brown RB, Bradley S, Opitz E, Cipriani D, Pieczarka R, Sands M. Surgical wound infections documented after hospital discharge. *Am J Infect Control*. 1987; 15:54–58.

PART III

Airborne Transmission

CHAPTER 14

Tuberculosis

Jacqueline S. Coberly and Richard E. Chaisson

INTRODUCTION

The ancient Greeks called it *phthisis*, the Romans *tabes*, the Hindus *rajayakshma*, and in Victorian England, it was *consumption*.[1] All of these different names referred to the wasting illness that is characteristic of the disease we now call *tuberculosis*. Tuberculosis is a complex communicable disease of humans caused by *Mycobacterium tuberculosis* and less commonly by the related bacteria *M. africanum* and *M. bovis*, collectively referred to as the *tubercle bacilli*.[2] With the advent of effective drug treatment in the 1950s and prophylaxis in the 1960s, many in the medical and public health communities, particularly in the industrialized countries, assumed that tuberculosis was conquered. This hubris led to several decades of neglect by the biomedical community, during which control efforts were ignored or deliberately weakened. Unfortunately, the economic, social, and public health factors that foster the propagation of tuberculosis had not been eliminated, not even from the industrialized nations. So, in the 1980s and 1990s, as the deterioration of control programs coincided with the HIV epidemic, tuberculosis rebounded. Numerous outbreaks were seen in the larger cities of the United States, which had the highest incidence of human immunodeficiency virus (HIV).[3] More serious, however, was that, in some areas of the developing world where tuberculosis and HIV are both

endemic, the incidence of tuberculosis doubled, and health care facilities were overwhelmed by the dual epidemic.

In 1999, The World Health Organization (WHO) ranked tuberculosis among the most serious health threats to the world. It is estimated that a third of the people in the world are latently infected with *M. tuberculosis*. In addition, 7 to 8 million new tuberculosis cases occur each year, and approximately 2 million people die from the disease.[4–6] In recent years, a renewed effort to promote tuberculosis control has been launched. Unfortunately, the wide distribution of the infection and its complex epidemiology and natural history, coupled with insufficient resources to adequately respond to the epidemic, will ensure that tuberculosis will be a serious public health problem for many more years.

THE ORGANISM

The family *Mycobacteriaceae*, of the order Actinomycetales, is composed of a number of slow-growing, acid-fast bacilli. Most are saprophytes, useful inhabitants of soil and water that help degrade organic material. Some are pathogens in animals and occasionally cause opportunistic infection in man.[7,8] Only four are highly pathogenic in humans: *Mycobacterium leprae,* which causes leprosy; and the tubercle bacilli, *M. tuberculosis*, *M. africanum,* and *M. bovis*, three closely related species that cause tuberculosis. Based on DNA homology and physical characteristics, two other species of mycobacteria, *M. microti* is sometimes grouped with the tubercle bacilli as *M. tuberculosis* complex but only rarely cause disease in humans.[1,2,8] With the advent of the HIV epidemic, several other mycobacteria, most notably *M. avium* complex (MAC), have become common opportunistic pathogens and cause illness in people infected with HIV, which is clinically similar to disseminated tuberculosis (Table 14–1).[2,7]

M. tuberculosis, M. africanum, and *M. bovis* are slender, slightly curved, rod-shaped bacteria averaging 4 by 0.3 mm.[2,7–10] *M. tuberculosis* is strictly aerobic, whereas *M. bovis* is microaerophilic and adapts more easily to nonpulmonary sites of infection. Like the other mycobacteria, they have an unusual concentration of high-molecular-weight lipids in their cell wall; accounting for approximately 50% of dry weight. This high lipid content makes these organisms hydrophobic and resistant to aqueous bactericidal agents and drying. It is also responsible for their characteristic acid-fastness, which is essentially synonymous with mycobacteria.[2,7]

Mycobacteria are slow-growing in culture, and because *M. tuberculosis* has a very long generation time (~24 hours), replication in culture is a slow process, often resulting in diagnostic delays. Traditionally, mycobacteria are grown on solid, enriched media, where colonies generally appear 4 to 6 weeks after inoculation. They can also be grown in liquid culture, where they form characteristic strings by light microscopy. Rapid liquid culture systems (e.g., BACTEC) have been adapted for use with mycobacteria and allow identification of organisms in as little as 9 to 16 days, depending on the concentration of microbes in the specimen being tested.[2,10] Use of DNA probes speeds speciation of organisms following growth. Alternatively, a number of biochemical tests can be used to speciate mycobacteria, though these are time consuming. Nucleic acid amplification procedures, such as polymerase chain reaction (PCR), are also used to diagnose tuberculosis, though these are not yet standardized.[2,11]

HISTORY

Evolution of the Tubercle Bacilli

Mycobacteria are ancient organisms that probably first appeared more than a million years ago in soil and water and gradually adapted to animal hosts during the Paleolithic period and later to man.[12,13] Skeletal remains of Neolithic man with deformities suggestive of tuberculosis have been found in Germany, France, Italy, Denmark, and Jordan and dated from 8,000 to 5,000 B.C.[1,14] It cannot be conclusively proved that these deformities are the result of infection with the tubercle bacillus because the organism cannot be cultured from the bone. The deformities themselves are strongly suggestive of spinal tuberculosis or Pott's disease, however.[1,12]

Traces of tuberculosis-like disease have also been identified in Egyptian mummies dating from 3,500 to 400 B.C.[2,13] One particularly well-preserved mummy of a young boy, who died from pulmonary disease around 1,000 B.C., was discovered with the lungs intact. Again, the causative organism could not be conclusively identified, but a diagnosis of tuberculosis was made based on the observation of pleural adhesion, blood in the trachea, and the presence of acid-fast bacilli in the lung tissue.[2] Egyptian artifacts from this period also begin to show people with the spinal deformities characteristic of Pott's disease.[2]

It is hypothesized that, once humans began domesticating cattle from about 7,000 to 4,000 B.C., they began to be frequently exposed to *M. bovis*. Initially, these exposures may have resulted in sporadic cases of spinal tuberculosis or, occasionally, isolated cases of intestinal or pulmonary disease.[12] These are the cases we see in the remains of Neolithic and Egyptian people. Eventually, however, *M. bovis* adapted itself to man and evolved into a new species, *M. tuberculosis,* which could spread between people via the aerosol route. This adaptation, combined with the increasing tendency of people to gather together in ever-larger populations, led to the es-

Table 14–1 Species of Mycobacteria

	Microbe	Reservoir	Clinical Manifestation
Always Pathogenic in Man	*Mycobacterium tuberculosis*	Man	Pulmonary and disseminated TB
	M. bovis	Man, cattle	TB-like disease
	M. leprae	Man, armadillo	Leprosy
	M. africanum	Man, monkey	Rarely TB-like pulmonary disease
Potentially Pathogenic in Man	*M. avium* complex	Soil, water, birds, fowl, swine, cattle, and environment	Disseminated and TB-like pulmonary disease
	M. kansasii	Water, cattle	TB-like disease
Uncommonly or Rarely Pathogenic in Man	*M. genavense*	Man?, pet birds?	Blood-borne disease with AIDS
	M. haemophilum	?	Subcutaneous nodules and ulcers primarily with AIDS
	M. malmoense	?, Environment	Adults: TB-like pulmonary disease; children: lymphadenitis
	M. marinum	Fish, water	Skin infections
	M. scrofulaceum	Soil, water	Cervical lymphadenitis
	M. simiae	Monkey, water	TB-like pulmonary disseminated disease with AIDS
	M. szulgai	?	TB-like pulmonary disease
	M. ulcerans	Man, environmental	Skin infections (Buruli ulcer)
	M. xenopi	Water, birds	TB-like pulmonary disease

Source: Adapted with permission from G.F. Brooks, J.S. Butel, and S.A. Morse, *Jawetz, Melnick & Adelberg's Medical Microbiology*, 21st ed., © 1998, The McGraw-Hill Companies.

tablishment of tuberculosis as an epidemic disease of humans.[1,12]

Global Evolution of the Epidemic

By the first century A.D., tuberculosis was well established in the Mediterranean states and Western Europe. It remained a relatively sporadic disease for centuries, until people began settling in larger communities.[12] The advent of the Industrial Revolution and the great migrations to the cities that followed created an ideal environment for the spread of tuberculosis.[13,15] In 1662, one of every six northern Europeans had tuberculosis; 100 years later, the figure had doubled.[2] Tuberculosis was so common that most of the population became infected, and 25% of all deaths were attributed to tuberculosis.[12] Thomas Sydenham was quoted in 1682 as saying that "Two thirds of those who die of chronic diseases . . . [are] . . . killed by phthisis."[15] The epidemic peaked in England in the 1780s and in Western Europe by 1800.[13]

Although sporadic, *M. bovis* infections were not uncommon in the largely agrarian societies of the New World; the English and European colonists are probably responsible for spreading *M. tuberculosis* throughout North America. Tuberculosis arrived on the Mayflower and was well established in the colonies by the early eighteenth century.[1,13] The epidemic passed through the United States in a wave pushing south and west with the spread of industrialization, and by the early twentieth century was endemic in North America.[13] Tuberculosis was also spread to South America by colonists but, because the Spanish quarantined consumptives in the seventeenth and eighteenth centuries, the disease was introduced a bit later there.[1] Tuberculosis also spread into Eastern Europe, Asia, and Africa from Western Europe. The epidemics in Russia came in the late nineteenth century and in Asia in the early twentieth century. Tuberculosis was still largely unknown in Africa at the beginning of the twentieth century and spread slowly through the interior with the colonizing Europeans.[1,12] The gradual spread of tuberculosis may help explain why the shape of the epidemic varies in different parts of the world today.

CLINICAL MANIFESTATIONS

As discussed in more detail later, tuberculosis begins with latent infection that can progress to active disease. Latent infection causes no symptoms, and most latently infected people are unaware that they harbor tubercle bacilli. Tuberculosis disease generally affects the lungs and respiratory tract but can strike nearly any organ system in the body. Both primary and reactivation tuberculosis disease can result in pulmonary or extrapulmonary manifestations. In immunocompetent people, about 80% of tuberculosis is pulmonary, and extrapulmonary disease is less common. Extrapulmonary disease is, however, much more common in immunodeficient individuals and children.[11,16] A small percentage of immunocompetent patients and many more immunodeficient ones develop both pulmonary and extrapulmonary tuberculosis.[16]

The onset of active tuberculosis is insidious, and the symptoms can be nonspecific. Pulmonary disease causes symptoms ranging from very mild to severe and can present with productive cough with or without bloody sputum, fatigue, anorexia and weight loss, fever, sweating and/or chills, and chest pain.[8,11,16] Extrapulmonary tuberculosis also causes fatigue and night sweats but generally other symptoms specifically related to the affected organ system will be prominent.[8,11,16,17] More frequent sites of extrapulmonary infection include the pleura, pericardium, larynx, lymph nodes, skeleton (particularly the spine), genitourinary tract, eyes, meninges, gastrointestinal tract, adrenal gland, and skin.[2,18] Systemic infection with tubercle bacilli occurs when hematogenous or lymphatic dissemination spreads the organism throughout the body, producing small nodules of infection in essentially every organ of the body. Early researchers named disseminated disease *miliary tuberculosis* because they thought that the tiny nodules resembled grains of millet, particularly when seen by chest radiography.[8,16,19] Miliary tuberculosis is especially common in children and in people with immunosuppression.[3,5,11]

DIAGNOSIS

Latent Tuberculosis Infection

Latent tuberculosis infection is asymptomatic; therefore, diagnosis is based on clinical tests that identify signs of infection or immunologic responses to tuberculosis antigens. In the past, tuberculosis infection was often diagnosed radiographically, with calcified lesions interpreted as evidence of infection.[2,20] This technique has been shown to lack both sensitivity and specificity and has been abandoned. Serologic diagnosis of tuberculosis infection has been extensively investigated but also lacks sensitivity because the number of tubercle bacilli in latent tuberculosis is very low, and antibody responses are limited.[21] Identification of specific cellular immune responses through the induction of delayed type hypersensitivity with tuberculin tests is now the most widely used method for diagnosing latent infection.[21,22] Tuberculin purified protein derivative (PPD) is a solution prepared from cultures of tubercle bacilli.[23,24] It was developed by Robert Koch in 1890 and touted as a cure for tuberculosis. The curative value of tuberculin was soon disproved, but further studies showed that it could be used to identify people with tuberculosis infection.[20,24,25] The Mantoux method of intracutaneous injection of a standardized dose of tuberculin has been widely validated, whereas other methods (i.e., the Tine test) have not. Individuals with a latent infection develop a zone of induration when a standardized amount of tuberculin is injected intracutaneously, whereas uninfected people react minimally or not at all. The result of the tuberculin skin test is reported as the width of induration that surrounds the test site 48 to 72 hours following injection.[22] The test is usually applied to the volar surface of the forearm and read by a trained observer, who measures induration by marking the edge of the hardened area of skin, either visually or by using a ballpoint pen to de-

marcate the border, and recording the distance across in millimeters. Induration of the injection site is the result of a delayed type hypersensitivity response in which activated T cells and macrophages migrate to the site of antigen injection and mount a localized cellular immune response. It is essential that at least 48 hours be allowed for this process to mature; earlier readings may produce falsely negative or positive results. Erythema of the site is nonspecific and should not be interpreted as a positive result. Positive results remain measurable for more than 1 week in most instances.

The performance characteristics of the tuberculin test were standardized in the 1940s in an important study led by Dr. Carroll Palmer, where varying concentrations of tuberculin were administered to a group of patients with active tuberculosis and to controls who were unlikely to have ever encountered tuberculosis in their lifetimes.[26] The currently used standard dose of 5 tuberculin units of PPD-S was found to elicit a reaction of greater than 10 mm of induration in almost 98% of tuberculosis patients and in less than 5% of controls. A smaller dose, 2 tuberculin units, of another preparation, RT-23 tuberculin, produces similar results.

Exposure to nontuberculous mycobacteria may induce cross-reactivity to tuberculin, which can result in a falsely positive response.[24] Similarly, vaccination against tuberculosis with bacillus Calmette-Guérin (BCG) vaccine can induce a response. The strength and durability of the reaction produced by BCG is less than with tuberculosis infection, and after 3 to 5 years, does not generally interfere with PPD testing.[11,27] Skin test results can also be falsely negative when the cellular immune system is impaired. People with active tuberculosis who are co-infected with HIV or have cancer or other immunosuppressive illnesses are frequently unable to mount a response to any skin test antigen, so tuberculin results in these people should be interpreted with some care.[17,18,24,26] Malnutrition also interferes with immunity and can inhibit response to tuberculin, as can acute viral infections such as measles.[8,20,22,28,29] In addition, between 10% and 25% of people with active tuberculosis fail to respond to tuberculin.[24,30] The size of the tuberculin response is not, however, associated with the patient's stage of disease because the size of reaction in active cases and their close contacts is similar.[18,24] Thus, the size of the reaction to tuberculin varies considerably, depending on the individual's exposure to the tubercle bacilli and other nontuberculous mycobacteria, BCG vaccination history, and immune status.[24]

Although the sensitivity and specificity of tuberculin testing can be evaluated in people with active tuberculosis, determining the accuracy of the test in people with latent infection is more difficult because no gold standard for diagnosis exists. In studies of U.S. Navy recruits undertaken in the 1950s and 1960s, a tuberculin reaction of >10 mm was strongly associated with the subsequent risk of tuberculosis. Nonetheless, because some people with negative tests develop tuberculosis and many people with positive tests do not, the interpretation of test results must be modified on the basis of clinical and epidemiologic knowledge. Perhaps more so than with most clinical tests, interpretation of the tuberculin test is highly dependent on prior probability of tuberculosis infection and clinical consequences of misreading the result. As shown in Table 14–2, the reaction size that is considered positive varies by the clinical status of the person being tested. For example, household contacts of an infectious tuberculosis patient have a high prior probability of infection; therefore, the cut-point for a positive test is 5 mm. Additionally, an HIV-infected person has a very high risk of developing active tuberculosis if infected, so a 5-mm reaction is considered positive because the consequences of misinterpreting the result are severe and because HIV infection suppresses the cellular immune response, which can diminish the size of the reaction to PPD.[31] For people who come from an area where tuberculosis is prevalent, a 10-mm response is considered positive, as is the case for people with medical conditions associated with increased tuberculosis risk (e.g., diabetes, steroid use, end-stage renal disease). For people with a low prior probability

of tuberculosis exposure and low risk of disease if infected, the cut-point for a positive test is 15 mm of induration.[24]

Active Tuberculosis Disease

In active tuberculosis, clinical signs and symptoms result from the replication of large numbers of tubercle bacilli and the ensuing inflammatory host response. Diagnosis of active tuberculosis is based on evaluation of epidemiologic assessment of tuberculosis risk, clinical findings and symptoms, and laboratory tests, including chest radiographs, tuberculin skin tests, and microscopic examination and culture of tissues, such as sputum or biopsy specimens.

The signs and symptoms of active tuberculosis are nonspecific and overlap with a number of other pulmonary and systemic diseases. Fever, sweats, and weight loss are prominent systemic findings and are usually of several weeks or months duration. Cough is a principal feature of pulmonary tuberculosis and can be associated with sputum production or hemoptysis. The symptoms of extrapulmonary tuberculosis are highly variable and depend on the specific organ involved.

Chest radiographs are critically important in diagnosing pulmonary tuberculosis. Classically, patients with reactivation tuberculosis have upper lobe, cavitary infiltrates or involvement of the superior segments of the lower lobes, whereas patients with primary tuberculosis have mostly lower or midlung infiltrates and hilar adenopathy. Recent studies using molecular epidemiologic techniques, however, have shown that both primary and reactivation tuberculosis can present with chest radiograph findings that are classic for the other form of disease. In the setting of clinical symptoms consistent with tuberculosis and an abnormal chest radiograph, specific diagnostic tests for tuberculosis should be undertaken. With HIV infection and tuberculosis, however, the chest radiography in some patients may be normal.

Diagnosis of tuberculosis is confirmed by identification of acid-fast bacilli by smear or by

Table 14–2 Cut-Points for Positive Tuberculin Skin Test

Category	*Cut-Point for Positive PPD**
Co-infected with HIV	≥5 mm
Close contacts of known cases	≥5 mm
Medical factors that increase risk for tuberculosis	≥10 mm
Residence in high-prevalence area	≥10 mm
Low risk for infection and disease	≥15 mm

*PPD, purified protein derivative.

Source: Adapted with permission from A. Fauci, *Harrison's Principles of Internal Medicine Companion Handbook*, 14th ed., © 1998, McGraw-Hill, Inc.

isolation of *M. tuberculosis* in cultures of sputum or other bodily fluid. Zeihl-Neelsen staining is the standard method used globally for microscopic identification of acid-fast bacilli. In this process, a fixed smear is exposed to hot carbol fushin dye for 2 to 3 minutes, rinsed, and decolorized with a dilute acid-alcohol solution. Mycobacteria absorb the carbol fushin dye but resist decolorization because of the high lipid content in their cell walls, hence the name *acid-fast bacilli*.[10] Fluorescent staining with auramine-rhodamine is a more sensitive but more expensive technique. Unfortunately, the number of tubercle bacilli present in sputum may be very low, particularly in noncavitary disease, so direct microscopic observation is a fairly insensitive way to diagnose tuberculosis. Only about 60% of culture-confirmed cases of tuberculosis are smear positive. Also, positive microscopy proves only the presence of acid-fast bacilli, which could include nonpathogenic species of mycobacteria or other acid-fast bacteria, such as *Nocardia*.[17,18]

Several types of tests, including nucleic acid amplification assays (e.g., PCR), mass spectrometry, or gas-liquid chromatography for tuberculostearic acid, and immunoassays for mycobacterial antigens and antibodies have been used to diagnose active tuberculosis with mixed results. Nucleic acid amplification tests have been approved in the United States for the diagnosis in patients with positive sputum smears. Both the positive and negative predictive values of these tests are high if the sputum smear is positive but in sputum smear-negative patients, the positive predictive value of nucleic acid amplification is only about 50%. The utility of this method may be improved with new generations of tests in the near future.

In many parts of the world where tuberculosis is endemic, culture and radiography are unavailable or are extremely limited. In these areas, diagnosis relies primarily on clinical history and microscopic examination of sputum. New, simple, rapid diagnostic techniques are desperately needed in these areas and would also be valuable in more industrialized areas.

Ultimately, the diagnosis of tuberculosis involves a synthesis of clinical and laboratory findings. The case definition of tuberculosis used for surveillance purposes accepts the diagnosis if there is a positive culture, a positive acid-fast smear with compatible clinical findings, or a characteristic illness with other evidence suggestive of tuberculosis and an appropriate response to antituberculosis therapy.

THERAPY

History of Therapy

The history of tuberculosis therapy is divided into three eras: the presanatorium, sanatorium, and chemotherapeutic eras. From earliest recognition of tuberculosis as a disease until the middle of the nineteenth century, therapy for tuberculosis was based on the presiding medical dogma.[31] When ill airs were thought to cause tuberculosis, patients were told to move to mild, mountain, or seaside climates. When imbalance of bodily humors was thought to be the cause of all disease, bloodletting was recommended for tuberculosis.[32] Rest or mild exercise and different variations in diet have also been recommended at various times. Although most of these treatments did the patient no harm, they also did little to deter the progress of the infection.

In the 1850s, a number of physicians observed that a prolonged rest in quiet, mountainous, rural areas had cured their patients of tuberculosis, and the sanatorium movement was born. The premise was that clean air, combined with rest or mild exercise and good food, would stimulate the body to heal itself. Therefore, patients were isolated in rural institutions built solely for the treatment of tuberculosis.[20,32] The first sanatorium was established by Brehmer in 1854 in the mountains of Germany, and as the idea took hold, sanatoria were built throughout Europe, the United States, and England.[20] Isolation of tuberculosis cases to the sanatorium, although perhaps no more beneficial to patients than extended rest at home, decreased the spread of tuberculosis in the community, contributing to the large decline in tuberculosis incidence seen in the late nineteenth and early twentieth centuries in Europe and the United States.[32] Developments in the basic sciences during the sanatorium movement also contributed to this decline. During this time, Koch discovered the causative agent of tuberculosis, and radiographic technology and surgical techniques were developed that greatly enhanced physicians' abilities to diagnose and treat tuberculosis.

Unfortunately, sanatorium care had its limitations, and in the early twentieth century, tuberculosis was still a major cause of death. In 1938, Rich and Follis showed that sulfanilamide inhibited the growth of *M. tuberculosis* in guinea pigs, and the search for effective chemotherapeutic agents for tuberculosis began.[32] Dapsone was tested against tuberculosis in 1940, and in 1943, streptomycin was found to have antituberculosis action. The identification of other antituberculosis drugs, including para-aminosalicylic acid (PAS) and isoniazid (INH), soon followed.[32]

The tradition of randomized clinical trials has a prominent place in the history of tuberculosis research. The scarcity of streptomycin in the early 1940s led the British Medical Research Council to perform the first multicenter, randomized, controlled clinical trial to estimate the efficacy of streptomycin against a placebo.[33] This elegant trial demonstrated the profound efficacy of streptomycin against the tubercle bacilli and the limitations of single drug therapy in the treatment of tuberculosis. More trials followed rapidly as new drugs were identified, each building on the information provided by earlier work. A series of trials over several decades proved the value of combination therapy for curing tuberculosis and preventing drug resistance, the efficacy of dual therapy with streptomycin and PAS,[34] the efficacy of combined therapy using INH,[35] the utility of multidrug therapy in shortening the duration of tuberculosis treatment, the minimum treatment time needed for effective cure of tuberculosis,[36–39] the optimum drug combination for therapy,[36–41] the efficacy of intermittent (twice or thrice weekly) treatment,[39,42–44] and the efficacy of treatment for tuberculosis in HIV-infected people.[45–48]

Current Therapy

The drugs most commonly used in treatment of tuberculosis today and their modes of action are shown in Table 14–3. Because the bacillary population in an infected person consists of actively growing, semidormant, and dormant mycobacteria,[49] effective chemotherapy is complex. Some drugs that kill actively growing bacilli cannot kill those in the latent, resting phase. Drug treatment must, therefore, continue for a minimum of 6 months to allow the majority of latent organisms to be exposed to the drugs during periods of metabolic activity, and be killed. Unfortunately, this long period of treat-

Table 14–3 First-Line Antituberculous Drugs and their Modes of Action

Drug (Abbreviation)	Mode of Action	Effect
Isoniazid (H)	bactericidal	kills metabolically active mycobacteria
Rifampicin (R)	bactericidal	kills metabolically active and semidormant mycobacteria
Pyrazinamide (Z)	bactericidal	kills mycobacteria at acid pH (within cells)
Streptomycin (S)	bacteriostatic	halts growth and reproduction, does not kill
Ethambutol (E)	bacteriostatic	halts growth and reproduction, does not kill
Thiacetazone (T)	bacteriostatic	halts growth and reproduction, does not kill

Source: Data from A.D. Harries and A.D. Maher, *TB/HIV: A Clinical Manual*, Copyright 1996, World Health Organization, and R.H. Alford, Antimycobacterial Agents, in *Principles and Practice of Infectious Diseases*, 3rd ed., pp. 350–360, G.L. Mandell, R.G. Douglas, Jr., and J.E. Bennett, eds., © 1990, Churchill Livingstone.

ment also allows sufficient time for mutant bacilli to emerge that are resistant to the drug being used for treatment. When a single drug is used for treatment of tuberculosis, mutants resistant to that drug rapidly emerge, eventually become the predominant bacilli, and therapy fails. Use of at least two drugs to which the organisms are susceptible reduces the probability of developing drug-resistant microbes to essentially zero.

Key to treatment success is adherence with the full drug regimen, which reduces the risk of treatment failure and the emergence of drug resistance. The Centers for Disease Control and Prevention (CDC) and the WHO recommend that directly observed therapy (DOT) be used for tuberculosis therapy. DOT implies that a health care worker monitors each tuberculosis patient closely and observes the patient taking each dose of antituberculosis medication. Historical analysis suggests that use of DOT contributes to reductions in tuberculosis incidence and dramatically reduces the incidence of drug-resistant tuberculosis. One randomized trial that compared DOT with self-administered therapy found no advantage to DOT; however, treatment outcomes in both groups were abominable, and the study was deeply flawed in other aspects.[50] DOT is generally accepted as a highly effective tuberculosis control strategy.

The WHO currently recommends a short-course DOT drug regimen (DOTS) for treatment of tuberculosis, which includes treatment with four drugs—generally, INH, rifampin, pyrazinamide, and ethambutol—for 2 months, followed by 4 months of treatment with INH and rifampin.[49] Review of many studies has shown that fewer than 6 months of drug therapy results in an unacceptably high treatment failure or relapse rates, whereas longer treatment regimens do not yield substantially better outcomes, with relapse rates of 5% or less.[37]

EPIDEMIOLOGY

Global Prevalence and Incidence

The magnitude of the global tuberculosis epidemic is staggering. One third of the world population, roughly 1.9 billion people, is infected with *M. tuberculosis*.[4,49] It is the seventh leading cause of death in the world and causes more deaths each year (~2 million) than all other infectious agents except HIV.[51,52]

Although tuberculosis re-emerged in the 1980s as a public health problem in the United States and other industrialized nations, 95% of all tuberculosis cases occur in the developing world (Figure 14–1).[51] Tuberculosis causes 25% of preventable adult deaths in the developing world,[4,49] and 75% of cases and 80% of deaths in these areas occur in adults aged 15 to 55, the most productive members of society.[4,29,49]

Approximately 7 to 8 million people develop tuberculosis each year.[4] Assuming that there are

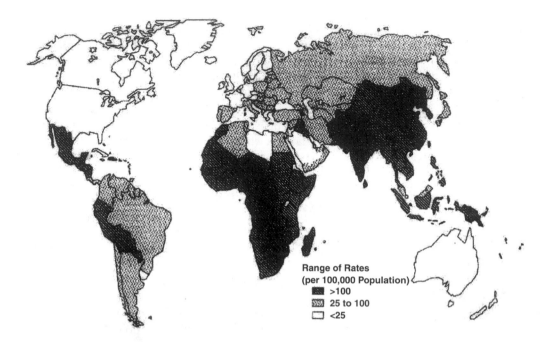

Figure 14–1 Estimated incidence of tuberculosis worldwide by country, 1997. *Source:* Reprinted with permission from M.C. Raviglione, D.E. Snider Jr, A. Kochi, Global Epidemiology of Tuberculosis, Morbidity and Mortality of a Worldwide Epidemic, *Journal of the American Medical Society*, Vol. 273, pp. 220–226, Copyright 1995, American Medical Society.

no significant improvements in prevention and control between 1999 and 2020, WHO estimates that in the first two decades of the twenty-first century, 1 billion people will acquire new tuberculosis infection, 200 million will develop active disease, and 70 million will die.[4,51]

Global Variation in Disease

In viewing tuberculosis incidence and mortality in the world in 1999, the pictures from Europe, the United States, South America, Asia, and Africa appear strikingly different (Figure 14–1). In the United States and Europe, incidence and mortality, except for pockets in large urban centers where HIV is modifying the course of the epidemic, are low in all age categories. Incidence and mortality is lowest in infancy and increases slowly but steadily throughout life. Rates are similar in men and women until

about 60 years of age and higher in men thereafter.[20]

In Latin America and the Caribbean, tuberculosis is much more prevalent, and incidence and mortality are higher than in Europe and the United States. Incidence and mortality curves show two peaks: in infancy, and in late adolescence and early adulthood. The first peak is higher in males and the second in females. As rates decline after the second peak, the incidence and mortality in males surpasses that in females (at about age 35) and remains higher until death.[13,53,54]

The prevalence of tuberculosis is higher still in Asia and Africa. As many as 60% to 70% of adults in some areas have evidence of latent infection. As in Latin America, incidence and mortality curves show two peaks, first in infancy when rates are higher in boys than girls. This differential equalizes later in childhood. In late adolescence, the curves again rise sharply, and this time, the rates in women exceed those in men. At about age 60, the rates flip once more, and the incidence in men again exceeds that in women.[13]

Natural History

The tubercle bacillus is only moderately infectious; about 20% to 30% of those exposed to an active case will become infected.[53] As with most other infectious diseases, development of clinical tuberculosis is a two-step process: infection of the host with the microorganism and development of active disease caused by unchecked microbial replication and the body's immune response. What is different about the tubercle bacillus is that after it infects tissues, it can remain dormant for 20 to 30 years before active disease develops.

In a classic infection, *M. tuberculosis* enters the body via minute droplet nuclei deposited in the air when a person with active tuberculosis coughs, talks, or sneezes.[22] The droplet nuclei travel through the airways and are deposited on the alveolar surface, where the microbe is ingested by alveolar macrophages and begins replication. Activated macrophages release cytokines, which, in turn, recruit more macrophages and activated T cells in an effort to control the infection.[7,8,16] At this point, either the inflammation-infection cycle continues and active primary tuberculosis develops (5% to 10% of people[32,52]) or the immune system contains the primary infection. A sizable but unknown proportion of the 90% to 95% of people whose immune system contains the primary infection develop latent infection.[8,32] In these people, the microbe can remain in macrophages and other cells for decades in a quiescent yet viable state. In 5% to 10% of people with a latent infection, some later waning of cellular immunity allows these dormant bacilli to begin growing again, resulting in an active infection, which is referred to as *reactivation tuberculosis*.[7,8,10]

The propagation of tuberculosis within a population can be viewed as a series of steps re-

lated to the natural history of tuberculosis infection in individuals, as illustrated in Figure 14–2. Within a population, a reservoir of tuberculosis exists within people with latent tuberculosis infection (Stage 1). Each year, a proportion of latently infected individuals develops active tuberculosis (Stage 2). Reactivation of latent tuberculosis is facilitated by recency of infection, malnutrition, immunosuppression, and other medical conditions that affect cellular immunity. Thus, in a population with a high prevalence of HIV infection, a large proportion of tuberculosis cases will be HIV infected (Figure 14–2, shaded area). People with reactivation tuberculosis transmit infection to their contacts, causing tuberculosis infection (Stage 3). Rapid diagnosis of infectious cases and effective therapy reduces the number of contacts who are infected, but even in the best of circumstances, an average of 10 contacts is infected before the case is sterilized with appropriate chemotherapy. Five to ten percent of these contacts will develop active tuberculosis within the next year or two (Stage 4) and will then pass active tuberculosis infection on to a number of their contacts (Stage 3). The remainder of the newly infected will enlarge the pool of latently infected individuals (Stage 1).

Mechanism of Transmission

Airborne transmission via the respiratory tract is the primary and most efficient mode of transmitting tuberculosis. People with active pulmonary or laryngeal tuberculosis discharge minute particles of sputum into the air when coughing, talking, sneezing, or singing.[13,22] These tiny droplets dry rapidly, leaving droplet nuclei, some of which contain a few mycobacteria. Large nuclei quickly drop out of the air, but smaller ones, 1 10 mm, are suspended in the air for long periods of time. Floating droplet nuclei are inhaled by uninfected people and lodge in the alveoli or terminal bronchioles to form the nidus of infection.[13,22] Pulmonary infection can spread systemically through the lymph or blood. The infectivity of an individual with pulmonary

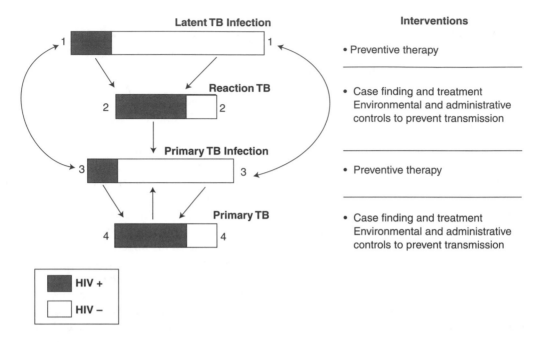

Figure 14–2 Dynamics of TB in a population with high HIV prevalence. *Source:* Reprinted with permission from K.M. De Cock and R.E. Chaisson, Tuberculosis Control in Countries with High Rates of HIV Infection, *International Journal of Tuberculosis and Lung Disease*, Vol. 3, pp. 457–465, © 1999, Churchill Livingstone.

tuberculosis is a function of the virulence of the bacteria, the frequency of cough, and the degree of pulmonary cavitation, which correlates with the bacterial load in the sputum.[13,18] Laryngeal tuberculosis is particularly infectious because all exhalations are forced through infected tissue.[22]

M. tuberculosis can also enter the body through mucous membranes in the gut, genitourinary tract, and conjunctiva or through abrasions or breaks in the skin. Infection via these routes generally produces an infection at the site of entry that may remain localized or may spread to other organs and tissues via the lymphatic or blood system.[10,22] Transmission through these portals is relatively rare, especially in industrialized areas, where the incidence of tuberculosis is low. These routes of infection are more common in developing countries, where the prevalence of

tuberculosis is higher, but respiratory transmission of tuberculosis is still the most efficient and common mode of transmission in all parts of the world.

Risk Factors Associated with Infection

As with other infectious diseases, risk factors for tuberculosis fall into two categories: those associated with infection and those associated with development of disease.[55] There have been very few studies that have directly examined risk factors associated with acquisition of tuberculosis infection. A classic study done by Chapman and colleagues[56] examined the environmental and social factors associated with acquisition of infection by children living in a household with one or more tuberculous adults. They found that the severity of disease in the index case was the strongest predictor of infection in the children. A clinical trial in Madras, India, offers further evidence that severity of disease is the primary risk factor for acquisition of infection.[53,57] This randomized trial compared the incidence of tuberculosis in household contacts of tuberculosis patients who were randomly allocated to receive 12 months of treatment at home or in a sanatorium. Household members were in daily contact with the patient for the duration of chemotherapy (home treatment) or saw the patient only at infrequent intervals during therapy (sanatorium treatment). The incidence of tuberculosis was essentially equal in both cohorts of contacts. Thus, when the risk of exposure to active bacilli is removed by sterilization of the index infection, the contact's risk of acquiring a new infection is eliminated.[55]

The earlier study by Chapman et al.[56] also showed that social factors, including crowding and poverty, were associated with infection but not as strongly as was severity of disease. They suggested that crowding and poverty acted only by modifying the environmental factors related to transmission. Studies in New York City[58] and Washington County, Maryland,[59] examined factors associated with prevalence of latent tuberculosis, as measured by a positive skin test reaction. These studies showed that latent tuberculosis infection was more common in impoverished areas, even after adjustment for age and, in the New York study, for race. These studies also suggest that it is the ills associated with poverty, such as crowding and substandard housing, that modify the risk of infection by increasing the probability of exposure to infectious sputum, should an individual have contact with a person with active tuberculosis.

It seems, therefore, that the risk of infection is a function of exposure to the tubercle bacilli, which, in turn, is controlled by the infectivity of the patient and the probability of contact with infectious organisms. Factors in the patient, such as severity of disease, frequency of cough, consistency of sputum, and initiation of chemo-

therapy, all affect the number and viability of the microbes expelled into the environment. Factors in the environment that increase the probability of contact with infected air, such as decreased ventilation, increased duration or intimacy of contact with the case, decrease in the amount of ultraviolet light available, and crowding, increase the risk of acquiring infection.[20,22,55] Fortunately, under normal household circumstances, tuberculosis is not highly infectious. The secondary attack rate for tuberculosis in 5- to 9-year-old household contacts was about 67%, substantially lower than that for measles, mumps, or pertussis.[55] The risk of infection increases dramatically in crowded conditions, such as prisons,[60] naval vessels,[61] and nursing homes,[62] and spread can be explosive in this type of confined setting.

Risk Factors Associated with Development of Disease

In the general population, only 5% to 10% of people infected with the tubercle bacillus develop active, clinical disease.[63] The risk factors that control progression from infection to disease are complex and intertwined but different from the extrinsic factors that control infection. Logically, these factors tend to be intrinsic because the time between infection and development of disease can vary significantly.[53]

Time Since Infection

Most cases of active tuberculosis develop within the first 2 years after infection, although the risk of infection is elevated through the fifth year after exposure.[53,64] In a Public Health Study of tuberculin-positive contacts of tuberculosis cases in the United States, the risk of developing tuberculosis was 1% in the first year after exposure, versus 0.07% 8 to 10 years later.[53] Similarly, in a cohort of tuberculin-negative, adult Norwegians followed longitudinally for tuberculin conversion and development of tuberculosis, radiographic changes associated with tuberculosis were observed in 130/272 (48%)

tuberculin converters, all within the first year after converting to a positive tuberculin reaction.[25] The question, however, is whether the time since infection is a true risk factor or a marker for another risk factor. Most likely, this is a marker for the true risk factors, which may include the virulence of the infecting strain of tuberculosis and the person's inherent susceptibility to developing active disease.

Fibrotic Lesions

The presence of healed fibrotic lesions increases the risk of tuberculosis, presumably from reactivation disease, although this is nearly impossible to prove. In studies of individuals with healed fibrotic lesions, the incidence of tuberculosis ranged from 2.0 to 4.0 cases per 1,000 person-years.[64,65] In a Danish study, reactors with calcified lesions were twice as likely to develop tuberculosis as were reactors without calcifications.

Age

The main question to be answered is whether the risk of developing active disease varies with age. It may seem logical to tackle this question by examining graphs plotting tuberculosis incidence and mortality by age in a specific population (Figure 14–3). Such graphs are cross-sectional, however, showing the rates of disease in many different birth cohorts at a particular instant in time, and the risk of tuberculosis can vary drastically for different birth cohorts. To clarify this issue, birth cohort analyses have been done in different populations to examine the risk of disease throughout life in cohorts of people born at the same time.[25,64] Figure 14–4 shows a cohort analysis done by Comstock from data collected and reported by the U.S. Public Health Service.[67] It shows that as a birth cohort ages, people susceptible to tuberculosis are eliminated by disease or mortality, eventually

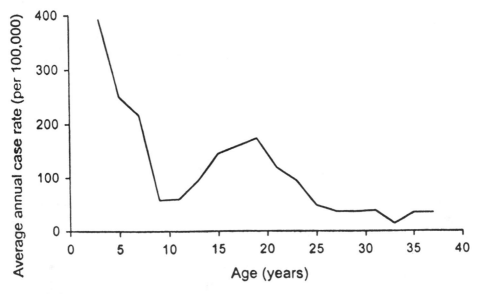

Figure 14–3 Standard tuberculosis incidence or mortality by age. *Source:* Reprinted with permission from G.W. Comstock, Frost Revisited: The Modern Epidemiology of Tuberculosis, *American Journal of Epidemiology*, Vol. 101, pp. 363–382, Copyright 1975. The Johns Hopkins University School of Hygiene and Public Health.

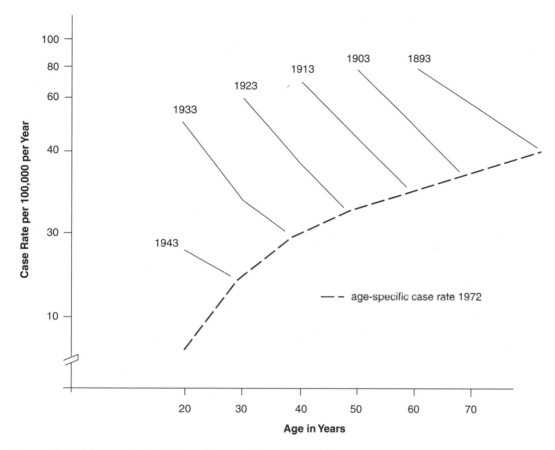

Figure 14–4 Cohort analysis of effect of age on tuberculosis incidence. *Source:* Reprinted with permission from G.W. Comstock, Frost Revisited: The Modern Epidemiology of Tuberculosis, *American Journal of Epidemiology*, Vol. 101, pp. 363–382, Copyright 1975, The Johns Hopkins University School of Hygiene and Public Health.

leaving a cohort that is more resistant to disease. Thus, the incidence of tuberculosis actually declines as a specific birth cohort ages. This elimination of susceptible people also has an effect on the overall susceptibility to tuberculosis in the community, eventually producing a community that is more resistant to disease. Thus, the risk of infection and consequently disease is lower for each successive birth cohort in the community. If you view the disease incidence cross-sectionally by age, the oldest birth cohorts, i.e., the oldest ages, have the highest incidence of infection.

This is because their risk of infection has been higher since birth, not because the incidence of tuberculosis increases with age. If you look instead at the tuberculosis incidence curve for each birth cohort, you will see that the risk of tuberculosis declines steadily over the lifetime of each cohort.

Sex

Numerous studies, both cross-sectional and longitudinal, have shown that the development of active tuberculosis varies by sex. In a prospective study in Puerto Rico, tuberculin-positive, tuberculosis-free people aged 1 to 19 years at enrollment were followed for over 18 years for the development of disease. In young children aged 1 to 6 years, the incidence of tuberculosis was higher in males than in females of the same age. After 6 years of age, however, the incidence was higher in females at all ages. This cohort was followed only until the oldest members were 40 years of age, however, so the authors could not comment on the risk of disease in older adults.[29] In a similar prospective study conducted in Banglore, India, a cohort of people were actively screened for tuberculosis annually for 8 years. The authors found that women aged 10 to 44 years had a 130% higher risk of developing tuberculosis than men of the same age, but that after age 44, the risk in men was as much as 250% higher than in women.[29] In a similar study in Gedde-Dahl, Norway, a cohort of tuberculin-negative adults was followed for tuberculin conversion and development of tuberculosis. The observed incidence of tuberculosis was equal in males and females under 19 years, 25% to 30% higher in women at age 20 to 39, and 17% to 25% higher in males than females after age 40. In the mass screening campaign in Denmark, investigators found that the incidence of tuberculosis was 71% higher in females than males at 24 to 34 years of age, 22% higher in females aged 35 to 44, and 67% higher in males over 45.[25,29,68] The effect of sex on development of disease was also studied in a population of Alaskan Inuits. Essentially, everyone in the population was tuberculin-positive by age 15. The investigators found that the incidence of tuberculosis was similar in males and females until about age 10, 25% higher in females from age 10 to 39, and similar in males and females 40 years of age and older.[29,54]

In summary, the risk of developing tuberculosis, given infection, appears to be higher in males than females during infancy and again after about age 45 to 60, and higher in females than males during adolescence and early adulthood. The reason for this divergence is not clear. The peak in women during reproductive years suggests that hormonal factors may be involved,[69] although pregnancy, in itself, does not seem to affect the risk of developing tuberculosis. It has also been suggested that the excess in men at older ages is due to increased immune suppression related to increased smoking and drinking, but the evidence for this is sketchy.[29]

Genetics

Genetic factors clearly play some role in the development of tuberculosis in humans, but the extent of the role is unclear. Lurie has shown there is some genetic basis for resistance to tuberculosis in rabbits,[70] and a variety of evidence suggests that the same is true for humans. The strongest evidence comes from twin studies, which examine the incidence of disease in pairs of monozygotic and dizygotic twins. Twin studies have shown that when one twin develops tuberculosis, the second in the pair is more likely to develop disease also if the twins share the exact same genome, i.e., if they are monozygotic. Many of these studies were done before the broad availability of computers made it possible to control for many factors at once, but Comstock was able to reanalyze the Prophit twin study data using multiple logistic regression.[71] He found that tuberculosis rates were more than two times higher in monozygotic than in dizygotic twins, even after adjustment for sex, age, infectivity of the index, type of tuberculosis, and years and closeness of contact. Although environment must play a role in the development of disease in twin pairs, it seems clear that monozygotic twins are at greater risk of disease than are dizygotes. If environment were the only factor controlling development of tuberculosis, the rates would be equal in both types of twins.

There have been other types of studies suggesting a genetic component in tuberculosis. In a well-done study by Overfield and Klauber,[72] the prevalence of a positive tuberculin response and active tuberculosis was correlated with ABO and MN blood types in a random sample of Alaskan Eskimos with a very high tuberculosis infection rate. She reported that people with blood types AB and B were three times more likely to have moderate to severe tuberculosis, compared with people with blood types O and A. In addition, individuals with type MM had 40% more moderate to severe disease than did those with types MN or NN, although the difference was not statistically significant. There also appears to be some correlation between development of tuberculosis and histocompatibility types.[13]

Edwards and colleagues[66] examined U.S. Navy recruits who had familial risk of tuberculosis. They found that men who had close, generally family, contact with a tuberculosis case were taller and thinner than were those without such exposure, regardless of their tuberculin status. This suggests that lean body build may be a marker for a familial risk for tuberculosis.[53,66] Studies have also drawn attention to the difference in tuberculosis incidence and prevalence in different races. For example, African Americans in the United States have historically had much higher rates of tuberculosis than have Caucasians. African Americans have also had higher rates of poverty, crowding, and malnutrition, however. All of these are factors that play a strong role in exposure to tuberculosis, so the difference in incidence may be related more to exposure than to genetics. Today, Hispanics, Asians, and other immigrant groups that are generally economically disadvantaged still have the highest risk of tuberculosis in industrialized areas, which are otherwise nearly free of disease. It seems likely, therefore, that much of the difference in tuberculosis incidence attributed to race may be due to differences in risk of infection, due to poor economic and living conditions, rather than to inherent genetic differences in the races. A recent study in the Yanomami Indians in Brazil suggests, however, that races that have been more recently exposed to tuberculosis as a whole may have less inherent immunity, e.g., herd immunity, than populations with a longer history of exposure.[30] This may help to explain the increased tuberculosis rates in people of African, Asian, and Hispanic descent because tuberculosis was introduced into these peoples by Europeans well after it had become epidemic in Europe. Two recent studies have also shown that genetic polymorphisms may be associated with tuberculosis risk. A case-control study in the Gambia found that allelic variation in the gene *nramp-1* was associated with tuberculosis risk, although wild-type alleles were present in the majority of cases and polymorphisms in a large proportion of controls.[73] Another study from Cambodia identified a specific HLA-DQ haplotype associated with tuberculosis.[74] The importance of genetic susceptibility to tuberculosis and specific gene markers for increased risk remains a controversial topic, and additional research on possible mechanisms for enhanced susceptibility is underway.

Stress

It has long been suggested that stress may affect the development of tuberculosis, perhaps by weakening the cell-mediated immune response that holds latent disease in check. A study in Denmark showed that among tuberculin reactors, the risk of developing active tuberculosis was lowest in married men, who presumably had the highest level of social support, intermediate in single and widowed men, and highest in divorced men who had the least social support. A similar but less dramatic trend was seen in women. In addition, married people who developed tuberculosis had less severe disease than did unmarried people.[13,69] Tuberculosis has also always been associated with poverty,[32,56,59] even after adjustment for other pertinent factors.[57] Chapman et al.[56] showed that poverty is probably a marker for increased risk of infection with tuberculosis, but it is possible that poverty imposes a psychologic stress on the body, reducing immune capacity and increasing the risk of reactivation or of development of disease, given exposure.

Nutrition

The association between poverty, crowding, and malnutrition is well established. It is no surprise, therefore, that tuberculosis, which is strongly associated with crowding and poverty, has also been associated with malnutrition.[20,32] A number of studies has examined the association of specific micronutrients with the development of tuberculosis. In one study, mean plasma vitamin A levels were lower in children with pulmonary tuberculosis than in those without it. More extensive or more severe disease was also associated with low vitamin A levels. High-dose treatment with vitamin A, however, had no effect on the course of the tuberculosis.[75] Low vitamin A and selenium levels have also been associated with an increased risk of developing tuberculosis in a cohort of HIV-infected, adult tuberculin reactors in Haiti.[76]

A study in tuberculin reactors found that reaction size increased as nutritional status improved, and severe malnutrition has also been associated with anergy to tuberculin skin test following BCG vaccination.[28] In times of war, food deprivation has also been associated with increased tuberculosis incidence and mortality, which disappeared when food became available again. This suggests that the deprivation caused an increase in reactivation disease, probably by inhibiting cell-mediated immunity.[20,25] There is also considerable literature suggesting that tall, thin men are more likely to develop tuberculosis than are shorter, heavier men.[66] Similarly, a study in Muscogee County, Georgia, measured the thickness of subcutaneous fat over the trapezius ridges in baseline photofluorograms of tuberculosis-free people. The investigators found that people with <5 mm of fat over the ridge were twice as likely to develop tuberculosis over the next 14 years as were people with 10 mm of fat or more.[53] It seems clear, therefore, that the risk of tuberculosis is higher in thinner people, but it is not clear whether thinness is the risk factor for disease or whether it is a marker of a genetic susceptibility. Edwards' studies in navy recruits suggest that thinness is more likely to be marker of genetic susceptibility to tuberculosis than to be a risk factor in and of itself.[53,66]

Occupation

Few studies have examined occupation as a risk factor for tuberculosis. The notable exception is exposure to silica in the work site. Silicosis has been shown to lower resistance to tuberculosis infection in animals, and tuberculosis is more common in people exposed to silica on the job than in those who are unexposed.[20] There also appears to be an interaction between silicosis, HIV infection, and tuberculosis in South African miners. Those with both silicosis and HIV are more likely to develop tuberculosis than are those with only one of the two risk factors. Inhalation therapists and funeral home workers have been found to have increased risk for tuberculosis infection and disease.[77,78] Health care workers, in general, however, appear to have varying rates of tuberculosis. In some settings the incidence is similar to or lower than rates in other occupational groups,[78] while in other instances, rates are actually increased.[79]

HIV Infection and AIDS

Infection with HIV has been identified as the most potent biologic risk factor for developing tuberculosis. In HIV-infected individuals with evidence of prior tuberculosis infection, the annual risk of reactivation is between 3% and 14%.[80] Among people already infected with HIV, newly acquired tuberculosis infection progresses to active disease within several months in a high proportion (~40%).[81] In areas where tuberculosis infection is common and HIV becomes prevalent, rapidly escalating rates of tuberculosis occur. In northern Thailand, for example, the incidence of tuberculosis doubled in one province over a 2-year period after HIV infection was introduced.[82] HIV-related immune deficiency compromises host response to tubercle bacilli, thereby raising the likelihood of reactivation of latent infection. Among HIV-infected people, the most important risk factors for reactivation of tuberculosis are a positive tuberculin skin test and a low CD4 lymphocyte count.[83] Although HIV infection can cause anergy to antigens such as tuberculin, a high proportion of HIV-infected patients with tuberculosis have a positive skin test, and the presence of a positive test is a powerful predictor of subsequent tuberculosis risk. Several early studies suggested that the anergy was associated with a very high risk of developing tuberculosis, and it was hypothesized that the lack of response to tuberculin indicated an inability of host immune responses to contain tubercle bacilli.[84,85] Subsequent studies have failed to confirm an association between anergy and reactivation tuberculosis,[86] and it has been suggested that anergy is a marker for severe immune deficiency that increases the risk of *primary* tuberculosis in areas where transmission of infection is common. As the CD4 count falls, the incidence of reactivation and primary tuberculosis rises, and extrapulmonary sites of disease become more frequent.[87] However, unlike most other opportunistic infections in HIV disease, tuberculosis can occur at a relatively high CD4 level and may be a first manifestation of HIV in many patients.[88] In addition, active tuberculosis can be transmitted by the airborne route between HIV-infected people, contributing to microepidemics of institutional and community outbreaks of disease.

The growth of the HIV infection over the past two decades has occurred largely in areas of the world where tuberculosis infection is endemic. As a result, tuberculosis has become one of the major opportunistic diseases associated with HIV infection and a leading cause of death in developing countries.[89] As discussed later, the HIV epidemic now seriously undermines tuberculosis control in many developing countries, and new and more aggressive strategies will be necessary to reduce the high incidence of tuberculosis seen in populations with high levels of HIV infection.

Other Factors

A variety of other factors, most of which have a negative impact on the immune system, is also known to increase the risk of developing tuberculosis. Those factors include malignancies, renal failure, gastrectomy, diabetes, jejunoileal bypass, corticosteroid treatment, and measles.[22,64]

BACILLUS CALMETTE-GUÉRIN

Tuberculosis was one of the first diseases for which a vaccine was developed. In 1921, Albert Calmette and Camille Guérin attenuated a virulent strain of *M. bovis* through serial passage on glycerinated bile potato media.[19,90,91] The final product, BCG, was tested in a human subject later that year and put into common use in France in 1924 to protect child contacts of active cases.[52,92,93]

Use of BCG in Europe soon became fairly common, but its efficacy was questioned by some, particularly in the United States. In 1930, 251 of 412 children vaccinated with BCG in Lubeck, Germany, contracted tuberculosis, and many died. It was subsequently shown that the children had accidentally been vaccinated with virulent tubercle bacilli from a culture stored in the same incubator as the BCG culture.[19,94] The Lubeck disaster, combined with the disruption of Europe during the World War II, discouraged the use of BCG for a time. Tuberculosis morbidity and mortality increased markedly during World War II,[25] however, and after the war, vaccination was quickly reinstituted in Europe and became the norm.[19] Today, BCG vaccine is one of the standard vaccines in the WHO Expanded Programme on Immunization[11] and is used in nearly every country in the world, with the notable exceptions of the United States and the Netherlands.

Bacillus Calmette-Guérin is one of the safest vaccines in use. It is given at birth to infants in more than 100 countries throughout the world and is recommended for some health care workers at risk of exposure to tuberculosis. The BCG vaccine is rarely given to healthy adult populations because the efficacy in this group is unclear. It is administered intradermally or percutaneously and generally causes a superficial, crusted ulcer at the site of administration. This heals in 2 to 3 months, generally leaving a 4- to 8-mm concave scar.[21] A small proportion of vaccinees gets suppurative axillary or cervical lymphadenopathy, which generally heals best without treatment. Persistent or disseminated BCG is a rare complication of vaccination that occurs in 3 to 6 infants per million vaccinations and in 1 to 14 cases per million vaccinations in people aged 1 to 20 years.[11,27] The risk is higher in immunocompromised individuals, e.g., those with HIV infection. Although the precise risk of disseminated BCG in HIV-infected individuals is unknown, BCG is contraindicated if HIV infection is present,[27] as well as in people with other forms of immune compromise and in those with skin infections or burns.[11,27]

Controlled studies to measure the efficacy of BCG have been ongoing since 1926 and have included observational and case-control studies and clinical trials. Case-control studies have been used to measure the efficacy of BCG vaccine in specific geographic regions. In these studies, the reported cases of tuberculosis in an area are matched to controls, and the efficacy is estimated from the tuberculosis incidence rate in vaccinated and unvaccinated cases and controls where:[95]

$$\% \text{ efficacy} = (1 - (R)) \times 100$$

$$\text{and R} = \frac{\text{incidence in the vaccinated}}{\text{incidence in the unvaccinated}}$$

The underlying assumption is that fewer than 80% of people have received vaccine; otherwise, there are too few unvaccinated cases and controls to estimate efficacy reliably.

Case-control studies have also been used to measure the relative efficacy of two different BCG vaccines given to the same population.[96,97] In these studies, it was possible to determine the relative efficacy of the different vaccines because they were given one after the other to the same population, using the same delivery methods. The efficacy for the time period covering each vaccine was estimated separately. Case-control studies are observational, and the lack of randomization means there is a potential for bias. The assumption in a case-control study is that, apart from the effect of the vaccine, the risk of developing tuberculosis is equal in the vaccinated and unvaccinated groups. If this is not true, the estimated efficacy may be incorrect.

In contact studies, cohorts of children living with newly diagnosed tuberculosis cases are followed for the development of tuberculosis. The incidence of tuberculosis is estimated in vaccinated and unvaccinated children, and vaccine efficacy is computed as in a case-control study.[19] As with the case-control studies, these cohort studies are not randomized, and results are questionable if the probability of vaccination varies with the risk of developing tuberculosis.

Many clinical trials, some randomized and some not, have also been done to determine the efficacy of BCG vaccine. At first glance, the results of these studies are confusing. The efficacy of BCG, as estimated in the different studies, ranges from –22% to +85%. The difficulty is that the studies have measured different products in different populations. The BCG vaccine was developed in 1921, during the infancy of microbiology. It came not from a single colony but from a culture of organisms and, thus, is not a strain in the strictest sense of the word.[19] The original strain of BCG was distributed to and subcultured in laboratories around the world producing a large number of daughter strains, some of them with very different characteristics from the original.[19] Thus, the organism used in the vaccination studies and trials has varied markedly. In addition, the route of administration and the dose of vaccine have varied; factors whose effect on efficacy are difficult to predict.[11] Furthermore, several studies have shown that exposure to nontuberculous mycobacteria may provide some protection against infection with *M. tuberculosis* and may reduce the efficacy of BCG.[63] To summarize, it appears that BCG provides some protection in infants against miliary disease and tuberculosis meningitis, but a good estimate of the efficacy is not available. It does not appear to confer good protection in adults and should probably be used only in extreme circumstances.

New, effective vaccines against tuberculosis are needed. Research in the field is expanding, and it is hoped that new candidate vaccines will be ready for testing in the next 10 to 15 years. Testing the new vaccines will be challenging. BCG vaccination is entrenched in developing countries, where the risk of tuberculosis is highest and the need for new tuberculosis vaccines is greatest. WHO has made a determined effort to ensure high coverage rates in infants in areas where tuberculosis is endemic. In these areas, where chemoprophylaxis is rare and treatment for tuberculosis can be problematic, it would be unethical to deprive infants of an available vaccine that provides even minimal protection against disseminated tuberculosis. Therefore, placebo-controlled efficacy trials will probably be impossible for the new vaccine(s), and studies will have to measure some as yet unknown biologic marker of protection, or compare the efficacy of the new vaccine against the efficacy of BCG and infer the relative efficacy of the two vaccines from those measurements.

TUBERCULOSIS CONTROL STRATEGIES

Case Finding and Treatment

In 1994, the WHO declared tuberculosis to be a global emergency and developed the DOTS program to combat the disease globally. Although DOTS is the cornerstone of the strategy, the WHO DOTS program is really a series of policies that are meant to result in effective tuberculosis control (Exhibit 14–1). The program aims to encourage governments to develop the political will to support tuberculosis control, a strong surveillance system that records and monitors cases, sufficient laboratory components to ensure diagnosis, effective short-course treatments that are at least partially observed, and a reliable supply of antituberculosis drugs.

The DOTS strategy aims for country programs to detect 70% of smear-positive tuberculosis cases and to treat 85% of those successfully. It is assumed that implementation of the DOTS strategy and achievement of these goals will make a substantial impact on tuberculosis incidence and will contribute to effective tuberculosis control. Indeed, when DOTs is implemented well in a country, large proportions of active tuberculosis cases can be treated and

Exhibit 14–1 Components of an Effective WHO DOTS Program

- A governmental commitment to tuberculosis control
- Case detection by microscopy, focusing on symptomatic patients who seek care
- Short-course therapy with at least the first 2 months of treatment supervised
- An administrative system for recording cases and assessing outcomes
- A reliable supply of antituberculosis drugs

cured, and drug resistance can be prevented.[98] Implementation of a DOTS program requires the establishment of a registration system, microscopy services, a stable drug supply, and adequate staffing to permit supervision of therapy for at least 2 months, and many countries with the greatest tuberculosis burden are the least able to undertake this kind of commitment. Although the per capita cost of effective tuberculosis treatment services is relatively low (e.g., $0.23 per year in Peru), mobilization of resources to create an integrated national program is understandably difficult. A larger problem, however, is the generation of political will to support tuberculosis control. Even in countries where substantial foreign assistance has been provided for tuberculosis services, control efforts frequently lag. Not surprisingly, the reasons for not making tuberculosis control a priority vary widely and include governmental disorganization and disruption, competing and urgent needs, and lack of interest or commitment in tuberculosis as a public health problem. Although the WHO notes that 76% of the world's population and 85% of tuberculosis patients live in countries that have adopted DOTS, for the most part, these countries have not implemented the DOTS strategy sufficiently to provide coverage for most patients, and only one third of tuberculosis cases worldwide are diagnosed and treated under the DOTS strategy. Among those countries that have fully implemented DOTS, virtually none has achieved 70% detection and 85% successful treatment. Operational research is needed to determine the best way to implement DOTS in different settings.

Epidemiologic Basis of Tuberculosis Control

Control of tuberculosis implies a reduction in the number of cases that occur each year within a community or population. In mathematical terms, tuberculosis control means that the reproductive rate of the disease must be less than 1.0; i.e., each case of tuberculosis must produce less than one secondary case. This simple and necessary goal of control has been largely overlooked in most international tuberculosis programming, which is largely focused on intermediary goals, such as case detection and cure rates. Although there is great medical and humanitarian value in finding, treating, and curing cases of tuberculosis, the perspective of public health requires that the principal aim of tuberculosis control be that the incidence of the disease is reduced.

The propagation of tuberculosis within a population can be viewed as a series of steps related to the natural history of tuberculosis infection in individuals, as illustrated in Figure 14–2.[99] The reservoir of tuberculosis in a community is the group of latently infected people at risk of developing tuberculosis (Stage 1). Some change in immunity in the latently infected allows the tubercle bacillus to begin active growth, and reactivation tuberculosis develops (Stage 2). These new cases are infectious, and each will infect a minimum of 8 to 15 contacts (Stage 3) before their infection is sterilized by appropriate chemotherapy. Rapid diagnosis and treatment of the new infectious cases reduces the number of infected contacts. Five to ten percent of these infected contacts will develop primary tuberculosis within 2 years (Stage 4), and the remainder will add to the pool of latently infected people (Stage 1).

A variety of factors moderates the dynamics of this model in a community. The most obvious is HIV infection. People co-infected with HIV and the tubercle bacillus have a dramatically increased risk of developing tuberculosis and contribute disproportionately to reactivation and new tuberculosis infections (Stages 2 and 3). In areas where HIV and tuberculosis are endemic, this increased risk of disease from reactivation and primary infection substantially increases the case rate (Stages 2 and 4). Other factors that prolong infectivity, such as poor case detection, lack of effective treatment, and drug resistance, also increase case rates.

Current Tuberculosis Control Strategies and Challenges

On a community level, tuberculosis can be controlled through the use of an effective vaccine, detection and treatment of infectious cases, and screening for and treatment of latent tuberculosis infection. In developing countries, control measures have emphasized BCG vaccination and case detection and treatment.[100] BCG vaccination of uninfected individuals is intended to provide protection against active tuberculosis infection and does not necessarily protect against reactivation of latent infection (Figure 14–2, Stage 3). Even when BCG vaccine is highly efficacious, new cases of tuberculosis will continue to arise from the latently infected pool until all at-risk individuals die. There is also increasing evidence that the efficacy of current BCG vaccines is attenuated. Thus, although BCG vaccination is widespread, the epidemiologic benefit gained from this intervention is limited.

Detection of tuberculosis cases and institution of effective chemotherapy is widely held to be the most important strategy for controlling tuberculosis and is the backbone of tuberculosis control. Rapid identification of cases and institution of effective treatment eliminates ongoing transmission of infection and limits the number of secondary cases, although an average of 8 to 15 contacts are infected before a newly identified infection can be sterilized with chemotherapy. It is, therefore, more accurate to state that case detection and treatment reduces but does not eliminate transmission of infection to susceptible individuals.

Chemoprophylaxis of latent tuberculosis infection with INH or other antituberculosis medications reduces the risk of subsequent tuberculosis by 60% to 90%.[101] Provision of chemoprophylaxis to people at high risk of developing tuberculosis is an important adjunct to case identification and treatment in reducing tuberculosis incidence in a community and has been used extensively in the United States and Europe. In the United States, INH preventive therapy is targeted at close contacts of infectious cases, individuals with HIV and latent tuberculosis infection, recent tuberculin converters, and other tuberculin-positive persons at high risk of developing active tuberculosis.[102] The use of chemoprophylaxis in resource-poor areas, however, is extremely limited and usually directed only at young children living in households with smear-positive cases. Unfortunately, the HIV epidemic has changed the dynamics of tuberculosis in many resource-poor areas, and some suggest that effective control of tuberculosis in these areas will require the implementation of chemoprophylaxis for people at high risk of developing tuberculosis. In addition, in Peru, a country with a high tuberculosis rate and little HIV infection, the implementation of a model DOTS program has improved treatment outcomes and lowered incidence initially, but does not appear to be continually lowering tuberculosis rates.[103] Thus, evidence that the DOTS strategy will be effective for long-term control of tuberculosis is equivocal, despite the evidence that it improves treatment outcomes and prevents emergence of drug resistance. DOTS may be the minimal level of tuberculosis control necessary, with additional strategies required for successful reduction in disease incidence.[104]

An additional problem limiting tuberculosis control efforts is the growing prevalence of drug-resistant disease. Between 1994 and 1997, a comprehensive global survey including 50,000 tuberculosis patients showed that the median prevalence of drug resistance was 9.9% for patients who had not had any prior therapy (primary resistance) and 35.6% for those with a history of previous therapy (acquired resistance).[105] Dramatic outbreaks of multidrug-resistant tuberculosis (MDR-TB) in HIV-infected patients and among health care workers in the United States in the early 1990s focused international attention on the emergence of strains of *M. tuberculosis* resistant to antimycobacterial drugs. Patients infected with strains resistant to multiple drugs are extremely difficult to cure, and the necessary treatment is much more toxic and expensive. As noted previously, good tuberculosis control programs prevent emergence of drug-resistant tuberculosis.

Currently there are a number of "hot spots" around the world where MDR-TB prevalence is high (Latvia, Estonia, Russia, Dominican Republic, Ivory Coast, China, India, and Argentina). In particular, prisoners in Russia have high rates of MDR-TB, and transmission within penal colonies is high.[106]

Aggressive tuberculosis control measures that include prevention of institutional transmission of infection, DOTS, screening, and prophylaxis can dramatically reduce the prevalence of MDR-TB. In New York City, for example, such an approach was extremely successful in reversing a disastrous epidemic of MDR-TB that affected that city in the early 1990s.[107] However, in other areas of the world, mobilization of resources to combat drug-resistant disease is more difficult, and community and institutional transmission of MDR strains will continue, resulting in escalating levels of resistant cases and more treatment failures and deaths.

CONCLUSION

Tuberculosis is one of the most prevalent and deadly infections on Earth. Because humans are the only reservoir of infection and transmission is via the aerosol route, elimination of tuberculosis is theoretically possible. Although recent advances in molecular epidemiology have improved our understanding of tuberculosis dynamics, the fundamental measures for controlling the disease have been known and available for decades. Despite this, tuberculosis control has never been worse. Recent threats to reducing the toll of tuberculosis include the HIV epidemic and drug resistance. Aggressive, comprehensive global efforts to control tuberculosis are an urgent priority.

REFERENCES

1. Haas F, Haas SS. The origins of *Mycobacterium tuberculosis* and the notion of its contagiousness. In: Rom WN, Garay SM, eds. *Tuberculosis*. New York: Little, Brown and Company; 1996:3–19.

2. Haas DW, des Prez RM. Mycobacterium tuberculosis. In: Mandell GL, Bennett JE, Dolin R, eds. *Mandell, Douglas and Bennett's Principles and Practice of Infectious Diseases*. 4th ed. New York: Churchill Livingstone; 1995:2213–2243.

3. Pitchenik AE, Cole C, Russell BW, Fischl MA, Spira TJ, Snider DE. Tuberculosis, atypical mycobacteriosis, and the acquired immunodeficiency syndrome among Haitian and non-Haitian patients in south Florida. *Ann Intern Med*. 1984;101:641–645.

4. *Global Tuberculosis Program*. Tuberculosis Fact Sheet No 104. <www.who.int/inf-fs/en/fact104.html> (2 December 1998). Accessed January 1999.

5. Raviglione MC, Snider DE, Kochi A. Global epidemiology of tuberculosis: morbidity and mortality of a worldwide epidemic. *JAMA*. 1995;273(3):220–226.

6. Dolin PJ, Raviglione MC, Kochi A. Estimates of future global tuberculosis morbidity and mortality. *MMWR*. 1993;42(49):961–964.

7. Brooks GF, Butel JS, Morse SA, eds. *Jawetz, Melnick & Adelberg's Medical Microbiology*. 21st ed. Stamford, CT: Appleton & Lange; 1998.

8. Robbins SL., Angell M, Kumar V, eds. *Basic Pathology*. 3rd ed. Philadelphia: W.B. Saunders Company; 1981:401–406.

9. Smith DW. Mycobacteria. In: Braude A, Davis CE, Fierer J, eds. *Infectious Disease and Medical Microbiology*. Philadelphia: W.B. Saunders Company; 1986.

10. Freeman BA. *Burrows Textbook of Microbiology*. 22nd ed. Philadelphia: W.B. Saunders Company; 1985.

11. American Academy of Pediatrics. Tuberculosis. In: Peter G, ed. *1997 Red Book: Report of the Committee on Infectious Diseases*. 24th ed. Elk Grove Village, IL: American Academy of Pediatrics; 1997:541–567.

12. Stead WW, Bates JH. Geographic and evolutionary epidemiology of tuberculosis. In: Rom WN, Garay SM, eds. *Tuberculosis*. New York: Little, Brown and Company; 1996:77–83.

13. Stead WW, Dutt AK. Epidemiology and host factors. In: Schlossberg D, ed. *Tuberculosis*. 3rd ed. New York: Springer-Verlag; 1994:1–16.

14. Formicola V, Milanesi Q, Scarsini C. Evidence of spinal tuberculosis at the beginning of the fourth millennium B.C. from Arene Candide Cave (Liguria, Italy). *Am J Phys Anthropol*. 1987;72:1–6.

15. Pesanti EL. A history of tuberculosis. In: Lutwick LI, ed. *Tuberculosis*. New York: Chapman & Hall; 1995.

16. Pitchenik AE, Fertel D, Block AB. Mycobacterial disease: epidemiology, diagnosis, treatment, and prevention. *Clin Chest Med*. 1988;9(3):425–441.

17. Cohen FL, Durham JD, eds. *Tuberculosis A Sourcebook for Nursing Practice*. New York: Springer Publishing Co.; 1995.

18. Isselbacher KJ, Braunwald E, Wilson JD, Martin JB, Fauci AS, Kasper DL. *Harrison's Principles of Internal Medicine Companion Handbook*. 13th ed. New York: McGraw-Hill: 1995.

19. ten Dam HG. BCG vaccination. In: Reichman LB, Hershfield ES, eds. *Tuberculosis: A Comprehensive International Approach*. New York: Marcel Dekker; 1993:251–274.

20. Comstock GW, O'Brien RJ. Tuberculosis. In: Evans AS, Brachman PS, eds. *Bacterial Infections of Humans, Epidemiology and Control*. 2nd ed. New York: Plenum Publishing; 1991:745–772.

21. Starke JR. Tuberculosis in children. *Curr Opin Pediatr*. 1995;7:268–277.

22. Benenson AS, ed. *Control of Communicable Diseases Manual*. 16th ed. Washington, DC: American Public Health Association; 1995.

23. Thomas CL, ed. *Taber's Cyclopedic Medical Dictionary*. Philadelphia: F.A. Davis; 1977.

24. Schein MF, Huebner RE. Tuberculin skin testing. In: Rossman MD, MacGregor RR, eds. *Tuberculosis Clinical Management and New Challenges*. New York: McGraw-Hill; 1995:73–88.

25. Sutherland I. Recent studies in the epidemiology of tuberculosis, based on the risk of being infected with tubercle bacilli. *Adv Tuberc Res*. 1976;19:1–63.

26. Furcolow ML, Hewell B, Nelson WE, Palmer CE. Quantitative studies of the tuberculin reaction. I. Titration of tuberculin sensitivity and its relation to tuberculosis infection. *Public Health Rep*. 1941;56:1082–1100.

27. Brewer TF, Wilson ME, Nardell EA. BCG immunization: review of past experience, current use, and future prospects. *Curr Clin Top Infect Dis*. 1995;15:253–270.

28. Kielmann AA, Oberoi IS, Chandra RK, Mehra VL. The effect of nutritional status on immune capacity and immune responses in preschool children in a rural community in India. *Bull WHO.* 1976;54:477–483.

29. Holmes CB, Hausler H, Nunn P. A review of sex differences in the epidemiology of tuberculosis. *Int J Tuberc Lung Dis.* 1998;2(2):96–104.

30. Sousa AO, Salem JI, Lee FK, et al. An epidemic of tuberculosis with a high rate of tuberculin anergy among a population previously unexposed to tuberculosis, the Yanomami Indians of the Brazilian Amazon. *Proc Natl Acad Sci.* 1997;94:13227–13232.

31. Johnson M, Coberly J, Clermont H, et al. Tuberculin skin test reactivity among adults infected with human immunodeficiency virus. *J Infect Dis.* 1992;166:194–198.

32. Dubos R, Dubos J. *The White Plague: Tuberculosis, Man and Society.* Boston: Little, Brown and Company; 1952.

33. British Medical Research Council. Streptomycin treatment of pulmonary tuberculosis. *Br Med J.* 1948;2:769–782.

34. British Medical Research Council. Treatment of pulmonary tuberculosis with streptomycin and p-aminosalicylic acid. *Br Med J.* 1950;2:1073–1078.

35. Hong Kong Chest Service/British Medical Research Council. Controlled trial of 4 three-times-weekly regimens and a daily regimen all given for 6 months for pulmonary tuberculosis; second report: the results up to 24 months. *Tubercle.* 1982;63:89–98.

36. Hong Kong Chest Service/Tuberculosis Research Centre Madras/British Medical Research Council. A controlled trial of 2-month, 3-month and 12-month regimens of chemotherapy for sputum-smear-negative pulmonary tuberculosis, results at 60 months. *Am Rev Respir Dis.* 1984;130:23–28.

37. Hong Kong Chest Service/Tuberculosis Research Centre, Madras/British Medical Research Council. A controlled trial of 3-month, 4-month and 6-month regimens of chemotherapy for sputum-smear-negative pulmonary tuberculosis, results at 5 years. *Am Rev Respir Dis.* 1989;139:871–876.

38. Singapore Tuberculosis Service/British Medical Research Council. Long-term follow-up of a clinical trial of six-month and four-month regimens of thermotherapy in the treatment of pulmonary tuberculosis. *Am Rev Respir Dis.* 1986;133:779–783.

39. Singapore Tuberculosis Service/British Medical Research Council. Five-year follow-up of a clinical trial of three 6-month regimens of chemotherapy given intermittently in the continuation phase in the treatment of pulmonary tuberculosis. *Am Rev Respir Dis.* 1988;137:1147–1150.

40. Azia A, Ishaq M, Jaffer NA, Akhwand R, Bhatti AH. Clinical trial of two short-course (6-month) regimes and a standard regimen (12-month) chemotherapy in retreatment of pulmonary tuberculosis in Pakistan. *Am Rev Respir Dis.* 1986;134:1056–1061.

41. Hong Kong Chest Service/British Medical Research Council. Five-year follow-up of a controlled trial of five 6-month regimens of chemotherapy for pulmonary tuberculosis. *Am Rev Respir Dis.* 1987;136:1339–1342.

42. Hong Kong Chest Service/British Medical Research Council. Controlled trial of 6-month and 8-month regimens in the treatment of pulmonary tuberculosis: the results up to 24 months. *Tubercle.* 1979;60:201–210.

43. East African/British Medical Research Councils Study. Controlled clinical trial of five short-course (4-month) chemotherapy regimens in pulmonary tuberculosis, second report of the 4th study. *Am Rev Respir Dis.* 1981; 123:165–170.

44. Castelo A, Jardim JRB, Goihman S, et al. Comparison of daily and twice-weekly regimens to treat pulmonary tuberculosis. *Lancet.* 1989;2:1173–1176.

45. Okwere A, Whalen C, Byckwaso F, et al. University-Case Western Reserve University research collaboration. *Lancet.* 1994;344:1323–1328.

46. Alwood K, Keruly JC, Moore-Rice K, Stanton DL, Chaulk P, Chaisson RE. Effectiveness of supervised, intermittent therapy for tuberculosis in HIV infected patients. *AIDS.* 1994;8:1103–1108.

47. Perriens JH, St. Louis ME, Mukadi YB, et al. Pulmonary tuberculosis in HIV-infected patients in Zaire: a controlled trial of treatment for either 6 or 12 months. *N Engl J Med.* 1995;332:779–784.

48. Chaisson RE, Clermont HC, Holt EA, et al. Six-month supervised intermittent tuberculosis therapy in Haitian patients with and without HIV infections. *Am J Respir Crit Care Med.* 1996;154:1034–1038.

49. Harries AD, Maher D. *TB/HIV: A Clinical Manual.* Geneva: World Health Organization (WHO); 1996.

50. Zwarenstein M, Schoeman JH, Vundule C, et al. Randomized controlled trial of self-supervised and directly observed treatment of tuberculosis. *Lancet.* 1998;352:1340–1343.

51. WHO, Global Tuberculosis Programme. *Global Tuberculosis Control. World Report 1999.* Geneva: WHO/CDS/CPC/TB/90.259.

52. Murray CJL, Styblo K, Rouillon A. Tuberculosis in developing countries: burden, intervention and cost. *Bull Int Union Tuberc Lung Dis.* 1990;65(1):1–20.

53. Comstock GW. Frost revisited: the modern epidemiology of tuberculosis. *Am J Epidemiol.* 1975;101:363–382.

54. Comstock G, Cauthen GM. Epidemiology of tuberculosis. In: Reichman LB, Hershfield ES, eds. *Tuberculosis:*

A Comprehensive International Approach. New York: Marcel Dekker; 1993:23–48.

55. Comstock GW. Epidemiology of tuberculosis. *Am Rev Respir Dis.* 1982;125(Suppl):8–15.

56. Chapman JS, Dyerly MD, Powell DR. Social and other factors in intrafamilial transmission of tuberculosis. *Am Rev Respir Dis.* 1964;90:48–60.

57. Kamat SR, Dawson JJY, Devadatta S, et al. A controlled study of the influence of segregation of tuberculous patients for one year on the attack rate of tuberculosis in a 5-year period in close family contacts in south India. *Bull WHO.* 1966;34:517–532.

58. Reichman LB, O'Day R. Tuberculous infection in a large urban population. *Am Rev Respir Dis.* 1978;117:705–712.

59. Kuemmerer JM, Comstock GW. Sociologic concomitants of tuberculin sensitivity. *Am Rev Respir Dis.* 1967;96:885–892.

60. Stead WW. Undetected tuberculosis in prison. *JAMA.* 1978;240:2544–2547.

61. Houk VN, Baker JH, Sorensen K, Kent DC. The epidemiology of tuberculosis infection in a closed environment. *Arch Environ Health.* 1968;16:26–35.

62. Stead WW, Lofgren JP, Warren E, Thomas C. Tuberculosis as an endemic and nosocomial infection among the elderly in nursing homes. *N Engl J Med.* 1985;312:1483–1487.

63. Comstock GW, Livesay VT, Woolpert SF. Evaluation of BCG vaccination among Puerto Rican children. *Am J Public Health.* 1974;64:283–291.

64. Rieder HL. Epidemiology of tuberculosis in Europe. *Eur Respir J.* 1995;20(Suppl):620–632.

65. IUAT Committee on Prophylaxis. Efficacy of various durations of isoniazid preventive therapy for tuberculosis: five years of follow-up in the IUAT trial. *Bull WHO.* 1982;60:555–564.

66. Edwards LB, Livesay VT, Acquaviva FA, Palmer CE. Height, weight, tuberculous infection, and tuberculous disease. *Arch Environ Health.* 1971;22:106–112.

67. Comstock GW. Frost revisited: the modern epidemiology of tuberculosis. *Am J Epidemiol.* 1975;101(5):363–382.

68. Horwitz O. Epidemiologic basis of tuberculosis eradication. 10. Lung studies on the risk of tuberculosis in the general population of a low-prevalence area. *Bull WHO.* 1969;41(1):95–113.

69. Horwitz O. Tuberculosis risk and marital status. *Am Rev Respir Dis.* 1971;104:22–31.

70. Lurie MB. *Resistance to Tuberculosis: Experimental Studies in Native Acquired Defensive Mechanisms.* Cambridge, MA: Harvard University Press; 1984:115–180.

71. Comstock GW. Tuberculosis in twins: a re-analysis of the Prophit survey. *Am Rev Respir Dis.* 1978;117:621–624.

72. Overfield T, Klauber MR. Prevalence of tuberculosis in Eskimos having blood group B gene. *Hum Biol.* 1980;52(1):87–92.

73. Bellamy R, Ruwende C, Corrah T, McAdam KP, Whittle HC, Hill AV. Variations in the *NRAMP1* gene and susceptibility to tuberculosis in West Africans. *N Engl J Med.* 1998;338(10):640–644.

74. Goldfeld AE, Delgado JC, Thim S, et al. Association of an HLA-DQ allele with clinical tuberculosis. *JAMA.* 1998;279:226–228.

75. Hanekom WA, Potgieter S, Hughes EJ, Malan H, Kessow G, Hussey GD. Vitamin A status and therapy in childhood pulmonary tuberculosis. *J Pediatr.* 1997;131(6):925–927.

76. Rwangabwoba JM, Humphrey J, Coberly J, Moulton L, Desormeaux J, Halsey N. *Vitamin A Status and Development of Tuberculosis and/or Mortality.* Vancouver, Canada: The XI International Conference on AIDS; July 1996.

77. McKenna MT, Hutton M, Cauthen G, Onorato IM. The association between occupation and tuberculosis: a population-based survey. *Am J Respir Crit Care Med.* 1996;154:587–593.

78. Geisseler JP, Nelson KE, Crispen RG, Moses VK. Tuberculosis in physicians: a continuing problem. *Am Rev Resp Dis.* 1986;133:773–778.

79. Barrett-Connor E. The epidemioilogy of tuberculosis in physicians. *JAMA.* 1979;241:33–38.

80. Hopewell PC, Chaisson RE. Tuberculosis and human immunodeficiency virus infection. In: Reichman LB, Hershfield E, eds. *Tuberculosis: A Comprehensive International Approach.* 2nd ed. New York: Marcel Dekker; 2000.

81. Daley CL, Small PM, Schecter GF, et al. An outbreak of tuberculosis with accelerated progression among persons infected with human immunodeficiency virus: an analysis using restriction-fragment-length polymorphisms. *N Engl J Med.* 1992;326:231–235.

82. Yinai H, Uthaivoravit W, Panich V, et al. Rapid increase in HIV-related tuberculosis, Ching Rai, Thailand, 1990–1994. *AIDS.* 1996;10:527–531.

83. Markowitz N, Hansen N, Hopewell PC, et al. Incidence of tuberculosis in the United States among HIV-infected patients. *Ann Intern Med.* 1997;126:123–132.

84. Selwyn PA, Sckell BM, Alcabes P, et al. High risk of active tuberculosis among intravenous drug users with cutaneous anergy. *JAMA.* 1992;268:504–509.

85. Antonucci G, Girardi E, Raviglione MC, Ippilito G. Risk factors for tuberculosis in HIV infected persons: a prospective cohort study. *JAMA.* 1995;274:143–148.

86. Caiaffa W, Graham NHM, Vlahov D, et al. Instability of delayed-type hypersensitivity (DTH) skin test anergy in human immunodeficiency infection. *Arch Int Med.* 1996;155:2111–2117.

87. Alwood K, Keruly JC, Moore-Rice K, et al. Effectiveness of supervised, intermittent therapy for tuberculosis in HIV-infected patients. *AIDS.* 1994;8:1103–1108.

88. Theuer CP, Hopewell PC, Elias D, et al. Human immunodeficiency virus infection in tuberculosis patients. *J Infect Dis.* 1990;162:8–12.

89. De Cock KM, Soro B, Coulibay IM, Lucas SB. Tuberculosis and HIV infection in sub-Saharan Africa. *JAMA.* 1992;268:1581–1587.

90. ten Dam HG. BCG vaccination: an old idea revisited. In: Rossman MD, MacGregor RR, eds. *Tuberculosis.* New York: McGraw-Hill; 1995:109–128.

91. Ayvazian LF. History of tuberculosis. In: Reichman LB, Hershfield ES, eds. *Tuberculosis: A Comprehensive International Approach.* New York: Marcel Dekker; 1993:1–22.

92. Fine PEM, Sterne JAC, Pönnighaus JM, Rees RJW. Delayed-type hypersensitivity, mycobacterial vaccines and protective immunity. *Lancet.* 1994;344:1245–1249.

93. Hawgood BJ. Doctor Albert Calmette 1863–1933: founder of antivenomous serotherapy and antituberculous BCG vaccination. *Toxicon.* 1999;37:1241–1258.

94. Comstock GW. Field trials of tuberculosis vaccines: how could we have done them better? *Controlled Clin Trials.* 1994;15:247–276.

95. Smith PG. Case-control studies of the efficacy of BCG against tuberculosis. In: *XXVIth IUAT World Conference1986.* Professional Postgraduate Services, International; 1987;73–79.

96. Shapiro C, Cook N, Evans D, et al. A case-control study of BCG and childhood tuberculosis in Cali, Colombia. *Int J Epidemiol.* 1985;14(3):441–446.

97. Sutrisna B, Utomo P, Komalarini S, Swatriani S. Penelitian efekitfitas vaksin GCG dan beberapa faktor lainnya pada anak yang menderita TBC berat di 3 Rumah sakit di Jakarta 1981–1982. *Medika.* 1983; 9:143–50.

98. Kenyon TA, Mwasekaga MJ, Huebner R, et al. Low levels of drug resistance amidst rapidly increasing tuberculosis and human immunodeficiency virus co-epidemics in Botswana. *Int J Tuberc Lung Dis.* 1999;3:4–11.

99. De Cock KM, Chaisson RE. Will DOTS do it? A reappraisal of tuberculosis control in countries with high rates of HIV infection. *Int J Tuberc Lung Dis.* 1999;3: 457–465.

100. International Union against Tuberculosis and Lung Disease (IUATLD). *Tuberculosis Guide for Low-Income Countries.* 3rd ed. Paris: IUATLD; 1994.

101. Ferebee SH. Controlled chemoprophylaxis trials in tuberculosis: a general review. *Adv Tuberc Res.* 1970; 17:28–106.

102. ATS/CDC. Control of tuberculosis in the United States. *Am Rev Respir Dis.* 1992;146:1623–1633.

103. *Tuberculosis in el Peru. Informe 1997.* Lima, Peru: Ministerio de Salud; 1998.

104. Chaisson RE, Coberly JS, De Cock KM. DOTS and drug resistance: a silver lining to a darkening cloud. *Int J Tuberc Lung Dis.* 1999;3:1–3.

105. WHO/IUATLD. *Anti-Tuberculosis Drug Resistance in the World.* Geneva: WHO/IUATLD; 1997.

106. Kimerling ME, Kluge H, Vezhnina N, et al. Inadequacy of the current WHO retreatment regimen in a central Siberian prison: treatment failure and MDR-TB. *Int J Tuberc Lung Dis.* 1999;3:451–453.

107. Freiden TR, Fujiwara PI, Washko RM, Hamburg PA. Tuberculosis in New York City: turning the tide. *N Engl J Med.* 1995;333:229–233.

CHAPTER 15

The Epidemiology of Acute Respiratory Infections

Neil M.H. Graham

INTRODUCTION

As recently as 1997, acute respiratory infections were termed a "forgotten pandemic."[1] These infections, which are composed of pneumonia, bronchitis, bronchiolitis, otitis media, sinusitis, pharyngitis, laryngitis, measles, and pertussis, continue to cause 19% of all deaths worldwide among children aged less than 5 years and 8.2% of all disability and premature mortality.[1] Children living in developing countries have especially high morbidity and mortality rates. Despite the pandemicity of acute lower respiratory infections, investigators of these illnesses receive only 0.15% of all health-related research and development dollars.[1] This translates to $0.51 per disability-adjusted life year (DALY), compared with $13 for asthma and $10 for rheumatic diseases.[1]

Although slow in coming, substantial gains in the battle against acute respiratory infections have been made with the public health approach to prophylaxis and treatment. Major advances have occurred to facilitate our understanding of the epidemiology and etiology of these infections. Data about risk factors continue to accumulate, with most information coming from the developed world, where funding, logistics, and infrastructure are available to support large multidimensional epidemiologic studies. Promising areas of epidemiologic investigation have been pursued since the 1980s, such as nutritional risk factors, the effects of indoor and outdoor air pollution, and the development of new vaccines. In this chapter, the impact on public health, etiology, and risk factors for acute respiratory infections are reviewed, and the major methodologic problems and requirements for future research are delineated.

IMPACT ON PUBLIC HEALTH

Developing Countries

Over the past 25 years, published data have indicated huge differences in mortality rates from acute respiratory infections between developing and developed countries. A World Health Organization (WHO) study in 1990 revealed that, in the world as a whole, the number of deaths attributable to respiratory infections was 12 times greater in developing countries than in developed countries (Table 15–1).[2] Leowski[3] has suggested that 25% to 33% of mortality in children aged less than 5 years is attributable to acute respiratory infections. If developed countries can be defined as those with infant mortality rates of ≤25 per 1,000, 98% of deaths from acute respiratory infections in infants and 99% of those in children aged 1 to 4 years can be expected to occur in less developed countries.[4] Conversely, countries with infant mortality of approximately 100 per 1,000 can be expected to contribute 58% of the deaths in infants and 66%

Table 15–1 World Health Organization Estimated Deaths from Respiratory Infections (Excluding Tuberculosis) in 1990

	Respiratory Infections		All Causes of Death
World	4,314,400	(8.6%)	49,971,100
Developed countries	330,000	(3.0%)	10,883,100
Developing countries	3,984,400	(10.2%)	39,088,000

Source: Data from C.J.L. Murray and A.D. Lopez, Global Comparative Assessments in the Health Sector, World Health Organization, 1994.

of those in children aged 1 to 4 years.[4] As these estimates are based on national mortality reporting systems of varying quality, underestimation of the true mortality rate is possible.

Pneumonia causes more deaths in children in the developing world (~3 million annually) than respiratory illness caused by pertussis and measles (~1 million).[1] According to Shann et al.,[1] this number is equivalent to the deaths that would occur if a jumbo jet carrying 400 children crashed every hour of every single day in a year. The Pan American Health Organization reported pneumonia deaths in Peru as being 37 times higher in infants and 43 times higher in children aged 1 to 4 years than rates in North America.[5] Infant deaths from pneumonia and influenza in 1977 were five times higher in Costa Rica, and 30 times higher in Paraguay, than in the United States.[6] In infants in the Philippines, pneumonia death rates have been reported to be 24 times higher than in Australian infants and 73 times higher than in Australian children aged 1 to 4 years.[7]

In contrast to these mortality data, acute respiratory infection–related morbidity appears to differ little between developing and developed countries. Among developing countries, mean episodes of respiratory illness per year have been reported as 7.3 in children aged less than 3 years and 6.2 in children aged 3 to 5 years in India,[8] 7.9 in children aged less than 3 years and 6.6 in children aged 3 to 5 years in Ethiopia,[9] and 4.9 and 5.7 in urban settings in Costa Rica.[10]

Similarly, in the developed world, data from the National Research Council studies of respiratory infection in young children in 12 countries suggest that the incidence in the first year of life ranges from five to nine episodes.[11] In the Seattle Virus Watch from 1965–1969, infants experienced four and one half mean episodes per year.[12] In Tecumseh, Michigan, infants experienced a mean of slightly more than six episodes of respiratory illness per year, and children aged 1 to 4 years experienced a mean of just more than five episodes per year.[13] It should be cautioned, however, that the studies from which these data were culled used widely differing methodologies and, thus, prevalence rates may not be directly comparable.

The incidence of chronic bronchitis (chronic obstructive pulmonary disease) is generally similar in developing and developed countries.[14] For example, Lai et al.[15] found 6.8% of an elderly group of Chinese living in Hong Kong to have chronic bronchitis, and pharmaceutical research indicated a 6.9% incidence in Taiwan.[14] However, Pandey[16] found a high incidence of chronic bronchitis (18%) in Nepal, with women and men equally affected. Indonesia also appears to have an especially high incidence of chronic bronchitis, although available data do not differentiate chronic bronchitis from acute bronchitis or account for multiple episodes during the observation period.[14] An age profile in a sample of nearly 250,000 persons in Indonesia noted the incidence of chronic bronchitis was

15.7% in those aged 30 to 39 years, 19.3% for those aged 40 to 54 years, and approximately 6% for those aged 55 years or older.[14]

Developed Countries

Acute respiratory infections are the leading cause of morbidity, accounting for 20% of medical consultations, 30% of absences from work, and 75% of all antibiotic prescriptions.[1] Of all the acute respiratory infections, pneumonia has been the most thoroughly studied. In 1900, pneumonia was the second most likely cause of death in the United States after tuberculosis.[17] Mortality rates per 100,000 population between 1910 and the present are shown in Figure 15–1.[17] In 1918, pneumonia mortality skyrocketed from the great influenza pandemic, which that year killed more than 540,000 Americans. Since that time, the pneumonia-related mortality rate has fallen significantly because of better hygiene practices and the availability of effective treatment, including antipneumococcal serum, sulfa drugs, penicillin, and other effective antibiotics. The slight increase in pneumonia-related deaths since 1990 is primarily because of the increase in the elderly population, who have a high pneumonia risk.[17] Currently, in the United States mortality rates from community-acquired pneumonia range from 1% to 5% in outpatients and from 15% to 30% in inpatients, making it the sixth leading cause of death.[18–20] Community-acquired pneumonia incurs hospitalization in 20% of patients and 65 million days of restricted activity.[21]

Figure 15–2 pinpoints where in the United States deaths from pneumonia occurred between 1979 and 1992.[17] Although it was long theorized that a higher mortality rate from pneumonia occurred during winter and that cold temperatures promote pneumonia, these ideas are not consistent with the pattern of mortality shown in Figure 15–2.[17] Indeed, no definitive pattern with regard to climate is apparent: California had the highest pneumonia-related mortality rates; Georgia and Massachusetts had high rates; and North Dakota had the third lowest rate. The fact that pneumonia-related deaths occurred least often in Florida is believed to be due to the "healthy retiree" effect; that is, the tendency of healthy older people to retire to places such as Florida, whereas less healthy people in the older age group remain at home.[17]

Hospital-acquired (nosocomial) pneumonia is the second most common nosocomial infection in the United States, but it is the type of nosocomial infection most frequently associated with a fatal outcome.[22] The annual incidence is 5 to 10 cases per 1,000 hospital admissions, and up to 20 times this figure in patients on ventilators.[22] Mortality rates run as high as 33% to 50% in patients on ventilators.[23,24] The availability of penicillin and other antibiotics to treat pneumonia has greatly reduced the mortality and morbidity associated with this infection.

Age-specific incidence rates of minor episodes of respiratory illness (primarily upper respiratory tract infections) in the United States have varied little since 1933, as indicated by the results of studies that evaluated populations of varying compositions and used differing study methodologies and definitions of acute respira-

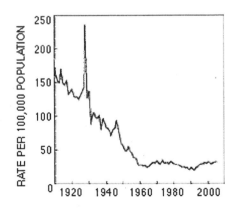

Figure 15–1 Rates in the graph are for the death registration area, which comprised 12 states in 1900 and 48 states by 1933. Alaska was added in 1959 and Hawaii in 1960. Not adjusted for changing age composition. *Source:* Roger Doyle © 2000.

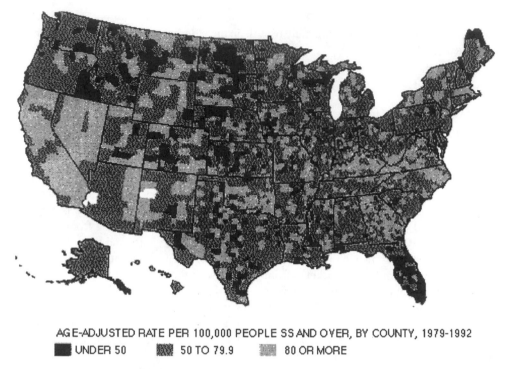

AGE-ADJUSTED RATE PER 100,000 PEOPLE 55 AND OVER, BY COUNTY, 1979-1992
■ UNDER 50   ▨ 50 TO 79.9   ▨ 80 OR MORE

Figure 15–2 Deaths from pneumonia in the United States. *Source:* Roger Doyle © 2000.

tory illness.[13,25–27] Over this period, however, pneumonia mortality rates have decreased in all age groups, except the elderly (Table 15–2). Indeed, since 1981, mortality rates have increased in pneumonia patients aged 55 years or older. It is unclear why this is occurring, although alterations in the types and pathogenicity of organisms causing pneumonia and changing host factors may be contributory factors.[28] Despite decreasing mortality rates for pneumonia and influenza in young children and infants, lower respiratory tract illness (croup, bronchitis, bronchiolitis, and pneumonia) remains an important cause of morbidity, annually affecting approximately 25% of children aged less than 1 year and 18% of children aged 1 to 4 years.[29–31] In 1989, Wright et al.[32] reported the cumulative incidence of first episodes of lower respiratory tract infection in infants to be 32.9% in children of families

participating in a prepaid health plan. This higher rate may have been seen because of differing diagnostic criteria compared with previous studies,[29–31] an active rather than a passive follow-up regimen, and increased physician attendance because of lack of a financial disincentive in a prepaid health plan. In older children and adults in the United Kingdom, acute respiratory infections accounted for almost one fourth of all primary care contacts, and one third of days taken off work were attributable to acute respiratory illness.[32] In a survey in Australia, 17% of patients aged 15 years or older and 43% of children aged less than 15 years consulted a doctor for respiratory symptoms during the 2 weeks presurvey.[33] A study in Adelaide, South Australia, showed that children younger than 5 years experienced a mean of seven episodes of respiratory illness per year, which prompted

Table 15-2 Age-Specific Mortality Rates from Pneumonia and Influenza in the United States, 1968–1996

Year	<1	1–4	5–14	15–24	25–34	35–44	45–54	55–64	65–74	75–84	≥85
					Age (years)						
1968	234.9	9.9	1.8	2.8	4.4	9.3	19.9	41.9	106.0	330.7	1,167.8
1970	180.8	7.6	1.6	2.4	3.8	8.5	17.3	36.2	90.2	272.8	814.5
1971	147.2	6.9	1.3	2.2	3.3	7.0	13.4	29.3	77.0	253.8	855.9
1973	115.7	5.9	1.4	2.0	3.1	6.9	14.5	31.6	82.1	295.6	910.4
1975	71.5	4.1	1.0	1.7	2.5	5.3	11.1	27.0	70.2	264.4	777.1
1977	53.2	3.1	0.9	1.3	2.0	4.4	9.6	21.9	58.5	236.2	731.2
1979	33.0	2.0	0.6	0.8	1.5	3.2	7.1	16.4	47.8	184.2	694.9
1981	22.6	1.8	0.5	0.8	1.5	3.3	7.4	18.4	52.5	209.3	845.8
1983	21.0	1.7	0.4	0.7	1.4	2.8	6.7	16.8	51.1	205.8	859.9
1986	17.6	1.4	0.4	0.7	1.7	3.6	7.0	18.6	58.6	242.8	1,032.1
1996	—	1.1	0.4	0.6	2.4[†]	2.4[†]	10.6[‡]	10.6[‡]	221.4[§]	221.4[§]	221.4[§]

[†]Ages 25 to 44 years grouped together this year.
[‡]Ages 45 to 64 years grouped together this year.
[§]Ages ≥65 years grouped together this year.

Source: Reprinted from Monthly Vital Statistics Report, U.S. Public Health Service, National Center for Health Statistics, 1968–1988, and National Vital Statistics Report 1998, Vol. 47, No. 9.

three doctor visits, 15 days of medication, and 52 days of respiratory symptoms annually.[34,35]

The incidence of chronic bronchitis is similar in the United States and Europe.[14] In 1994, Enright et al.[36] reported that 5.1% to 5.4% of the middle-aged to elderly population in the United States have chronic bronchitis, with a lower prevalence in nonsmokers. In Europe, chronic bronchitis has been reported to affect 3.7% of people in Denmark,[37] 4.5% in Norway,[38] 6% and 6.4% in Barcelona and Valencia, Spain, respectively,[39,40] and 6.7% in Sweden.[41]

In the United States in 1998, community-acquired pneumonia accounted for an estimated $3.6 billion for treating patients aged less than 65 years and $4.8 billion for treating patients aged 65 years or older.[42] In 1999, costs associated with acute exacerbations of chronic bronchitis were $419 million in patients aged less than 65 years and three times that much ($1.2 billion) for patients aged 65 years and older.[43]

CLASSIFICATION OF ACUTE RESPIRATORY INFECTIONS

Two basic systems are most commonly used to classify acute respiratory infections: (*a*) the case-management classification system, and (*b*) the "traditional" clinical classification system (Table 15–3).

Case-Management Classification

In an effort to reduce pneumonia-related mortality, the World Health Organization has developed a simple case-management approach to be followed by village health care workers. Before 1988, simplified case classifications, as used in India,[44] Papua New Guinea,[45] and other developing countries,[46] were applied successfully by health workers to determine when children should be given antibiotics or referred to secondary or tertiary level care. Adherence with these classifications resulted in reductions in both pneumonia-related mortality and in overall mortality. The simplified case definitions were based on respiratory rates recorded among chil-

dren with symptoms of respiratory infections. The sensitivity and specificity of increased respiratory rate were determined using clinically confirmed or chest radiograph–confirmed pneumonia (or, "lower respiratory tract infection") as the putative "gold standard." For example, using receiver operating characteristic (ROC) curves, Cherian et al.[47] showed that higher respiratory rates were more sensitive and specific for infants than for older children aged less than 5 years (Figure 15–3).

In 1988, changes were made to improve the specificity of case-management guidelines.[46,48–50] Although the primary focus remained on pneumonia, classification and management of syndromes causing stridor and wheezing were directly addressed, and otitis media was classified separately (Table 15–3). Other major differences from the earlier classification were in the less than 2-month-old age group, about whom the newer classification recognized that a respiratory rate greater than 50 breaths/minute and some chest indrawing could be considered normal,[48] with regard to cough, which is often absent in neonates with pneumonia, the newer classification specified that this sign is not sufficiently sensitive to be used as an indicator of severe disease. The newer case-management classification recommended that signs of general sepsis should be sought (i.e., fever, feeding problems, drowsiness, convulsions, abdominal distention, hypothermia) as well as more specific signs of pneumonia (respiratory rate >60 breaths/minute, severe chest indrawing, respiratory grunt) when determining whether to prescribe antibiotics and to hospitalize.[48]

Clinical Classification

Acute respiratory infections can be classified by the site of primary pathology (Table 15–3). This system is preferred by most physicians, and it is compatible with the International Classification of Diseases system. However, such classification can lead to some confusion because infections are not always limited to one part of the respiratory tract. Moreover, clinicians may dis-

Table 15–3 Classification of Acute Respiratory Infection Clinical Syndromes

Case-Management Classification (children aged 2 months to 4 years)			"Traditional" Classification
Stridor	*Wheezing*	*No Wheezing*	
Mild	Mild	Mild	Upper respiratory tract syndromes
Hoarseness plus "barking" cough; no stridor when calm = mild croup	Improves with bronchodilator; respiratory rate <50/min = mild bronchiolitis or asthma	Cough; nasal obstruction; respiratory rate <50/min = URI,* cold	Common cold; URI* Acute otitis media Pharyngitis/tonsillitis Acute sinusitis
Home care; no antibiotic	Oral salbutamol	No antibiotic; home care	
	Moderate	Moderate	Middle respiratory tract syndromes
	Improves with bronchodilator; respiratory rate 50–70/min = mild bronchiolitis or asthma	Respiratory rate >50/min; no chest indrawing = pneumonia	Croup Laryngotracheo-bronchitis Epiglottitis Laryngitis Tracheitis
	Consider antibiotic; oral salbutamol; home care	Antibiotic; home care	
Severe	Severe	Severe	Lower respiratory tract syndromes
Stridor when calm; chest indrawing = severe croup or epiglottis	No improvement with bronchodilator; respiratory rate >70/min = severe bronchiolitis or asthma	Respiratory rate >50/min; chest indrawing = severe pneumonia	Bronchiolltls Bronchitis Pneumonia
Admit; antibiotic; manage airway	Admit; bronchodilators; consider oxygen and antibiotics	Admit; antibiotic	
	Very severe	Very Severe	
	Cyanosis or inability to drink = very severe bronchiolitis or asthma	Cyanosis or inability to drink = very severe pneumonia	
	Admit; bronchodilators; oxygen and consider antibiotic	Antibiotic; admit; oxygen	

*URI, upper respiratory infection.

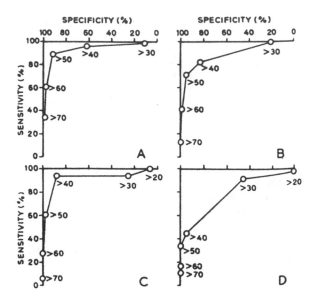

Figure 15–3 Receiver operating characteristic (ROC) curves for respiratory rates as indicators of lower respiratory tract infections in infants and children. *Source:* Reprinted with permission from T. Cherian et al., Evaluation of Simple Clinical Signs for the Diagnosis of Acute Lower Respiratory Tract Infection, *The Lancet*, Vol. 2, pp. 125–128, © by The Lancet Ltd., 1998.

agree on whether an acute respiratory infection can be termed "upper," "middle," and "lower." Stridor-causing conditions often have been classified as upper respiratory tract infections, thus suggesting mild disease, which can be a misleading assumption. As stridor can cause severe, and possibly fatal, respiratory distress, consideration has been given to classifying stridor-causing conditions as acute lower respiratory infections.[51]

PATHOGENS RESPONSIBLE FOR ACUTE RESPIRATORY INFECTIONS

In a large percentage of patients with acute respiratory infections, the pathogens responsible for infection are not known. This problem is especially notable with regard to community-acquired pneumonia, for which the causative organism is unknown in approximately 98% of those treated as outpatients and 50% to 60% of those treated as hospital inpatients.[52,53]

Viruses

Upper respiratory viral infections in children and adults are caused by rhinoviruses (30% to 50%) or coronaviruses (5% to 20%), with the remainder (30% to 65%) due to influenza virus, parainfluenza virus, respiratory syncytial virus, adenoviruses, and certain enteroviruses.[54,55] These infections are generally mild, self-limiting, and do not involve respiratory distress.

In children, viral causes of the acute lower respiratory tract infections, pneumonia, bronchiolitis, and croup generally appear to be similar in both developed and developing countries,[56–65] the primary pathogens being respiratory syncytial virus; parainfluenza virus types 1, 2, and 3; influenza virus types A and B; adenoviruses; and enteroviruses. Respiratory syncytial virus is most commonly associated with bronchiolitis, and parainfluenza virus (especially type 1) is more often associated with croup.[66–69] In developing countries, measles contributes to croup and serious morbidity in other lower respiratory infections more than it does in the developed world.[70,71] Approximately 90% of cases of acute bronchitis are caused by viruses, including influenza virus, parainfluenza virus, and rhinovirus.[72]

In adults, viral causes of pneumonia are generally less important than nonviral causes. However, influenza has been associated with a significant proportion of cases in adults, perhaps causing as many as half of all virus-associated cases, and approximately 8% to 10% of all pneumonias in general.[28,73] Respiratory syncytial virus and parainfluenza also have been identified in some adult cases of pneumonia, but these viruses are less commonly implicated than influenza.[74] In developed countries, influenza epidemics in elderly patients (≥65 years of age) are associated with especially high mortality and hospitalization rates from acute respiratory infections; thus, influenza poses a major health risk to this age group.[75] More than 50% of excess hospitalizations and more than 80% of influenza-related deaths occur in persons aged 65 years and older, in whom mortality is 30 to 50 times greater than in younger adults.[76] In developing countries, viral causes of adult lower respiratory tract infections have not been widely studied. No indication is seen that viral pathogens are implicated to any greater degree in pneumonia cases in developing countries than they are in developed countries, although the mode of transmission in the poorer nations (unwashed hands, contaminated water) can differ from those in the developed world (day-care facilities, contaminated aerosols).[76]

Most epidemiologic studies have been hampered by the limited laboratory techniques available to isolate viral pathogens. Isolation of virus from 20% to 25% of specimens has been the maximal rate in several well-conducted studies.[31,67,77–79] Recent improvements in these techniques might be expected to result in higher isolation rates being more common. When combinations of viral culture and immunofluorescence techniques were used in one study of lower respiratory infections in infants to identify viral pathogens from throat and nasopharyngeal swabs, a 66% isolation rate was reported.[32]

Bacteria

Some studies of the bacterial causes of pneumonia have been marred by the methodologic problem of contamination of sputum specimens by nasopharyngeal and oropharyngeal organisms.[80] Therefore, sputum cultures may be of limited value. As bronchoscopic and transtracheal aspirates are also at risk of contamination,[81,82] most investigators rely on percutaneous needle lung aspirates and blood culture for accurate diagnosis of pneumonia.[83]

Developing Countries

Bacteria-caused lower respiratory infections are more common in children in developing countries than in the developed world, where viral infections are more often encountered.[29,31] Reliable data regarding pathogens responsible for pneumonia in adults in developing countries have come chiefly from hospital studies.[73] *Streptococcus pneumoniae* is by far the most important cause of pneumonia in adults: it is associated with up to 70% of cases in which a pathogen is isolated,[73,84] with *Haemophilis influenzae* and *Staphylococcus aureus* being relatively less important in adults than in children (together accounting for ~10% of cases). *Streptococcus pyogenes* and *Corynebacterium diphtheriae* most commonly cause pharyngitis/tonsillitis. Acute epiglottitis is caused chiefly by *H. influenzae* type B, and whooping cough by *Bordetella pertussis*.[55,85,86] In otitis media, *S. pneumoniae* and *H. influenzae* are the most commonly isolated bacteria,[87] but *Moraxella catarrhalis* has been isolated in 27% of patients in some series.[88] *S. pneumoniae* and *H. influenzae* are also important in acute sinusitis in children[89] and in adults.[90,91]

Berman and McIntosh[55] have reviewed studies of bacteria isolated from children in developing countries using lung aspiration techniques. The most frequently isolated pathogens were *H. influenzae*, *S. pneumoniae* (together accounting for 54% of isolates), and *S. aureus* (accounting for 17% of isolates). A subsequent study in Zimbabwe found a similar pattern of pathogens responsible for lower respiratory infections.[92]

Developed Countries

The key bacterial pathogens responsible for community-acquired pneumonia in the developed world appear to be the same as those in developing countries. A literature review of 15 published reports from North America showed the most common bacterial pathogens to be *S.*

pneumoniae (20% to 60% of isolates) and *H. influenzae* (3% to 10%) (Table 15–4). A meta-analysis of 122 published studies between 1966 and 1995 (*N* = 7,057) indicated that *S. pneumoniae* was responsible for 66% of deaths in community-acquired pneumonia cases.[93] A review of nosocomial pneumonia indicated that gram-negative bacteria account for 50% to 70% of cases (Table 15–5).[93] The most frequently isolated pathogen is *Pseudomonas aeruginosa*, followed by a diverse array of *Enterobacteriaceae*. These bacteria reach the lower airways by aspiration of gastric contents.

Approximately 50% to 75% of infective exacerbations of chronic bronchitis are bacterial in origin.[14] Studies conducted in the Northern Hemisphere have consistently shown *H. in-*

Table 15–4 Pathogens Most Commonly Involved with Community-Acquired Pneumonia

Microbial Agents	Literature Review* (%)	The British Thoracic Society[†] (%)	Meta-analysis[‡] Cases (%)	Deaths (%)
Bacteria				
–*Streptococcus pneumoniae*	20–60	60–75	65	66
–*Haemophilus influenzae*	3–10	4–5	12	7
–*Staphylococcus aureus*	3–5	1–5	2	6
–Gram-negative bacilli	3–10	Rare	1	3
–Miscellaneous agents[§]	3–5	(Not included)	4	9
Atypical pathogens	10–20	—	12	6
–*Legionella* sp.	2–8	2–5	4	5
–*Mycoplasma pneumoniae*	1–6	5–18	7	1
–*Chlamydia pneumoniae*	4–6	(Not included)	1	<1
Viral	2–15	8–16	3	≤1
Aspiration pneumonia	6–10	(Not included)	—	—
No diagnosis	30–60	—	—	—

* Based on analysis of 15 published reports from North America.[92] Low and high values are deleted.

[†] Estimates are based on analysis of 453 adults in prospective study of community-acquired pneumonia in 25 British hospitals.[92]

[‡] Meta-analysis of 122 published studies of community-acquired pneumonia in the English language literature 1966 to 1995; data are limited to 7,057 patients who had an etiologic diagnosis.[92] Percentage of death column refers to percentage of all deaths attributed to the designated pathogen.

[§] Includes *Moraxella catarrhalis*, group A streptococcus, and *Neisseria meningitidis* (each 1% to 2%).

Source: Reprinted with permission from J.G. Bartlett, Approach to the Patient with Pneumonia, In *Infectious Diseases*, 2nd Ed., pp. 553–564, © 1998, W.B. Saunders Company.

Table 15–5 Pathogens Most Commonly Involved in Nosocomial Pneumonia

Pathogen	%
Bacterial	
–Gram-negative bacilli	50–70
—*Pseudomonas aeruginosa**	
—*Enterobacteriaceae**	
–*Staphylococcus aureus**	15–30
–Anaerobic bacteria	10–30
–*Haemophilus influenzae*	10–20
–*Streptococcus pneumoniae*	10–20
–*Legionella**	4
Viral	10–20
–Cytomegalovirus	
–Influenza virus*	
–Respiratory syncytial virus*	
Fungal	<1
–*Aspergillus**	

*May cause nosocomial epidemics.

Source: Reprinted with permission from J.G. Bartlett, Approach to the Patient with Pneumonia, In *Infectious Diseases*, 2nd Ed., pp. 553–564, © 1998, W.B. Saunders Company.

fluenzae to be the major pathogen and *M. catarrhalis* to be the second most common pathogen.[72]

Other Pathogens

Mycoplasma pneumoniae, *Chlamydia* species, *Legionella* species, and *Pneumocystis carinii* are the nonviral respiratory pathogens most frequently responsible for pneumonia and acute bronchitis in both children and adults.[31,68,94,95] *M. pneumoniae* can also cause upper respiratory infections.[94,96] Of the *Chlamydia* species, *C. trachomatis* is implicated more in cases of pneumonia in young infants,[97] and *C. pneumoniae* (also called TWAR, based on the names of the first two isolates, TW-183 and AR-39) is responsible primarily for pneumonia cases among older children and adults.[97–99] Most of the cases of *P. carinii* pneumonia that have been reported since the early 1980s have been in patients with the acquired immune deficiency syndrome (AIDS). *P. carinii* pneumonia occurs as an opportunistic infection in patients with AIDS most frequently when their CD4+ lymphocyte counts fall below 200 cells/mm^3. Approximately 60% to 80% of AIDS patients will develop *P. carinii* pneumonia at some stage during the course of their illness.[100,101] In developed countries, both children and adults with AIDS and other conditions associated with immunosuppression are at significant risk of *P. carinii* pneumonia. In developing countries, AIDS-associated *P. carinii* pneumonia is less common, but the reasons for this are unclear.[102] Human immune deficiency virus (HIV)–infected patients have a greater incidence of community-acquired pneumonia caused by the intracellular bacterial pathogens *Salmonella* and *Legionella* than patients not infected with HIV.[103]

RISK FACTORS

The risk factors for community-acquired pneumonia and nosocomial pneumonia are summarized in Exhibits 15–1 and 15–2, respectively.[104] Specifics pertaining to key risk factors are provided below.

Demographic Factors

Age

The incidence of viral respiratory illness peaks in infancy and early childhood and steadily decreases with age because of changes in patterns of exposure and age-related acquisition of specific immunity to an increasing number of virus types encountered over time (Table 15–6).[12,25–27,105] On examination of markers of more severe conditions (e.g., pneumonia and influenza mortality rates), a different pattern of age-related change is observed. Although infants are at greater risk from pneumonia than older children and young to middle-aged adults, mortality rates are highest in the elderly (Table 15–2). Elderly patients have reduced vital capacity and respiratory muscle strength, and impaired local and general immune defenses, all of

Table 15–6 Acute Respiratory Infection Morbidity Rates in Four U.S. Cohort Studies

Investigators	Years	Population	Mean Incidence per Year by Age Group (years)											
			<1	1–2	3–4	5–9	10–14	15–19	20–24	25–29	30–39	40–49	50–59	≥60
van Volkenburgh and Frost[25]	1924	Public health service families		3.0		2.7	1.9	1.4		2.0*	1.8†	1.6‡	1.4§	
	1928–1929	Baltimore, MD, families		4.5		3.5	3.5	2.4	2.8		2.7	2.4	1.7	
	1929–1930	Baltimore, MD, families		4.5		3.8	2.8	2.3	2.7		2.6	2.3	2.1	
Gwaltney et al.[26]	1963–1966	Insurance company employees						2.5		2.1	2.2	1.7		
Fox et al.[27]	1965–1969	Seattle, WA, families	5.1	5.8	5.8	3.8	2.3							
Monto and Ullman[13]	1969–1971	Tecumseh, MI, families	6.1	5.7	4.7	3.5	2.7	2.4	2.8	2.7	2.3	1.7	1.6	1.3

* 25–34 years of age.
† 35–44 years of age.
‡ 45–54 years of age.
§ ≥55 years of age.
¶ ≥45 years of age.

Source: Reprinted with permission from N.M.H. Graham, The Epidemiology of Acute Respiratory Infection in Children and Adults: A Global Perspective, *Epidemiologic Reviews*, Vol. 12, pp. 149–178, © 1990, Oxford University Press.

Exhibit 15–1 Risk Factors of Community-Acquired Pneumonia

1. Old age
2. Smoking (>20 cigarettes a day)
3. Air pollution
4. Chronic diseases (e.g., diabetes, chronic hepatopathies, renal, cardiac, respiratory failure)
5. Malnutrition, precarious social and economic situations
6. Acute and chronic alcoholism
7. Chronic obstructive pulmonary disease
8. Primitive ciliary dyskinesia, bronchiectasis, cystic fibrosis
9. Congestive cardiomyopathies
10. Neuromuscular diseases
11. Dementia
12. Autoimmune diseases (LES, rheumatoid arthritis and other collagen diseases)
13. Malignancy
14. Immunodeficiencies
15. Splenectomy
16. Immunosuppressive therapies
17. Drug addiction
18. Inadequate use of antibiotics

Source: Reprinted with permission from F. Ginesu and P. Pirina, Etiology and Risk Factors of Adult Pneumonia, *Journal of Chemotherapy*, Vol. 7, pp. 277–285, © 1995.

which make them more susceptible than younger adults to severe acute lower respiratory infection. Pneumonia and influenza mortality rates, in particular, have increased in the elderly population over the past 15 years (Table 15–2). The most likely explanation for this is that many more at-risk persons (e.g., those with cardiovascular disease and chronic airways obstruction) are surviving into old age and suffering pneumonia as a terminal event. It is also possible that some of these deaths may have been attributable to changing virulence of respiratory pathogens and increased cumulative exposures to environmental factors, such as smoking and air pollution.

In developing countries, data on pneumonia-related mortality rates over the entire age range are sparse because many nations, especially those in Africa and Asia, do not report information to the World Health Organization.[106] However, Costa Rica and Cuba have contributed data, and both developing countries show an excess burden of mortality in infants and young children (Table 15–7).[6] Mortality rates in older children and young adults in Costa Rica are not much higher than those in the United States. As in the United States, mortality rates rise rapidly in the elderly in Costa Rica and Cuba, the rise being especially pronounced in Cuba.

Gender

The incidence of acute respiratory infections has been known to vary according to gender since the 1920s. In Baltimore, between 1928 and 1930, van Volkenburgh and Frost[25] reported higher rates of acute respiratory infections in boys aged younger than 9 years, and the reverse pattern above that age. Similar findings were reported by Monto and Ullman,[13] with higher rates of infection in boys aged less than 3 years, but lower rates in older age groups. Gwaltney et al.[26] found that young women aged 16 to 24 years experienced more upper respiratory tract illness than did young men of similar age, even after adjusting for number of children and smoking status, with no differences being seen in patients aged more than 24 years. A review of pneumonia cases between 1979 and 1992 showed men to be at greater risk of pneumonia than women; this was considered partly due to men being more susceptible because of increased exposure to two key pneumonia risk factors—alcoholism and nicotine.[17]

Fox et al.[27] found that mothers in Seattle families experienced more upper respiratory illness than did their husbands, but not more lower respiratory illness. This could have been due to the mothers' more frequent exposure to young children. However, a subsequent study of viral chest infections in infants found no differences in incidence by sex.[32] Pneumonia-related mortality rates in older adults are higher in men than in

Exhibit 15–2 Risk Factors for Nosocomial Pneumonia

1. Advanced age (>65 y)
2. Chronic diseases (e.g., diabetes, cardiopathies, chronic obstructive pulmonary disease, chronic hepatopathies, chronic alcoholism, respiratory, cardiac, renal failure, obesity)
3. Malignancy
4. Prolonged immobilization (stroke, neuromuscular diseases)
5. Immunosuppressive therapies (cytotoxics, steroids)
6. Immunodeficiencies
7. Thoracic and abdominal surgery
8. Burns
9. Traumas (thorax and abdomen, multiple, rib fractures, pulmonary contusions, pneumothorax, hemothorax)
10. Treatment with antacids and/or H2 blockers
11. Antibiotic therapy and prophylaxis
12. Increase in number of hospitalized patients susceptible to infections
13. Increase in invasive techniques for diagnosis and therapy
14. Mechanical ventilation (MV):
    –Reintubation
    –MV duration (> 3 d)
    –Positive end-expiratory pressure
    –Persistence of coma during MV
    –Severity of underlying disease
    –Gastric content aspiration
    –Oropharyngeal aspiration
    –Intensive care unit
15. Airway instrumentation
16. Previous intubations and endotracheal prostheses
17. Ultrasound nebulizers and humidifier systems
18. Increase in number of staff members caring for the patient
19. Visitors, relatives, friends, and so on
20. Moving the patient inside the hospital
21. Health staff not adequately educated to prevent nosocomial infections
22. Inadequate hospital structures and facilities
23. Organ transplantation
24. Periodontitis, dental caries, gingivitis

Source: Reprinted with permission from F. Ginesu and P. Pirina, Etiology and Risk Factors of Adult Pneumonia, *Journal of Chemotherapy,* Vol. 7, pp. 277–285, © 1995.

women (Table 15–7), although this is not the case with mortality rates from upper respiratory tract infection. The reason for this greater susceptibility of older men is not certain, but it may be because of their generally higher rates of cardiovascular disease and chronic airway obstruction than are seen in women.

Outdoor Air Pollution

Outdoor air pollution has been known to affect the incidence of acute respiratory infections since the early 1930s. Episodes of acute, severe, particulate air pollution in the Meuse Valley, Belgium (1930), Donora, Pennsylvania (1948), New York City (1953 and 1962), and greater London, England (1948, 1952, and 1956), were associated with increases in all-cause mortality,

primarily because of more deaths from pneumonia and cardiovascular disease.[107–113] An estimated 4,000 excess deaths were reported in the disastrous London fog of 1952.[107] The elderly and very elderly in greater London were the groups most greatly affected.

These studies prompted research to evaluate the effects of much lower levels of air pollution on the outcomes of acute respiratory illnesses. The components of air pollution most widely studied have been suspended respirable particulates, sulfur dioxide, nitrogen dioxide, and ozone. Although studies in the 1960s and 1970s provided somewhat contradictory results,[114] they were instrumental in changing the focus on outcomes from mortality to both mortality and morbidity. Indeed, morbidity was considered a more sensitive outcome measure than mortality in

Table 15–7 Pneumonia Mortality Rates (per 100,000 Population) by Age and Sex in the United States, Costa Rica, and Cuba, 1987

Country	Sex	Age (years)									
		<1	1–4	5–14	15–24	25–34	35–44	45–54	55–64	65–74	≥75
United States	Male	19.2	1.4	0.3	0.8	2.3	4.7	9.2	23.6	78.8	505.2
	Female	15.7	1.2	0.3	0.6	1.2	2.2	4.7	12.0	48.6	360.1
Costa Rica	Male	206.6	10.0		0.3		2.8	1.1	3.2	46.5	464.3
	Female	127.6	5.2	0.3		0.4	1.4	2.1	6.1	28.4	383.4
Cuba	Male	115.0	4.7	0.9	1.5	3.0	3.2	9.5	34.1	139.2	943.1
	Female	102.9	4.3	0.6	1.7	2.2	3.6	7.9	28.4	89.8	766.8

Source: Reprinted with permission from World Health Statistics Annual, p. 105, © 1989, World Health Organization.

studies of relatively low levels of air pollution. In 1964, Toyama[115] reported a correlation between bronchitis mortality and level of suspended particulates in all ages. He also found that respiratory morbidity rates were higher for all age groups, and ventilatory function poorer, in children in air-polluted cities compared with relatively nonpolluted rural areas. Lunn et al.[116,117] studied respiratory illness patterns in children exposed to relatively high and low levels of particulate matter (smoke) and sulfur dioxide in Sheffield, United Kingdom. These investigators found a relationship between exposure to high levels of particles and sulfur dioxide in air and repeated episodes of acute upper and lower respiratory tract illness, after adjusting for socioeconomic status. Conversely, Colley and Reid[118] found a relationship between air pollution (urban/rural comparison) and acute lower, but not upper, respiratory illness in children. This effect was most marked in the lower social classes. Cassel et al.[119] also found no relationship between air pollution and upper respiratory illness. In infants in England and Wales who were examined and followed between 1958 and 1964, pneumonia and respiratory disease mortality were strongly associated with air pollution.[120] Lawther et al.,[121] in 1970, related acute exacerbations of chronic bronchitis to daily variations in smoke and sulfur dioxide.

Health effects in adults have been estimated to occur above 500 µg/m³ of sulfur dioxide and 250 µg/m³ of smoke in adults, and 180 µg/m³ and 120 µg/m³, respectively, in children older than age 4 years.[114] A weaker but still significant relationship was also seen in children aged 1 to 4 years. In the Great Salt Lake Basin and the Rocky Mountains, high levels of sulfur dioxide and suspended sulfate were associated with excess reports of croup in children (age-, sex-, social class–adjusted rates) who resided in a high pollution area for more than 3 years.[122] Durham[123] found that upper respiratory symptoms reported by Los Angeles college students presenting to campus health centers were significantly correlated with sulfur dioxide and nitrogen dioxide

levels independent of the effects of age, weather, and smoking levels. Levy et al.[124] found that high levels of sulfur dioxide and particulate matter, but not nitrogen dioxide, carbon monoxide, or pollen, predicted hospital admission for acute respiratory disease in children and adults, after adjusting for the effects of temperature. In Chicago, acute upper and lower respiratory tract illness attack rates were reported to be higher in both adults and children, but in New York only lower respiratory tract illness attack rates were significantly higher in residents of high pollution areas.

Studies in the 1980s sought to examine the effects of air pollution at much lower levels than earlier studies and have tried to determine which components of air pollution were of primary importance. Studies designed to allow concurrent comparisons of similar demographic areas and adjustment for confounding factors (e.g., the Six Cities Study[125]) were instrumental in clarifying the role of outdoor air pollution in increasing susceptibility to acute respiratory illness. Ware et al.[125] found that between-city annual mean differences in particulate and suspended sulfate concentrations as low as 80 µg/m³ doubled the risk of acute cough and substantially increased risk of bronchitis and other lower respiratory illness in children. These investigators also found significant, but weaker, associations with sulfur dioxide. Mean monthly peaks of sulfur dioxide did not exceed a range of 80 to 200 µg/m³. In a study by Pope,[126] 24-hour fine-particulate levels as low as 50 µg/m³ were associated with significantly increased hospitalization rates in children and adults for acute respiratory disease. The associations were stronger for bronchitis and asthma than for pneumonia and pleurisy, and persisted when adjustments were made for meteorologic variables. Derriennic et al.[127] observed that sulfur dioxide levels, but not levels of particulates or nitrogen dioxide, predicted deaths from respiratory disease in adults aged more than 65 years. Other studies have confirmed the importance of the association between particulates, sulfur dioxide, and respiratory symptoms in children.[128,129] The evidence is now supportive of the hypothesis that suspended particulates, suspended sulfates, and sulfur dioxide at levels currently being measured in ambient air significantly increase the risk of morbidity from acute respiratory illness in adults and children. Because most studies do not include virologic sampling, it is unclear whether morbidity is chiefly caused by bronchial reactivity and respiratory tract irritation or by infection. Studies supported by virologic culture and serology are needed to answer this question.

Ozone exposures below the U.S. ambient air quality standard have been associated with acute changes in ventilatory function[130] and increased risk of cough and lower respiratory illness.[131] The importance of ambient levels of nitrogen dioxide as a risk factor for respiratory illness is less clear.[128,132]

Indoor Air Pollution

Indoor air pollution from passive smoke, nitrogen dioxide from gas cooking or heating, and smoke from biomass fuels have been investigated for their impact on acute respiratory infections. A 1999 review of studies published during the 1990s showed that the incidence of respiratory illnesses and middle ear infection was greater in children living in homes where either parent smoked, with odds ratios between 1.2 and 1.6.[133] The odds ratios were much higher in preschool than in school-aged children. For sudden infant death syndrome, the odds ratio for maternal smoking was about two. Exposure to maternal cigarette smoke approximately doubles the risk of lower respiratory tract infection in children aged less than 2 years.[134,135] Paternal smoking seems less contributory to infection rates, possibly because fathers are generally around their children less than mothers during their children's first 2 years of life.[136,137] Passive smoking is believed to increase respiratory infection rates in children by reducing mucociliary clearance.[133] Although negative studies have also been reported,[138–140] these either involved

small numbers of patients[140] or did not report on smoking effects in children aged less than 2 years.[138,139]

In studies linking maternal smoking during pregnancy with respiratory infections in infants, prenatal smoking was found to be a stronger risk factor for bronchitis in infants than postnatal smoking.[141,142] As the number of women who change their smoking habit during or after pregnancy is few, it is difficult to identify sufficiently large comparison groups to fully settle this question.

Heating stoves and natural gas cooking increase exposure of household members to nitrogen dioxide.[143,144] However, studies designed to investigate a relationship between the low levels of nitrogen dioxide and enhancement of risk of acute respiratory illness have yielded equivocal results.[132,145–149] One study showed that children in Adelaide who lived in homes using gas heating were more likely to develop acute respiratory illness than those living in homes with electric heating, but the level of significance was marginal (odds ratio [OR] = 1.6; 95% confidence interval [CI] 1.0–2.6).[150] Based on current data, any effects attributable to nitrogen dioxide exposures are likely to be very small, if they exist at all.[151]

In developing countries, the negative public health impact of smoke from biomass fuels used for cooking is well established. Exposure to firewood or other biomass smoke during cooking can occur in up to 50% of the world's households.[152] Woodsmoke, in particular, is thought to be responsible for almost 50% of all cases of obstructive airways disease.[14] In 1996, a multivariate analysis of a case-control study in Colombia found woodsmoke to be more highly associated (OR, 3.43) with development of chronic bronchitis in women than either tobacco use or passive smoking (ORs, 2.22 and 2.05, respectively).[153] Children in many developing countries are exposed to respirable particles from these fuels at peak and daily indoor concentrations approximately 20 times greater than the levels present in developed countries where two packs of cigarettes are smoked per day[151] (a level at which the risk of many respiratory symptoms approximately doubles[135]). In a study in Nepal, Pandey et al.[154] found a relationship between hours per day spent near a stove and episodes of severe acute lower respiratory tract illness in children aged less than 2 years. However, this study was flawed by the lack of adjustment made for confounding factors, such as parental smoking. In a small, poorly controlled study, Kossove[155] found that Zulu infants presenting to a medical clinic with acute lower respiratory illness were more likely to be exposed to cooking smoke at home than children without respiratory illness. Campbell et al.[156] reported that children carried on their mother's back during cooking periods were at a 2.8 times greater risk of an episode of "fast or difficult breathing" (predictive of acute lower respiratory infection) than children who were not carried in this way.[157] All of these studies had methodologic problems because they were conducted in high acute respiratory infection incidence areas where exposure to indoor smoke is universally high and exposure dose was not measured. Intervention studies in high incidence areas need to be conducted to evaluate respiratory infection rates in persons living in homes using wood fuel compared with those living in homes using smokeless fuel or fluted stoves.

In the developed world, one U.S. study of children from homes with wood-burning stoves were found to experience more acute upper and lower respiratory tract illness than children from homes without such stoves.[158,159] Levels of the many gases, chemicals, and respirable particulates in wood smoke were not reported, which would have been desirable to assess the stove–illness connection in more detail. However, the greater incidence of respiratory illness was not explained by social class, smoking, or other indoor sources of air pollution. Another study in the United States, using a retrospective design, found no relationship between wood smoke exposure and respiratory illness in school-aged children.[159] By inference, this suggests that preschool children may be more at risk of acute respiratory infection in living environments heated by wood-burning stoves than are older children.

Smoking

A relationship between smoking and acute respiratory infection was first established in several prospective studies conducted in the late 1950s.[161–167] These data indicated that smokers were at increased risk of dying from pneumonia and influenza, their overall pneumonia:influenza mortality ratio being 1.4 (range, 0.7 to 2.6). Four subsequent studies showed that smoking is associated with increased severity and incidence of influenza.[168–171] Kark et al.[171] reported that the attributable proportion of influenza ascribable to smoking was 31% for all influenza cases and 41% for severe influenza cases. Tobacco smoking is undoubtedly the most common cause of chronic bronchitis.[14] In the Tecumseh family-based study, Monto et al.[172] assessed the incidence of respiratory illness in smokers and nonsmokers. In otherwise healthy index cases, both male and female smokers experienced more episodes of acute respiratory illness than nonsmokers. Studies in adolescents and young adults have also reported more respiratory symptoms in smokers than nonsmokers.[173–175] Reingold[176] found that smoking significantly increased the incidence of pneumonia and pneumonia-related mortality, and that smoking is an important independent risk factor for Legionnaires' disease. Lipsky et al.[177] found that smoking independently increased the risk of pneumococcal infections fourfold in their study of "high risk" adults. Petitti and Friedman[178] also found smokers to be at greater risk of pneumonia and influenza, but the risk was lower in those smoking low-tar cigarettes. Conversely, Simberkoff et al.[179] found no relationship between pneumonia mortality and smoking in patients at high risk. In a community-based study in which the prevalence of smoking was assessed among patients with pneumonia, Woodhead et al.[180] reported that 100 of 236 patients with pneumonia (42%) were current smokers, and that 175 of them (74%) had smoked "at some time." However, a control group was not used in this study to see if smoking was associated with higher pneumonia rates.

In the American Cancer Society's 25-state study from 1959 to 1965, male smokers were at greater risk of dying from influenza and pneumonia (International Classification of Diseases, 7th revision, codes 480–481, 490–493) than male nonsmokers (relative risk [RR] = 1.82; 95% CI, 1.45–2.27).[181] This study did not show female smokers to be at increased risk. However, in the 50-city study in 1982–1986, risk of mortality from pneumonia and other respiratory disease (International Classification of Diseases, 9th revision, codes 010–012, 480–489, 493) was significantly increased in current female smokers (RR = 2.18; 95% CI, 1.60– 2.97) as well as current male smokers (RR = 1.99; 95% CI, 1.52–2.61) aged 35 years and older.[181]

Crowding

Crowding favors the propagation of respiratory infections, as it does all contagious diseases. As early as 1927, a highly significant correlation was seen between the proportion of overcrowded houses in a borough (two or more persons per room) and pneumonia mortality in England and Wales.[182] The strongest correlation was in the age group 0 to 5 years, although an effect was also seen in the age groups 45 to 64 and 65 to 74 years. Pneumonia epidemics were observed in crowded living conditions in South African mining camps, during the construction of the Panama Canal, and in Civilian Conservation Corps barracks.[183] In 1945, Payling-Wright and Payling-Wright[184] showed strong correlations between crowding (persons per room and number of children per family) and mortality from bronchopneumonia in children aged less than 2 years. Another study demonstrated a significant correlation between crowding and

death from bronchopneumonia in infants, although the investigators cautioned that the relationship was confounded by indices of air pollution, social class, and educational status.[120]

Family Size

Since the 1970s, studies have focused on family size as a measure of crowding. The number and age of siblings in families predict the rates of acute lower respiratory tract infection in infants,[140] incidence of bronchitis and pneumonia in infants,[185] and rates of acute respiratory illness in older children and adults.[186] In developing countries, given the extreme level of confounding between malnutrition and crowding as risk factors for acute respiratory infection, it is difficult to separate out the relative contribution of each.

Day-Care Centers

In developed countries, increased reliance on day-care centers for children has led to another type of crowding. Children attending group day-care centers are at increased risk of acute upper and lower respiratory tract infections.[140,187] In particular, day-care attendance greatly increases the risk of acute otitis media in children.[188–191]

Refugee Camps

During the 1990s, acute respiratory infections, along with measles and diarrrheal disease, were the most frequent causes of death among refugees who escaped Somalia during the 1992–1993 famine[192] and among Bhutanese refugees emigrating into southeastern Nepal during 1991–1992 to escape ethnic persecution.[193]

Marfin et al.[193] examined the morbidity and mortality among 73,500 Bhutanese refugees who emigrated into southeastern Nepal (six refugee camps) between February 1991 and June 1992 to escape ethnic persecution in Bhutan. Crude mortality rates up to 1.15 per 10,000 deaths per day were reported during the first 6 months of surveillance. The leading causes of death were measles, diarrhea, and acute respiratory infections.

Nutrition

As malnutrition is so closely correlated with poverty, crowding, poor housing, and poor education in developing countries, it has proved difficult to identify an independent effect of this factor on risk for respiratory infection.[194–196] Nevertheless, epidemiologic studies evaluating certain nutritional interventions (vitamin A and breastfeeding) have shown that malnutrition is at least contributory to respiratory health.

In a study in Costa Rica, James[10] assessed the relationship of malnutrition (comparison of weight with standard measures) and respiratory illness in poor children under the age of 5 years. His unadjusted analysis indicated that malnourished children experienced 2.7 times more bronchitis and 19 times more pneumonia, and they were far more likely to be hospitalized than well-nourished children. Children of low weight experienced no more upper respiratory illness than did children of normal weight, but their episodes lasted longer. Tupasi et al.[196] reported 27-fold increased relative risk for pneumonia-related mortality in hospitalized children with third-degree malnutrition, with relative risks of 11.3 and 4.4 for second- and first-degree malnutrition, respectively. However, their multivariate analyses indicated that malnutrition was not related to incidence of respiratory morbidity, possibly because of strong confounding from socioeconomic status. Berman et al.[70] found a significant relationship between malnutrition and pneumonia, but not between malnutrition and bronchitis or tracheobronchitis, in children attending health centers in Cali, Colombia. Escobar et al.[57] observed that in children hospitalized with lower respiratory illness, mortality increased in relation to the level of malnutrition (weight for age).

In a case-control study reported in 1996, Fonseca et al.[197] used a risk factor questionnaire to determine key factors contributing to childhood pneumonia among 650 children aged less than 2 years living in urban poor areas of Forteleza, Brazil. Age-matched controls were recruited from the neighborhood where the children with pneumonia lived. Malnutrition was the most important risk factor, although low birthweight, non-breastfeeding, attendance at a day-care center, crowding, high parity, and incomplete vaccination status each posed a significant risk. Children who had suffered from previous episodes of wheezing or who had been hospitalized for pneumonia had a greater than threefold increased risk of contracting the disease. Pneumonia risk in this study was not influenced by socioeconomic status or by environmental variables.

In the early 1980s, vitamin A deficiency in children was found to be a risk factor associated with both increased morbidity from respiratory infection and increased overall mortality.[198,199] In Thailand, children with deficient serum retinol were four times more likely to experience respiratory morbidity than children who were not deficient.[200] This study also found that supplementation with vitamin A offered some protection against respiratory illness; however, this varied by age and length of follow-up, probably because of small sample size. In well-nourished children in Adelaide, Pinnock et al.[201,202] conducted two placebo-controlled vitamin A intervention studies. In the first study, respiratory morbidity in children with a history of frequent respiratory illness was reduced by 19% in those taking the supplement.[201] However, in the second study, vitamin A supplementation did not affect respiratory morbidity significantly in children aged 2 to 7 years who had an episode of bronchiolitis in the first year of life and who were followed for 12 months.[202] In view of the disparate findings between retinol-deficient and well-nourished children, the beneficial effects of vitamin A supplementation are likely to be limited to populations whose diets are significantly deficient.

In developing countries, breastfeeding has shown a protective effect against respiratory infections. In Brazil, for instance, breastfeeding reduced the incidence of upper respiratory morbidity, otitis media, and pneumonia in young infants in one study,[203] and respiratory infection mortality in children in another.[204] It is unclear whether the protective effect of breast milk was from its conferred antiinfective properties,[205] from improved hygiene, or from nutritional factors *per sé*. Similarly, in Rwanda, mortality from acute lower respiratory infection in hospitalized children aged less than 2 years was lower in those who were breastfed.[206] In developed countries, breastfeeding appears to be clearly protective against the risk of acute otitis media,[205,206] but perhaps not against other types of respiratory morbidity. Many studies in which bivariate analyses were conducted have reported that breastfed babies were at significantly lower risk of respiratory illness, but the relationship was not seen after adjustments were made for confounding factors.[207–211]

Certain other nutritional factors have been suggested as possibly influencing respiratory health, although the link is weak or inconclusive. Obesity was reported to be associated with increased incidence of respiratory illness in infants in one study,[212] but these findings were confounded by the fact that the normal weight comparison group was of higher socioeconomic status and had been breastfed much longer. Although vitamin C supplementation has been suggested to prevent or to treat upper respiratory tract infections, the results of placebo-controlled trials have been too unimpressive to prompt a global recommendation for use of this vitamin.[213–215]

Lower Respiratory Tract Infection in Early Infancy

Several studies have reported a relationship between acute lower respiratory tract infection in the first 2 years of life and the development in adulthood of chronic cough,[174,216] reduced ventilatory function,[217–220] and increased bronchial reactivity.[217–220] In a case-control study in 1985,[150] young children who experienced high levels of respiratory illness morbidity were 11 times more likely to have experienced an episode of bronchitis, bronchiolitis, or pneumonia in the first year of life than children who had experienced low levels of morbidity (controls). The relationship remained strong (OR, 9.5; 95% CI, 5.5–

16.6) even after adjustments were made for number of siblings, use of child care, sex, parental history of respiratory illness, breastfeeding, maternal stress levels, exposure to gas heating, parental occupational status, and low birthweight. In a 3-year study of pneumococcal vaccine in young children, the strongest predictor of acute respiratory morbidity (recorded in respiratory-symptom diaries by the mothers) in any 6-month period was the level of morbidity the previous 6 months.[201,221] In England and Wales, Barker and Osmond[222] found an increased incidence of mortality among people with chronic bronchitis who had a history of childhood respiratory infection.

It is unclear whether lower respiratory infection in early life acts as a true risk factor by causing long-term damage to the lower respiratory tract or whether it acts as an early marker for genetically preprogrammed subsequent respiratory morbidity (chronic or acute). It will be difficult to determine which factor is more important until an effective intervention is available (e.g., a vaccine for respiratory syncytial virus). If previous respiratory morbidity predicts the level of subsequent morbidity from respiratory infections, implications also are seen for statistical analyses of these types of data. For autocorrelation of this type, a need is seen to control or adjust for repeated episodes of acute lower respiratory illness; alternatively, the first episode can be used as the outcome for analysis. In prospective studies, Kaplan-Meier curves and Cox regression analysis are then often used to estimate "survival time."[32] Where frequent outcomes occur, as with upper respiratory tract infections, use of the first episode as an outcome would result in loss of too much data. Autoregression techniques,[223] which have not been widely used in studies of acute respiratory infections, allow adjustment for autocorrelated variables in multivariate models.

Psychosocial Factors

The relationship between psychosocial factors and respiratory infections has been investigated in cross-sectional and retrospective studies,[223–229] in prospective epidemiologic studies,[230–232] and in experimental settings.[233–235] Upper respiratory infections or illnesses were the outcomes of interest in these studies, and no data regarding lower respiratory illness were presented. Two cross-sectional studies reported a relationship between respiratory infection and social isolation, life changes, illness behavior, maladaptive coping, and unresolved role crisis.[226,227] However, these studies did not address the effect of psychosocial factors on respiratory infection rates. Another cross-sectional study indicated a relationship between anxiety and upper respiratory illness, but it was unclear how the outcome was measured.[223] In a longitudinal study that controlled for the effects of age, sex, race, family income, and family size in the analyses by Boyce et al.,[226] high life-event scores and strict family routines were associated with increased duration and severity of acute respiratory illness in children. However, these investigators did not measure stress levels or rigidity of family routines until the end of the study. Other cross-sectional studies have found relationships between poor family functioning and doctor visits for acute respiratory infections in children,[229] type A personality and respiratory illness in college students,[227] and maternal stress and bronchitis in children.[228] None of these three studies controlled for confounding factors, nor did they address the temporal relationship between psychosocial factors and respiratory illness.

Several prospective studies have shown that psychosocial factors can increase susceptibility to upper respiratory tract infections.[231–236] Kasl et al.[231] evaluated the relationship between a combination of high motivation and poor academic performance with clinical infectious mononucleosis in U.S. Military Academy cadets at West Point, New York. Over a 4-year period, cadets who seroconverted to Epstein-Barr virus were monitored, and those with high motivation, a poor academic record, and an "overachieving" father were significantly more likely to have clinical infectious mononucleosis than a sub-

clinical infection. Poor academic record and high motivation interacted in this study to increase the risk of clinical disease significantly. Disease severity was confirmed by ascertaining the heterophil antibody titers in the clinical and subclinical cases. In a series of studies involving experimentally induced colds at the Common Cold Unit in the United Kingdom, introversion was associated with higher symptom and virus-shedding scores and certain life changes that resulted in decreased activity predicted virus shedding; cognitive dissonance was associated with increased symptoms.[233–235] Although patients who appear to be more introverted and those reporting higher stress or anxiety levels might be expected to report more symptoms, the finding that these factors were also associated with virus shedding in two of the studies substantiates objective validation of a psychosocial–illness relationship. Graham et al.[230] studied the relationship between stress and upper respiratory tract infection in a prospective study in Adelaide. In a blinded fashion, episodes of illness were divided into definite, uncertain, and doubtful, which were confirmed, where possible, by a study nurse, virologic culture, or both. To optimize the precision of stress measurement, a combination of three measures (major life events, minor life events, and psychological distress) was used in the initial analyses. Prestudy stress variables predicted nurse-confirmed episodes and symptom days in "definite" episodes even after adjusting for a range of confounding factors. Prestudy stress levels also predicted both episodes and symptom days of respiratory illness. Finally, in a longitudinal study of 16 families ($N = 100$), Meyer and Haggerty[232] reported that stressful life events in families were four times more likely to precede an episode of streptococcal pharyngitis than to follow it. High stress levels were also significantly associated with rises in antistreptolysin O titer in this study. Although no adjustments were made for confounding factors, the objective outcome measures and prospective design were strengths of this study.

Two mechanisms have been suggested to account for why stress and anxiety might predispose to respiratory infection.[4] First, because psychological stress and other psychological factors appear to suppress many components of immune function,[236] this may lead to increased susceptibility to respiratory infection. However, it is possible that the immune function fluctuations observed to be associated with psychological factors may not have high clinical relevance. Second, high stress levels or anxiety may lead to reduced adherence to normal hygiene measures (e.g., handwashing and use of tissues) usually used to reduce transmission of respiratory viruses.[237–239] This mechanism is questionable, however, because in experimental cold studies, transmission factors were controlled.[233–235]

Socioeconomic Status

In general, socioeconomic status, whether measured by rankings of occupational prestige,[118,174] level of income,[184] or educational status,[120] appears to be associated with increased susceptibility to acute lower, but not upper, respiratory tract infections. Gardner et al.[140] used a combined measure of family income, insurance status, and parental educational level to measure socioeconomic status, which they found to be related only to lower respiratory illness. Measures of proportion of families with incomes below the poverty line and of occupational prestige have been linked with increased mortality from bronchitis and pneumonia in children,[184] as has educational status.[120] The differentials in pneumonia and influenza mortality observed between economically developing and developed countries (Table 15–7) reflect the association of low socioeconomic development with susceptibility to pneumonia, in particular. However, the relatively similar levels of upper respiratory illness reported in developing and developed countries lends support to findings in developed countries that low socioeconomic status does not increase the risk of these conditions.[8–13,25–27]

The results of a retrospective study by Schenker et al.[240] differ from those of the studies mentioned above. These investigators found a relationship between low socioeconomic status (occupational status or educational level of parents) and severe chest illness in the first 2 years of life, as well as with chronic respiratory symptoms, but not with pneumonia or bronchitis. The disparity between the conclusions of this study and the others may be attributed to its presentation of differential symptom reporting rates by lower and high educational groups. This illustrates how differently alternate measures of socioeconomic status can behave in predicting respiratory illness; it may also indicate that lower social class could be a stronger risk factor for lower rather than upper respiratory illness. Tupasi et al.[196] confirmed that low socioeconomic status within developing countries also strongly predicts risk of acute respiratory infection. However, these investigators did not differentiate between upper and lower tracts of respiratory infection, nor did they separate out the effects of factors such as crowding, malnutrition, and immunization status. This adjustment is very important in analyzing the results from epidemiologic studies investigating socioeconomic risk factors. Indeed, bivariate analyses performed in a study in Adelaide showed that children of parents of lower occupational status had increased susceptibility to respiratory illness.[241] However, after adjusting for factors such as sex, maternal smoking, number of siblings, parental history of respiratory illness, breastfeeding, use of child care, and maternal stress levels, the relationship between social class and increased risk of respiratory infection was no longer observed.

Meteorologic Factors

Epidemics of acute respiratory infections have correlated best with low temperature, humidity, precipitation, or all of those factors, which are associated with increased time spent indoors, either at home or at school.[242–244] Any situation in which crowding is present facilitates efficient viral transmission. It is not clear whether meteorologic factors alone cause increased host susceptibility or enhanced viral integrity, or whether crowding must be a concomitant. The effects of low temperature or "chilling" on host susceptibility has been well studied.[245–247] In studies conducted in the United States and the United Kingdom, volunteers experimentally infected with rhinoviruses and exposed to combinations of cold temperatures, wet clothes, and fatigue had no greater than normal susceptibility to infection.[245–247] Studies as early as the 1920s suggested a correlation between low temperatures and increases in mortality from pneumonia and bronchitis[184,248]; however, the results of these studies were confounded by increased time spent indoors (resulting in crowding) and higher levels of air pollution during winter. The latter factor may be an important contributor to respiratory illness. After all, in the Northern Hemisphere, peak levels of respirable particulate air pollution occur in midwinter, presumably because condensation, cloud cover, and precipitation prevent dispersal of particulates and gases; thus, trapped pathogens in the ambient air would be more likely. In a study by Pope,[126] low temperature was the meteorologic variable most closely correlated with hospitalization for respiratory disease, and together with mean fine particulate levels explained 83% of the variance in total monthly hospital admissions for respiratory disease.

Humidity could also be a meteorologic factor contributing to respiratory morbidity. As rhinoviruses survive better at higher humidities, Gwaltney[249] has postulated that rhinovirus-caused infections may be more easily transmitted in places where, or in seasons when, humidity is high. As high humidity is often associated with the rainy season in temperate or warm climates, meteorologic studies investigating a humidity–respiratory infection correlation would need to factor the effect of crowding into analyses, as more of the study population would be expected to stay indoors to avoid the rain, thus confounding study results.

Care-Seeking Behavior

The care-seeking behavior of families and their expectations regarding appropriate treat-ment affect the morbidity and mortality associated with acute respiratory infections.[250] Factors influencing the choice of provider are the mother's perceptions of the cause of illness, distance from a provider, cost of care, availability and accessibility of a provider, and past experience with that provider. Some families demonstrate a "wait-and-see attitude" because of limited funds, distance from a health provider, not recognizing the severity of the illness, waiting for home remedies to work, or local custom prohibiting a mother to leave her home for any purpose.[251–253] In developing countries, patients can seek care from several different people (e.g., physicians, healers, shamans), making assessment of treatment difficult.

Human Immunodeficiency Virus Infection

Human immunodeficiency virus infection predisposes people to several different types of acute respiratory infections, the most common of which is *Pneumocystis carinii* pneumonia.[254] In 60% of newly diagnosed cases of AIDS, *P. carinii* pneumonia is the initial AIDS-defining illness, and an additional 20% of patients with AIDS will develop *P. carinii* pneumonia during the course of their illness.[100,101] Children with AIDS are also at risk from *P. carinii*, but at a slightly lower rate than adults.[255–257] *P. carinii* pneumonia does not appear to be an important pulmonary complication of AIDS in Africa.[102] This lack of association in Africa may, in part, be because of the difficulty of diagnosing this condition when bronchoscopy is not readily available.[100] However, introduction of sputum induction techniques currently used in developed countries[258] may prove useful in improving the diagnostic accuracy of studies in Africa. This should lead to a more definitive picture of the incidence of *P. carinii* pneumonia in HIV-infected persons on that continent. Adults and children infected with HIV are also at increased risk from bacterial pneumonia.[100,259] *Streptococcus pneumoniae* and *Haemophilus influenzae* are the most commonly isolated organisms in community-acquired, HIV-associated bacterial pneumonia. Risk of pneumonia appears to be increased in HIV-infected patients with and without AIDS.[260–264] The most common viral pulmonary infection found in both adults and children with AIDS is cytomegalovirus.[100,256,257] However, the pathogenicity of this virus in the lung is not always entirely clear, because it is sometimes isolated in the absence of histologic evidence of cytopathic change to lung parenchyma.[265] The causative agents of acute lower respiratory tract infections in HIV-infected patients in Africa have yet to be completely elucidated. In general, gastrointestinal and dermatologic complications are more common in Africa than in the United States, where pulmonary complications most often manifest.[102] In one study, only 14% of HIV-infected Africans living in Europe had *P. carinii* pneumonia.[266] The most common pulmonary complication of HIV infection in Africa appears to be tuberculosis,[267,268] although few studies have used appropriate microbiologic techniques to establish accurate estimates of risk in comparison with other organisms. It seems likely that HIV-infected children and adults in Africa will be at greatly increased risk from pneumonia caused by pyogenic bacteria such as *S. pneumoniae*, *H. influenzae*, and *Staphylococcus aureus*, because these organisms are already important causes of pneumonia in that part of the world.

Whether HIV infection is associated with increased susceptibility to upper respiratory tract infections or respiratory viruses in general, is not known. It is also not known whether these less serious conditions can predispose to secondary bacterial invasion and pneumonia in patients with AIDS. If immune system activation is important in the pathogenesis of AIDS, as has been postulated, another issue that needs to be explored is whether viral respiratory infections play a role in accelerating disease progression.

Low Birthweight

Low birthweight may be an important risk factor for acute respiratory infections, as evidenced by the higher mortality rates of low-birthweight infants compared with normal-weight infants in developing countries in the first year of life.[6] Drillien[269] reported that low-birthweight babies (<4 lb, 8 oz [<2,000 g]) experienced higher rates of respiratory illness in the first 2 years of life. This relationship persisted when this investigator stratified by a "maternal care" index, although what was meant by maternal care was not well defined. After stratification by quality of housing and maternal care, low birthweight did not predict respiratory illness. In a 7-year birth cohort study, Chan et al.[270] found that low birthweight (<2,000 g) was associated with subsequent chronic cough, but not wheeze. However, as acute respiratory symptoms were not reported in this study, the effect of low birthweight on respiratory infection rate could not be assessed. Victora et al.[271] found that a birthweight of less than 2,500 g was associated with increased mortality from respiratory infections, and this relationship persisted after adjustment for parental employment status, income, and education. In a study in India, Datta et al.[272] observed that, during the first year of life, low-birthweight infants (<2,500 g) had the same respiratory illness attack rate as normal-weight infants (4.65 vs 4.56 episodes), but a much higher case fatality rate (24.6 vs 3.2 per 100 episodes of moderate or severe respiratory illness). These data suggest that low-birthweight children may experience more severe respiratory infections; however, these infections are no more frequent than in normal-weight control populations. As low birthweight is associated with crowding, poverty, and poor nutritional status, these factors may cause too much confounding to allow any conclusions about the independent contribution of low birthweight on respiratory health.

Overprescribing of Antibiotics and Misuse of Medication

Shann et al.[1] have estimated that 75% of antibiotic prescriptions are written for acute respiratory infections. Most of these prescriptions are probably unnecessary because the infections treated are predominantly viral in origin and, therefore, are unresponsive to drugs directed against bacterial pathogens. The annual costs incurred by inappropriate antibiotic prescribing is estimated at $8 billion worldwide.[1] Overprescribing of antibiotics poses a public health risk because it hastens the development of antibiotic resistance.

In developing countries, overprescribing of antibiotics by unqualified medical practitioners is especially common.[250] Self-medication with drugs that can mask the symptoms of respiratory infections, inappropriate courses of medication prescribed by health care providers, and premature discontinuation of therapy also contribute to increased morbidity in cases of acute respiratory infections.[251,273-275] In China, herbal remedies are still commonly used to treat these infections. Liu and Douglas[276] identified 27 articles published primarily in Chinese language journals between 1985 and 1996 that described favorable effects of herbal remedies for acute respiratory infections. These authors found limitations in the study design and data presentation of the clinical trials. They believed that definitive conclusions about efficacy could not be made in view of insufficient information on randomization and baseline comparisons, the use of outcome measures that were either complicated or of doubtful validity, the use of poorly defined terms to connote efficacy (e.g., "effect rate"), and inadequate or missing statistical analysis. Therefore, it is possible that millions of Chinese are currently receiving inadequate treatment of acute respiratory infections.

Increasing Resistance to Antibiotics

Clinical response to antibiotics, especially penicillins and oral cephalosporins, has been greatly affected by the rise of antibiotic resistance since the 1980s. Resistance rates of *H. influenzae* to penicillin and amoxicillin have been reported to be 30% to 40% in Singapore, Indonesia, Thailand, Taiwan, Hong Kong, and the Philippines, and 15% in Malaysia and Korea.[14] In Latin America, the prevalence of amoxicillin resistance to *H. influenzae* varies greatly among countries. It has been reported to be almost 50% in hospital isolates in Guatemala, 25% to 30% in the general population of Argentina and Venezuela, 10% in Colombia and Uruguay, and 2.5% in Ecuador.[14] Pneumococcal resistance is more than 70% among patients in hospitals in Manila, Philippines, 30% to 40% in Hong Kong, Korea, and Taiwan, and 10% to 20% in Singapore and Malaysia.[14] The prevalence of pneumococcal resistance is generally lower in Latin America than Southeast Asia, although it has reached 15% to 25% in some areas.[14]

Other Host Factors

Primarily uncontrolled studies have mentioned many other factors as possibly increasing the risk of pneumonia in adults. In high-risk outpatients, Simberkoff et al.[179] found that chronic pulmonary, cardiac, and renal disease predicted the incidence of pneumonia, but they did not observe an association with hepatic disease, alcoholism, or diabetes mellitus. Lipsky et al.[177] noted that dementia, cerebrovascular disease, and institutionalization independently predicted pneumonia. They also confirmed that increasing age, smoking, chronic obstructive lung disease, and congestive cardiac failure increased pneumonia risk, but that diabetes mellitus, malignancy, or heavy alcohol use did not.

Maternal antibodies to respiratory syncytial and influenza viruses in cord blood appear to be protective against subsequent infection in infants.[277,278] If maternal immunity can be passively transferred to infants, it would be expected that vaccination of pregnant women would be beneficial in protecting the infant against these viruses. A family history of asthma is associated with increased risk of bronchiolitis in infancy, and it appears to strongly interact with exposure factors such as presence of an older sibling in the house and passive smoking.[279] The contribution of genetic factors to the risk of respiratory infection in children appears to be supported by other studies reporting increased rates of wheeze-related respiratory infection in infants with higher virus-specific immunoglobulin E responses to respiratory syncytial,[280] and parainfluenza viruses,[281] and in those with small airway diameters.[282]

EFFICIENT METHODS OF DATA COLLECTION TO EVALUATE RESPIRATORY EPIDEMIOLOGY

No standardized questionnaires exist for collection of acute respiratory infection symptom data, although standardized instruments developed by the American Thoracic Society[283] and the British Medical Research Council[284] are available to measure chronic respiratory symptomatology. As the focus of the latter questionnaires is set on symptoms of airway reactivity and allergy, they cannot be readily adapted for studies of acute respiratory infections. This situation has prompted many researchers to create and use either nonstandardized respiratory symptom diaries (Figure 15–4) or recall questionnaires. Respiratory diaries have three advantages over questionnaires: (*a*) they practically eliminate recall bias; (*b*) they are useful in studies where specific symptom complexes are important; and (*c*) they are more likely to be accurate records of symptom duration. The main drawback of respiratory symptom diaries is that they require daily recording by the study participant, which could be viewed by participants as such a burden that they may stop making entries, as happens especially in multiyear studies.

Alternatively, research assistants can call or visit study participants on a weekly or biweekly basis to inquire via a questionnaire about symptom frequency and duration in the preceding period. Although this approach has all the problems associated with recall data, it has advantages of sustainability over long periods and the ability of the interviewer to define symptoms more clearly than would otherwise be possible using a diary approach. Questionnaires, which are easier to standardize than symptom diaries, have been shown to be associated with higher compliance rates over a 2-year period in patients with lower respiratory infections.[285,286]

Standardized questionnaires are especially needed in developing countries.[287] Often, the clinical and laboratory expertise and facilities are not available to confirm a diagnosis, and many difficulties exist regarding standardizing measures of exposure between studies. The National Research Council's project in 12 countries[11] was a major attempt to standardize data collection and study protocols. Although some variation in methods was inevitable, these data are probably the most comparable of any collected to date. Much effort has been given to developing criteria for identifying acute lower respiratory infections from simple clinical signs. Several studies have now shown that tachypnea and a history of fast breathing[45,287–288] are highly sensitive and specific predictors of lower respiratory tract infections in both community[289] and hospital settings.[45,287,288] The sensitivity and specificity of tachypnea as a diagnostic criterion is improved when chest indrawing is considered.[289] Campbell et al.[290] reported that the best predictors of lobar pneumonia in infants were temperature above 38.5°C and a respiratory rate greater than 60 per minute. Diagnoses more specific than "acute lower respiratory infection," such as severe pneumonia, may not be predictable based only on the presence of a respiratory rate of more than 50 per minute. Nevertheless, to conduct epidemiologic studies in developing countries, the high sensitivity and specificity of maternal history of fast breathing as a predictor of acute lower respiratory tract infection is still very valuable.

CONCLUSION

The epidemiology of acute respiratory infections is well understood today primarily because of research that has been conducted during the past three decades. Clear associations between acute respiratory infections and chronic disease in adults, direct smoking, passive smoking, crowding, and breastfeeding have been well documented. The relatively higher in-

CHILD'S NAME ID RESPIRATORY EVENTS IN EARLY CHILDHOOD

DECEMBER 1998	1	2	3	4	5	6	7	8	9	10	11	12	13	14	15	16	17	18	19	20	21	22	23	24	25	26	27	28	29	30 31
Is he/she completely well? Y=Yes N = No																														
Do you think he/she has a cold? Y or N																														
Record each symptom he/she experiences each day. Mark with X.																														
Runny nose																														
Stopped-up nose																														
Hoarse throat																														
Wheezy/noisy breathing																														
Moist cough																														
Dry cough																														
Fever (feels hot)																														
Pulling at ears																														
Medication given (M)*																														
* Doctor visits (D)*																														
Hospital visits (V)/ Hospital stays (S)* (*more details on back)																														
OTHER ILLNESSES (give brief details)																														

Figure 15–4 Example of an acute respiratory illness symptom diary used in a 2-year cohort study of infants in Adelaide, Australia, 1988–1990. *Source:* Reprinted with permission from N.M.H. Graham, The Epidemiology of Acute Respiratory Infection in Children and Adults: A Global Perspective, *Epidemiologic Reviews*, Vol. 12, pp. 149–178, © 1990, Johns Hopkins University School of Hygiene and Public Health.

cidence of acute respiratory infections in developing countries compared with the developed world results from a combination and interaction of factors associated with poverty and lower social status—large family size, crowded living conditions, less access to medical care, higher smoking rates, potential for nutritional deficit, lower breastfeeding rates, exposure to environmental pollutants (tobacco smoke, wood smoke, urban air pollution), and stressful living environments.

In developed countries, certain issues remain to be better defined, including the relationship between air pollution and acute respiratory infections, the relation between maternal antibody levels and passive immunity in infants, and the reasons for the increase in pneumonia mortality in older age groups. Standardization of acute symptom questionnaires and symptom diaries still needs to be done to facilitate more complete and thorough epidemiologic studies in both developing and developed countries.

REFERENCES

1. Shann F, Woolcock A, Black R, et al. Introduction: acute respiratory tract infections—the forgotten pandemic. *Clin Infect Dis*. 1999;28:189–191.

2. Murray CJL, Lopez AD. *Global Comparative Assessments in the Health Sector*. Geneva: WHO; 1994.

3. Leowski J. Mortality from acute respiratory infections in children under 5 years of age: global estimates. *World Health Stat Q*. 1986;39:138–144.

4. Graham NMH. The epidemiology of acute respiratory infection in children and adults: a global perspective. *Epidemiol Rev*. 1990;12:149–178.

5. Pan American Health Organization. Acute respiratory infections in the Americas. *Epidemiol Bull*. 1980;1:1–4.

6. Pio A, Leowski J, ten Dam HG. The magnitude of the problem of acute respiratory infections. In: Douglas RM, Kerby-Eaton E, eds. *Acute Respiratory Infections: Proceedings of an International Workshop*. Adelaide, South Australia: University of Adelaide; 1985:3–16.

7. Douglas RM. *Acute Respiratory Infections*. (WHO/WPR/RC30/TP/1). Manila, Philippines: World Health Organization; 1979.

8. Kamath KR, Feldman RA, Sundar Rao PSS, et al. Infection and disease in a group of South Indian families. II. General morbidity patterns in families and family members. *Am J Epidemiol*. 1969;89:375–383.

9. Freij L, Wall S. Exploring child health and its ecology. The Kirkos study in Addis Ababa. An evaluation of procedures in the measurement of acute morbidity and a search for causal structure. *Acta Paediatr Scand Suppl*. 1977;267:1–18.

10. James JW. Longitudinal study of the morbidity of diarrheal and respiratory infections in malnourished children. *Am J Clin Nutr*. 1972;25:690–694.

11. Berman S. Epidemiology of acute respiratory infections in children of developing countries. *Rev Infect Dis*. 1991;13(suppl 6):S454–462.

12. Fox JP, Cooney MK, Hall CE. The Seattle virus watch. V. Epidemiologic observations of rhinovirus infections, 1965–1969, in families with young children. *Am J Epidemiol*. 1975;101:122–143.

13. Monto AS, Ullman B. Acute respiratory illness in an American community. *JAMA*. 1974;227:164–169.

14. Ball P, Make B. Acute exacerbations of chronic bronchitis. An international comparison. *Chest*. 1998;113(Suppl 3):199S–204S.

15. Lai CKW, Ho SC, Lau J, et al. Respiratory symptoms in elderly Chinese living in Hong Kong. *Eur Respir J*. 1995;8:2055–2061.

16. Pandey MR. Domestic smoke pollution and chronic bronchitis in a rural community of the hill region in Nepal. *Thorax*. 1984;39:337–339.

17. Doyle R. *U.S. deaths from pneumonia*. http://www.sciam.com/0297issue/0297scicit6.html.

18. Meeker DP, Longworth DL. Community-acquired pneumonia: an update. *Cleve Clin J Med*. 1996;63:16–30.

19. Fine MJ, Chowdhry T, Ketema A. Outpatient management of community-acquired pneumonia. *Hosp Pract (Off Ed)*. 1998;3:123–133.

20. Marrie TJ. Community-acquired pneumonia: epidemiology, etiology, treatment. *Infect Dis Clin North Am*. 1998;13:723–740.

21. Farber MO. Managing community-acquired pneumonia. Factors to consider in outpatient care. *Postgrad Med*. 1999;105:106–114.

22. Mandell LA, Campbell GD Jr. Nosocomial pneumonia guidelines. An international perspective. *Chest*. 1998;113(Suppl 3):188S–193S.

23. Fagon JY, Chastre J, Hance A, et al. Nosocomial pneumonia in ventilated patients: a cohort study evaluating attributable mortality and hospital stay. *Am J Med*. 1993;94:281–288.

24. American Thoracic Society. Hospital-acquired pneumonia in adults: diagnosis, assessment of severity, initial antimicrobial therapy, and preventative strategies. *Am J Respir Crit Care Med.* 1996;153:1711–1725.

25. van Volkenburgh VA, Frost WH. Acute minor respiratory diseases prevailing in a group of families residing in Baltimore, Maryland, 1928–1930. Prevalence, distribution and clinical description of observed cases. *Am J Hygiene.* 1933;17:122–153.

26. Gwaltney JM Jr, Hendley JO, Simon C, et al. Rhinovirus infections in an industrial population. I. The occurrence of illness. *N Engl J Med.* 1966;275:1261–1268.

27. Fox JP, Hall CE, Cooney MK, et al. The Seattle virus watch. II. Objectives, study population and its observation, data processing and summary of illnesses. *Am J Epidemiol.* 1972;96:270–285.

28. Bates JH. Microbiologic etiology of pneumonia. *Chest.* 1989;95(Suppl 5):194S–197S.

29. Glezen W, Denny FW. Epidemiology of acute lower respiratory disease in children. *N Engl J Med.* 1973;288:498–505.

30. Henderson FW, Clyde WA, Collier AM, et al. The etiologic and epidemiologic spectrum of bronchiolitis in pediatric practice. *J Pediatr.* 1979;95:183–190.

31. Denny FW, Clyde WA. Acute lower respiratory tract infections in non-hospitalized children. *J Pediatr.* 1986;108:635–646.

32. Wright AL, Taussig LM, Ray CC, et al. The Tucson children's respiratory study. II. Lower respiratory tract illness in the first year of life. *Am J Epidemiol.* 1989;129:1232–1246.

33. Cole P, Wilson R. Host-microbial interrelationships in respiratory infection. *Chest.* 1989;95(Suppl):217S–221S.

34. Australian Bureau of Statistics. *Australian Health Survey.* Preliminary bulletin no. 1. Canberra, Australia: Australian Bureau of Statistics; 1977.

35. Douglas RM. ARI—the Cinderella of communicable diseases. In: Douglas RM, Kerby-Eaton E, eds. *Acute Respiratory Infections in Children.* Proceedings of an international workshop. Adelaide, South Australia: University of Adelaide; 1985:1–2.

36. Enright PL, Krumla RA, Higgins MW, et al. Prevalence and correlates of respiratory symptoms in the elderly. *Chest.* 1994;106:827–834.

37. Lange P, Groth S, Nyboe J, et al. Chronic obstructive lung disease in Copenhagen: cross-sectional epidemiological aspects. *J Intern Med.* 1989;226:25–32.

38. Bakke PS, Baste V, Hanoa R, et al. Prevalence of obstructive lung disease in a general population: relation to occupational title and exposure to some airborne agents. *Thorax.* 1991;46:863–870.

39. Alonso J, Anto JM. *Encuesta de salut de Barcelona. 1986* (government publication). Barcelona; 1989.

40. Brotons B, Perez JA, Sanchez-Toril F, et al. Prevalencia de la enfermedad obstructiva cronica y el asma: estudio transversal. *Arch Bronconeumol.* 1994;103:481–484.

41. Lundback B, Nystrom L, Rosenhall L, et al. Obstructive lung disease in northern Sweden: respiratory symptoms assessed by postal questionnaire. *Eur Respir J.* 1991;4:257–266.

42. Niederman MS, McCombs JS, Unger AN, Kumar A, Popovian R. The cost of treating community-acquired pneumonia. *Clin Ther.* 1998;20:820–837.

43. Niederman MS, McCombs JS, Unger AN, Kumar A, Popovian R. Treatment cost of acute exacerbations of chronic bronchitis. *Clin Ther.* 1999;21:576–591.

44. McCord C, Kielmann AA. A successful programme for medical auxiliaries treating childhood diarrhea and pneumonia. *Trop Doct.* 1978;8:220–225.

45. Shann FA, Hart K, Thomas D. Acute lower respiratory tract infections in children: possible criteria for selection of patients for antibiotic therapy and hospital admission. *Bull World Health Organ.* 1984;62:749–753.

46. World Health Organization. *Case Management of Acute Respiratory Infections in Children: Intervention Studies.* (WHO/ARI/88.2). Geneva, Switzerland: World Health Organization; 1988.

47. Cherian T, John TJ, Simoes E, Steinhoff MC, John M. Evaluation of simple clinical signs for the diagnosis of acute lower respiratory tract infection. *Lancet.* 1988;2:125–128.

48. World Health Organization. *ARI Programme Report. 1988.* (WHO/ARI/89.3). Geneva, Switzerland: World Health Organization; 1989.

49. World Health Organization. Programme of acute respiratory infections. *Report of the Fourth Meeting of the Technical Advisory Group.* (WHO/ARI/89.4). Geneva, Switzerland: World Health Organization; 1989.

50. World Health Organization. *Case Management of Acute Respiratory Infections in Children in Developing Countries.* (WHO/RSD/85.151). Geneva, Switzerland: World Health Organization; 1985.

51. World Health Organization. *Proposal for the Classification of Acute Respiratory Infections and Tuberculosis for the Tenth Revision of the International Classification of Diseases.* (WHO/RSD/88.25). Geneva, Switzerland: World Health Organization; 1985.

52. Bartlett JG, Breiman RF, Mandell G, et al., for the Infectious Diseases Society of America. Community-acquired pneumonia in adults: guidelines for management. *Clin Infect Dis.* 1998;26:811–838.

53. Reimer LG, Caroll KC. Role of the microbiology laboratory in the diagnosis of lower respiratory tract infections. *Clin Infect Dis.* 1998;26:742–748.

54. Reed SE. The etiology and epidemiology of common colds and the possibilities of prevention. *Clin Otolaryngol.* 1981;6:379–387.

55. Berman S, McIntosh K. Selective primary healthcare: strategies for control of disease in the developing world. XXI. Acute respiratory infections. *Rev Infect Dis.* 1985; 7:674–691.

56. Berman S, Duenas A, Bedoya A, et al. Acute lower respiratory tract illnesses in Cali, Colombia: a two-year ambulatory study. *Pediatrics.* 1983;71:210–218.

57. Escobar JA, Dover AS, Duenas A, et al. Etiology of respiratory tract infections in children in Cali, Colombia. *Pediatrics.* 1976;57:123–130.

58. Shann F, Gratten M, Germer S, et al. Aetiology of pneumonia in children in Goroka Hospital, Papua New Guinea. *Lancet.* 1984;2:537–541.

59. Sobeslavsky O, Sebikari SRK, Harland PSEG, et al. The viral etiology of acute respiratory infections in children in Uganda. *Bull World Health Organ.* 1977;55:625–631.

60. Ogunbi O. Bacterial and viral etiology of bronchiolitis and bronchopneumonia in Lagos children. *J Trop Med Hyg.* 1970;73:138–140.

61. Monto AJ, Johnson KM. Respiratory infections in the American tropics. *Am J Trop Med Hyg.* 1968;17:867–874.

62. Chanock R, Chambon L, Chang W, et al. WHO respiratory disease survey in children: a serological study. *Bull World Health Organ.* 1967;37:363–369.

63. Spence L, Barratt N. Respiratory syncytial virus associated with acute respiratory infections in Trinidadian patients. *Am J Epidemiol.* 1968;88:257–266.

64. Kloene W, Bang FB, Chakraborty SM, et al. A two-year respiratory virus survey in four villages in West Bengal, India. *Am J Epidemiol.* 1970;92:307–320.

65. Olson LC, Lexomboon U, Sithisarn P, et al. The etiology of respiratory tract infections in a tropical country. *Am J Epidemiol.* 1973;97:34–43.

66. Belshe RB, Van Voris LP, Mufson MA. Impact of viral respiratory diseases on infants and young children in a rural and urban area of southern West Virginia. *Am J Epidemiol.* 1983;117:467–474.

67. Foy HM, Cooney MK, Maletzky AJ, et al. Incidence and etiology of pneumonia, croup and bronchiolitis in preschool children belonging to a prepaid medical care group over a four-year period. *Am J Epidemiol.* 1973; 97:80–92.

68. Mufson MA, Krause HE, Mocega HE, et al. Viruses, *Mycoplasma pneumoniae* and bacteria associated with lower respiratory tract disease among infants. *Am J Epidemiol.* 1970;91:192–202.

69. Murphy TF, Henderson FW, Clyde WA Jr, et al. Pneumonia: an eleven-year study in a pediatric practice. *Am J Epidemiol.* 1981;113:12–21.

70. Berman S, Duenas A, Bedoya A, et al. Acute lower respiratory tract illnesses in Cali, Colombia: a two-year ambulatory study. *Pediatrics.* 1983;71:210–218.

71. Wesley AG. Indications for intubation in laryngotracheobronchitis in black children. *S Afr Med J.* 1975;49:1126–1128.

72. Bariffi F, Sanduzzi A, Ponticiello A. Epidemiology of lower respiratory tract infections. *J Chemother.* 1995; 7:263–276.

73. MacFarlane JT. Treatment of lower respiratory infections. *Lancet.* 1987;2:1446–1449.

74. Marrie TJ, Durant H, Yates L. Community-acquired pneumonia requiring hospitalization: 5 year prospective study. *Rev Infect Dis.* 1989;11:586–599.

75. Clezen WP. Serious morbidity and mortality associated with influenza epidemics. *Epidemiol Rev.* 1982;4:25–44.

76. Hayden FG. Respiratory viral infections. In: Federman DD, ed. *Scientific American Medicine.* New York: Scientific American, Inc.; 1997:1–12.

77. Monto AS, Napier JA, Metzner HL. The Tecumseh study of respiratory illness. I. Plan of study and observations on syndromes of acute respiratory disease. *Am J Epidemiol.* 1971;94:269–279.

78. Monto AS, Cavallaro JJ. The Tecumseh study of respiratory illness. II. Patterns of occurrence of infection with respiratory pathogens. 1965–1969. *Am J Epidemiol.* 1971;94:280–289.

79. Maletzky AJ, Cooney MK, Luce R, et al. Epidemiology of viral and mycoplasma agents associated with childhood lower respiratory illness in a civilian population. *J Pediatr.* 1971;78:407–414.

80. Barrett-Connor E. The nonvalue of sputum culture in the diagnosis of pneumococcal pneumonia. *Am Rev Resp Dis.* 1971;103:845–848.

81. Davidson M, Tempest B, Palmer DL. Bacteriologic diagnosis of acute pneumonia: comparison of sputum, transtracheal aspirates and lung aspirates. *JAMA.* 1976; 235:158–163.

82. Halperin SA, Suratt PM, Gwaltney JM Jr, et al. Bacterial cultures of the lower respiratory tract in normal volunteers with and without experimental rhinovirus infection using a plugged double catheter system. *Am Rev Respir Dis.* 1982;125:678–680.

83. Silverman M, Stratton D, Diallo A, et al. Diagnosis of acute bacterial pneumonia in Nigerian children. Value of needle aspirations of lung and counter current electrophoresis. *Arch Dis Child.* 1977;52:925–931.

84. Macfarlane JT, Finch RG, Ward MJ, et al. Hospital study of adult community acquired pneumonia. *Lancet.* 1982;2:255–258.

85. Molleni RA. Epiglottitis: incidence of extraepiglottic infection. Report of 72 cases and review of the literature. *Pediatrics*. 1976;58:526–531.

86. Miller DL, Alderslade R, Ross EM. Whooping cough and whooping cough vaccine: the risks and benefits debate. *Epidemiol Rev*. 1982;4:1–24.

87. Howie VM, Ploussard JH, Lester RL Jr. Otitis media: a clinical and bacteriological correlation. *Pediatrics*. 1970;45:29–35.

88. Engelhardt D, Cohen D, Strauss N, et al. Randomized study of myringotomy, amoxycillin/clavulanate or both for acute otitis media in infants. *Lancet*. 1989;2:141–143.

89. Wald ER, Milmoe GJ, Bowen A, et al. Acute maxillary sinusitis in children. *N Engl J Med*. 1981;304:749–754.

90. Evans FO, Sydnor JB, Moore WEC, et al. Sinusitis of the maxillary antrum. *N Engl J Med*. 1975;293:735–739.

91. Hamory BH, Sande MA, Snydor A, et al. Etiology and antimicrobial therapy of acute maxillary sinusitis. *J Infect Dis*. 1979;139:197–202.

92. Ikeogu MO. Acute pneumonia in Zimbabwe: bacterial isolates by lung aspirations. *Arch Dis Child*. 1988;63:1266–1267.

93. Bartlett JG. Approach to the patient with pneumonia. In: Gorbach SL, Bartlett JG, Blacklow NR, eds. *Infectious Diseases*. 2nd ed. Philadelphia: WB Saunders Co.; 1998.

94. Grayston JT, Alexander E, Kenny G, et al. *Mycoplasma pneumoniae* infections. *JAMA*. 1965;19:369–374.

95. Jansson E, Wager O, Stenstrom R, et al. Studies on Eaton PPLO pneumonia. *Br Med J*. 1964;1:142–145.

96. Komaroff AL, Aronson MD, Pass TM, et al. Serologic evidence of chlamydia and mycoplasma pharyngitis in adults. *Science*. 1983;222:927–929.

97. Stagno S, Brasfield DM, Brown MB, et al. Infant pneumonitis associated with cytomegalovirus, chlamydia, pneumocystis and ureaplasma. *Pediatrics*. 1981;68:322–329.

98. Grayston JT, Kuo CC, Wang SP, et al. A new *Chlamydia psittaci* strain, TWAR, isolated from acute respiratory tract infections. *N Engl J Med*. 1986;315:161–168.

99. Marrie TJ, Grayston JT, Wang SP, et al. Pneumonia associated with TWAR strain of chlamydia. *Ann Intern Med*. 1987;106:507–511.

100. Murray JF, Felton CP, Garay SM, et al. Pulmonary complications of the acquired immunodeficiency syndrome. Report of a National Heart, Lung, and Blood Institute workshop. *N Engl J Med*. 1984;310:1682–1688.

101. Centers for Disease Control. Update: acquired immunodeficiency syndrome—United States. *MMWR*. 1985;34:245–248.

102. Quinn TC, Mann JM, Curran JW, et al. AIDS in Africa: an epidemiologic paradigm. *Science*. 1986;234:955–963.

103. Cunha BA. Community-acquired pneumonia in human immunodeficiency virus-infected patients. *Clin Infect Dis*. 1999;28:410–411.

104. Ginesu F, Pirina P. Etiology and risk factors of adult pneumonia. *J Chemother*. 1995;7:277–285.

105. Fox JP, Cooney MK, Hall CE, et al. Rhinoviruses in Seattle families, 1975–1979. *Am J Epidemiol*. 1985;122:830–846.

106. World Health Organization. *World Health Statistics Annual*. Geneva, Switzerland: World Health Organization, 1989.

107. Logan WPD. Mortality in the London fog incident, 1952. *Lancet*. 1953;1:336–338.

108. Firket J. The cause of the symptoms found in the Meuse Valley during the fog of December, 1930. *Bull Acad R Med Belg*. 1931;11:683–741.

109. Gore AT, Shaddick CW. Atmosphere pollution and mortality in the county of London. *Br J Prev Soc Med*. 1958;12:104–113.

110. Ciocco A, Thompson DJ. A follow-up of Donora ten years after: methodology and findings. *Am J Public Health*. 1961;51:155–164.

111. Greenberg L, Jacobs MB, Droletti BM, et al. Report of an air pollution incident in New York City, November. 1953. *Public Health Rep*. 1962;77:7–16.

112. Greenberg L, Erhardt C, Field F, et al. Intermittent air pollution episodes in New York City, 1962. *Public Health Rep*. 1963;78:1061–1064.

113. Daley C. Air pollution and causes of death. *Br J Prev Soc Med*. 1959;13:14–27.

114. Holland WW, Bennett AE, Cameron IR, et al. Health effects of particulate air pollution: reappraising the evidence. *Am J Epidemiol*. 1979;110:527–659.

115. Toyama T. Air pollution and its effects in Japan. *Arch Environ Health*. 1964;8:153–173.

116. Lunn JR, Knowelden J, Handyside AJ. Patterns of respiratory illness in Sheffield infant school children. *Br J Prev Soc Med*. 1967;21:7–16.

117. Lunn JE, Knowelden J, Roe JW. Patterns of respiratory illness in Sheffield infant school children. *Br J Prev Soc Med*. 1970;24:223–228.

118. Colley JRT, Reid DD. Urban and social origins of childhood bronchitis in England and Wales. *Br Med J*. 1970;2:213–217.

119. Cassel EJ, Lebowitz M, McCarroll JR. The relationship between air pollution, weather, and symptoms in an urban population. *Am Rev Respir Dis*. 1972;106:677–683.

120. Collins JJ, Kasap HS, Holland WW. Environmental

factors in child mortality in England and Wales. *Am J Epidemiol*. 1971;93:10–22.

121. Lawther PJ, Waller RE, Henderson M. Air pollution and exacerbations of bronchitis. *Thorax*. 1970;25:525–539.

122. French JC, Lowrimore C, Nelson WC, et al. The effect of sulphur dioxide and suspended sulphates on acute respiratory disease. *Arch Environ Health*. 1973;27:129–133.

123. Durham WH. Air pollution and student health. *Arch Environ Health*. 1974;28:241–254.

124. Levy D, Gent M, Newhouse MT. Relationship between acute respiratory illness and air pollution levels in an industrial city. *Am Rev Respir Dis*. 1977;116:167–173.

125. Ware JH, Ferris BC, Dockery DW, et al. Effects of ambient sulphur oxides and suspended particles on respiratory health of preadolescent children. *Am Rev Respir Dis*. 1986;133:834–842.

126. Pope CA. Respiratory disease associated with community air pollution and a steel mill, Utah Valley. *Am J Public Health*. 1989;79:623–628.

127. Derriennic F, Richardson S, Mollie A, et al. Short-term effects of sulphur dioxide pollution on mortality in two French cities. *Int J Epidemiol*. 1989;18:186–187.

128. Dockery DW, Speizer FE, Stram DO, et al. Effects of inhalable particles on respiratory health of children. *Am Rev Respir Dis*. 1989;139:587–594.

129. Dales RE, Spitzer WO, Suissa S, et al. Respiratory health of a population living downwind from natural gas refineries. *Am Rev Respir Dis*. 1989;139:595–600.

130. Kinney PL, Ware JH, Spangler JD, et al. Short-term pulmonary function change in association with ozone levels. *Am Rev Respir Dis*. 1989;139:56–61.

131. Schwartz J, Dockery DW, Wypii D, et al. Acute effects of air pollution on respiratory symptom reporting in children [abstract]. *Am Rev Respir Dis*. 1989;139 (Suppl):A27.

132. Goings SAJ, Kulla TJ, Bascom R, et al. Effect of nitrogen dioxide exposure on susceptibility to influenza A virus infection in healthy adults. *Am Rev Respir Dis*. 1989;1075–1081.

133. Cook DG, Strachan DP. Summary of effects of parental smoking on the respiratory health of children and implications for research. *Thorax*. 1999;54:357–366.

134. Fergusson DM, Horwood LJ, Shannon FT. Parental smoking and respiratory illness in infancy. *Arch Dis Child*. 1980;55:358–361.

135. Ferris BG, Ware JH, Berkey CS, et al. Effects of passive smoking on health of children. *Environ Health Perspect*. 1985;62:289–295.

136. Colley JRT, Holland WW, Corkhill RT. Influence of passive smoking and parental phlegm on pneumonia

and bronchitis in early childhood. *Lancet*. 1974;2:1031–1034.

137. Fergusson DM, Horwood LJ. Parental smoking and respiratory illness during early childhood: a six-year longitudinal study. *Pediatr Pulmonol*. 1985;1:99–106.

138. Lebowitz MD, Burrows B. Respiratory symptoms related to smoking habits of family adults. *Chest*. 1976;69:48–50.

139. Love GJ, Lan S, Shy CM, et al. The incidence and severity of acute respiratory illness in families exposed to different levels of air pollution, New York metropolitan area, 1971–2. *Arch Environ Health*. 1981;36:66–73.

140. Gardner G, Frank AL, Taber L. Effects of social and family factors on viral respiratory infection and illness in the first year of life. *J Epidemiol Community Health*. 1984;38:42–48.

141. Taylor B, Wadsworth J. Maternal smoking during pregnancy and lower respiratory tract illness early in life. *Arch Dis Child*. 1987;62:786–789.

142. Comstock GW, Meyer MB, Helsing KJ, et al. Respiratory effects of household exposures to tobacco smoke and gas cooking. *Am Rev Respir Dis*. 1981;124:143–148.

143. Melia RJW, Florey C duV, Darby SC, et al. Differences in NO_2 levels in kitchens with gas or electric cookers. *Atmospheric Environ*. 1978;12:1379–1381.

144. Spangler JD, Duffy CP, Letz R, et al. Nitrogen-dioxide inside and outside 137 homes and implications for ambient air quality standards and health effects research. *Environ Sci Technol*. 1983;17:164–168.

145. Ware JH, Dockery DW, Spiro A, et al. Passive smoking, gas cooking and respiratory health of children living in six cities. *Am Rev Respir Dis*. 1984;129:366–374.

146. Melia RJ, Florey C duV, Altman DC, et al. Association between gas cooking and respiratory disease in children. *Br Med J*. 1977;2:149–152.

147. Melia RJ, Florey C duV, Chinn S. The relation between respiratory illness in primary school children and the use of gas for cooking. I. Results from a national survey. *Int J Epidemiol*. 1979;8:333–338.

148. Keller MD, Lanese RR, Mitchell RI, et al. Respiratory illness in households using gas and electricity for cooking. I. Survey of incidence. *Environ Res*. 1979;19:495–503.

149. Keller MD, Lanese RR, Mitchell RI, et al. Respiratory illness in households using gas and electricity for cooking. II. Symptoms and objective findings. *Environ Res*. 1979;19:504–515.

150. Graham NMH. *Psychosocial Factors in the Epidemiology of Acute Respiratory Infection* [MD thesis].

Adelaide, South Australia: University of Adelaide; 1987.

151. Samet JM, Marbury MC, Spangler JD. Health effects and sources of indoor air pollution. Part 1. *Am Rev Respir Dis*. 1987;136:1486–1508.

152. Smith KR, Aggarwal AL, Dave RM. Air pollution and rural biomass fuel in developing countries: a pilot study in India and implications for research and policy. *Atmospheric Environ*. 1983;17:2343–2362.

153. Dennis RJ, Maldonado D, Norman S, et al. Wood-smoke exposure and risk for obstructive airways disease among women. *Chest*. 1996;109:115–119.

154. Pandey MR, Boleij JSM, Smith KR, et al. Indoor air pollution in developing countries and acute respiratory infection in children. *Lancet*. 1989;1:427–429.

155. Kossove D. Smoke-filled rooms and lower respiratory disease in infants. *S Afr Med J*. 1982;61:622–624.

156. Campbell H, Armstrong JRM, Byass P. Indoor air pollution in developing countries and acute respiratory infection in children. *Lancet*. 1989;1:1012.

157. Campbell H, Byass P, Greenwood BM. Simple clinical signs for the diagnosis of acute respiratory infections. *Lancet*. 1988;2:742–743.

158. Honicky RE, Osborne JS, Akpom CA. Symptoms of respiratory illness in young children and the use of wood-burning stoves for indoor heating. *Pediatrics*. 1985;75:587–593.

159. Osborne JS III, Honicky RE. Chest illness in young children and indoor heating with wood [abstract]. *Am Rev Respir Dis*. 1989;139(Suppl):A29.

160. Tuthill RW. Woodstoves, formaldehyde, and respiratory disease. *Am J Epidemiol*. 1984;120:952–955.

161. Doll R, Hill AB. Lung cancer and other causes of death in relation to smoking. *Br Med J*. 1956;2:1071–1081.

162. Hammond EC, Horn D. Smoking and death rates: report on forty-four months of follow-up on 187,783 men. I. Total mortality. *JAMA*. 1958;166:1159–1172.

163. Hammond EC, Horn D. Smoking and death rates: report on forty-four months of follow-up on 187,783 men. II. Death rates by cause. *JAMA*. 1958;166:1294–1308.

164. Dorn HF. The mortality of smokers and nonsmokers. *Am Stat Assoc Proc Soc Stat Sect*. 1958;1:34–71.

165. Dunn JE, Linden G, Breslow L. Lung cancer mortality experience of men in certain occupations in California. *Am J Public Health*. 1960;50:1475–1487.

166. Bes EWR, Josie GH, Walker CB. A Canadian study of mortality in relation to smoking habits, a preliminary report. *Can J Public Health*. 1961;52:99–106.

167. US Public Health Service. *Smoking and Health*. Report of the advisory committee to the Surgeon General of the Public Health Service. Atlanta, GA: US Department of Health, Education and Welfare, Public Health Service, Centers for Disease Control; 1964 (PHS publication no. 1103).

168. Finklea JF, Sandifer SH, Smith DD. Cigarette smoking and epidemic influenza. *Am J Epidemiol*. 1969;90:390–399.

169. Mackenzie JS, Mackenzie IM, Holt PG. The effect of cigarette smoking on susceptibility to epidemic influenza and on serological responses to live attenuated and killed subunit influenza vaccines. *J Hyg (Camb)*. 1976;77:409–417.

170. Kark JD, Lebuish M. Smoking and epidemic influenza-like illness in female military recruits: a brief survey. *Am J Public Health*. 1981;71:530–532.

171. Kark JD, Lebuish M, Rannon L. Cigarette smoking as a risk factor for epidemic a (h1n1) influenza in young men. *N Engl J Med*. 1982;307:1042–1046.

172. Monto AS, Higgins MW, Ross HW. The Tecumseh study of respiratory illness. VIII. Acute infection in chronic respiratory disease and comparison groups. *Am Rev Respir Dis*. 1975;111:27–36.

173. Holland WW, Elliott A. Cigarette smoking, respiratory symptoms and antismoking propaganda. *Lancet*. 1968;1:41–43.

174. Colley JRT, Douglas JWB, Reid DD. Respiratory disease in young adults: influence of early childhood lower respiratory tract illness, social class, air pollution and smoking. *Br Med J*. 1973;3:195–198.

175. Rush D. Respiratory symptoms in a group of American secondary school students: the overwhelming association with cigarette smoking. *Int J Epidemiol*. 1974;3:153–165.

176. Reingold AL. Role of *Legionellae* in acute infections of the lower respiratory tract. *Rev Infect Dis*. 1988;10:1018–1028.

177. Lipsky BA, Boyko EJ, Inui TS, et al. Risk factors for acquiring pneumococcal infections. *Arch Intern Med*. 1986;146:2179–2185.

178. Petitti DB, Friedman GD. Respiratory morbidity in smokers of low and high yield cigarettes. *Prev Med*. 1985;14:217–225.

179. Simberkoff MS, Cross AP, Al-Ibrahim M, et al. Efficacy of pneumococcal vaccine in high risk patients. Results of a Veterans Administration cooperative study. *N Engl J Med*. 1986;315:1318–1327.

180. Woodhead MA, MacFarlane JT, McCracken JS, et al. Prospective study of the aetiology and outcome of pneumonia in the community. *Lancet*. 1987;1:671–674.

181. US Department of Health and Human Services. *Reducing the Consequences of Smoking; 25 Years of Progress*. Atlanta, GA: US Department of Health and Human Services, Public Health Service, Centers for

Disease Control; 1989 (DHHS publication no. (CDC)89–8411).

182. Woods HM. The influence of external factors on the mortality from pneumonia in childhood and later adult life. *J Hyg (Camb)*. 1927;26:36–43.

183. Finland M. Pneumococcal infections. In: Evans AS, Feldman HA, eds. *Bacterial Infections in Humans. Epidemiology and Control*. New York: Plenum; 1982.

184. Payling-Wright G, Payling-Wright H. Etiological factors in broncho-pneumonia amongst infants in London. *J Hyg (Camb)*. 1945;44:15–30.

185. Leeder S, Corkhill R, Irwig LM, et al. Influence of family factors on the incidence of lower respiratory illness during the first year of life. *Br J Prev Soc Med*. 1976; 30:203–212.

186. Monto AS, Ross HW. Acute respiratory illness in the community: effect of family composition, smoking and chronic symptoms. *Br J Prev Soc Med*. 1977;31:101–108.

187. Strangert K. Respiratory illness in preschool children with different forms of day care. *Pediatrics*. 1976; 57:191–196.

188. Bell DM, Gleiber UW, Mercer AA, et al. Illness associated with child day care: a study of incidence and cost. *Am J Public Health*. 1989;79:479–484.

189. Strangert K. Otitis media in young children in different types of day-care. *Scand J Infect Dis*. 1977;9:113–123.

190. Vinther B, Pederson CB, Elbrond O. Otitis media in childhood. Sociomedical aspects with special reference to day care conditions. *Clin Otolaryngol*. 1984;9:3–8.

191. Silipa M, Karma P, Pukander J, et al. The Bayesian approach to the evaluation of risk factors in acute and recurrent otitis media. *Acta Otolaryngol*. 1988;106:94–101.

192. Moore PS, Marfin AA, Quenomoen LE, et al. Mortality rates in displaced and resident populations of central Somalia during the famine of 1992. *Lancet*. 1993; 341:935–938.

193. Marfin AA, Moore J, Collins C, et al. Infectious disease surveillance during emergency relief to Bhutanese refugees in Nepal. *JAMA*. 1994;272:377–381.

194. Aaby P, Bukh J, Lisse IM, et al. Decline in measles mortality: nutrition, age at infection or exposure. *Br Med J*. 1988;296:1226–1228.

195. Aaby P. Malnutrition and overcrowding/intensive exposure in severe measles infection: review of community studies. *Rev Infect Dis*. 1988;10:478–491.

196. Tupasi TE, Velmonte MA, Sanvictores MEG, et al. Determinants of morbidity and mortality due to acute respiratory infections: implications for intervention. *J Infect Dis*. 1988;157:615–623.

197. Fonseca W, Kirkwood BR, Victora CG, Fuchs SR, Flores JA, Misago C. Risk factors for childhood pneumonia among the urban poor in Fortaleza, Brazil: a case-control study. *Bull World Health Organ*. 1996; 74:199–208.

198. Sommer A, Tarwotjo I, Hussaini G, et al. Increased mortality in mild vitamin A deficiency. *Lancet*. 1983; 2:585–588.

199. Sommer A, Katz J, Tarwotjo I. Increased risk of respiratory disease and diarrhea in children with pre-existing mild vitamin A deficiency. *Am J Clin Nutr*. 1984; 40:1090–1095.

200. Bloem MW, Wedel M, Egger RJ, et al. Mild vitamin A deficiency and risk of respiratory tract diseases and diarrhea in preschool and school children in northeastern Thailand. *Am J Epidemiol*. 1990;131:332–339.

201. Pinnock CB, Douglas RM, Badcock NR. Vitamin A status in children who are prone to respiratory tract infections. *Australian Paediatric J*. 1986;22:95–99.

202. Pinnock CB, Douglas RM, Martin AJ, et al. Vitamin A status of children with a history of respiratory syncytial virus infection in infancy. *Aust Paediatr J*. 1988; 24:286–289.

203. Forman MR, Gravbard BI, Hoffman HJ, et al. The Pima infant feeding study: breast feeding and respiratory infections in the first year of life. *Int J Epidemol*. 1984;13:447–453.

204. Victora C, Smith PG, Vaughan JP, et al. Evidence of protection by breast feeding against infant deaths from infectious diseases in Brazil. *Lancet*. 1987;2:319–322.

205. Saarinen UM. Prolonged breast feeding as a prophylaxis for recurrent otitis media. *Acta Paediatr Scand*. 1982;71:567–571.

206. Teele DW, Klein JO, Rosner B, et al. Epidemiology of otitis media during the first seven years of life in children in greater Boston: a prospective cohort study. *J Infect Dis*. 1989;160:83–94.

207. Pullan CR, Toms GL, Martin AJ, et al. Breast feeding and respiratory syncytial virus infection. *Br Med J*. 1980;281:1034–1036.

208. Watkins CJ, Leeder SR, Corkhill RT. The relationship between breast and bottle feeding and respiratory illness in the first year of life. *J Epidemiol Community Health*. 1979;33:180–182.

209. Taylor B, Wadsworth J, Golding J, et al. Breast-feeding, bronchitis, and admissions for lower respiratory illness and gastroenteritis during the first five years. *Lancet*. 1982;1:1227–1229.

210. Fergusson DM, Horwood LJ, Shannon FT, et al. Infant health and breast feeding during the first 16 weeks of life. *Austr Paediatr J*. 1978;14:254–258.

211. Fergusson DM, Horwood LJ, Shannon FT, et al. Breast feeding, gastrointestinal and lower respiratory illness in the first two years. *Austr Paediatr J*. 1981;17:191–195.

212. Tracey VV, De NC, Harper JR. Obesity and respiratory

infection in infants and young children. *Br Med J.* 1971;1:16–18.

213. Wright AL, Holberg CJ, Martinex FD, et al. Breast feeding and lower respiratory tract illness in the first year of life. *Br Med J.* 1989;229:946–949.

214. Tyrell DAJ, Wallace-Craig J, Meade TW, et al. A trial of ascorbic acid in the treatment of the common cold. *Br J Prev Soc Med.* 1977;31:189–191.

215. Pitt HA, Costrini AM. Vitamin C prophylaxis in marine recruits. *JAMA.* 1979;241:908–911.

216. Strachan DP, Anderson HR, Bland JM, et al. Asthma as a link between chest illness in childhood and chronic cough and phlegm in young adults. *Br Med J.* 1988; 296:890–893.

217. Weiss ST, Tager IB, Muñoz A, et al. The relationship of respiratory infections in early childhood to the occurrence of increased levels of bronchial responsiveness and atrophy. *Am Rev Respir Dis.* 1985;131:573–578.

218. Woolcock AJ, Leeder SR, Pear JK, et al. The influence of lower respiratory illness in infancy and childhood and subsequent cigarette smoking on lung function in Sydney school children. *Am Rev Respir Dis.* 1979; 120:5–14.

219. Kattan M, Keens TG, Lapierre JG, et al. Pulmonary function abnormalities in symptom-free children after bronchiolitis. *Pediatrics.* 1977;59:883–888.

220. Mok JYQ, Simpson H. Outcome for acute bronchitis, bronchiolitis, and pneumonia in infancy. *Arch Dis Child.* 1984;59:306–309.

221. Douglas RM, Miles HB. Vaccination against *Streptococcus pneumoniae* in childhood: lack of a demonstrable benefit in young Australian children. *J Infect Dis.* 1984;149:861–869.

222. Barker DJP, Osmond C. Childhood respiratory infection and adult chronic bronchitis in England and Wales. *Br Med J.* 1986;293:1271–1275.

223. Belfer ML, Shader RI, DiMascio A, et al. Stress and bronchitis. *Br Med J.* 1968;3:805–806.

224. Jacobs MA, Spilken AZ, Norman MM, et al. Life stress and respiratory illness. *Psychosom Med.* 1970;32:233–242.

225. Belfer ML, Shader RI, DiMascio A, et al. Stress and bronchitis. *Br Med J.* 1968;3:805–806.

226. Boyce WT, Jensen EW, Cassel JC, et al. Influence of life events and family routines on childhood respiratory tract illness. *Pediatrics.* 1977;60:609–615.

227. Stout CW, Bloom LJ. Type A behavior and upper respiratory infections. *J Human Stress.* 1981;8:4–7.

228. Hart H, Bax M, Jenkins S. Health and behavior in preschool children. *Child Care Health Dev.* 1984;10:1–16.

229. Foulke FG, Reeb KG, Graham AV, et al. Family func-

tion, respiratory illness and otitis media in urban black infants. *Fam Med.* 1988;20:128–132.

230. Graham NMH, Douglas RM, Ryan P. Stress and acute respiratory infection. *Am J Epidemiol.* 1986;124:389–401.

231. Kasl SV, Evans AS, Niederman JC. Psychosocial risk factors in the development of infectious mononucleosis. *Psychosom Med.* 1979;41:445–466.

232. Meyer RJ, Haggerty RJ. Streptococcal infections in families: factors altering susceptibility. *Pediatrics.* 1962:29:539–549.

233. Totman R, Kiff J, Reed SE, et al. Predicting experimental colds in volunteers from different measures of life stress. *J Psychosom Res.* 1950;24:155–163.

234. Totman R, Reed SE, Craig JW. Cognitive dissonance, stress and virus-induced common colds. *J Psychosom Res.* 1977;21:51–61.

235. Broadbent DE, Broadbent MHP, Philpotts RJ, et al. Some further studies on the prediction of experimental colds in volunteers by psychological factors. *J Psychosom Res.* 1984;28:511–523.

236. Kiecolt-Glaser JK, Glaser R. Psychological influences on immunity. *Psychosomatics.* 1986;27:621–624.

237. Dick EC, Houssain, SV, Mink KA, et al. Interruption of transmission of rhinovirus colds among human volunteers using virucidal paper handkerchiefs. *J Infect Dis.* 1986;153;352–356.

238. Gwaltney JM, Moskolski PB, Hendley JO. Hand-to-hand transmission of rhinovirus colds. *Ann Intern Med.* 1978;88:463–467.

239. Gwaltney JM Jr, Hendley JO. Transmission of experimental rhinovirus infection by contaminated surfaces. *Am J Epidemiol.* 1982;116:828–833.

240. Schenker MB, Samet JM, Speizer FE. Risk factors for childhood respiratory disease. The effect of host factors and home environmental exposures. *Am Rev Respir Dis.* 1983;128:1038–1043.

241. Graham NMH, Woodward AJ, Ryan P, et al. Acute respiratory illness in Adelaide children. II. The relationship of maternal stress, social supports and family functioning. *Int J Epidemiol.* 1990;19:937–944.

242. Dingle JM, Badger GF, Jordan WS Jr. *Illness in the Home. A Study of 25,000 Illnesses in a Group of Cleveland Families.* Cleveland, OH: Western Reserve University; 1964.

243. Beem MO. Acute respiratory illness in nursery school children: a longitudinal study of the occurrence of illness and respiratory viruses. *Am J Epidemiol.* 1969; 90:30–44.

244. Hendley JO, Gwaltney JM Jr, Jordan WS Jr. Rhinovirus infections in an industrial population. IV. Infections within families of employees during two fall peaks of respiratory illness. *Am J Epidemiol.* 1969;89:184–196.

245. Douglas RG Jr, Lindgram KM, Cough RB. Exposure to cold environment and rhinovirus cold. Failure to demonstrate an effect. *N Engl J Med*. 1968;279:742–747.

246. Christie AB. *Infectious Diseases: Epidemiology and Clinical Practice*. Edinburgh, Scotland: Churchill Livingstone; 1974.

247. Jackson GG, Muldoon RL, Johnson GC, et al. Contribution of volunteers to studies of the common cold. *Am Rev Respir Dis*. 1963;88(Suppl):120–127.

248. Young M. The influence of weather conditions on the mortality from bronchitis and pneumonia in children. *J Hyg*. 1924;23:151–175.

249. Gwaltney JM. Epidemiology of the common cold. *Ann N Y Acad Sci*. 1980;353:54–60.

250. D'Souza RM. Care-seeking behavior. *Clin Infect Dis*. 1999;28:234.

251. D'Souza RM. *Household Determinants of Childhood Mortality: Illness Management in Karachi Slums*. Canberra, Australia: National Centre for Epidemiology and Population Health, The Australian National University; 1997:316.

252. Kundi MZM, Anjum M, Mull DS, Mull JD. Maternal perceptions of pneumonia and pneumonia signs in Pakistani children. *Soc Sci Med*. 1993;37:649–660.

253. Rahaman MM, Aziz KMS, Munshi MH, Patwari Y, Rahman M. A diarrhea clinic in rural Bangladesh: influence of distance, age and sex on attendance and diarrheal mortality. *Am J Public Health*. 1982;72:1124–1128.

254. Hughes WT. *Pneumocystis carinii* pneumonia. *N Engl J Med*. 1987;317:1021–1023.

255. Rubinstein A, Sicklick M, Gupta A, et al. Acquired immunodeficiency with reversed T4/T8 ratios in infants born to promiscuous and drug addicted mothers. *JAMA*. 1983;249:2350–2356.

256. Oleske J, Minnefar AB, Cooper B, et al. Immune deficiency syndrome in children. *JAMA*. 1983;249:2345–2349.

257. Scott GB, Buck BE, Leterman JG, et al. Acquired immunodeficiency syndrome in infants. *N Engl J Med*. 1984;310:76–81.

258. Leigh TR, Parsons P, Hume C, et al. Sputum induction for diagnosis of *Pneumocystis carinii* pneumonia. *Lancet*. 1989;2:205–206.

259. Bernstein LJ, Krieger BZ, Novick B, et al. Bacterial infection in the acquired immunodeficiency syndrome. *Pediatr Infect Dis J*. 1985;4:472–475.

260. Schlamm HT, Yancowitz SR. *Haemophilus influenzae* pneumonia in young adults with AIDS, ARC, or risk of AIDS. *Am J Med*. 1989;86:11–14.

261. Rolston KVI, Uribe-Botero G, Mansell PWA. Bacterial infections in adult patients with the acquired immune deficiency syndrome (AIDS) and AIDS-related complex. *Am J Med*. 1987;83:604–605.

262. Witt DJ, Craven DE, McCabe WR. Bacterial infections in adult patients with the acquired immune deficiency syndrome (AIDS) and AIDS-related complex. *Am J Med*. 1987;82:900–906.

263. White S, Tsou E, Waldhorn RE, et al. Life-threatening bacterial pneumonia in male homosexuals with laboratory features of the acquired immunodeficiency syndrome. *Chest*. 1985;87:486–488.

264. Selwyn PA, Feingold AR, Martel D, et al. Increased risk of bacterial pneumonia in HIV-infected intravenous drug users without AIDS. *AIDS*. 1988;2:267–272.

265. Murray JF, Garay SM, Hopewell PC, et al. Pulmonary complications of the acquired immunodeficiency syndrome: an update. *Am Rev Respir Dis*. 1987;135:504–509.

266. Biggar RJ, Bouvet E, Ebbeen P, et al. Clinical features of AIDS in Europe. *Eur J Cancer Clin Oncol*. 1984;20:165–167.

267. Hira SK, Ngandu N, Wadhawan D, et al. Clinical and epidemiological features of HIV infection at a referral clinic in Zambia. *J Acquir Immune Defic Syndr*. 1990;3:87–91.

268. Piot P, Laga M, Ryder R, et al. The global epidemiology of HIV infection: continuity, heterogeneity, and change. *J Acquir Immune Defic Syndr*. 1990;3:403–412.

269. Drillien CM. A longitudinal study of the growth and development of prematurely and maturely born children. Part IV. Morbidity. *Arch Dis Child*. 1959;14:210–217.

270. Chan KN, Elliman A, Bryan E, et al. Respiratory symptoms in children of low birth weight. *Arch Dis Child*. 1989;64:1294–1304.

271. Victora CG, Smith PG, Barros FC, et al. Risk factors for deaths due to respiratory infections among Brazilian infants. *Int J Epidemiol*. 1989;18:918–925.

272. Datta N, Kumar V, Kumar L, et al. Application of a case management approach to the control of acute respiratory infections in low birth weight infants: a feasibility study. *Bull World Health Organ*. 1987;65:77–82.

273. Caldwell JC, Reddy PH, Caldwell P. The social component of mortality decline: an investigation in South India employing alternative methodologies. *Population Studies*. 1983;37:185–205.

274. Abosede OA. Self-medication: an important aspect of primary health care. *Soc Sci Med*. 1984;19:699–703.

275. Colson AC. The differential use of medical resources in developing countries. *J Health Soc Behav*. 1971;12:226–237.

276. Liu C, Douglas RM. Chinese herbal medicine in the treatment of acute respiratory tract infections: review

of randomized and controlled clinical trials. *Clin Infect Dis*. 1999;28:235–236.

277. Puck JM, Glezen WP, Frank AL, et al. Protection of infants from infection with influenza A virus by transplacentally acquired antibody. *J Infect Dis*. 1980;142: 844–849.

278. Glezen WP, Paredes A, Allison JE, et al. Risk of respiratory syncytial virus infection for infants from low income families in relationship to age, sex, ethnic group and maternal antibody level. *J Pediatr*. 1981;98:708–715.

279. McConnochie KM, Roghmann KJ. Parental smoking, presence of older siblings and family history of asthma increase risk of bronchiolitis. *Am J Dis Child*. 1986; 140:806–812.

280. Welliver RC, Wong DT, Sun M, et al. The development of respiratory syncytial virus specific IgE and the release of histamine in nasopharyngeal secretions after infection. *N Engl J Med*. 1981;305:841–846.

281. Welliver RC, Wong DT, Middleton E, et al. Role of parainfluenza virus specific IgE in pathogenesis of croup and wheezing subsequent to infection. *J Pediatr*. 1982;101:889–896.

282. Martinez FD, Morgan WJ, Wright AL, et al. Diminished lung function as a predisposing factor for wheezing respiratory illness in children. *N Engl J Med*. 1988; 319:1112–1117.

283. Speizer F, Comstock G. Recommended respiratory disease questionnaires for use with adults and children in epidemiological research. *Am Rev Respir Dis*. 1978; 118:7–53.

284. Fletcher CM. Standardized questionnaire on respiratory symptoms. A statement prepared for and approved by the Medical Research Council's Committee on the Etiology for Chronic Bronchitis. *Br Med J*. 1960; 2:1665.

285. Gold DR, Weiss ST, Tager IB, et al. Comparison of questionnaire and diary methods in acute childhood respiratory illness surveillance. *Am Rev Respir Dis*. 1989;139:847–849.

286. Miller DL. *Some Problems in the Classification of Acute Respiratory Infection in Young Children and Questionnaire Design*. (WHO/RSD/81.8). Geneva, Switzerland: World Health Organization; 1981.

287. Leventhal JM. Clinical predictors of pneumonia as a guide to ordering chest roentgenograms. *Clin Pediatr*. 1982;21:730–734.

288. Cherian T, John TJ, Simoes E, et al. Evaluation of simple clinical signs for the diagnosis of acute lower respiratory tract infection. *Lancet*. 1988;2:125–128.

289. Campbell H, Byass P, Greenwood BM. Simple clinical signs for the diagnosis of acute lower respiratory infections. *Lancet*. 1988;2:742–743.

290. Campbell H, Byass P, Lamont AC, et al. Assessment of clinical criteria for identification of severe acute lower respiratory tract infections in children. *Lancet*. 1989; 1:297–299.

CHAPTER 16

Epidemiology and Prevention of Influenza

Mark C. Steinhoff

INTRODUCTION

Influenza virus has a unique epidemiology of annual epidemics of respiratory disease with attack rates of 10% to 30% in all regions of the world. It is also the classical emerging infection, causing global pandemics when new antigenic variants emerge. Influenza viruses are epizootic in avian and animal species, and recent analyses of nucleic acid sequences indicate that human influenza A viruses derive from avian influenza viruses. The antigenic mutability of this virus is the key to its ability to cause annual epidemics and periodic pandemics. The genetic and molecular aspects of mutability will be described in relation to the unique epidemiology of this virus. Because antigenic change is random and not predictable, the influenza virus will continue to cause widespread epidemics, although many aspects of the epidemiology and mutability of this virus are understood and effective antivirals and vaccines are available. Current control strategies require re-evaluation to achieve a true reduction in the toll of influenza morbidity and mortality, and enhanced pandemic preparedness is essential.

THE VIRUS

Influenza virus was one of the first human viruses to be cultured and studied. In 1933, Smith, Andrews, and Laidlaw first isolated human influenza A virus from a ferret (infected by secretions from an ill W. Smith). Burnet developed the technique of culture in hens' eggs in 1936, which enabled study of the viruses and development of vaccines. Influenza B virus was isolated in 1940, and type C virus in 1947.[1]

Influenza type A and B viruses contain eight segments of single-stranded RNA that code for ten separate proteins. Influenza type C has seven RNA segments and a single surface glycoprotein. Table 16–1 summarizes the gene segments and their associated proteins. The hemagglutinin (HA) and neuraminidase (NA) are surface glycoproteins that are important in both pathogenesis and immune protection from infection. The HA functions as the attachment protein, mediating attachment to sialic acid-containing glycoproteins on columnar epithelial cells of the respiratory tract. HA has a binding site that is highly conserved and surrounded by five specific antigenic epitopes that manifest rapid changes. Specific antibody to these HA epitopes prevent attachment and entry of influenza viruses into host cells. HA specificity for receptor binding is a determinant of which species can be infected, or host range. The HA is also a virulence determinant. The HA protein must be cleaved into H1 and H2 proteins by host proteases to create a hydrophobic tail necessary for fusion of viral and host cell membranes. The host proteases are found in human respiratory and avian enteric tissues. In avian viruses, the introduction of basic

Table 16–1 The Genes of Influenza A Virus and Their Protein Products

RNA Segment Number	Gene Product	Protein	Proposed Functions of Protein
1	PB1	Polymerase	RNA transcriptase
2	PB2	Polymerase	RNA transcriptase
3	PA	Polymerase	RNA transcriptase
4	HA	Hemagglutinin	Viral attachment to cell membranes; major antigenic and virulence determinant
5	NA	Neuraminidase	Release from membranes; major antigenic determinant
6	NP	Nucleoprotein	Encapsidates RNA, type-specific antigen
7	M1	Matrix	Surrounds viral core; involved in assembly and budding
	M2	Ion channel	
8	NS1	Nonstructural	RNA binding
	NS2	Nonstructural	Unknown

amino acids near the HA cleavage site permits cleavage by proteases of other tissues, which allows viral infection of vascular, central nervous system, and other tissues (pantropism) and a dramatic increase in virulence.[2] For example, a 1983 epidemic of chicken influenza in Pennsylvania changed from mild disease to a lethal disease after a mutation at the cleavage site. In contrast, the NA cleaves sialic acid residues, to allow virus release from the host epithelial cell; specific anti-NA antibody presumably diminishes release of virons from host cells.

The subtypes of influenza A virus are determined by these two surface antigens. Among influenza A viruses that infect humans, three different HA subtypes have classically been described—H1, H2, and H3. H5 has also recently been shown to infect humans.

NOMENCLATURE

The nomenclature of influenza viruses is somewhat complex because of the need to name all new strains. Virus strains are named with (*a*) the virus type, (*b*) the geographic site of first identification of the specific virus, (*c*) the strain number from the isolating laboratory, (*d*) the year of virus isolation, and (*e*) the virus subtype (for influenza A). For example, one of the viruses in the influenza vaccine that was recently recommended is A Beijing/32/96(H3N2). This refers to a type A virus first isolated in Beijing in

1996, as laboratory strain number 32, which is subtype H3N2.

CLINICAL FEATURES OF THE DISEASE

The word "influenza" is from the Italian (derived from Latin *influentia),* referring to the influence of the stars, from before the modern understanding of the causation of influenza epidemics. The clinical disease influenza is familiar, because everyone has been infected. It is characterized by an abrupt onset of fever and respiratory symptoms, including rhinorrhea, cough, and sore throat. Myalgia and headache are more common with influenza than with other respiratory viral infections, and the malaise and prostration of this disease are well known. Gastrointestinal symptoms are not common in adults, but 50% of infants and children may have vomiting, abdominal pain, and diarrhea with influenza. Influenza disease is usually self-limited, lasting for 3 to 5 days, but complications, which are more frequent in the elderly and persons with chronic illnesses, can prolong illness. Some patients may develop an influenza viral pneumonia, which can be fatal. More commonly, a secondary bacterial pneumonia may occur up to 2 weeks after the acute viral infection. In infants and children, otitis media and croup are common complications. Other less frequent complications include myocarditis, myositis, and encephalitis. Reye's syndrome, a hepatic and CNS complication seen in children, is associated with the use of aspirin and other salicylates.

Influenza virus spreads through respiratory secretions of infected persons, which may contain up to 10^5 virus particles/mL. An infected person generates infectious aerosols of secretions during coughing, sneezing, and talking. In addition, infectious secretions are spread by direct (by kissing) or indirect (by nose-finger-doorknob) contact with respiratory mucosa. The inhaled virus attaches to columnar epithelial cells of the upper respiratory tract and initiates a new infection in the host. The incubation period is from 1 to 4 days, and infected hosts are capable of transmitting the virus from shortly before the onset of clinical disease up to the fourth or fifth day of illness.

Diagnosis

Because of the clinical similarity of influenza virus infection to the manifestations of other respiratory viral infections, influenza virus infection cannot be reliably diagnosed from clinical signs and symptoms. Although some clinicians and many laypersons use the term "flu" or "influenza" to describe respiratory illness, only viral culture or serology can prove the presence of influenza virus. Culture requires nasal or throat secretions obtained within 3 days of onset, which are then cultured in embryonated hens' eggs or tissue culture. Viral growth occurs in 2 to 3 days, after which the virus is identified using reagents for type and subtype. Influenza virus can also be identified rapidly within 1 day in clinic settings using rapid antigen detection methods, such as immunofluorescence or enzyme-linked immunosorbent assay (ELISA) and other techniques. Infection is proven by serology to show a fourfold increase in antibodies to influenza virus and requires acute and convalescent blood specimens obtained approximately 3 weeks apart. Standard techniques for detection of influenza antibodies include hemagglutination inhibition (HI), complement fixation (CF), and ELISA techniques.

EPIDEMIOLOGY

Epidemics and Pandemics

The influenza virus causes annual epidemics of disease, and it has caused three global pandemics in the 20th century ("pandemic" from the Greek: *pan* = all, *demos* = people). Pandemics of febrile respiratory disease that resemble influenza have been described since the days of Hippocrates (Table 16–2). The characteristic pattern of an influenza pandemic is initiation from a single geographic focus (often in Asia) and rapid spread, often along routes of travel. High attack rates of all age groups are observed. Although

Table 16–2 A Century of Antigenic Shifts of Influenza A Virus (See Figure 16–5)

Years	Virus Description	Antigenic Change (Source)	Pandemic
1889	H3N2*	Not known	Severe
1900	H3N8*	Not known	Moderate
1918→56	H1N1 "Spanish"*	HA, NA (? swine)	Major; 20 million deaths in first year
1957→68	H2N2 "Asian"	New HA, NA, PB1 (avian)	Severe
1968→	H3N2 "Hong Kong"	New HA,[†] PB1 (avian)	Moderate
1977→	H1N1 "Russian"	Apparently identical with 1956 H1N1[‡]	Relatively mild[§]

* Data derived from serology; pandemic virus not available for study because influenza virus was first cultured in 1933.

   [†] New human H3 HA varied by only six amino acids from parent avian H3 HA, with all changes at sites important for receptor binding and antigenicity.

   [‡] May have escaped from a laboratory.

   [§] Those aged more than 22 years had antibody from 1918–1956 H1N1 strain.

case fatality rates are usually not increased substantially, because of the very large number of infections and cases, the number of hospitalizations and deaths are unusually high. In a pandemic, multiple waves of infections can sweep through a community, each wave infecting sectors of the population different from those affected in the initial pandemic episode.

The 1918 "Spanish influenza" pandemic had an attack rate of 20% to 30% in adults, and 30% to 45% in children. The case fatality rate in adults was as high as 15% to 50%, with an unusual occurrence of deaths in young adults (Figure 16–1). It is estimated that at least 20 to 40 million persons died in this global pandemic, many of them young adults (See text box, "Influenza Pandemic").

Annual local epidemics follow a fairly predictable pattern (Figure 16–2).[3] In North America, epidemics usually occur between November and March, manifested first by high rates of school and industrial absenteeism, followed by an increase in visits to health care facilities, an increase in pneumonia and influenza hospital admissions, and finally an increase in deaths from pneumonia or influenza.[3] In any single locality, epidemic influenza often begins abruptly, reaches a peak within 3 weeks, and usually ends by 8 weeks. A city or region can experience two sequential or overlapping epidemics with different strains of viruses in a single winter (Figure 16–3 and Table 16–4). Epidemics in the Southern Hemisphere usually occur in the May to September winter season; in some cases, they are caused by the new strain of epidemic virus that will cause epidemics in the Northern Hemisphere the following winter. In the tropics, disease seasonality can be associated with monsoons, or a year-round isolation of influenza virus may be observed. Virus spread during the winter season is said to be favored by the fact that virus survives better in environments of lower temperature and humidity. In tropical areas, spread during the monsoon suggests that indoor crowding caused by weather may be a more important factor.

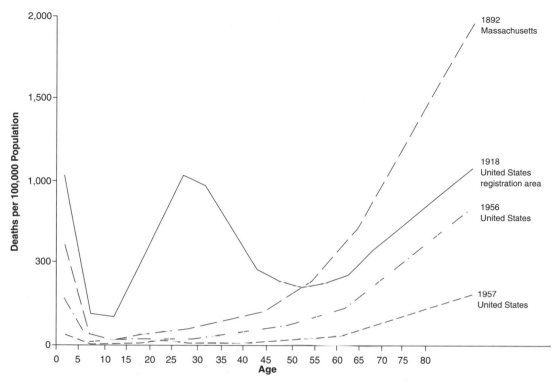

Figure 16–1 Age distribution of mortality for selected influenza epidemics in the United States. Note the difference between the 1918 pandemic with high young adult mortality rates and other epidemics with higher mortality at the extremes of the age spectrum. *Source:* Reprinted with permission from C.C. Dauer and R.E. Sterling, 1961, Mortality from Influenza, *American Review of Respiratory Diseases*, Vol. 82, Supplement, pp. 15–26. Official Journal of the American Thoracic Society, © American Lung Association.

In general, rates of infection in infants and children are higher than those of adults, although the rates of hospitalization are lower in children. Families with school-aged children have the highest rates of infection. These observations suggest that relatively immunologically naive children are important in the spread of epidemic strains. Table 16–3 summarizes recent U.S. data on rates for hospitalization for influenza.

Each epidemic and pandemic varies in size and impact, determined by the degree of the antigenic variation of the new virus, its virulence, and the level of existing protective immunity in the infected population. (See Table 16–2, noting the association between the degree of antigenic

difference and the size of the pandemic.) During average epidemics in North America, attack rates are often 10% to 20% in large populations, although certain population groups (e.g., school children or nursing home residents) and local outbreaks can have attack rates of 40% to 50%. More than 20,000 influenza-associated excess deaths occurred in the United States during each of nine epidemics between 1972 and 1991, and more than 40,000 deaths occurred during three of them. Persons aged more than 65 years account for 90% of the excess deaths associated with annual epidemics. Although pandemics cause many deaths over one or two winters, the cumulative deaths during successive epidemics

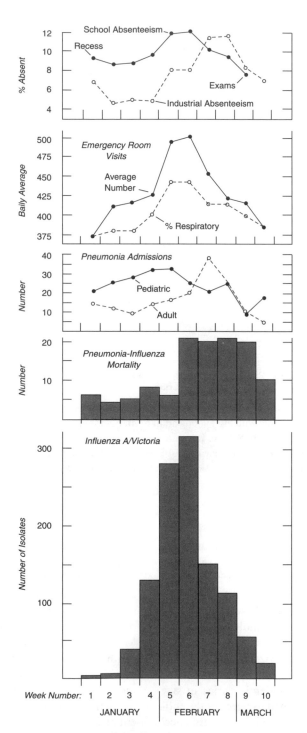

Figure 16–2 Pattern of 1976 influenza epidemic in Houston. *Source:* Reprinted with permission from W.P. Glezen and R.B. Couch, Interpandemic Influenza in the Houston Area, 1974–1976, *The New England Journal of Medicine*, Vol. 298, pp. 587–592. Copyright © 1978 Massachusetts Medical Society. All rights reserved.

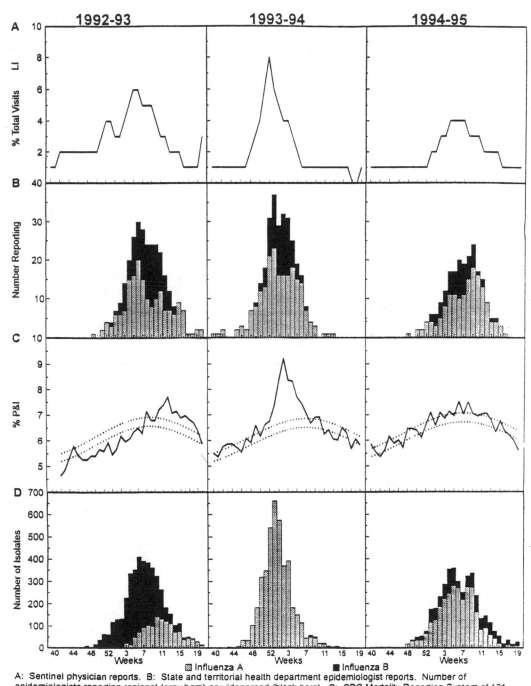

A: Sentinel physician reports. B: State and territorial health department epidemiologist reports. Number of epidemiologists reporting regional (gray bars) or widespread (black bars). C: CDC Mortality Reporting System of 121 Cities. D: Proportion of influenza B to influenza A isolated during the season by WHO collaborating laboratones.

Figure 16–3 Pattern of influenza disease reports and viral cultures for the United States, synopsis of 1992–95 surveillance data from the Centers for Disease Control and Prevention. *Source:* Reprinted from Centers for Disease Control and Prevention.

Table 16–3 Influenza Disease by Age Group

Age (years)	Rate of Hospitalization/100,000	
	Normal	High Risk
0–4	100	500
5–14	20	200
15–44	20–30	40–60
45–64	20–40	80–400
≥65	200	≥1,000

Source: Reprinted from MMWR, Vol. 45, RR-4, 1999, Centers for Disease Control and Prevention.

during an inter-pandemic period can exceed the total pandemic deaths. For example, it has been estimated that the H3N2 virus in its first pandemic in 1968–1969 caused 34,000 deaths in the United States, and it caused more than 300,000 deaths in the annual epidemics from 1969–1970 until the early 1990s. Since the 1990s, influenza has been associated with an average of 148,000 hospitalizations per year in the United States.

Surveillance for influenza disease and for specific influenza viruses is necessary to track epidemic disease, to detect pandemics, and to determine virus serotypes for vaccine policy. In the United States, the Centers for Disease Control and Prevention (CDC) uses four surveillance systems.

1. A sentinel physician surveillance network, utilizing a simple clinical definition of influenza-like illness (ILI): Fever greater than 100°F, plus cough or sore throat. Approximately 260 family practice physicians each week from October through May record the total number of patient visits for the week, and the num-

Table 16–4 Characteristics of Vaccine and Epidemic Influenza Viruses (1992–1995)*

Epidemic Season	Influenza Vaccine Composition	Proportion Circulating Type/Subtype[†]	Predominant Strain within Type/Subtype[†]
1992–93	A/Texas/36/91 (H1N1)	1	A/Texas/36/91[‡]
	A/Beijing/353/89 (H3N2)	30	A/Beijing/32/92
	B/Panama/45/90	69	B/Panama/45/90
1993–94	A/Texas/36/91 (H1N1	0	A/Texas/36/91[‡]
	A/Beijing/32/92 (H3N2)	98	A/Beijing/32/92
	B/Panama/45/90	2	B/Panama/45/90
1994–95	A/Texas/36/91 (H1N1)	1	A/Texas/36/91[‡]
	A/Shangdong/9/93 (H3N2)	61	64% A/Shangdong/09/93 36% A/Johannesburg/33/94[§]
	B/Panama/45/90	38	25% B/Panama/45/90 75% B/Beijing/184/93[§]

* See Figure 16–3
† Percent of isolates reported to CDC by collaborating laboratories of south Atlantic region of the United States.
‡ Or, the closely related A/Taiwan/01/86.
§ Fifty percent of winter epidemic virus isolates did not match the vaccine strains: (0.36 × 0.61 = 22% of type A(H3) isolates) plus (0.38 × 0.75 = 28% type B isolates).

Source: Reprinted from Centers for Disease Control and Prevention.

ber of patients examined for influenza-like illness by age group, and report this information electronically to CDC.

2. The collaborating laboratory surveillance system: 70 World Health Organization (WHO) collaborating laboratories and 50 other laboratories in the United States from October through May report the total number of specimens received for respiratory virus testing and the number of positive isolates of influenza virus.

3. The 122 cities mortality reporting system: Selected cities with a population of more than 100,000 provide data on the percent of deaths that are listed with pneumonia as the underlying cause or as associated with influenza. These data are graphically summarized in the *Morbidity and Mortality Weekly Report* (MMWR) from CDC.

4. State and territorial epidemiologists' reports of influenza activity levels: Each state epidemiologist reports the estimated level of influenza activity as no activity or sporadic (sporadically occurring cases of ILI or culture confirmed influenza [CCI] without school or institutional outbreaks), regional (outbreaks of ILI or CCI in counties that total <50% of the state population), or widespread activity (outbreaks of ILI or CCI in counties that are >50% of the total state population). These influenza data from all sources are summarized and reported periodically in MMWR. See Figure 16–3 for recent data from these four surveillance systems, and observe their correlation.

MECHANISMS OF ANTIGENIC VARIATION

Because most epidemic and all twentieth century pandemic infections by influenza virus are type A, the following discussion will focus on type A influenza. Although indistinguishable from type A in an individual patient, type B influenza disease is usually less severe, and it does not appear to cause pandemics. Type C disease is generally mild and not associated with widespread epidemics or pandemics.

The mutability or antigenic variation of influenza virus has been described as "antigenic drift," denoting minor antigen changes, and "antigenic shift" to describe major genetic and antigenic changes.

Antigenic drift describes the frequent minor antigenic changes in the HA and NA surface antigens, which account for the annual epidemics. Antigenic drift is ascribed to the relatively high rate of spontaneous mutation in RNA viruses. RNA polymerase is a low fidelity transcription enzyme without a proofreading function. The high rate of replication of these viruses with low fidelity will generate many new amino acid substitutions in surface glycoproteins, some of which will be advantageous to the virus, allowing it to become an epidemic strain. Studies have shown that from 1968 to 1979, 7.9 nucleotide and 3.4 amino acid changes occurred per year, equivalent to an approximate annual 1% change in the amino acid composition of the HA. Most antigenic change is observed in the five specific epitopes of HA that surround the binding site; as noted previously, the binding site itself demonstrates little sequence variation. It is assumed that antibody binding to these epitopes sterically block access to the binding site, preventing attachment to and infection of host cells. Amino acid sequencing has shown that drift variants are sequential, suggesting selective pressure. For example, H3 sequential drift variants from 1968 to 1988 had four or more amino acid differences in at least two antigenic sites. The H1N1 virus strain (which was the first cultured influenza) shows substantial genetic drift from the 1918 H1N1 pandemic strain. It is also possible that changes in nonsurface proteins may influence replication, transmission, or tissue tropism (virulence), conferring a selective advantage to a specific strain. It is thought that after 10 to 30 years of circulation of a specific subtype most members of the population will have antibody to that subtype, increasing the selection pressure for a new shift variant.

INFLUENZA PANDEMIC: SPANISH FLU AND AWAKENINGS; SWINE FLU AND ADVERSE REACTIONS

The influenza pandemic of 1918–1919, referred to as the "Spanish flu" caused more deaths globally than any pandemic since the Black Death (bubonic plague) of the 14th century.[26,27] Estimates of the total number of deaths worldwide vary, but most sources estimate the pandemic caused at least 20 to 40 million deaths. This estimate is an obvious underestimate because deaths in Asia and Africa were only crudely estimated by colonial authorities. Influenza illness was first reported among American troops in the midwestern United States, spread across the Atlantic with the movement of 1.5 million U.S. forces to the Western Front and then around the world.

Influenza was reported in March 1918 from Ft. Riley, Kansas. In April, relatively mild influenza disease with low mortality was reported in troops in New York City and elsewhere on the East Coast. By the 15th of April, U.S. troops in France were reporting influenza illnesses, as were troops in Britain. It is likely that crowding increased attack rates and mortality in the military. The U.S. Navy estimated that 40% of its seamen became ill. There were 54,000 battle deaths among U.S. forces in Europe and 43,000 influenza and pneumonia deaths. Battle lines were no barrier; German troops reported "blitzkatarrh" shortly after U.S. troops reported influenza, and German commanders complained that the disease disrupted their attack plans.

By May and June 1918, most of Europe was experiencing the epidemic. Disease was reported in Africa in May, in India and China in July and August—influenza had circled the world in 5 months. During the summer, the character of the disease changed, characterized by higher rates of pneumonia in young adults with case fatality rates of 50% reported. Some authorities suggest that the virus had mutated into a more virulent form.

Ships brought the epidemic to islands. For example, in Tahiti 10% of the population died within 25 days of the onset of the epidemic.

Similarly, in Western Samoa in November 1918, 20% of the population of 38,000 died within a 2-month period. On the other hand, the isolated Tristan da Cunha islands, isolated in the South Atlantic, did not experience the pandemic.

Beginning in August 1918, a second wave of severe disease swept the eastern coast of the United States, which was called "Spanish flu" because it was brought by ship from Europe. (Because of wartime censorship, British, French, German, and U.S. authorities did not report epidemic disease; Spain was neutral, reported the epidemic, and was rewarded with paternity in name.) This time the United States experienced the severe influenza disease with higher case fatality rates seen in the European Western Front. A common description is of cyanosis and death from pneumonia within 2 to 3 days of illness onset.

Surveys in the United States showed that 280/1,000 persons had clinical influenza symptoms. An estimated 550,000 excess deaths occurred in the United States, meaning approximately 1 of 200 persons died of influenza during the winter of 1918–1919. Philadelphia reported the highest mortality rate: 12,897 influenza and pneumonia deaths in October and November of 1918, with a peak of 700 deaths/day in late October. In these two months, 1 of every 130 persons in Philadelphia died of Spanish flu, a 2-month mortality rate of 0.77%, leading to disruption of civic life, including a shortage of coffins.

Desperate medical and public health authorities recommended many remedies and preventive actions now regarded as ineffective, including the use of gauze face masks, aerosol sprays, garlic or camphor necklaces, and legislation against public spitting. Uniquely, death rates were highest in the healthy 20 to 30 year age group, which usually experiences the lowest mortality in influenza pandemics; pregnant women were unusually susceptible. Reported death rates

continues

were lower in military and civilian African Americans than in whites, but approximately 2% of all Native Americans died during the epidemic.

The Spanish influenza epidemic of 1918 has been substantially ignored by historians, perhaps because it occurred at the end of World War I. Oliver Sack's book, *Awakenings*, and the movie based on the book describe encephalitis lethargica, associated with the 1918 influenza epidemic and the post encephalitic catatonic state some patients experienced. New cases of both encephalitis lethargica and classical catatonic syndrome have been rare since the 1920s. Katherine Ann Porter's novel, *Pale Horse, Pale Rider*, describes the experiences and feelings of young Americans during the pandemic.

Earlier retrospective analysis had suggested the Spanish flu was an H1N1 strain derived from swine sources (which in turn had been derived from avian strains). When in January 1976 a similar swine H1N1 strain (A/New Jersey/76) was isolated in an ill soldier who died at Fort Dix, NJ, some United States public health authorities feared another pandemic and advised expanded immunization. Although not supported by all experts, a decision was reached to initiate mass immunization against swine flu, and the Swine Flu Program was announced in March 1976. A new national surveillance program for influenza disease and for vaccine adverse events was implemented. When liability issues were raised by the manufacturers, a special Swine Flu Tort Claims bill was passed by Congress, which specified that any claim arising from the swine flu program should be filed against the federal government. Vacci-

nation started in October 1976, although no cases of swine flu disease were reported, and only one other country (The Netherlands) planned mass immunization. When, in December 1976, more than 500 cases of Guillain-Barré disease were reported following swine flu immunization, the vaccination program was suspended. Criticism based on hindsight abounded: The *New York Times* published an editorial, "The Swine Flu Fiasco," which excoriated government and public health officials. Although the incumbent President Ford received the vaccine, his victorious challenger Jimmy Carter declined it; the swine flu program was not invoked by either party during the 1976 election.

The two major architects of the program, the Director of the CDC and the Assistant Secretary for Health of HEW resigned, and the credibility of their agencies was reduced. A total of 48 million Americans received the swine flu vaccine, but only six cases of "swine flu" H1N1 disease were recorded, which suggests that the A/New Jersey/76 strain was not transmitted efficiently. More than 500 cases of Guillain-Barré syndrome were reported, apparently associated with influenza vaccine, for which the federal government assumed liability and paid damages. Analysis suggested the risk of Guillain-Barré syndrome in 1976 vaccinees was seven to ten times increased over background risk, to about ten cases for every million vaccine recipients. A recent evaluation of Guillain-Barré syndrome associated with current influenza vaccine suggests a relative risk of 1.7, approximately one case per million vaccinees.[18] This suggests the 1976 H1N1 vaccine had a unique association with Guillain-Barré syndrome.

Antigenic shift describes the major changes of HA, NA, or both of the surface antigens that create a new subtype. If the HA and NA determinants are novel, no antibody protection is present in human populations, and the stage may be set for a pandemic.

Viruses with segmented genomes can generate new variants rapidly by the random reassort-

ment of the RNA segments. Co-infection of a single host cell by two influenza strains, each with a different eight-segmented genome, theoretically can generate 2^8 or 254 variants. It is thought that the "mixing vessel" host for influenza is likely swine, which are in contact with birds and humans, although humans can also serve this role. Most new variants will not have a survival advantage and will die out. However, if a shift variant (*a*) retains the ability to replicate well in humans, (*b*) is efficiently transmissible between humans, and (*c*) has new surface HA or NA determinants that evade existing influenza antibody profiles in the human population, a pandemic may ensue. Historically, serology and virology reveal that three antigenic shifts occurred during the 20th century, leading to three pandemics. Table 16–2 summarizes antigenic shifts of influenza A virus over the last century. Figure 16–4 demonstrates details of the antigenic shift of 1968, and Figure 16–5 shows all pandemics.

To summarize the pandemics of the 20th century: In 1918, the pandemic of influenza A H1N1 "Spanish flu" killed 20 to 40 million people in the first year; 500,000 in the United States alone. In 1957, a major shift occurred with both new avian HA and NA (H1N1 to H2N2). In 1968, a new HA (H2N2 to H3N2) from an avian source was introduced, leading to a moderately severe pandemic. In 1977, the old 1951 H1N1 strain reappeared (perhaps having escaped from a laboratory), causing attack rates of more than 50% in younger members of the population, who had been born after 1968 and, therefore, had no antibody to the antecedent

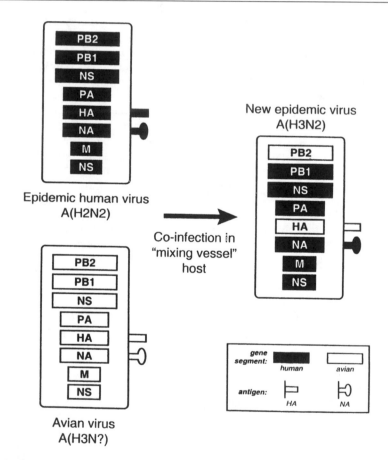

Figure 16–4 Diagram showing the last antigenic shift in 1968, when a new avian gene was acquired. Gene segments are color-coded to represent avian or human species origin and their associated surface proteins. *Source:* Copyright © Mark C. Steinhoff.

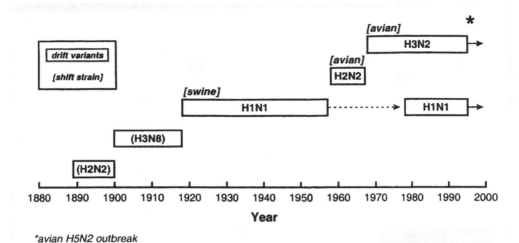

Figure 16–5 Twentieth century history of influenza antigenic shifts and pandemics, and inter-pandemic antigenic drift. *Source:* Reprinted from Centers for Disease Control and Prevention.

H1N1 subtype. Since 1977, both H1N1 and H3N2 subtypes co-circulate worldwide (Table 16–2 and Figure 16–5).

In summary, influenza viruses with new surface antigens emerge, cause a pandemic, and become established in human populations. As the proportion of persons with antibodies against the specific pandemic strain increases within the population, the circulating influenza virus subtype must change or die out. Antigenic drift allows a specific influenza subtype to persist in the human population. It is assumed that annual epidemics occur in the inter-pandemic period because drift variant viruses with new minor antigenic changes can infect some members of the population. A new pandemic occurs after an antigenic shift. The shift can result from genetic reassortment between human and animal influenza viruses or from direct transmission of an animal strain to humans, as was documented with influenza A (H5N1) in Hong Kong in the winter of 1997–1998.[4,5] This virus isolated from humans had only avian genes, with no evidence of reassortment with human viruses. It is apparent that the novel avian influenza A (H5N1) virus did cause disease in at least 18 humans in Hong Kong (6 of whom died), but did not efficiently transmit from human to human, hence did not become pandemic. It must be remembered that this avian virus may at any time reassort with human-adapted viruses and acquire efficient transmissibility and, thus, could cause a pandemic in the near future. For this reason, public health authorities have begun development of H5 vaccines. The 1998 Hong Kong experience and the swine influenza 1976 episode show that surface antigens, virulence, and transmissibility all vary independently and unpredictably. Not all new shift viruses with novel antigens will cause a pandemic, unless the criteria of transmissibility and human infectivity are met also.

Genetic reassortment also occurs frequently in egg or tissue culture. The vaccine manufacturers use this viral characteristic to rapidly develop new vaccine strains. Two viruses are selected: a wild virus with the epidemic NA and HA antigens, and a laboratory-adapted virus with the characteristics of vigorous growth in egg culture. Eggs are infected simultaneously with both viruses and the reassortant progeny virus that exhibits both the epidemic HA and NA and the property of good growth in eggs is selected as the vaccine strain for production.

EPIZOOTIC INFECTIONS AND EVOLUTIONARY HISTORY

The current working hypothesis developed by Webster and others[6,7] is that avian influenza strains are the source for all influenza viruses seen in birds and mammals. Analysis of molecular relationships suggests that all A subtypes are descended from a primordial avian influenza virus. All the known 14 HA and 9 NA influenza subtypes have been isolated from avian sources, which is likely their natural habitat, but only certain subtypes are found in mammalian species including swine, horses, seals, whales, and mink. Infection of feral (ducks, geese, gulls, terns, and shearwaters) or domestic (turkeys, chickens, geese, ducks, quail, and pheasants) avian species is usually asymptomatic, but occasionally has resulted in epidemics of avian disease.[2] Ducks excrete up to $10^{8.7}$ virus particles/gram of feces, and influenza virus is found in waters where ducks reside. The rate of antigenic drift is low in birds, suggesting stable adaptation between virus and avian host. It has been found that pigs have epithelial cell receptors for both human and avian HA. Pigs are thought to be the "mixing vessels," intermediate hosts of avian and mammalian influenza virus, providing an opportunity for antigenic shift. Although the virus of the 1918 pandemic has not been cultured, pandemic viral RNA from bodies buried in permafrost in Alaska and from autopsy material from the military has been analyzed and shows that the pandemic strain was unique and related to early swine strains. Further analysis of the RNA sequence is being carried out to determine if a genetic explanation for its high virulence can be obtained.[8] It is of note that the avian equivalent of H1N1 is still circulating in avian species. The role of avian carriage of virus during annual water fowl migration from the Northern to the Southern Hemisphere in the spread of new influenza variants is being investigated.

PREVENTION STRATEGIES AND TREATMENT

Vaccines to prevent infection, and use of antiviral drugs either prophylactically or for treatment are the currently available strategies to reduce influenza disease. This section will describe the recommended use of inactivated influenza vaccine, and of amantadine or rimantadine; new vaccines and treatment modalities will be discussed in a later section.

Vaccines

Vaccines were developed soon after influenza virus was shown to grow in embryonated hens' eggs. An early vaccine trial in 1943 showed that a killed virus vaccine was effective in young adults. The current inactivated vaccine is derived from virus grown on chorioallantoic membranes of embryonated eggs. The allantoic fluids are ultracentrifuged to purify the virus particles, and the viruses are inactivated by formaldehyde or beta-propriolactone. Some manufacturers disrupt the virus particles to produce a "split virus vaccine" using tween, detergents, or ether. The potency is assessed by measuring HA antigen, and vaccines are standardized to contain 15 to 20 µg of HA antigen per dose. Egg-grown influenza viruses have been shown to have antigenic variation from the parent human strain, which may account for the variable protection of inactivated vaccines. Some workers have shown that growth of human-derived influenza virus in human cell lines produces HA antigens with identical amino acid sequences to the parent strain. Vaccines are immunogenic in adults after a single dose, but require two doses in infants and children who are immunologically naive. Current inactivated vaccines are 50% to 80% effective in preventing disease when the epidemic influenza virus matches the vaccine strains.

The current vaccine strategy in the United States is to provide protection for persons at high risk for adverse outcomes from influenza virus infection.[9] In brief, these groups include those at increased risk for influenza complications (see Exhibit 16–1), persons who can transmit influenza to those at high risk, as well as other special groups including persons infected with HIV,[10] travelers, and members of the population who wish to avoid influenza infection. Exhibit 16–1 summarizes influenza vaccine recommendations for the United States.

Pregnancy was associated with excess mortality in the 1918 influenza pandemic. Recent evaluations have shown a relative risk of 4.7 for influenza-related hospitalization of pregnant women in the third trimester, compared with postpartum controls.[11] It is estimated that the rate of hospitalization for pregnant women is about 250/100,000, and that 1,000 influenza vaccinations would prevent one to two hospitalizations of pregnant women.

Exhibit 16–1 Persons Who Should Receive Influenza Vaccine

- Older than 65 or residents of long-term care facilities.
- Persons older than 6 months with chronic disorders of pulmonary or cardiac systems, metabolic, renal or hemoglobinpathy disorders, or with immunosuppression.
- Children 6 months to 18 years on long-term aspirin therapy (for rheumatoid arthritis).
- Women who will be more than 14 weeks' pregnant during winter epidemic season.
- Persons who can transmit influenza to any of the above (health care providers, employees of long-term care facilities, or family members).
- Special groups: HIV-infected persons, travelers, students, essential community service providers, or anyone who wishes to avoid influenza.

Source: Adapted from Centers for Disease Control and Prevention.

Virus mutability with antigenic shift and drift means a new vaccine must be produced each year, to counter the new antigenic variants that continually arise. Each year in January a review of circulating viruses in the Northern and Southern Hemispheres is undertaken by WHO, using data from a global network of surveillance laboratories, and the most likely epidemic influenza A (H1N1, H3N2) and a B strain are selected. The vaccine seed viruses are produced and distributed to manufacturers for production in eggs, clinical testing, licensing, packaging, and distribution by October before the winter influenza season. The four U.S. vaccine manufacturers produce 70 to 80 million doses each year between February and October. This complex process is repeated annually, and is remarkably effective. Table 16–4 shows the varying match between vaccine strains and epidemic viruses for recent years in the United States.

This vaccine strategy is relatively effective in preventing disease and mortality in vaccinated persons in those years in which the vaccine composition closely matches the epidemic virus. It is unlikely to have any impact on the overall epidemic pattern, however, because only a small proportion of the susceptible population (ie, those at high risk) is vaccinated. A vaccine strategy to vaccinate healthy persons has some merit, and had been used in Japan until the early 1990s. Recent studies suggest that influenza immunization of healthy children will reduce all otitis media episodes by 40%[12,13] and of healthy adults will reduce reported respiratory illness by 20% and absenteeism by 36%.[14–16] Strategies to vaccinate a large proportion of the population have the potential to disrupt epidemic transmission and protect many persons.[17] Since recent data have suggested the importance of school-aged children in transmission during an epidemic, some authorities believe they should be targeted as vaccine recipients in order to control epidemics.

The inactivated influenza vaccines that are currently recommended and commercially available do not contain live viruses and cannot cause influenza disease. The most frequent side effect of vaccination is local soreness at the vaccination site, which can last for 1 or 2 days. Symptoms of fever, malaise, and myalgia have been infrequently reported, most often in persons who have had no exposure to influenza vaccine (e.g., young children). Allergic anaphylactic reactions, which can occur rarely after influenza vaccination, are related to hypersensitivity to residual egg protein in these vaccines or to thimerosal. The 1976 swine influenza vaccine was associated with an increased frequency of Guillain-Barré syndrome of ascending paralysis. Recently, the association has been evaluated with current vaccines, and it is estimated to occur in approximately one case per million vaccines—far less than the risk of severe influenza complications if not vaccinated (Table 16–3).[18]

Antiviral agents, amantadine and rimantadine, inhibit the replication of type A influenza viruses (but have no effect on type B) by interfering with the M2 protein, which forms an ion channel. When taken prophylactically, these drugs have been shown to be 70% to 90% effective in preventing illness during influenza A epidemics. In addition, if begun within 48 hours of illness onset in healthy adults, these drugs can reduce the severity and duration of influenza A illness. Both drugs have CNS side effects of nervousness, anxiety, difficulty in concentrating, and light-headedness in approximately 6% of those taking rimantadine prophylactically and 14% of those taking amantadine prophylactically. Up to 3% of subjects experienced nausea and anorexia when taking these drugs. These drugs are advised for children only above the age of 1 year, and the dosages are summarized in Table 16–5.[19]

NEW MODALITIES OF PREVENTION AND TREATMENT

Live attenuated influenza viruses have been shown to be as effective as the inactivated virus vaccines.[20] Most promising is the cold-adapted attenuated influenza virus that is derived from an epidemic strain and an attenuated cold-adapted virus. The cold-adapted virus does not replicate effectively at 37°C, hence it can infect humans, but does not cause disease.[20] After reassortment of the two viruses, progeny with the epidemic surface antigens and the characteristic of low growth in humans are selected and produced. These vaccine strains have been extensively tested in adults and children, and demonstrate protective efficacy and excellent safety characteristics.[16,20,21] Their chief advantage is that they can be administered as nose drops or aerosol, and, therefore, are more acceptable to patients

---

Table 16–5 Antiviral Agents for Influenza Treatment and Prophylaxis

	Amantadine	Rimantadine	Zanamivir	Oseltamivir
Types of influenza viruses inhibited	Influenza A	Influenza A	Influenza A and B	Influenza A and B
Route of administration	Oral (tablet, capsule, syrup)	Oral (tablet, syrup)	Oral inhalation*	Oral (capsule)
Ages for which treatment is approved	>=1 year	>=14 years	>=12 years	>=18 years
Ages for which prophylaxis is approved	>=1 year	>=1 year	Not approved for prophylaxis	Not approved for prophylaxis

*Zanamivir is administered by plastic oral inhalation device.

Source: Adapted from MMWR, Vol. 48, RR14, 1999, Centers for Disease Control and Prevention.

and do not require medical personnel for administration. The cold-adapted influenza vaccines are not yet licensed (in 1999) for use in the United States, but it is expected that they will be approved in the near future. The ease of administration of these vaccines and their ready acceptance may allow new evaluation of strategies of population vaccination to avert an epidemic, rather than the current strategy of immunizing only persons at high risk.[22]

A number of new antiviral drugs for treatment of influenza have been evaluated in humans, including those that block receptor sites on host cells or inhibit NA activity.[23,24] An NA inhibitor, zanamivir (a sialic acid analogue), reduces disease duration by 1 or more days and prevents both type A and B disease with 67% to 82% effectiveness when taken prophylactically. Zanamivir (or Relenza) was licensed in the United States in July 1999 as inhalation therapy for persons older than 12 years. An oral NA inhibitor, oseltamivir, has been shown to be effective for prophylaxis and treatment for influenza[25] and was licensed for use in adults in October 1999.

PREPARING FOR THE PANDEMIC

Many experts predict that a new pandemic with a unique influenza shift virus is inevitable and can occur at any time. The appearance of the H5N1 virus in humans in Hong Kong has led to a reassessment of pandemic planning in the United States and globally. In its review of preparedness, the CDC has estimated that a new virus would arrive in the United States within 1 to 6 months of its appearance elsewhere, and would likely initiate the pandemic at many cities with international airports. It is unlikely that any existing vaccine would be useful, and stocks of antivirals would not be adequate to treat the large number of cases expected in a naive population. As in previous pandemics, health care workers will likely be at increased risk, affecting the care of the ill. Current estimates are that the United States would have 200 million cases, up to 800,000 hospitalizations, and as many as 300,000 influenza deaths within the 3- to 4-month period of the first sweep of the pandemic. (See www.cdc.gov/vd/nvpo/pandemicflu.htm for the current planning guide.) Current plans include improved surveillance and monitoring of the emergence of new viruses, stockpiling of antiviral drugs, development of a drug distribution system, strategic planning to develop and distribute new vaccines, and improved communications between WHO and national and local authorities.

The WHO has strengthened the FluNet, a global surveillance system with laboratories in 83 countries, and has sped up the process of identifying possible new shift viruses (those that are not typed with existing antisera). Some experts have suggested that closer monitoring of avian and swine influenza viruses and epidemic diseases may assist in prediction of new pandemic human influenza strains. Virologists are working on techniques to adapt a newly arising influenza virus for rapid production of a vaccine. Because the onset of a new pandemic or the characteristics of a new pandemic virus cannot be predicted reliably, preparation to speed the response to the pandemic may be the best approach.

REFERENCES

1. Murphy BR, Webster RG. Orthomyxovirus. In: Fields BN, Knipe DM, Howley PM, Chanock RM, Melnick JL, Monath TP, Roizman B, Straus SE, eds. *Virology.* 3rd ed. Philadelphia: Lippincott-Raven Publishers; 1996: 1409–1432.

2. Webster RG. Influenza virus: transmission between species and relevance to emergence of the next human pandemic. *Arch Virol.* 1997;13(suppl):105–113.

3. Couch RB, Kasel WP, Glezen TR, et al. Influenza: its control and person and populations. *J Infect Dis.* 1986; 153:431–440.

4. Subbarao K, Klimov A, Katz J, et al. Characterization of an avian influenza A (H5N1) virus isolated from a child with fatal respiratory illness. *Science.* 1998;279:393–396.

5. Claas EC, Osterhaus AD, van Beek R, et al. Human in-

fluenza A H5N1 virus related to a highly pathogenic avian influenza virus. *Lancet.* 1998;351:472–477.

6. Glezen WP. Emerging infections: pandemic influenza. *Epidemiol Rev.* 1996;18:64–76.

7. Webster RG. Influenza: an emerging microbial pathogen. In: Krause RM, ed. *Emerging Infections.* New York: Academic Press; 1998:275–300.

8. Reid AH, Fanning TG, Hultin JV, Taubenberger JK. Origin and evolution of the 1918 "Spanish" influenza virus hemagglutinin gene. *Proc Natl Acad Sci USA.* 1999;96:1651–1656.

9. Prevention and control of influenza: recommendations of the Advisory Committee on Immunization Practices (ACIP). *MMWR.* 1999;48(RR4):1–28.

10. Tasker SA, Treanor JJ, Paxton WB, Wallace MR. Efficacy of influenza vaccination in HIV-infected persons: a randomized, double-blind, placebo-controlled trial. *Ann Intern Med.* 1999;131:430–433.

11. Neuzil KM, Reed GW, Mitchel EF, Simonsen L, Griffin MR. Impact of influenza on acute cardiopulmonary hospitalizations in pregnant women. *Am J Epidemiol.* 1998; 148:1094–1102.

12. Heikkinen T, Ruuskanen O, Waris M, Ziegler T, Arola M, Halonen P. Influenza vaccination in the prevention of acute otitis media in children. *Am J Dis Child.* 1991; 145:445–448.

13. Clements DA, Langdon L, Bland C, Walter E. Influenza A vaccine decreases the incidence of otitis media in 6- to 30-month-old children in day care. *Arch Pediatr Adolesc Med.* 1995;1490:1113–1117.

14. Nichol KL, Lind A, Margolis KL, et al. The effectiveness of vaccination against influenza in healthy, working adults. *N Engl J Med.* 1995;333:889–893.

15. Wilde JA, McMillan J, Serwint J, Butta J, O'Riordan MA, Steinhoff MC. Effectiveness of influenza vaccine in health care professionals: a randomized controlled trial. *JAMA.* 1999;281:908–913.

16. Nichol KL, Mendelman PM, Mallon KP, et al. Effectiveness of live, attenuated intranasal influenza virus vaccine in healthy, working adults: a randomized controlled trial. *JAMA.* 1999;282:137–144.

17. Patriarca PA. New options for prevention and control of influenza. *JAMA.* 1999;282:75–77.

18. Lasky T, Terracciano GJ, Magder L, et al. The Guillain-Barré syndrome and the 1992–1993 and 1993–1994 influenza vaccines. *N Engl J Med.* 1998;339:1797–1802.

19. Douglas RG Jr. Prophylaxis and treatment of influenza. *N Engl J Med.* 1990;322:443–450.

20. Steinhoff MC, Halsey NA, Fries LF, et al. The A/Mallard/6750/78 avian-human, but not the A/Ann Arbor/6/60 cold-adapted, Influenza A/Kawasaki/86 (H1N1) reassortant virus vaccine retains partial virulence for infants and children. *J Infect Dis.* 1991;163:1023–1028.

21. Belshe RB, Mendelman PM, Treanor J, et al. The efficacy of live attenuated, cold-adapted, trivalent, intranasal influenza virus vaccine in children. *N Engl J Med.* 1998;338:1405–1412.

22. Barnett ED. Influenza immunization for children. *N Engl J Med.* 1998;338:1459–1461.

23. Hayden FG, Osterhaus ADME, Treanor JJ, et al for the GG167 Influenza Study Group. Efficacy and safety of the neuraminidase inhibitor zanamivir in the treatment of influenza virus infections. *N Engl J Med.* 1997; 337:874–880.

24. Monto AS, Robinson DP, Herlocher ML, Hinson JM Jr., Elliott MJ, Crisp A. Zanamivir in the prevention of influenza among healthy adults: a randomized controlled trial. *JAMA.* 1999;282:31–35.

25. Hayden FG, Treanor JJ, Fritz S, et al. Use of oral neuraminidase inhibitor oseltamivir in experimental human influenza. Randomized controlled trials for prevention and treatment. *JAMA.* 1999;282:1240–1246.

26. Crosby AW. *America's Forgotten Epidemic, the influenza of 1918.* New York: Cambridge University Press; 1989.

27. Neustadt RE, Fineberg HV. *The Swine Flu Affair: Decision-making on a Slippery Disease.* Washington, DC: U.S. Dept of Health, Education, and Welfare; 1978.

SUGGESTED INTERNET RESOURCES

CDC Influenza Web Page URL: http://www.cdc.gov/ncidod/diseases/flu/fluvirus/htm.

WHO Influenza Web page URL: http://who.int/emc/diseases/flu/index.html. (Interactive maps of global flu data are at: http://oms/b3e/jussieu/fr/flunet.)

Part IV

Diarrheal Diseases

CHAPTER 17

Diarrheal Diseases

Robert E. Black

Diarrheal diseases are an important global problem, causing high rates of morbidity and mortality in developing countries.[1] Although mortality from infectious diarrheal diseases has been reduced to a low rate in more economically developed countries, substantial morbidity and associated costs continue.[2-4] In addition, high rates of diarrhea in some settings (e.g., hospitals and day-care centers) and outbreaks of foodborne diarrhea have resulted in increased concern.

Diarrheal diseases occur most frequently in the conditions of poor environmental sanitation and hygiene, inadequate water supplies, poverty, and limited education that are found especially in developing countries. As these conditions improved over the last century in the now more economically developed countries, the problems with diarrheal diseases have greatly diminished.[5] Likewise, many developing countries are undergoing a similar economic, social, and epidemiologic transition with decreasing rates of diarrheal diseases. Unfortunately, nearly all countries in the world have populations still living in poor environmental conditions and poverty. These populations may continue to have high rates of diarrhea and even diarrheal mortality.

From the beginning of the 1980s, substantial global efforts were directed at reduction of diarrheal disease mortality.[6] It was recognized that dehydration from diarrhea played a substantial part in the fatal illnesses and that this dehydration could be prevented or treated with oral fluid and electrolyte replacement, along with continued feeding. Such efforts possibly make effective therapy more widely available through national diarrheal disease control programs in developing countries. Similar clinical approaches have also improved the management of diarrhea in the United States. These programs have resulted in improved therapy and a reduction in diarrhea-related mortality. With the consequent reduction in diarrheal deaths from dehydration, attention has been directed at dysentery and persistent diarrhea, which are also major causes of diarrhea-related mortality. In addition, increased efforts are being directed at prevention of diarrhea, making an understanding of the etiology and epidemiology, including patterns of transmission, of diarrheal diseases an essential basis for potential prevention measures.

GENERAL EPIDEMIOLOGY

Definitions

Diarrhea is a symptom complex characterized by stools of decreased consistency and increased number. Although diarrhea can be defined as the occurrence of these symptoms, simply in comparison to that individual's prior bowel pattern, epidemiologic studies usually have used a more precise definition.[7] Most studies now consider diarrhea to be present when three or more liquid stools are passed during a 24-hour period. At least 2 days free of diarrhea are usually required to define an episode as terminated. Dysentery is a diarrheal disease defined by the presence of blood in liquid stools.

Although most diarrheal episodes resolve within a week, a small proportion continues for 2 weeks or more.[8] Studies in many countries show that the distribution of episode durations is continuous, but skewed toward the longer durations. Thus, any definition of "persistent" diarrhea is arbitrary; however, having a definition is useful for research and disease control purposes. The World Health Organization (WHO) defines persistent diarrhea operationally as an episode that lasts for at least 14 days. It has also been reported that this definition of persistent diarrhea identifies children who tend to have a very high prevalence of diarrhea from both acute and persistent episodes.[9,10] The term "persistent diarrhea," as used by WHO, encompasses episodes that begin acutely and continue for longer than their expected duration, and it is not intended to include infrequent diarrheal disorders, such as hereditary syndromes, gluten-sensitive enteropathy, or other noninfectious conditions.

Data Sources

Data to describe the epidemiology of diarrheal diseases come from three main sources: prospective studies in households or health facilities, passive or active surveillance systems, and outbreak investigations. Surveys may also provide limited types of information.

Prospective studies in households in developing countries have generally used visits by health workers at an interval of no more than 1 week to collect data on symptoms and to obtain specimens of stool for causative testing. Such studies in more developed countries often use a combination of household visits and telephone contacts. Prospective studies in health facilities can be done in general outpatient clinics, hospital wards, or special populations (e.g., studies of nosocomial infections in newborn nurseries).

Passive surveillance is an approach in which health care workers routinely report the occur-

rence of a specified disease to public health officials, whereas active surveillance generally involves the seeking of specific diseases by contact with health workers or laboratories. Passive surveillance, which can be done on a wide scale, is relatively inexpensive, but its value may be limited by reporting that is incomplete, biased, and delayed. Active surveillance of selected diseases might be appropriate if a need is seen for more complete and timely information. In general, developing countries do not have useful passive or active surveillance systems for diarrheal diseases. In the United States, surveillance systems exist for only a limited number of diarrheal diseases or pathogens that are reported through laboratory-based passive surveillance.

Investigation of outbreaks of diarrheal diseases can be very useful to rapidly develop information on the risk factors, transmission patterns, and control measures for enteric pathogens. Such investigations can lead to controls to contain that outbreak, as well as help develop measures to prevent future outbreaks.

In developing countries, surveys are commonly conducted to get information about health conditions and the use of health services. Although information on the presence of diarrhea in the respondent on the day of survey can be reported accurately, it is not possible to determine the true incidence of diarrheal diseases from the survey because of problems with reporting such a frequent and commonly mild illness, as well as the potential distortions introduced by seasonal variation in diarrheal incidence. Surveys can provide information on more clear and memorable events such as hospitalization or death from diarrheal diseases in a relatively recent time period or medical care received for current episodes.

Incidence

A summary of prospective, community-based studies in developing countries concluded that the median annual incidence of all cases of diarrhea in children aged less than 5 years was 2.6 episodes. Diarrheal incidence has varied in the different settings in which it has been studied (Table 17–1). This variation could be caused by methodologic differences, such as the definition of diarrhea or surveillance techniques used in the study. In the summary of the community-based studies, findings were that the incidence was highest in studies with a small number of children under surveillance and with more frequent home visiting, which suggests that the other studies may have found lower rates because of underreporting.[1] At the same time, it is likely that actual differences exist in the incidence of diarrhea in different populations because of different environmental and host risk factors, as well as the relative frequency of various enteropathogens. Both methodologic and setting-specific differences can also affect the distribution of diarrheal episode durations. Studies that have the most intensive and frequent surveillance are most likely to identify mild and short-duration episodes that might not otherwise be reported with less intensive case finding.

In developing countries, the incidence of diarrhea varies greatly with age.[11] Generally the first 2 years of life have the highest incidence followed by a decline with increasing age. Peak incidence is often at age 6 to 7 months (Figure 17–1). The incidence in boys and girls is generally similar; however, in some countries boys may more often be taken to health facilities, giving the appearance of higher rates of diarrhea.

In the United States, the Centers for Disease Control and Prevention has estimated that 21 to 37 million episodes of diarrhea occur each year in children aged less than 5 years with approximately 10% of these illnesses leading to a visit to a physician.[3] It has also been estimated that foodborne disease, which is predominantly a diarrheal disease, accounts for more than 80 million illnesses each year in the United States.[12] A prospective community-based study found an annual incidence rate of diarrhea in persons of all ages of 0.63 episodes per person-year of observation.[13] The highest incidence was in infants who had a rate of 1.43 episodes per person-year. In developed countries, the elderly may be another group at particular risk of diarrheal diseases. Adults in long-term care facilities have a greater problem with diarrheal diseases. Children attending day-care centers have a higher incidence because of person-to-person transmission within these settings.

Another group of individuals from developed countries who are at increased risk of diarrhea are those who travel to developing countries.[14] Numerous studies have demonstrated that about half of such travelers will develop diarrhea during a trip of approximately 2 weeks.

IMPACT OF DIARRHEA

It is well appreciated that diarrheal diseases are important causes of death in developing countries. It has been estimated that approxi-

Table 17–1 Diarrhea Incidence and Duration in Children Aged <6 Years in Community-Based Studies in Developing Countries

Study	Age Group (months)	Episodes	Diarrheal Incidence (per 100 child-years)	Diarrheal Duration (days)		
				1–7	8–14	≥15
Bangladesh	0–59	941	557	66	21	14
Brazil	0–71	519	600	82	15	3
India	0–71	471	61	35	55	10
Brazil	0–60	2896	1140	76	13	11
Peru	0–35	5302	807	88	9	3
Bangladesh	0–59	2609	455	71	22	7
Bangladesh	0–71	1074	195	50	27	23

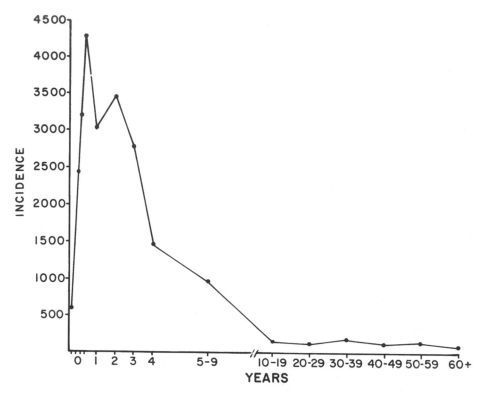

Figure 17–1 Annual age-specific incidence of diarrhea per 1,000 person-years assessed by household surveillance. *Source:* Reprinted with permission from R.E. Black et al., Incidence and Severity of Rotavirus and *Escherichia coli* Diarrhea in Rural Bangladesh, *Lancet,* Vol. 1, p. 142, © by The Lancet Ltd., 1981.

mately 3.3 million deaths occur each year in these settings from diarrheal diseases.[1] The diarrheal mortality rate is highest in the first year of life with about 20 deaths per 1,000 children. Although the rate of approximately 5 deaths per 1,000 children in the 1- to 4-year age group is lower, this group still accounts for approximately half of the diarrheal deaths in childhood.

The case fatality rates in children in developing countries have been reported to range from 0.1% to 0.5% in settings as diverse as urban Central African Republic, rural Egypt, rural North India, and rural Indonesia. It has been estimated that overall the diarrheal case fatality rate in children under age 5 years in developing countries is 0.2%. The case fatality rate is highest in the youngest children. In rural India, the case fatality rate for persistent diarrhea was re-

ported to be 20 times higher than that for acute diarrhea.[15]

In more developed countries, the diarrheal mortality rate and the illness case fatality rate are very low.[2,3] Although the highest incidence of diarrheal disease is in children, it is likely that fewer than 200 child deaths occur per year from diarrheal disease in the United States. Nearly all of the estimated 10,000 deaths per year from diarrheal diseases in the United States are in adults, with two thirds of these being in the elderly.

In developing countries, the infectious diseases of childhood have an adverse effect on growth. Diarrheal diseases have the greatest effect of all the infectious diseases, possibly because of reduction in appetite, altered feeding practices, and decreased absorption of nutrients, along with the very high prevalence of diarrhea in young children in these settings.[16] The magnitude of the effect of diarrheal diseases on growth seems to be modified by a number of factors. Continued breastfeeding and continued feeding during diarrhea can prevent weight faltering. In addition, children who consume a good diet will both better withstand the illness and have the potential to grow more rapidly after the illness to recover from any weight loss. Because most children in developed country settings usually have appropriate treatment and are receiving an adequate diet, the growth effects of diarrhea, especially given the low prevalence of the illness, is probably very small.

Diarrheal diseases are an economic burden because of the costs of medical care, medications, and lost work. Because the illnesses can largely be managed by fluid and nutritional therapy, much of the medication use (i.e., antibiotics and so-called antidiarrheal drugs) is an unnecessary expense and is potentially hazardous. In the United States, it is estimated that the economic burden of foodborne diseases for treatment and lost work of ill individuals is more than $28 billion per year.[12] Endemic childhood diarrhea costs many billions more.

MICROBIAL ETIOLOGIES

Relative Importance of Enteropathogens

Many bacterial, viral, and parasitic agents have been associated with diarrhea in both developing and developed countries. Because the highest rates of diarrheal diseases and the most severe consequences are generally in young children, most studies have focused on this age group. Older children and adults can become ill from the same enteropathogens, but the proportions of illness due to these organisms can vary because of immunity acquired from prior infection or from differential exposure to the various pathogens.

Community-based studies are those in which household visits are made to identify cases of diarrhea and to collect fecal specimens for identification of enteropathogens. These studies best represent the overall incidence of diarrheal disease, regardless of severity or care-seeking. Based on a review of 24 studies with comprehensive microbiology from 13 developing countries, enterotoxigenic *Escherichia coli* (ETEC), with a median of 14%, caused the most diarrheal episodes (Table 17–2). The next most commonly found organism is *Giardia lamblia*. *Campylobacter* species and rotavirus are both identified in 6% of these diarrheal episodes. *Cryptosporidium parvum* and *Shigella* species were both found in 4% of episodes. Other organisms were found less frequently. The relative importance of these organisms was variable in the different studies.

Studies in health facilities, either outpatient clinics or hospital wards, are done in a more selected group of patients for whom care was sought, often because of an illness of greater severity. A review of 73 studies conducted in health facilities in 33 developing countries found that rotavirus was the most frequently found enteropathogen, with a median of 20% (Table 17–3). However, these studies demonstrated that bacterial pathogens predominated overall, accounting for more than 30% of illnesses. Of these, the most common was ETEC. As illustrated in the range of percentage identification in Table 17–3, each of these bacterial pathogens can be found frequently in some settings. Among the parasites, *C. parvum* was the most common and *G. lamblia* and *Entamoeba histolytica* were less frequently identified.

In general, community-based studies identified an enteropathogen in approximately 50% of the episodes and the health facility–based studies in about 70%. The detection tests for many of the enteropathogens do not have optimal sensitivity, which may lead to underestimating the importance of the enteropathogen. In addition, other known enteropathogens were evaluated in most of these studies. Although it is likely that these enteropathogens individually account for only a small proportion of the episodes, collectively they likely cause most of the episodes not associated with one of the more common enteropathogens.

Table 17–2 Percentage Identification of Selected Enteropathogens in Children with Diarrhea in Community-Based Studies in Developing Countries

Enteropathogen	Number of Studies	Median	Range
Aeromonas sp	9	2	<1–13
Campylobacter sp	18	6	1–24
Cryptosporidium parvum	7	4	2–7
Entamoeba histolytica	17	<1	<1–9
Enterotoxigenic *Escherichia coli*	22	14	2–41
Giardia lamblia	18	10.5	<1–24
Rotavirus	22	6	2–29
Salmonella sp	23	1	0–6
Shigella sp	24	4	1–27
Vibrios	14	<1	0–3

Among the possible enteropathogens are viral agents, such as adenovirus, astrovirus, coronavirus, and Norwalk virus (Table 17–4). In addition, there are other 27-nm viruses similar to Norwalk virus that can also cause illnesses with diarrhea, vomiting, or both. The identification of an enteropathogen from feces during diarrhea does not necessarily mean that that organism is causing the illness. In fact, studies performing comprehensive microbiology often find two or more enteropathogens simultaneously, making it often impossible to ascertain which is causing the illness. These mixed infections could occur because the individual is exposed simultaneously or sequentially to more than one enteropathogen.

Asymptomatic enteric infections are common in developing countries and less so in developed country settings. In community-based studies, children often have been evaluated for enteropathogens on a routine basis, as well as when they had diarrhea. In health facility–based studies, controls were often evaluated (e.g., children who came to the same facility for a reason other than diarrhea). Community-based studies often find a similar rate of identification of entero-

Table 17–3 Percentage Identification of Selected Enteropathogens in Children with Diarrhea in Health Facilities in Developing Countries

Enteropathogen	Number of Studies	Median	Range
Aeromonas sp	22	2.5	<1–42
Campylobacter sp	56	7	0–32
Cryptosporidium parvum	10	4	1–12
Entamoeba histolytica	42	1	0–7
Enterotoxigenic *Escherichia coli*	51	11	1–54
Giardia lamblia	43	2	0–28
Rotavirus	58	20	5–49
Salmonella sp	71	4	0–38
Shigella sp	72	5	0–33
Vibrios	40	1	0–33

Table 17–4 Percentage Identification of Possible Viral Enteropathogens in Children with Diarrhea in Developing Countries

Virus	Number of Studies	Median	Range
Adenovirus	19	3	0–6
Astrovirus	5	2	<1–14
Coronavirus	3	3	0–3
Norwalk virus	5	3	<1–5

pathogens in children when they have diarrhea and when they do not. For example, in nine community-based studies in developing countries, the median identification of *Campylobacter* species in patients during diarrhea was 8% and during times when they did not have diarrhea it was 7% (Table 17–5). Some enteropathogens (e.g., rotavirus) can have a higher rate of identification in these studies during diarrhea, compared with times when the child is well. In health facility–based studies, often the distinction between diarrhea and control in regard to the percentage with enteropathogens is more clear (Table 17–5).

The pathogenicity (i.e., the number of infections with diarrhea per the total number of infections) varies by enteropathogen and in some cases by age (Table 17–6). For example, the pathogenicity of rotavirus is lower in the first 6 months of life than in the second 6 months, presumably because of passive protection from maternally derived antibody in early infancy.[17] On the other hand, some pathogens, such as *Shigella*

species, may have a higher pathogenicity early in childhood. This may occur because the initial infection induces some immunity that protects more against subsequent illness than against infection.

The virulence (i.e., the number of severe illnesses per the total number of illnesses) can also vary by enteropathogen. This can be illustrated by the propensity of the organism to cause an illness that leads to dehydration. In community-based studies in Bangladesh,[11,18] children with rotavirus diarrhea or cholera are most likely to develop dehydration (Table 17–7). Those with ETEC had a modestly increased rate of dehydration compared with all other types of diarrhea.

In the United States, the relative importance of the various enteropathogens differs from that in developing countries. In studies done in health facilities, rotavirus is the most prevalent enteropathogen associated with diarrhea, as it is in developing countries.[19] Table 17–8 shows the percentage of selected enteropathogens in children with diarrhea (and controls) attending an outpatient clinic in the United States. In general, the bacterial causes are less important in developed counties, although *Aeromonas*, *Campylobacter*, and *Salmonella* species may be important in some settings. This pattern may be shifted closer to a developing country pattern in certain higher-risk populations. For example, residents of Indian reservations in the United States have had higher rates of diarrhea than the general population, although good access to medical care has now reduced the diarrheal mortality to a very low level.[20,21] In such settings (Table 17–9),

Table 17–5 Median Percentage Identification of *Campylobacter* sp and Rotavirus from Cases of Diarrhea and Controls without Diarrhea in Community-Based Studies in Developing Countries

Enteropathogen	Community-Based Studies			Health Facility–Based Studies		
	(N)	Diarrhea	Control	(N)	Diarrhea	Control
Campylobacter sp	9	8	7	29	7	2
Rotavirus	11	4	1	31	21	4

Table 17–6 Pathogenicity of Selected Enteropathogens by Age Group in Peruvian Infants in Community-Based Study

Enteropathogen	Age 0–5 Months			Age 6–11 Months		
	Infections with Diarrhea (N)	Total Infections	Patho-genicity	Infections with Diarrhea (N)	Total Infections	Patho-genicity
Campylobacter sp	73	177	0.41	65	188	0.35
Enterotoxigenic *Escherichia coli*	42	119	0.35	40	103	0.39
Rotavirus	18	33	0.55	23	28	0.82
Shigella sp	14	17	0.82	16	34	0.47

rotavirus is still the most important pathogen, but other organisms such as ETEC and *Campylobacter* species may play a more prominent role than they do in the general population in the United States.

In the United States, approximately 500 outbreaks of foodborne disease are reported to the Centers for Disease Control and Prevention annually. Of those with a cause identified (40%), a bacterial organism has been found in 75%. Traditionally, *Salmonella* species, *Staphylococcus aureus*, and *Clostridium perfringens* have been considered the main responsible organisms, and they continue to be important. A number of other organisms, commonly spread by the foodborne route, notably *Campylobacter* species and *E. coli* O157:H7, have also caused substantial morbidity. In the five states participating in the U.S. Foodborne Diseases Active Surveillance Net-

work in 1998, the incidence rate of *Campylobacter* was 21.7 per 100,000 population, *Salmonella* 12.7 per 100,000, and *E. coli* O157:H7 2.8 per 100,000. A small percentage of annual outbreaks in the United States are caused by viruses (e.g., caliciviruses) or parasitic organisms (e.g., *Cryptosporidium* or *Cyclospora*). The incidence of *Cryptosporidium* ranged from 0.6 per 100,000 in Maryland to 3.7 to 100,000 in Minnesota. *S. aureus* was not part of this case surveillance. When investigating an outbreak of diarrhea that is possibly related to consumption of contaminated food, it is important to consider the different clinical presentations of these pathogens.[22] For example, staphylococcal illness often has severe vomiting along with diarrhea, does not usually present with fever, and generally lasts about a day. *C. perfringens* usually has diarrhea without fever and also lasts less than a

Table 17–7 Percentage of Children <5 Years Experiencing Dehydration during Diarrheal Episodes by Enteropathogen in Two Community-Based Studies in Rural Bangladesh

Enteropathogen	Episodes (N)	Dehydration (N)	Dehybration (%)
Rotavirus	78	28	36
Vibrio cholerae	3	1	33
Enterotoxigenic *Escherichia coli*	322	17	5
Other	843	17	2
Total	1246	63	76

Table 17–8 Percentage Identification of Selected Enteropathogens in Children with Diarrhea and Controls Attending an Outpatient Clinic in the United States

Enteropathogen	Diarrhea Cases (N = 246)	Controls (N = 155)
Adenovirus (enteric)	4	0
Aeromonas sp	6	7
Campylobacter sp	<1	<1
Cryptosporidium parvum	<1	0
Enterotoxigenic *Escherichia coli*	0	0
Giardia lamblia	<1	0
Rotavirus	22	10
Salmonella sp	5	0
Shigella sp	0	—
Vibrios	<1	0

Source: Adapted with permission from K.L. Kotloff et al., Acute Diarrhea in Baltimore Children Attending an Outpatient Clinic, *Pediatric Infectious Disease Journal*, Vol. 7, No. 11, pp. 753–759, Copyright © 1988, Lippincott Williams & Wilkins.

day. *Salmonella* infection often has diarrhea, vomiting, and fever and may last for several days. The incubation period of the causes of infectious foodborne diarrhea also differs. *Staphylococcus* has an incubation period of 2–7 hours, whereas *C. perfringens* has an incubation of 8–14 hours and *Salmonella* of 2–3 days.

SPECIFIC ENTEROPATHOGENS

Bacterial Agents

Campylobacter jejuni or *E. coli* cause watery diarrhea and sometimes dysentery, especially in young children.[23] Immunity acquired from campylobacter infections is the likely explanation

Table 17–9 Percentage Identification of Selected Enteropathogens in Children with Diarrhea in Different Settings on a U.S. Indian Reservation

Enteropathogen	Home	Outpatient Clinic (N = 535)	Hospital (N = 488)
Adenovirus	2	3	5
Aeromonas sp	1	1	2
Campylobacter sp	5	4	3
Enterotoxigenic *Escherichia coli*	5	5	14
Rotavirus	8	6	24
Salmonella sp	<1	1	1
Shigella sp	7	6	5
Vibrios	0	0	<1

Source: Adapted with permission from R.B. Sack et al., *Journal of Diarrhoeal Disease Research*, March 13 (1), pp. 12–17, © 1995, International Centre for Diarrhoeal Disease Research.

for the low rate of illness in adults and the high prevalence of asymptomatic infection occurring in developing countries. In the United States, *Campylobacter* species infection occurs in all age groups with peak incidences the first year of life and later in young adults. The higher rate of disease in young adults is said to be related to food handling errors made by these individuals when cooking. A summer seasonality is seen with *Campylobacter* species infections.

Escherichia coli can produce diarrhea by a variety of mechanisms.[24] Although *E. coli* organisms are part of the normal flora of the intestine, this organism can also possess a variety of virulence properties. The diarrheagenic potential of *E. coli* was recognized decades ago with the so-called enteropathogenic *E. coli* (EPEC).[25] These organisms were identified by the serotypes of *E. coli* that were implicated in diarrheal outbreaks. This nomenclature has now been superseded. Diarrheagenic *E. coli* are designated based on the demonstration of virulence properties or on laboratory characteristics felt to be associated with virulence properties. Some of the strains previously referred to as enteropathogenic have been found to produce "attaching and effacing" lesions in the intestine and patterns of adherence in tissue culture assays.[24,26] The pathogenic role of subgroups of these adherent *E. coli* in acute or persistent diarrhea has been well established, whereas the role of others is still in question.[27,28]

Other strains of enterotoxigenic *E. coli* produce a heat-labile toxin (LT), a heat-stable toxin (ST), or both. A number of assays can now be used to evaluate these organisms for toxin production or the genetic capability to produce these toxins.[24] Although these assays are not optimally sensitive because they require testing of a small number of organisms in the feces, ETEC are still the most frequent cause of diarrheal illnesses in children in developing countries. It has been demonstrated further that many ETEC produce colonization factors that are important in pathogenesis, indicating that not all toxin-producing *E. coli* are necessarily pathogens.[24] This may be a partial explanation for the high fre-

quency of asymptomatic infections with ETEC in developing country settings; it is also clear, however, that acquired immunity can protect from illness, but not from colonization.[29] An enteroinvasive type of *E. coli* has been described to result in dysentery and to have a pathogenesis similar to that found with *Shigella* species.[24] These organisms occasionally cause outbreaks, but they do not appear to be frequent causes of endemic diarrheal diseases.

In the early 1980s, *E. coli* O157:H7 was identified as an important cause of hemorrhagic colitis.[30] These organisms produce exotoxins, which resemble the Shiga toxin of *Shigella dysenteriae* type 1. These enterohemorrhagic *E. coli* (EHEC) have developed into a major public health problem in the United States and Canada, but appear to be rare in developing country settings. Large outbreaks of EHEC have occurred in which some patients developed hemolytic uremic syndrome or other serious complications, which can lead to death in approximately 2% of patients.[31] The primary reservoir for EHEC is cattle and transmission to humans has been most commonly related to consumption of undercooked ground beef or unpasteurized milk. Outbreaks have also been traced to other foods and person-to-person transmission, and predominates in day-care centers and other types of institutions.

Salmonella species continue to be an important public health problem in developed countries, but their importance varies in developing countries. In the United States, the highest attack rate for salmonellosis is in infants, but elderly and immunosuppressed individuals are also at high risk.[32] *Salmonella* species have animal hosts, especially poultry. In fact, *S. enteritidis* can colonize the ovaries of egg-laying hens, which can result in infection of the egg before it is laid.[33] The rates of salmonellosis have increased in developed countries in the last decade, all of which is from foodborne transmission. Salmonellosis often has a summer seasonality.

Four serogroups of *Shigella* exist. In developing countries, *S. flexneri* is the most common followed by *S. sonnei*, *S. boydii*, and *S. dysenteriae;* however, outbreaks of *S. dysenteriae* type 1 (or Shiga's bacillus) have occurred in many countries.[34,35] The resulting illnesses are often severe, resulting in high case fatality, and these organisms may be resistant to most commonly used antibiotics. In the United States and most developed countries, *S. sonnei* is the most common serogroup with *S. flexneri* accounting for most of the remainder.[36] In endemic situations, shigellosis is primarily a disease of children, reflecting the likelihood of fecal-oral transmission in this age group. Foodborne and waterborne outbreaks occur occasionally, but the predominant route of transmission is from person to person. Shigellosis has a seasonality predominantly in the warm months, although in developing countries this may also be influenced by the availability of water and changes in the level of personal hygiene.

Cholera is a diarrheal illness caused by infection of the small intestine with *Vibrio cholerae*. It has been feared for centuries because cholera epidemics can result in high mortality and social disruption.[37] A series of global pandemics of cholera have occurred. The seventh pandemic, which is still continuing, is generally thought to have begun in 1961. This pandemic, caused by the *V. cholerae*, biotype El Tor, spread from Sulawesi throughout Asia, the Middle East, the Soviet Union, Africa, and into a few countries of Europe. North America has had no indigenous cases of cholera in this century until a single case was detected in Texas in 1973. It has subsequently been discovered that *V. cholerae* El Tor is endemic in the Gulf Coast area of Texas and Louisiana; cases have sporadically occurred in that area. Latin America had been spared from cholera epidemics since the end of the last century; however, cholera reappeared in Peru in 1991. It subsequently spread throughout much of South and Central America, with some cases being imported into the United States.[38]

All previous cholera pandemics have been caused by *V. cholerae* serotype O1 until 1992 when cases of cholera associated with a *V. cholerae* strain that did not agglutinate with O1 antisera were reported from India and Bangladesh. This strain, subsequently designated serotype O139, caused epidemic disease throughout India and Bangladesh and cases in a number of other countries of Asia.[39] After the initial outbreaks due to this organism, the rates of disease have decreased, but the strain persists along with *V. cholerae* O1. These outbreaks demonstrate the potential for strains of *V. cholerae*, other than serotype O1, to cause epidemic cholera and may represent the beginning of a new pandemic.

In endemic areas, cholera predominantly affects children aged 2 to 5 years, but can cause a large proportion of severe watery diarrheal diseases in adults during the season of transmission.[37] Immunity develops after initial infection, although asymptomatic infections can still occur. In areas that have not had previous exposure to *V. cholerae*, the entire population is susceptible, resulting in high outbreak attack rates in children and adults. *Vibrio cholerae* may have an environmental reservoir in marshes and rivers and is commonly spread by seafood, as well as directly by water.

A number of other vibrios can cause diarrhea, as well as bacteremia and other serious illness.[40] *V. parahemolyticus* can cause diarrhea, including outbreaks. These illnesses occur with low frequency in most countries, but in Japan *V. parahemolyticus* is a frequent cause of diarrhea and outbreaks.[41] In North America, as well as other countries, *V. vulnificus* and non-O1 *V. cholerae* also cause diarrhea and systemic infection.[40,42]

Aeromonas hydrophila, often, and *Plesiomonas shigelloides*, less frequently, are found during episodes of diarrhea in developing countries.[43,44] These organisms appear much less frequently in developed country settings. At least for *A. hydrophila*, the higher rate of isolation of the organism during diarrhea compared with controls suggests a causative role.[45] However, the importance of these organisms and the mechanisms by which they can cause diarrhea are unknown.

Yersinia enterocolitica can cause diarrhea and other abdominal symptoms. It is a common cause of disease in Western Europe and outbreaks have occurred in the United States, primarily from contaminated meat and milk.[46] This organism has been sought in studies of diarrhea etiology in a number of developing countries, but has been rarely found in cases of diarrhea.[47]

Clostridium difficile causes colitis associated with the use of a variety of antibiotics. Although this organism can be found in acute diarrhea, the causative relationship is unclear.[48]

A number of other bacterial enteropathogens are associated with diarrheal diseases. These organisms are primarily involved in foodborne disease outbreaks, but can also cause sporadic cases of diarrhea. *Bacillus cereus* has been associated with outbreaks related to consumption of cooked rice and *Clostridium perfringens* is usually associated with outbreaks in which the spores of the organism germinate in anaerobic conditions after meat has been cooked, resulting in the production of the toxin that causes diarrhea.[49] *Staphylococcus aureus* outbreaks of diarrhea are often caused by a food handler contaminating a food, resulting in production by the organism of a heat-stable enterotoxin. Ingestion of this pre-formed toxin causes the illness.

Strains of *Bacteroides fragilis* that produce an enterotoxin have recently been associated with diarrheal diseases, both in the United States and in Bangladesh.[50,51] Because of limited availability of the diagnostic assay, the importance of this enteropathogen is unknown.

Viral Agents

Rotaviruses are the most important viral agent causing diarrheal diseases. Illness largely occurs in the first 2 years of life throughout the world.[11,52,53] Rotavirus diarrhea has a winter seasonality in most developed countries, but the seasonality in developing countries is less marked with disease occurring throughout the year. In addition to the role of rotavirus as an endemic enteropathogen, outbreaks have occurred in day-care centers and hospitals. The organism may be a cause of a small proportion of disease in adults, such as caregivers for small children and in travelers from developed countries to developing countries.

Enteric adenoviruses (serotypes 40 and 41) are the second most important cause of viral diarrhea.[54,55] These organisms appear to occur worldwide. The Norwalk agent and related 27-nm caliciviruses (e.g., Hawaii and Snow Mountain agents) cause watery diarrhea, vomiting, or both.[56] Although no diagnostic test for these agents using feces is readily available, sero-epidemiologic studies indicate that these agents occur worldwide. Several studies indicate that the Norwalk agent alone may account for 2% to 5% of childhood diarrheas in developing countries.[57] It may have a similar importance in the United States. The importance of the other caliciviruses is unknown, they likely cause an additional fraction of diarrheal episodes.

Other viruses or viruslike particles have been proposed as causes of diarrhea.[58,59] Coronaviruses, astroviruses, and small, round viruslike particles have been found during diarrhea. Pestivirus has also been reported in association with diarrhea.[60] The causative role of these agents and their importance is unknown.

Parasitic Agents

Cryptosporidium parvum, a coccidian parasite, is likely the most important parasitic cause of diarrheal diseases.[61] It has a global distribution as an endemic disease, but may also occur in outbreaks, including large waterborne outbreaks from municipal water systems. Cryptosporidial cysts are very resistant to chlorine and must be removed from drinking water by filtration. Related organisms of the true coccidia, such as *Isospora belli* can cause diarrhea, but they appear to be uncommon except possibly in association with AIDS.[62] Diarrhea associated with microsporidia also occurs with AIDS, but the role of this organism in immunocompetent individuals is not described.[63]

Cyclospora cayetanensis, previously referred to as "cyanobacterium-like bodies" and other names, is a newly described enteropathogen.[64] These coccidian parasites have been found in a number of developing countries and may be of comparable importance to *C. parvum*. In developed countries, these organisms have been known to cause diarrheal disease in AIDS patients and in travelers to developing countries.[65,66] Outbreaks have been reported from consumption of imported raspberries.

Giardia lamblia is a common protozoan with a very high carriage rate in populations in many developing countries, particularly in children.[67] It does not appear to be an important diarrheal pathogen in most developing country settings.[68,69] In developed countries, *G. lamblia* may be a frequent parasitic cause of diarrhea.[70] Infections are passed from person to person and are common in day-care centers and other institutions. Water- or foodborne outbreaks have also occurred. As with *C. parvum*, prevention of waterborne giardiasis depends on adequate water filtration to remove the parasitic cysts.

Entamoeba histolytica can cause amebiasis, and it may be associated with extra-intestinal complications, such as liver abscess.[71,72] This parasite appears to be a less frequent cause of childhood diarrhea or dysentery in developing countries and is rare in developed countries. Other protozoan infections can be associated with diarrhea, including those caused by *Balantidium coli* and *Chilomastix mesnili. Blastocystis hominis* is of uncertain pathogenicity.[73]

Most intestinal helminthic infections are not associated with diarrhea, but dysentery and even rectal prolapse has been associated with severe *Trichuris trichiura* infections and diarrhea with other intestinal parasites.[74]

TRANSMISSION ROUTES

General Factors

Diarrheal diseases result from exposure of a susceptible host to a pathogenic organism. Nearly all enteropathogens are transmitted by direct contact with human feces or indirectly through contact with feces through water, food, or eating utensils. Some enteropathogens have an animal or environmental reservoir and contact with the pathogen from these sources can then result in infection. It is clear that populations of lower socioeconomic status or educational level may have a higher exposure to enteropathogens because of living in poorer environmental conditions or having less hygienic practices, particularly in child care.

Water

Waterborne transmission has been documented for most enteropathogens.[75] For some, such as *V. cholerae* and Norwalk virus, this may be the predominant form of transmission, but even for these pathogens foodborne transmission also may be common. The use of contaminated sources of water for bathing, washing, swimming, cleaning, and washing feeding utensils has been implicated in both transmission and consumption of contaminated water.[76]

In developing country settings without access to tap water in the home, poor handling practices of water stored in the house, mainly by introduction of contaminated hands or utensils into water containers, have been linked to an increased risk for diarrheal diseases.[77] Studies have now documented that water quantity in many situations is more important than water quality for diarrheal diseases.[75] This is because water availability is important for hygienic behaviors that would prevent much of the transmission by person to person or through food.

Food

Breastfeeding, especially exclusively, protects against diarrheal diseases.[78,79] This is in part because breastfed children are less exposed to enteropathogens that might be in food or water. Furthermore, breast milk may provide passive immunologic protection against some of the organisms. Especially in developing countries, the incidence of diarrheal diseases increases sharply with the introduction of weaning foods.[80] These foods are often heavily contaminated; studies have demonstrated the relationship between consumption of more contaminated foods and illness related to organisms such as ETEC.[81] The level of bacterial contamination can vary by the type of food and by food handling practices. It is strongly influenced by the storage time between initial preparation and consumption because many of the bacterial enteropathogens can multiply in the food during storage at ambient temperature.[81] Food can be contaminated in the home or before it reaches the home. In developing countries, most foods are assumed to be contaminated. This applies even to uncooked fruits and vegetables that might become contaminated from irrigation with sewage or through improper handling. In the United States and other developed countries, some foods (e.g., chicken) are also assumed to be contaminated with *Salmonella* and *Campylobacter* species.[49] In addition, the recent outbreaks of *E. coli* O157:H7 suggest that all ground beef must be considered potentially contaminated with this organism. Until further control of these infections in the reservoir and at the processing level are implemented, the primary control is proper cooking.

In developing countries, much of the food production is still done in small scale at the local level. In contrast, in developed countries an increasing trend is seen toward large-scale production and distribution of food. These production and slaughtering techniques (e.g., of poultry) make contamination with enteropathogens much more widespread. In addition, developed countries are increasingly importing food from all over the world.[49] This means that consumers are at risk of exposure to contaminated fruits and vegetables, as well as other products.

Feeding Utensils

In developing countries, baby bottles, bottle nipples, cups, spoons, and food containers are frequently contaminated with fecal bacteria, as well as with specific enteropathogens.[17,82] These utensils are difficult to keep clean in unhygienic environments. Although boiling or the use of sterilizing solution is effective in eliminating contamination, these methods may be used inconsistently. The risk of feeding utensils, water, and food contamination makes breastfeeding

that much more desirable in settings with poor environmental sanitation.

Animals

Animals can be the reservoir for a variety of enteropathogens.[31,83,84] Poultry is the primary source for *C. jejuni* and *Salmonella* species, whereas an important animal reservoir for *E. coli* O157:H7 is cattle. *C. perfringens* is also commonly associated with animals and *Y. enterocolitica* commonly with pigs and cows. Shellfish can be a reservoir for *V. cholerae* and other vibrios.

Flies

A variety of enteropathogens have been isolated from flies, including bacterial, viral, and parasitic.[85] The organisms can be carried on the external surface of the fly or ingested, in which case the bacteria survival can be prolonged. Conceivably, flies could contaminate food or even water in the house, but the evidence for flies as a means of transmission is inconclusive.[85] Intervention studies have shown that fly control at a military camp in Israel resulted in reduced diarrhea and particularly shigellosis.[86] These findings need to be confirmed in populations that are more typical of developing countries lacking adequate water and sanitation and with poor hygiene before fly control can be promoted as a major public health intervention in those areas.

Hygiene

Personal hygiene practices are closely linked with person-to-person transmission of diarrhea.[87] Of hygiene practices, handwashing is probably the most widely studied. The increased risk of diarrhea with inadequate handwashing, in particular after defecation or cleaning a child, has been documented. Intervention studies have confirmed this by demonstrating a reduction in the incidence of diarrhea with proper handwashing.[88,89] Handwashing with soap is effective in eliminating fecal contamination, even viruses. In developing countries where soap may not be available, handwashing with mud, ash, or other agents that facilitate removal of contaminants from the hands has also been found to be effective, but rinsing with water alone less so.[90]

Another important hygiene behavior is proper disposal of fecal material. In developing countries with poor sanitation, defecation in the yard or in open areas and nonhygienic methods of feces disposal are demonstrated risk factors for diarrhea. Crawling infants who may come in contact with the feces on the ground are at particular risk.[91] A transmission risk may also exist in unhygienic latrines or school toilets.

HOST RISK FACTORS

Nutrition

Malnutrition and diarrheal diseases are often found together in developing countries because they coexist in children living in poor socioeconomic and environmental conditions. In addition, malnutrition can be a direct risk factor for diarrheal diseases through compromised immunologic function and tissue regenerative capability. Malnourished children in developing countries have been found to have a risk of diarrhea increased by up to 70%.[92–94] Other studies, however, found no increase in diarrheal incidence in malnourished children.[95] Nearly all studies show that malnourished children have diarrheal episodes of longer duration and often greater severity.[95]

Micronutrient Deficiencies

In addition to general malnutrition, specific micronutrient deficiencies can result in either a higher incidence or greater severity of diarrhea. Vitamin A deficiency is associated with more severe diarrhea; in deficient populations, vitamin A supplementation reduced diarrheal mortality.[96,97] Zinc deficiency is also related to diarrhea. Zinc supplementation in populations presumed to be deficient reduced the incidence and duration of diarrheal episodes.[98] Other micronutrients may be related to diarrhea as well. As with malnutrition in general, these specific micronutrient deficiencies can result in immunologic compromise or reduced ability to repair damaged intestinal mucosa.

Gastric Acid

The acidic contents of the stomach are an important barrier to ingested enteropathogens, especially many of the bacterial agents. Hypochlorhydria can increase the likelihood that an adequate quantity of the pathogen would reach the small intestine and cause infection.[99] Thus, medical conditions that reduce gastric acid or medications that neutralize the acid may lead to a greater frequency or severity of diarrheal diseases. Furthermore, *Helicobacter pylori* infection in the stomach is common in children in developing countries.[100] Because this infection can cause hypochlorhydria, it may result in a greater risk of diarrhea.

Genetic Factors

Some genetic predisposition to diarrheal diseases exists, but current evidence is very limited. Persons of blood group O have a greater risk of developing cholera and have more severe illness than persons of other blood groups.[101] Few studies have been done to examine such a relationship between blood group and other enteropathogens, but limited data do not demonstrate a strong relationship for ETEC or vibrios other than *V. cholerae* O1.[102,103]

IMMUNITY

Immunity plays an important role in susceptibility to enteropathogens. Maternal antibody is provided to the infant through breast milk, which protects against a variety of enteric infections. Transplacental antibody may also play a role in some infections. Immunity is actively acquired by the individual who has a diarrheal disease or, in some cases, even an asymptomatic infection.

Some evidence indicates that the immune system can be compromised by micronutrient deficiencies, reducing the resistance to enteric infection. Studies have shown that depressed cell-mediated immunity is associated with an increase in both acute and persistent diarrhea.[93,94] Immunocompetence in a child can be compromised by previous viral infections, such as measles or influenza, or by other infections, such as tuberculosis or typhoid fever. These infections, along with micronutrient deficiencies could place individuals at a greater risk of diarrhea or of more severe illness through alteration in immune function or by other mechanisms.

A vaccine is currently available for cholera. A parenteral cholera vaccine provides approximately 50% protection lasting for less than 6 months. New killed or live *V. cholerae* vaccines may offer greater efficacy and duration of protection. An oral vaccine consisting of killed vibrios resulted in 52% efficacy for preventing cholera during a 3-year period in Bangladesh. Addition of the B subunit of cholera toxin to the vaccine to stimulate antitoxic immunity did not enhance protection during this period. A live attenuated strain of *V. cholerae* that has shown high efficacy in volunteer studies is being evaluated in a large field trial.

A vaccine for rotavirus has recently been licensed in the United States and some countries in Europe. This oral attenuated vaccine has been recommended for routine use in early infancy, but use has been suspended in the United States due to reported cases of intussuception following vaccination. Vaccines for many other important enteropathogens, such as campylobacter, ETEC, and *Shigella*, are also in development and being evaluated.

ANTIMICROBIAL RESISTANCE

A progressive increase in resistance to antibiotics has been seen among the bacterial enteropathogens.[104] For some of the enteropathogens for which there is an animal reservoir, this resistance may be the result of large-scale use of antimicrobial agents to prevent or treat infections in

the animals, including provisional low-dose antibiotics in animal feed.[105] Certainly, extensive use of antibiotics for human infections also plays a part in the development of antimicrobial resistance. Especially problematic is the extensive use of antibiotics in developing countries without prescription or medical supervision.[106] This has resulted in outbreaks caused by organisms such as *V. cholerae* and *Shigella dysenteriae* type 1, which are resistant to most commonly used antibiotics. Unfortunately, in developing countries alternative antibiotics are often unavailable or unaffordable.

STRATEGIES FOR CONTROL

Reduction of mortality from diarrheal diseases by appropriate treatment is the mainstay of diarrheal disease control programs.[6] Correction of dehydration by oral rehydration therapy, or intravenous therapy if necessary, and maintenance of nutrition by continued feeding during illness have played an important role in reducing diarrheal disease mortality throughout the world. Antibiotic therapy of dysentery as presumed shigellosis and of cholera will reduce the illness severity and case fatality rate; a few of the parasitic agents can also be specifically treated with antimicrobial agents.

For developing countries, reduction in the incidence of diarrheal diseases is a continuing challenge. Reviews of intervention research concluded that promotion of breastfeeding and improved weaning practices are a high priority for diarrheal prevention. It was estimated that successful breastfeeding promotion programs could reduce diarrheal incidence early in infancy and childhood diarrheal mortality rates by up to 9%.[107] Improved weaning practices could have the added advantage of improving the nutritional content of the diet as well as decreasing microbial contamination.[108,109]

Vitamin A supplementation has been shown to reduce diarrheal mortality in children ages 6 to 59 months old, and zinc supplementation was found in randomized controlled trials to reduce diarrhea prevalence by 25%.[110] Improved water supply, sanitation, and hygiene behaviors would also be expected to reduce diarrheal incidence. If both water supply and sanitation are improved in a typical developing country setting, it was estimated that diarrheal incidence and mortality could be reduced by about 25%.[75] Hygiene education may further enhance the impact. In fact, handwashing education programs have been found to reduce diarrheal incidence by 14% to 48%.[87] It may be expected that programs combining water supply, sanitation, and hygiene education may reduce diarrheal morbidity by 25% to 50%.

Measles immunization, which is currently being widely implemented in developing countries, would likely result in a slight reduction in diarrheal incidence and a more substantial reduction in diarrheal mortality.[111] Improved cholera vaccines may have a role for control of this disease in selected populations.[112] A vaccine for rotavirus could potentially have widespread applicability in developing countries because rotavirus may be responsible for 5% of all diarrheal episodes and 20% of diarrheal deaths.[112] A

highly efficacious vaccine that can be administered early in infancy will be necessary for this to be successfully used as a control strategy. Because rotavirus diarrhea is also an important cause of morbidity and health care costs in developed countries, a vaccine would likely be a cost-effective preventive strategy in these settings as well.[4]

Whereas reduction in the incidence of diarrhea and its complications will follow from general economic development and improved environmental conditions, it is clear that particular interventions could speed the progress in this regard. Although efforts must continue to provide effective case management for diarrhea, increasing emphasis should be given to prevention of diarrheal morbidity. This is feasible, even in developing country settings, through improved feeding practices and nutrition and an enhanced water supply, sanitation, and hygiene. Because numerous enteropathogens cause diarrhea, especially in the developing countries, and because vaccines protect only against specific organisms, these more general control measures are essential.

REFERENCES

1. Bern C, Martines J, de Zoysa I, Glass RI. The magnitude of the global problem of diarrheal disease: a ten-year update. *Bull World Health Organ.* 1992;70:705–714.

2. Kilgore PE, Holman RC, Matthew MS, et al. Trends of diarrheal disease–associated mortality in US children, 1968 through 1991. *JAMA.* 1995;274:1143–1148.

3. Glass RI, Lew JF, Gangarosa RE, et al. Estimates of morbidity and mortality rates for diarrheal disease in American children. *J Pediatr.* 1991;118:27–33.

4. Smith JC, Haddix AC, Teutsch SM, Glass RI. Cost-effectiveness analysis of a rotavirus immunization program for the United States. *Pediatrics.* 1995;96:609–615.

5. Newsholme A. *Fifty Years in Public Health.* London: George Allen and Unwin; 1939:321–360.

6. Claeson M, Merson MH. Global progress in the control of diarrheal diseases. *Pediatr Infect Dis J.* 1990;9:345–355.

7. Baqui AH, Black RE, Yunus MD, Hoque ARA, Chowdhury HR, Sack RB. Methodological issues in diarrhoeal diseases epidemiology: definition of diarrhoeal episodes. *Int J Epidemiol.* 1991;20:1057–1063.

8. Black RE. Persistent diarrhea in children of developing countries. *Pediatr Inf Dis J.* 1993;12:751–761.

9. McAuliffe JF, Shields DS, de Souza MA, Sakell J, Schorling J, Guerrant RL. Prolonged and recurring diarrhea in the northeast of Brazil: examination of cases from a community-based study. *J Pediatr Gastroenterol Nutr.* 1986;5:902–906.

10. Baqui AH, Black RE, Sack RB, Yunus MD, Siddique AK, Chowdhury HR. Epidemiological and clinical characteristics of acute and persistent diarrhea in rural Bangladeshi children. *Acta Paediatr.* 1992;381(Suppl):15–21.

11. Black RE, Merson MH, Huq I, Alim ARMA, Yunus MD. Incidence and severity of rotavirus and *Escherichia coli* diarrhoea in rural Bangladesh. *Lancet.* 1981;1:141–143.

12. Archer DL, Kvenberg JE. Incidence and cost of foodborne diarrheal disease in the United States. *J Food Protect.* 1985;48:887–894.

13. Monto AS, Koopman JS. The Tecumseh Study: XI occurrence of acute enteric illness in the community. *Am J Epidemiol.* 1980;112:323–333.

14. Black RE. Epidemiology of travelers' diarrhea and relative importance of various pathogens. *Rev Infect Dis.* 1990;12(Suppl 1):S73–S79.

15. Bhan MK, Arora NH, Ghai KR, Khoshoo V, Bhandari N. Major factors in diarrhoea related mortality among rural children. *Indian J Med Res.* 1986;83:9–12.

16. Black RE. Would control of childhood infectious diseases reduce malnutrition? *Acta Paediatr Scand Suppl.* 1991;374:133–140.

17. Black RE, Lopez de Romana G, Brown KH, Bravo N, Bazalar OG, Kanashiro HC. Incidence and etiology of infantile diarrhea and major routes of transmission in Huascar, Peru. *Am J Epidemiol.* 1989;129:785–799.

18. Black RE, Brown KH, Becker S, Abdul Alim ARM, Huq I. Longitudinal studies of infectious diseases and physical growth of children in rural Bangladesh. II. Incidence of diarrhea and association with known pathogens. *Am J Epidemiol.* 1982;115:315–324.

19. Kotloff KL, Wasserman SS, Steciak JY, et al. Acute diarrhea in Baltimore children attending an outpatient clinic. *Pediatr Infect Dis J.* 1988;7:753–759.

20. Sack RB, Santosham M, Reid R, et al. Diarrhoeal diseases in the White Mountain Apaches: clinical studies. *J Diarrhoeal Dis Res.* 1995;13:12–17.

21. Santosham M, Sack RB, Reid R, et al. Diarrheal diseases in the White Mountain Apaches: epidemiologic studies. *J Diarrhoeal Dis Res.* 1995;13:18–28.

22. Horwitz MA. Specific diagnosis of foodborne diseases. *Gastroenterology.* 1977;73:375–381.

23. Nachamkin I, Blaser MJ, Tompkins LS, eds. *Campylobacter jejuni: Current Status and Future Trends.* Washington, DC: American Society for Microbiology; 1992.

24. Levine MM. *Escherichia coli* that cause diarrhea: enterotoxigenic, enteropathogenic, enteroinvasive, enterohemorrhagic, and enteroadherent. *J Infect Dis.* 1987; 155:377–388.

25. Robins-Browne RM. Traditional enteropathogenic *Escherichia coli* of infantile diarrhea. *Rev Infect Dis.* 1987;9:28–53.

26. Clausen CR, Christie DL. Chronic diarrhea in infants caused by adherent enteropathogenic *Escherichia coli.* *J Pediatr.* 1982;100:358–361.

27. Korzeniowski OM, Dantas W, Trabulsi LR, Guerrant RL. A controlled study of endemic sporadic diarrhea among adult residents of southern Brazil. *Trans R Soc Trop Med Hyg.* 1984;84:363–369.

28. Lanata CF, Black RE, Gilman RH, Lazo F, Del Aquila R. Epidemiologic, clinical, and laboratory characteristics of acute vs. persistent diarrhea in periurban Lima, Peru. *J Ped Gastroenterol Nutr.* 1991;12:82–88.

29. Black RE, Merson MH, Rowe B, et al. Enterotoxigenic *Escherichia coli* diarrhoea: acquired immunity and transmission in an endemic area. *Bull World Health Organ.* 1981;59:263–268.

30. Riley LW, Remis RS, Helgerson SD, et al. Hemorrhagic colitis associated with a rare *Escherichia coli* serotype. *N Engl J Med.* 1983;308:681.

31. Griffin PM, Tauxe RV. The epidemiology of infections caused by *Escherichia coli* O157:H7, other enterohemorrhagic *E. coli*, and the associated hemolytic uremic syndrome. *Epidemiol Rev.* 1991;13:60–98.

32. Chalker RB, Blaser MJ. A review of human salmonellosis: III. Magnitude of salmonella infections in the United States. *Rev Infect Dis.* 1987;7:111–124.

33. Gast RK, Beard CW. Production of *Salmonella enteritidis* contaminated eggs by experimentally infected hens. *Avian Dis.* 1990;34:438–446.

34. Khan MU, Roy NC, Islam R, Huq I, Stoll B. Fourteen years of shigellosis in Dhaka: an epidemiological analysis. *Int J Epidemiol.* 1985;14:607–613.

35. Ebright JR, Moore EC, Sanborn WR, Schaeberg D, Kyle J, Ishida K. Epidemic shiga bacillus dysentery in Central Africa. *Am J Trop Med Hyg.* 1984;33:1192–1197.

36. Lee LA, Shapiro CN, Hargrett-Bean N, et al. Hyperendemic shigellosis in the United States: a review of surveillance data for 1967–1988. *J Infect Dis.* 1991;164:894–900.

37. Glass RI, Black RE. The epidemiology of cholera. In: Barua D, Greenough III WB, eds. *Cholera.* New York: Plenum Medical Book Company; 1992:129–154.

38. Ries AA, Vugia DJ, Beingolea L, et al. Cholera in Piura, Peru: a modern urban epidemic. *J Infect Dis.* 1992;166:1429–1433.

39. Cholera Working Group, International Centre for Diarrhoeal Diseases Research, Bangladesh. Large epidemic of cholera-like disease in Bangladesh caused by *Vibrio cholerae* O139 synonym Bengal. *Lancet.* 1993;342:387–390.

40. Black PA, Weaver RE, Hollis DG. Diseases of humans (other than cholera) caused by vibrios. *Annu Rev Microbiol.* 1980;34:341.

41. Fukami T, Saku K. Clinical epidemiology of infectious enteritis of outpatients at Tokyo Metropolitan Bokuto General Hospital. In: Saito M, Nakaya R, Matsubara Y, eds. *Infectious Enteritis in Japan.* Tokyo: Saikon Publishing; 1986:211–220.

42. Levine WC, Griffin PM, and the Gulf Coast Working Group. Vibrio infections on the Gulf Coast: results of first year of regional surveillance. *J Infect Dis.* 1993; 167:479–483.

43. Holmberg SD, Farmer III JJ. *Aeromonas hydrophila* and *Plesiomonas shigelloides* as causes of intestinal infections. *Rev Infect Dis.* 1984;6:633–639.

44. Rennels MB, Levine MM. Classical bacterial diarrhea:

perspectives and update—salmonella, shigella, *Escherichia coli*, aeromonas, and plesiomonas. *Pediatr Infect Dis.* 1986;5(Suppl 1):S91–S100.

45. Gracey M, Burke V, Robinson J. Aeromonas-associated gastroentertis. *Lancet.* 1982;2:1304–1306.

46. Black RE, Jackson RJ, Tsai TF, et al. Epidemic *Yersinia enterocolitica* infection due to contaminated chocolate milk. *N Engl J Med.* 1978;298:76–79.

47. Samadi AR, Wachsmuth K, Huq MI, Mahbub M, Agbonlahor DE. An attempt to detect *Yersinia enterocolitica*. *Trop Geograph Med.* 1982;34:151–154.

48. Torres JF, Cedillo R, Sánchez J, Dillman C, Giono S, Muñoz O. Prevalence of *Clostridium difficile* and its cytotoxin in infants in Mexico. *J Clin Microbiol.* 1984;20: 274–275.

49. Bean NH, Griffin PM. Foodborne disease outbreaks in the United States, 1973–1987: pathogens, vehicles and trends. *J Food Protect.* 1990;53:804–817.

50. Sack RB, Myers LL, Almeido-Hill J, et al. Enterotoxigenic *Bacteroides fragilis*: epidemiologic studies of its role as a human diarrhoeal pathogen. *J Diarrhoeal Dis Res.* 1992;10:4–9.

51. Sack RB, Albert MJ, Alam K, et al. Isolation of enterotoxigenic *Bacteroides fragilis* from Bangladeshi children with diarrhea: a controlled study. *J Clin Microbiol.* 1994;32:960–963.

52. Yolken RH, Wyatt RG, Zissis G, et al. Epidemiology of human rotavirus types 1 and 2 as studied by enzyme-linked immunosorbent assay. *N Engl J Med.* 1978; 299:1156.

53. Black RE, Merson MH, Rahman ASMM, et al. A two year study of bacterial, viral, and parasitic agents associated with diarrhea in rural Bangladesh. *J Infect Dis.* 1980;142:660–664.

54. Gary Jr GW, Hierholzer JC, Black RE. Characteristics of noncultivable adenoviruses associated with diarrhea in infants: a new subgroup of human adenoviruses. *J Clin Microbiol.* 1979;10:96–103.

55. Uhnoo I, Wadell G, Svensson L, Johansson ME. Importance of enteric adenoviruses 40 and 41 in acute gastroenteritis in infants and young children. *J Clin Microbiol.* 1984;20:365–372.

56. Greenberg HB, Valdesuso J, Kapikian AZ, et al. Prevalence of antibody to the Norwalk virus in various countries. *Infect Immun.* 1979;26:270–273.

57. Black RE, Greenberg HB, Kapikian AZ, Brown KH, Becker S. Acquisition of serum antibody to Norwalk virus and rotavirus and relation to diarrhea in a longitudinal study of young children in rural Bangladesh. *J Infect Dis.* 1982;145:483–489.

58. Tiemessen CT, Wegerhoff FO, Erasmus MJ, Kidd AH. Infection by enteric adenoviruses, rotaviruses, and other agents in a rural African environment. *J Med Virol.* 1989;28:176–182.

59. Kurtz JB, Lee TW, Pickering D. Astrovirus associated gastroenteritis in a children's ward. *J Clin Path.* 1977; 30:948–952.

60. Yolken R, Dubovi E, Leister F, et al. Infantile gastroenteritis associated with excretion of pestivirus antigens. *Lancet.* 1989;1:517–520.

61. Current WL, Garcia LS. Cryptosporidiosis. *Clin Microbiol Rev.* 1991;4:325–358.

62. Guerrant RL, Bobak DA. Bacterial and protozoal gastroenteritis. *N Engl J Med.* 1991;325(5):327–340.

63. Shadduck JA. Human microsporidiosis and AIDS. *Rev Infect Dis.* 1989;11:203–207.

64. Ortega YR, Sterling CR, Gilman RH, Cama VA, Diaz F. *Cyclospora* species: a new protozoan pathogen of humans. *N Engl J Med.* 1993;328:1308–1312.

65. Shlim DR, Cohen MT, Eaton M, et al. An alga-like organism associated with an outbreak of prolonged diarrhea among foreigners in Nepal. *Am J Trop Med Hyg.* 1991;45:383–389.

66. Elder GH, Hunter PR, Codd GA. Hazardous freshwater cyanobacteria (blue-green algae). *Lancet.* 1993;341: 1519–1520.

67. Stevens DP. Selective primary health care: strategies for control of disease in the developing world. XIX. Giardiasis. *Rev Infect Dis.* 1985;7:530–535.

68. Gilman RH, Marquis GS, Miranda E, Vestegui M, Martinez H. Rapid reinfection of *Giardia lamblia* after treatment in hyperendemic third world community. *Lancet.* 1988;1:343–345.

69. Sullivan PS, DuPont HL, Arafat RR, et al. Illness and reservoirs associated with *Giardia lamblia* infection in rural Egypt: the case against treatment in developing world environments of high endemicity. *Am J Epidemiol.* 1988;127:1272–1281.

70. Flanagan PA. Giardia—diagnosis, clinical course and epidemiology: a review. *Epidemiol Infect.* 1992;109:1–22.

71. Wanke C, Butler T, Islam M. Epidemiologic and clinical features of invasive amebiasis in Bangladesh: a case control comparison with other diarrheal diseases and postmortem findings. *Am J Trop Med Hyg.* 1988; 38:335–341.

72. Nanda R, Bavaja U, Anand BS. *Entamoeba histolytica* cyst passers: clinical features and outcome in untreated subjects. *Lancet.* 1984;2:301–303.

73. Casemore DP. Foodborne protozoal infection. *Lancet.* 1990;336:1427–1443.

74. Genta RM. Diarrhea in helminthic infections. *Clin Infect Dis.* 1993;16(Suppl 2):S122–S129.

75. Esrey SA, Feachem RG, Hughes JM. Interventions for the control of diarrhoeal diseases among young children: improving water supplies and excreta disposal facilities. *Bull World Health Organ.* 1985;63:757–772.

76. Hughes JM, Boyce JM, Levine RJ, et al. Epidemiology of El Tor cholera in rural Bangladesh: importance of surface water in transmission. *Bull World Health Organ.* 1982;60:395–404.

77. Swerdlow DL, Mintz ED, Rodriguez M, et al. Waterborne transmission of epidemic cholera in Trujillo, Peru: lessons for a continent at risk. *Lancet.* 1992;340:28–33.

78. Brown KH, Black RE, Lopez de Romaña G, Creed de Kanashiro H. Infant-feeding practices and their relationship with diarrheal and other diseases in Huascar (Lima), Peru. *Pediatrics.* 1989;83:31–40.

79. Popkin BM, Adair L, Akin JS, Black R, Briscoe J, Flieger W. Breast-feeding and diarrheal morbidity. *Pediatrics.* 1990;86:874–882.

80. Barrell RAE, Rowland MGM. Infant foods as a potential source of diarrhoeal illness in rural West Africa. *Trans R Soc Trop Med Hyg.* 1979;73:85–90.

81. Black RE, Brown KH, Becker S, Abdul Alim ARM, Merson MH. Contamination of weaning foods and transmission of enterotoxigenic *Escherichia coli* diarrhoea in children in rural Bangladesh. *Trans R Soc Trop Med Hyg.* 1982;76:259–264.

82. Cherian A, Lawande RV. Recovery of potential pathogens from feeding bottle contents and teats in Zaria, Nigeria. *Trans R Soc Trop Med Hyg.* 1985;79:840–842.

83. Rodrigue DC, Tauxe RV, Rower B. International increase in *Salmonella enteritidis*: a new pandemic? *Epidemiol Infect.* 1990;105:21–27.

84. Blaser MJ, LaForce FM, Wilson NA, Wang WL. Reservoirs for human campylobacteriosis. *J Infect Dis.* 1980;141:665–669.

85. Esrey SA. *Interventions for the Control of Diarrhoeal Diseases among Young Children: Fly Control.* Geneva: World Health Organization; 1991. WHO/CDD/91.37.

86. Cohen D, Green M, Block C, et al. Reduction of transmission of shigellosis by control of houseflies (*Musca domestica*). *Lancet.* 1991;337:993–997.

87. Feachem RG. Interventions for the control of diarrhoeal diseases among young children: promotion of personal and domestic hygiene. *Bull World Health Organ.* 1984;62:467–476.

88. Black, RE, Dykes AC, Anderson KE, et al. Handwashing to prevent diarrhea in day-care centers. *Am J Epidemiol.* 1981;113:445–451.

89. Khan MU. Interruption of shigellosis by hand washing. *Trans R Soc Trop Med Hyg.* 1982;76:164–168.

90. Hoque BA, Briend A. A comparison of local handwashing agents in Bangladesh. *J Trop Med Hyg.* 1991;94:61–64.

91. Zeitlin MF, Guldan G, Klein RE, Ahmad N, Ahmad K. *Sanitary Conditions of Crawling Infants in Rural Bangladesh.* Report to the USAID Asia Bureau and to the HHS Office of International Health, Bangladesh.

92. Sepúlveda J, Willett W, Muñoz A. Malnutrition and diarrhea. A longitudinal study among urban Mexican children. *Am J Epidemiol.* 1988;127:365–376.

93. Black RE, Lanata CF, Lazo F. Delayed cutaneous hypersensitivity: epidemiologic factors affecting and usefulness in predicting diarrheal incidence in young Peruvian children. *Pediatr Infect Dis J.* 1989;8:210–215.

94. Baqui AH, Black RE, Sack RB, Chowdhury HR, Yunus M, Siddique AK. Malnutrition, cell-mediated immune deficiency and diarrhea: a community-based longitudinal study in rural Bangladeshi children. *Am J Epidemiol.* 1993;137:355–365.

95. Black RE, Brown KH, Becker S. Malnutrition is a determining factor in diarrheal duration, but not incidence, among young children in a longitudinal study in rural Bangladesh. *Am J Clin Nutr.* 1984;37:87–94.

96. Sommer A, Katz J, Tarwotjo I. Increased risk of respiratory disease and diarrhea in children with preexisting mild vitamin A deficiency. *Am J Clin Nutr.* 1984;40:1090–1095.

97. Sommer A, Dijunaedi E, Loeden AA, et al. Impact of vitamin A supplementation on childhood mortality. *Lancet.* 1986;1169–1173.

98. Sazawal S, Black RE, Bhan MK, et al. Efficacy of zinc supplementation in reducing the incidence and prevalence of acute diarrhea—a community-based, double-blind, controlled trial. *Am J Clin Nutr.* 1997;66:413–418.

99. Schiraldi O, Benvestito V, Di Bari C, et al. Gastric abnormalities in cholera: epidemiological and clinical considerations. *Bull World Health Organ.* 1974;51:349–352.

100. Sullivan PB, Thomas JE, Wight DGD, et al. *Helicobacter pylori* in Gambian children with chronic diarrhoea and malnutrition. *Arch Dis Child.* 1990;65:189–191.

101. Glass RI, Holmgren J, Haley CE, Khan, et al. Predisposition for cholera of individuals with O blood group. Possible evolutionary significance. *Am J Epidemiol.* 1985;121:791–796.

102. Black RE, Levine MM, Clements ML, Hughes T, O'Donnell S. Association between O blood group and occurrence and severity of diarrhoea due to *Escherichia coli. Trans R Soc Trop Med Hyg.* 1987;81:120–123.

103. van Loon FPL, Clemens JD, Sack DA, et al. ABO blood groups and the risk of diarrhea due to enterotoxigenic *Escherichia coli. J Infect Dis.* 1991;163:1243–1246.

104. Lederberg J, Shope RE, Oaks SC Jr, eds. *Emerging Infections: Microbial Threats to Health in the United States.* National Academy Press; 1992.

105. Cohen ML, Tauxe RV. Drug-resistant salmonella in the United States: an epidemiologic perspective. *Science.* 1986;234:964.

106. Harris S, Black RE. How useful are pharmaceuticals in managing diarrhoeal diseases in developing countries? *Health Policy and Management.* 1991;6:141–147.

107. Feachem RG, Koblinsky MA. Interventions for the control of diarrhoeal disease among young children: promotion of breast-feeding. *Bull World Health Organ.* 1984;62:271–291.

108. World Health Organization. Research on improving Infant feeding practices to prevent diarrhoea or reduce its severity: memorandum from a JHU/WHO meeting. *Bull World Health Organ.* 1989;67:27–33.

109. Ashworth A, Feachem RG. Interventions for the control of diarrhoeal diseases among young children: weaning education. *Bull World Health Organ.* 1985; 63(6):1115–1117.

110. Zinc investigators' collaborative group prevention of diarrhea and pneumonia by zinc supplementation in children in developing countries: Pooled analysis of randomized controlled trials. *J Pediatr.* (in press).

111. Feachem RG, Koblinsky MA. Interventions for the control of diarrhoeal diseases among young children: measles immunisation. *Bull World Health Organ.* 1983;61:641–652.

112. de Zoysa I, Feachem RG. Interventions for the control of diarrhoeal diseases among young children: rotavirus and cholera immunization. *Bull World Health Organ.* 1985;63:569–583.

PART V

Blood and Body Fluid as a Reservoir of Infectious Diseases

Review of the Epidemiology of Human Immunodeficiency Virus Infection and Acquired Immune Deficiency Syndrome

Neil M.H. Graham

INTRODUCTION

The acquired immune deficiency syndrome (AIDS) has metamorphosed from an epidemic in the 1980s to a pandemic in the 1990s. Through the end of 1997, AIDS has been responsible for the deaths of 5.1 million men, 3.9 million women, and 2.7 million children globally—approximately the same number of deaths due to malaria over this period.[1] The possibility of a novel type of viral infection that could progressively destroy the immune system was first suspected in 1981, when there was a sharp increase in the number of reports of the opportunistic illnesses *Pneumocystis carinii* pneumonia (PCP) and Kaposi's sarcoma in relatively young, previously healthy homosexual males and a comparable increase in the number of cases of PCP in young children of mothers who were injection drug users (IDUs).[2] In 1983, hemophiliacs who had received transfusions of Factor VIII were identified as a third group in whom the incidence of immunodeficiency and PCP was increasing.[2] The unusual escalation in PCP cases in all of these populations resulted in an increase in the number of requests received by the Centers for Disease Control (CDC) for the anti-*Pneumocystis* drug pentamidine.[3]

Investigations to uncover the cause of an infectious process manifested by the progressive destruction of the immune system led to the discovery and isolation in 1983 of the pathogen responsible for AIDS, the human immunodeficiency virus (HIV).[2] Since then, this retrovirus has been detected in more than 99% of patients diagnosed with AIDS.[4] Exhibit 18–1 contains a brief time line of major events that have occurred in AIDS diagnosis and treatment since the beginning of the epidemic.

Molecular epidemiologic data indicate that both HIV type 1 (HIV-1) and type 2 (HIV-2) infections were zoonotic in origin. HIV-1 evolved from the *Pan troglodytes troglodytes* subspecies of chimpanzee and has been present in that subspecies for centuries.[5] HIV-2 is very similar genetically to the simian immunodeficiency virus that is endemic among sooty mangabeys.[6] HIV-1 was most likely transmitted from chimpanzees to humans by contamination of a person's open wound with the infected blood of a chimpanzee that had been butchered for the purposes of consumption.[7] Conversely, HIV-2 may have been transmitted through the handling of "bush meat" from the sooty mangabey, a traditional source of nutrition in sub-Saharan Africa.[8]

The purpose of this chapter is to describe the epidemiology of HIV/AIDS. In so doing, the key viral characteristics of HIV, the risk factors of the epidemic, the geographic distribution of AIDS cases, and the impact of therapeutics and preventive measures on HIV-related morbidity and mortality are discussed.

Exhibit 18–1 Milestones in the Diagnosis and Treatment of HIV Infection

1981:	Recognition of an immune deficiency syndrome producing Kaposi's sarcoma and PCP in homosexual men
1982:	Immune deficiency syndrome identified in injection drug users
1983:	AIDS reported in hemophiliacs and in infants of drug-addicted mothers; HIV isolated by Robert Gallo (National Cancer Institute) and Luc Montagnier (Pasteur Institute, France)
1984:	Transfusion-associated AIDS reported; AIDS noted in heterosexual population in Zaire
1985:	Tests to detect the virus became available
1987:	The reverse transcriptase inhibitor, zidovudine (azidothymidine; AZT) became the first drug to treat HIV-1 infection
1995–96:	The first protease inhibitors became available
1996:	Combination antiretroviral therapy using reverse transcriptase inhibitors and protease inhibitors became the standard
1998:	The first HIV vaccine clinical trials were conducted in the United States

HIV CHARACTERISTICS

HIV attacks the immune system and undermines its function, allowing the opportunistic infections and malignancies that are the hallmarks of AIDS to occur.[9] The virus is classified as a lentivirus, a subfamily of the retroviruses. By definition, retroviruses are RNA viruses that contain the reverse transcriptase enzyme. Reverse transcriptase catalyzes the synthesis of DNA from an RNA template. As its name implies, reverse transcriptase causes the "reverse" of the usual transcription process, which involves the synthesis of RNA from a DNA template. All retroviruses have a diploid genome containing two single strands of RNA. Following infection with the HIV virus, the viral reverse transcriptase produces a haploid double-stranded DNA provirus. This provirus gets inserted into the chromosomal DNA of the host cell. Once it is integrated, the provirus may remain latent, especially in resting lymphocytes. However, if the cells are activated, transcription and translation occur, allowing the assembly of viral proteins necessary for the production of virions that are released to infect other cells.[10]

HIV has a high replication rate, with approximately 10 billion viral particles produced each day.[11–13] The generation time of HIV averages 2.6 days, with the half-life of the virus lasting no more than 6 hours and the half-life of an infected cell measuring 1.3 days. Using these figures, it has been calculated that 140 generations of HIV are produced each year in an infected patient. A second, slower decay phase has also been described involving latently infected CD4+ T lymphocytes.

Just as HIV has a high replication rate, it also has a high mutation rate of 3×10^{-5} nucleotides per replication cycle. The HIV genome contains 10^4 nucleotides. Based on the mutation rate, this means that every possible single mutation is generated daily.[11] This has implications for the generation of resistant mutants that may be selected for by antiretroviral therapy.

Figure 18–1 shows the organization and structure of the HIV genome and virion.[14] As with other retroviruses, HIV-1 contains the three key coding regions *pol, gag,* and *env. Pol* encodes reverse transcriptase, integrase, and protease, which are necessary for replication of HIV-1. *Gag* encodes the capsid proteins. *Env* encodes

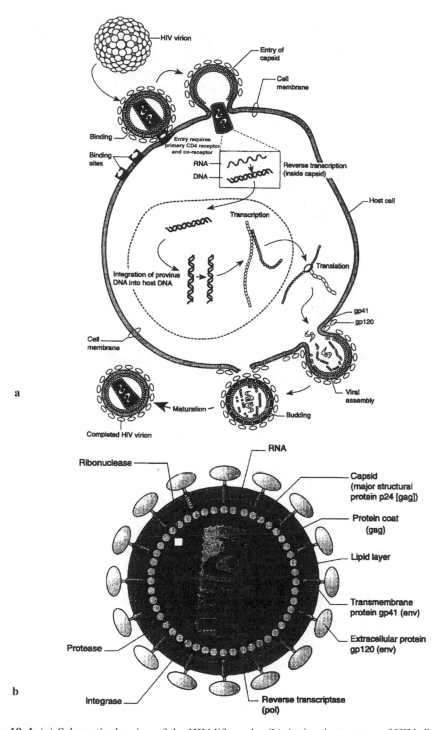

Figure 18–1 (**a**) Schematic drawing of the HIV life cycle; (**b**) Antigenic structure of HIV. *Source:* Reprinted with permission from HIV/AIDS Learning System, Section 2.3, *The Prime Deceiver: HIV*, Figures 14 and 15, © Glaxo Wellcome, Inc.

for the external glycoprotein that attaches to cell receptors to initiate infection. Other proteins encoded for by HIV-1 regulate gene expression, promote propagation of the virus, and increase the complexity of the virus. Some of the major HIV-1 proteins include gp120, gp41, p16/p14, p19, p27/p25, and p24. The gp120 and gp41 proteins are external envelope proteins that bind to the receptors of CD4 cells. These proteins are found in the plasma membrane and envelope region of the virus. The p16/p14 *tat* proteins, found mostly in the nucleus and nucleolus of infected cells, function as an activator of viral transcription. The p19 *rev* protein is responsible for the transport and stability of viral RNA. This protein travels between the cytoplasm and the

nucleolus of the infected cell. The p27/p25 *nef* proteins are active in the downregulation of CD4 cells. They reside in the plasma membrane as well as the cytoplasm. The p24 *gag* protein functions in the core capsid and is found in the virion.

HIV NATURAL HISTORY

Course of Disease

HIV infection is characterized by three phases: acute (primary) infection, clinical latency, and chronic infection (including development of symptomatic disease and, eventually, AIDS) (Figure 18–2).[15] Acute infection (acute seroconversion) occurs soon after a person has

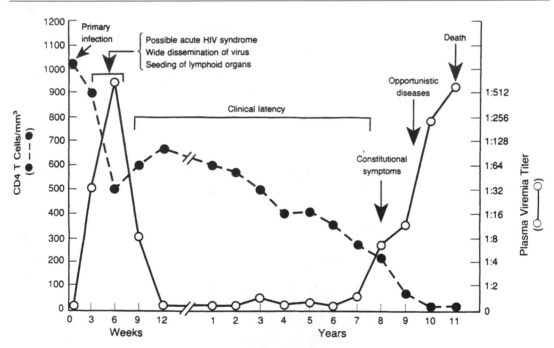

Figure 18–2 Typical course of HIV infection in persons who receive no treatment. Following primary infection, a chain of events occurs over the next decade of the person's life—widespread dissemination of HIV in peripheral blood accompanied by an abrupt fall in CD4⁺ T lymphocytes; a clinical latency period lasting about 5 years; further declines in CD4 cells marked progressively by constitutional symptoms, opportunistic diseases, and death. *Source:* Reprinted with permission from G. Pantaleo et al., Mechanisms of Disease: The Immunopathogenesis of Human Immunodeficiency Virus Infection, *New England Journal of Medicine*, Vol. 328, pp. 327–335. Copyright © 1993, Massachusetts Medical Society. All rights reserved.

been infected with the virus. During this phase, which may last for years, HIV levels in plasma are high; immune response is active and usually sufficient to reduce the amount of virus in the circulation and shift it into the lymphatic system. Cytotoxic cells, complement, and neutralizing antibodies are activated in the acute infection phase, although neutralizing antibodies do not reach detectable levels for 2–3 months after infection. Patients frequently (i.e., about 30% of cases) present with a viral syndrome consisting of fever (97% of cases), adenopathy (77%), pharyngitis (73%), rash (70%), and myalgia or arthralgia (58%).

During the clinical latency phase of HIV infection, outward clinical signs and symptoms are absent. Nevertheless, viral replication continues unabated within the lymphatic system. The patient's immune response is able to sequester the virus, resulting in increased lymphocyte production. However, the immune system eventually begins to break down, and plasma virus levels rise as a consequence.

In the chronic infection phase, there is progressive, symptomatic clinical disease due to severe immune dysfunction, elevated plasma HIV levels, and decreased CD4 lymphocyte cell counts to below $200/mm^3$. This includes non-AIDS-defining conditions, such as oral candidiasis, rash, and herpes simplex eruption. Later in the course of infection, opportunistic illnesses occur, at which time the patient is said to have AIDS. Prior to the availability of antiretroviral therapy, these opportunistic illnesses and immunodeficiency-related wasting were often the primary causes of death in patients with AIDS. Table 18–1 shows the pattern of opportunistic illnesses that were observed between 1992 and 1997 among HIV-infected patients in 11 U.S. cities.[16] Evaluation of trends shows that *P. carinii* pneumonia continues to be the most frequently observed opportunistic illness; other trends that are occurring are increases in the incidence of esophageal candidiasis and wasting syndrome, and decreases in the incidence of *Mycobacterium avium* complex and pulmonary tuberculosis.

Factors Associated with Disease Progression

Several factors influence the susceptibility of the host to HIV infection (Table 18–2).[17] For example, the presence of the CCR5-Δ32 homozygous mutation can render people highly resistant to infection by macrophage-tropic HIV strains. Much research has been done on people with HIV-1 infection who never develop AIDS. These individuals, termed *nonprogressors*, constitute about 5–10% of all HIV-1-infected persons. HIV-1 replication is 4–20 times lower in the peripheral blood mononuclear cells and lymph nodes of nonprogressors than in HIV-1-infected persons with progressive disease. Immune response against HIV-1 in nonprogressors is more vigorous and specific than that in progressors. This response is characterized by specific neutralizing antibodies to genetically diverse strains of HIV-1 and HIV-specific cytotoxic activity against HIV *env* and *gag* proteins. Persons with long-term nonprogressive HIV infection have preserved lymphoid tissue with reduced formation of germinal centers and reduced HIV trapping. Some nonprogressors may be infected with a less virulent strain of HIV-1.

HIV Detection and Monitoring

HIV is detected in plasma by use of the enzyme-linked immunosorbent assay (ELISA). Staging of HIV infection is based on criteria established by the CDC. Two surrogate marker laboratory values are crucial in estimating morbidity and mortality in HIV-infected persons: plasma viral load (the number of HIV-1 RNA copies in 1 mL of plasma) and CD4 count (the total number of circulating lymphocytes that bear the CD4 marker).

In most persons with HIV infection, as plasma levels of HIV-1 RNA increase, CD4 cell counts decrease as a hallmark of progressive damage to the immune system (Figure 18–2). However, discordance between trends in HIV-1 RNA levels and CD4 counts have been observed in up to 20% of patients.[18] The risk of progression to AIDS or death appears to increase about 50% for

Table 18–1 Percentage* of Persons with at Least One Acquired Immunodeficiency Syndrome-Defining Opportunistic Illness (OI) for Whom a Given OI Occurred First, by Disease and Year of Diagnosis—Adult/Adolescent Spectrum of HIV Disease Project,[†] 1992–1997

Disease	Total (N = 12,982)	1992 (N = 3,023)	1993 (N = 2,804)	1994 (N = 2,648)	1995 (N = 2,107)	1996 (N = 1,602)	1997 (N = 798)	Trends[‡]
Pneumocystis carinii pneumonia	35.9	36.6	35.0	34.7	34.7	38.1	42.6	none
Esophageal candidiasis	12.4	11.5	11.4	11.2	14.1	14.8	15.0	increasing
Kaposi's sarcoma	11.6	11.1	12.0	11.6	13.2	9.5	10.7	none
Wasting syndrome	7.8	10.5	6.1	5.8	7.2	8.4	12.2	increaasing
Mycobacterium avium complex	6.4	5.7	5.7	8.2	7.2	5.6	4.8	decreasing
Pulmonary tuberculosis	5.0	6.4	5.9	5.2	3.7	2.6	3.6	decreasing
Extrapulmonary cryptococcosis	4.3	4.0	5.0	3.8	4.6	4.3	3.8	none
HIV encephalopathy	4.2	3.8	4.7	4.1	3.5	5.1	3.6	none
Cytomegalovirus retinitis	3.7	3.4	3.8	4.3	3.5	4.0	2.6	none
Cytomegalovirus disease	3.2	3.7	2.7	3.1	4.0	3.3	1.1	none
Toxoplasmosis of brain	3.0	2.9	3.0	3.0	3.1	3.3	2.6	none
Chronic cryptosporidiosis	2.7	1.8	3.2	3.2	3.1	2.8	1.5	none
Recurrent pneumonia	2.5	2.1	2.7	2.5	2.5	2.8	3.0	none
Extrapulmonary tuberculosis	2.1	2.6	2.4	2.0	1.8	1.2	0.9	decreasing
Chronic herpes simplex	2.1	2.4	3.1	1.7	1.8	1.3	0.5	decreasing
Immunoblastic lymphoma	1.5	1.2	1.4	2.3	0.8	2.1	1.9	increasing
Progressive multifocal leukoencephalopathy	1.0	0.5	0.7	1.5	1.3	1.6	0.7	increasing
Invasive cervical cancer[§]	0.9	1.1	0.5	1.5	1.1	0.1	0.9	none
Disseminated histoplasmosis	0.7	0.9	0.7	0.7	0.7	0.3	1.0	none
Burkitt's lymphoma	0.7	0.6	0.7	0.7	0.4	0.9	1.5	none
Other disseminated Mycobacterium	0.6	1.2	0.6	0.4	0.3	0.5	0.4	decreasing
Primary brain lymphoma	0.4	0.6	0.3	0.6	0.3	0.3	0.1	none
Pulmonary candidiasis	0.3	0.2	0.6	0.4	0.2	0.2	0.2	none
Disseminated coccidioidomycosis	0.1	0.0	0.1	0.0	0.0	0.4	0.7	increasing
Recurrent Salmonella septicemia	0.1	0.1	0.1	0.1	0.0	0.2	0.0	none
Chronic isosporiasis	0.0	0.0	0.1	0.0	0.0	0.0	0.1	none

* Data for each opportunistic illness are standardized to national acquired immunodeficiency syndrome surveillance cases by age, race, country of birth, sex, and human immunodeficiency virus (HIV) exposure mode. Data from all cities are weighted equally.
† A CDC-sponsored surveillance project that collects data at selected sites in 11 U.S. cities.
‡ The direction of change is given for trends that were significant (p<0.05), based on the stratified (HIV exposure mode, race, sex, age, metropolitan area, and country of birth) Cochran-Mantel-Haenszel statistic.
§ Restricted to women.

Source: Reprinted from the Centers for Disease Control and Prevention.

Table 18–2 Factors that Can Affect Host Susceptibility to HIV Infection

Factor	Mechanism
CCR5-Δ32 homozygous mutation	Absence of cell-surface expression of HIV coreceptor CCR5 due to a homozygous 32-base pair deletion renders individuals highly resistant to infection by macrophage-tropic HIV strains.
HIV-specific helper T-cell responses	T-helper cells that proliferate or secrete interleukin-2 in response to HIV antigens may stimulate CTL or other potentially protective immune responses.
Specific HLA polymorphisms	Different HLA molecules present HIV peptides with varying efficiency, which may affect the strength of immune responses. Antibodies or T cells that recognize epitopes cross-reactive between HLA and HIV-proteins or non–cross-reactive foreign alloantigens may inhibit HIV virions or destroy infected cells.
Mucosal HIV-specific IgA and IgG antibodies	Antibodies may inhibit HIV at the mucosal surfaces and prevent or clear HIV infection of the host cells.
β-chemokine production	At increased concentrations, β-chemokines MIP-1α, MIP-1β, and RANTES may bind efficiently to CCR5 and prevent entry of macrophage-tropic HIV strains into host $CD4^+$ cells.
$CD8^+$ T-lymphocyte antiviral factor (CAF)	CAF inhibits replication of HIV-1 and HIV-2 in infected $CD4^+$ cells, probably at the level of transcription.
HIV-specific cytotoxic T-cell responses	$CD8^+$ and/or $CD4^+$ CTL kill HIV-infected cells, which present viral peptides associated with HLA molecules.

CTL, cytotoxic T cells; HLA, human leukocyte antigen; Ig, immunoglobulin.

Source: Adapted from K.A. Buchacz et al, Genetic and Immunological Host Factors Associated with Susceptibility to HIV-1 Infection, *AIDS*, 1998;12(suppl A):S87–S94, © 1998, Lippincott Williams & Wilkins.

every threefold increase in plasma HIV-1 RNA.

CD4 counts, which are normally about 750 ± 250 cells/mm³, are usually reduced by about 40–50% early in HIV infection. Vulnerability to opportunistic infections increases markedly when CD4 cell counts fall below 200/mm³ (Figure 18–3).[19] The relationship between baseline HIV-1 RNA levels measured in a large multicenter AIDS cohort study of HIV-infected adults (n = 1604) and their subsequent rate of CD4 cell decline are shown in Figure 18–4.[20] Progressive loss of CD4 cells is observed in all strata of baseline plasma HIV RNA levels, with much more rapid rates of CD4 cell decline seen in persons with higher baseline HIV-1 RNA levels.

This study also shows a clear gradient in risk for disease progression and death with increasing baseline plasma HIV RNA levels.[21–23]

RELATIONSHIP OF HIV TYPE AND EPIDEMICITY

HIV Types

Two types of HIV exist: HIV-1, discovered in 1983; and HIV-2, discovered in 1986.[13] HIV-1 and HIV-2 have similar genetic structures, except that HIV-2 has a *vpx* gene instead of a *vpu* gene. The nucleotide and amino acid homology between the viruses is about 60% for the more

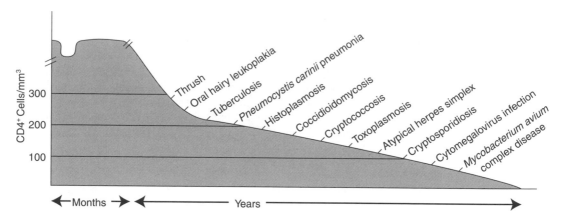

Figure 18–3 Occurrence of opportunistic illnesses that typically occur as the CD4+ lymphocyte count in peripheral blood progressively decreases over time in an untreated HIV-infected patient. *Source:* Schooley RT, Acquired Immunodeficiency Syndrome. *Scientific American Medicine*, Vol. 2. Dale DC, Federman DD, Eds. Scientific American, Inc., New York, 1998. All rights reserved.

conserved *gag* and *pol* genes, and 30–40% for the other viral genes, including *env*. HIV-1 and HIV-2 share the same modes of transmission. However, HIV-1 is spread worldwide, and its prevalence is rising in most countries. Conversely, HIV-2 is confined primarily to West Africa (especially Gambia, Senegal, Côte d'Ivoire, Guinea-Bissau) and India, and its prevalence is relatively stable in these countries. HIV-1 is associated with a higher mother-to-child transmission rate (20–35% vs. 0–4%), attacks a younger age group (peak age 20–34 years vs. 45–55 years), and produces higher excess mortality (10-fold vs. twofold).[24] The lower efficiency of heterosexual transmission of HIV-2 is also believed to be due to lower concentration of this virus type in cervicovaginal secretions. In a study in Côte d'Ivoire of dually infected female commercial sex workers (n = 205), only 3% shed HIV-2 in their cervicovaginal secretions, compared with 26% who shed HIV-1.[25] Similar results were observed in two studies in Dakar, Senegal.[26,27] Comparative studies of viral shedding in semen have yet to be done. The lower transmissibility of HIV-2 infection could be due to the possibility of HIV-2 requiring a wider range of coreceptors than does HIV-1 to enter host cells.[28–30]

The clinical manifestations of HIV-2 disease are similar to those of HIV-1,[31,32] although HIV-2-infected patients have shown a lower frequency of Kaposi's sarcoma.[33] Like infection with HIV-1, HIV-2 infection can lead to CD4 cell decline, opportunistic infections, HIV-associated malignancies, and early death. However, the median time from infection to AIDS with HIV-2 infection is longer than it is with HIV-1 infection. Thus, in a cohort of women in Senegal (n = 131), the incidence of AIDS was 0.95 per 100 person-years of observation (pyo) in HIV-2-infected women, compared to 5.6 pyo in HIV-1-infected women.[34] An incubation period of 14 years is not uncommon in HIV-2-infected patients, and a relatively larger proportion of HIV-2 patients than HIV-1 patients is categorized as nonprogressors.[35,36] In a community-based study in Guinea-Bissau in which adjustments were made for patient age and a 9-year follow-up period was observed, the mortality rate of HIV-2-infected patients was twice as high as that in HIV-negative persons.[37] In contrast, a study in a rural area of Uganda reported a mortality rate 9.7 times higher in HIV-1-infected persons than in HIV-negative persons.[38] The highest incidence of HIV-2 is in Guinea-Bissau, where it affects 7–9% of the population.[39,40] About 4.3% of all

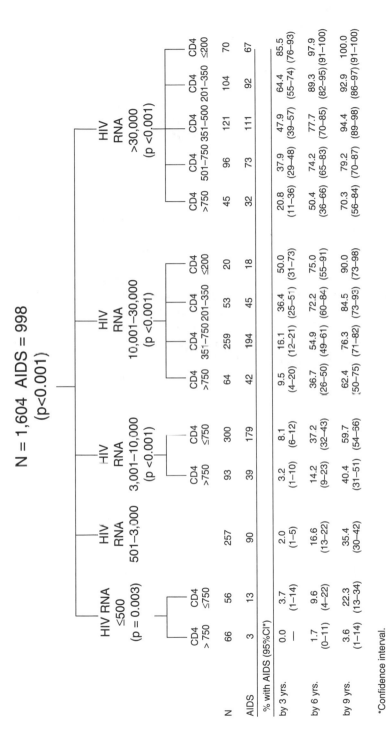

Figure 18–4 Probability of AIDS by baseline HIV-1 RNA and CD4+ cell count. *Source:* Reprinted with permission from Mellors et al., Plasma Viral Load and CD4+ Lymphocytes as Prognostic Markers of HIV-1 Infection, *Annals of Internal Medicine,* Vol. 126, pp. 946–954, © 1997, American College of Physicians–American Society of Internal Medicine.

pregnant women living in the capital city, Bissau, are HIV-2-positive.[41] HIV-2 has not gotten a strong foothold in North America (67 cases reported through 1999) or Europe (<100 cumulative cases in most countries). Dual infection with HIV-2 and HIV-1 follows a clinical course similar to that of HIV-1 infection.[42]

Cohen[43] postulated in 1995 that HIV-2 could possibly act as an "attenuated" HIV-1, thereby providing protection against subsequent HIV-1 infection. This hypothesis has been supported by laboratory studies that showed indications of HIV-2 infection prompting immune or other responses against HIV-1.[44,45] However, cohort studies have yielded diverse results regarding an HIV-2 protective effect. In favor of the hypothesis, Travers et al[46] studied a cohort of 756 female commercial sex workers in Senegal from 1985 to 1994. HIV-1 incidence in HIV-2-positive women was less than half that of HIV-2-negative women (1.06 per 100 pyo vs. 2.53 per 100 pyo). After adjusting for calendar year, gonorrhea infection status, age, nationality, and years of registered prostitution, the incidence rate ratio (IRR) was 0.32 (95% confidence interval, 0.20–0.59), suggesting a protective effect against HIV-1 infection of 68% by preceding HIV-2 infection. In later updates of this cohort, the protective effect was reported as 74% (1996)[47] and 58% (1997).[48] This study has been criticized because of possible selection bias.[24]

Arguing against the HIV-2 protection hypothesis are the findings of three studies from West Africa showing a higher incidence of HIV-1 infection in HIV-2-infected persons.[24,49,50] These studies included 242 female commercial sex workers in Gambia evaluated during 1988–1995 (crude IRR, 1.7),[50] 729 low-risk men and women in Bissau (IRR, 10.1) (unpublished data [O. Larsen et al][24]), and 406 women in Côte d'Ivoire (risk ratio, 2.91).[49] Although increased risk of HIV-1 infection in these three studies may have been due to residual confounding, it could also have been due to HIV-2-induced damage to the immune system, facilitating HIV-1 infection.[24] The issue of HIV-2 protection versus facilitation of HIV-1 infection still needs to be clarified, and

to do this will require longitudinal studies in populations with a high HIV-2 baseline prevalence.

HIV Subtypes (Clades)

HIV is characterized by great genetic variability. HIV-1 has been classified into at least 10 genetic subtypes, designated A to J, in the major group (group M), and into a minor group of highly heterogeneous strains, designated O. An additional minor group, designated N, has been described recently. Particular subtypes are found more often in certain countries and regions of the world (Table 18–3). Recombination between subtypes has also been reported. A B/C recombinant is in evidence in Southern China and an A/B recombinant is circulating in Russia. As people mix within and between countries, it is expected that many subtypes of HIV-1 will start appearing in most countries. Subtype B predominates in industrialized Western countries, where most transmission is among homosexual men (termed *men who have sex with men* [MSM] from here on) and IDUs.[51] Subtypes A, C, D, and E predominate in Asia and Africa, where most transmission is among heterosexuals. Two studies suggest that subtype E may be more efficiently transmitted heterosexually than subtype B.[52,53] In view of the latter, Anderson et al[54] speculated that introduction of non-B subtypes in the West could result in more extensive heterosexual transmission. In a surveillance study involving 2104 HIV-1-infected patients in Thailand, HIV-1 subtypes B and E were found to produce similar degrees of immunosuppression and a comparable spectrum of opportunistic illnesses.[55]

Differences in transmissibility have been the focus of considerable epidemiologic interest. In in vitro studies involving Langerhans' cells, subtypes E and C have shown higher replication than subtype B viruses.[52] Results of a cross-sectional study of heterosexual couples in Thailand suggest a higher risk of heterosexual transmission of subtype E than that of subtype B.[53] However, there is also evidence against major bio-

Table 18–3 Worldwide Geographic Distribution of HIV-1 Subtypes and HIV-2

Geographic Region	HIV-1 Subtypes										HIV-2
	Group M									O	
	A	B	C	D	E	F	G	H	I		
Africa	+	+	+	+	+	+	+	+		+	+
Europe	+	+	+	+		+	+	+		+	+
Asia		+	+		+						
India	+	+	+								+
Australia		+									
North America		+									+
South America		+	+		+						
Middle East									+		

Source: Reprinted with permission from W.D. Hardy Jr., The Human Immunodeficiency Virus, *Medical Clinics of North America*, Vol. 80, pp. 1239–1261, © 1996, W.B. Saunders Company.

logic differences of different HIV-1 subtypes. For example, the presence of many subtypes other than B in Europe is occurring without any indication of a major spread in heterosexuals. Furthermore, studies of maternal–infant transmission of HIV-1 in different regions of the world suggest similar rates of vertical transmission among the different HIV-1 subtypes.[51]

MODES OF TRANSMISSION AND RISK BEHAVIORS

HIV infection is spread by sexual intercourse, IDU, perinatal transmission, transfusion of blood and blood products, organ transplantation, and occupational exposure to HIV-contaminated blood or body fluids.

Sexual Transmission

Unprotected receptive anal intercourse is the most effective mode of sexual transmission of HIV.[56] Among MSM, the biggest HIV risk factor is a combination of receptive anal intercourse and a high number of male sexual partners.[57–61] History of anogenital rectal gonorrhea or other ulcerative sexually transmitted diseases (STDs)

(herpes simplex, syphilis), rectal trauma due primarily to the practice of fisting (one partner positioning his fist into the other's anorectal region), and rectal douching also enhance the likelihood of HIV infection in this high-risk group.[57,60–62] Receptive oral sex is associated with only a small risk.[63,64] The probability of encountering an infected sexual partner is increased in MSM who frequent sex clubs or bathhouses for sex and those who have sexual contact with partners from cities with a high prevalence of AIDS.[65,66]

Lesbians represent fewer than 1% of all cases of HIV infection. No clinical or statistical evidence of female-to-female transmission has been reported among exclusively homosexual women.[67] Of lesbian cases reported to the CDC to date, most have occurred among IDUs, and the rest have been attributable to receipt of contaminated blood or blood products. Indeed, of the 164 cases of AIDS reported in exclusively homosexual women from June 1980 to June 1991, 93% were attributed to IDU and 7% to blood transfusion.[68] The low incidence of female-to-female HIV transmission is due primarily to the small number of women who are homosexual or bisexual (3–4%).[69,70] Traumatic sex has been reported anecdotally to result in HIV transmission between women.[71,72] Bisexual women are more likely to be HIV-positive than are exclusively lesbian or heterosexual women and are more likely to exchange sex for money.[67]

Vaginal-penile heterosexual intercourse is an inefficient mode of HIV transmission, especially from an infected woman to a man.[73,74] HIV risk in heterosexuals is enhanced when other well-defined risk factors are involved, including multiple sex partners,[75] sex with a partner with STDs characterized by genital ulcers (allowing direct exposure to HIV-laden blood),[76–80] engaging in receptive anal intercourse,[81] and having sex with persons from areas of high HIV infection or high-risk behaviors (eg, IDUs). Nonulcerating gonorrhea and *Chlamydia* infections have also been reported in some heterosexual HIV cases.[82,83] Factors that facilitate transmission among heterosexuals include genital trauma and exposure to blood during intercourse (eg, sex during the time of menses),[84] lack of male circumcision, and the use of IUDs and oral contraceptives.[82,85,86] Sexual transmission is more likely when the infected partner has advanced disease, such as those manifesting AIDS, when high viral loads are present both in their blood and genital fluids.[79,87] Use of alcohol or other recreational drugs that impair judgment may lead to unsafe sex and, therefore, are considered risk factors. Use of crack, a form of cocaine that can be smoked, has been linked with increased sexual activity, exchange of sex for money or drugs, and increased rates of STDs, all of which contribute to a greater likelihood of spreading HIV.

Use of Condoms and Other Protective Agents. Latex condoms have been shown in in vitro permeability tests to block the passage of HIV.[88–91] In behavioral studies, the consistent and correct use of condoms has reduced the risk of HIV among heterosexual couples, MSM, and prostitutes.[88,90,92–95] In serodiscordant couples (one HIV-positive partner and one HIV-negative partner), one study showed HIV transmission to be prevented in all cases,[92] and another study showed a 90% risk reduction.[95]

Topical microbicides are being developed to kill HIV or to prevent HIV contact with the genital mucosa.[96] In a double-blind, placebo-controlled trial in Cameroon, 1292 HIV-negative female sex workers were assigned to use either a film containing 70 mg of nonoxynol-9 (N9) or a placebo film, inserted into the vagina before intercourse. All of the women were provided with latex condoms and were instructed to have their male sexual partners use them. At monthly follow-up visits, women were tested for HIV infection, genital lesions were examined by colposcope, and endocervical specimens were tested for gonorrhea and *Chlamydia* infection with DNA probes. The rates of HIV infection (cases per 100 woman-years) were *not* different between the N9 (6.7) and the placebo groups (6.6) (rate ratio, 1.0; 95% CI, 0.7–1.5). The rates of *Chlamydia* infection and gonorrhea also were not significantly different. A slightly higher rate of genital lesions was observed in the N9 group, compared with placebo (42.2 vs. 33.5 cases per 100 woman-years), possibly due to irritation with the microbicide. The Joint United Nations Programme on HIV/AIDS (UNAIDS) is currently conducting a multicenter, placebo-controlled, triple-blind trial assessing the effect of 53.5 mg of N-9 vaginal gel on HIV transmission in female sex workers in South Africa, Thailand, Benin, and Côte d'Ivoire (COL-1492). Because microbicides can cause epithelial inflammation, there is controversy about whether the consequent increased vascularity may counter the antiviral effect of these preparations.

Transmission among Injecting Drug Users

Injection drug use continues to be a major risk factor for HIV transmission, and in some areas of the world, it is responsible for a higher number of cases of HIV infection than is sex. Drug injection practices, sexual behavior, STDs, and the increase in cocaine use are all factors that contribute to HIV transmission among drug users. IDUs frequently share needles, syringes, and other drug paraphernalia. During "booting"— the practice of drawing a small amount of blood back into the syringe prior to injection—HIV and other blood-borne infectious agents can be transmitted to others using the same syringe or needle. The "cooker" (equipment used to prepare the drugs) may be contaminated with HIV-infected blood. Thus, when it is shared, further HIV transmission is facilitated. During "front-loading," the needle is removed from the recipient syringe and replaced with a new needle from a donor syringe. This practice allows solution to be transferred from the donor to the recipient syringe.[97] In "backloading," the syringe is used to mix drugs and to measure out shares of drug to other IDUs by squirting drug solution into their syringes. With the practice of "skinpopping," drugs are inserted into a muscle or under the skin. Once an IDU becomes HIV-infected, the infection can be spread by unsafe injection practices, through sexual intercourse, or perinatally to the unborn child.

In the United States, information concerning drug-using behaviors has been obtained chiefly from drug users in treatment programs. Among IDUs, the risk of HIV infection increases with the number of different needle-sharing partners, frequency of drug injection, frequency of sharing equipment, use of unsterilized needles, use of cookers, frequency of frontloading and backloading, use of "shooting galleries," use of cocaine and cocaine/heroin combinations ("speedball"), and frequency of receptive anal intercourse among men.[97–107] The risk of HIV infection among people who inject cocaine is greater than that among heroin injectors because cocaine has a short half-life, necessitating more frequent injections and, hence, more exposure to HIV.[108] In the United States, HIV seroprevalence surveys show a higher proportion of HIV-positive cases among black than among white IDUs.[109,110]

Many IDUs engage in risky sexual behaviors, and these are characteristically males who do not use condoms and who have partners who are not IDUs.[111] As with other high-risk groups, crack and alcohol use increases the probability of unsafe sexual practices[112] and, thus, the likelihood of contracting HIV infection. The longevity of active drug use has not been proven to be a consistent factor to progression to AIDS.[113–116] Among IDUs, HIV infection progresses more rapidly to AIDS with increasing age.[113,114,117]

Perinatal (Vertical) Transmission

HIV can be transmitted vertically from mother to fetus in utero, intrapartum, or postpartum to an infant by breastfeeding. In the United States, most infants acquire HIV in utero or intrapartum because breastfeeding is discouraged among HIV-infected women. Although the timing of maternal-fetal transmission is uncertain, HIV has been isolated in fetal tissue during the early to late stages of pregnancy, from placental tissue during the first trimester,[118,119] and from cord blood of infants at delivery.[120] However, most experts believe that 65% to 80% of transmission occurs during the intrapartum (delivery) period in nonbreastfeeding populations.

Caesarean section appears to reduce the risk of HIV transmission.[121–124] A meta-analysis that included data from 8533 mother-child pairs from 15 international cohort studies of non-breastfeeding women showed that, after adjusting for receipt of antiretroviral therapy, maternal disease stage, and infant birth weight, elective Caesarean section decreased the likelihood of HIV transmission by approximately 50% (adjusted odds ratio, 0.43; 95% CI, 0.33–0.56).[125] When elective Caesarean section was combined with receipt of zidovudine (azidothymidine [AZT]) during the antepartum, intrapartum, and neonatal periods, HIV transmission was reduced by about 85%, compared with other modes of delivery and no zidovudine administration (adjusted odds ratio, 0.13; 95% CI, 0.09–0.19).[125]

The incidence of HIV infection among infants born to HIV-infected mothers has been reported to be 14% in Europe, 20–30% in the United States, and 45% in Kenya.[120–122,126] These variations in transmission rates may be attributable to differences in obstetric and breastfeeding practices, inherent factors of the study population, and virulence characteristics of the virus.[127] In mothers who become infected during late pregnancy or lactation, the risk of HIV transmission though breast milk may be as high as 50%, due to the very high viral load seen at the early stage of infection.[128] However, the rate of postnatal transmission of HIV-1 from mothers who have been HIV-positive throughout their pregnancy is lower (5–15%).[129] Research artifacts, such as incomplete follow-up and varying diagnostic precision, can also explain some of the differences in rates that have been observed.

Maternal-fetal transmission is facilitated by advanced HIV disease (when high viral load is present in the mother), CD4 cell counts less than 400/mm³, high CD8 cell counts, lack of maternal neutralizing antibody, maternal p24 antigenemia, and placental membrane inflammation.[120,126,130–133] A greater risk has been reported in premature infants, compared with full-term infants and in first-born twins, compared with second-born twins.[123,134,135] The presence of maternal anti-gp 120 was reported to be associated with a lower likelihood of transmission in one study but not in another.[136–138] Zidovudine, administered during gestation and/or labor and delivery, reduces HIV transmission, even in women with low CD4 counts.[132,139] In ACTG Protocol 076, zidovudine, administered to a selected group of HIV-infected women during pregnancy, labor, and delivery and to their newborns, decreased the risk of perinatal HIV transmission by about two thirds, compared with mothers who received placebo.[139] Because of this, the Public Health Service made a recommendation that zidovudine be given to pregnant HIV-infected women and their newborns.[140]

Transmission by Blood Transfusion, Administration of Blood Products, and Organ Transplantation

In most developed countries, HIV transmission by blood transfusion is very infrequent because of current practices of HIV antibody testing of all donated blood and plasma, increased sensitivity of contemporary HIV-antibody enzyme immunosorbent assays (EIA), improved donor interviewing about risk behaviors associated with HIV infection, self-deferral by potential donors aware of their HIV status, and maintenance of deferral lists of donors who have tested HIV-seropositive in the past. Also, nucleic acid amplification of all donations in the United States has been implemented recently to detect HIV-infected ELISA-negative specimens from donors who were in the window period at the time of donation. Moreover, as clotting factor now undergoes heat treatment to inactivate HIV, the transmission of HIV to recipients of clotting factor is unlikely. However, HIV transmission occurs in over 90% of recipients of HIV-infected blood and cellular blood components.[141]

Before HIV screening became available, 75–90% of recipients of factor VIII concentrate and 30% of all factor IX recipients were infected.[142] The risk of HIV transmission from a whole organ of an HIV-infected donor is nearly 100%.[143] Fresh-frozen, unprocessed bone from a donor who is HIV-positive is at high risk for HIV infection if marrow elements and adherent tissue are not removed. Relatively avascular solid tissue poses a lower risk for HIV transmission, especially it if has been processed by techniques that might inactivate HIV.[144] It is possible for persons to become infected by receipt of blood, organs, and tissues from donors who were recently HIV-infected but who tested seronegative because they were within the 4- to 26-week period that spans primary infection to seroconversion.[143,145] However, more sensitive third-generation EIAs have decreased the duration of the seronegative window period to three to six weeks. Alternatively, multiple blood transfusions just prior to organ donation may dilute the anti-HIV antibody titer in the donor below a detectable level. After the licensure of the HIV ELISA antibody screening test, the risk of transfusion-acquired infection declined. However, Ward et al from CDC reported 9 cases of persons with AIDS who had been infected by screened HIV-negative blood. These persons were infected by donors who were in the window period soon after infection.[146] At this time there was great concern about the frequency of transfusion-transmitted HIV from donors who tested ELISA-negative but were infected.[147]

Therefore, two prospective studies were funded by NIH to evaluate the frequency of transmission from HIV-seronegative donors. One study evaluated more than 12,000 cardiac surgery patients who had been transfused with about 120,000 units of blood or blood products. These patients were tested for HIV antibodies prior and six months after their transfusions. Two infections were detected, a rate of 1 per 60,000 donations.[148] Another study involved testing pools of 50 blood specimens from ELISA seronegative donors by culture and nucleic acid amplification by PCR. This study found one PCR-positive specimen in about 160,000 donors.[149] These two studies were reassuring in that they showed that transfusion-transmitted infection from HIV-seronegative donors was very rare. Since this time, more effective recruitment of low-risk donors, especially repeat donors, and more sensitive screening assays have further reduced the risk of transfusion-transmitted HIV in the United States.

It has been estimated that the acquisition of HIV infection through receipt of an HIV-contaminated unit of blood that tests false-negative for HIV antibody occurs at a rate of 26 per million.[146,147] Approximately 6 per 100,000 blood donations collected by the American Red Cross in 1993 tested positive for HIV antibody.[150] One in 450,000 to one in 660,000 donations per year, or about 18–27 annual donations, were infectious for HIV but were not detected by current screening tests.[151]

In August 1995, the FDA recommended that safe blood supplies be maintained by having all blood and plasma donations screened for p24 antigen.[152] Tests for p24 antigen can detect HIV infection earlier than can an EIA antibody test in persons in the acute period of HIV infection.[152] Screening for p24 has been shown to reduce the infectious window period.[153] It is estimated that, in the United States, p24 antigen screening could remove 4–6 infectious donations from the 12 million done annually that would otherwise not be detected by other screening tests.[152] In order to decrease the risk of transfusion-transmitted HIV due to a false negative ELISA when a donor is in the window period, all blood donations in the United States are now tested by PCR to detect HIV RNA. This nucleic acid testing has virtually eliminated the risk of transfusion-transmitted HIV infection.

Transmission to Health Care Workers

HIV infection is a risk for health care workers and laboratory personnel who handle sharp instruments or body fluids from HIV-infected patients. Needle-stick accidents pose a far greater risk than does intact skin or mucous membrane exposure to HIV-contaminated blood or body fluids. A 0.4% HIV seroconversion rate has been reported in health care workers who had percutaneous injuries with HIV-contaminated surgical instruments.[154,155] Most of these injuries have occurred in emergency situations involving resuscitation attempts and during surgery. The risk of HIV infection is greatest when the health care worker has been exposed to a large quantity of blood from patients with advanced HIV disease and very high viral loads. Single exposure of mucosal and nonintact skin to HIV-contaminated body fluids accounts for a lower infection risk (less than 0.1%) than does penetrating exposures.[156] One large prospective study evaluating 2,712 intact cutaneous exposures detected no infections.[157] Nevertheless, there have been reports of HIV transmission in cases where there was prolonged cutaneous exposure to HIV-contaminated fluids or blood splashes.[158]

An HIV-infected dentist was reported to be responsible for HIV spread to six of his patients.[159,160] However, later it was found that some of these patients had other identified HIV risk factors. Nevertheless, after genetic sequencing of the viruses from several of the infected patients, it was concluded that the viruses in the patients and the dentist were from the same source. In one case where a patient was originally believed to have been infected by an HIV-seropositive surgeon, the patient was later discovered to be an IDU and, thus, at risk of HIV infection. In hospitals in the developing world, inadequate infection control practices regarding contaminated syringes and needles have resulted in HIV transmission to patients.

Environmental and Casual Contact Transmission

Environmental transmission of HIV is not believed to occur. Although extensive study of HIV survival in the environment revealed that HIV could be recovered by tissue-culture techniques 1–3 days after drying,[161] the clinical relevance of these samples was dubious because they were several thousand-fold more concentrated than were blood samples normally seen in persons with HIV infection. However, environmental contamination could pose a risk for persons working in a research laboratory where concentrated virus preparations exist. In fact, at least one transmission has occurred in this setting. Environmental spread of HIV is also unlikely because the rate of inactivation of HIV is very rapid. CDC studies have demonstrated that drying causes HIV concentrations to decrease by 90–99% within several hours.[162] No one has been infected with HIV due to contact with an environmental surface because HIV is unable to reproduce, spread, or maintain infectivity outside its living host.[163] There is no evidence to support the possibility of HIV transmission by insects.[164–167]

Household transmission of HIV in the absence of sexual or percutaneous exposure is rare. HIV has not been shown to be transmitted through the sharing of household items, such as towels, plates, sheets, glasses, toilet, or bath or shower facilities that have been soiled by feces, saliva, urine, or tears.[168] Studies in the United States and Europe of nonsexual, non–needle-sharing household contacts of persons with HIV infection have indicated no evidence of infection among family members.[169–172] No familial cases of HIV infection were seen in 17 studies involving 1,167 nonsexual household contacts.[172] The rate of transmission from these studies was estimated to be only 0–0.2 infections per 100 person-years.[172] HIV transmission has been reported in households where needles were shared

for medical injections at home and where there was mucocutaneous exposure to blood or other body substances during home health care.[173–178] In one unusual case reported to the CDC involving HIV transmission between two brothers with hemophilia, the putative spread of infection was due to sharing the same razor for shaving.[172]

Social and Cultural Factors

Urbanization has been associated with a higher prevalence of STDs in many parts of the world because bringing people closer together increases the likelihood of sexual encounters.[179,180] In the United States, HIV/AIDS has been observed more frequently in urban than in rural areas. Sexual mixing patterns can define how rapidly HIV-1 spreads in a population.[181,182] In cities with a high male/female ratio, such as Nairobi, Bombay, and Harare, the rate of casual and commercial sex is increased. This has led to high HIV-1 prevalence rates in sex workers and their clients, and ultimately an increased incidence of HIV infection in the general population of these cities. Sexual practices may vary in frequency between countries and regions of the world. For example, unprotected receptive anal intercourse is unusual in sub-Saharan Africa, whereas it plays a significant role in the spread of HIV in the United States, Latin America, and some Caribbean countries.[183,184] Bisexuality appears to be more common in Latin America than in many other Western countries.[184] In most developing countries, expression of a homosexual lifestyle is repressed; therefore, MSM in these countries may be more hesitant in surveys to admit to anal intercourse.

Significant rural-to-urban migration is occurring throughout the developing world. The use of migrant labor exposes the worker to long absences, increasing the possibility of family breakdown and turning to other sexual partners.[185] Higher HIV incidence is seen among women who are poor and who have few options to make money.[179] Poverty predisposes to commercial sex, homelessness in adults, the presence of street children, poor education, and migration, all of which may enhance the possibility of spreading HIV infection.

UNAIDS and the World Health Organization (WHO) conducted an international study in 1998 to evaluate the effect of literacy on HIV incidence.[186] In 161 countries for which literacy and HIV data were available, the higher the rate of literacy, the lower was the rate of HIV infection. The study coordinators suggested that these results were found because better educated people have greater access to information about HIV, how it is spread, and how it can be avoided. However, in sub-Saharan Africa, the opposite literacy-HIV incidence pattern has emerged.[186] It is possible that, in this region, the rapid social changes that have accompanied education have prompted behaviors that increase the risk of HIV infection. Higher-paying jobs among the educated in this region have apparently served to support these behaviors. Education has emancipated many women of sub-Saharan Africa, resulting in their greater social mobility and increased likelihood of being involved in more sexual relationships.

GLOBAL EPIDEMIOLOGIC TRENDS

UNAIDS and WHO work together with networks of AIDS researchers and national AIDS programs around the world to track and model HIV infection. Their efforts have resulted in improvement in provision of information on HIV infection and AIDS in many countries. Very specific data are now being culled from numerous observational databases, including the Multicenter AIDS Cohort Study, the HIV Epidemiology Research Study, the Western Australian HIV Cohort Study, and the Johns Hopkins HIV Clinical Practice Cohort. Improved data collection has made it possible to build models not only on a regional basis, but for 90 individual countries, as well. Serosurveys that have been done mainly in rural areas have provided better indications of the likely relationship between urban and rural HIV infection patterns.

The WHO has reported that, as of December 1997, 30.6 million people in the world were living with HIV/AIDS, of whom 12.1 million were women and 1.1 million were children younger than 15 years of age. Approximately 11.7 million people have died of AIDS, 2.3 million in 1997 alone (Table 18–4).[186] More than 70% of the cumulative cases of HIV infection have occurred in Africa (Figure 18–5). In 1997, nearly 5.8 million people became infected.[187] Most new infections were reported from sub-Saharan Africa, India, and Southeast Asia. The regional distribution of AIDS is shown in Table 18–5. By the year 2000, it is expected that a minimal cumulative total of 40 million cases of HIV infection and 10 million adult AIDS cases will be seen, of whom about 90% will be from developing countries.

Europe

In Western Europe, HIV infection rates have decreased.[186] New infections are concentrated among IDUs in the southern countries of the continent, especially Greece and Portugal. Approximately 30,000 Western Europeans were found to be newly infected with HIV in 1997. Fewer than 500 children under 15 years old were infected with HIV in 1997, and this low number was thought to be due to the use of antiretroviral drugs given to women during pregnancy and the standard of using safe alternatives to breast-feeding.

In Eastern Europe, HIV infection was seldom reported until 1994. At the start of 1995, all of Eastern Europe had approximately 30,000 infections among its 450 million people, an infection rate one-fifteenth that seen in Western Europe at that time.[186] However, by the end of 1997, the incidence of HIV infection increased sixfold, with 190,000 adults currently infected. Since 1995, the largest increases in HIV infection have been reported in the countries of the former Soviet Union, Belarus, Moldova, the Russian Federation, and Ukraine. Ukraine is the most heavily affected country in this region, with 70 times as many HIV-positive people in 1998 as in 1994. There are currently almost four times as many HIV infections in the Ukraine

Table 18–4 Global Summary of the HIV/AIDS Epidemic as of December 1997

People newly infected with HIV in 1997	Total	5.8 million
	Adults	5.2 million
	Women	2.1 million
	Children <15 yr	590,000
No. of people living with HIV/AIDS	Total	30.6 million
	Adults	29.5 million
	Women	12.1 million
	Children <15 yr	1.1 million
AIDS deaths in 1997	Total	2.3 million
	Adults	1.8 million
	Women	820,000
	Children <15 yr	460,000
Total no. of AIDS deaths since the beginning of the epidemic	Total	11.7 million
	Adults	9.0 million
	Women	4.0 million
	Children <15 yr	2.7 million
Total no. of AIDS orphans* since the beginning of the epidemic		8.2 million

*Defined as HIV-negative children who lost their mothers or both parents to AIDS when they were under the age of 15 yr. *Source:* Reprinted with permission from *Report on the Global HIV/AIDS Epidemic*, June 1998, © World Health Organization.

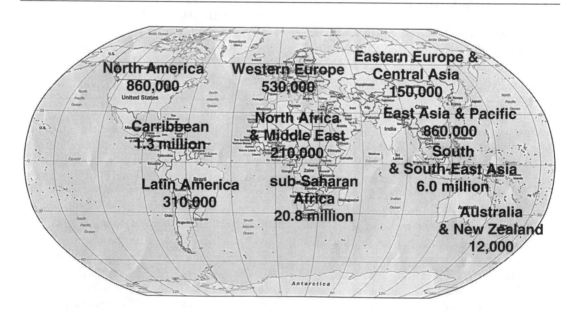

Figure 18–5 Total number of adults and children living with HIV/AIDS at the end of 1997. *Source:* Reprinted with permission from *Report on the Global HIV/AIDS Epidemic*, June 1998, © WHO and UNAIDS.

Table 18-5 Regional HIV/AIDS Statistics and Features as of December 1997

Region	Epidemic Started	Adults and Children Living with HIV/AIDs	Adult Prevalence Rate* (%)	Cumulative No. of Orphans+	Percentage of HIV-Positive Adults Who Are Women (%)	Main Mode(s) of Transmission for Adults Living with HIV/AIDS
Sub-Saharan Africa	Late 1970s–early 1980s	20.8 million	7.4	7.8 million	50	Heterosexual
North Africa and Middle East	Late 1980s	210,000	0.13	14,200	20	IDU, Heterosexual
South and Southeast Asia	Late 1980s	6.0 million	0.6	220,000	25	Heterosexual, IDU
East Asia and Pacific	Late 1980s	440,000	0.05	1,900	11	IDU, Heterosexual, MSM
Latin America	Late 1970s–early 1980s	1.3 million	0.5	91,000	19	MSM, IDU, Heterosexual
Caribbean	Late 1970s–early 1980s	310,000	1.9	48,000	33	Heterosexual, MSM
Eastern Europe and Central Asia	Early 1990s	150,000	0.07	30	25	IDU, MSM
Western Europe	Late 1970s–early 1980s	530,000	0.3	8,700	20	MSM, IDU
North America	Late 1970s–early 1980s	860,000	0.6	70,000	20	MSM, IDU, Heterosexual
Australia and New Zealand	Late 1970s–early 1980s	12,000	0.1	300	5	MSM, IDU
Total		30.6 million	1.0	8.2 million	41	

MSM, men who have sex with men; IDU, injection drug users

* The proportion of adults living with HIV/AIDS in the adult population (15–49 years of age)

+ Orphans are defined as HIV-negative children who lost their mothers or both parents to AIDS when they were under age 15

Source: Reprinted with permission from Joint United Nations Programme on HIV/AIDS (UNAIDS)/World Health Organizations, *Report on the Global HIV/AIDS Epidemic: Fact Sheet*, Geneva: UNAIDS/WHO, © 1997, World Health Organization.

alone as there were in all of Eastern Europe in 1995.

Similarly, in the Russian Federation, 158 people were found to be HIV-positive in 1994, and this number increased to 4,399 by 1997.[186] Eighty percent of these cases have been related to unsafe injection of illicit drugs. It is estimated that, in the Russian Federation, there are six people living with HIV for every one who has been tested. Therefore, current figures of HIV prevalence are likely to be much lower than the actual numbers. Sex partners of IDUs provide a conduit for the spread of the virus into the general population. In Kalingrad, a third of sex workers are IDUs living with HIV, and four of five women with HIV make a living from sex. The economic collapse of the Russian Federation has contributed to these high-risk behaviors. Another factor that has facilitated HIV transmission is the rising incidence of syphilis, which has increased 100-fold to over 250-fold in the Russian Federation, as well as in Ukraine, Moldova, and Belarus.

Middle East

In the Middle East and Northern Africa, approximately 210,000 people (<1% of the world total) were living with HIV/AIDS at the end of 1997.[186] Less is known about HIV infection rates in these areas than elsewhere in the world. Some countries with large populations of immigrant workers do mass screening for HIV. None has estimated the infection rate at greater than one adult in 100. The conservative social and political attitudes in the Middle East and Northern Africa have impeded government evaluation of HIV risk behavior. Community and nongovernmental organizations have been more effective in instituting programs for sex workers to reduce the risk of HIV spread.

Africa

AIDS is now the most serious public health problem in Africa. Higher mother-to-child transmission has been observed in Africa (30–40%)

than in the Western world.[188] Africa has a high incidence of tuberculosis, malaria, and vitamin A deficiency, all of which have been shown to increase the risk of HIV transmission.[189–191] Although sub-Saharan Africa contains only 10% of the world's population, it harbors two thirds of all persons currently infected with HIV.[192,193] Twenty million adults and children are infected. More than 90% of adults in sub-Saharan Africa have been infected through heterosexual contact, and most children acquire the infection from their mothers. Because of AIDS-related mortality, the population growth rate in sub-Saharan Africa is expected to decline from an average of 3% to less than 2% per year by 2000.[194]

The incidence of HIV in Africa varies by region and country. In Southern Africa, severe HIV epidemics have been ongoing for a long time in Malawi, Zambia, and Zimbabwe. More recently, epidemics have been observed in South Africa, Botswana, and Lesotho.[192] Urban areas of Zambia and Zimbabwe have prevalence rates among adults ranging from 20% to 45% in persons aged 20–30 years old.[193,195] The South African government estimated that, in 1997, 6% of the population (2.4 million people) were living with HIV, a 33% increase over 1995 figures. Although HIV was rare in Botswana in the mid-1980s, 43% of pregnant women in its capital city, Francistown, are now HIV-positive.

HIV infection in East Africa had spread rapidly in the late 1970s and early 1980s. As a result, 15–30% of pregnant women in urban areas of East Africa are HIV-positive. About 36% of all HIV-infected persons live in East Africa. The movement of people along the trans-African highway is a major factor driving the epidemic in East Africa. HIV prevalence rates continue to increase in Kenya, but they have plateaued at high levels in certain areas of East Africa and decreased in some urban areas of Uganda.[194,196] Prevention efforts are thought to be responsible for HIV reduction in Uganda.[196]

The HIV epidemic started later in West Africa than in East Africa. The economic upswing in Côte d'Ivoire prompted considerable migration from neighboring countries.[192,194,197] By 1996, prevalence rates of 10–15% were found among pregnant women in Abidjan, smaller towns and rural areas, and some neighboring countries (notably, Burkina Faso). Conversely, the incidence of HIV has stabilized at the lower level of 2–3% in Senegal. West Africa also has the greatest number of HIV-2 infections in the world, with the epicenter in Guinea-Bissau, where more than 7% of pregnant women are infected with HIV-2.[198–200]

In North Africa, the rates of HIV among the general population are less than 1%, and the modes of transmission include heterosexual and homosexual contact and IDU.[192,194] Although Central Africa has been less affected than have the other regions of Africa, HIV infection rates of approximately 5% have been reported among pregnant women.

Latin America

In Latin America and the Caribbean, HIV/AIDS is monitored mainly through AIDS case reporting and analysis. Also, HIV sentinel surveillance programs are ongoing. The epidemic spread of HIV infection in Latin America and the Caribbean appears to have begun in the late 1970s, just as it did in North America. At the end of 1997, about 1.6 million people were living with HIV/AIDS in these countries. Approximately 580,000 had died of AIDS since the start of the epidemic (see Table 18–5).

HIV prevalence rates in Latin American countries have been culled from scattered studies involving marginalized or neglected populations. Unlike in North America, where HIV has been spread primarily through homosexual contact, in Latin America and the Caribbean, the major mode of HIV transmission has been heterosexual contact and IDU since the mid-1980s.[201–203] Nevertheless, rates of HIV infection in MSM remain high. Indeed, in 1993 and 1994, the incidence of HIV among MSM in Costa Rica was reported to be 5% and more than 30% in Mexico City.[194] In Brazil, the relative proportion of cases in MSM has decreased from about 70% in 1980–1986 to about 30% at the end of 1997

because of the steadily rising number of cases due to heterosexual contact (>40% of cases) and IDU. In Brazil, MSM commonly are bisexual and frequently have female sexual partners, facilitating transmission beyond the MSM population. Rates of HIV infection among IDUs range from 5–11% in Mexico to about 50% in Brazil and Argentina.[187,194] As in the United States, HIV infection and AIDS cases are being seen increasingly in women.

In the Caribbean, more diverse epidemic patterns are evident. The main mode of HIV transmission in Martinique, Barbados, and Trinidad and Tobago is MSM, whereas more HIV infection in Guyana and the Bahamas is due to heterosexual transmission. In 1992, the prevalence rate in pregnant women was 7% in Guyana and 4% in the Bahamas.[204]

Asia

In Asia, the spread of HIV began in the late 1980s. Surveillance systems in Asia are limited because the HIV epidemic is a more recent phenomenon than in other parts of the world. Therefore, application of results from limited studies performed to date to the entire populations of Asian countries may be unreliable. At the end of 1997, approximately 6 million people were estimated to be living with HIV/AIDS in South and Southeast Asia, 3–5 million in India, and 440,000 in East Asia and the Pacific, excluding Australia and New Zealand (Table 18–5).[187] India has by far the greatest number of HIV infections in the world and, according to current trends, it is likely to experience a doubling of these numbers in the next few years.[187] At least 750,000 have died of AIDS. In view of the large Asian and Indian populations currently HIV-infected and their inability to afford treatment, a far greater effect of the HIV epidemic on morbidity and mortality is expected during the early years of the twenty-first century.

The initial spread of HIV is thought to be due to the rapid increase in IDU that occurred in the 1980s in South and Southeast Asia,[205] especially in areas of Thailand, Malaysia, Myanmar, Vietnam, India, China, and Cambodia. Seroprevalence levels reached as high as 50% in IDUs by the early 1990s.[206–211] Following this wave of transmission among IDUs, heterosexual transmission rapidly increased; it is now the major mode of HIV transmission in Asia. The first indication of a rapid increase in heterosexual transmission was seen among female prostitutes in Thailand and in Bombay, India. Prevalence rates skyrocketed from 0% in 1987 to more than 20% in 1991 in Bombay,[194,212,213] and from 15% to 40% in northern Thailand during approximately this same period.[194,207,214,215] By 1993, rates of HIV infection in Thailand reached 4%, with the highest rates in the northern provinces (up to 20%).[216] In view of the magnitude of these HIV rates and the morbidity caused by them, the Thai government initiated the 100% Condom Use Program.[217] The program focused on decreasing sex with commercial or unknown partners and increasing the use of condoms during these types of sexual encounters. As a result, the incidence in young Thai men has decreased since 1993.[218–220] However, this reduction in HIV incidence has not yet been observed in pregnant women, in whom HIV seropositivity has stabilized at about 2%.

In China, the national government estimated that approximately 200,000 people were living with HIV/AIDS at the end of 1996; by the end of 1997, this number doubled, due to two major HIV epidemics—one among IDUs in the mountain areas of southwest China, along the southern borders with Myanmar, Laos, and Vietnam, and the other among heterosexuals along the eastern seaboard, where prostitution has re-emerged.[221] The rising rate of STDs in the latter region of China poses an additional risk factor that is facilitating more rapid heterosexual transmission of HIV.

HIV prevalence in Southeast Asia is diverse. Several Southeast Asian countries have low rates of HIV infection, despite the presence of well-developed commercial sex industries. Thus, infection rates of <0.5% have been reported in Singapore, the Philippines, and Indonesia.[222] Conversely, in Cambodia, sentinel HIV surveillance has shown that about 5% of pregnant women, 6% of soldiers and policemen, and 50% of sex workers have tested HIV-positive.[223] The high incidence of HIV infection in Cambodia is believed to be due to the frequent visits that Cambodian men have with commercial sex workers (75% of the military and police force and 40% of students visit a sex worker at least annually). Interestingly, the high rate of HIV infection among Cambodian men is occurring despite the dramatic rise in condom sales over the past few years, with 1 million units currently being sold each month. In Myanmar and Vietnam, the incidence of HIV infection is increasing rapidly, especially among IDUs. In Myanmar, HIV positivity has been reported in 2% of pregnant women in the general population and in 67% of IDUs. Among commercial sex workers, the incidence of HIV infection increased from 4% in 1992 to >20% in 1996.[194,224] Several countries in Asia and Southeast Asia are experiencing major epidemics of HIV among IDUs; these countries include Myanmar, Thailand, Vietnam, China, India, and Malaysia.

Australia and New Zealand

In Australia, the annual numbers of AIDS cases has decreased from a peak of 946 cases in 1994 to 809 cases in 1995, 690 cases in 1996, and 432 cases in 1997.[225] Similarly, the AIDS Epidemiology Group has reported that the incidence of AIDS is decreasing in New Zealand to a degree similar to that seen in the United Kingdom, Germany, and Sweden.[226]

EPIDEMIOLOGIC TRENDS IN THE UNITED STATES

Overall Incidence

In the United States, 688,200 cases of AIDS have been reported to the CDC since 1981.[227] The incidence of AIDS escalated steadily between 1985 and 1993, after which time it began to fall, due to the availability of antiretroviral therapy, increasing use of prophylactic regimens against opportunistic infections, and improvements in medical care that allowed patients with HIV to remain AIDS-free (Figure 18–6). The expansion of the case definition of AIDS in 1993 to include CD4 counts under 200/mm³ as an "AIDS-defining" condition accounted for the abrupt increase in incidence observed that year. This artificial increase required statistical adjustments to interpret AIDS incidence data properly. In 1998, an estimated 297,135 persons were living with AIDS, a 10% increase from 1997 (Figure 18–7). The latter increase is due to improved survival of AIDS patients who have received treatment and decreases in the number of deaths.

Mortality Rate in the United States

Between 1981 and 1998, approximately 410,800 people in the United States died of AIDS, including 50% of all adults (405,862) and 58% of children (4,938) who were HIV-seropositive.[227] The incidence of AIDS-related

deaths rose steadily between 1985 and 1995. Thereafter, the AIDS-related mortality rate decreased, due primarily to the standard of pharmacotherapy changing to combination antiretroviral therapy regimens that included protease inhibitors and reverse transcriptase inhibitors. Although the annual number of AIDS-related deaths has decreased, AIDS remains a leading cause of death among persons 25–44 years old.

Exposure Category Trends

Men Who Have Sex with Men

Between 1985 and 1998, MSM had the highest overall incidence of AIDS in the United States (Figure 18–8). However, the proportion of MSM AIDS cases decreased over this period, from a high of >60% in 1985 to 35% in 1998. MSM who inject illicit drugs have the fourth highest incidence of AIDS in the United States. Of more than 16,000 MSM AIDS cases reported to the CDC in 1998, 23% were IDUs.

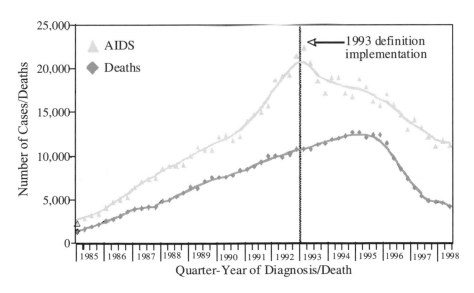

Figure 18–6 Estimated incidence of AIDS and deaths of adults with AIDS in the U.S. between 1985 and June 1998. *Source:* Reprinted from Centers for Disease Control and Prevention.

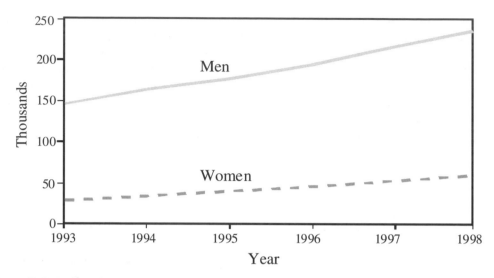

Figure 18–7 Estimated number of persons living with AIDS in the U.S. between 1993 and 1998, by sex. *Source:* Reprinted from Centers for Disease Control and Prevention.

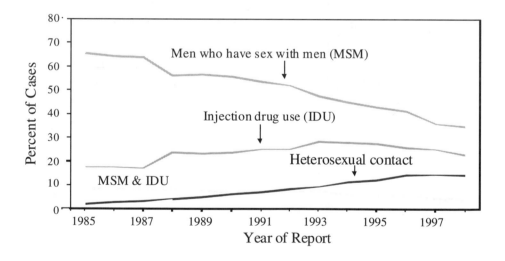

Figure 18–8 Cases of AIDS reported in the United States between 1985 and 1998, by exposure category. Excludes cases with other or unreported risk pending medical record review and reclassification. *Source:* Reprinted from Centers for Disease control and Prevention.

Injection Drug Users

The second highest incidence of AIDS in the United States between 1985 and 1998 was in IDUs.[227] The number of AIDS cases rose steadily until 1993, after which a decline occurred. In 1998, IDUs accounted for 23% of all adult AIDS cases. More than half of IDU-associated cases are heterosexual males, 21% are females, 13% are MSM who inject drugs, and 12% are heterosexual partners of an IDU.

Heterosexual Contact

Heterosexual contact was the third most frequent cause of AIDS in the United States between 1985 and 1998.[227] In contrast to the trend for reduced numbers of AIDS cases among MSM, the proportion of AIDS cases among heterosexuals has increased in the United States from <5% in 1985 to 21% in 1998. Many of these heterosexuals have acquired the HIV infection through sexual contact with an infected IDU.

Blood Product Transmission

The incidence of AIDS in transfusion recipients (1%) and hemophilia cases (<1%) is the lowest it has ever been, due presumably to preventive measures that have been taken to ensure HIV-free blood and factor VIII.[227] The low rates of infection reflect the success of prevention measures through donor deferral and screening of the blood supply.

Perinatal Transmission

Exposure categories have changed over the past 17 years in mothers who transmit HIV to their children.[227] In the early 1980s, most of these women were exposed to HIV through IDU, and only 10–15% of the women were reported without a risk (Figure 18–9).[227] In 1997, IDU accounted for fewer maternal cases (27%), and the risk-unspecified category was much higher (38%). Most risk-unspecified cases will be reclassified into the recognized risk categories as further information becomes available. The proportion of women exposed to HIV by a heterosexual partner who is HIV-infected or who has a known risk has increased from 22% in 1980 to 36% in 1997. These trends parallel those seen among women with AIDS.

Nearly 40% of children with perinatally acquired AIDS were diagnosed within the first

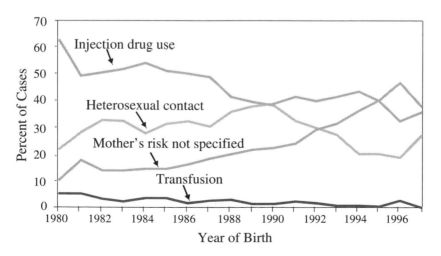

Figure 18–9 Perinatally acquired AIDS cases reported in the United States between 1980 and 1997, by mother's exposure category. *Source:* Reprinted from Centers for Disease Control and Prevention.

year of life; 22% were diagnosed within the first 6 months. The CDC suggests that this distribution may change if more HIV-infected child-bearing women become aware of their HIV status and seek medical care early in their infants' lives, when treatment could prevent HIV disease progression. The incidence of perinatally acquired AIDS was highest in 1992 and has declined since then, due largely to the use of zidovudine by pregnant HIV-infected women and their newborns and the implementation of Public Health Service guidelines for universal counseling and voluntary HIV testing of pregnant women (Figure 18–10).[227]

Age and Gender Trends

Most of the HIV infections in the United States between 1981 and 1998 have been in persons 20–39 years old (74%), whereas most cases of AIDS have been reported in persons 30–49 years old (71%) (Figure 18–11).[227] The latter trend probably reflects the time needed for AIDS to become manifest after an HIV diagnosis is made. Data from the 33 areas that conducted

HIV surveillance in 1998 showed that 41% of persons diagnosed with HIV were under 30 years of age, compared with approximately 18% of AIDS cases (Table 18–6). The CDC suggest that these findings reinforce the need for HIV data to describe the "front end" of the epidemic, where prevention should be focused. Among persons who were HIV-positive, 16% of men and 21% of women were in their twenties, and 26% of men and 21% of women were in their forties.

Nearly all newly infected children acquire HIV perinatally from their mothers. Since the start of the AIDS epidemic, 8,461 children have been reported with AIDS, 91% of whom acquired it perinatally. In 1998, 382 children were reported to CDC with AIDS, and perinatal transmission was responsible for 89% of these cases. Four percent of children in the United States acquired HIV from a blood or blood product transfusion, and 3% because of their hemophilia. For 2% of children, the CDC lists the source of infection as "other or not reported exposure." Of these, 150 had an unidentified risk, 2 were exposed to HIV-infected blood in a household set-

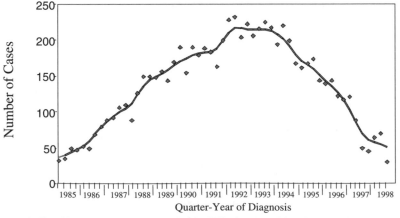

*Adjusted for reporting delays and redistribution of NIRs, data reported through March 1999

Figure 18–10 Perinatally acquired AIDS cases reported in the United States between 1985 and 1998, by quarter-year of diagnosis. *Source:* Reprinted from Centers for Disease Control and Prevention.

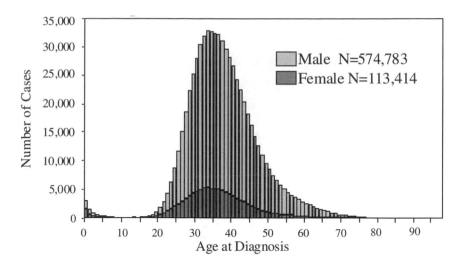

Figure 18–11 Number of AIDS cases reported in the United States between 1981 and 1998, by age and sex. *Source:* Reprinted from Centers for Disease control and Prevention.

ting, and 10 children had sexual contact with an adult with or at high risk for HIV infection.

In 1998, 728 adolescents were reported with HIV infection, and 297 adolescents were re-

Table 18–6 Age at Diagnosis of HIV Infection or AIDS Reported through 1998, United States

Age	HIV*		AIDS	
	Number	Percent	Number	Percent
<12	1,875	2	8,461	1
13–19	4,161	4	3,423	<1
20–29	36,820	35	117,718	17
30–39	41,448	39	310,197	45
40–49	16,800	16	176,239	26
50+	5,471	5	72,162	11
	106,575		688,200	

*Data from 33 areas with confidential HIV infection surveillance

Source: Reprinted from Centers for Disease Control and Prevention.

ported with AIDS nationwide and from the 30 areas that conduct confidential HIV infection surveillance (Figure 18–12).[227] In most areas with HIV surveillance, the number of adolescents reported with HIV was greater than the number reported with AIDS.

Eighty-four percent of the 688,200 cases of AIDS reported to the CDC since 1981 have been in men; in 1998, the percentage had fallen to 77%. Of all cases of AIDS reported since 1981, 45% of men and 44% of women were 30–39 years of age at diagnosis. Adolescent cases have occurred in a slightly greater proportion of females than males (1% vs 0.4%), although in 1998, AIDS was diagnosed in a similar number of female and male adolescents in the United States (150 vs 147).

Although the number of AIDS cases is rising in both men and women, the proportion of female cases is increasing faster.[227] Since 1995, an average of approximately 12,500 cases of AIDS has been diagnosed in women each year. Over 16,000 women 15–34 years old, who were considered to be of childbearing age and who have

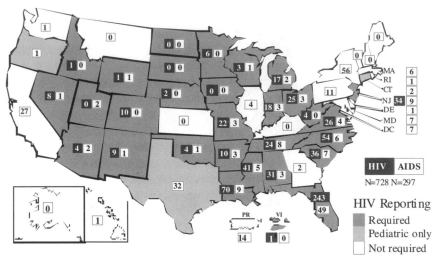

*For areas with confidential HIV surveillance. Includes 34 persons who were residents of areas
 without HIV infection surveillance but who were reported by areas with HIV surveillance.
aHIV Surveillance initiated in July 1998.
bHIV Surveillance initiated in December 1998.

Figure 18–12 Cases of HIV infection and AIDS in 13– to 19–year-olds reported in the United States in 1998.
Source: Reprinted from Centers for Disease Control and Prevention.

the highest fertility, were reported to be living with AIDS in the United States at the end of 1998—20% of all persons living with AIDS in the United States. An additional 13,298 women of this age group were reported living with HIV infection from the 30 areas that conduct confidential HIV infection surveillance. From 1981 to 1998, 43% of female AIDS cases in the United States were attributed to IDU; in 1998, 29% of female cases were IDUs (Figure 18–13).[227] The proportion attributed to heterosexual contact appears stable; however, many of the cases with an unreported risk may be due to heterosexual contact. Overall, heterosexual transmission accounted for 38% of AIDS cases reported among women in 1998. Eleven percent of these women reported heterosexual contact with an IDU, and the other 26% reported sexual contact with men of unspecified or other risks, such as men who have sex with men and women. The proportion of female AIDS cases related to hemophilia has not changed, and the proportion attributed to the receipt of blood products and transfusions has

declined from 3% to 1% of cases. Twenty-nine percent of cases in women were attributed to IDU and 1% to transfusions. The remainder of cases, 32%, were due to other or unidentified modes of exposure, including many cases that are pending further medical record review and investigation.

Race and Ethnicity Trends

Since 1985, the proportion of AIDS cases among whites has decreased, whereas it has increased among blacks and Hispanics (Figure 18–14).[227] Figure 18–15 depicts the proportionately higher distribution of AIDS cases reported in 1998 among racial/ethnic groups (n = 48,269), compared with the general population in the United States, Puerto Rico, and U.S. territories. Thirty-three percent of the cases were among white persons (down from 46% in 1993), whereas 71% of the population was white. Forty-five percent of cases reported were among black persons (up from 35% in 1993), although

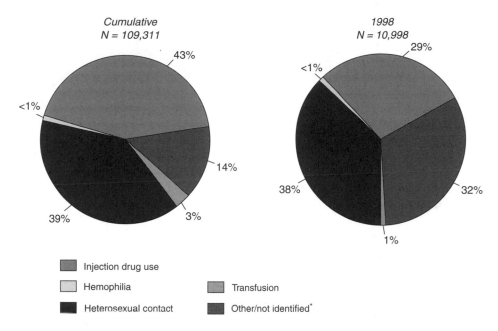

*Includes patients whose medical record review is pending; patients who died, were lost to follow-up, or declined interview; and patients with other or undetermined modes of exposure.

Figure 18–13 AIDS cases in adult/adolescent women reported in the United States between 1981 and 1998, by exposure category. *Source:* Reprinted from Centers for Disease Control and Prevention.

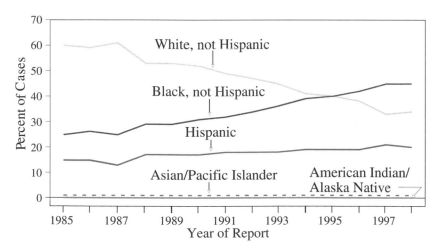

Figure 18–14 Proportion of AIDS cases in each major race/ethnicity category reported in the United States between 1985 and 1998. *Source:* Reprinted from Centers for Disease Control and Prevention.

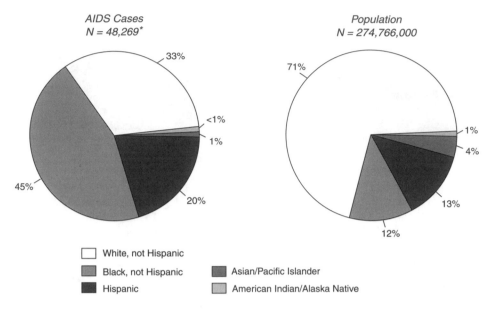

Figure 18–15 Proportion of AIDS cases in each major race/ethnicity category reported in the United States in 1998, compared with the proportion of the United States population in each category. *Source:* Reprinted from Centers for Disease Control and Prevention.

only 12% of the population was black. Twenty percent of cases were Hispanic, compared with 13% of the population. Overall, over half of the AIDS cases reported in the United States were among blacks and Hispanics. Only small changes have been observed in proportions of the other racial/ethnic groups during the 1990s. The proportion of Asian/Pacific Islander and Native American/Alaska Native persons living with AIDS has remained approximately 1% and <1%, respectively, since 1993 (Figure 18–14). Between 1993 and 1998, the number of AIDS cases increased among Asian/Pacific Islanders from approximately 1,284 to 2,320 persons, and among Native American/Alaska Natives from approximately 559 to 971 persons.

With regard to differentiating the incidence in minorities by gender, over 570,000 cases of AIDS have been reported among adult/adolescent men since 1981. Of these, about a third

were black men, and 18% were Hispanic men.[227] Although the number of AIDS cases reported in 1998 was similar for white and black men, the AIDS population rate was nearly seven times higher for black men than for white men (125 vs 18 per 100,000 men). Similarly, the AIDS population rate was over three times higher for Hispanic men than for white men (58 vs 18 per 100,000 men). The CDC speculates that the disproportionately higher number of AIDS cases among blacks and Hispanics is due to a greater prevalence of risk behaviors in these groups. Approximately 57% of men reported with AIDS were MSM, 22% were IDUs, and 8% were MSM who injected drugs of abuse. The distribution of risk varies by racial/ethnic group; among white men, 75% of cases were among MSM, and only 9% were IDU. Comparable figures were observed for Asian/Pacific Islander men. Among black men, 38% were MSM, and nearly as many (35%) were IDU. Among Hispanic men, a similar pattern was apparent: 43% MSM and 36% IDU. Among Native American/Alaska Native American men, 57% of reported cases were MSM, and 17% were IDU.

Black and Hispanic women have also been disproportionately affected by the AIDS epidemic.[227] Over 100,000 cases of AIDS have been reported among women since 1981. Fifty-seven percent of the cases were among black women, and 20% were among Hispanic women. More than half of the nearly 11,000 AIDS cases reported among women in 1998 were among black women. The AIDS population rate has been reported to be 12–26 times higher among black women than among white women (varying by state in the United States), and 8.5 times higher in Hispanic women than in white women. Few AIDS cases were reported in 1998 among Native American/Alaska Native women and Asian/Pacific Islander women. Nevertheless, the AIDS population rate among Native American/Alaska Native women was twice that of white women.

In 43% of the women reported with AIDS, HIV infection was attributed to IDU, and in 39%, it was attributed to heterosexual contact with either an IDU, a bisexual male, a person with hemophilia, a transfusion recipient with HIV, or an HIV-infected person. The proportion of white, black, and Native American/Alaska Native women in each risk group was similar, with 42–47% of cases among IDU, 37–40% due to heterosexual contact, and 15–18% due to heterosexual contact with an IDU. More Hispanic and Asian/Pacific Islander women acquire AIDS by heterosexual contact (47%). Of these, 22% of Hispanic women and 13% of Asian/Pacific Islander women reported sexual contact with an IDU. Asian/Pacific Islander women had the greatest proportion of cases without a reported or identified risk (36%), compared with the other racial/ethnic groups (13–19%). This may reflect language or cultural barriers impeding the acquisition of information pertaining to risk.

Between 1981 and 1998, there were 4,911 reported cases of AIDS among persons with hemophilia or coagulation disorders and 8,382 cases attributed to the receipt of blood transfusions, blood components, or tissue. These cases have included persons of all racial and ethnic groups, and no differences according to race/ethnicity have been apparent.

Geographic Trends

Between 1993 and 1998, the estimated number of persons living with AIDS increased in all regions of the United States, with a proportional increase of 34–37% in the South, and a proportional decrease from 23% to 20% in the West (Figure 18–16).[227] Only about 9,000 persons with AIDS (3% of the total) live in the U.S. dependencies, possessions, and associated nations. Figure 18–17 shows AIDS rates per 100,000 population in each state, the District of Columbia, Puerto Rico, and the Virgin Islands for 1998.[227] The highest rates were reported in New York, Puerto Rico, Maryland, and Florida. Most reports of AIDS cases came primarily from large metropolitan cities (population >500,000) in the South or the Northeast; reports of AIDS from smaller metropolitan and rural areas came chiefly from states in the North Central region and the South.

Most of the adolescents with HIV infection and AIDS live in the Southern and East Coast states, Texas, California, and some Midwestern states. More women reported IDU than heterosexual contact as an AIDS risk in the Northeast (where over half of the female cases were IDUs), in contrast to the other regions. In the other three regions, cases were nearly equally distributed between the two main risk exposures.

The highest state-specific AIDS rates for whites in 1998 were in Hawaii, California, Florida, New York, Texas, Washington, DC, and other states in the Northeast and Southwest.[227] The rates for whites were considerably lower than those for blacks or Hispanics, with an overall U.S. rate of 9.9 per 100,000 population, compared with 86.3 for blacks and 39.1 for Hispanics. The incidence of AIDS for black, white, and Hispanic women was highest in the Northeast, compared with the other U.S. regions, with

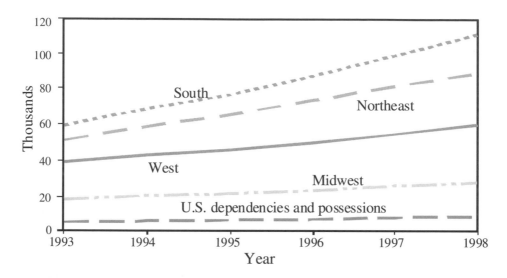

Figure 18–16 Estimated number of persons in the United States living with AIDS, by geographic region. *Source:* Reprinted from Centers for Disease Control and Prevention.

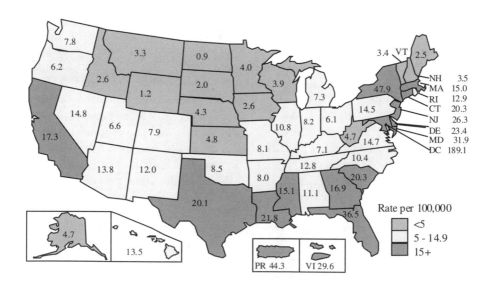

Figure 18–17 AIDS rates per 100,000 population reported in the United States in 1998, by state. *Source:* Reprinted from Centers for Disease Control and Prevention.

the next highest incidence in the South. State-specific AIDS rates for blacks in 1998 ranged from 17.4 in Iowa to 183.5 in Florida. Rates were highest in states in the Northeast that generally have high AIDS counts, such as New York, New Jersey, Maryland, Delaware, Massachusetts, and Connecticut. Rates among Hispanic women were higher than among white women in each region, especially the Northeast. The distribution of state-specific AIDS rates for Hispanics was similar to that for blacks, with rates highest in the Northeastern states and lower in the North Central states. Too few women Asian/Pacific Islanders and American Indians/ Alaska Natives were reported with AIDS in 1998 to allow for stable rate calculations when stratified by region of residence.

IMPACT OF ANTIRETROVIRAL THERAPY ON EPIDEMICITY

Before antiretroviral treatment became available, all patients with AIDS were considered highly likely to develop a new AIDS-defining illness or to die within 2 years. Over the last 17 years, much progress has been made in improving the quality and duration of life of persons with HIV infection. In 1987, the reverse transcriptase inhibitor zidovudine was the first anti-AIDS treatment to become available. Over the ensuing years, other reverse transcriptase inhibitors were marketed and were used as monotherapy or duotherapy. However, resistance to these regimens developed over a short time, limiting their long-term efficacy.

During the 1990s, extraordinary progress was made in developing highly active triple combination antiretroviral therapies (HAART), as well as continuing progress in preventing and treating individual opportunistic infections. Protease inhibitors became available in 1995, and their combination with reverse transcriptase inhibitors was found to extend life significantly in patients with AIDS. Palella et al.[228] studied over 1,000 patients with AIDS (CD4 cell counts <100 cells/mm^3) in the CDC-sponsored HIV Outpatient Study (HOPS) between 1994 and mid-1997. In patients who started taking HAART combination regimens in 1996, marked declines were observed, from 29.4 deaths per 100 person-years in 1995 to 8.8 deaths per 100 person-years in the second quarter of 1997 (Figure 18–18). Reduction in the number of opportunistic infections was also observed. Similar

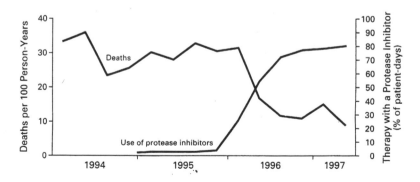

Figure 18–18 Mortality in patients with CD4 cell counts <100/mm^3 and use of antiretroviral therapy, including a protease inhibitor among patients in the HOPS cohort study in the United States, 1994–97. *Source:* Reprinted with permission from Palella et al, Declining Morbidity and Mortality among Patients with Advanced Human Immunodeficiency Virus Infection, *The New England Journal of Medicine*, Vol. 338, pp. 853–860. Copyright © 1998, Massachusetts Medical Society. All rights reserved.

findings were also reported in the European study EuroSIDA, with a decline in mortality of 23.7 deaths per 100 person-years from March to September 1995 (pre-HAART) to 4.1 per 100 person-years from September 1997 to March 1998 (post-HAART).[229]

The goal of instituting potent combination antiretroviral therapy is to maximally suppress HIV replication to below the levels of detection of sensitive plasma HIV RNA assays (eg, <50 copies/mL in the Roche PCR assay) to limit the potential for selection of antiretroviral-resistant HIV variants. The National Institutes of Health (NIH) recommends that combination antiretroviral therapy be started in HIV-infected persons who are symptomatic or show signs of AIDS (unexplained fever, thrush), regardless of their CD4 cell count or HIV-1 RNA level.[230] Treatment should also be initiated in asymptomatic HIV-infected patients if their CD4 cell counts are below 500/mm^3 or their plamsa HIV-1 RNA levels are >20,000 (RT-PCR assay) or >10,000 (bDNA assay) copies/mL.

Although combination antiretroviral drug therapy is highly effective, its usefulness is limited if patients do not adhere to their regimens. Paterson et al[231] found that viral suppression to <400 copies/mL is achievable in 81% of patients only if they are >95% adherent to taking all doses of their protease inhibitor-containing regimens and doing so at the recommended times. Such viral suppression is achievable in only 25% of patients if they are only 70–80% adherent and in 6% of those who are <70% adherent. Unfortunately, adherence can be difficult because many antiretroviral regimens are complicated, involving the taking of 13–60 pills per day in two or three divided doses.[232] The patient also may have to observe dietary and fluid requirements. Forgetting, being at an unfortuitous location at the time of dosing, and fear of adverse events may all contribute to nonadherence. Simplification of regimens, using twice-daily over thrice-daily regimens, and using regimens that reduce the number of pills that need to be taken by giving dosage forms that combine two medications (eg, the lamivudine/zidovudine combination tablet)

have been shown to aid adherence to treatment and, thus, increase the likelihood of lowering viral burden.[232,233] Because the annual cost of antiretroviral treatment is $12,000–$15,000, patients who have no way of paying for treatment either do not get it or may get it only sporadically. In any case, expense of medication contributes to nonadherence, and it is a major reason for such treatment being inaccessible to HIV-infected patients in the developing world. Thus, only a small portion of all of the HIV-infected persons in the world actually receive antiretroviral drug therapy.

Prophylaxis against opportunistic infections (especially PCP, toxoplasmosis, *M. avium* complex disease, and bacterial infections) has reduced morbidity and mortality due to these types of infections. Although HAART has lowered the need for some prophylactic regimens, HIV-infected patients who develop multiple resistance to antiretroviral agents will ultimately need prophylaxis against opportunistic infections. Trimethoprim/sulfamethoxazole has been shown to reduce not only the incidence of PCP but also of toxoplasmosis and bacterial infections. More recently, atovaquone, dapsone, and aerosolized pentamidine have been introduced as alternatives for the many patients who cannot tolerate trimethoprim/sulfamethoxazole.

IMPACT OF PUBLIC HEALTH/ PREVENTION PROGRAMS ON EPIDEMICITY

Several measures have been implemented to halt the spread of HIV infection that, if properly executed, can be highly effective. These measures include education and behavior modification, the promotion and provision of condoms, the treatment of other sexually transmitted diseases, methadone maintenance programs for IDUs, needle-exchange programs, and the use of antiretroviral drugs to prevent the transmission of HIV from mother to infant.[234]

In the United States and France, the Pediatric AIDS Clinical Trials Group (PACTG) protocol 076 demonstrated in 1994 that a three-part zidovudine regimen administered during pregnancy (100 mg orally five times daily, starting at 14–34 weeks gestation), intrapartum (2 mg/kg intravenous loading dose, followed by 1 mg/kg/h by continuous infusion), and to the neonate (2 mg/kg orally, four times daily) could reduce the risk of transmission by 68% (from 25.5% in the placebo group to 8.3% in the zidovudine group).[235] Use of this regimen in the United States and other industrialized countries has resulted in marked reduction in perinatal transmission rates. However, the complexity and cost of the regimen have limited its applicability in developing countries, where most perinatal transmission occurs.[236] A less complicated zidovudine regimen was evaluated in a placebo-controlled trial in Thailand in 1998.[237] In this regimen, zidovudine 300 mg orally twice daily is started at 36 weeks gestation, and 300 mg orally is given every 3 hours intrapartum. Neonates did not receive zidovudine in this study, and this may have accounted for the efficacy (reduction in risk of perinatal transmission, 51%) being lower than was reported in PACTG 076. In both PACTG 076 and the Thailand short-course, women were advised not to breastfeed. Thus, if either regimen were to be followed in developing countries where breastfeeding is common, efficacy in preventing perinatal transmission would be expected to be lower.

Most of 16 studies evaluating needle-exchange programs have shown that program participation reduces drug-related HIV risk in IDUs.[238] However, they have not shown any reduction in the rates of HIV sex risk behavior.

IMPACT OF AIDS ON FERTILITY

The possibility that HIV-positive women could have lower fertility than uninfected women first became apparent in 1994 with the publication of a Uganda population survey.[239] Since then, other population surveys in sub-Saharan Africa have indicated a 25–40% lower fertility rate among HIV-infected women and a larger reduction in incidence of pregnancies.[240–244]

Several reasons account for lower fertility among women in this region.[245] Some of the women may have been subfertile naturally, which may have increased marital instability, leading to more rapid partner change and increased risk of HIV infection. Women at advanced stages of HIV infection are more likely to be amenorrheic and anovulatory. They also experience spontaneous abortion more often. Indeed, a metanalysis found that summary odds ratios for spontaneous abortion and stillbirth were 4.05 and 3.91, respectively, among HIV-infected women, compared with noninfected women.[246–248]

HIV-infected women who have other STDs, such as syphilis, are at a greater risk of miscarrying. Part of the reduced fertility in sub-Saharan women could be due to male sex partners who are at more advanced stages of HIV infection and, therefore, have reduced spermatozoa production.[245] Zaba and Fregson[242] have estimated that lower fertility in HIV-positive women currently causes a population-attributable reduction in total fertility on the order of 0.4% for each percentage point of HIV prevalence in the general female population.

THE FUTURE OF THE HIV/AIDS EPIDEMIC

HIV infection/AIDS is currently the fourth leading cause of death worldwide. As of 1999, about 16,000 new HIV infections occurred every day.[8,249] More than 95% of all new infections are being reported from developing countries; this trend will occur at least over the next decade. By the new millennium, more than 40 million people will likely be infected with HIV. The HIV epidemic is staggering in terms of both human tragedy and ruin to the growth and economy of countries in the developing world. Prevention and treatment alone currently cost $14 billion annually.[250]

The pool of skilled workers and managers is diminishing in many African countries, reversing gains in development that had been seen in the 1980s. The United Nations Population Division predicts that by 2010–2015, life expectancy in the nine African countries with the highest prevalence of HIV infection will decrease by an average of 16 years.[251] Political instability between and within these countries is also expected to occur as a result of loss of a substantial part of the workforce. Because most infected mothers in sub-Saharan Africa die within 5–10 years of giving birth, the number of maternal orphans will increase in this century.

In contrast, the numbers of new AIDS diagnoses and deaths in the developed world will decrease over the next decade. This trend is already evident; in the United States, the age-adjusted

Table 18–7 Methods To Decrease HIV Transmission

Risk Group	Methods

1. Sexual Contact	a. Reduce number of partners
	b. Condom use
	c. Female diaphragm
	d. Microbicide (vaginal/rectal*)
	   Non-oxynol 9 (?)
	   Pro-2000
	   PMPA
	   Others (?)
	e. Detection and treatment of STDs
	f. Reduce/avoid excess alcohol use

2. Injection Drug Use	a. Avoid/reduce needle sharing b. Needle exchange c. Methadone treatment d. Bleach or alcohol disinfection of paraphernalia* e. Safe sex
3. Perinatal	a. Identify and treat HIV+ mothers with antiretrovirals b. Cesarean section c. Prevent/treat chorioamnionitis d. Avoid internal fetal monitoring e. Detect/treat STDs in mother f. Avoid long labor
4. Transfusion Recipients	a. Avoid use of paid donors b. Use of repeat donors (vs first-time donors) c. Use of female volunteer donors d. Screen donors with risk behavior questionnaires e. Test blood for HIV ELISA f. Test blood for p24 antigen g. Test blood for HIV RNA by PCR h. Heat treatment (pasteurization) of plasma pools/derivatives i. Avoid unnecessary transfusion or use of blood products

* These methods have not been shown to be protective in controlled clinical trials

death rate from AIDS fell 48% between 1996 and 1997,[252] and similar decreases were observed in western Europe and Australia.[253,254] Further gains in terms of decreased morbidity and mortality and enhanced quality of life among HIV-infected persons are likely as research in the developing world uncovers new antiretroviral drug treatments, expertise of health professionals regarding HIV infection grows, access to health care is improved, and prevention efforts aimed at reducing high-risk behaviors are uniformly instituted in schools and communities. Methods that have been proposed and evaluated to prevent HIV infection by sexual, parenteral drug use, transfusion, and perinatal transmission are listed in Table 18–7.

Research for the development of a vaccine to prevent HIV infection will continue at an aggressive pace over the next few years. At the NIH, funding for HIV vaccine research increased from $100.5 million in fiscal year 1995 to $194.1 million in fiscal year 1999.[8] Presently, over 3,000 uninfected volunteers are enrolled in over 50 HIV vaccine studies sponsored by the NIH.[8] The ultimate control or elimination of HIV infection and AIDS will occur only through the synergy of research efforts among the pharmaceutical industry, the government, and academia.

REFERENCES

1. Schwartländer B, Sittitrai W. Commentary: HIV/AIDS in the 1990s and beyond. *Bull WHO*. 1998;76:437–443.

2. Essex ME. Origin of acquired immunodeficiency syndrome. In: DeVita VT Jr, et al, eds. *AIDS: Biology, Diagnosis, Treatment and Prevention*. 4th ed. New York: Lippincott-Raven Publishers; 1997.

3. Shilts R. *And the Band Played On*. New York: Penguin Books; 1988.

4. Hirsch MS, Kaplan JC. The biomedical impact of the AIDS epidemic. In: Broder S et al, eds. *Textbook of AIDS Medicine;* Baltimore: Williams & Wilkins; 1994.

5. Gao F, Bailes E, Robertson DL, et al. Origin of HIV-1 in the chimpanzee *Pan troglodytes troglodytes*. *Nature*. 1999;397:436–341.

6. Hirsch VM, Olmsted RA, Murphey-Corb M, Purcell RH, Johnson PR. An African primate lentivirus (SIVsm) closely related to HIV-2. *Nature*. 1989;339:389–392.

7. Weiss RA, Wrangham RW. From *Pan* to pandemic. *Nature*. 1999;397:385–386.

8. Fauci AS. The AIDS epidemic—Considerations for the 21st century. *N Engl J Med*. 1999;341:1046–1050.

9. Saag MS. Natural history of HIV-1 disease. In: Broder S et al, eds. *Textbook of AIDS Medicine*. Baltimore: Williams & Wilkins; 1994.

10. Weiss RA. The virus and its target cells. In: Broder S et al, eds. *Textbook of AIDS Medicine*. Baltimore: Williams & Wilkins; 1994.

11. Mansky LM, Temin HM. Lower in vivo mutation rate of human immunodeficiency virus type 1 than that predicted from the fidelity of purified reverse transcriptase. *J Virol*. 1995;69:5087–5094.

12. Perelson AS, Neumann AU, Markowitz M, Leonard JM, Ho DD. HIV-1 dynamics *in vivo*: virion clearance rate, infected cell life span, and viral generation time. *Science*. 1996;271:1582–1586.

13. Perelson AS, Essunger P, Cao YZ, et al. Decay characteristics of HIV-1–infected compartments during combination therapy. *Nature*. 1997;387:188–191.

14. Pavlakis GN. The molecular biology of human immunodeficiency virus type 1. In: DeVita VT Jr, et al, eds. *AIDS: Biology, Diagnosis, Treatment and Prevention*. 4th ed. New York: Lippincott-Raven Publishers; 1997.

15. Centers for Disease Control and Prevention (CDC). Report of the NIH Panel to define principles for therapy of HIV infection and guidelines for the use of antiretroviral agents in HIV-infected adults and adolescents. *MMWR*. 1998;47(no RR-5):1–82.

16. CDC. 1999 USPHS/IDSA guidelines for the prevention of opportunistic infections in persons infected with human immunodeficiency virus: U.S. Public Health Service (USPHS) and Infectious Diseases Society of America (IDSA). *MMWR*. 1999;48(no RR-10):1–66.

17. Buchacz KA, Wilkinson DA, Krowka JF, Koup RA, Padian NS. Genetic and immunological host factors associated with susceptibility to HIV-1 infection. *AIDS*. 1998;12(suppl A):S87–S97.

18. Raboud JM, Montaner JSG, Conway B, et al. Variation in plasma RNA levels, CD4 cell counts, and p24 antigen levels in clinically stable men with human immunodeficiency virus infection. *J Infect Dis*. 1996;174:191–194.

19. Schooley RT. Acquired immunodeficiency syndrome. In: Cassel CK et al, eds. *Scientific American Medicine*. New York: Scientific American, Inc: 1998;2:sec. XI, 1–7.

20. Mellors JW, Muñoz A, Giorgi JV, et al. Plasma viral load and CD4+ lymphocytes as prognostic markers of HIV-1 infection. *Ann Intern Med.* 1997;126:946–954.

21. Mellors JW, Kingsley LA, Rinaldo CR, et al. Quantitation of HIV-1 RNA in plasma predicts outcome after seroconversion. *Ann Intern Med.* 1995;122:573–579.

22. O'Brien TR, Blattner WA, Waters D et al. Serum HIV-1 RNA levels and time to development of AIDS in the Multicenter Hemophilia Cohort Study. *JAMA.* 1996; 276:105–110.

23. O'Brien TR, Rosenberg PS, Yellin F, Goedert JJ. Longitudinal HIV-1 RNA levels in a cohort of homosexual men. *J AIDS Hum Retrovirol.* 1998;18:155–161.

24. van der Loeff MF, Aaby P. Towards a better understanding of the epidemiology of HIV-2. *AIDS.* 1999;13(suppl A):S69–S84.

25. Ghys PD, Fraqnsen K, Diallo MO, et al. The associations between cervicovaginal HIV shedding, sexually transmitted diseases and immunosuppression in female sex workers in Abidjan, Côte d'Ivoire. *AIDS.* 1997; 11:F85–F93.

26. Samb ND, Seck K, Samb B, et al. Cervico-vaginal shedding of HIV and STD among prostitutes and AIDS patients in Senegal. *Xth International Conference on AIDS and STD in Africa, Abidjan, Côte d'Ivoire.* 1997. Abstract B.178.

27. Sankale JL, Mboup S, Essex ME, Kanki PJ. Genetic characterization of viral quasispecies in blood and cervical secretions of HIV-1 and HIV-2 infected women. *12th World AIDS Conference.* Geneva. 1998. Abstract 60652.

28. Guillon C, van der Ende ME, Boers PH, Gruters RA, Schutten M, Osterhaus AD. Coreceptor usage of human immunodeficiency virus type 2 primary isolates and biological clones is broad and does not correlate with their syncytium-inducing capacities. *J Virol.* 1998;72:6260–6263.

29. Owen SM, Ellenberger D, Rayfield M, et al. Genetically divergent strains of human immunodeficiency virus type 2 use multiple coreceptors for viral entry. *J Virol.* 1998;72:5425–5432.

30. McKnight A, Dittmar MT, Moniz-Periera J, et al. A broad range of chemokine receptors are used by primary isolates of human immunodeficiency virus type 2 as coreceptors with CD4. *J Virol.* 1998;72:4065–4071.

31. Grant AD, Djomand G, De Cock KM. Natural history and spectrum of disease in adults with HIV/AIDS in Africa. *AIDS.* 1997;11(suppl B):S43–S54.

32. Greenberg AE, Kadio A, Grant AD, et al. Clinical manifestations of advanced HIV disease using hospital surveillance, clinical and autopsy data in Abidjan, Côte d'Ivoire. *12th World AIDS Conference.* Geneva. 1998. Abstract 12146.

33. Ariyoshi K, Schim van der Loeff M, Cook P, et al. Kaposi's sarcoma in the Gambia, West Africa is less frequent in human immunodeficiency virus type 2 than in human immunodeficiency virus type 1 infection despite a high prevalence of human herpes virus 8. *J Hum Virol.* 1998;1:193–199.

34. Marlink R, Kanki P, Thior I, et al. Reduced rate of disease development after HIV-2 infection as compared to HIV-1. *Science.* 1994;265:1587–1590.

35. Ancelle R, Bletry O, Baglin AC, Brun-Vezinet F, Rey MA, Godeau P. Long incubation period for HIV-2 infection. *Lancet.* 1987;1:688–689. Letter.

36. Mota-Miranda A, Gomes MH, Serrao MR, et al. Long term nonprogressive HIV-2 infection. *XI International Conference on AIDS.* Vancouver, Canada. 1996. Abstract We.C.3469.

37. Poulsen AG, Aaby P, Larsen O, et al. 9-year HIV-2-associated mortality in an urban community in Bissau, West Africa. *Lancet.* 1997;349:911–914.

38. Nunn AJ, Mulder DW, Kamali A, Ruberantwari A, Kengeya-Kayondo JF, Whitworth J. Mortality associated with HIV-1 infection over five years in a rural Ugandan population: cohort study. *Br Med J.* 1997;315: 767–771.

39. Poulsen AG, Kvinesdal B, Aaby P, et al. Prevalence of and mortality from human immunodeficiency virus type 2 in Bissau, West Africa. *Lancet.* 1989;1:827–831.

40. Wilkins A, Ricard D, Todd J, Whittle H, Dias F, Paulo Da Silva A. The epidemiology of HIV infection in a rural area of Guinea-Bissau. *AIDS.* 1993;7:1119–1122.

41. Norrgren H, Andersson S, Dias F, Naucler A, Biberfeld G. Trends of incidence and prevalence of HIV-1 and HIV-2 in Guinea-Bissau. *Xth International Conference on AIDS and STD in Africa, Abidjan, Côte d'Ivoire.* 1997. Abstract B.045.

42. Wiktor S, Sassan-Morokko M, Abouya L, et al. HIV-1 plasma viral load in tuberculosis patients with single HIV-1 and dual HIV-1/2 infections, Abidjan, Côte d'Ivoire. *12th World AIDS Conference.* Geneva. 1998. Abstract 13328.

43. Cohen J. Can one type of HIV protect against another type? *Science.* 1995;268:1566.

44. Weiss RA, Clapham PR, Weber JN, et al. HIV-2 antisera cross-neutralize HIV-1. *AIDS.* 1988;2:95–100.

45. Bottiger B, Karlsson A, Andreasson PA, et al. Envelope cross-reactivity between human immunodeficiency virus types 1 and 2 detected by different serological methods: correlation between cross-neutralization and reactivity against the main neutralizing site. *J Virol.* 1990; 64:3492–3499.

46. Travers K, Mboup S, Marlink R, et al. Natural protection against HIV-1 infection provided by HIV-2. *Science.* 1995;268:1612–1615.

47. Kanki PJ, Eisen G, Travers KU, et al. HIV-2 and natural protection against HIV-1 infection. *Science.* 1996;272: 1959–1960.

48. Travers K, Eisen G, Hsieh C, et al. HIV-2 provides natural protection against HIV-1 infection. *Xth International Conference on AIDS and STD in Africa, Abidjan, Côte d'Ivoire.* 1997. Abstract A.072.

49. Ekpini ER, Wiktor SZ, Satten GA, et al. Late postnatal mother-to-child transmission of HIV-1 in Adidjan, Côte d'Ivoire. *Lancet.* 1997;349:1054–1059.

50. Ariyoshi K, Schim van der Loeff M, Sabally S, Cham F, Corrah T, Whittle H. Does HIV-2 infection provide cross-protection against HIV-1 infection? *AIDS.* 1997; 11:1053–1054. Letter.

51. Mastro TD, Kunanusont C, Dondero IJ, Wesi C. Why do HIV-1 subtypes segregate among persons with different risk behaviors in South Africa and Thailand? *AIDS.* 1997;11:113–116.

52. Soto-Ramirez LE, Renjifo B, McLane MF, et al. HIV-1 Langerhans' cell tropism associated with heterosexual transmission of HIV. *Science.* 1996;271:1291–1293.

53. Kunanusort C, Foy HM, Kreiss JK, et al. HIV-1 subtypes and male-to-female transmission in Thailand. *Lancet.* 1995;345:1078–1083.

54. Anderson RM, Schwartländer B, McCutchan F, Hu D. Implications of genetic variability in HIV for epidemiology and public health. *Lancet.* 1996;347:1778–1779.

55. Amornkul PN, Tansuphasawadikul S, Limpakarnjanarat K, et al. Clinical disease associated with HIV subtype B' and E infection among 2104 patients in Thailand. *AIDS.* 1999;13:1963–1969.

56. Detels R, English P, Visscher BR, et al. Seroconversion, sexual activity, and condom use among 2915 HIV seronegative men followed up for up to 2 years. *J AIDS.* 1989;2:77–83.

57. Winkelstein W, Lyman DM, Padian N, et al. Sexual practices and risk of infection by the human immunodeficiency virus: the San Francisco Men's Health Study. *JAMA.* 1987;257:321–325.

58. Caussy D, Goedert J. The epidemiology of human immunodeficiency virus and acquired immunodeficiency syndrome. *Semin Oncol.* 1990;17:244–250.

59. Kingsley LA, Detels R, Kaslow R, et al. Risk factors for seroconversion to human immunodeficiency virus among male homosexuals: results from the Multicenter AIDS Cohort Study. *Lancet.* 1987;1:345–349.

60. Moss AR, Osmond D, Bacchetti P, et al. Risk factors for AIDS and HIV seropositivity in homosexual men. *Am J Epidemiol.* 1987;125:1035–1047.

61. Cecares CF, van Griensven GJP. Male homosexual transmission of HIV-1. *AIDS.* 1994;8:1051–1061.

62. Chmiel JS, Detels R, Kaslow RA, et al. Factors associated with prevalent human immunodeficiency virus (HIV) infection in the Multicenter AIDS Cohort Study. *Am J Epidemiol.* 1987;126:568–577.

63. Samuel M, Hessol N, Shiboski S, et al. Factors associated with human immunodeficiency virus seroconversion in homosexual men in three San Francisco cohort studies, 1984–1989. *J AIDS.* 1993;6:303–312.

64. Keet IPM, Albrecht van Lent N, Sanfort REM, et al. Orogenital sex and the transmission of HIV among homosexual men. *AIDS.* 1992;6:223–226.

65. Jeffries E, Willoughby KB, Boyko W, et al. The Vancouver lymphadenopathy-AIDS study: 2. Seroepidemiology of HTLV-III antibody. *Can Med Assoc J.* 1985; 132:1373–1377.

66. Melbye M, Biggar R, Ebbesen PE, et al. Seroepidemiology of HTLV-III antibody in Danish homosexual men: prevalence, transmission, and disease outcome. *Br Med J.* 1984;289:573–575.

67. Bevier PJ, Chiasson MA, Hefferman RT, Castro KG. Women at a sexually transmitted disease clinic who reported same-sex contact: their HIV seroprevalence and risk behaviors. *Am J Public Health.* 1995;85:1366–1371.

68. Chu SY, Hammett TA, Buehler JW. Update: epidemiology of reported cases of AIDS in women who report sex only with other women, United States, 1980–1991. *AIDS.* 1992;6:518–519.

69. McCombs SB, McCray E, Wendell DA, Sweeney PA, Onorato IM. Epidemiology of HIV-1 infection in bisexual women. *J AIDS.* 1992;5:850–852.

70. Petersen LR, Doll L, White C, Chu S, HIV Blood Donor Study Group. No evidence for female-to-female HIV transmission among 960,000 female blood donors. *J AIDS.* 1992;5:853–855.

71. Marmor M, Weiss L, Lynden M, et al. Possible female-to-female transmission of human immunodeficiency virus. *Ann Intern Med.* 1986;105:969.

72. Monzon OT, Capellan JM. Female-to-female transmission of HIV. *Lancet.* 1987;1:40–41.

73. Johnson AM, Laga M. Heterosexual transmission of HIV. *AIDS.* 1988;2(suppl 1):S49–S56.

74. Holmberg SD, Horsburgh CR Jr, Ward JW, et al. Biological factors in the sexual transmission of human immunodeficiency virus. *J Infect Dis.* 1989;160:116–125.

75. Centers for Disease Control. The second 100,000 cases of acquired immunodeficiency syndrome—United States, June 1991. *MMWR.* 1992;41:28–29.

76. Glasel M. High-risk sexual practices in the transmission of AIDS. In: DeVita VT, ed. *AIDS: Etiology, Diagnosis, Treatment, and Prevention.* 2nd ed. Philadelphia: JB Lippincott, 1988.

77. Cameron DW, Simonsen JN, D'Costa LJ, et al. Female to male transmission of human immunodeficiency virus

type 1: risk factors for seroconversion in men. *Lancet.* 1989;2:403–407.

78. Plummer FA, Simonsen JN, Cameron DW, et al. Cofactors in male-female sexual transmission of human immunodeficiency virus type 1. *J Infect Dis.* 1991;163: 233–239.

79. Nolte S, Sohn MA, Koons B. Prevention of HIV infection in women. *J Obstet Gynecol.* 1993;2:128–134.

80. Padian N, Shiboski S, Jewell N. Female-to-male transmission of human immunodeficiency virus. *JAMA.* 1991;266:1554–1558.

81. Padian N, Marquis L, Francis D, et al. Male-to-female transmission of human immunodeficiency virus. *JAMA.* 1987;258:788–790.

82. Greenspan A, Castro KG. Heterosexual transmission of HIV infection. *SIECUS Report.* 1990;19:1–8.

83. Cameron DW, Padian NS. Sexual transmission of HIV and the epidemiology of other sexually transmitted diseases. *AIDS.* 1990;4(suppl 1):S99–S103.

84. Lifson AR. The epidemiology of AIDS and HIV infection. *AIDS.* 1990;4(suppl 1):S23–S28.

85. Jeffries E, Willoughby KB, Boyko W, et al. The Vancouver lymphadenopathy-AIDS study: 2. Seroepidemiology of HTLV-III antibody. *Can Med Assoc J.* 1985; 132:1373–1377.

86. Saracco A, Musicco M, Nicolosi A, et al. Man-to-woman sexual transmission of HIV: Longitudinal study of 343 steady partners of infected men. *AIDS.* 1993;6: 497–502.

87. Melbye M, Biggar R, Ebbesen PE, et al. Seroepidemiology of HTLV-III antibody in Danish homosexual men: Prevalence, transmission, and disease outcome. *Br Med J.* 1984;289:573–575.

88. Moss AR, Osmond D, Bacchetti P, et al. Risk factors for AIDS and HIV seropositivity in homosexual men. *Am J Epidemiol.* 1987;125:1035–1047.

89. Centers for Disease Control. Update: Barrier protection against HIV infection and other sexually transmitted diseases. *MMWR.* 1993;42:589–591, 597.

90. Keeling RP. HIV disease: Current concepts. *J Counseling Dev.* 1993;71:261–274.

91. Centers for Disease Control. *Facts about Condoms and Their Use in Preventing HIV Infection and other STDs.* Atlanta, Ga: January 1995.

92. Saracco A, Musicco M, Nicolosi A, et al. Man-to-woman sexual transmission of HIV: longitudinal study of 343 steady partners of infected men. *AIDS.* 1993;6: 497–502.

93. Padian NS. Prostitute women and AIDS epidemiology. *AIDS.* 1988;2:413–419.

94. European Study Group on Heterosexual Transmission of HIV. Comparison of female to male and male to fe-male transmission of HIV in 563 stable couples. *Br Med J.* 1992;304:809–813.

95. De Vincenzi I, European Study Group on Heterosexual Transmission of HIV. Heterosexual transmission of HIV in a European cohort of couples. *IXth International Conference on AIDS.* Berlin: June 1993. Abstract WSCO2–1.

96. Van Damme L, Rosenberg ZF. Microbicides and barrier methods in HIV prevention. *AIDS.* 1999;13(suppl A):S85–S92.

97. Jose B, Friedman SR, Neaigus A, et al. Syringe-mediated drug-sharing (backloading): A new risk factor for HIV among injecting drug users. *AIDS.* 1993;7:1653–1660.

98. Anthony JC, Vlahov D, Nelson KE, Cohn S, et al. New evidence on intravenous cocaine use and the risk of infection with the human immunodeficiency virus. *Am J Epidemiol.* 1991;134:1179–1184.

99. Sasse H, Salmas S, Conti S, et al. Risk behaviors for HIV-1 infection in Italian drug users: report from a multicenter study. *J AIDS.* 1989;2:486–496.

100. Vlahov D, Munoz A, Anthony JC, Cohen S, Celentano DD, Nelson KE. Association of drug-injection patterns with antibody to human immunodeficiency virus type 1 among intravenous drug users in Baltimore, Maryland. *Am J Epidemiol.* 1990;132:847–856.

101. Chaisson RE, Moss AR, Onishi R, Osmond D, Carlson J. Human immunodeficiency virus infection in heterosexual intravenous drug users in San Francisco. *Am J Public Health.* 1987;77:169–172.

102. Van de Hoek JA, Coputinho RA, Van Haastrecht JHA, van Zadelhoff AW, Goudsmit J. Prevalence and risk factors of HIV infections among drug users and drug-using prostitutes in Amsterdam. *AIDS.* 1988;2:55–60.

103. Marmor M, Des Jarlais DC, Cohen H, et al. Risk factors for infection with human immunodeficiency virus among intravenous drug abusers in New York City. *AIDS.* 1987;1:39–44.

104. Battjes RJ, Pickens RW, Haverkos HW, Sloboda Z. HIV risk factors among injecting drug users in five US cities. *AIDS.* 1994;8:681–687.

105. Schoenbaum EE, Harter D, Selwyn PA, et al. Risk factors for human immunodeficiency virus infection in intravenous drug users. *N Engl J Med.* 1989;321:874–879.

106. Nelson KE, Vlahov D, Solomon L, Cohn S, Munoz A. Temporal trends of HIV infection in a cohort of injecting drug users in Baltimore, Maryland. *Ann Int Med.* 1995;155:1305–1311.

107. Vlahov D. HIV seroconversion studies among intravenous drug users. *AIDS.* 1994;8:263–265.

108. Karan LD. Primary care for AIDS and chemical dependence. *West J Med.* 1990;152:538–542.

109. Centers for Disease Control. *National HIV Serosurveillance Summary. Results through 1992.* Vol 3. Atlanta, Ga: US Dept Health Human Services; 1994.

110. Hahn RA, Onorato IM, Jones TS, et al. Prevalence of HIV infection among intravenous drug users in the United States. *JAMA.* 1989;18:2677–2684.

111. Brundage JF. Epidemiology of HIV infection and AIDS in the United States. *Dermatol Clin.* 1991;9: 442–452.

112. Moss AR, Vranizan K, Gorter R, et al. HIV seroconversion in intravenous drug users in San Francisco, 1985–1990. *AIDS.* 1994;8:223–231.

113. Ronald PJM, Robertson JR, Elton RA. Continued drug use and other cofactors for progression to AIDS among injecting drug users. *AIDS.* 1994;8:339–343.

114. The Italian seroconversion study. Disease progression and early predictors of AIDS in HIV-seroconverted injecting drug users. *AIDS.* 1992;6:421–426.

115. Selwyn PA, Alcabes P, Hartel D, et al. Clinical manifestations and predictors of disease progression in drug users with human immunodeficiency virus infection. *N Engl J Med.* 1992;327:1697–1703.

116. Phillips AN, Sabin CA, Mocroft A. Active drug injecting and progression of HIV infection. *AIDS.* 1994;8: 385–386.

117. Phillips AN, Lee CA, Elford J, et al. More rapid progression to AIDS in older HIV-infected people: the role of CD4+ T-cell counts. *J AIDS.* 1991;4:970–975.

118. Jovaisas E, Koch MA, Schafer A, Stauber M, Lowenthal D. LAV/HTLV-III in a 20 week fetus. *Lancet.* 1985;2:1129.

119. Sprecher S, Soumenkoff G, Puissant F, et al. Vertical transmission of HIV in 15-week fetus. *Lancet.* 1986; 2:288

120. Ryder R, Nsa W, Hassig S, et al. Perinatal transmission of the human immunodeficiency virus type 1 to infants of seropositive women in Zaire. *N Engl J Med.* 1989; 320.1637–1642.

121. Blanche S, Rouzioux C, Guihard Moscato ML, et al. A prospective study of infants born to women seropositive for human immunodeficiency virus type 1. *N Engl J Med.* 1989;320:1643–1648.

122. European Collaborative Study. Mother-to-child transmission of HIV infection. *Lancet.* 1988;2:1039–1043.

123. European Collaborative Study. Risk factors for mother-to-child transmission of HIV-1. *Lancet.* 1992; 339:1007–1012.

124. Hutto C, Parks WP, Lai SH, et al. A hospital-based prospective study of perinatal infection with human immunodeficiency virus type 1. *J Pediatr.* 1991;118: 347–353.

125. The International Perinatal HIV Group. The mode of delivery and the risk of vertical transmission of human immunodeficiency virus type 1: a meta-analysis of 15 prospective cohort studies. *N Engl J Med.* 1999; 340:977–987.

126. ACOG issues report on HIV infection in women. *AFP Family Phys.* 1992;46(2):579–585.

127. Von Seidlein L, Bryson YJ. Maternal-fetal transmission of the human immunodeficiency virus type 1. *Semin Pediatr Infect Dis.* 1994;5(1):78–86.

128. Van de Perre P, Simonon A, Msellati P, et al. Postnatal transmission of human immunodeficiency virus type 1 from mother to infant. *N Engl J Med.* 1991;325:593–598.

129. Wiktor SZ, Ekpini E, Nduati RW. Prevention of mother-to-child transmission of HIV-1 in Africa. *AIDS.* 1997;11(suppl B):S79–S87.

130. Caussy D, Goedert J. The epidemiology of human immunodeficiency virus and acquired immunodeficiency syndrome. *Semin Oncol.* 1990;17:244–250.

131. St Louis ME, Kamenga M, Brown C, et al. Risk for perinatal HIV-1 transmission according to maternal immunologic, virologic and placental factors. *JAMA.* 1993;269:2853–2859.

132. Boyer PJ, Dillon M, Navaie M, et al. Factors predictive of maternal-fetal transmission of HIV-1: Preliminary analysis of zidovudine given during pregnancy and/or delivery. *JAMA.* 1994;271:1925–1930.

133. Scarlatti G, Albert J, Rossi P, et al. Mother-to-child transmission of human immunodeficiency virus type 1: correlation with neutralizing antibodies against primary isolates. *J Infect Dis.* 1993;168:207–210.

134. Goedert JJ, Duliege AM, Amos CI, et al. High risk of HIV-1 infection for first-born. The International Registry of HIV-exposed Twins. *Lancet.* 1991;338:1471–1475.

135. Duliege AM, Amos CI, Felton S, et al. HIV-1 infection rate and progression of disease in 1st and 2nd born twins born to HIV infected mothers: hypothesis regarding in utero and perinatal exposers. *IX International Conference AIDS.* Berlin. 1993. Abstract WS-C10–4.

136. Goedert JJ, Mendez H, Drummond JE, et al. Mother-to-infant transmission of human immunodeficiency virus type 1: association with prematurity or low anti-gp120. *Lancet.* 1989;2:1351–1354.

137. Rossi P, Moschese V, Broliden PA, et al. Presence of maternal antibodies to human immunodeficiency virus 1 envelope glycoprotein gp120 epitopes correlates with the uninfected status of children born to seropositive mothers. *Proc Natl Acad Sci USA.* 1989;86:8055–8058.

138. Halsey NA, Markham R, Wahren B, et al. Lack of association between maternal antibodies to V3 loop peptides and maternal infant HIV-1 transmission. *J AIDS.* 1992;5:153–157.

139. Connor EM, Sperling RS, Gelber R, et al. Reduction of maternal-infant transmission of human immunodeficiency virus type 1 with zidovudine treatment. *N Engl J Med.* 1994;331:1173–1180.

140. Centers for Disease Control. Recommendations of the U.S. Public Health Service task force on the use of zidovudine to reduce perinatal transmission of human immunodeficiency virus. *MMWR.* 1994;43(no RR-11).

141. Donegan E, Stuart M, Niland JC, et al. Infection with human immunodeficiency virus type 1 (HIV-1) among recipients of antibody-positive blood donations. *Ann Intern Med.* 1990;113:733–739.

142. Caussy D, Goedert J. The epidemiology of human immunodeficiency virus and acquired immunodeficiency syndrome. *Semin Oncol.* 1990;17:244–250.

143. Simonds RJ, Holmberg SD, Hurwitz RL, et al. Transmission of human immunodeficiency virus type 1 from a seronegative organ and tissue donor. *N Engl J Med.* 1992;326:726–732.

144. Centers for Disease Control. Guidelines for preventing transmission of human immunodeficiency virus through transplantation of human tissue and organs. *MMWR.* 1994, 43(no RR-8).

145. Patijn GA, Strengers PFW, Persijn HM. Prevention of transmission of HIV by organ and tissue transplantation. *Trans Int.* 1993;6:165–172.

146. Ward JW, Holmberg SD, Allen JR, et al. Transmission of human immunodeficiency virus (HIV) by blood transfusions screened as negative for HIV antibody. *N Engl J Med.* 1988;318:473–478.

147. Cumming PD, Wallace EL, Schorr JB, Dodd RY. Exposure of patients to human immunodeficiency virus through transfusion of blood products that test antibody negative. *N Engl J Med.* 1989;321:941–946.

148. Nelson KE, Donahue JG, Munoz A, et al. Transmission of retroviruses from seronegative donors by transfusion during cardiac surgery: a multicenter study of HIV and HIV I/II infections. *Ann Intern Med.* 1992; 117:554–559.

149. Busch MP, Ehler BE, Khayam-Bashi N, et al. Evaluation of screened blood donations for human immunodeficiency virus type 1 infection by culture of DNA amplification of pooled cells. *N Engl J Med.* 1991; 325:2–5.

150. Centers for Disease Control. *National HIV Serosurveillance Summary: Results through 1992.* Vol 3. Atlanta, Ga: US Department of Health and Human Services; 1994.

151. Lackritz EM, Satten GA, Aberle-Grasse J, et al. Estimated risk of transmission of the human immunodeficiency virus by screened blood in the United States. *N Engl J Med.* 1995;333:1721–1725.

152. Centers for Disease Control. US Public Health Service guidelines for testing and counseling blood and plasma donors for human immunodeficiency virus type 1 antigen. *MMWR.* 1996;45(no RR-2).

153. Busch MP, Lee LLJ, Satten GA, et al. Time course of detection of viral and serologic markers preceding human immunodeficiency virus type 1 seroconversion: implications for screening of blood and tissue donors. *Transfusion.* 1995;35:91–97.

154. Tokars JI, Marcus R, Culver DH, Schable CA, et al. Surveillance of HIV infection and zidovudine use among health care workers after occupational exposure. *Ann Intern Med.* 1993;118:913–919.

155. Centers for Disease Control. Public Health Service statement on management of occupational exposure to human immunodeficiency virus, including considerations retarding zidovudine postexposure use. *MMWR.* 1990;39(no RR-1), whole pamphlet.

156. Ippolito G, Puro V, De Carli G. The risk of occupational human immunodeficiency virus infection in health care workers: the Italian Study Group on Occupational Risk of HIV infection. *Arch Intern Med.* 1993; 153:1451–1458.

157. Henderson DK, Fahey BJ, Willy M, et al. Risk for occupational exposure transmission of human immunodeficiency virus type 1 (HIV-1) associated with clinical exposures. A prospective evaluation. *Ann Intern Med.* 1990;113:740–746.

158. Caussy D, Goedert J. The epidemiology of human immunodeficiency virus and acquired immunodeficiency syndrome. *Semin Oncol.* 1990;17:244–250.

159. Centers for Disease Control. Investigations of patients who have been treated by HIV-infected health-care workers—United States. *MMWR.* 1993;42:329–331, 337.

160. Gooch B, Marianos D, Ciesielski C, et al. Lack of evidence for patient-to-patient transmission of HIV in a dental practice. *JAMA.* 1993;124:38–44.

161. Resnik L, Veren K, Salahuddin SZ, Tondreau S, Markham PD. Stability and inactivation of HTLV-III/LAV under clinical and laboratory environments. *JAMA.* 1986;255:1887–1891.

162. Centers for Disease Control. Recommendations for prevention of HIV transmission of health-care settings. *MMWR.* 1987;36(no 2S).

163. Centers for Disease Control. Facts about the human immunodeficiency virus and its transmission. Atlanta, Ga; February 1993.

164. Webb PA, Happ CM, Maupin GO, et al. Potential for insect transmission of HIV: experimental exposure of *Cimex hemipterus* and *Toxorbynchites amboinensis* to human immunodeficiency virus. *J Infect Dis.* 1989; 160:970–977.

165. Srinivasan A, York D, Bohan C. Lack of HIV replication in arthropod cells. *Lancet.* 1987;1:1094–1095.

166. Jupp PG, Lyons SF. Experimental assessment of bedbugs (*Cimex lectularius* and *Cimex hemipterus*) and mosquitoes (*Aedes aegypti formosus*) as vectors of human immunodeficiency virus. *AIDS.* 1987;1:171–174.

167. Castro KG, Lieb S, Jaffe HW, et al. Transmission of HIV in Belle Glade, Florida. Lessons for other communities in the United States. *Science.* 1988;239:193.

168. Levy JA. Pathogenesis of human immunodeficiency virus infection. *Microbiol Rev.* 1993;57:183–289.

169. Friedland G, Kahl P, Saltzman B, et al. Additional evidence for lack of transmission of HIV infection by close interpersonal casual contact. *AIDS.* 1990;4:639–644.

170. Friedland GH, Salthzman BR, Rogers MF, et al. Lack of transmission of HTLV-III/LAV infection to household contacts of patients with AIDS or AIDS-related complex with oral candidiasis. *N Engl J Med.* 1986;314:344–349.

171. Rogers MF, White C, Sanders T, et al. Lack of transmission human immunodeficiency virus from infected children to their household contacts. *Pediatrics.* 1990;84:210–214.

172. Centers for Disease Control. HIV transmission between two adolescent brothers with hemophilia. *MMWR.* 1993;42:948–951.

173. Wahn V, Kramer H, Voit T, et al. Horizontal transmission of HIV infection between two siblings. *Lancet.* 1986;2:694.

174. Koenig RE, Gautier T, Levy JA. Unusual intrafamilial transmission of human immunodeficiency virus. *Lancet.* 1986;2:627.

175. Fitzgibbon JE, Gaur S, Frenkel LD, et al. Transmission from one child to another of human immunodeficiency virus type 1 with a zidovudine-resistance mutation. *N Engl J Med.* 1993;329:1835–1841.

176. Centers for Disease Control. HIV infection in 2 brothers receiving intravenous therapy for hemophilia. *MMWR.* 1992;41:228–231.

177. Centers for Disease Control. Apparent transmission of human T-lymphotrophic virus type III/lymphadenopathy associated virus from a child to a mother providing health care. *MMWR.* 1986;35:76–79.

178. Centers for Disease Control. Human immunodeficiency virus transmission in household settings—United States. *MMWR.* 1994;43:347–356.

179. Over M, Piot P. HIV infection and sexually transmitted diseases. In: Jamison DT, Mosley WH, eds. *Disease Control Priorities in Developing Countries.* Washington, DC: World Bank; 1993.

180. Hira SR. Sexually transmitted diseases: a menace to mothers and children. *World Health Forum.* 1986;7:243–247.

181. Larson A. Social context of HIV transmission in Africa: historical and cultural bases of east and central African sexual relations. *Rev Infect Dis.* 1989;11:71–73.

182. Boily MC, Anderson RM. Sexual contact patterns between men and women and the spread of HIV-1 in urban centres in Africa. *IMA J Math Appl Med Biol.* 1991;8:221–247.

183. Quinn TC, Mann JM, Curran JW, et al. AIDS in Africa: an epidemiological paradigm. *Science.* 1986;16:516–519.

184. Parker RG, Tawil O. Bisexual behavior and HIV transmission in Latin America. In: Tielman R, Carballo M, Hendriks A, eds. *Bisexuality and HIV/AIDS.* New York: Prometheus Press; 1991.

185. Hunt CW. Migrant labor and sexually transmitted disease: AIDS in Africa. *J Health Soc Behav.* 1989;30:353–373.

186. UNAIDS/WHO. *Report on the Global HIV/AIDS Epidemic.* June 1998.

187. Joint United Nations Programme on HIV/AIDS (UNAIDS)/World Health Organization (WHO). *Report on the Global HIV/AIDS Epidemic: Fact Sheet.* Geneva: UNAIDS/WHO; 1997.

188. Working Group on Mother-to-Child Transmission of HIV. Rates of mother-to-child transmission of HIV-1 in Africa, America and Europe: results from 13 perinatal studies. *J AIDS.* 1995;8:506–510.

189. Shafer RW, Montoya JG. Tuberculosis. In: Merigan TC, et al, eds.: *Textbook of AIDS Medicine.* 2nd ed. Baltimore: Williams & Wilkins; 199:261–284.

190. Bioland PB, Wirima JJ, Steketee RW, Chillma B, Hightower A, Breman JG. Maternal HIV infection and infant mortality in Malawi: Evidence for increased mortality due to placental malaria infection. *AIDS.* 1995;9:721–726.

191. Mofenson LM, Fowler MG. Interruption of maternofetal transmission. *AIDS.* 1999;13(suppl A):S205–S214.

192. Tarantola D, Schwartländer B. HIV/AIDS epidemics in sub-Saharan Africa: Dynamism, diversity and discrete declines? In: Laga M, De Cock K, Kaleeba N, eds. *AIDS in Africa.* 2nd ed. London: Rapid Science; 1997:S5–S21.

193. Tarantola D, Mann J. Global overview: A powerful HIV/AIDS pandemic. In: Mann J, Tarantola D, eds. *AIDS in the World II.* New York: Oxford University Press; 1996:5–40.

194. United States Bureau of the Census. Recent HIV seroprevalence levels by country: January 1997. Washing-

ton DC: Population Division, US Bureau of the Census; 1997.

195. Fylkesnes K, Musonda RM, Kasumba K, et al. The HIV epidemic in Zambia: socio-demographic prevalence patterns and indications of trends among childbearing women. *AIDS.* 1997;11:339–345.

196. Asiimwe-Okiror G, Opio AA, Musinguzi J, et al. Change in sexual behaviour and decline in HIV infection among young pregnant women in urban Uganda. *AIDS.* 1997;11:1757–1763.

197. Djomand G, Greenberg A, Sassan-Morokro M, et al. The epidemic of HIV/AIDS in Abidjan, Côte d'Ivoire: a review of data collected by project RETRO-CI from 1987 to 1993. *J AIDS Hum Retrovirol.* 1995;10:358–365.

198. De Cock KM, Adjorlolo G, Ekpini E, et al. Epidemiology and transmission of HIV-2: why there is no HIV-2 pandemic. *JAMA.* 1993;270:2083–2086.

199. Kanki PJ, Peeters M, Guéye-Ndiaye A. Virology of HIV-1 and HIV-2: implications for Africa. *AIDS.* 1997;11(suppl B):S33–S42.

200. Anderson S, Albert J, Norrgen H, et al. Trends of incidence and prevalence of HIV-1 in Guinea-Bissau, West Africa, and preliminary data on subtypes. Presented at the 11th International Conference on AIDS, Vancouver, 1996. Abstract Mo.C.1480.

201. Quinn TC, Narrain JP, Zacarias FRK. AIDS in the Americas: a public health priority for the region. *AIDS.* 1990;4:709–724.

202. Hospedales J, White F, Gayle C, et al. Epidemiology of HIV/AIDS in the Caribbean. In: Lamptey P, White F, Figueroa FP, et al, eds. *The Handbook for AIDS Prevention in the Caribbean.* Research Triangle Park, NC: Family Health International; 1992:1–23.

203. Basset D, Narain J. Changing pattern of HIV transmission in the Caribbean. In: *AIDS: Profile of an Epidemic.* Scientific publication no. 514. Pan American Health Organization; 1988:200–204.

204. Joint United Nations Programme on HIV/AIDS (UNAIDS)/World Health Organization (WHO). *HIV/AIDS/STD Epi Fact Sheet: Caribbean.* Geneva: UNAIDS/WHO; 1997.

205. Li PCK, Yeoh EK. Current epidemiological trends of HIV infection in Asia. *AIDS Clin Rev.* 1992;1–24.

206. Des Jarlais DC, Friedman SR, Chooanya K, et al. International epidemiology of HIV and AIDS among injecting drug users. *AIDS.* 1992;6:1053–1068.

207. Weniger BG, Limpakarnjanarat K, Ungchusok K, et al. The epidemiology of HIV infection and AIDS in Thailand. *AIDS.* 1991;5(suppl 2):S71–S85.

208. Ford N, Koetsawang S. The socio-cultural context of the transmission of HIV in Thailand. *Soc Sci Med.* 1991;33:405–414.

209. Naik TN, Sarkar S, Singh HL, et al. Intravenous drug users: a new high risk group for HIV infection in India. *AIDS.* 1991;5:117–118.

210. Sarkat S, Mokerjee P, Roy A, et al. Descriptive epidemiology of intravenous heroin users: a new risk group for transmission of HIV in India. *J Infect Dis.* 1991; 23:201–207.

211. Zhang JP. An epidemiological study on HIV infection in Ruili County, Yennan Province. *Chung Hua Liu Hsing Ping Hsueh Tsa Chih.* 1991;12:9–12.

212. Bhave GG, Wagle UD, Tripathy SP. HIV sero-surveillance in promiscuous females in Bombay, India. Presented at the 6th International Conference on AIDS, San Francisco. 1991. Abstract FC 612.

213. Boonchalaksi W, Guest P. *Prostitution in Thailand.* Institute for Population and Social Research publication no. 171. Bangkok: Mahidol University; 1994.

214. Siraprapasiri T, Thanprasertsuk S, Rodklay A, et al. Risk factors for HIV among prostitutes in Chiangmai, Thailand. *AIDS.* 1991;5:579–582.

215. Ministry of Health, Thailand. *Surveillance Report.* Bangkok: Ministry of Health; 1997.

216. Nelson KE, Celentano DD, Suprasept S, et al. Risk factors for human immunodeficiency virus infection among young adults in northern Thailand. *JAMA.* 1993;270:955–960.

217. Rojanapithayakorn W, Hanenberg R. The 100% Condom Program in Thailand: editorial review. *AIDS.* 1996;10:1–7.

218. Nelson K, Celentano D, Eiumtrakol S, et al. Changes in sexual behavior and a decline in HIV infection among young men in Thailand. *N Engl J Med.* 1996;335:297–303.

219. Brody S. Decline in HIV infections in Thailand. *N Engl J Med.* 1996;335:1998–1999.

220. Brown T, Sittitrai W, Vanichseni S, et al. The recent epidemiology of HIV and AIDS in Thailand. *AIDS.* 1994;8(suppl 2):S131–S141.

221. Mastro TD, Zhang KL, Pandu S, Nelson KE. HIV infection and AIDS in Asia. In: Pizzo P, Wilfort CM, eds. *Pediatric AIDS,* 3d ed. Baltimore, Md: Williams and Wilkins; 1998.

222. World Health Organization (WHO), Regional Office for the Western Pacific. *STD, HIV, and AIDS Surveillance Report, Issue 10; and Report on the Global Epidemic.* Geneva: UNAIDS; 1997.

223. National AIDS Programme. *Report of the National AIDS Programme, Cambodia.* Phnom Penh: National AIDS Programme; 1997.

224. National AIDS Prevention and Control Programme. *Report of the National AIDS Prevention and Control Programme, Myanmar.* Rangoon: National AIDS Prevention and Control Programme; 1997.

225. National Centre in HIV Epidemiology and Clinical Research. *HIV/AIDS and Related Diseases in Australia: Annual Surveillance Report 1998*. Sydney, Australia: NCHECR, UNSW; 1998.

226. Sharples KJ, Dickson NP, Paul C, Skegg DCG. HIV/AIDS in New Zealand: an epidemic in decline. *AIDS*. 1996;10:1273–1278.

227. Centers for Disease Control and Prevention. *HIV Surveillance*. <www.cdc.gov/nchstp/hiv_aids> August 9, 1999.

228. Palella FJ, Delaney KM, Moorman AC, et al. Declining morbidity and mortality among patients with advanced human immunodeficiency virus infection. *N Engl J Med*. 1998;338:853–860.

229. Mocroft A, Vella S, Benfield TL, et al. Changing patterns of mortality across Europe in patients infected with HIV-1. *Lancet*. 1998;352:1725–1730.

230. National Institutes of Health: Report of the NIH panel to define principles of therapy of HIV infection and guidelines for the use of antiretroviral agents in HIV-infected adults and adolescents <www.hivatis.org/guidelines/AAMay599.pdf>. Last accessed 15 January 2000.

231. Paterson D, Swindells S, Mohr J, et al. How much adherence is enough? A prospective study of adherence to protease inhibitor therapy using MEMSCaps. *6th Conference on Retroviruses and Opportunistic Infections*. January 31–February 4, 1999, Chicago, Ill. Abstract 92.

232. von Bargen S, Moorman A, Holmberg S. How many pills do patients with HIV infection take? *JAMA*. 1998;280:29.

233. Williams A, Friedland G. Adherence, compliance, and HAART. *AIDS Clin Care*. 1997;9:51–56.

234. Coates TJ, Collins C. Preventing HIV infection. *Sci Am*. 1998;279:96–97.

235. Connor EM, Sperling RS. Gelber R, et al. Reduction of maternal-infant transmission of human immunodeficiency virus type 1 with zidovudine treatment. *N Engl J Med*. 1994;331:1173–1180.

236. Mofenson LM, Fowler MG. Interruption of materno-fetal transmission. *AIDS*. 1999;13(suppl A):S205–S214.

237. Centers for Disease Control. Administration of zidovudine during late pregnancy and delivery to prevent perinatal transmission—Thailand, 1996–1998. *MMWR*. 1998;47:151–154.

238. Public Health Impact of Needle Exchange Programs in the United States and Abroad, 1993. <www.caps.ucsf.edu>.

239. Sewankambo NK, Wawe MJ, Gray RH, et al. Demographic impact of HIV infection in rural Rakai District, Uganda: results of a population-based cohort study. *AIDS*. 1994;8:1707–1713.

240. Gray R, Wawer MJ, Serwadda D, et al. Population-based study of fertility in women with HIV-1 infection in Uganda. *Lancet*. 1998;351:98–103.

241. Carpenter LM, Nakiyingi JS, Ruberantwari A, et al. Estimates of the impact of HIV-1 infection on fertility in a rural Ugandan population cohort. *Health Trans Rev*. 1997;7:113–126.

242. Zaba B, Gregson S. Measuring the impact of HIV on fertility in Africa. *AIDS*. 1998;12(suppl 1):S41–S50.

243. Kilian A, Gregson S, Ndyanabangi B, et al. Reductions in risk behaviour provide the most consistent explanation of declining HIV-1 prevalence in Uganda. *AIDS*. 1999;13:391–398.

244. Fylkesnes K, Ndhlovu Z, Kasumba K, et al. Studying dynamics of the HIV epidemic: population-based data compared with sentinel surveillance in Zambia. *AIDS*. 1998;12:1227–1234.

245. Gregson S, Zaba B, Garnett GP. Low fertility in women with HIV and the impact of the epidemic on orphanhood and early childhood mortality in sub-Saharan Africa. *AIDS*. 1999;13(suppl A):S249–S257.

246. D'Ubaldo C, Pezzotti P, Rezza G, et al. Association between HIV-1 infection and miscarriage: a retrospective study. *AIDS*. 1998;12:1087–1093.

247. Brocklehurst P, French R. The association between maternal HIV infection and perinatal outcome: a systematic review of the literature and meta-analysis. *Br J Obstet Gynaecol*. 1998;105:836–848.

248. Desigrees du Lou A, Mseellati P, Ramon R, et al. HIV-1 infection and reproductive history: a retrospective study among pregnant women: Abidjan, Cote d'Ivoire, 1995–1996. *Int J STD AIDS*. 1998;9:452–456.

249. WHO. *AIDS Epidemic Update: December 1998*. Geneva: Joint United Nations Programme on HIV/AIDS (UNAIDS), World Health Organization; 1998.

250. WHO. *Removing Obstacles to Healthy Development*. Geneva: World Health Organization; 1999.

251. Department of Economic and Social Affairs of the United Nations Secretariat. *The Demographic Impact of HIV/AIDS*. New York: United Nations; 1999.

252. Hoyert DL, Kochanek KD, Murphy SL. Deaths: final data for 1997. *Natl Vital Stat Rep*. 1999;47(19):1–104.

253. Mocroft A, Vella S, Benfield TL, et al. Changing patterns of mortality across Europe in patients infected with HIV-1. *Lancet*. 1998;352:1725–1730.

254. Dore GJ, Brown T, Tarntola D, Kaldor JM. HIV and AIDS in the Asia-Pacific region: an epidemiological overview. *AIDS*. 1998;12(suppl B):S1–S10.

CHAPTER 19

Viral Hepatitis

Kenrad E. Nelson and David L. Thomas

INTRODUCTION

Hepatitis is inflammation of the liver, which may be caused by viral or other infections, toxins, and a number of other conditions. This chapter considers the epidemiology of the five viruses that have been identified as causing hepatitis as their primary clinical syndrome. These include hepatitis A virus (HAV) and hepatitis E virus (HEV), which are transmitted by fecal-oral exposures from an infected to a susceptible individual, and hepatitis B virus (HBV), hepatitis C virus (HCV), and hepatitis delta virus (HDV), which are transmitted by blood, sexual, or perinatal contact.

Other viruses, such as cytomegalovirus (CMV), Epstein-Barr virus (EBV), yellow fever virus, Lassa fever virus, Ebola virus, and other agents may also infect the liver and cause hepatitis (Exhibit 19–1). However, their clinical manifestations usually reflect infection of other tissues, so they are not considered to be hepatitis viruses.

As early as the seventeenth century, epidemics of jaundice and other manifestations of liver disease were associated with military campaigns and were especially problematic during World War II.[1] Hepatitis following use of glycerinated human lymph to prevent smallpox was described in 1885.[2] Outbreaks of jaundice related to the administration of pooled human serum to prevent mumps[3] or to prepare a yellow fever vaccine[4] suggested that a transmissible agent was present in human blood. Blood transmission of hepatitis was also suggested by the frequent recognition of hepatitis in syphilis patients treated in clinics where injection equipment was not sterilized between patients.[5] Conversely, hepatitis was uncommon in patients attending clinics with good infection control practices.[5]

Along with the appreciation that human blood could transmit hepatitis came the recognition that many cases of hepatitis, including epidemics of the disease, did not follow blood exposure. The suspicion that there were at least two different epidemiologic types of hepatitis virus was confirmed by studies of Krugman et al.[6] at the Willowbrook State School in New York. These studies showed that viruses that he labeled *MS-2 strains* were exclusively transmitted parenterally, whereas other MS-1 strains could be transmitted orally. Furthermore, heat-inactivated convalescent sera obtained after MS-2 infection could prevent MS-2 infection. These studies laid the basis for the classification of hepatitis into serum hepatitis (MS-2 viruses) and infectious hepatitis (MS-1 viruses). In the 1950s and 1960s, there were numerous attempts to isolate the virus(es) or infect experimental animals with the agents responsible for hepatitis. However, in 1965, the Australia antigen was isolated from the blood of Australian aboriginals by Blumberg and associates.[7] This antigen was subsequently found to be the hepatitis B surface antigen (HBsAg).[8] Within a decade of this discovery, the HBV virus and its major antigens had been fully

Exhibit 19–1 Conditions that Cause Hepatitis in Humans

Hepatitis viruses
  Hepatitis A virus
  Hepatitis B virus
  Hepatitis C virus
  Hepatitis D virus
  Hepatitis E virus

Other viruses
  Epstein-Barr Virus
  Human immunodeficiency virus
  Lassa fever virus
  Yellow fever virus
  Adenovirus
  Herpes simplex virus
  Human herpes-6 virus
  Ebola virus

Nonviral infectious agents
  Pneumococcal pneumonia
  Leptospirosis
  Syphilis
  Coxiella burnetti
  Toxoplasmosis

Noninfections
  Alcohol
  Medications (Dilantin, isoniazid, ritonavir, chlorpromazine, rifampin, etc.)
  Anesthesia (halothane)

characterized, and serologic tools became available for epidemiologic studies.

After the introduction of the routine screening of blood donors for HBsAg in 1973, the incidence of posttransfusion hepatitis decreased by about 50%. Posttransfusion hepatitis that was not due to hepatitis B indicated that another parenterally transmitted hepatitis virus existed.[9] HCV was discovered in 1989 and was shown to be the primary etiologic agent of parenterally transmitted non-A, non-B (PT-NANB) hepatitis worldwide.[10–12] The hepatitis delta virus (HDV) was discovered by Rizzetto in 1977 and was initially described as a new antigen detectable in patients with HBV-associated chronic liver disease.[13] Studies in chimpanzees subsequently es-

tablished that HDV was a unique RNA virus that was transmissible but dependent on the presence of active HBV infection to cause infection in humans.[14]

Viral particles of HAV were identified in stool samples of patients with infectious hepatitis in 1973.[15] Over the next several years, the immunologic and virologic aspects of HAV and its natural history were more clearly defined. In 1979, HAV was first grown in tissue culture[16]; subsequently, vaccines were developed from cell culture-derived virus and shown to be effective.[17,18]

Large epidemics of water-borne hepatitis, most notably a very large epidemic that occurred in New Delhi, India, in 1955, were found not to be due to HAV when convalescent sera from persons who were infected during this large epidemic were tested after HAV antibody tests became available.[18] This condition was referred to as enterically transmitted non-A, non-B hepatitis.[19]

Viruslike particles were identified in the feces of patients by immune electron microscopy in the early 1980s. This hepatitis virus, called *hepatitis E virus* (HEV), was an enterically transmitted non-A, non-B hepatitis (ET-NANB) virus. Subsequently, an animal model of hepatitis E was developed in cynomolgus monkeys.[19,20]

Biologic Basis for Transmission

These five viruses differ markedly in their genetic composition and biology (Table 19–1). It is not known why each of these viruses principally infects the liver and causes hepatic inflammation. However, it is assumed that receptors allow entry of hepatitis viruses into hepatocytes where replication principally occurs. The inability of HBV, HCV, and HDV to be transmitted through fecal-oral exposures relates to their lipid envelopes that are unstable in the biliary excretory tract, rendering these viruses noninfectious in stool. HAV and HEV do not have envelopes, are infectious in stool, and are relatively stable under environmental conditions.

The capability of hepatitis viruses to be spread by blood relates to the total time that the virus

Table 19–1 Characteristics of Hepatitis Viruses

Virus	Nucleic Acid	Routes of Transmission	Mortality	Risk of Chronic Illness
HAV	Unenveloped single-stranded RNA	Fecal-oral	Low	None
HBV	Enveloped double-stranded DNA	Parenteral (sex, perinatal)	Mod–high	High
HCV	Enveloped single-stranded RNA	Parenteral (sex, perinatal)	Mod–high	High
HDV	Enveloped single-stranded RNA	Parenteral (sex)	High	High
HEV	Unenveloped single-stranded RNA	Fecal-oral	Low–mod	None

exists in the blood and, thus, the size of the transmission reservoir. All hepatitis viruses can cause infection if they are percutaneously inoculated. However, HAV and HEV exist in blood for very brief intervals and, thus, only rarely contaminate percutaneous transmission vehicles, such as blood products or needles. In contrast, HBV, HCV, and HDV may be detected in the blood of asymptomatic carriers for decades.

Clinical Syndrome

All hepatitis viruses may cause the same general syndrome (Exhibit 19–2). After exposure, there is an incubation period of from 2 to 10 weeks for HAV and HEV, from 4 to 10 weeks for HCV, and from 6 to 20 weeks for HBV. This may be followed by a flulike prodromal illness with fever, chills, anorexia, vomiting, and fatigue. A few patients with HBV infection will develop a urticarial rash, arthralgia, arthritis, or glomerulonephritis during the acute illness, due to immune complexes. As the systemic symptoms improve, jaundice may occur, followed by a period of convalescence. The hallmark of hepatitis is an elevation in the blood of levels of enzymes contained in the liver, specifically alanine aminotransferase (ALT) and aspartate ami-

Exhibit 19–2 Clinical Course of Viral Hepatitis

Incubation	Time from exposure to first symptoms, ranging from 2–4 weeks for HAV to 6–12 weeks for HBV.
Prodrome	A flulike illness that can precede jaundice.
Icterus	Jaundice (dark urine and yellow discoloration of sclera) occurs variably in adults, most with HAV and least with HCV infection.
Convalescence	Period of resolution of jaundice.
Recovery or persistence	In the months after HCV, HBV, and HDV infections, it becomes evident whether an infection will persist or resolve; HAV and HEV infections always resolve and never become chronic.

notransferase (AST). The blood bilirubin may also rise, with levels greater than 3.0 mg/dL producing jaundice. Rarely, patients will develop acute fulminant hepatic necrosis and liver failure. This is more frequent with HAV, HDV, and HEV than with HCV infection.

HEPATITIS A VIRUS

Virology

The hepatitis A virus (HAV) is a small (27-nm) nonenveloped RNA virus belonging to the family *Picornaviridae*. The virus, which has icosohedral symmetry and contains about 2,500 nucleotides, is composed of at least four major structural polypeptides, VP1 to VP4. The genomic organization and replication of HAV is similar to that of polio virus and other picornaviruses. However, HAV has little nucleotide or amino acid homology with other enteroviruses, and there is less evidence that HAV replicates in intestinal tissues. HAV was originally classified in the genus enterovirus but it is now classified in a separate genus, designated *Hepatovirus*.

HAV is quite stable in the environment after it is shed in the feces, retaining infectivity for at least 2 to 4 weeks at room temperatures. The virus is resistant to nonionic detergents, chloroform, or ether and retains infectivity at pH 1.0 at 38°C for 90 minutes. It is only partially inactivated at 60°C for 1 hour. Temperatures of 85° to 95°C for 1 minute are required to inactivate HAV in shellfish. It is also relatively resistant to free chlorine, especially when the virus is associated with organic matter. These features explain the occurrence of HAV outbreaks from consumption of shellfish and other foods or beverages and outbreaks associated with swimming pools.

HAV exists as a single serotype, and HAV infection—whether symptomatic or not—confers life-long immunity in people infected with strains from any location worldwide. Only man and several nonhuman primates (e.g., marmosets, tamarins, owl monkeys, and chimpanzees) are known to be naturally infected with HAV.

In 1979, HAV was cultured in fetal rhesus monkey kidney cells after the virus had been passaged multiple times in marmosets.[16] Since then, HAV has been cultivated directly from clinical or environmental samples but adaptation periods of 4 to 10 weeks have been required for detection of significant amounts of HAV antigen in infected cells. Generally, HAV isolates do not produce cytopathology in tissue cultures, although cytopathic variants have been isolated that produce plaques in cell culture.

The isolation of the virus has allowed comparative virologic studies to be done and diagnostic reagents to be developed to confirm current or past infection and immunity. Recently, inactivated vaccines have been developed, and their demonstrated safety and efficacy has resulted in licensure by the Food and Drug Administration.[17,18] Research on the development of a live attenuated HAV vaccine is continuing in the hope that a less expensive, easier-to-administer vaccine can be developed because HAV infections are important globally.

Clinical Features and Diagnosis

In the individual, the clinical features of acute HAV infection are not sufficiently distinctive to allow differentiation from other types of acute viral hepatitis. However, prodromal symptoms, including anorexia, nausea, abdominal discomfort, diarrhea, and fever may be more prominent than in patients infected with HBV or HCV, and they often begin abruptly. Rarely, arthritis, urticarial rash, arteritis, or aplastic anemia has been reported in patients with acute HAV infection. HAV infection can cause 2.0% to 27% of cases of acute fulminant hepatitis in developed countries.[21,22] Unlike HBV and HCV infections, there is no evidence that HAV causes chronic hepatitis. However, about 10% to 15% of patients with acute HAV have a relapse of their illness within a few weeks of their recovery. These relapses have been shown to be accompanied by excretion of virus in the stool, suggestions that such patients are infectious during a clinical relapse.[23]

An important clinical feature of HAV infection is the inverse correlation of symptoms with the age of the patient. Most infants and children under age 6 have mild, often nonspecific symptoms or, more commonly, their acute infection is completely asymptomatic. Among children under age 3, only about 5% develop jaundice. The rate of icteric disease is about 10% in children 4 to 6 years of age. In contrast, most adolescents and adults develop jaundice, and 75% develop characteristic prodromal symptoms. The public health importance of HAV infections in developed countries is related to the high rates of morbidity, which can persist for a few weeks. As noted above, some patients will have a recurrence of symptoms that prolongs morbidity.

The specific diagnosis of HAV infection is confirmed by testing a serum specimen for IgM antibodies to HAV. The antibody assay is highly sensitive and specific. Antibodies of the IgM class usually develop by the time the patient is symptomatic and persist for 3 to 6 months. Total Ig or IgG antibodies in the absence of IgM antibodies usually signify previous infection. Most patients, even those who are not icteric, will have elevated serum ALT and AST levels during the acute infection. Although HAV is present in the stool in the presymptomatic and pre-icteric phases of the illness, viral cultures are not generally done because of the difficulty in isolation of this virus in tissue culture.

Transmission Routes

The principal means of HAV transmission is by ingestion of infectious feces. Infection can occur by direct person-to-person transfer of virus on hands or fomites, or by consumption of contaminated food or water. In addition, blood-borne transmission occurs rarely because HAV is present in the blood from the middle of the incubation period until early in the clinical illness. Infectivity titers in the stool are very high, i.e., up to 10^8 infectious units per gram of feces in the late incubation period and first week of the illness.[25] Viremia also occurs but persists for a shorter period than does the virus in the feces.

Virus can also be present in saliva at 10^4 lower levels than are present in the serum.[26]

Household or sexual contact with a person with hepatitis is the most common exposure reported by patients with HAV infections reported to the Centers for Disease Control and Prevention (CDC), accounting for about 22% of cases (Figure 19–1).[27] To be counted as a secondary case, the most recent exposure to a case of hepatitis should have been 2 to 6 weeks before onset of illness. Transmission among homosexual men has been well documented; whether this occurs through sexual contact or simply by nonsexual intimate contact is not clear.[28,29]

Transmission of HAV by blood occurs infrequently.[30,31] However, a large outbreak of parenterally transmitted HAV has recently occurred in European hemophiliacs related to contaminated pooled clotting factor concentrates.[32] This outbreak was due to the use of a large pool of plasma donors; the highly purified pooled product, which did not include neutralizing antibodies; and the absence of a virus inactivation process effective against HAV in the preparation of the concentrate.[33] Injection drug users are believed to be at increased risk of infection, but whether this is due to parenteral or fecal-oral transmission from poor hygienic practices is uncertain.[28,34,35]

Common-source outbreaks have occurred from contamination of food and water supplies.[36,37] Food-borne outbreaks usually result from contamination of food by an infected food handler who is asymptomatic or is in the incubation period. The usual foods responsible for food-borne outbreaks are those eaten uncooked, such as salads, fruit, lettuce, sandwiches, glazed or iced pastries, and some dairy products.[38,39] Some food-borne outbreaks have involved consumption of shellfish harvested from sewage-contaminated waters that have been eaten with little or no cooking.[40,41] Bivalve mollusks, e.g., clams, oysters, and mussels, are at particular high risk of transmission of HAV because they filter large volumes of water and concentrate infectious HAV and other viruses in their digestive system.[42] In addition, outbreaks of HAV have

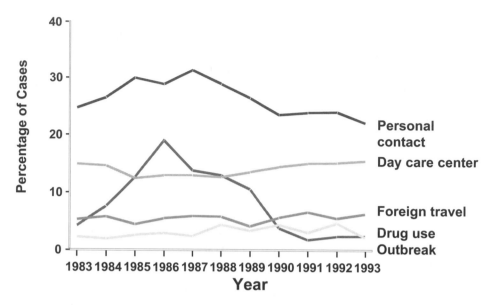

Figure 19–1 Sources of hepatitis A virus infection by mutually exclusive groups, United States, 1983–1993. *Source:* Reprinted from Viral Hepatitis Surveillance Program, Centers for Disease Control and Prevention.

been reported from consumption of foods contaminated at the time of harvest or processing that were subsequently served raw, such as lettuce, strawberries, and raspberries.[38,39] Nevertheless, hepatitis traced to contaminated food or water accounts for only about 8% of HAV cases reported to the CDC.[43,44]

Transmission in the day-care setting has been studied, especially in Maricopa County (Phoenix), Arizona. Studies in this area in the late 1970s identified a twofold increase in HAV cases; most of the increase could be traced to direct or indirect contact with an infected child or employee in a day-care center.[45–47]

In centers enrolling children in diapers, hepatitis A outbreaks may be common. In this setting, HAV may be spread not only among children but also to adult contacts in the center, at home, or in the community. Infected infants and young children are rarely jaundiced but they may transmit HAV to adult contacts, who are likely to become symptomatic. Adult contacts of 1- to 2-year-old children are at highest risk of infection. In centers not enrolling children in

diapers, outbreaks are much less common.[45] In addition to the absence of symptoms in infected children, prolonged viral secretion in infants has been linked to transmission in day-care centers and hospitals. Over 15% of all HAV infections reported to the CDC were related to day-care center transmission (Figure 19–1).

International travel to developing countries with contaminated food or water supplies may also result in HAV infection. The risk of HAV infection during international travel is highest among long-term residents of developing countries, such as missionaries, Peace Corps volunteers, and military and peace-keeping force personnel.[48–50] Although short-term tourists are at increased risk of HAV, the risk is not great.

Worldwide Epidemiology

The epidemiology of HAV infections varies greatly in different populations throughout the world. Seroprevalence studies in various countries have been used to define levels of endemicity to classify areas into those with high, intermediate, or low endemicity. Areas with high endemicity for HAV include countries in Africa, Asia, Central and South America, and the Middle East (Figure 19–2). In these areas, the prevalence of HAV antibody reaches 90% among adults, and most children become infected by age 10. However, persons of upper socioeconomic class may not become infected until they reach adolescence or adulthood.

In more developed countries in Europe and Asia, the endemicity of HAV is intermediate, and the prevalence of HAV antibody varies widely. In countries such as Italy, Greece, Thailand, Taiwan, and Korea, the prevalence of HAV antibody in adults reaches 80% or higher, but in children under age 10, antibody prevalence is only 20% to 30%, and the major increase in antibody occurs in persons between the ages of 10 and 20 (Figure 19–3).[51–54] These data indicate a cohort effect in which older adults belong to cohorts that were infected in childhood. Paradoxically, this delay in the occurrence of infection actually increases morbidity, because

early childhood infection is usually asymptomatic.[51]

In Europe and the United States, HAV antibody prevalence in adults varies from 30% to 50% but is less than 10% in children under age 10. However, low socioeconomic status is associated with high rates of infection.[55]

In some northern European countries and in Japan, HAV infection has become quite unusual. The antibody prevalence is well below 10% in children and adolescents. However, adults over age 40 have antibody prevalence of 30% to 60%, indicating a cohort effect when HAV infections were more common.

In countries with high endemicity of HAV infection, most acute hepatitis in children under age 15 is due to HAV; however, HAV is rarely the cause of hepatitis in adults. In areas of intermediate endemicity, studies have shown that a relatively high proportion (50% to 80%) of adult cases of hepatitis are due to HAV. In low endemicity areas in Western Europe and the United States, the majority of acute hepatitis cases in

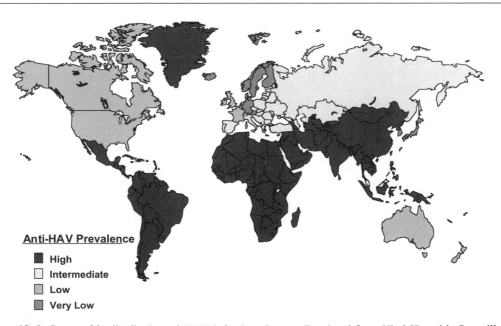

Anti-HAV Prevalence

■ High
□ Intermediate
▨ Low
▨ Very Low

Figure 19–2 Geographic distribution of HAV infection. *Source:* Reprinted from Viral Hepatitis Surveillance Program, Centers for Disease Control and Prevention.

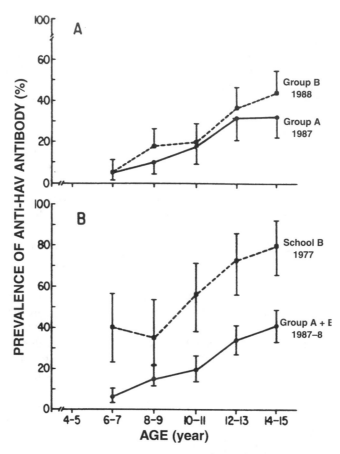

Figure 19–3 Age-specific hepatitis A (HAV) antibody prevalence (with 95% confidence intervals) among schoolchildren in Bangkok: A, rates measured in 1987 (group A) and 1988; B, combined antibody prevalence rates for groups A and B contrasted to those in the group B school in 1977. *Source:* Reprinted with permission from B.L. Innis, R. Snitbhan, and C.H. Hoke et al., The Declining Transmission of Hepatitis A in Thailand, *Journal of Infectious Diseases*, Vol. 163, pp. 989–995, Copyright 1991, University of Chicago Press.

children is caused by HAV, but in adults, the proportion varies from 10% to 50%.[55]

Despite the fact that the United States is considered to be a country where the endemicity of HAV is low, there is considerable geographic variation among HAV incidence rates within the country. In the United States, counties having more than 10% of the population classified as American Indian have HAV incidence rates 3.5 times higher than other counties.[55,56] Similarly, counties with 15% or more of the population

classified as Hispanic have average rates 2.1 times higher than other counties. The incidence rate by age is highest in persons under age 40.

In the United States and many other countries with low or intermediate endemicity, HAV incidence is cyclical, with 7- to 10-year peaks in the number of reported cases (Figure 19–4). The most recent peak year in the United States was in 1989, when almost 36,000 cases were reported.[43,57] The cyclical pattern of HAV is also apparent in Shanghai, China (Figure 19–5).

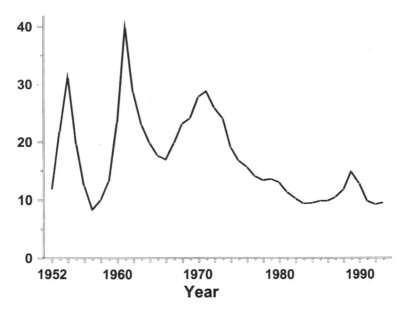

Figure 19–4 Incidence of hepatitis A, United States, 1952–1993. *Source:* Reprinted from National Notifiable Diseases Surveillance System, Centers for Disease Control and Prevention.

However, an epidemic of HAV involving 300,000 cases from consumption of contaminated raw clams occurred in Shanghai in 1989.[41] This large food-borne epidemic illustrates the potential for spread of HAV in a country where the endemicity has been reduced in recent years by improvements in the hygienic qualities of the food and water supply and the accumulation of a large susceptible adult population.

Prevention

Improved environmental sanitation to prevent fecal contamination of food and water has been the most important means of preventing infection.[51–54]

Until recently, passive immunization with pooled human immunoglobulin (IG) has been the only means of providing post- or pre-exposure prophylaxis against hepatitis A. IG is highly effective in preventing symptomatic HAV infections if given before or within 2 weeks after exposure to the virus.[58,59] If given prior to expo-

sure, IG is nearly 100% effective in preventing symptomatic infection. However, depending on the dose, this protection may last for 1 to 6 months. If given after exposure, IG is only 75% to 85% effective[60]; HAV infection may occur but symptoms are rare, and fecal shedding of the virus is limited. The decreased symptoms in patients who receive IG after infection may be due to limitations in the spread of HAV within the liver until a protective immune response is mounted, and is often called passive-active immunization.[36]

For postexposure prophylaxis of adult household contacts of acute cases, the usual recommended dose of IG is 0.02 ml/kg, or about 1.5 to 2.0 ml given intramuscularly. IG is often not recommended or is ineffective in common-source food-borne or water-borne outbreaks when exposure is identified too late for infection to be prevented.[61,62] Prior to the licensure of effective HAV vaccines, repeated pre-exposure prophylaxis with IG was recommended at 6-month intervals for persons who continued to be at high

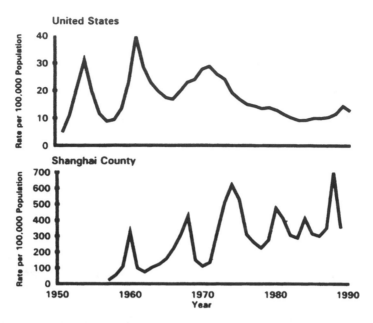

Figure 19–5 Incidence patterns of reported cases of hepatitis A, United States and Shanghai County, People's Republic of China. *Source:* Reprinted with permission from A.S. Evans and R.A. Kaslow, *Viral Infections of Humans*, p. 269, © 1997, Plenum Publishing Corporation.

risk of exposure, such as Peace Corps volunteers and medical missionaries.[60] However, active immunization is now a much preferable preventive strategy. Two inactivated HAV vaccines have been licensed in the United States. These vaccines were tested in 1- to 16-year-olds in Thailand[18] and in 2- to 16-year-olds living in a Hassidic Jewish community in New York state.[17] Both vaccines are highly effective. Although the long-term efficacy of these vaccines is uncertain, the high efficacy in preventing acute HAV raises the possibility that HAV morbidity could be reduced dramatically with selective vaccination of high-risk populations.

HEPATITIS B VIRUS

Virology

Hepatitis B virus is a partially double-stranded DNA virus that is a member of the family *Hepadnaviridae*. This family includes several other animal viruses, including woodchuck hepatitis virus, duck hepatitis virus, and ground squirrel hepatitis virus. The HBV genome has about 3,200 nucleotides and replicates through an RNA intermediate that is transcribed by a gene product with reverse transcriptase activity. The proteins encoded by the HBV genome are the envelope, the nucleocapsid, the X protein, and a DNA polymerase.

The envelope proteins encoded by the HBV genome include pre-S, pre-S2, and the HBsAg, which is a glycosylated lipoprotein that contains the major site for binding of neutralizing antibody. HBsAg can circulate as a part of the complete virion, i.e., the Dane particle, or independently of viral particles. Four subtypes of HBsAg have been identified, which are designated *adw, ayw, adr* and *ayr*. The "a" epitope, which is common to all HBsAg subtypes, is the binding epitope for neutralizing antibodies.

Therefore, antibodies to HBsAg are protective for all subtypes.[63] However, occurrence of the other subtype determinants varies geographically, such that HBsAg subtyping has been used in epidemiologic studies to establish patterns of transmission.[64] The subtypes do not appear to differ in infectivity or virulence. Nonlethal mutations can also occur in the S gene, sufficiently altering expression of this protein to permit viral escape from neutralizing antibodies.

HBV encodes nucleocapsid proteins, which include HBeAg and HBV core antigen (HBcoreAg). HBeAg is a marker for current active viral replication. However, mutations can occur that truncate expression of e antigen without substantially altering virion production. The resultant viral phenotype results in clinical infection with HBV DNA and HBsAg but no detectable HBeAg in the blood. Some individuals infected with these HBeAg-negative mutant viruses have developed fulminant hepatitis.[65–68] The HBcoreAg is the major nucleocapsid protein and is not detected in the serum but is present in the liver. The cellular immune response to HBcoreAg in the liver is believed by some investigators to be responsible for hepatic necrosis associated with chronic liver disease in HBV carriers.[69–72] Persons infected with HBV form antibodies to HBcoreAg that are persistent and useful in the diagnosis of current or previous infection. Humans are the only natural host for HBV infection. The chimpanzee is the primary experimental model for infection but the disease has also been studied in gibbons, marmosets, and other primates.[73] HBV can retain infectivity for at least 1 month at room temperature and much longer when frozen. Heating to 90°C for 1 hour renders HBV noninfectious.

Clinical Features and Diagnosis

The clinical features of HBV infection are similar to those of other hepatitis viruses and range from asymptomatic infection to jaundice following a flulike prodromal illness. However, persons with acute HBV infection are more likely to develop a serum sickness–like illness

(arthritis, arthralgia, urticarial rash), and chronic infection is associated with glomerulonephritis or vasculitis resembling periarteritis nodosa.[74]

As with HAV infection, a direct relationship exists between the age of the patient and the likelihood that an acute HBV infection will be symptomatic. Infections in infants and children rarely cause jaundice and are usually completely asymptomatic, whereas 10% to 20% of children over age 6 and 40% to 50% of adults develop jaundice with acute HBV infection.[75]

The probability that chronic infection will develop is inversely related to the rates of jaundice during acute infection. In infants born to a mother who is an HBeAg-positive carrier, the risk of infection with chronic carriage (defined as carriage for over 1 year) is about 80% to 90%.[76–78] The risk of chronic infection decreases with increasing age. By age 6, chronic infection occurs in 5% to 10% of individuals. The risk of chronic infection in adolescents and adults is 1% to 5%. Persons who are immunosuppressed, such as patients on dialysis, oncology or transplant patients, or persons with HIV infection or AIDS, have high rates of chronic carriage of HBV after acute infection.

Most persons with persistent HBV infection do not develop chronic liver disease, and a spectrum of histologic disease has been described.[78–80] Some patients have normal liver biopsies; chronic persistent hepatitis is diagnosed in patients with low-grade focal inflammation, and chronic active hepatitis is characterized by diffuse active inflammation with bridging necrosis between hepatic lobules. Cirrhosis is characterized by scarring, diffuse necrosis, and regeneration and disruption of hepatic lobular architecture.

The probability of clinically significant chronic liver disease is higher in persons infected as infants or children than when infection occurs during adult life.[81] Prospective studies in Taiwan have estimated that 25% of persons infected as infants or children who become chronic HBV carriers develop primary hepatocellular carcinoma (PHC) during their lifetime.[81–85]

Hepatitis B Virus and Primary Liver Cancer

In the last 30 years, considerable evidence has been published describing chronic HBV infection as a cause of PHC in humans. The evidence includes ecologic data that indicate geographic areas where the HBV carrier rates are highest (Figure 19–6), as well as the areas where PHC is most common. More persuasive are several prospective cohort studies of infection with HBV and the subsequent development of PHC. In the largest and most comprehensive of these studies, Beasley et al.[83] studied 22,707 male civil servants between the ages of 40 and 59 in Taiwan between March 15, 1976, and June 3, 1978. These men were all healthy and free of liver cancer at baseline. By December, 1985, 151 of these men experienced incident PHC in a cumulative 186,000 person-years of follow-up, an average of 8.2 years per 100 person-years. Overall, 141 of the men who developed PHC were HBsAg carriers at baseline; the rate of PHC in HBsAg carriers was 505 per 100 person-years of follow-up. Among non-HBsAg carriers, the rate of PHC was only 5.3 per 100 person-years. The relative risk of PHC for HBsAg carriers was 104.

Additional prospective studies of the risk of PHC in areas where this neoplasm is common have shown similar strong associations with chronic HBV infection.[82] The risk is especially high in China, and prospective studies suggest that 40% of Chinese males with chronic HBV infection will die from PHC.[83] The World Health Organization has estimated that 80% of all PHC cases in the world occur in persons with chronic HBV infection.[82]

Although the precise molecular mechanism of carcinogenesis is not known, HBV DNA is often clonally integrated into the cellular DNA of carcinoma cells, indicating that these tumors have arisen by a clonal expansion of a cell with HBV integration.[84–86] The biologic plausibility of the oncogenic potential of HBV is supported by data from studies of carcinogenesis of other animal hepadnaviruses. Chronic hepatitis and liver cancer have been documented in wood-

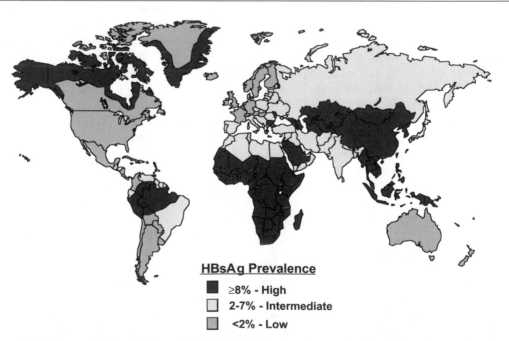

HBsAg Prevalence

■ ≥8% - High
□ 2-7% - Intermediate
▨ <2% - Low

Figure 19–6 Geographic distribution of chronic HBV infection. *Source:* Reprinted from Centers for Disease Control and Prevention.

chucks in the United States and in ducks in China that are infected with other hepadnaviruses closely related to HBV. The association of PHC with persistent hepadnavirus infections in woodchucks and the Beachey ground squirrel is even stronger than the association between HBV and PHC in humans. In fact, the risk of liver cancer in animals who have carried these hepadnaviruses for 3 years or more approaches 100%.[87–91] However, it is also possible that HBV induces PHC indirectly by increasing cell turnover, because PHC occurs with many other chronic liver diseases.

From a public health perspective, the most encouraging data linking HBV infection to PHC is the reduction in the incidence of PHC associated with immunization for HBV in Taiwan.[92] A nationwide hepatitis B vaccination program of all newborn infants of HBsAg carrier mothers began in July 1984. The program was expanded to include all newborns in 1987, then to include children and adults who were HBV-uninfected between 1987 and 1990. The rates of primary liver cancer reported to the tumor registry among 6- to 9-year-olds fell from 0.52 per 100,000 (82 cases among 15,739,570 children) born between July 1978 and June 1984, prior to the immunization program, to 0.13 per 100,000 (3 cases among 2,281,106 children) in those born between July 1984 and June 1986. This significant decrease was not seen for other neoplasms and strongly suggests that HBV immunization of newborns prevented subsequent liver cancer in this cohort of immunized children.

Diagnosis

The diagnosis of HBV infection is usually confirmed using serologic tests. The glycoprotein coat of HBV contains HBsAg, which is produced in excess and can circulate independent of the virus. Detection of HBsAg has evolved from first-generation immunodiffusion methods to third-generation methods, including reverse passive hemagglutination (RPHA) and more sensitive methods that utilize radioimmunoassay (RAI) or enzyme immunoassay (EIA).

The presence of HBsAg indicates active HBV infection but testing for IgM antibody to hepatitis B core (anti-HBc) is needed to determine whether the HBV infection is acute or chronic. Detection of HBsAg is possible in acute infections during the incubation period prior to the increase in liver enzymes or the appearance of jaundice and for several weeks thereafter (Figure 19–7). In persons who develop chronic HBV infection, HBsAg persists in the serum (Figure 19–8).

Antibody to HBsAg (anti-HBs) appears with recovery from acute infection and after immunization with HBV vaccine, which is prepared from purified HBsAg. Anti-HBs titers have been measured to document the levels of protective antibodies after immunization, and anti-HBs of 10 IU/mL or more are felt to be protective. Commonly, anti-HBs levels may not rise for several months after acute HBV infection, and initially they complex with HBsAg and may be undetectable.

Hepatitis B core antigen (HBcAg) is part of the viral nucleocapsid. No serologic test for HBcAg is available because this antigen doesn't circulate but is localized within hepatic cells. However, antibodies to HBcAg (anti-HBc) are commonly used to diagnose current or past HBV infection. Anti-HBc develops soon after HBV infection and persists for the lifetime of an individual.[93,94] Therefore, it is a good marker of past HBV infection. IgM anti-HBc persists for the first 3 to 6 months after an acute HBV infection and is a good marker of acute infection. Antibodies to HBgAg (anti-HBg) can be useful in measuring infection after HBV vaccine, because the vaccine will produce only anti-HBs. Anti-HBc testing has also been used to screen blood donors since 1987, because these antibodies were found to be a useful surrogate marker for hepatitis C virus infection (HCV) prior to the licensure of specific antibody tests for HCV in 1990.[95,96] Screening of blood donors for anti-HBc has continued, despite the development of sensitive tests for HCV because donors who are anti-HBc positive also are believed to be at somewhat higher risk of being in the window period of HIV infection. However, with the de-

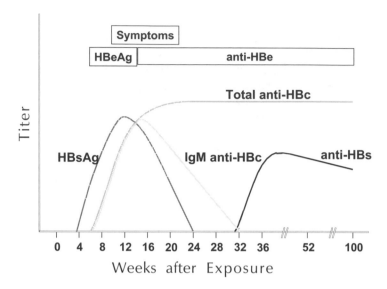

Figure 19–7 Acute hepatitis B virus infection with recovery. *Source:* Reprinted from Centers for Disease Control and Prevention.

velopment and implementation of nucleic acid testing of blood donors for HIV infection using PCR methods, some authorities have recommended that anti-HBc testing of blood donors be discontinued.

Although the diagnosis of recent HBV infection is generally made by detecting HBsAg and/or IgM anti-HBc, other methods also can be used to document active HBV infection. A third antigen–antibody system involves HBeAg, which is a soluble conformational antigen that consists of a portion of the HBcAg. HBeAg is found in the blood during acute or chronic HBV infection and is a marker of infectivity. For example, 90% of pregnant women whose blood is positive for HBeAg at the time of delivery will transmit HBV to their newborn infants in the absence of the administration of immunoglobulin or vaccine to the infant.[76] However, because infants whose mothers are HBsAg-positive but HBeAg-negative at delivery may become infected, decisions to use HBV vaccine for prevention of transmission are not based on the HBeAg status of the mother. On the other hand, the potential infectivity of health care personnel and subsequent work restrictions are judged largely by

HBeAg results. The enzyme HBV-DNA polymerase can also be measured in the serum and, like HBeAg, is a marker of active replication of HBV.

In addition to the serologic methods described above, HBV-DNA can be detected in serum by nucleic acid hybridization or PCR amplification. Although these diagnostic methods are primarily available in research laboratories, monitoring of HBV-DNA can be a useful method of following patients receiving antiviral therapy and for screening for HBsAg mutants (see above). HBV-DNA can be detected in tissue by *in situ* hybridization or PCR amplification. HBV does not replicate reliably to high titers in cell cultures. The dynamics of the appearance of HBV antigens and antibody responses to infection are depicted in Figures 19–7 and 19–8.

Transmission Routes

HBV can be transmitted by percutaneous blood exposure, sexual intercourse, and from a mother to her infant. The risk of parenteral transmission of HBV in developed countries has been greatly reduced in recent years by the screening

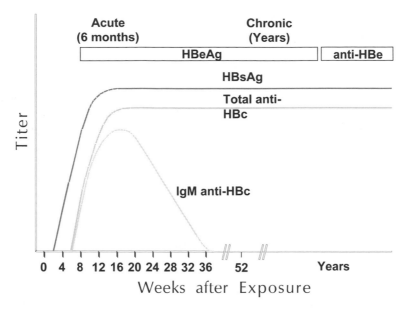

Figure 19–8 Progression to chronic hepatitis B virus infection. *Source:* Reprinted from Centers for Disease control and Prevention.

of blood donors for HBsAg and the use of sterile disposable injection equipment. However, parenteral transmission still occurs in some situations. Persons who inject illicit drugs commonly share injection equipment and have a very high prevalence and incidence of HBV infection.[97,98] Persons receiving pooled blood products also have high rates of HBV infection because very large pools may include a rare donor who was in the seronegative window period or had a false-negative test for HBsAg at the time of donation.

In many developing countries, where the HBsAg carrier rate is very high, i.e., 10% or higher, in the general population and disposable injection equipment is not available, HBV transmission by medical injections continues to be common. Also, parenteral exposures, such as acupuncture, tattoos, and body piercing, are risks for HBV transmission.

Because of the very high concentration of virus, up to 10^{10} virions/mL, in some persons with acute or chronic HBV infection, exposures to minute amounts of blood that occur from activities such as sharing of toothbrushes, razors,

wash cloths, or towels and the presence of eczematous skin lesions that exude serum result in transmission in the household setting.[99–101] HBV transmission has also been demonstrated to children or teachers in a classroom.[102] Other populations who are at high risk of HBV infection include clients of institutions for the developmentally disabled and prisoners.

HBV is also transmitted by sexual intercourse. Numerous studies in various populations have shown that the prevalence of HBV increases with the number of sex partners.[103–105] Populations with large numbers of partners, such as commercial sex workers and both homosexuals and heterosexuals with multiple partners have very high prevalence of HBV infection.[103–105] In households, the sexual partners of an HBsAg carrier are at much greater risk of HBV infection than are others in the household.[99,103,104] Virologic studies have shown that HBV is present in semen and other secretions, although at levels 100- to 1,000-fold lower than in the blood.

In many parts of the world, HBV infection is commonly acquired during the perinatal period or in early childhood. Infants born to a mother who is an HBsAg carrier and is HBeAg-positive have a 90% risk of acquiring an HBV infection if they are not given hepatitis B immunoglobulin or HBV vaccine.[76] Infants of women who are HBsAg positive but HBeAg negative have a lower (but still elevated) risk.

Worldwide Epidemiology

The prevalence of HBV infection varies greatly worldwide. In some areas of the world, HBV infections are highly endemic, and 8% or more of the total population are chronic carriers of HBsAg. These areas constitute 45% of the global population and include China and Southeast Asian countries, sub-Saharan Africa, and several areas in the Arctic, including Alaska, Northern Canada, and Greenland (Figure 19–6). In most of these areas, primary liver cancer is also very common and is often the most frequent cancer in adult males. Nearly all HBV infections occur during the perinatal period or in early childhood in these areas. Because acute HBV infections in infancy and early childhood result in a high rate of chronic carriage, the high endemicity is perpetuated from one generation to the next.

In developed countries of North America, Western Europe, Australia, and some areas of South America, the rates of HBV infection are much lower. Less than 2% of the population are chronic carriers, and the overall infection rate, measured by the prevalence of anti-HBc antibodies, is 5% to 20% (Figure 19–6). In these areas, which constitute 12% of the global population, the frequency of perinatal or early childhood infection is low; however, they may account for a disproportionately high number of chronic HBV infections. Also, immigrants from highly endemic areas may contribute substantially to the subset of HBV infections that are transmitted during the perinatal and early childhood period.[103,104] In these areas, most infections occur among high-risk adult populations, including injection drug users; homosexual men; persons with multiple sex partners; patients with

multiple exposures to pooled blood products, such as hemophiliacs; and health care workers.[103]

The remaining parts of the world, which constitute about 43% of the global population, have an intermediate rate of HBV infection (Figure 19–6). The prevalence of HBsAg positivity ranges from 2% to 8%, and serologic evidence of past infection is found in 20% to 60% of the population. In these areas, there are mixed patterns of infant, early childhood, and adult transmission.

The CDC has estimated the risk factors for acute hepatitis B virus infection by detailed epidemiologic assessment of the behaviors associated with infection in the sentinel counties study of viral hepatitis in several representative U.S. counties. The CDC estimate of the proportion of persons with acute HBV infections associated with known risk factors in 1992–1993 was as follows: heterosexual contact, 41%; injection drug use, 15%; homosexual activity, 9%; household contact, 2%; health care employment, 1%; others, 1%; and unknown, 31% (Figure 19–9). It is likely that the relative contribution of injection drug use to HBV infections may be much higher in large inner city populations in the United States.

The number of chronic carriers of HBV in the United States has probably increased in recent years. It is estimated that at least 5% of the U.S. population has been infected with HBV, based on testing the sera obtained in the national health and nutrition survey in 1978–1980, which is a probability sample of the U.S. population.[105,106] However, the black population was found to have a fourfold greater risk of infection than did whites in this study. Also, persons who have immigrated from China or Southeast Asia have much higher rates of HBV infections than do other residents of the United States.[103] Other countries also have subpopulations with higher rates of HBV infections. Eskimo populations in Canada and the United States have high rates of HBV, and immigrants to Israel from Africa have high rates.[107,108] The endemicity of HBV is high in residents of the Amazon basin in South

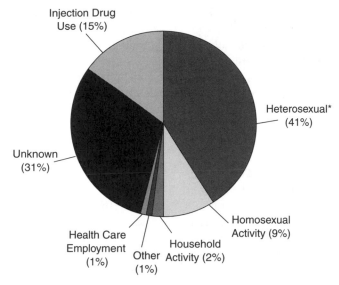

Injection Drug
Use (15%)

Heterosexual*
(41%)

Unknown
(31%)

Homosexual
Activity (9%)

Health Care
Employment
(1%)

Other
(1%)

Household
Activity (2%)

*Includes sexual contact with acute cases, carriers, and multiple partners.

Figure 19–9 Risk factors for acute hepatitis B, United States, 1992–1993. *Source:* CDC Sentinel Counties Study of Viral Hepatitis. Reprinted from Sentinel Counties Study of Viral Hepatitis, Centers for Disease Control and Prevention.

America, whereas it is lower in other areas of South America.[109]

The increased rates of chronic HBV infection in the United States in recent years is related to a number of factors. Among them are an increase in the sizes of the populations of injection drug users, an increase in the population with multiple sex partners, increased immigration from Southeast Asia, where HBV carrier rates are high, and the influence of the AIDS epidemic, with increased rates of chronic carriage of HBV in persons who are immunosuppressed.[103] Also, there has been some transmission in the health care setting. Outbreaks of hepatitis B were common among hemodialysis patients during the 1960s and 1970s, related to percutaneous exposures to blood. Health care workers have been infected from needle sticks from contaminated needles used in infected patients for blood drawing or suturing and dental procedures.[110,111] Laboratory workers or phlebotomists who have frequent contact with blood are at relatively high risk of infection. Rarely, infected health care workers have transmitted HBV to their patients.[111–113] However, transmission in the hospital setting has become much less common with the implementation of HBV vaccination of staff and patients, institution of "universal precautions" for infection control, and testing and isolation of HBsAg carriers in some settings, e.g., dialysis. Despite the recent decrease in the risk of HBV transmission in the health care setting in the United States, the risk of nosocomial transmission in developing countries where HBV is highly endemic remains significant.

The risk of transfusion-transmitted HBV infections in the United States has declined substantially in the last few decades. Screening of blood donors for HBsAg was instituted in 1973. More effective screening of blood donors for drug use or sexual risk behavior and exclusion of male homosexual donors was implemented to reduce the risk of HIV transmission in the early 1980s.

A recent study of the incidence of hepatocellular carcinoma in the United States has estimated that the disease has increased by 46% between 1976–1980 and 1991–1995.[114] This increased incidence of liver cancer probably reflects the combined effects of an increased rate of chronic HBV and HCV infections, combined with the effects of alcohol use among carriers of these viruses.

Prevention

Studies of strategies to prevent HBV infection began in the 1970s. Krugman et al.[115] showed that heat-inactivated whole virus preparations from HBV carriers could prevent infection. Also, it was shown that immunoglobulin containing high titers of antibodies to surface antigen was effective in preventing infection after acute exposure.

The initial vaccines were prepared from the plasma of persons chronically infected with HBV. The plasma was treated to inactivate adventitious viruses with chemical-physical inactivation steps, and HBsAg was purified. These plasma-derived vaccines were found to be highly effective and safe.[116,117] The overall preventive efficacy was 92%; however, nearly 100% of subjects who developed anti-HBs above 10 MIU/ml were protected, especially from developing chronic HBV infection.[116]

Subsequently, hepatitis B vaccines were produced using recombinant DNA technology to express HBsAg in yeast or mammalian cells. These new subunit vaccines were found to be comparable to plasma-derived vaccines in preventing acute and chronic infections and were highly purified and free of other viral antigens.[118–120] This was the first successful use of molecular genetic methods to produce a human vaccine.

Pre-exposure vaccination requires three or more doses to induce a protective immune response. HBV vaccines provide good long-term protection—for at least 10 years—among persons who respond to the initial vaccine series (Table 19–2). In persons whose level of antibody declines, exposure to HBV rarely results in clinically apparent acute or chronic infection. However, some individuals will develop anti-HBc, and a few will develop HBsAg (Table 19–3). Although it is currently not known whether HBV vaccine will provide life-long immunity to infections, available data suggest that persons who respond well to vaccine are protected for at least 10 years.[121]

HBV vaccines are poorly immunogenic if given subcutaneously rather than by the intramuscular route.[122,123] Also, when HBV vaccines are frozen, their immunogenicity declines.

Table 19–2 Estimates of Acute and Chronic Disease Burden for Viral Hepatitis, United States

	HAV	HBV	HCV	HDV
Acute infections (× 1000)/year*	125–200	140–320	35–180	6–13
Fulminant deaths/year	100	150	?	35
Chronic infections	0	1–1.25 million	3.5 million	70,000
Chronic liver disease deaths/year	0	5,000	8–10,000	1,000

*Range based on estimated annual incidence, 1984–1994.

Source: Reprinted from Centers for Disease Control and Prevention.

Table 19–3 Long-Term Protection from Hepatitis B Virus Infection among Cohorts of Children and Adults Known to Have Responded to Hepatitis B Vaccination

| | Follow-up | | Anti-HBs | HBV Infections | |
Study Group	No.*	(yr)	Loss† (%)	Anti-HBc (+)	HBsAg (+)
Postexposure immunoprophylaxis: infants of HBeAg-positive mothers					
Passive–active					
Taiwan	199	5	3	0	0
Taiwan	654	5	9	46	4
United States	315	4–11	12	30	0
Active					
China	55	5	17	6	1
Routine pre-exposure immunization of infants/children					
Senegal	100	6	22	8	4
Alaska	600	10	17	4	0
Venezuela	280	6	29	6	0
Pre-exposure immunization of adults					
Homosexual men	634	9	54	48	4
Homosexual men	127	11	61	26	0
Alaskan Eskimos	272	10	38	6	0

*Number of cases; some studies used person-years of follow-up.
†Less than 10 MIU/mL of anti-HBs.

Source: Reprinted with permission from A.S. Evans and R.A. Kaslow, Viral Infections of Humans, p. 385, © 1997, Plenum Publishing Corporation.

Therefore, it is important that HBV vaccine be administered in the deltoid area in adults to ensure that the vaccine is given intramuscularly. Even with proper handling and administration, some persons respond poorly to HBV vaccines, based on genetic factors. One study found that persons who were homozygous for a certain major histocompatibility haplotype (HLA-B8, SCO1, DR 3) responded poorly to HBV vaccines.[124] Although most persons responded to vaccine; up to 50% of vaccine responders have anti-HBs titers less than 10 MIU/ml several years later. These true responders are protected against disease but years later are difficult to distinguish from nonresponders. Thus, when checking vaccine response, it is necessary to measure anti-HBs titers about 2 months after the third vaccine dose.

Strategies for the use of HBV vaccines to prevent HBV infections must consider the epidemiology of the infection and populations in whom the risk of infection is greatest. In many developing countries, especially in Asia, where the endemicity of HBV is high and perinatal infection accounts for a large proportion of HBV infections, vaccine should be given soon after birth. Where the rate of HBeAg positivity among pregnant women is low and perinatal transmission is less of a risk, the first dose of HBV vaccine can be given to newborns, or the vaccine series can be started with the series of diphtheria-tetanus-pertussis vaccine (see Chapter 10).

The World Health Organization has recommended that HBV vaccines be included with the vaccines given in the expanded program of immunization (EPI) for countries having high or moderate endemicity of hepatitis B virus infection.[125] Unfortunately, many countries in sub-Saharan Africa have not yet included HBV vaccine in their EPI programs because of economic constraints and lack of appreciation of the sequelae of chronic HBV infections in their countries.

Initially, in the United States, HBV vaccine was used selectively in high-risk adults and children. However, this strategy did not substantially affect the incidence of HBV infection because it proved to be very difficult to identify and immunize persons who were at risk. Recently, the strategy has been changed to include HBV vaccine in the regular childhood immunization schedule, in addition to targeted immunization of persons at higher risk, such as illicit drug users, persons with multiple sex partners, and health care workers. An economic analysis of the routine use of HBV vaccine for the immunization of infants found this strategy to be cost-effective in the United States over a wide range of assumptions.[126] There is some evidence that the incidence of HBV has declined in the United States in the past few years. The decline may not be due entirely to a change in vaccination policy but also to a wider implementation of methods to prevent the sexual and parenteral transmission of HBV infectious diseases.

It is particularly important periodically to screen persons who are chronic HBV carriers for PHC. A tumor marker, alpha fetoprotein (AFP) has been found to be elevated in persons with liver cancer. Neither the sensitivity nor specificity of the test is ideal for early detection of PHC. Nonetheless, a program of periodic AFP screening of chronic HBsAg carriers, followed by ultrasound evaluation of those with elevated levels and resection of hepatic tumors, has lowered the mortality from hepatitis B–associated liver cancer.[127]

Treatment

Infection can be suppressed or eradicated in some chronic carriers. Treatment of carriers with alpha interferon for 4 months or more has been reported to suppress HBV-DNA levels in 25% to 40% of carriers.[128,129] However, at least half of those treated patients will rebound after the treatment is stopped. Because alpha interferon is expensive and associated with significant side effects, its use has been limited, especially in developing nations.

Recently, other antiviral drugs have been evaluated to treat chronic HBV carriers. In a study of 358 Chinese patients who were chronic hepatitis B carriers with significant hepatic fibrosis or necrosis at baseline, treatment with lamivudine (3TC) for 1 year was associated with a reduction of the severity of liver pathology in about half of the patients.[130] More recently, a study of lamivudine treatment of chronic carriers in the United States reported favorable virologic and histologic responses in about half of the patients.[131] Unfortunately, relapses can occur after discontinuation of lamivudine and resistant mutants can emerge in those maintained on treatment. The biology of HBV, which includes hepatic integration of viral DNA, suggests that the development of effective antiviral treatment may be difficult.

Orthotopic liver transplantation has also been used for the treatment of chronic carriers; however, the transplanted liver is almost always reinfected, and this is not an option for most persons worldwide. It is a major public health challenge to implement the delivery of effective HBV vaccines to prevent chronic infections and their serious sequelae in the populations that need them.

DELTA HEPATITIS

Virology

Hepatitis delta virus (HDV) was discovered by Rizzetto and colleagues in Italy in 1977.[13] The virus was originally described as a new antigen in patients with chronic HBV infection. The virus could be transmitted to chimpanzees only if they were infected with HBV.[14] Also, HDV infections can be established in other species, i.e., woodchucks, ducks, and ground squirrels, that are chronically infected with their respective hepadnaviruses. However, natural HDV infections have not been identified in these animals.

The HDV is a 35- to 38-nm enveloped particle that contains a small circular single-stranded RNA; the internal protein is the delta antigen, and the outer coat is the HBsAg. The virus appears to be related to some disease-causing viruses of plants. Only one serotype of HDV is known to occur. However, three genotypes have been described, based on nucleic acid homology of isolates from different locations: one from North America, Europe, and Asia; one from Japan; and one from tropical South America.

Clinical Features and Diagnosis

The clinical features of acute and chronic HDV infection are similar to those with other forms of hepatitis. However, persons who are co-infected with HBV and HDV from the same source may have more severe acute hepatitis than persons who have only HBV infection.[132] Anicteric hepatitis occurs in only 20% to 30% of adult patients with HBV and HDV co-infections but in over 50% of adults who are infected with HBV alone.[133] Also, some persons who are co-infected with HDV and HBV may have a biphasic illness.[133] Fulminant hepatitis may occur in some persons who are co-infected with these two viruses and appears to be much more common than in persons infected with only HBV.

Superinfection occurs in persons chronically infected with HBV who are exposed to HDV. Jaundice and further elevation in the liver enzymes may occur very soon after HDV superinfection in a person who is a chronic HBsAg carrier. However, serologic evidence of HDV infection may not occur for 2 to 6 weeks (Figure 19–10). Jaundice precedes serologic evidence of infection, due to the fact that liver cells are already infected with HBV. Such patients generally develop chronic infection and are at high risk of severe chronic liver disease.[134] Some data suggest that patients who are co-infected with HDV have a higher risk of developing primary liver cancer than do those with HBV infection alone; however, the risk of liver cancer in such patients has not been clearly defined.

HDV infection can be diagnosed serologically. Enzyme immunoassay tests are available for testing for HDV antigen and antibodies in serum. Persons who are co-infected will be posi-

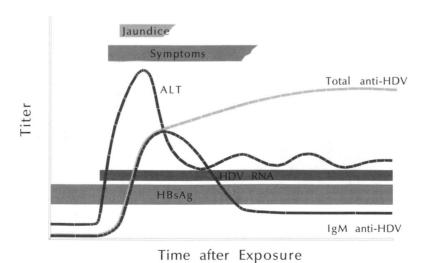

Figure 19–10 HBV-HDV superinfection. *Source:* Reprinted from Centers for Disease Control and Prevention.

tive for anti-IgM anti-HBc and a marker of delta infection. Although delta antigen is detectable in liver tissue, it is not always observed in blood. Likewise, anti-HDV can be undetectable in some instances of acute self-limited infection. Antibodies to HDV appear soon after acute HDV infection, so co-infected patients may also be HDV antibody-positive.

HDV superinfection of HBsAg carriers will be HDV antigen- or antibody-positive and IgM anti-HBc-negative. HDV antigen is usually cleared, but HDV antibody can persist for years. Also, patients infected with HDV will have HDV RNA in their serum.

Transmission Routes

HDV transmission can occur either by parenteral exposure to blood from HDV-infected persons or by sexual contact with a carrier. Outbreaks of HDV have been reported among injection drug users in Los Angeles and Worcester, Massachusetts.[135] Indirect exposure to infected blood may account for most of the cases in the epidemic areas of South America.[136] Sexual transmission is much less efficient, and HDV infections are uncommon in homosexual men who are HBsAg carriers.

Worldwide Epidemiology

Infections with HDV have been reported throughout the world, but generally correspond to areas where HBV is highly endemic, with some exceptions (Figure 19–11). The regions with the highest prevalence of HDV are in northern Columbia, Venezuela, the Amazon basin of Brazil, parts of Africa, Romania, and Southern Italy. The prevalence of HDV is low in the United States and Western Europe but is higher among some populations of injection drug users in these areas. The prevalence of HDV is very low in China and Southeast Asia, despite the high level of HBV endemicity in this region.

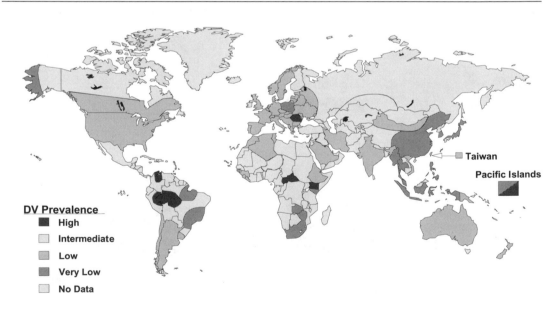

Figure 19–11 Geographic distribution of HDV infection. *Source:* Reprinted from Centers for Disease Control and Prevention.

Prevention

Methods for the control and prevention of HDV infection are the same as those used to prevent hepatitis B virus infection. Successful immunization with HBV vaccine of persons at risk for HBV would also prevent HDV. In addition, the risk of HDV superinfection should be a major incentive for injection drug users who are HBsAg carriers to avoid further high-risk exposures. All HBsAg carriers should be counseled to avoid parenteral or sexual exposure to possible HBV-HDV carriers.

HEPATITIS C VIRUS

Virology

HCV is a spherical, enveloped, RNA virus approximately 50 nm in diameter that contains a positive-sense, single-stranded genome approximately 9.7 kb in length.[137,138] HCV is a member of the family *Flaviviridae*, classified within its own *Hepacivirus* genus. The RNA contains a single large (~3,000 aa) open reading frame (ORF) flanked by highly conserved 5' and 3' untranslated regions.[139] The ~9.0 kb ORF encodes a polyprotein that is cotranslationally processed into at least 10 proteins. These include,

from the amino terminus, structural proteins (the viral nucleocapsid or "core" protein, the envelope proteins E1 and E2, and a short, possibly transmembrane protein, p7 or NS2A) and six nonstructural proteins that are involved in replication of the viral RNA (Figure 19–12).

The liver is presumed to be the primary source of virus present in blood, because HCV-specific antigens and both negative- and positive-strand HCV RNA have been identified within hepatocytes.[137,140,141] Some data suggest that the virus may also replicate within peripheral mononuclear cells of lymphoid or perhaps bone marrow origin.[142,143] However, when assays are done with strand-specific rTth, Lanford et al.[144] have shown that extra hepatic replication is insufficient to explain HCV RNA detected in blood. Mathematical models of viral kinetics suggest a half-life of approximately 2.5 hours for virions in the bloodstream and that up to 1.0×10^{12} virions are produced each day in a chronically infected human.[145] This rate exceeds comparable estimates of the production of HIV by more than an order of magnitude. The high level of virion turnover, coupled with the absence of proofreading by the NS5B RNA polymerase, results in relatively rapid accumulation of mutations within the viral genome. Multiple HCV variants can be recovered from the plasma and liver of an

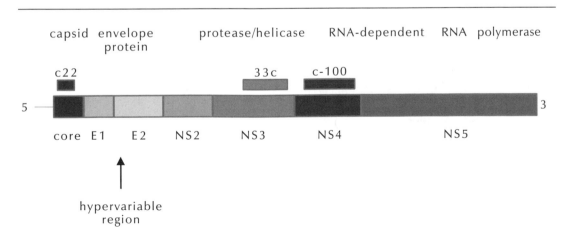

Figure 19–12 Hepatitis C virus. *Source:* Reprinted from Centers for Disease Control and Prevention.

infected individual at any time. Thus, like many RNA viruses, HCV exists in each infected person as a quasispecies, or "swarm" of closely related but distinct genetic sequences.[146,147] For example, in the blood of a recently infected individual, up to 85% of cDNA clones recovered from viral RNAs may represent unique genetic variants.[148]

HCV infections are often persistent (see below), indicating that the virus has evolved mechanisms to escape immune surveillance. Because of limitations in experimental models and the infrequent recognition of natural acute infection, these mechanisms are poorly understood. It has been proposed that the quasispecies nature of the infection is responsible for persistence, and individuals with a more complex infection were more likely to have persistence infection in one study.[149] However, because single clone infections of chimpanzees can persist, viral complexity is clearly not necessary and could be a result of persistence, rather than the cause.[150] One paradox is that HCV persistence occurs despite a broad humoral and cellular immune response. It has been suggested that HCV sequence variation may contribute to viral persistence. Mutations may alter the amino acid sequences of critical epitopes, leading to the escape of a new quasispecies variant from a previously suppressive immune response, either cellular or humoral.[151–153] Viral escape from a cytotoxic lymphocyte clone has been reported in a persistently infected chimpanzee and was shown to correlate with a single NS3 amino acid substitution.[153]

HCV transmission requires that infectious virions contact susceptible cells that sustain replication. It is difficult to ascertain which body fluids contain infectious hepatitis C virions. Using sensitive techniques, HCV RNA can be detected in blood (including serum and plasma), saliva, tears, seminal fluid, ascitic fluid, and cerebrospinal fluid.[154–158] HCV RNA-containing blood is infectious when administered intravenously, for example, by transfusion or experimental inoculation of chimpanzees. In addition, one chimpanzee was infected by intravenous inoculation of saliva.[159] However, there is very little information regarding the potential infectivity of other nonblood body fluids, both because the experiments have not been performed and because accidental percutaneous exposures to nonblood body fluids are rare.

The second requirement for transmission is contact of infectious virions with a susceptible cell. HCV replication occurs in the hepatocyte and possibly elsewhere. There are some data to suggest that HCV interacts with CD81 molecules.[160] However, their role as an HCV receptor is not established, and very little is known about cellular susceptibility to HCV infection. For example, seminal fluid may contain HCV RNA, but sexual transmission is uncommon. Whether this discrepancy is due to a paucity of infectious virions in seminal fluid or insufficient numbers of susceptible cells in the genital mucosa is unknown.

HCV diversity can be exploited for epidemiologic research. The nucleotide sequence corresponding to the HCV envelope and some nonstructural proteins is highly variable, and at least six distinct HCV genotypes have been described.[161,162] The genetic heterogeneity of HCV strains is sufficiently high that detection of the same or nearly identical nucleotide sequences in two individuals is strong evidence for a common source of infection. These comparisons have been used to demonstrate HCV transmission between sexual partners, within families, among patients, and from health care workers to patients.[163–166] HCV genotype/subtype classification also may be used epidemiologically but is less specific than is nucleotide sequence analysis.

Clinical Features and Diagnosis

Acute HCV infection is usually unnoticed. Fewer than one fifth of persons will have jaundice or sufficient symptoms to seek medical care. When symptoms do occur, they are indistinguishable from those caused by other hepatitis viruses. After the acute infection, 85% of persons will have persistent viremia, and more than half will have elevated levels of liver enzymes.[167-170] HCV infection may persist over 10 to 50 years without symptoms or with symptoms such as malaise that are too general to be attributed to HCV infection. From 2% to 25% of individuals with persistent HCV infection will develop life-threatening cirrhosis and/or liver cancer.[170-173] Cirrhosis can cause liver failure, which manifests as esophageal varices, ascites, hypoprothrombinemia, and hepatic encephalopathy. HCV infection is also associated with vasculitis (essential mixed cryoglobulinemia),[174,175] membranoproliferative glomerulonephritis,[175,176] and sporadic porphyria cutanea tarda.[177,178] Approximately 10,000 persons die of HCV infection each year in the United States.[179]

The laboratory diagnosis of HCV infection is based principally on detection by enzyme immunoassay of antibodies to recombinant HCV peptides.[180-182] The sensitivity of the latest, third-generation, HCV antibody assay is estimated to be 97%, and it can detect HCV antibody within 6 to 8 weeks of exposure.[183,184] These assays are measures of HCV infection, not immunity. Assays for IgM HCV antibodies are not clinically useful.

The U.S. Food and Drug Administration (FDA) has licensed the recombinant immunoblot assay (RIBA) (Ortho Diagnostic Systems, Raritan, NJ) as a supplemental test to the enzyme immunoassay.[185,186] The RIBA generally identifies the specific antigens to which antibodies are reacting in the EIA and may be positive (≥2 antigens), indeterminate (1 antigen), or negative. EIA- and RIBA-positive sera usually contain HCV RNA, as indicated by direct detection and by look-back studies of donations that caused infection after transfusion.[185,187,188] EIA-positive, RIBA-indeterminate sera may also contain HCV RNA, especially if the reactivity was to core or NS3 antigens (the c22–3 and c33-c bands). The RIBA assay is useful to confirm the specificity of a positive EIA test, especially if it is weakly positive. In populations at low risk of HCV infection, such as healthy blood donors, many weakly positive EIA tests are HCV specific.[186]

HCV RNA can be detected in plasma and serum by reverse transcription polymerase chain reaction (PCR) and by branched DNA (bDNA) assays. Detection of HCV RNA indicates ongoing infection, whereas clearance of serum HCV RNA, either spontaneously or following treatment, correlates with ALT normalization and improvement in liver histology. As of November 1999, no RNA detection assays had yet been approved by the FDA for diagnosis of HCV infection, and their reliability has been questioned. In one study, only 16% of 31 laboratories accurately identified all samples in a standardized panel.[189] Thus, HCV infection is usually diagnosed by detection of HCV antibody by enzyme immunoassay, followed by either detection of HCV RNA or supplemental (RIBA) antibody testing.

There are several methods for HCV RNA quantification but none is FDA approved as of November 1999.[190-192] Various methods have been utilized to determine the genotype of a viral strain. The most commonly used tests detect subtype-specific point mutations in PCR-amplified cDNA. These include the line probe assay (LIPA), which is based on reverse dot-blot hybridization (Innogenetics, Zwijnaarde, Belgium), restriction fragment-length polymorphism assays, and PCR using subtype-specific primers.[193-196] Phylogenetic analysis of cDNA sequence is the gold standard for evaluating HCV genotypes.

Transmission Routes

Transfusion of Blood Products

Transfusion of HCV RNA-containing blood or organs almost always results in transmission.[188,197-200] Prior to screening blood donations for HCV antibodies and surrogate markers, approximately 17% of HCV infections in the United States were caused by transfusion.[201] With screening, the risk of transfusion transmission of HCV has been reduced substantially.[202,203] In 1987, routine screening of blood donors for elevations in the liver enzyme, alanine aminotransferase (ALT), and antibodies to

HBcAg were instituted primarily to decrease the risk of transmitting hepatitis C virus. It is estimated that these surrogate markers for HCV infection reduced the risk of transfusion transmission of HCV by about 50%.[96] In May 1990, the first-generation two-antigen serologic test for HCV was licensed and used to screen all blood donors in the United States. The use of this specific HCV screening test further reduced the risk of the transmission of HCV by blood products. The probable rate of transmission of viral infections by transfusion was estimated by calculating the number of donors who were in the seronegative window period at the time of donation in 1991–1993, by modeling data from seroconverters among repeat donors at five large Red Cross blood banks. This study estimated that about 1 in 63,000 donors who were HBV infected and 1 in 103,000 who were HCV infected were in the seronegative window period at the time of their donation.[204] Transfusion transmission may still occur from donors with recent infection who have not yet developed antibodies and possibly from others who lose or never develop HCV antibody.[205] However, this risk is estimated to be less than 1 in 100,000.[206] Accordingly, blood transfusion now causes less than 4% of HCV infections in the United States.[201]

HCV also has been transmitted by intravenous administration of contaminated blood products, including immunoglobulin (IG) and clotting factors, as illustrated in several large outbreaks.[206–209] Current IG viral inactivation procedures and recombinant clotting factor use should diminish the risk of further transmission by these products.

HCV can also be transmitted by percutaneous needle sticks, as occur among illicit injection drug users and inadvertently in the practice of medicine. From a single needle-stick exposure, the risk of HCV transmission to a susceptible person is approximately 3%, intermediate between HBV (30%) and HIV (0.3%). Because of multiple needle-stick exposures, 50% to 95% of persons acknowledging drug use have HCV infection.[210–215] Injection drug users acquire HCV infection by sharing contaminated needles and

drug-use equipment, sometimes among groups of persons, such as in "shooting galleries." New initiates into drug use are at highest risk for HCV infection.[216] HCV infection that occurs in the context of drug use but without acknowledged injection use may be due to other blood exposures (such as sharing straws for intranasal ingestion of cocaine).[217] However, unacknowledged injection use is difficult to exclude, and the extent to which HCV transmission can occur through intranasal cocaine use remains an important area of research.

HCV transmission occurs in 3% to 8% of health care workers who experience needle-stick exposures to HCV-infected patients.[218–220] Whereas hollow-bore needle-stick exposures account for most transmission from patients to health care workers, HCV infection has also been reported from blood splashed on the conjunctiva and a solid bore needle stick.[221] Nonetheless, the occurrence of HCV infection among dental and medical health care workers is commonly less than or similar to the general population, demonstrating that long-term infection is uncommon after such exposures.[222–228]

Other forms of blood-borne nosocomial transmission also occur. Patient-to-patient HCV transmission has been documented. In one example, two patients acquired HCV infection 8 to 10 weeks after a colonoscopic procedure, which was performed with the same colonoscope as had been used hours earlier on an HCV-infected patient.[163] HCV isolates from all three patients had high nucleotide identity in a variable HCV genomic segment, essentially proving a common source of infection. Nosocomial HCV transmission also has been suggested by identification of clusters of untransfused patients with similar HCV nucleotide sequences. In one Swedish hematology ward, five clusters of identical or closely related viruses were found. All patients in each cluster had overlapping hospitalizations but not common sources of blood.[166] Similarly, there is evidence of patient-to-patient HCV transmission in several dialysis centers.[229–232]

Nosocomial transmission of HCV is rare in developed countries, where recent receipt or provision of health care is not commonly acknowledged by patients with new HCV infections.[233] However, in developed countries, traditional and nontraditional medical practices are probably the leading source of HCV transmission (discussed below). Breaks in infection control practices have been detected in some instances of nosocomial HCV transmission and are impossible to exclude in others. Strict adherence to these guidelines must be vigorously maintained, especially when mucosal barriers frequently are broken, such as in dialysis units.

HCV has also been transmitted from health care providers to patients, although this is rare. In one instance, HCV infection was detected in six patients after cardiac surgery.[164] Blood donors for these patients were HCV-negative. Five of six patients had a genetically similar, unusual HCV strain that later also was found in the surgeon. No infection control breaches were identified. However, percutaneous injuries occurred occasionally when the surgeon tied wires to close the sternum.

HCV can be transmitted by other unusual percutaneous exposures. Tattooing has been associated with HCV infection.[234,235] A human bite and folk remedies such as acupuncture and scarification rituals have also been associated with HCV infection (see below).[236]

HCV is probably infrequently transmitted by sexual intercourse. Biologic plausibility exists for sexual transmission, as evidenced by detection of HCV RNA in semen and saliva.[154,156,157] However, as mentioned above, we do not know whether these fluids contain infectious virions in sufficient quantity to transmit infection or whether the mucosal barrier is protective. Evidence for sexual transmission is indirect. High rates of HCV infection have been found in persons with multiple sexual partners and commercial sex workers,[165,237–241] and acute HCV infection has been reported in instances where sexual, but not other exposures, are recognized.[242,243] In studies of families of HCV-infected patients, sexual partners are generally the only contacts at increased infection risk, a risk that increases with the duration of the relationship.[244–247] High

nucleotide identity is often found in the HCV strains of the sexual partners.[165,245,247,248]

Sexual transmission could explain these findings. However, it is virtually impossible to exclude other common exposures, such as sharing razors, other subtle percutaneous exposures, or unacknowledged drug use. The importance of the "indirect" nature of the evidence is underscored by other evidence suggesting that sexual transmission is rare. Studies of long-term sexual partners of HCV-infected hemophiliacs and transfusion recipients generally show little or no HCV transmission, even if there had been frequent unprotected sexual intercourse.[249–252] HCV prevalence rates among homosexual men also are generally lower than for other infections, such as HIV, HBV, and syphilis, for which sexual transmission is well established.[253–256]

Although the risk of transmission attributable to intercourse per se may never be precisely defined, individuals with HCV-positive sexual partners and especially those with multiple partners generally are at increased risk of infection. Individuals in long-term monogamous relationships should be informed of the low risk of transmission and may elect not to use barrier precautions.

Perinatal Transmission

HCV infection occurs in 2% to 8% of infants born to HCV-infected mothers.[257–263] Because of passive transfer of maternal HCV antibody, infant HCV infection must be diagnosed through detection in infant serum of HCV RNA or HCV antibody after 18 months of age. HIV co-infection has been associated with more frequent transmission of HCV from mother to infant in some studies.[260,264] Higher maternal HCV viral load also has been associated with transmission of HCV from mother to infant.[259,265–268] The effect of maternal HIV on perinatal HCV transmission may be through increasing the HCV viral load.[269–272] HCV RNA has been detected in breast milk,[259,273,274] but the risk of transmission does not appear to be substantially increased in breastfeeding infants.[275]

Worldwide Epidemiology

It is estimated that there are more than 170 million persons infected with HCV worldwide.[276] Through August 1997, 130 countries had reported HCV prevalence rates to the World Health Organization or in the literature in at least one population. HCV infection was found in all but three countries, and it is difficult to imagine that infection would not be found there with further investigation. In developed nations, general population HCV prevalence rates are generally less than 3%, whereas, among volunteer blood donors, they are less than 1%.

There are several highly endemic regions. In most, HCV infection is prevalent among persons over 40 years of age but uncommon in those less than 20 years of age.[277–280] This cohort effect suggests a time-restricted exposure that, in many instances, appears to have been receipt of a medical procedure. In Egypt, HCV prevalence rates from 10% to 30% have been found.[281–286] Although not yet confirmed, in Egypt, it is suspected that a national campaign to treat schistosomiasis infections was responsible. Up until the 1970s, parenteral antischistosomiasis therapies were administered to entire villages, and needles were frequently reused. Similarly, in several areas in Italy and Japan, a high HCV prevalence among older persons was linked to receipt of medical care.[277,278,280,287,288] In the isolated Arahiro region of Japan, 45% of individuals over 41 years of age had HCV infection,[289] whereas, in another area, the same-age prevalence was 2%. Folk remedies, such as acupuncture and cutting of skin with nonsterilized knives, were identified as likely transmission modes. Percutaneous folk practices have occurred for thousands of years and probably account for the worldwide distribution of HCV.

High rates of HCV infection also have been reported in urban areas of developed countries. In urban Baltimore, Maryland, HCV infection was found in 18% of patients attending an inner-city emergency department and 15% attending a nearby clinic for sexually transmitted diseases.[238,290] Injection drug use, not medical procedures, is chiefly responsible for transmission in this setting.

The epidemiology of HCV infection has been carefully studied in several developed nations, including the United States and France. In the United States, the yearly incidence of HCV infection has declined since the 1980s.[179,291] At least two thirds of community-acquired HCV infections are related to injection drug use. Injection drug use in the 6 months prior to infection is acknowledged by approximately 38% of subjects.[233,292] However, noninjection drug use and other indicators of injection use are acknowledged by another 44%. Sexual or household exposure to HCV is detected in approximately 10% of individuals with acute HCV infection, whereas transfusions, occupational exposures, and other factors are infrequently (<4%) identified.

The epidemiology and overall burden of HCV infection in the United States has been further characterized using the Third National Health and Nutrition Examination (NHANES) data.[293] A total of 23,527 persons, who were representative of the general population of the United States, were tested for HCV infection. Antibodies to HCV were detected in 1.8%, or almost 4 million persons. Active infection (HCV RNA) was detected in 74%, suggesting that 2.7 million persons in the United States have ongoing infection. Illegal drug use and high-risk sexual exposures were associated with HCV infection, as were low socioeconomic indices, low levels of education, and poverty. This large-scale "representative" sampling was a major breakthrough in our understanding of the burden and distribution of infection. However, it also points to the difficulty of ascertaining risk, because some of the factors identified, such as marijuana use and low education, represent unmeasured exposures (residual confounding). Furthermore, because a history of the injection of illicit drugs was not included in the NHANES interview, it is difficult to estimate the contribution of current or remote drug injection to the HCV prevalence in this sample.[294]

Prevention

HCV prevention is chiefly accomplished through efforts to prevent exposure. There are no vaccines available to prevent HCV infection. Vigorous vaccine development efforts are ongoing but the complexity of the infection and poor understanding of the immune response complicate this work. Postexposure administration of immunoglobulin to prevent HCV infection is not currently recommended because there is little evidence that it was effective in the past and even more reason to doubt the effectiveness of the newer products that do not contain HCV antibody.[179]

The incidence of HCV infection has declined in the United States. One reason is the practice of screening blood donations for HCV antibody and surrogate markers. In some but not all studies, use of needle exchange programs has also been associated with reductions in HCV incidence.[295,296] However, HCV incidence has declined in areas where there are no needle exchange programs. Because most HCV infections in developed nations are due to illicit injection drug use, expanded efforts to treat drug dependence are urgently needed. In developing nations, it is urgent to begin programs to alter attitudes regarding blood exposures and to improve the safety of necessary percutaneous practices.

HEPATITIS E VIRUS

Virology

Hepatitis E virus (HEV) is a single-strand, positive sense RNA virus, approximately 32 nm in diameter.[297–299] The virus is relatively sensitive, being inactivated by CsCl, freeze-thawing, and pelleting. Like HAV, HEV lacks an envelope, making it stable in bile and, thus, transmissible by ingestion of fecally contaminated water. HEV is resistant to the pH extremes of the gastrointestinal tract, although it is assumed that water chlorination decreases infectivity.

The HEV genome is approximately 7.2 kb and consists of three ORFs. Recombinant antigens synthesized from the second and third ORFs are used in diagnostic assays. HEV isolates may have as little as 75% homology and three serotypes have been identified. Isolates collected in the Western hemisphere are especially heterogeneous but phylogenetically cluster with a highly related virus from swine.[300] HEV shares certain morphologic and biophysical properties with caliciviruses, yet its genomic organization is notably different from others in this family.[301] Currently, HEV remains unclassified, although recent genomic analyses may prompt the formation of a new family of single-strand, polyadenylated RNA viruses.

Although HEV does not proliferate well in cell culture, animal models have been developed. Most experiments have been conducted in nonhuman primate species using the cynomolgus macaque, *Macaca fascicularis*.[302] Laboratory infections of chimpanzees, tamarins, owl monkeys, rhesus monkeys, and even rats have also been reported.[303,304] Especially interesting is natural recovery of an HEV-like agent from swine.[299]

Clinical Features and Diagnosis

Clinically, HEV is impossible to distinguish from other hepatitis virus infections. As with HAV infection, the disease is self-limiting, and most patients recover completely without complications or sequelae. No chronic or carrier state has been demonstrated after hepatitis E infection. The typical incubation period ranges from 15 to 60 days (mean 40 days) from the time of exposure.[305] The liver is probably the main site of HEV replication in infected humans. HEV infection is rarely fatal in the general population. However, fulminant hepatic failure can occur, especially in pregnant women.[306–308] During a 1993–1994 Pakistan HEV outbreak, attack rates of icteric hepatitis increased by trimester of pregnancy.[307]

As with all hepatitis virus infections, viremia can be detected before the onset of symptoms or liver enzyme elevations. HEV RNA is detectable in blood for 14 to 28 days in most patients with clinical disease, although it may be prolonged.[305,309] HEV has been detected in stool up to 9 days prior to the icteric phase of disease and typically lasts 7 to 14 days thereafter.[305,310]

The serologic course of HEV infection has been determined using nonhuman primate models, human volunteer studies, and outbreak investigations. Both IgG and IgM antibody responses occur soon after HEV infection, with peak antibody titers occurring 2 to 4 weeks after inoculation or infection.[305,311] The HEV IgM titers decline rapidly within 3 months after infection. Published data on the persistence of anti-HEV IgG are somewhat conflicting. A study of Egyptian children noted the disappearance of anti-HEV IgG within 6 to 12 months after infection,[312] and in Indonesia, 28% of persons involved in an HEV outbreak lost anti-HEV over 2 years of follow-up.[313] On the other hand, in some persons, IgG anti-HEV persists for 15 or more years.[311,314,315] Discrepancies in these results may relate to the laboratory tests, as demonstrated by Mast and colleagues who found that synthetic peptide-based EIAs were less sensitive for the detection of remote infections, when compared with recombinant antigen assays.[314]

HEV diagnosis can be complicated by what appears to be serologic cross-reactivity with another unrecognized condition/infection. In one study, approximately 20% of blood donors from Maryland, New York, and California had IgG anti-HEV, although only one human HEV infection has ever been demonstrated to originate in the United States.[316] Given the lack of familiarity of most laboratories with HEV testing, a practical approach is to collect sera, store at −20°C in a cryovial, and contact a local reference laboratory for assistance. In the United States, practitioners with patients having unexplained acute jaundice and negative tests for HAV, HBV, and HCV should contact the hepatitis branch of the CDC at (404) 639-3048 for assistance.

Transmission Routes

The possible routes of HEV transmission are the same as with HAV. However, HEV infection appears to be more frequently linked to ingestion of contaminated water. In many Asian countries, epidemics of HEV infection have occurred during periods of monsoon rains.[317] Because there is a brief period of viremia, blood-borne transmission is also possible with HEV.[318] Similarly, mother-to-infant transmission has been reported.[319]

Direct comparisons of the efficiency of person-to-person transmission of HEV and HAV are difficult, because, in most areas of the world where HEV infections occur, the majority of persons have already been infected with HAV by 10 years of age. However, person-to-person HEV transmission seems to be less efficient than HAV, as indicated by the lower secondary attack rates.[320] The propensity to cause "large-scale" outbreaks is associated more with HEV than HAV but may be an artifact of the more extensive population-wide immunity from HAV in areas where large outbreaks have been reported. Fecal contamination of water supplies from a variety of causes is a frequent finding in evaluations of HEV outbreaks and probably explains the tendency for outbreaks to occur following the rainy season.

The reservoir for HEV infections is an area of renewed interest. Humans are the only proven reservoir for HEV. However, a highly related virus has been found in swine.[300,321] This HEV-like swine virus can cause infection of nonhuman primates, and HEV can infect swine.[321] Moreover, antibody that cross-reacts with HEV antigens (and in some cases, neutralizes HEV) has been detected in swine, rats, and other animals.[322] These findings may explain the serologic evidence of HEV infection found in non-endemic areas. However, more research is needed to determine how extensive this family of viruses is and to what extent these viruses infect humans.

Worldwide Epidemiology

HEV infections are rare in developed countries. Only one case of HEV infection has been documented to have originated in the United States; others have been imported by travel-

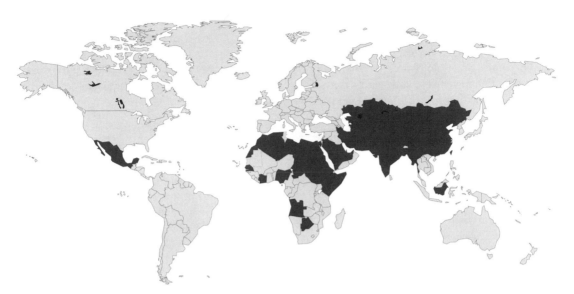

Figure 19–13 Geographic distribution of hepatitis E outbreaks or confirmed infection in >25% of sporadic non-ABC hepatitis. *Source:* Reprinted from Centers for Disease Control and Prevention.

ers.[323] As mentioned above, a far greater proportion of those living in developed nations may have serologic reactivity to HEV. However, this seroreactivity was not correlated with a history of jaundice or, for that matter, traditional markers of blood-borne or sexually transmitted infectious diseases.[316]

Like HAV, HEV is endemic in many developing countries (Figure 19–13). However, interesting epidemiologic differences have been observed between those two enterically transmitted viruses. A striking increase in the age-specific HEV clinical attack rate is seen, beginning in the third decade of life.[324,326] In contrast, HAV infection is almost universal in developing nations by the age of 10 years. This difference could be explained by less frequent transmission of HEV and, thus, postponement of infection for years, when it is clinically apparent (similar to what has happened with HAV infections in countries undergoing economic transition). The difference could also be explained if HEV infection of children did not result in durable immunity.

Development of serologic tests for HEV infection has not completely resolved this issue.

Although HEV infection has been demonstrated in children,[312] in many studies, the seroprevalence is low until the third decade of life.[326–329] On the other hand, others have demonstrated substantially higher seroprevalence rates of HEV infection in children.[330] Thus, the conventional wisdom that HEV infection is less common in children may relate to differences in the tools used to measure infection. No matter what the explanation, HEV remains unique among enteric viruses in this peak in clinical attack rate, beginning in the third decade of life.

Prevention

Because HEV infection rarely occurs in developed countries, the most important control measures involve improvements in hygiene, especially in the development of an uncontaminated water supply.

There is emerging data that indicate HEV infection can be prevented (or at least disease modified) by vaccination and immunoglobulin administration.[331–335] However, at present, there are no available vaccines to prevent HEV infection.

OTHER VIRUSES

For 5% to 20% of persons with acute hepatitis syndromes, no etiology is found (non-A to E hepatitis). Other viruses, such as GB virus C (or the hepatitis G virus), TTV virus, and SEN-V virus, have been discovered in this context.[336-338] However, some of these recently described viruses (e.g., GB-C, TTV) may not usually cause hepatitis. Nevertheless, other viral agents likely are responsible for some cases of hepatitis.

REFERENCES

1. Zuckerman AJ. The history of viral hepatitis from antiquity to the present. In: Deinhardt F, Deinhardt J, eds. *Viral Hepatitis Laboratory and Clinical Science.* New York: Marcel Dekker; 1983:3–32.

2. Lürman A. Eine icterus epidemic. *Berl Klin Worchenschr.* 1885;22:20–23.

3. Beeson PB, Chainey G, McFarlan AM. Hepatitis following injection of mumps convalescent plasma. *Lancet.* 1944;1:814–821.

4. Sawyer WA, Meyer KF, Eaton WD, et al. Jaundice in army personnel in the western region of the United States and its relation to vaccination against yellow fever. *Am J Hyg.* 1944;39:334.

5. MacCallum FO. Jaundice in syphilitics. *Br J Vener Dis.* 1943;19:63.

6. Krugman S. Giles JP, Hammond J. Infectious hepatitis: evidence for two distinctive, clinical, epidemiological and immunological types of infections. *JAMA.* 1967; 200:365–373.

7. Blumberg BS, Alter HJ, Visnich S. A "new" antigen in leukemia sera. *JAMA.* 1965;191:541–546.

8. Prince AM. An antigen detected in the blood during the incubation period of serum hepatitis. *Proc Natl Acad Sci USA.* 1968;60:814–821.

9. Feinstone SM, Kapikian AZ, Purcell RH, Alter AJ, Holland PV. Transfusion-associated hepatitis not due to viral hepatitis type A or B. *N Engl J Med.* 1975;292:767–770.

10. Alter HJ, Purcell RH, Shih JW, Melpolder JC, Houghton M, Choo QL, Kuo G. Detection of antibody to hepatitis C in prospectively followed transfusion recipients with acute and chronic non-A, non-B hepatitis. *N Engl J Med.* 1989;321:1494–1500.

11. Choo QL, Koo G, Weiner AJ, Overby LR, Bradley DW, Houghton M. Isolation of a cDNA clone derived from a blood borne non-A, non-B viral hepatitis genome. *Science.* 1989;244:351–362.

12. Kuo G, Choo QL, Alter HJ, et al. An assay for circulating antibodies to a major etiologic virus of human non-A, non-B hepatitis. *Science.* 1989;244:362–364.

13. Rizzetto M, Canese MC, Arico S, et al. Immunofluorescence detection of a new antigen-antibody system associated to the hepatitis B virus in the liver and in the serum of HBsAg carriers. *Gut.* 1977;18:997–1003.

14. Rizzetto M, Canese MC, Gerin JC, et al Transmission of the hepatitis virus associated delta antigen to chimpanzees. *J Infect Dis.* 1980;141:590–601.

15. Feinstone SM, Kapikian AZ, Purcell RH. Hepatitis A: detection by immune electron microscopy of a virus-like antigen association with acute illness. *Science.* 1973; 182:1026–1028.

16. Provost PJ, Hilleman MR. Propagation of human hepatitis A virus in cell culture in vitro. *Proc Soc Exp Biol Med.* 1979;160:213.

17. Werzberger A, Mensch B, Kuter B, et al. A controlled trial of formalin-inactivated hepatitis A vaccine in healthy children. *N Engl J Med.* 1992;327:453–457.

18. Innis BL, Snitbban R, Kunasol P, et al. Protection against hepatitis A by an inactivated vaccine. *JAMA.* 1994;271:1328–1334.

18. Wong DL, Purcell RH, Sreentvasan MA, Prasad SR, Parri KM. Epidemic and endemic hepatitis in India: evidence for non A/non B hepatitis virus etiology. *Lancet.* 1980;2:876–878.

19. Bradley DW, Krawczynski K, Cook EH, McCaustland KA, Humphrey CD, Spelbring JG, Myint H, Maynard JE. Enterically transmitted non-A, non-b hepatitis: serial passage of disease in cynomolgus monkeys and tamarins, and discovery of disease associated with 27 to 34 nm virus-like particles. *Proc Natl Acad Sci USA.* 1987; 84:6277–6281.

20. Kane MA, Bradley DW, Shrestha SM, et al. Epidemic non-A, non-B hepatitis in Nepal: recovery of a possible etiologic agent and transmission to marmosets. *JAMA.* 1984;252:3140–3145.

21. Acute Hepatic Failure Study Group. Etiology and prognosis in fulminant hepatitis. *Gastroenterology.* 1979; 77:A33.

22. Mathieson CR, Skinholj P, Nielsen JO, Purcell RH, Wong DC, Ranek C. Hepatitis A, B and non-A, non-B in fulminant hepatitis. *Gut.* 1980;21:72–77.

23. Sjogren MH, Tanneh, Fay O, et al. Hepatitis A virus in stool during clinical relapse. *Ann Intern Med.* 1987; 106:221.

24. Andre FE, D'Hondt E, Delem A, Safary A. Clinical assessment of the safety and efficacy of an inactivated hepatitis A vaccine. Rationale and summary of findings. *Vaccine*. 1992;10(Suppl. 1):S160–S163.

25. Conlepis AG, Locarnini SA, Lehmann NC, Gust D. Detection of hepatitis A virus in the feces of patients with naturally acquired infections. *J Infect Dis*. 1980; 141:151.

26. Cohen JL, Feinstone S, Purcell RH. Hepatitis A virus infection in a chimpanzee: duration of viremia and detection of virus in saliva and throat swabs. *J Infect Dis*. 1989;180:887.

27. Shapiro CN, Coleman PJ, McQuillan GM, Alter MJ, Margolis HS. Epidemiology of hepatitis A: seroepidemiology and risk groups in the USA. *Vaccine*. 1992; 10:S59–S62.

28. Villano SA, Nelson KE, Vlahov D, et al. Hepatitis-A among homosexual men and injection drug users: more evidence for vaccination. *Clin Infect Dis*. 1997;25:726–728.

29. Corey L, Holmes HK. Sexual transmission of hepatitis A in homosexual men. *N Engl J Med*. 1980;302:345–438.

30. Noble RC, Kane MA, Reeves SA, Roeckel I. Post transfusion hepatitis A in a neonatal intensive care unit. *JAMA*. 1984;252:2711–2715.

31. Rosenblum LS, Villarino ME, Nainan OV, et al. Hepatitis A outbreak in a neonatal intensive care unit: risk factors for transmission and evidence of prolonged viral excretion among preterm infants. *J Infect Dis*. 1991;164:476–482.

32. Mannucci PM, Gdorin S, Gringeri A, et al. Transmission of hepatitis A to patients with hemophilia by factor VIII concentrates treated with organic solvent and detergent to inactivate viruses. *Am Intern Med*. 1994;120:1–10.

33. Lemon SM, Murphy PC, Smith A, et al. Removal/neutralization of hepatitis A virus during manufacture of high pruity, solvent/detergent factor VIII concentrate. *J Med Virol*. 1994;43:44–48.

34. Widell A, Hansson BG, Moestrup T, Nordenfelt E. Increased occurrence of hepatitis A with cyclic outbreaks among drug addicts in a Swedish community. *Infection*. 1983;11:198–204.

35. Centers for Disease Control. Hepatitis A among drug users. *MMWR*. 1988;37:297.

36. Lemon SM. Type A viral hepatitis. New developments in an old disease. *N Engl J Med*. 1985;313:1059–1067.

37. Bergeisen GH, Hinds MW, Skaggs JW. A waterborne outbreak of hepatitis A in Meade County, Kentucky. *Am J Public Health*. 1985;75:161–168.

38. Niu Mt, Polish LB, Robertson BH, et al. A multi-state outbreak of hepatitis A associated with frozen strawberries. *J Infect Dis*. 1992;166:518–529.

39. Rosenblum LS, Mirkin IR, Allen DT, Safford S, Hadler SC. A multi-focal outbreak of hepatitis A traced to commercially distributed lettuce. *Am J Public Health*. 1990; 80:1075–1079.

40. Desenclos JA, Klontz KC, Wilder MH, Nainan OV, Margolis HS, Gunn RA. A multi-state outbreak of hepatitis A caused by the consumption of raw oysters. *Am J Public Health*. 1991;81:1268–1272.

41. Halliday ML, Kang L, Lao Y, et al. An epidemic of hepatitis A attributable to the ingestion of raw claims in Shanghai, China. *J Infect Dis*. 1991;164:852–859.

42. Enriquez R, Frosner GG, Hochstein-Montzel V, Riedemann S, Reinhardt G. Accumulation and persistence of hepatitis A virus in mussels. *J Med Virol*. 1992;37:174–179.

43. Centers for Disease Control. *Hepatitis Surveillance Report*. 1994;55:1–35.

44. Shapiro CM, Shaw FE, Mendel EI, Hadler SC. Epidemiology of hepatitis in the United States. In: Hollinger FB, Lemon SM, Margolis HS, eds. *Viral Hepatitis and Liver Disease*. Baltimore: Williams & Wilkins; 1991:214–220.

45. Hadler SC, McFarland L. Hepatitis in day care centers. Epidemiology and prevention. *Rev Infect Dis*. 1985; 8:548–557.

46. Hadler SC, Webster HM, Erben JJ, et al. Hepatitis A in daycare centers. A community-wide assessment. *N Engl J Med*. 1980;302:1222–1230.

47. Gingrich GA, Hadler SC, Elder HA, Asleko. Serologic investigation of an outbreak of hepatitis A in a rural daycare center. *Am J Public Health*. 1983;83:1190–1198.

48. Lange WR, France JD. High incidence of viral hepatitis among American missionaries in Africa. *Am J Trop Med Hyg*. 1990;43:527–533.

49. Steffen R. Risk of hepatitis A in travelers. *Vaccine*. 1992;30:569–572.

50. Bancroft WH, Lemon SM. Hepatitis A from the military perspective. In: Gerety RJ, ed. *Hepatitis A*. New York: Academic Press; 1984:81–100.

51. Innis BL, Snithban R, Hoke CH, Muniudhorn W, Laorakpongse T. The declining transmission of hepatitis A in Thailand. *J Infect Dis*. 1991;163:989–995.

52. Hsu HY, Chang MH, Chen DS, Lee CY, Sung JL. Changing seroepidemiology of hepatitis A virus infection in Taiwan. *J Med Virol*. 17:297–301.

53. Kremastinis J, Kalapothaki V, Trichopoulos D. The changing epidemiologic pattern of hepatitis A infection in urban Greece. *Am J Epidemiol*. 1984;120:203–206.

54. Stroffolini T, Decrescenzo L, Giammacco A, et al. Changing patterns of hepatitis virus infection in children in Palermo, Italy. *Eur J Epidemiol*. 1990;6:84–87.

55. Shapiro CN, Coleman PJ, McQuillan GM, Alter HJ,

Margolis HS. Epidemiology of hepatitis A: seroepidemiology and risk groups in the USA. *Vaccine.* 1992; 10:S59–S62.

56. Shaw FGJ, Shapiro CN, Welty TK, Dill W, Reddington J, Hadler SC. Hepatitis transmission among the Sioux Indians of South Dakota. *Am J Public Health.* 1990; 80:1091–1094.

57. Centers for Disease Control. *Hepatitis Surveillance Report.* 1996;56:15–27.

58. Krugman S, Ward R, Giles JP, Jacobs AM. Infectious hepatitis, study on effect of gammaglobulin and on the incidence of apparent infection. *JAMA.* 1960;174:823–883.

59. Winokur PC, Stapleton JT. Immunoglobulin prophylaxis for hepatitis A. *Clin Infect Dis.* 1992;14:580–586.

60. Advisory Committee on Immunization Practices CDC. Recommendations for protection against viral hepatitis. *MMWR.* 1985;34:315–316.

61. Carl M, Francis DP, Maynard JE. Food-borne hepatitis: recommendations for control. *J Infect Dis.* 1983.

62. Centers for Disease Control. Protection against viral hepatitis: recommendation of the immunization practices advisory committee. *MMWR.* 1990;39:5–27.

63. Szmuness W, Stevens CE, Harley EJ, et al. Hepatitis B vaccine in medical staff on hemodialysis units: efficacy and subtype cross-protection. *N Engl J Med.* 1982; 307:1481–1486.

64. Coursaget-Pauty AM, Plancoa A, Soulier JP. Distribution of HBsAg subtypes in the world. *Vox Sang.* 1983; 44:197–211.

65. Brown JC, Carman WF, Thomas HC. The clinical significance of molecular variation within the hepatitis B virus genome. *Hepatology.* 1992;15:144–148.

66. Hawkins AE, Gilson RJC, Beath SV, et al. Novel application of a point mutation assay: evidence for transmission of hepatitis B viruses with precore mutations and their detection in infants with fulminant hepatitis B. *J Med Virol.* 1994;44:13–21.

67. Fingerote RJ, Bain VG. Fulminant hepatic failure. *Am J Gastroenterol.* 1993;88:1000–1010.

68. Terazawa S, Kojsma M, Yamanaka T, et al. Hepatitis B virus mutants with pre-core region defects in two babies with fulminant hepatitis and their mothers positive for antibodies to hepatitis B e antigen. *Pediatr Res.* 1991; 29:5–9.

69. Penna A. Chisani FV, Bertolotti A, et al. Cytotoxic T lymphocytes recognize an HLA-DZ-restricted epitope within the hepatitis B virus nucleocapsid antigen. *J Exp Med.* 1991;174:1568–1570.

70. Ando K, Moriyama T, Guidotti LG, et al. Mechanism of class I restricted immunopathology. A transgenic mouse model of fulminant hepatitis. *J Exp Med.* 1993;178: 1541–1554.

71. Yoakum GH, Korba BE, Lechner JR, et al. High-frequency transfusion and cytopathology of hepatitis B virus core antigen gene in human cells. *Science.* 1983; 22:385–389.

72. Pignattelli M, Waters J, Brown D, et al. HLA class I antigens on hepatocyte membrane during recovery from acute hepatitis B virus infection and during interferon therapy in chronic hepatitis B virus infection. *Hepatology.* 1986;6:349–355.

73. Deinhardt F. Hepatitis in primates. In: Lauffer M, ed. *Advances in Virus Research.* Vol. 20. New York: Academic Press; 1976:113–157.

74. Deinstag JL. Immunogenesis of the extra hepatic manifestation of hepatitis B virus infection. *Springer Semin Immunopathol.* 1981;3:461–475.

75. McMahon BJ, Alward WLM, Ball DB, et al. Acute hepatitis B virus infection: relation of age to the clinic expression of disease and subsequent development of the carrier state. *J Infect Dis.* 1985;157:599–603.

76. Stevens CE, Neurath RA, Bensley RP, Szmuness W. HBeAg and anti-HBe detection by radioimmunoassay: correlation of vertical transmission of hepatitis B virus in Taiwan. *J Med Virol.* 1979;3:237–241.

77. Ganem D. Persistent infection of human with hepatitis B virus, mechanisms and consequences. *Rev Infect Dis.* 1982;4:1026–1047.

78. Hoofnagle JH, Shafritz DA, Popper H. Chronic type B hepatitis and the "healthy" HBsAg carrier state. *Hepatology.* 1987;7:758–763.

79. McMahon BJ, Alberts SR, Wainwright RB, Bulkow L, Lanier AP. Hepatitis B related sequelae. Prospective study in 1400 hepatitis B surface antigen positive Alaska native carriers. *Arch Intern Med.* 1990; 150:1051–1054.

80. Beasley RP, Hwang LY, Stevens CE, et al. Efficacy of hepatitis B immunoglobulin for prevention of perinatal transmission of the hepatitis B virus: final report of a randomized double-blind, placebo-controlled trial. *Hepatology.* 1983;3:135–141.

81. Hsieh CC, Tzonoa A, Zaritsanos K, Kalaman E, Lan SJ, Trichopulos D. Age at first establishment of chronic hepatitis B virus infection and hepatocellular carcinoma risk. A birth order study. *Am J Epidemiol.* 1992;136: 1115–1121.

82. Beasley RP. Hepatitis B virus. The major etiology of hepatocellular carcinoma. *Cancer.* 1988;61:1942–1956.

83. Beasley RP, Hwong LY, Lin CC, Chicu CS. Hepatocellular carcinoma and hepatitis B virus. A prospective study of 22,207 men in Taiwan. *Lancet.* 1981;2:1129–1133.

84. Aoki N, Robinson WS. Hepatitis B virus in cirrhosis and hepatocellular carcinoma nodules. *Mol Biol Med.* 1989; 6:398–408.

85. Shih C, Burke K, Chou MJ, et al. Tight clustering of human hepatitis B virus integration sites in hepatomas near a triple-stranded region. *J Virol.* 1987;61:3491–3498.

86. Safritz DA, Shoural D, Sherman H, Hadziyannis S, Kew M. Integration of hepatitis B virus DNA into the genome of liver cells in chronic liver disease and hepatocellular carcinoma. *N Engl J Med.* 1981;305:1067–1075.

87. Gerin JL. Experimental WHV infection of woodchucks: an animal model of hepadnavirus-induced liver cancer. *Gastroenterol Jpn.* 1990;25(Suppl):38–42.

88. Korba BE, Weks FU, Baldwin B, et al. Hepatocellular carcinoma in wood chuck hepatitis virus-infected woodchucks: presence of viral DNA in tumor tissue from known carriers and animals serologically recovered from acute infections. *Hepatology.* 1989;9:465–470.

89. Marion PL, Van Davelano MJ, Knight SS, et al. Hepatocellular carcinoma in ground squirrels persistently infected with ground squirrel hepatitis virus. *Proc Natl Acad Sci USA.* 1983;33:4543–4546.

90. Popper HJ, Roth L, Purcell RH, Tennant BC, Gerin JH. Hepatocarcinogenicity of the woodchuck hepatitis virus. *Proc Natl acad Sci USA.* 1987;84:855–870.

91. Popper HJ, Shih JW, Gerin JH, et al. Woodchuck hepatitis and hepatocellular carcinoma: correlation of histologic with virologic observations. *Hepatology.* 1981;1:91–98.

92. Chang M-H, Chen C-J, Lai M-S, et al. Universal hepatitis B vaccination in Taiwan and the incidence of hepatocellular carcinoma in children. *N Engl J Med.* 1997;336:1855–1859.

93. Hoofnagle JH, Di Bisceglie AM. Serologic diagnosis of acute and chronic hepatitis. *Semin Liver Dis.* 1991;11:73–83.

94. Seeff LB, Beebe BW, Hoofnagle JH, et al. A serologic follow-up of the 1942 epidemic of post-vaccination hepatitis in the United States Army. *N Engl J Med.* 1987;316:965–970.

95. Koziol DE, Holland PV, Allong DW, et al. Antibody to hepatitis B core antigen as a paradoxical marker for non-A, non-B hepatitis agents in donated blood. *Annals Intern Med.* 1986;104:488–495.

96. Donahue JG, Munoz A, Ness PM, et al. The declining risk of post-transfusion hepatitis C virus infection. *N Engl J Med.* 1992;327:369–373.

97. Levine OS, Vlahov D, Nelson KE. Epidemiology of hepatitis B virus infections among injecting drug users: seroprevalence, risk factors and viral interactions. *Epidemiol Rev.* 1994;16:418–436.

98. Garfein R, Vlahov D, Galai N, Doherty MC, Nelson KE. Prevalence of hepatitis C virus, hepatitis C virus, hepatitis B virus, human immunodeficiency virus and human T-lymphotrophic virus infections in short term injection

drug users. *Am J Public Health.* 1996;86:655–661.

99. Bernier RH, Sampliner R, Gerety R, Tabor E, Hamilton F, Nathanson N. Hepatitis B infection in households of chronic carriers of hepatitis B surface antigen: factors associated with prevalence of infection. *Am J Epidemiol.* 1982;116:199–211.

100. Franks AL, Berg CJ, Kane MA, et al. Hepatitis B infection among children born in the United States to Southeast Asian refugees. *N Engl J Med.* 1089;321:1301–1305.

101. Hurie MB, Mart EE, Davis JP. Horizontal transmission of hepatitis B virus infection to United States-born children of Hmong refugees. *Pediatrics.* 1992;89:269–274.

102. Williams I, Smith MG, Sinha D, et al. Hepatitis B virus transmission in an elementary school setting. *JAMA.* 1997;278:2167–2169.

103. Margolis AS, Alter MJ, Hadler SC. Hepatitis B: evolving epidemiology and implications for control. *Semin Liver Dis.* 1991;11:84–92.

104. Alter MJ, Hadler SC, Judson FN, et al. The changing epidemiology of hepatitis B in the United States: need for alternative vaccination strategies. *JAMA.* 1990;263:1218–1222.

105. McQuillan GM, Coleman PJ, Kruszon-Maran D, Moyer LA, Lambert SB, Margolis HS. Prevalence of hepatitis B virus infection in the United States: the national health and nutrition examination surveys, 1976 through 1994. *Am J Public Health.* 1999;89:14–18.

106. McQuillan GM, Townsend TR, Fields HA, et al. The seroepidemiology of hepatitis B virus in the United States 1976–89. *Am J Med.* 1989;87:5–10.

107. Bogomolski-Yaholow V, Granot E, Linder N, et al. Prevalence of HBsAg carriers in native and immigrant pregnant female populations in Israel and passive/active vaccination against HBV of newborns at risk. *J Med Virol.* 1991;34:217–222.

108. McMahon BJ, Schoenberg S, Bulkow L, et al. Seroprevalence of hepatitis B viral markers in 52,000 Alaskan natives. *Am J Epidemiol.* 1993;138:544–549.

109. Fay OH, Hadler SC, Maynard JE, Pinherro F. Hepatitis in the Americas. *Bull Pan Am Health Org.* 1985;19:401–408.

110. Feldman RE, Schiff ER. Hepatitis in dental professionals. *JAMA.* 1975;232:1228–1230.

111. Mosley JW, Edwards VM, Casey G, Redeker AG, White E. Hepatitis B virus infection in dentists. *N Engl J Med.* 1975;293:729–734.

112. Carl M, Blakey DL, Francis DP, Maynard JE. Interruption of hepatitis B transmission by modification of gynecologists surgical technique. *Lancet.* 1982;1:731–733.

113. Shaw FE Jr, Barrett CI, Hamm R, et al. Lethal outbreak of hepatitis B in a clinical practice. *JAMA*. 1986;255: 3260–3264.

114. El-Serag HB, Mason AC. Rising incidence of hepatocellular carcinoma in the United States. *N Engl J Med*. 1999;340:745–750.

115. Krugman S, Giles JP, Hammond J. Hepatitis virus effect of heat on the infectivity and antigenicity of MS-1 and MS-2 strain. *J Infect Dis*. 1970;122:423–436.

116. Szmuness W, Stevens CE, Harley EJ, et al. Hepatitis B vaccine: demonstration of efficacy in a controlled clinical trial in a high risk population in the United States. *N Engl J Med*. 1980;303:833–841.

117. Francis DP, Hadler SC, Thompson SE, et al. Prevention of hepatitis B with vaccine. Report from the Centers for Disease Control multi-center efficacy trial among homosexual men. *Ann Intern Med*. 1982;97: 362–366.

118. Yu ZY, Liu CB, Francis DP, et al. Prevention of perinatal acquisition of hepatitis B virus carriage using vaccine: preliminary report of a randomized double-blind placebo-controlled and comparative trial. *Pediatrics*. 1985;76:713–718.

119. Pooduotawan Y, Sanpayat S, Pongpuniert W. Protective efficacy of a recombinant DNA hepatitis B vaccine in neonates of HBe antigen-positive mothers. *JAMA*. 1989;261:3278–3281.

120. Stevens CE, Taylor PR, Tong MJ, et al. Yeast-recombinant hepatitis B vaccine. Efficacy with hepatitis B immunoglobulin in prevention of perinatal hepatitis B virus transmission. *JAMA*. 1987;257:2612–2616.

121. Centers for Disease Control and Prevention. Update: recommendations to prevent hepatitis B virus transmission—United States. *MMWR*. 1995;44:574–575.

122. Ukena T, Esber H, Bessette R, et al. Site of injection and response to hepatitis B vaccine. *N Engl J Med*. 1985;313:579–580.

123. Centers for Disease Control. Suboptimal responses to hepatitis B vaccine given by injection in the buttock. *MMWR*. 1985;34:105–108.

124. Alper CA, Kruskall MS, Marcus-Bagley D, et al. Genetic prediction of non response to hepatitis B vaccine. *N Engl J Med*. 1989;321:708–712.

125. World Health Organization. Progression the control of viral hepatitis: memorandum from WHO meeting. *Bull WHO*. 1988;66:443–455.

126. Margolis HS, Coleman PJ, Brown RG, Mart EE, Sheingold SH, Arevelo JA. Prevention of hepatitis B virus transmission by immunization: an economic analysis of current recommendation. *JAMA*. 1995; 274:1201–1208.

127. McMahon BJ, Lanier A, Wainwright RB, Kilkenny JJ. Hepatocellular carcinoma in Alaska Eskimos: epidemiology, clinical features and early detection. *Prog Liver Dis*. 1990;9:643–55.

128. Korenman J, Baker R, Waggoner J, Everhart JE, Di Bisceglie AM, Hoofnagle JH. Long-term remission in chronic hepatitis B after alfa-interferon therapy. *Ann Intern Med*. 1991;114:629–634.

129. Perrillo RP, Schiff ER, Davis GL. A randomized controlled trial of interferon alfa-2b alone and after prednisone withdrawal for the treatment of chronic hepatitis B. *N Engl J Med*. 1990;323:295–301.

130. Lai CL, Chien R-N, Leung NWY. A one-year trial of Lamivudine for chronic hepatitis B. *N Engl J Med*. 1998;339:61–68.

131. Dienstag JL, Schiff ER, Wright TL, et al. Lamivudine initial treatment for chronic hepatitis B in the United States. *N Engl J Med*. 1999;341:1256–1263.

132. Fields HA, Hadler SC. Delta hepatitis: a review. *J Clin Immunoassay*. 1986;9:128–142.

133. Arico S, Aragona M, Rizzetto M, et al. Clinical significance of antibody to the hepatitis delta virus in symptomless HBsAg carriers. *Lancet*. 1985;2:356–357.

134. Caredda F, Antinoni S, Re T, Pastechia C, Moroni M. Course and prognosis of acute HDV hepatitis. *Prog Clin Biol Res*. 1987;234:267–276.

135. Lettau L, McCarthy JG, Smith MH, et al. An outbreak of severe hepatitis due to delta and hepatitis B virus in injection drug users and their contacts. *N Engl J Med*. 1987;317:1256–1261.

136. Hadler SC, De Monson M, Ponzotto A, et al. Delta virus infection and severe hepatitis: an epidemic in the Yupca Indians of Venezuela. *Ann Intern Med*. 1984; 100:339–344.

137. Shimizu YK, Feinstone SM, Kohara M, Purcell RH, Yoshikura H. Hepatitis C virus: detection of intracellular virus particles by electron microscopy. *Hepatology*. 1996;23:205–209.

138. Kaito M, Watanabe S, Tsukiyama-Kohara K, et al. Hepatitis C virus particle detected by immunoelectron microscopic study. *J Gen Virol*. 1994;75:1755–1760.

139. Choo QL, Richman KH, Han JH, et al. Genetic organization and diversity of the hepatitis C virus. *Proc Natl Acad Sci USA*. 1991;88:2451–2455.

140. Negro F, Pacchioni D, Shimizu Y, et al. Detection of intrahepatic replication of hepatitis C virus RNA by in situ hybridization and comparison with histopathology. *Proc Natl Acad Sci USA*. 1992;89:2247–2251.

141. Krawczynski K, Beach MJ, Bradley DW, et al. Hepatitis C antigens in hepatocytes. Immuno-morphologic detection and identification. *Gastroenterology*. 1992; 103:622–629.

142. Lerat H, Berby F, Trabaud MA, Vidalin O, Major M, Trépo C, Inchauspé G. Specific detection of hepatitis C

virus minus strand RNA in hematopoietic cells. *J Clin Invest.* 1996;97:845–851.

143. Shimizu YK, Igarashi H, Kanematu T, et al. Sequence analysis of the hepatitis C virus genome recovered from serum, liver, and peripheral blood mononuclear cells of infected chimpanzees. *J Virol.* 1997;71:5769–5773.

144. Lanford RE, Chavez D, Von Chisari F, Sureau C. Lack of detection of negative-strand hepatitis C virus RNA in peripheral blood mononuclear cells and other extrahepatic tissues by the highly strand-specific rTth reverse transcriptase PCR. *J Virol.* 1995;69:8079–8083.

145. Neumann AU, Lam NP, Dahari H, et al. Hepatitis C viral dynamics in vivo and the antiviral efficacy of interferon-alpha therapy. *Science.* 1998;282:103–107.

146. Martell M, Esteban JI, Quer J, et al. Hepatitis C virus (HCV) circulates as a population of different but closely related genomes: quasispecies nature of HCV genome distribution. *J Virol.* 1992;66:3225–3229.

147. Kato N, Ootsuyama Y, Tanaka T, et al. Marked sequence diversity in the putative envelope proteins of hepatitis C viruses. *Virus Res.* 1992;22:107–123.

148. Wang Y, Ray SC, Laeyendecker O, Ticehurst JR, Thomas DL. Assessment of hepatitis C virus sequence complexity by the electrophoretic mobility of both single- and double-stranded DNA. *J Clin Micro.* 1998;36:2982–2989.

149. Ray SC, Wang YM, Laeyendecker O, Ticehurst J, Villano SA, Thomas DL. Acute hepatitis C virus structural gene sequences as predictors of persistent viremia: hypervariable region 1 as decoy. *J Virol.* 1998;73:2938–2946.

150. Major ME, Mihalik K, Fernandez J, et al. Long-term follow-up of chimpanzees inoculated with the first infectious clone for hepatitis C virus. *J Virol.* 1999;73:3317–3325.

151. Weiner AJ, Geysen HM, Christopherson C, et al. Evidence for immune selection of hepatitis C virus (HCV) putative envelope glycoprotein variants: potential role in chronic HCV infections. *Proc Natl Acad Sci USA.* 1992;89:3468–3472.

152. Shimizu YK, Hijikata M, Iwamoto A, Alter HJ, Purcell RH, Yoshikura H. Neutralizing antibodies against hepatitis C virus and the emergence of neutralization escape mutant viruses. *J Virol.* 1994;68:1494–1500.

153. Weiner A, Erickson AL, Kansopon J, et al. Persistent hepatitis C virus infection in a chimpanzee is associated with emergence of a cytotoxic T lymphocyte escape variant. *Proc Natl Acad Sci USA.* 1995;92:2755–2759.

154. Liou TC, Chang TT, Young KC, Lin XZ, Lin CY, Wu HL. Detection of HCV RNA in saliva, urine, seminal fluid, and ascites. *J Med Virol.* 1992;37:197–202.

155. Chen M, Yun Z-B, Sällberg M, et al. Detection of hepatitis C virus RNA in the cell fraction of saliva before and after oral surgery. *J Med Virol.* 1995;45:223–226.

156. Wang JT, Wang TH, Sheu JC, Lin JT, Chen DS. Hepatitis C virus RNA in saliva of patients with posttransfusion hepatitis and low efficiency of transmission among spouses. *J Med Virol.* 1992;36:28–31.

157. Fiore RJ, Potenza D, Monno L, et al. Detection of HCV RNA in serum and seminal fluid from HIV-1 co-infected intravenous drug addicts. *J Med Virol.* 1995;46:364–367.

158. Mendel I, Muraine M, Riachi G, et al. Detection and genotyping of the hepatitis C RNA in tear fluid from patients with chronic hepatitis C. *J Med Virol.* 1997;51:231–233.

159. Abe K, Inchauspe G. Transmission of hepatitis C by saliva. *Lancet.* 1991;337:248.

160. Pileri P, Uematsu Y, Campagnoli S, et al. Binding of hepatitis C virus to CD81. *Science.* 1998;282:938–941.

161. Bukh J, Miller RH, Purcell RH. Genetic heterogeneity of hepatitis C virus: quasispecies and genotypes. *Semin Liver Dis.* 1995;15:41–63.

162. Simmonds P, Holmes EC, Cha T-A, et al. Classification of hepatitis C virus into six major genotypes and a series of subtypes by phylogenetic analysis of the NS-5 region. *J Gen Virol.* 1993;74:2391–2399.

163. Bronowicki JP, Venard V, Botté C, et al. Patient-to-patient transmission of hepatitis C virus during colonoscopy. *N Engl J Med.* 1997;337:237–240.

164. Esteban JI, Gómez J, Martell M, et al. Transmission of hepatitis C virus by a cardiac surgeon. *N Engl J Med.* 1996;334:555–560.

165. Thomas DL, Zenilman JZ, Alter HJ, Shih JW, Galai N, Quinn TC. Sexual transmission of hepatitis C virus among patients attending Baltimore sexually transmitted diseases clinics—an analysis of 309 sexual partnerships. *J Infect Dis.* 1995;171:768–775.

166. Allander T, Gruber A, Naghavi M, et al. Frequent patient-to-patient transmission of hepatitis C virus in a haematology ward. *Lancet.* 1995;345:603–607.

167. Villano SA, Vlahov D, Nelson KE, Cohn S, Thomas DL. Persistence of viremia and the importance of long-term follow-up after acute hepatitis C infection. *Hepatology.* 1999;29:908–914.

168. Inglesby TV, Rai R, Astemborski J, et al. A prospective, community-based evaluation of liver enzymes in individuals with hepatitis C after drug use. *Hepatology.* 1999;29:590–596.

169. Farci P, Alter HJ, Wong D, et al. A long-term study of hepatitis C virus replication in non-A, non- B hepatitis. *N Engl J Med.* 1991;325:98–104.

170. Alter MJ, Margolis HS, Krawczynski K, et al. The

natural history of community acquired hepatitis C in the United States. *N Engl J Med*. 1992;327:1899–1905.

171. Tong MJ, El-Farra NS, Reikes AR, Co RL. Clinical outcomes after transfusion-associated hepatitis C. *N Engl J Med*. 1995;332:1463–1466.

172. Kiyosawa K, Sodeyama T, Tanaka E, et al. Interrelationship of blood transfusion, non-A, non-B hepatitis and hepatocellular carcinoma: analysis by detection of antibody to hepatitis C virus. *Hepatology*. 1990;12: 671–675.

173. Kenny-Walsh E. Clinical outcomes after hepatitis C infection from contaminated anti-D immune globulin. Irish Hepatology Research Group. *N Engl J Med*. 1999;340:1228–1233.

174. Agnello V, Chung RT, Kaplan LM. A role for hepatitis C virus infection in Type II cryoglobulinemia. *N Engl J Med*. 1992;327:1490–1495.

175. Misiani R, Bellavita P, Fenili D, et al. Hepatitis C virus infection in patients with essential mixed cryoglobulinemia. *Ann Intern Med*. 1992;117:573–577.

176. Johnson RJ, Gretch DR, Yamabe H, et al. Membranoproliferative glomerulonephritis associated with hepatitis C virus infection [see comments]. *N Engl J Med*. 1993;328:465–470.

177. Fargion S, Piperno A, Cappellini MD, et al. Hepatitis C virus and porphyria cutanea tarda: evidence of a strong association. *Hepatology*. 1992;16:1322–1326.

178. DeCastro M, Sanchez J, Herrera JF, et al. Hepatitis C virus antibodies and liver disease in patients with porphyria cutanea tarda. *Hepatology*. 1993;17:551–557.

179. Centers for Disease Control and Prevention. *Recommendations for Prevention and Control of Hepatitis C Virus Infection and HCV-Related Chronic Disease*. 47(no. RR-19), 1–39. 10–16–1998.

180. McHutchinson JG, Person JL, Govindarajan S, et al. Improved detection of hepatitis C virus antibodies in high-risk populations. *Hepatology*. 1992;15:19–25.

181. Nakatsuji Y, Matsumoto A, Tanaka E, Ogata H, Kiyosawa K. Detection of chronic hepatitis C virus infection by four diagnostic systems: first-generation and second-generation enzyme-linked immunosorbent assay, second-generation recombinant immunoblot assay and nested polymerase chain reaction analysis. *Hepatology*. 1992;16:300–305.

182. Chien DY, Choo QL, Tabrizi A, et al. Diagnosis of hepatitis C virus (HCV) infection using an immunodominant chimeric polyprotein to capture circulating antibodies: reevaluation of the role of HCV in liver disease. *Proc Natl Acad Sci USA*. 1992;89:10011–10015.

183. Couroucé A-M, Le Marrec N, Girault A, Ducamp S, Simon N. Anti-hepatitis C virus (anti-HCV) seroconversion in patients undergoing hemodialysis: com-

parison of second- and third-generation anti-HCV assays. *Transfusion*. 1994;34:790–795.

184. Vallari DS, Jett BW, Alter HJ, Mimms LT, Holzman R, Shih JW. Serological markers of posttransfusion hepatitis C viral infection. *J Clin Micro*. 1992;30:552–556.

185. van der Poel CL, Cuypers HTM, Reesink HW, et al. Confirmation of hepatitis C virus infection by new four-antigen recombinant immunoblot assay. *Lancet*. 1991;337:317–319.

186. Buffet C, Charnaux N, Laurent-Puig P, et al. Enhanced detection of antibodies to hepatitis C virus by use of a third-generation recombinant immunoblot assay. *J Med Virol*. 1994;43:259–261.

187. McGuinness PH, Bishop GA, Lien A, Wiley B, Parsons C, McCaughan GW. Detection of serum hepatitis C virus RNA in HCV antibody-seropositive volunteer blood donors. *Hepatology*. 1993;18:485–490.

188. Vrielink H, van der Poel CL, Reesink HW, et al. Lookback study of infectivity of anti-HCV ELISA-positive blood components. *Lancet*. 1995;345:95–96.

189. Zaaijer HL, Cuypers HTM, Reesink HW, Winkel IN, Gerken G, Lelie PN. Reliability of polymerase chain reaction for detection of hepatitis C virus. *Lancet*. 1993;341:722–724.

190. Bresters D, Cuypers HT, Reesink HW, et al. Comparison of quantitative cDNA-PCR with the branched DNA hybridization assay for monitoring plasma hepatitis C virus RNA levels in haemophilia patients participating in a controlled interferon trial. *J Med Virol*. 1994;43:262–268.

191. Gretch DR, Dela Rosa C, Carithers RL, Jr., Willson RA, Williams B, Corey L. Assessment of hepatitis C viremia using molecular amplification technologies: correlations and clinical implications. *Ann Intern Med*. 1995;123:321–329.

192. Miskovsky EP, Carella AV, Gutekunst K, Sun C, Quinn TC, Thomas DL. Clinical characterization of a competitive PCR assay for quantitative testing of hepatitis C virus. *J Clin Microbiol*. 1996;34:1975–1979.

193. Stuyver L, Rossau R, Wyseur A, et al. Typing of hepatitis C virus isolates and characterization of new subtypes using a line probe assay. *J Gen Virol*. 1993; 74:1093–1102.

194. Stuyver L, Wyseur A, Van Arnhem W, Hernandez F, Maertens G. Second-generation line probe assay for hepatitis C virus genotyping. *J Clin Microbiol*. 1996; 34:2259–2266.

195. Thiers V, Jaffredo F, Tuveri R, Chodan N, Bréchot C. Development of a simple restriction fragment length polymorphism (RFLP) based assay for HCV genotyping and comparative analysis with genotyping and serotyping tests. *J Virol Methods*. 1997;65:9–17.

196. Widell A, Shev S, Mansson S, et al. Genotyping of hepatitis C virus isolates by a modified polymerase chain reaction assay using type specific primers: epidemiological applications. *J Med Virol.* 1994;44:272–279.

197. Esteban JI, Lopez-Talavera JC, Genesca J, et al. High rate of infectivity and liver disease in blood donors with antibodies to hepatitis C virus. *Ann Intern Med.* 1991;115:443–449.

198. Pereira BJG, Milford EL, Kirkman RL, et al. Prevalence of hepatitis C virus RNA in organ donors positive for hepatitis C antibody and in the recipients of their organs. *N Engl J Med.* 1992;327:910–915.

199. Terrault NA, Wright TL. Hepatitis C virus in the setting of transplantation. *Semin Liver Dis.* 1995;15:92–100.

200. Pereira BJG, Milford EL, Kirkman RL, Levey AS. Transmission of hepatitis C virus by organ transplantation. *N Engl J Med.* 1991;325:454–460.

201. Centers for Disease Control and Prevention. Public Health Service interagency guidelines for screening blood, plasma, organs, tissue and semen for evidence of hepatitis B and C. *MMWR.* 1991;40:1–23.

202. Donahue JG, Munoz A, Ness PM, et al. The declining risk of post-transfusion hepatitis C virus infection. *N Engl J Med.* 1992;327:369–373.

203. Blajchman MA, Bull SB, Feinman SV. Post-transfusion hepatitis: impact of non-A, non-B hepatitis surrogate tests. *Lancet.* 1995;345:21–25.

204. Schreiber GB, Busch MP, Kleinman SH, Korelitz JJ. The risk of transfusion-transmitted viral infections. *N Engl J Med.* 1996;334:1685–90.

205. Widell A, Elmud H, Persson MH, Jonsson M. Transmission of hepatitis C via both erythrocyte and platelet transfusions from a single donor in serological window-phase of hepatitis C. *Vox Sang.* 1996;71:55–57.

206. Yap PL, McOmish F, Webster ADB, et al. Hepatitis C virus transmission by intravenous immunoglobulin. *J Hepatol.* 1994;21:455–460.

207. Bjoro K, Froland SS, Yun Z, Samdal HH, Haaland T. Hepatitis C infection in patients with primary hypogammaglobulinemia after treatment with contaminated immune globulin. *N Engl J Med.* 1994;331:1607–1611.

208. Power JP, Lawlor E, Davidson F. *Lancet.* 1994; 344:1166–1167.

209. Bresee JS, Mast EE, Coleman FJ, et al. Hepatitis C virus infection associated with administration of intravenous immune globulin—a cohort study. *JAMA.* 1996; 276:1563–1567.

210. Thomas DL, Vlahov D, Solomon L, et al. Correlates of hepatitis C virus infections among injection drug users in Baltimore. *Medicine.* 1995;74:212–220.

211. Bolumar F, Hernandez-Aguado I, Ferrer L, Ruiz I, Aviñó M, Rebagliato M. Prevalence of antibodies to hepatitis C in a population of intravenous drug users in Valencia, Spain, 1990–1992. *Int J Epidemiol.* 1996; 25:204–209.

212. Girardi E, Zaccarelli M, Tossini G, Puro V, Narciso P, Visco G. Hepatitis C virus infection in intravenous drug users: prevalence and risk factors. *Scand J Infect Dis.* 1990;22:751–752.

213. Bell J, Batey RG, Farrell GC, Crewe EB, Cunningham AL, Byth K. Hepatitis C virus in intravenous drug users. *Med J Aust.* 1990;153:274–276.

214. Van Ameijden EJ, van den Hoek JA, Mientjes GH, Coutinho RA. A longitudinal study on the incidence and transmission patterns of HIV, HBV and HCV infection among drug users in Amsterdam. *Eur J Epidemiol.* 1993;9:255–262.

215. Patti AM, Santi AL, Pompa MG, et al. Viral hepatitis and drugs: a continuing problem. *Int J Epidemiol.* 1993;22:135–139.

216. Garfein RS, Doherty MC, Brown D, et al. Hepatitis C virus infection among short-term injection drug users. *J AIDS.* 1998;18:S11–S19.

217. Conry-Cantilena C, Vanraden MT, Gibble J, et al. Routes of infection, viremia, and liver disease in blood donors found to have hepatitis C virus infection. *N Engl J Med.* 1996;334:1691–1696.

218. Kiyosawa K, Sodeyama T, Tanaka E, et al. Hepatitis C in hospital employees with needlestick injuries [see comments]. *Ann Intern Med.* 1991;115:367–369.

219. Ridzon R, Gallagher K, Ciesielski C, et al. Simultaneous transmission of human immunodeficiency virus and hepatitis C virus from a needle-stick injury. *N Engl J Med.* 1997;336:919–922.

220. Mitsui T, Iwano K, Masuko K, et al. Hepatitis C virus infection in medical personnel after needlestick accident. *Hepatology.* 1992;16:1109–1114.

221. Sartori M, La Terra G, Aglietta M, Manzin A, Navino C, Verzetti G. Transmission of hepatitis C via blood splash into conjunctiva. *Scand J Infect Dis.* 1993;25: 270–271.

222. Thomas DL, Gruninger SE, Siew C, Joy ED, Quinn TC. Occupational risk of hepatitis C infections among general dentists and oral surgeons in North America. *Am J Med.* 1996;100:41–45.

223. Thomas DL, Factor S, Kelen G, Washington AS, Taylor E, Quinn TQ. Hepatitis B and C in health care workers at the Johns Hopkins Hospital. *Arch Intern Med.* 1993;153:1705–1712.

224. Gerberding JL. Incidence and prevalence of human immunodeficiency virus, hepatitis B virus, hepatitis C virus, and cytomegalovirus among health care person-

nel at risk for blood exposure: final report from a longitudinal study. *J Infect Dis*. 1994;170:1410–1417.

225. Kuo MY, Hahn LJ, Hong CY, Kao JH, Chen DS. Low prevalence of hepatitis C virus infection among dentists in Taiwan. *J Med Virol*. 1993;40:10–13.

226. Campello C, Majori S, Poli A, Pacini P, Nicolardi L, Pini F. Prevalence of HCV antibodies in health-care workers from northern Italy. *Infection*. 1992;20:224–226.

227. Polish LB, Tong MJ, Co RL, Coleman PJ, Alter MJ. Risk factors for hepatitis C virus infection among health care personnel in a community hospital. *Am J Infect Control*. 1993;21:196–200.

228. Puro V, Petrosillo N, Ippolito G, et al. Occupational hepatitis C virus infection in Italian health care workers. *Am J Public Health*. 1995;85:1272–1275.

229. Schvarcz R, Johansson B, Nyström B, Sönnerborg A. Nosocomial transmission of hepatitis C virus. *Infection*. 1997;25:74–77.

230. Munro J, Biggs JD, McCruden EAB. Detection of a cluster of hepatitis C infections in a renal transplant unit by analysis of sequence variation of the NS5a gene. *J Infect Dis*. 1996;174:177–180.

231. Stuyver L, Claeys H, Wyseur A, et al. Hepatitis C virus in a hemodialysis unit: molecular evidence for nosocomial transmission. *Kidney Int*. 1996;49:889–895.

232. Sampietro M, Badalamenti S, Salvadori S, et al. High prevalence of a rare hepatitis C virus in patients treated in the same hemodialysis unit: evidence for nosocomial transmission of HCV. *Kidney Int*. 1995;47:911–917.

233. Alter MJ. Epidemiology of hepatitis C. *Hepatology*. 1997;26:62S–65S.

234. Ko YC, Ho MS, Chiang TA, Chang SJ, Chang PY. Tattooing as a risk of hepatitis C virus infection. *J Med Virol*. 1992;38:288–291.

235. Sun DX, Zhang FG, Geng YQ, Xi DS. Hepatitis C transmission by cosmetic tattooing in women. *Lancet*. 1996;347:541.

236. Dusheiko GM, Smith M, Scheuer PJ. Hepatitis C virus transmission by human bite. *Lancet*. 1990;336:503–504.

237. van Doornum GJJ, Hooykaas C, Cuypers MT, van Der Lind MMD, Coutinho RS. Prevalence of hepatitis C virus infections among heterosexuals with multiple partners. *J Med Virol*. 1991;35:22–27.

238. Thomas DL, Cannon RO, Shapiro C, Hook EWI, Alter MJ, Quinn TC. *J Infect Dis*. 1994;169:990–995.

239. Petersen EE, Clemens R, Bock HL, Friese K, Hess G. Hepatitis B and C in heterosexual patients with various sexually transmitted diseases. *Infection*. 1992;20:128–131.

240. Nakashima K, Kashiwagi S, Hayashi J, et al. Sexual transmission of hepatitis C virus among female prostitutes and patients with sexually transmitted diseases in Fukuoka, Kyushu, Japan. *Am J Epidemiol*. 1992;136:1132–1137.

241. Utsumi T, Hashimoto E, Okumura Y, et al. Heterosexual activity as a risk factor for the transmission of hepatitis C virus. *J Med Virol*. 1995;46:122–125.

242. Capelli C, Prati D, Bosoni P, et al. Sexual transmission of hepatitis C virus to a repeat blood donor. *Transfusion*. 1997;37:436–440.

243. Healey CJ, Smith DB, Walker JL, et al. Acute hepatitis C infection after sexual exposure. *Gut*. 1995;36:148–150.

244. Akahane Y, Kojima M, Sugai Y, et al. Hepatitis C virus infection in spouses of patients with type C chronic liver disease [see comments]. *Ann Intern Med*. 1994;120:748–752.

245. Kao JH, Chen PJ, Yang PM, et al. Intrafamilial transmission of hepatitis C virus: the important role of infections between spouses. *J Infect Dis*. 1992;166:900–903.

246. Kao JH, Hwang YT, Chen PJ, et al. Transmission of hepatitis C virus between spouses: the important role of exposure duration. *Am J Gastroenterol*. 1996;91:2087–2090.

247. Chayama K, Kobayashi M, Tsubota A, et al. Molecular analysis of intraspousal transmission of hepatitis C virus. *J Hepatol*. 1995;22:431–439.

248. Piazza M, Sagliocca L, Tosone GM, et al. Sexual transmission of the hepatitis C virus and efficacy of prophylaxis with intramuscular immune serum globulin—a randomized controlled trial. *Arch Intern Med*. 1997;157:1537–1544.

249. Bresters D, Mauser-Bunschoten ED, Reesink HW, et al. Sexual transmission of hepatitis C. *Lancet*. 1993;342:210–211.

250. Everhart JE, Di Bisceglie AM, Murray LM, et al. Risk for non-A, non-B (Type C) hepatitis through sexual or household contact with chronic carriers. *Ann Intern Med*. 1990;112:544–555.

251. Brettler DB, Mannucci PM, Gringeri A, et al. The low risk of hepatitis C virus transmission among sexual partners of hepatitis C infected hemophilic males: an international, multicenter study. *Blood*. 1992;80:540–543.

252. Gordon SC, Patel AH, Kulesza GW, Barnes RE, Silverman AL. Lack of evidence for the heterosexual transmission of hepatitis C. *Am J Gastroenterol*. 1992;87:1849–1851.

253. Melbye M, Biggar RJ, Wantzin P, Krogsgaard K, Ebbesen P, Becker NG. Sexual transmission of hepatitis C virus: cohort study (1981–1989) among European homosexual men. *Br Med J*. 1990;301:210–212.

254. Osmond DH, Charlebois E, Sheppard HW, et al. Comparison of risk factors for hepatitis C and hepatitis B virus infection in homosexual men. *J Infect Dis.* 1993; 167:66–71.

255. Bodsworth NJ, Cunningham P, Kaldor J, Donovan B. Hepatitis C virus infection in a large cohort of homosexually active men: independent associations with HIV-1 infection and injecting drug use but not sexual behaviour. *Genitourin Med.* 1996;72:118–122.

256. Donahue JG, Nelson KE, Munoz A, et al. Antibody to hepatitis C virus among cardiac surgery patients, homosexual men, and intravenous drug users in Baltimore, Maryland. *Am J Epidemiol.* 1991;134:1206–1211.

257. Roudot Thoraval F, Pawlotsky JM, Thiers V, et al. Lack of mother-to-infant transmission of hepatitis C virus in human immunodeficiency virus-seronegative women: a prospective study with hepatitis C virus RNA testing. *Hepatology.* 1993;17:772–777.

258. Reinus JF, Leikin EL, Alter HJ, et al. Failure to detect vertical transmission of hepatitis C virus. *Ann Intern Med.* 1992;117:881–886.

259. Ohto H, Terazawa S, Nobuhiko S, et al. Transmission of hepatitis C virus from mothers to infants. *N Engl J Med.* 1994;330:744–750.

260. Zanetti AR, Tanzi E, Paccagnini S, et al. Mother-to-infant transmission of hepatitis C virus. *Lancet.* 1995; 345:289–291.

261. Lam JPH, McOmish F, Burns SM, Yap PL, Mok JYQ, Simmonds P. Infrequent vertical transmission of hepatitis C virus. *J Infect Dis.* 1993;167:572–576.

262. Novati R, Thiers V, Monforte AD, et al. Mother-to-child transmission of hepatitis C virus detected by nested polymerase chain reaction. *J Infect Dis.* 1992; 165:720–723.

263. Wejstal R, Widell A, Mansson A-S, Hermodsson S, Norkrans G. Mother-to-infant transmission of hepatitis C virus. *Ann Intern Med.* 1992;117:887–890.

264. Weintrub PS, Veereman Wauters G, Cowan MJ, Thaler MM. Hepatitis C virus infection in infants whose mothers took street drugs intravenously. *J Pediatr.* 1991;119:869.

265. Thomas DL, Villano SA, Reister K, et al. Perinatal transmission of hepatitis C virus from human immunodeficiency virus type 1-infected individuals. *J Enfect Dis.* 1998;177:1480–1488.

266. Matsubara T, Sumazaki R, Takita H. Mother-to-infant transmission of hepatitis C virus: a prospective study. *Eur J Pediatr.* 1995;154:973–978.

267. Lin H-H, Kao J-H, Hsu H-Y, et al. Possible role of high-titer maternal viremia in perinatal transmission of hepatitis C virus. *J Infect Dis.* 1994;169:638–641.

268. Moriya T, Sasaki F, Mizui M, et al. Transmission of hepatitis C virus from mothers to infants: its frequency and risk factors revisited. *Biomed Pharmacother.* 1995;49:59–64.

269. Telfer PT, Brown D, Devereux H, Lee CA, Dusheiko GM. HCV RNA levels and HIV infection: evidence for a viral interaction in haemophilic patients. *Br J Haematol.* 1994;88:397–399.

270. Sherman KE, O'Brien J, Gutierrez G, et al. Quantitative evaluation of hepatitis C virus RNA in patients with concurrent human immunodeficiency virus infections. *J Clin Microbiol.* 1993;31:2679–2682.

271. Eyster ME, Fried MW, Di Bisceglie AM, Goedert JJ. Increasing hepatitis C virus RNA levels in hemophiliacs: relationship to human immunodeficiency virus infection and liver disease. *Blood.* 1994;84:1020–1023.

272. Thomas DL, Shih JW, Alter HJ, et al. Effect of human immunodeficiency virus on hepatitis C virus infection among injecting drug users. *J Infect Dis.* 1996; 174:690–695.

273. Ogasawara S, Kage M, Kosai K, Shimamatsu K, Kojiro M. Hepatitis C virus RNA in saliva and breastmilk of hepatitis C carrier mothers. *Lancet.* 1993; 341:561.

274. Ohto H, Okamoto H, Mishiro S. Vertical transmission of hepatitis C virus. Reply. *N Engl J Med.* 1994; 331:400.

275. Lin H-H, Kao J-H, Hsu H-Y, et al. Absence of infection in breast-fed infants born to hepatitis C virus-infected mothers. *J Pediatr.* 1995;126:589–591.

276. World Health Organization. Hepatitis C: global prevalence. *Weekly Epidemiological Record.* Geneva: WHO;1997:341–348.

277. Osella AR, Misciagna G, Leone A, Di Leo A, Fiore G. Epidemiology of hepatitis C virus infection in an area of southern Italy. *J Hepatol.* 1997;27:30–35.

278. Chiaramonte M, Stroffolini T, Lorenzoni U, et al. Risk factors in community-acquired chronic hepatitis C virus infection: a case-control study in Italy. *J Hepatol.* 1996;24:129–134.

279. Nakashima K, Ikematsu H, Hayashi J, Kishihara Y, Mitsutake A, Kashiwagi S. Intrafamilial transmission of hepatitis C virus among the population of an endemic area of Japan. *JAMA.* 1995;274:1459–1461.

280. Guadagnino V, Stroffolini T, Rapicetta M, et al. Prevalence, risk factors, and genotype distribution of hepatitis C virus infection in the general population: a community-based survey in southern Italy. *Hepatology.* 1997;26:1006–1011.

281. Arthur RR, Hassan NF, Abdallah MY, et al. Hepatitis C antibody prevalence in blood donors in different governorates in Egypt. *Trans R Soc Trop Med Hyg.* 1997;91:271–274.

282. Abdel-Wahab MF, Zakaria S, Kamel M, et al. High

seroprevalence of hepatitis C infection among risk groups in Egypt. *Am J Trop Med Hyg.* 1994;51:563–567.

283. Kamel MA, Ghaffar YA, Wasef MA, Wright M, Clark LC, Miller FD. High HCV prevalence in Egyptian blood donors [letter; comment] [see comments]. *Lancet.* 1992;340:427.

284. Darwish MA, Raouf TA, Rushdy P, Constantine NT, Rao MR, Edelman R. Risk factors associated with a high seroprevalence of hepatitis C virus infection in Egyptian blood donors. *Am J Trop Med Hyg.* 1993;49:440–447.

285. Hibbs RG, Corwin AL, Hassan NF, et al. The epidemiology of antibody to hepatitis C in Egypt [letter]. [Review]. *J Infect Dis.* 1993; 168:789–790.

286. El-Sayed NM, Gomatos PJ, Rodier GR, et al. Seroprevalence survey of Egyptian tourism workers for hepatitis B virus, hepatitis C virus, human immunodeficiency virus, and *Treponema pallidum* infections: association of hepatitis C virus infections with specific regions of Egypt. *Am J Trop Med Hyg.* 1996;55:179–184.

287. Prati D, Capelli C, Silvani C, et al. The incidence and risk factors of community-acquired hepatitis C in a cohort of Italian blood donors. *Hepatology.* 1997;25:702–704.

288. Noguchi S, Sata M, Suzuki H, Mizokami M, Tanikawa K. Routes of transmission of hepatitis C virus in an endemic rural area of Japan—molecular epidemiologic study of hepatitis C virus infection. *Scand J Infect Dis.* 1997;29:23–28.

289. Kiyosawa K, Tanaka E, Sodeyama T, et al. Transmission of hepatitis C in an isolated area in Japan: community-acquired infection. *Gastroenterology.* 1994;106:1596–1602.

290. Kelen GD, Green GB, Purcell RH, et al. Hepatitis B and hepatitis C in emergency department patients [see comments]. *N Engl J Med.* 1992;326:1399–1404.

291. Alter MJ. Epidemiology of hepatitis C in the West. *Semin Liver Dis.* 1995;15:5–14.

292. Alter MJ, Hadler SC, Judson FN, et al. Risk factors for acute non-A, non-B hepatitis in the United States and association with hepatitis C virus infection. *JAMA.* 1990;264:2231–2235.

293. Alter MJ, Kruszon-Moran D, Nainan OV, et al. The prevalence of hepatitis C virus infection in the United States, 1988 through 1994. *N Engl J Med.* 1999;341:556–562.

294. Letter to NEJM Regarding NHANES Study of HEV.

295. Hagan H, Jarlais DCD, Friedman SR, Purchase D, Alter MJ. Reduced risk of hepatitis B and hepatitis C among injection drug users in the Tacoma syringe exchange program. *Am J Public Health.* 1995;85:1531–1537.

296. Hagan H, McGough JP, Thiede H, Weiss NS, Hopkins S, Alexander ER. Syringe exchange and risk of infection with hepatitis B and C viruses. *Am J Epidemiol.* 1999;149:203–213.

297. Reyes GR, Purdy MA, Kim JP, et al. Isolation of a cDNA from the virus responsible for enterically transmitted non-A, non-B hepatitis. *Eur J Biochem.* 1990; 247:1335–1339.

298. Ticehurst J. Identification and characterization of hepatitis E virus. In: Hollinger FB, ed. *Viral Hepatitis and Liver Disease.* Baltimore: Williams & Wilkins; 1991: 501–513.

299. Bradley DW. Hepatitis E virus: a brief review of the biology, molecular virology, and immunology of a novel virus. *J Hepatol.* 1995;22(Suppl. 1):140–145.

300. Meng XJ, Purcell RH, Halbur PG, et al. A novel virus in swine is closely related to the human hepatitis E virus. *Proc Natl Acad Sci USA.* 1997;94:9860–9865.

301. Scharschmidt BF. Hepatitis E: a virus in waiting. *Lancet.* 1995;346:519–520.

302. Longer CF, Denny SL, Caudill JD, et al. Experimental hepatitis E: pathogenesis in cynomolgus macaques (*Macaca fascicularis*). *J Infect Dis.* 1993;168:602–609.

303. Maneerat Y, Clayson ET, Myint KS, Young GD, Innis BL. Experimental infection of the laboratory rat with the hepatitis E virus. *J Med Virol.* 1996;48:121–128.

304. Bradley DW, Krawczynski K, Cook EH, et al. Enterically transmitted non-A, non-B hepatitis: serial passage of disease in cynomolgus macaques and tamarins and recovery of disease-associated 27 to 34 nm viruslike particles. *Proc Natl Acad Sci USA.* 1987;84:6277–6281.

305. Chauhan A, Jamell S, Dilawari JB, Chawla YK, Kaur U, Ganguly NK. Hepatitis E transmission to a volunteer. *Lancet.* 1993;341:149–150.

306. Nanda SK, Yalcinkaya K, Panigrahi AK, Acharya SK, Jameel S, Panda SK. Etiological role of hepatitis E virus in sporadic fulminant hepatitis. *J Med Virol.* 1994; 42:133–137.

307. Rab MA, Bile MK, Mubarik MM, et al. Water-borne hepatitis E virus epidemic in Islamabad, Pakistan: a common source outbreak traced to the malfunction of a modern water treatment plant. *Am J Trop Med Hyg.* 1997;57:151–157.

308. Acharya SK, Dasarathy S, Kumer TL, et al. Fulminant hepatitis in a tropical population: clinical course, cause, and early predictors of outcome [see comments]. *Hepatology.* 1996;23:1448–1455.

309. Nanda SK, Ansari IH, Acharya SK, Jameel S, Panda SK. Protracted viremia during acute sporadic hepatitis E virus infection. *Gastroenterology.* 1995;108:225–230.

310. Ticehurst J, Popkin TJ, Bryan JP, et al. Association of hepatitis E virus with an outbreak of hepatitis in Pakistan: serologic responses and pattern of virus excretion. *J Med Virol.* 1992;36:84–92.

311. Bryan JP, Tsarev SA, Iqbal M, et al. Epidemic hepatitis E in Pakistan: patterns of serologic response and evidence that antibody to hepatitis E virus protects against disease. *J Infect Dis.* 1994;170:517–521.

312. Goldsmith R, Yarbough PO, Reyes GR, et al. Enzyme-linked immunosorbent assay for diagnosis of acute sporadic hepatitis E in Egyptian children. *Lancet.* 1992;339:328–331.

313. Corwin A, Jarot K, Lubis I, et al. Two years' investigation of epidemic hepatitis E virus transmission in West Kalimantan (Borneo), Indonesia. *Trans R Soc Trop Med Hyg.* 1995;89:262–265.

314. Mast EE, Alter MJ, Holland PV, Purcell RH. Evaluation of assays for antibody to hepatitis E virus by a serum panel. Hepatitis E Virus Antibody Serum Panel Evaluation Group. *Hepatology.* 1998;27:857–861.

315. Khuroo MS, Kamili S, Dar MY, Moecklii R, Jameel S. Hepatitis E and long-term antibody status [letter]. *Lancet.* 1993;341:1355.

316. Thomas DL, Yarbough PO, Vlahov D, et al. Seroreactivity to hepatitis E virus in areas where the disease is not endemic. *J Clin Microbiol.* 1997;35:1244–1247.

317. Labrique AB, Thomas DL, Stoszck SK, Nelson KE. Hepatitis E: new emerging infectious disease. *Epidemiol Rev.* 1999;21:162–178.

318. Wang CH, Flehmig B, Moeckli R. Transmission of hepatitis E virus by transfusion? [letter]. *Lancet.* 1993; 341:825–826.

319. Khuroo MS, Kamili S, Jameel S. Vertical transmission of hepatitis E virus. *Lancet.* 1995;345:1025–1026.

320. Aggarwal R, Naik SR. Hepatitis E: intrafamilial transmission versus waterborne spread. *J Hepatol.* 1994; 21:718–723.

321. Meng XJ, Halbur PG, Shapiro MS, et al. Genetic and experimental evidence for cross-species infection by swine hepatitis E virus. *J Virol.* 1998;72:9714–9721.

322. Kabrane-Lazizi Y, Fine JB, Elm J, et al. Evidence for widespread infection of wild rats with hepatitis E virus in the United States. *Am J Trop Med Hyg.* 1999; 61:331–335.

323. Kwo PY, Schlauder GG, Carpenter HA, et al. Acute hepatitis E by a new isolate acquired in the United States. *Mayo Clin Proc.* 1997;72:1133–1136.

324. Wong DC, Purcell RH, Sreenivasan MA, Prasad SR, Parvi KM. Epidemic and endemic hepatitis in India: evidence for non-A, non-B hepatitis virus etiology. *Lancet.* 1980;2:876–878.

325. Khuroo MS. Study of an epidemic of non-A, non-B hepatitis: possibility of another human hepatitis virus distinct from post-transfusion non-A, non-B type. *Am J Med.* 1980;68:818–824.

326. Thomas DL, Mahley RW, Badur S, Palaoglu KE, Quinn TQ. Epidemiology of hepatitis E virus infection in Turkey. *Lancet.* 1993;341:1561–1562.

327. Clayson ET, Shrestha MP, Vaughn DW, et al. Rates of hepatitis E virus infection and disease among adolescents and adults in Kathmandu, Nepal. *J Infect Dis.* 1997;176:763–766.

328. Arankalle VA, Tsarev SA, Chadha MS, et al. Age-specific prevalence of antibodies to hepatitis A and E viruses in Pune, India, 1982 and 1992. *J Infect Dis.* 1995;171:447–450.

329. Lee SD, Wang YJ, Lu RH, Chan CY, Lo KJ, Moeckli R. Seroprevalence of antibody to hepatitis E virus among Chinese subjects in Taiwan. *Hepatology.* 1994; 19:866–870.

330. Aggarwal R, Shahi H, Naik S, Yachha SK, Naik SR. Evidence in favour of high infection rate with hepatitis E virus among young children in India [letter]. *J Hepatol.* 1997;26:1425–1426.

331. Meng J, Pillot J, Dai X, Fields HA, Khudyakov YE. Neutralization of different geographic strains of the hepatitis E virus with anti-hepatitis E virus-positive serum samples obtained from different sources. *Virology.* 1998;249:316–324.

332. Bryan JP, Tsarev SA, Iqbal M, et al. Epidemic hepatitis E in Pakistan: patterns of serologic response and evidence that antibody to hepatitis E virus protects against disease. *J Infect Dis.* 1994;170:517–521.

333. Arankalle VA, Chadha MS, Chobe LP, Nair R, Banerjee K. Cross-challenge studies in rhesus monkeys employing different Indian isolates of hepatitis E virus. *J Med Virol.* 1995;46:358–363.

334. Tsarev SA, Tsareva TS, Emerson SU, et al. Successful passive and active immunization of cynomolgus monkeys against hepatitis E. *Proc Natl Acad Sci USA.* 1994;91:10198–10202.

335. Tsarev SA, Emerson SU, Tsareva TS, et al. Variation in course of hepatitis E in experimentally infected cynomolgus monkeys. *J Infect Dis.* 1993;167:1302–1306.

336. Simons JN, Leary TP, Dawson GJ, et al. Isolation of novel virus-like sequences associated with human hepatitis. *Nature Med.* 1995;1:564–569.

337. Alter HJ, Nakatsuji Y, Melpolder JC, Wages J, Wesley R, Shih J, Kim J. The incidence and disease implications of transfusion associated hepatitis G virus infection. *N Engl J Med.* 1997;336:747–754.

338. Linnen J, Wages J Jr, Zhang-Keck ZY, et al. Molecular cloning and disease association of hepatitis G virus: a transfusion-transmissible agent. *Eur J Biochem.* 1996;271:505–508.

CHAPTER 20

Sexually Transmitted Diseases

Jonathan M. Zenilman

In the United States, 12 million new cases of sexually transmitted diseases (STDs) occur annually, with an estimated direct economic impact of $10 billion a year.[1] Sexually transmitted infections include more than 25 organisms and their accompanying syndromes that are transmitted through sexual activity, some of which are presented in Exhibit 20–1. This chapter reviews the epidemiology of STDs and assesses the personal risk factors and the community factors that contribute to STD morbidity. A number of specific diseases will be reviewed in detail, focusing on the most common organisms including *Neisseria gonorrhoeae, Chlamydia trachomatis, Treponema pallidum* (syphilis), *Hemophilus ducreyi* (chancroid), *Trichomonas vaginalis*, bacterial vaginosis, and chronic viral infections, including herpes simplex and human papillomavirus. STDs result in direct medical consequences and also cause long-term sequelae, such as pelvic inflammatory disease (PID) and malignancies. STDs are also a major cause of perinatal complications that can result either through transplacental or perinatal transmission (Table 20–1).

Understanding the pathophysiology and epidemiology of STDs is a critical first step in developing rational control strategies. Traditional approaches have included clinic-based screening and partner notification. New approaches to community-based STD control include behavioral counseling interventions, use of computerized disease surveillance systems, geographic mapping, and use of noninvasive new diagnostic techniques and population-based screening in the nonclinical setting. The chapter concludes with a focus on special topics, especially the relationship between STDs and contraception and human immunodeficiency virus (HIV) infection.

TRANSMISSION MODE: THE DEFINITION OF A SEXUALLY TRANSMITTED DISEASE

Sexually transmitted diseases are transmitted through sexual intercourse. Sexual intercourse is defined as sexual contact, including vaginal intercourse, oral intercourse (ie, fellatio or cunnilingus), or rectal intercourse. Sexually transmitted diseases can be transmitted between heterosexual or homosexual partners. Different types of sexual activity may result in increased risks. Receptive rectal intercourse and vaginal intercourse carry the highest risks of STD transmission.

Unique in the infectious disease world, STDs are completely dependent on behavioral factors for transmission. Abstinent individuals will not contract an STD. Acquisition of an STD is also dependent on the probability of coming into contact with an STD-infected partner, susceptibility of the host, and efficiency of transmission of the organism through sexual intercourse.[2] These factors are critical for understanding an STD epidemiologic model.

Exhibit 20–1 Sexually Transmitted Diseases

A. *Bacterial*
   Gonorrhea (*Neisseria gonorrhoeae*)
   Syphilis (*Treponema pallidum*)
   Chlamydia (*Chlamydia trachomatis*)
   Chancroid (*Haemophilus ducreyi*)
   Granuloma inguinale (*Calymmatobacte-rium granulomatis*)
   Lymphogranuloma venereum (*Chlamydia trachomatis* LGV serovars)
   Bacterial vaginosis (vaginal flora ecologic disturbance)

B. *Viral*
   Genital herpes (*Herpes simplex* type 1 and type 2)
   Human papillomavirus infection
   Hepatitis B infection
   Human immunodeficiency virus
   Human T-cell lymphotropic virus type 1 (HTLV-1)
   Cytomegalovirus

C. *Parasitic*
   Trichomonas
   Scabies
   Pediculosis

The incidence of STDs is highest in adolescents and young adults. For gonorrhea and chlamydial infections, for which the largest bodies of data are available, more than 95% of incident infections occur in individuals between the ages of 15 and 39 years.[3] Highest rates of incidence are seen in adolescent women, aged 15 to 19 years, and in men who are aged 20 to 24 years.[4] These findings correlate very closely with sexual behavior patterns. For example, sexual partner turnover is highest in the adolescent and young adult age groups. Not only is the absolute number of sexual partners important, but also the type of sexual partner contributes to potential infection risk. Individuals with partners who are more likely to be infected with STDs (eg, those involved in commercial sex work or drug use) are much more likely to contract an STD than individuals who do not have high risk sexual partners. Similarly, persons with serial partners (but only having one sexual partner at a time) are less likely to spread STDs than persons who have multiple concurrent sex partners.[5]

STDs AS A COMPONENT OF REPRODUCTIVE HEALTH CARE

Sexually transmitted diseases need to be evaluated within the context of overall morbidity attributable to unprotected sexual behavior.[6,7] Reproductive health care has been balkanized through the development of categorical public health programs that deal with pregnancy (family planning clinics, federal support of birth control) and separate disease-oriented programs (eg, for STDs and HIV). This approach is inefficient because risky sexual behavior patterns also result in morbidity such as unintended pregnancy, low birth weight infants, the cost of pregnancy terminations, STDs, direct costs attributable to STD care, and the long-term STD costs, including complications of STDs (eg, pelvic inflammatory disease and ectopic pregnancy), HIV, and STD-facilitated HIV transmission.

Developing effective prevention control strategies requires understanding patterns of sexual behavior, which include:

- The age of sexual debut: Individuals with younger age at first coitus are at greater risk for STD.[7]
- Number of partners, including delineation between serial partners (serial monogamy) or number of concurrent partners. Individuals with multiple concurrent partners are much more likely to spread STDs than individuals with serial partners.[8]
- Use of barrier protection methods, including condom use patterns.[9]
- Other comorbidities, especially drug use, socioeconomic status, commercial sex work, and travel to areas where STDs are highly endemic. In parts of the world, such as Western Europe where STD rates are low, travelers to highly endemic areas account for over half of the new bacterial STD infections.[10]

Table 20–1 Perinatal Complications of Sexually Transmitted Diseases

Organism	Complication
Gonorrhea, chlamydia	Ophthalmia Pneumonia Low birth weight
Syphilis	Congenital syphilis
Trichomonas Bacterial vaginosis	Premature rupture of membranes, premature delivery
Herpes simplex	Congenital herpes syndrome
Human papillomavirus	Laryngeal papillomatosis
Hepatitis B	Perinatal transmission
Human immunodeficiency virus	Perinatal transmission

SEXUAL BEHAVIOR ASSESSMENT

Assessing sexual behavior, which is difficult, is usually done by cross-sectional survey. The National Survey of Family Growth[11] has found that between 1970 and 1988, 26.7% and 46.0% of white and black, respectively, teenage women had had premarital sexual intercourse. By 1988, this had increased to 51% and 59% for whites and blacks, respectively.[12] These data indicate that a large proportion of the adolescent population was at risk for STDs. Condom use patterns were below 50% for both groups in 1988. A more recent survey found that 75% of respondents used condoms, with higher rates of condom use being seen among the African American populations.

A survey of adolescents conducted in 1995 and 1997 by the Centers for Disease Control and Prevention (the Youth Risk Factor Surveillance Survey)[13] found that the proportion of those sexually active decreased from 53% to 48%. Of those sexually active in 1997, 16% had four or more partners and 57% had used condoms at last intercourse (Figure 20–1). Condom use rate in African American respondents was 64%. Twenty-five percent of all participants had used either alcohol or drugs at last intercourse, which presents a critical problem in developing prevention strategies.

COVARIATES

Socioeconomic factors have been associated with the increased incidence of STDs.[14] These factors include higher rates of STDs in impoverished areas. Socioeconomic status has been linked to increased incidence of STDs in a number of different settings, including rural and urban areas in the United States and developing countries.[15] Areas in which available health services have decreased, especially preventive health services, have also seen an increased incidence of STDs. Furthermore, increases in STD incidence have also been linked to the imposition of fees for previously free public health clinical services.[16] In Eastern Europe, which has experienced tremendous social disruption, disin-

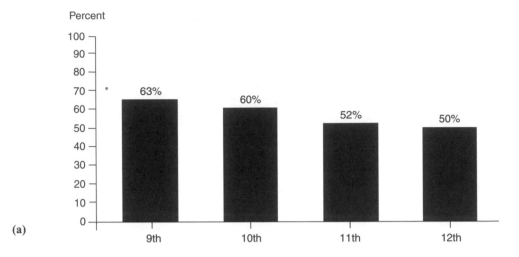

(a)

*Among currently sexually active students.

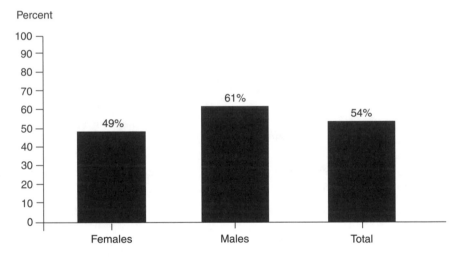

(b)   *Among currently sexually active students.

Figure 20–1 (a) Percentage of high school students who used a condom during last sexual intercourse,* by grade, and **(b)** Percentage of high school students who used a condom during last sexual intercourse,* by sex. *Source:* Reprinted from Youth Risk Behavior Surveillance—United States, 1995, *MMWR*, September 27, 1996, 45 (Supplement SS-4), Centers for Disease Control and Prevention.

tegration of the health system and loosening of travel restrictions have led to the development of a very large STD epidemic.[17]

Urbanization in developing countries has been strongly associated with increased STD rates.[18] Because of economic development in urban areas, men are attracted to the cities for job opportunities. In the absence of regular female partners, they avail themselves of commercial sex. These contacts, in turn, provide social networks that readily spread sexually transmitted diseases.[19] When the men return home for holiday, they spread STDs to their spouses or other regular sexual partners. The ramifications of these patterns were particularly demonstrated in India where monogamous women were at risk for STD and HIV infection through the behaviors of their spouses.[20]

In the United States, illicit drug use and its associated sexual behaviors are associated with STD incidence, especially syphilis.[21-24] In part, this is related to the direct pharmacologic activities of the drugs themselves (eg, cocaine can stimulate increased sexual activity); however, more important are the behaviors associated with drug use and the marketing of drugs, including prostitution.

In the United States, when STD incidence is examined by race or ethnicity, very wide discrepancies are demonstrated between racial/ethnic groups.[25] For example, in 1995, overall gonorrhea rates for African Americans were 1,087/ 100,000 compared with 29/100,000 for whites and 91/100,000 for Hispanics. The highest rates were seen in African American women aged between 15 and 19 years; the gonorrhea rate in this age group was 4,772/100,000 (overall U.S. rate for women aged 15 to 19 = 897/100,000), and in African American men aged 20 to 24 years the rate was 5,496/100,000 (overall U.S. rate for men aged 20 to 24 = 745/100,000). African Americans accounted for 79% of the total reported cases of gonorrhea and 86% of all reported cases of primary and secondary syphilis. Race and ethnicity in the United States often correlate with other more fundamental determinants of health status such as socioeconomic status, access to good quality medical care, and efforts to receive good quality medical care. Reporting biases may also play a role, although these differences occur even when these biases are controlled.

GONORRHEA

In 1996, 325,883 cases of gonorrhea were reported to the Centers for Disease Control and Prevention by local and state health departments[26]; this figure represented the lowest rate in more than 25 years. An additional one to two cases are thought to occur for every reported case. Although the incidence of gonorrhea has decreased by nearly 70% since the peak of the gonorrhea epidemic in the mid-1970s, the infection has become increasingly prevalent in inner-city areas (Figure 20–2).

The incidence of gonorrhea in the United States is approaching the year 2000 objective (rate of 100/100,00), but it is still higher than in most other developed countries. In the United States, the disease has become increasingly a disease of poverty, especially among African Americans. Gonorrhea is associated with increased numbers of sex partners, having a recent new sexual partner, and lower rates of barrier contraceptive use.

The overall population-based rates for gonorrhea are deceptive. Rates among adolescents, the group at highest risk for STDs, are five to ten times higher, and in African American adolescents the rates are 20 to 30 times higher than the national rate.

Gonorrhea is caused by *Neisseria gonorrhoeae,* a fastidious gram-negative coccus.[27] In men, urethritis is the most common syndrome.[28] Discharge or dysuria usually appears within 1 week of exposure, although as many as 5% to 10% of patients never have signs or symptoms.[29] Asymptomatic disease can exist in men up to several weeks after infection. Some controversy exists about whether asymptomatic disease represents presymptomatic disease or true asymptomatic infection. Nevertheless, the organism is potentially transmissible to sexual partners from infected persons who are asymptomatic.

In women, gonorrhea typically causes cervical disease (cervicitis). Women with untreated gonococcal cervicitis develop upper genital tract infection, that is, PID.[30-33] Semantically, PID represents infection of the soft tissue upper genital tract structures, and includes endometritis, salpingitis, oophoritis, and pelvic peritonitis. Fatalities from PID are rare. However, severe acute PID can lead to tubo-ovarian abscess and the ne-

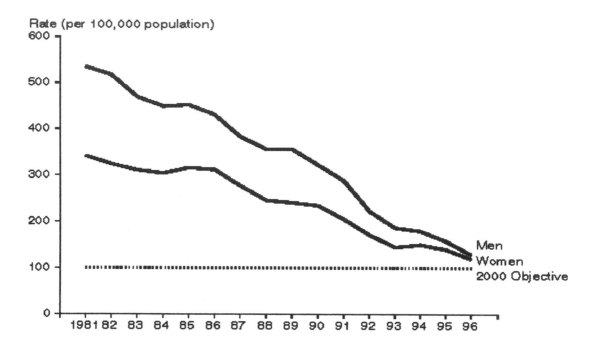

Figure 20–2 Gonorrhea—rates by gender: United States, 1981–1996 and the Healthy People year 2000 objective. *Source:* Reprinted from Division of STD Prevention, Sexually Transmitted Disease Surveillance, 1996, DHHS-PHS, Centers for Disease Control and Prevention, p. 17, 1997.

cessity, at times, for hysterectomy. The chronic complications are more common. Women with a previous history of PID are more likely to have tubal-factor infertility and are at higher risk for ectopic pregnancy.[34,35] The overall direct economic impact of PID in the United States was estimated to be $4.2 billion in 1990.[36]

Estimates of PID incidence vary, and they are made difficult by the lack of prospective studies. Early studies suggested that PID occurs in approximately 30% of women with untreated gonorrhea.[37] In the United States, approximately 200,000 cases of PID were estimated to have required hospitalization in 1988, with a total burden of cases estimated at more than 500,000.[38]

Symptomatic anorectal gonococcal disease occurs in persons with a history of receptive rectal intercourse.[39] Approximately 50% have symptoms that include rectal pain, discharge, constipation, and tenesmus. Because rectal gon-

orrhea in men implies a history of unprotected rectal intercourse, surveillance of rectal gonorrhea has been useful as a surrogate marker for HIV risk in gay men. For example, early in the acquired immunodeficiency syndrome (AIDS) epidemic, the rate of rectal gonorrhea declined.[40] Similarly, troubling trends of an increase of gonorrhea in homosexual men were reported in 1997, which correlated with observed increases in HIV-risk behavior among homosexual adolescents.[41]

Gonococcal pharyngitis[42,43] occurs in men or women after oral sexual exposure. The disease is clinically indistinguishable from any other bacterial pharyngitis, and it is asymptomatic in as many as 60% of cases. Disseminated gonococcal infection (gonococcal septicemia) occurs in approximately 0.1% to 0.5% of total gonococcal cases.[44,45] Occasionally, disseminated gonococcal infection can lead to endocarditis[46] or meningitis, both of which can be particularly devastating.

Perinatal Disease

Although perinatal infection is relatively rare in the United States, it is still often found in the developing world. Perinatal gonococcal disease is transmitted by direct exposure to an infant passing through the birth canal of an infected cervix.[47,48] Gonococcal ophthalmia, which is a severe public health problem in the developing world, is effectively prevented by inexpensive prophylaxis.[49] The incidence of gonococcal ophthalmia is estimated to be 42% among infants exposed to an infected cervical canal.[50] These infants develop a purulent conjunctivitis that can then rapidly progress to keratitis and subsequently to corneal blindness. Ophthalmia is also occasionally seen in adults—usually as a result of self-inoculation.

Diagnosis and Treatment

Traditionally, gonorrhea has been diagnosed by bacterial culture. In the past 3 years, major advances in both DNA and RNA amplification have allowed the development of nucleic acid amplification techniques. The most commonly used and recently licensed tests in the United States include polymerase chain reaction and ligase chain reaction.[51] Both techniques are at least as sensitive as culture and may be more sensitive in certain situations. Furthermore, the high sensitivity of these techniques has allowed them to be used in urine.[52] The use of urine as a diagnostic technique has facilitated expansion of gonorrhea screening efforts,[53] especially in populations where clinical service provision is difficult or inadequate.

Treatment[54] for mucosal gonorrhea infections is based on providing single-dose regimens, preferably oral antibiotics that are effective against most or all of the known resistant determinants. Current single-dose oral regimens include ciprofloxacin (500 mg), ofloxacin (400 mg), and cefixime (400 mg). All patients treated for gonorrhea should also be treated for chlamydia, with either azithromycin (1 g [single dose]) or doxycycline (100 mg [twice daily for 1 week]).

Antimicrobial Resistance

For 30 years after World War II, penicillin was the antimicrobial therapy of choice.[55] In 1976, the first case of penicillinase-producing *Neisseria gonorrhoeae* (PPNG) was reported. PPNG rapidly developed into a major public health problem and made the penicillin class of antibiotics obsolete by the mid-1980s.[56] Chromosomally mediated resistance to penicillin[57] (CMRNG) was described in the early 1980s; high level plasmid-mediated tetracycline resistance (TRNG) developed in 1985[58]; and, more recently, quinolone resistance[59] (QRNG) has been described in a number of cities in the United States as well as in Southeast Asia. Development of standardized effective gonococcal treatment strategies[60] has required accurate surveillance, which has occurred since the mid-1980s with the implementation of the national gonorrhea surveillance network[61] (GISP). This multisite surveillance system has provided standardized mechanisms for determining antimicrobial resistance. Baseline behavioral and treatment data are also collected. As a byproduct of that system, recently, the GISP described increased incidence of anorectal infection in the GISP cohort, suggesting that risky practices were beginning to develop within the homosexual community served by the GISP program.

Control

Appreciating the clinical and epidemiologic characteristics of gonorrhea is important in developing control strategies. Partner notification has been extraordinarily ineffective in controlling gonococcal infection because of the short incubation period,[62] estimated to be between 1 and 2 days. In this context, it is therefore impossible to "surround" an epidemic focus of gonococcal disease and capture and treat the infected partners. In contrast, screening strategies, traditionally oriented toward women, have had a significant impact in lowering disease prevalence. With the availability of new noninvasive urine diagnostic tests, screening strategies for men in high-risk settings have become a practical option.

CHLAMYDIA

Chlamydia trachomatis infection is the most common STD in the United States, with approximately four million cases estimated annually.[63–65] The clinical syndromes of chlamydia infection are similar to those seen in gonorrhea; however, they tend to be less acute but cause a significant number of complications. In men, the most common syndrome is chlamydia urethritis, which in the United States accounts for approximately 40% of all cases of nongonococcal urethritis.[66,67] Urethritis in men typically presents as a mucoid discharge, associated often with dysuria. Asymptomatic infection occurs in more than 30% of cases.[68–70] The time from infection to development of symptoms is longer than that for gonorrhea, usually about 7 to 14 days.

In women, cervical infection is the most commonly reported syndrome. More than half of women with cervical infection are asymptomatic.[71] When symptoms occur, they can manifest as vaginal discharge or poorly differentiated abdominal or lower abdominal pain.[72,73] At clinical examination, often no clinical signs are present. When they are present, they include mucopurulent cervical discharge, friability, and edema. Although cervical ectopy traditionally has been associated with chlamydia, studies by the author's group have demonstrated that cervical ectopy, when clinically strictly defined, is actually not more significantly found in adolescent women with chlamydia infections than in uninfected women.[74]

Left untreated, approximately 30% of women with chlamydial infection will develop pelvic inflammatory disease.[75] The PID of chlamydia is associated with lower rates of clinical symptoms than the PID seen in gonorrhea. However, this subacute PID is associated with higher rates of subsequent infertility.[76] Chlamydia induces an inflammatory reaction characterized by fibrosis.

Rectal chlamydia[77] infection occurs predominantly in homosexual men who have had receptive rectal intercourse. Rectal infection also occurs in heterosexual women where similar exposures are reported. Oropharyngeal chlamydial infection appears not to be a clinically important entity.

The epidemiology of chlamydia is interesting because a number of artifacts are seen in the reporting scheme. Reported chlamydia infections are more common in women than in men and rates have increased substantially since 1984 (Figure 20–3). Both of these trends are artifacts. The large rate difference between women and men results from different ascertainment practices.[78] Women are typically diagnosed with a chlamydial infection on the basis of a chlamydia screening test performed at a routine physical examination. Clinical practice guidelines strongly recommend routine chlamydia screening for asymptomatic sexually active women aged less than 25 years. Risk factors for chlamydia infection include a history of multiple sex partners, a recent new sex partner, low rates of barrier contraceptive use, and a history of an STD. Epidemiologic predictive models have been widely studied as potential tools to help target screening and intervention efforts. Chlamydial infection is also consistently associated with lower socioeconomic status and younger age. Clinical features, such as cervical friability, seen more often in younger women, are highly associated with chlamydial infection. However, the practical utility of these models is problematic because even the most sophisticated ones do not capture one third of cases. For example, a large recent study in Baltimore of high-risk adolescents found that chlamydial incidence was 17% per year.[79] However, no single risk factor was predictive. Population-based screening programs have demonstrated high rates of asymptomatic infection. A recent large study of U.S. Army military recruits found a chlamydial prevalence of 9%, with some evidence of regional variation.[80] Studies of men in emergency departments and adolescent clinics have demon-

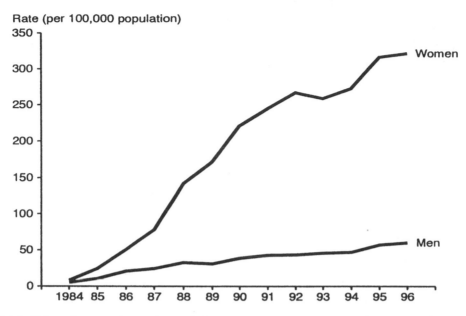

Figure 20–3 Chlamydia—rates by gender: United States, 1984–1996. *Source:* Reprinted from Division of STD Prevention, Sexually Transmitted Disease Surveillance, 1996, DHHS, PHS, Centers for Disease Control and Prevention, p. 9, 1997.

strated asymptomatic infection rates as high as 6% to 9%.

Chlamydia screening of women has also been incorporated recently into quality assurance guidelines for managed care organizations, such as the Health Employer Data Information Set (HEDIS).[81] In contrast, men often are treated for chlamydia infection on the basis of presentation of a syndrome of urethritis or as a contact to a woman with a chlamydia infection and a definitive etiologic diagnosis is not made.[82] Therefore, many infections among men do not meet the surveillance definition and are never reported.

The trend of increasing incidence of infection, with the most recent number of cases, 490,080, reported to CDC in 1996, results from increased screening activity and increased reporting. For example, in 1985 fewer than 10 states required reporting of chlamydia infections; this number has since increased to 40 states with reporting requirements. A true estimate of chlamydia prevalence, therefore, is not known, which presents major problems in evaluating trends.

Advances in chlamydia screening technology since the early 1980s have resulted in increased availability of chlamydia screening tests. Before 1984 chlamydia testing was available only by tissue culture, which is expensive and cumbersome. In 1984, the first antigen detection tests, based on either fluorescent antibody or enzyme-linked immunosorbent assay (ELISA) technologies, were licensed and became widely available in the United States. These tests have been replaced by genetic probe technologies, and more recently, by DNA and other nucleic acid amplification technologies that can be performed both on anogenital specimens and urine.[83,84] The development of new, noninvasive urine-based nucleic acid–based technologies will result in substantial expansion of screening activities because of the reduced need to perform clinical examinations.

The rates of chlamydia are highest in adolescent women and drop off steeply after the early 20s. For example, the reported rate of infection of women aged between 15 and 19 years is 2,069/100,000 and 531/100,000 for women aged 25 to 29. Some authorities believe that this steep drop off in incidence may not be related only to behavior but also to the development of partial immunity to clinical infection through periodic repeated exposures.

Chlamydia screening programs have proved to be effective.[85,86] Implementation of chlamydia screening resulted in an initial increase in chlamydia prevalence among women tested, followed by a nearly 50% decrease over 4 subsequent years. These data demonstrate that a screening intervention alone can have an impact on chlamydia prevalence by removing infected individuals from the population after they are detected and treated.

A more rigorous demonstration of the screening and treatment effect on population incidence was published in 1997. In this study, the Group Health Cooperative of Puget Sound, which has longitudinal tracking ability of all of its clients, demonstrated that periodic chlamydia screening resulted in a 44% reduction in incident PID among the managed care population.[87] Partner notification has not been evaluated.

GENITAL ULCER DISEASES—SYPHILIS

Syphilis[88] is a multistaged disease caused by the bacterium *Treponema pallidum*. *T. pallidum* is a spirochete, which has a number of microbiologic characteristics that have an impact on the epidemiology and clinical management of infection. *T. pallidum* cannot be grown in culture. Therefore, clinical or serologic diagnosis of syphilis is the primary means of detection. Understanding the clinical staging of syphilis is important in developing epidemiologic approaches.

Syphilis is classified into three clinical stages: primary, secondary, and late (including tertiary

and late benign syphilis). Latent syphilis is a serologic diagnosis where symptoms are not apparent and which is differentiated into early (infection duration < 1 year) or late (infection duration > 1 year). Infectious disease specialists are often called on to consider syphilis in consultation on patients with genital ulcers, in an acute febrile patient with vasculitis symptoms, to advise in the management of complications of late syphilis, especially neurosyphilis, and in the interpretation of syphilis serological test results.

Epidemiology

Syphilis typically is seen in situations wherein exist multiple opportunities for large numbers of anonymous sex partners, such as the recent association of syphilis with homosexual bathhouses or drug "crack houses." In 1996, 11,387 cases of syphilis were reported, which was the lowest number of cases since 1959 in the United States. Syphilis is predominantly seen in minority communities, especially in the South. In addition, studies of syphilis in the late 1980s and early 1990s have demonstrated that syphilis is associated with illicit drug behaviors, especially the use of crack cocaine.[89]

The epidemiology of syphilis presents a fascinating overview of changing demographics of STD epidemiology (Figure 20–4). A steady decline in cases has been seen since the introduction of penicillin at the end of World War II. From 1976 to 1981, a 50% increase in reported cases of syphilis occurred, predominantly among white gay men. These findings reflected the increases in STDs among gay men overall, as well as the gay liberation movement and the use of bathhouse establishments with increases in anonymous sex with multiple partners. Between 1981 and 1984, a precipitous drop in the incidence of syphilis occurred, which was largely driven by a greater than 90% decrease of syphilis incidence in gay men, in response to the HIV epidemic. However, from 1984 to 1989, a greater than 100% increase in syphilis was reported. This increase was accounted for by a

Rate (per 100,000 population)

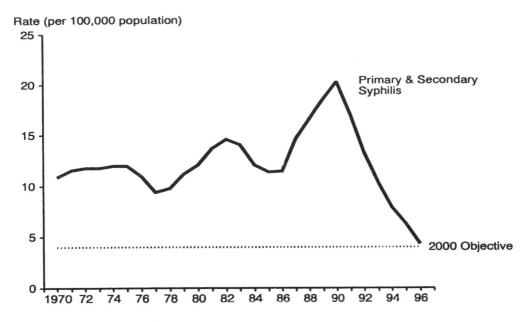

Figure 20–4 Primary and secondary syphilis—reported rates: United States, 1970–1996 and the Healthy People year 2000 objective. *Source:* Reprinted from Division of STD Prevention, Sexually Transmitted Disease Surveillance, 1996, DHHS, PHS, Centers for Disease Control and Prevention, p. 23, 1997.

change in the characteristics of the epidemic from that involving primarily homosexual men to a predominance of minority heterosexual individuals. The male-to-female ratio during this period dropped from 4:1 to nearly 1:1, which was followed by a large upsurge in congenital syphilis cases in 1989–1990. However, trends have decreased since that time, with the exception of several geographic areas, including Baltimore, Maryland, and a variety of counties in the Southeast. Syphilis occurs in settings characterized by high sex partner turnover, such as among prostitutes, transients, and "sex for drugs" exchange situations among drug users. In developed countries, syphilis has been associated with a variety of social and behavioral factors, including bathhouses frequented by homosexual men, prostitution related to drug abuse, and poor access to health care. In the developing world, more important issues are prostitution, transience, and poor access to health care.

Clinical Course

Initial infection with *Treponema pallidum* occurs through sexual contact involving a mucosal membrane.[90] The incubation period ranges between 10 and 30 days. Transmission of syphilis is relatively inefficient. Studies have demonstrated that the transmission efficiency of syphilis between an infected and uninfected partner is only about 20% per sexual contact. After the initial exposure, a latency period of 3 weeks takes place prior to the development of the initial symptoms. During this latency period (or in epidemiologic terms "critical period"), a newly infected individual is not infectious to his or her sexual partners. This time period is crucial in the control of syphilis, because effective antibiotic treatment at this time will prevent transmission. Preventive therapy of exposed partners is widely used to control the spread of infectious syphilis. After the development of the initial genital ulcerative lesion, or chancre, the patient becomes infectious.

The chancre is a painless lesion with an indurated border, with associated painless lymphadenopathy. A dark-field microscopic examination of the ulcer reveals characteristic motile treponemes. Syphilis is a systemic disease. Even in primary syphilis, systemic dissemination can occur. Of patients in some studies with early primary syphilis, 10% to 15% have cerebral spinal fluid (CSF) abnormalities,[91] which is of special concern in treating patients who also have an HIV infection.

Left untreated, the chancre will heal spontaneously within 2 to 3 weeks; however, 4 to 8 weeks later, the secondary syphilis syndrome develops. Secondary syphilis is a systemic vasculitis caused by high levels of *T. pallidum* in the blood and associated immunologic responses. The most characteristic findings are dermatologic, including the classic palmar or plantar rash. Other manifestations include alopecia (hair loss), mucosal lesions and visceral involvement, which can include granulomatous hepatitis, nephrotic syndrome, optic neuritis, and rarely, meningovascular syphilis. Left untreated, the secondary syphilis syndrome will spontaneously resolve, usually within 1 to 2 months of onset.

The late complications of syphilis (eg, neurosyphilis), cardiovascular syphilis, and gummatous syphilis do not develop until 10 to 20 years after the resolution of early syphilis. In patients who are infected with HIV, case reports have suggested that late complications can occur much earlier.[92]

Early latent syphilis is a serologic diagnosis in which a fourfold increase in titer (ie, two dilutions, see below) occurs within 1 year, with previous documentation of the earlier serology. Late latent syphilis is a serologic diagnosis of syphilis occurring more than 1 year after a baseline diagnosis.

Diagnosis of Primary Syphilis

Dark-field microscopic examination of the ulcer exudate establishes the diagnosis. Unfortu-nately, dark-field microscopy is not available in most clinical settings. False-negative results can occur if patients apply bactericidal creams to the lesions. Therefore, diagnosis is most often clinically established by the presence of a lesion in association with positive serologic findings.

Serology

Serologic diagnosis of syphilis is a two-step procedure.[93] Initially, a nontreponemal screening test is performed. The most widely used tests are the venereal disease research laboratory (VDRL) and the rapid plasma reagin (RPR) test. Results of these tests are reported as titers (ie, the dilutions required to achieve a negative reaction using standard reagents). Patients with a positive nontreponemal test should have a confirmatory test such as the fluorescent treponemal antibody-absorbed (FTA-ABS) or microhemagglutination (MHATP or HATS) tests. Up to 20% of patients with positive nontreponemal tests will have negative confirmatory tests. These are termed biologic false-positive (BFP) results. Most frequently, these are seen in patients with past series of intravenous drug abuse, pregnancy, systemic disorders such as lupus erythematosus, and rheumatoid arthritis and other infectious processes such as Lyme disease. BFPs with titers greater than 1:16 are extremely unusual. In primary syphilis, the sensitivity of serologic testing is 85%. Some false-negative findings occur because seroconversion occasionally takes longer to develop than the genital ulcer. In secondary syphilis, sensitivity of serologic diagnosis approaches 100% and the titers can be extremely high. In fact, we can see a "prozone phenomenon" where true positivity can only be detected when the specimen is tested at a higher dilution.

Syphilis in HIV-Infected Patients

Studies in STD clinics have demonstrated that HIV prevalence in patients with syphilis is up to three times greater than in non-syphilis patients in these settings.[94] Studies conducted in inner-city clinics in Baltimore[95] (309 patients) and the Bronx[96] (50 patients) suggest that patients with HIV may be more likely to present with secondary syphilis. However, the serologic manifestations and serologic response to treatment are not affected by HIV status.

Because of initial reports of treatment failure in patients with HIV infections, many experts believed that all patients with syphilis, and especially patients with coexistent HIV infection, should be treated more aggressively than other patients. Prospective studies done by CDC investigators have demonstrated that this is rarely necessary.

Congenital Syphilis

Vertical transmission of syphilis can also occur. The transmission rate among pregnant women with syphilis is estimated to be more than 60%. Infection in the infant is often manifest either as stillbirth or as the stigmata of congenital syphilis, which include clinical syndromes at birth, such as osteoformative abnormalities, including "saber shins," Hutchinson's incisors, and mulberry molars. In women who have untreated primary or secondary syphilis, the vertical transmission rate is estimated to be 75% to 95%. Late congenital syphilis is rarely seen in the antibiotic era.

Transmission occurs transplacentally. Screening during the first and third trimesters and treatment for congenital syphilis during pregnancy effectively prevent this disorder. Cases of congenital syphilis should be considered "sentinel events" and should initiate an intensive investigation of the public health prevention program. Cases are often associated with no prenatal care and with drug use, especially crack cocaine, during pregnancy. The diagnosis of congenital syphilis is complex because of the passively acquired antibody in the immediate postpartum period. For example, infants whose mothers have been successfully treated for syphilis often have positive syphilis serologic tests. The development of surveillance definitions is oriented to-

ward differentiating those with active infection compared with those with inactive infection.

Treatment

Treatment[97] of primary, secondary, and early latent syphilis is recommended with benzathine penicillin. For patients allergic to penicillin, doxycycline can be used according to the regimen shown in Exhibit 20–1. Treatment of patients with late latent syphilis, late syphilis, or syphilis of unknown duration (serologic syphilis in which an initial benchmark cannot be defined) should be treated with benzathine penicillin (2.4 million units) intramuscularly for 3 weeks. Patients with neurosyphilis should be treated with high-dose intravenous penicillin (24 million units) for 10 days. Pregnant women with syphilis should be treated only with penicillin-based regimens.

Intervention Approaches

Intervention approaches to syphilis control have long capitalized on the unique clinical aspects of the disease. These include:

1. After treatment, an individual is noninfectious to sexual partners. With the advent of penicillin therapy, this has become a major tool in developing intervention strategies.
2. The long latency period from time of infection to time of infectiousness offers an opportunity for reducing secondary spread contacts. This has been the basis of syphilis control programs based on partner notification and screening programs.
3. The availability of an inexpensive diagnostic screening test (the syphilis serologic test) allows widespread screening opportunities.
4. Demonstration that treatment during pregnancy prevents vertical transmission has also resulted in the establishment of prenatal screening and treatment programs.

Syphilis presents the prototype disease for the use of partner notification and presumptive treatment of partners.[98] Although the empiric evidence strongly suggests that this has been an effective approach in syphilis control, no randomized trials have been performed to demonstrate the efficacy of this strategy. Furthermore, partner notification is complicated in situations where large numbers of anonymous sex partners are the secondary contacts. This has been an important issue in evaluating disease intervention approaches in homosexual bathhouses and crack cocaine-associated epidemics.[99] In these situations, many public health intervention strategies have revolved around aggressive screening and presumptive treatment of partners.

CHANCROID

Chancroid is a genital ulcer disease caused by the organism *Haemophilus ducreyi*. Chancroid is primarily seen in developing countries and in subtropical areas of the developing world, such as the southern United States. In 1996, 338 cases were reported mostly from New York, Texas, and Louisiana. The causative organism is exceedingly difficult to cultivate. Despite advances in technology, cultures are only about 80% sensitive even in the most efficient laboratory settings. The fastidious growth characteristics of *H. ducreyi* render easily accessible diagnostic evaluation difficult. In the United States, cases are usually associated with prostitution and illicit drug use.[100–102]

The incubation period of chancroid is between 4 and 7 days. The ulcer develops initially as a tender papule with erythema.[103] The ulcer typically is undermined and, in contrast to syphilis, it is often painful and indurated, and it has a purulent exudate. Painful large adenopathy is seen in up to 50% of patients. These can develop into large purulent nodes, which can then develop into buboes and spontaneously rupture, forming sinus tracts. Chancroid does not disseminate or cause systemic disease. Oddly enough, chancroid is not vertically transmitted and has not been associated with major perinatal or neonatal complications.

The classic identifying features of chancroidal ulcers are a short incubation period; painful, tender ulcerations with undermined, beefy appearance; purulent exudate; and rapid resolution with appropriate antimicrobial treatment.

Diagnosis of chancroid is difficult because the organism grows only on special media at 33°C. Culture media are not widely available outside of infectious disease reference centers. Newer diagnostic tests using DNA amplification techniques of ulcer exudate[104,105] have been developed, but they are not yet widely available.

In the United States, chancroid should be considered as a potential cause of genital ulcer in the following groups:

1. Patients with genital ulcers in an area where chancroid is known to be endemic. Outbreaks over the past 10 years have occurred in New York, Philadelphia, South Florida, Southern California, and Mississippi.
2. Patients with genital ulcer disease who have recently traveled or been exposed to an individual who has traveled to developing countries.
3. If any doubt about the diagnosis exists, presumptive treatment may be an option, as it is extremely effective.

Chancroid is effectively treated with antimicrobial therapy.[106] Current treatment regimens include third-generation cephalosporins, the quinolones, and azithromycin. Development of resistance does occur, and evidence suggests that resistance determinants can be shared between *Haemophilus ducreyi* and *Neisseria gonorrhoeae*. This was especially evident in the early 1980s with the penicillin-resistant determinants found in gonorrhea (PPNG).

Epidemiology

Chancroid is the most common genital ulcer disease in many developing parts of the world, especially Sub-Saharan Africa. It has been con-clusively demonstrated to be a facilitator or co-factor for HIV transmission, and HIV has been successfully cultivated from the base of chan-croidal ulcers. Vertical transmission does not appear to occur with *Haemophilus ducreyi*. In the United States, outbreaks of chancroid gener-ally have been associated with heterosexual, drug-using activity. No homosexually related epidemics have been reported in the United States. In addition, other risks factors that appear to play a role in the epidemiology of chancroid include alcohol use, intravenous drug use, and sex with commercial sex workers. Chancroid should also be considered in travelers to en-demic areas who present with a genital ulcer.

Epidemiologic approaches in chancroid con-trol are based on detection of disease and aggres-sive treatment. No studies have been performed to demonstrate the effectiveness of partner noti-fication. In addition, the issue of diagnosis is a major problem. Therefore, surveillance of cases of genital ulcer disease that do not respond to traditional therapies is useful for detecting the emergence of chancroid within a defined popu-lation. Subsequent to identification, aggressive partner notification and even presumptive treat-ment approaches have been successful in reduc-ing outbreaks in the United States.

Chancroid can be differentiated from both syphilis and herpes in that the genital ulcers do not respond to penicillin or to antiviral drugs; the genital ulcers do not resolve spontaneously; and the ulcer responds very rapidly to ceftriaxone and to other recommended antichancroid thera-pies. In the United States, chancroid should be considered whenever an epidemiologic investi-gation discloses travel of patients or their part-ners to endemic areas in developing tropical countries.

GENITAL HERPES INFECTION

Herpes simplex infections are characterized by life-long infection, latency, and recurrences. Genital herpes infection is almost exclusively

sexually transmitted.[107] Approximately 90% of genital herpes is caused by herpes simplex type 2 (HSV-2); 10% is caused by HSV-1. This ratio of HSV-1 to HSV-2 is reversed in cases of orofacial herpes. Orofacial herpes caused by herpes simplex type 1 is transmitted as an upper respiratory tract infection, usually in early child-hood. HSV-1 and HSV-2 cause similar clinical syndromes at the respective mucosal sites. Be-cause of the high degree of DNA homology be-tween the two viral subtypes, serologic differen-tiation is difficult.[108]

Acute infection with herpes simplex occurs after inoculation of virus to the mucosal site. Pri-mary infection is often asymptomatic.[109] When symptomatic cases occur, a mucosal or epider-mal ulcer develops. Simultaneously, viral par-ticles enter the sensory nerve roots supplying the area and travel cephalad along the nerve axons to the dorsal root ganglia (DRG) where latency develops. For genital herpes, latency develops in the lumbosacral dorsal root ganglia, and for orofacial herpes in the trigeminal ganglia. When recurrences occur, viral particles begin replica-tion in the DRG, travel centripetally to the pe-riphery, exit at the mucosa or skin surface, and cause a repeat genital ulceration. Because of prior immunologic priming of the humoral and cellular immune systems, recurring outbreaks are typically shorter than the primary infection.

Clinical Features

Genital herpes can occur at any exposed mu-cosal site (genitalia, rectum, mouth). In primary disease, the ulceration develops 5 to 10 days after exposure; systemic signs,[110] such as fever, myalgia, headache, and occasionally meningeal irritation, may also be associated with the in-fection. Recurrent herpes can develop at any time after the primary infection. In many set-tings, patients report a prodrome, which can consist of low-grade fever, pruritis, or tingling at the site of recurrence. Patients often report that they are able to feel the recurrence devel-oping with nonspecific signs and symptoms, which is most likely related to irritation of the peripheral nerve roots.

Because many patients have asymptomatic primary infection, differentiation of a *clinical first episode* into primary disease or recurrence (in patients who have had an asymptomatic primary episode) is often not possible. In the research setting, *primary* infections are defined as an initial clinical episode with no serologic evidence of prior infection. Most patients, however, presenting with their initial episode, actually have serologic evidence of prior infection.[111] This is termed *first clinical episode of recurrent disease.* This is often a very confusing point to clinicians, and is made more difficult by the unavailability of accurate serologic tests.

Symptomatic recurrences are less symptomatic and heal faster than the primary episode. Recurrences occur most frequently within the first year after primary infection and the frequency decreases thereafter. The factors involved in inducing recurrent episodes are not well characterized. Physical and physiologic stresses have been classically cited as important cofactors, but few well-controlled studies have elucidated these relationships. Methodologically, these investigations are difficult and, therefore, most of the associations are based on anecdotal reports.

Asymptomatic shedding plays a major role in transmission of HSV. Asymptomatic shedding occurs between clinical outbreaks, especially in the first few years after diagnosis. Initial culture studies of women with a recent diagnosis of primary herpes found that asymptomatic shedding occurred approximately 1% of the time.[112] The asymptomatic culture-diagnosed shedding definitely represents a potential infectious inoculum ($\sim 10^4$ viral particles). Further recent work with polymerase chain reaction (PCR) demonstrated that the shedding detectable by PCR occurred almost on a daily basis. From a transmission and public health standpoint, the implications of the PCR data are not fully understood. Asymptomatic shedding rates are increased in persons with HIV or other immunodeficiencies. For example, women with HSV- and HIV-induced immuno-suppression (CD4<200) had asymptomatic shedding 22% of the time.[113] The asymptomatic shedding issue presents particularly thorny problems in recommending disease-control strategies.

Epidemiology

Genital herpes is widely prevalent in the adult population in the United States. Because of the difficulty in differentiating recurrences from new infection, accurate incidence data are difficult to enumerate. The numbers of first-office consultation visits for genital herpes, which has been used as a surrogate, have been increasing since the late 1970s[114] (Figure 20–5). Periodic cross-sectional seroprevalence studies of HSV-2 have been useful. Once an individual is seropositive for HSV-2, that person is positive for life. Therefore, epidemiologic studies have focused on understanding the prevalence of infection. Incident infection is much harder to diagnose because of the requirement for documented seronegativity followed by seroconversion. Seropositivity for genital herpes begins to increase at 14 years of age (Figure 20–6). Seropositivity has been associated with increased numbers of sexual partners, minority race, and lower socioeconomic status. Interestingly, even when adjusting for reporting artifacts due to socioeconomic differences, African Americans still have substantially higher rates of HSV-2 seropositivity than other ethnic groups.

Seroprevalence studies using type-specific research grade assays have demonstrated that approximately one of six married, sexually active Americans (40 million) is infected with the herpes simplex virus,[115,116] most of whom are asymptomatic. Individuals who are asymptomatic shedders comprise the majority of primary HSV source contacts, ie, the patient from whom people with acute primary genital herpes got their disease.[117] Although asymptomatic shedding occurs only 1% to 2% of the time, the large numbers of infected individuals increase the attributable fraction of disease transmitted by asymptomatic shedders.

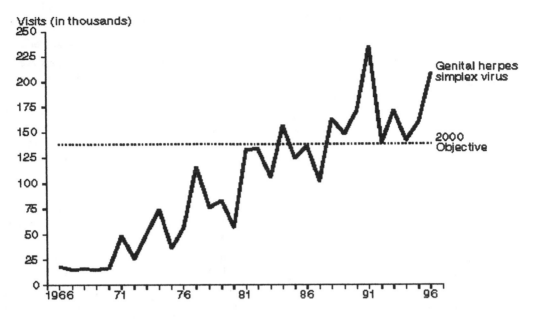

Figure 20–5 Genital herpes simplex virus infections—initial visits to physicians' offices: United States, 1966–1996 and the Healthy People year 2000 objective. *Source:* Reprinted from National Disease and Therapeutic Index (IMS America, Ltd.).

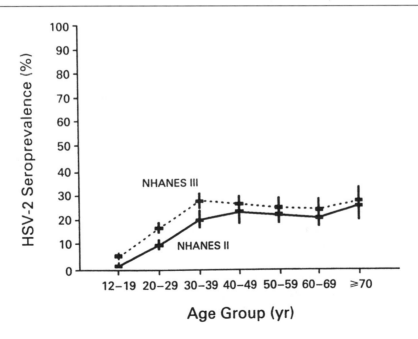

Figure 20–6 Herpes simplex virus (HSV)-2 seroprevalence according to age in NHANES II (1976 to 1980) and NHANES III (1988 to 1994). Bars indicate 95% confidence intervals (CIs). *Source:* Reprinted with permission from Fleming et al, Herpes Simplex Virus Type 2 in the United States, 1976 to 1994, *New England Journal of Medicine*, Vol. 337, pp. 1105–1111, Copyright © 1997, Massachusetts Medical Society. All rights reserved.

The epidemiology is determined by the natural history of the disease. Herpes simplex virus is the causative agent of genital herpes. Most genital infections are caused by HSV-2; however, in parts of the world, especially the United Kingdom, HSV-1 has been increasingly implicated as a causative agent for genital herpes. Nevertheless, the HSV-2 serostatus of individuals has been useful as a marker of sexual activity.

Clinical Manifestations

Classically, the ulcers have soft borders, are exquisitely painful, and are less than half a centimeter in diameter. The range of symptoms and signs includes small painless ulcerations that can be confused with folliculitis to large giant ulcerations, which can be confused with chancroid. In women, genital herpes can occur on the labium majora, labium minora, or the mucosal surfaces of the introitus. Vesicular and hemorrhagic cervicitis may also be seen, which can cause vaginal burning, discharge, and lower abdominal pain. Herpes occurs in the rectum and perirectal areas in individuals who have had receptive rectal intercourse. Because of involvement of the dorsal root ganglia, approximately 10% of patients will have lesions on adjacent dermatomes (such as L1, L2) in which lesions may be seen on the buttocks or lateral thighs.[118] These generally are due to referred or sympathetic lesions.

Diagnosis

Culture or other direct viral-specific tests, such as a direct fluorescent antibody or DNA probe, make the virologic diagnosis of herpes. Directly obtained specimens are easily typed into HSV-1 and HSV-2 using monoclonal antibody reagents. Serologic diagnosis of herpes previously had not been possible.[119] However, an ELISA assay (POC-it, HSV-2, Diagnology Inc, Research Triangle Park, NC), based on antibodies to glycoprotein G of HSV-2, has been licensed recently by the FDA, and is reported to be specific for HSV-2 infection.

Herpes Simplex in Pregnancy

Recurrent herpes during pregnancy[120] is not a severe clinical problem unless lesions are present in the birth canal at the time of delivery, which is an indication for a caesarean section. Another approach advocated by some obstetricians and perinatologists is routine cultures of the birth canal at parturition. If herpes simplex is diagnosed (which usually occurs by culture within 1 to 2 days), the infant can be started on prophylactic antiviral therapy.

The major risk in pregnant women is development of primary herpes during the last trimester of pregnancy. In those cases, up to one third of infants will be born with the neonatal herpes syndrome that can be fatal or lead to disability.[121] Fetal infection is presumed to occur transplacentally. Primary infection during pregnancy can occur *only* if the pregnant woman was previously uninfected and has an infected male partner. This is the type of setting where serologic diagnoses of previously unrecognized HSV would be useful.

Treatment

In acute primary or recurrent genital herpes, treatment with nucleoside analogs results in more rapid healing of symptoms and more rapid resolution of both viral shedding and the ulcer. Treatment, however, is not curative. Acyclovir, which has been used for treatment since 1982, has a long track record of efficacy and safety; it has recently become available in generic formulations. New recently approved drugs for the treatment of genital herpes include famciclovir and valacyclovir, both of which offer the advantages of less frequent dosing.

Suppressive Therapy

In individuals who have more than six recurrences of genital herpes per year, or who are profoundly immunosuppressed or have recurrent disease (such as those with advanced HIV disease, transplant recipients, or patients undergoing chemotherapy), suppressive therapy is indicated. Suppressive regimens are more than 90% protective in preventing recurrences.[122]

Intervention Strategies

From an epidemiologic and control perspective, a number of factors are associated with increased HSV transmission:

1. Asymptomatic viral shedding. Asymptomatic viral shedding is actually implicated in more than half of the cases of new primary herpes transmission. Therefore, patients, who are under the impression that if they are asymptomatic they are unlikely to shed virus, can present a clinical and public health problem by spreading HSV to their sexual partners.
2. Misclassification of herpes symptoms with those of other infections. Especially in women, herpes recurrences are confused with other vaginal infections, especially "yeast infections." Therefore, in situations where hepatic vaginitis is misdiagnosed, individuals who are symptomatic because of HSV-2 infection may spread HSV to their partners.
3. Studies in monogamous couples in which one partner is infected and the other uninfected (discordant) indicate that approximately 11% of partners will seroconvert per calendar year of exposure.[123] Studies have demonstrated that seroconversion is less likely to occur in the face of antiviral therapy. However, studies to document this are still under way and, even if implemented, this intervention would be extremely expensive.

HSV-2 has also been implicated in the transmission of HIV. Prospective and retrospective studies in the United States and abroad have demonstrated the presence of HSV-2, after adjusting for other behavioral and clinical risk factors, is an independent predictor of increased HIV seroconversion. These findings were demonstrated in large prospective studies conducted among Thai military recruits in the early 1990s as part of a generalized overall prevention campaign.[124] No evidence exists to suggest that HSV-2 transmission can be prevented by condoms. However, studying this issue is difficult because of the difficulty in documenting HIV-2 incidence, relatively low rates of seroconversion, and the need for a 100% condom use to prevent transmission, an objective that is seldom achieved consistently.

HUMAN PAPILLOMAVIRUS INFECTION

Human papillomaviruses (HPVs)[125,126] are small RNA viruses that have the unique capacity to cause chronic infection; they can cause malignant transformation, and they cannot be cultured in vitro, making diagnosis of subclinical infection difficult.[127]

More than 80 subtypes of HPV exist. The HPV types that most commonly infect the genital tract are HPV-6, -11, -16, and -18. HPV-6 and -11 have been termed low-risk types, as they are seldom associated with malignancy and, instead, occur on external surfaces of the vulva, anus, and vagina. In contrast, HPV-16 and -18 are frequently found in invasive cervical and other epithelial cancers and, thus, are classified as high-risk types.

The vast majority of HPV infections are asymptomatic. The genital HPV, which are transmitted sexually,[128] have been identified in skin as well as genital secretions. The incubation period is not well defined, although most authorities estimate that it is approximately 3 months, with a reported range of 3 weeks to 8 months. A small proportion of patients infected with genital subtypes will develop *condyloma acuminata*, or genital warts. These lesions are fleshy, nonvascular warts, caused by proliferation of the keratinized epithelium, that can occur anywhere on the external genitalia. In women, cervical warts are occasionally observed; in men, lesions may be present on the penis or inside the urethra.

Treatment for condylomata is based on tissue-destructive therapy. Genital warts are a proliferative epithelial process caused by HPV stimulation. In most cases, the proliferative epithelial lesion is benign and therapy for warts is mostly cosmetic. An eradication of HPV-containing tissue is impossible because grossly and histologically normal appearing tissues can be infected with HPV and cannot be detected unless specifically probed by DNA analysis. Therefore, the treatment of HPV genital wart lesions by traditional destructive methods such as liquid nitrogen or surgery has been associated with substantial recurrence rates because HPV infection is often present in the normal surgical margins.

It is estimated that approximately 1% of the sexually active population in the United States has clinically apparent genital warts; in STD clinic populations the percentage is much higher.[129] Trend data collected by the CDC suggest that the incidence has increased over the past 30 years. Studies that use colposcopic or cytologic examination as the basis for diagnosis yield higher prevalence estimates. Estimates of infection range from 20% to above 90%, depending on the specific populations studied, with college students,[130] adolescents,[131,132] and commercial sex workers demonstrating the highest rates. These prevalence data, therefore, strongly suggest that in many cases HPV infection will spontaneously resolve because prevalence decreases with age.

Over the past 20 years, HPV, especially subtypes HPV-16 and HPV-18,[133] have been strongly associated with the development of epithelial squamous cell carcinomas.[134–136] The sexually transmitted epithelial cancers include cervical carcinoma, vulvar carcinoma, some oral carcinomas, penile carcinoma, and anal carcinoma. Sexually transmitted HPV-associated anal and oral carcinomas are seen predominantly in homosexual men, and they are associated with HIV infection.[137]

In cervical cancer, HPV infection of the transition zone can cause a number of changes leading to malignant transformation. The hallmark of HPV infection is koilocytosis, a ballooning of the nuclear portion of the cervical epithelial cells. Left unchecked, this can lead to cervical atypia, early cervical malignant dysplasia, or frank malignant transformation. The latency period, especially in an immunocompetent host, from development of HPV infection to development of early cervical cancer is often 5 to 10 years. Advanced cervical cancer cases often take more than 20 years to develop. Therefore, clinical recommendations are focused more on reducing the risk of cervical cancer than on HPV infection, in large part because of the high prevalence of HPV infection. Furthermore, cervical cancer occurs in only a small minority of patients infected with HPV (Figure 20–7). However, HPV infection occurs early after sexual activity and is neither necessary nor sufficient for oncogenesis. Other risk factors for cervical cancer include early age at HPV infection, immunodeficiency, especially HIV infection, and smoking.[138] Hormonal con-

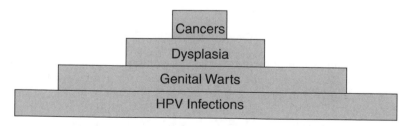

Figure 20–7 Human papillomavirus (HPV) pyramid

traceptives do not appear to play a major role in the development of cervical cancer.[139]

A continuum of HPV infection is seen, which includes asymptomatic HPV infection, development of genital warts, and development of malignancies. The continuum may have discontinuities in many patients. For example, it is not uncommon for patients who have never developed genital warts to develop cervical cancer. Similarly, most patients with genital warts do not progress to develop cervical cancer.

Clinical Screening for HPV—The Pap Smear Approach

Nearly all squamous cervical cancer is associated with HPV. Because of the long latency period, and the slow, local progression of squamous cell cervical cancer, screening for the disease is an effective prevention measure. Development of advanced cervical cancer should be considered a sentinel event of preventive screening and cause one to evaluate the cancer prevention program.

The CDC and the American Cancer Society recommend Pap smear screening every 3 years.[140] These programs have been found to be extremely effective in reducing the population-based morbidity and mortality from cervical cancer, but they are expensive interventions and require access to highly trained cytotechnologists. In HIV-infected women, screening is recommended every 6 months because of the more aggressive disease seen in these patients.[141] If cervical abnormalities are found, then further evaluation can be done, including colposcopy and, possibly, biopsy. External genital wart presence alone is not an indication for colposcopy. Although nucleic acid technologies are available, the utility of these tests in practice has yet to be shown.

Within a sexually active couple, implementing HPV prevention presents a number of important logistical and technical challenges. First, the infection in the male is not well characterized. Penile cancer is caused by HPV, but in the United States and other developed countries it

occurs at very low frequency. Asymptomatic infection in the male is common, and no clinical evidence exists to support routine screening, either using acetic acid techniques or other tissue-based techniques. Therefore, we are left with recommendations for consistent condom use, which may not be a practical option in couples who are monogamous and in a stable relationship.

VAGINAL INFECTIONS

When evaluating individuals with vaginal infections or vaginal discharge, it is imperative to differentiate primary vaginal infections from cervical infections presenting as vaginitis. Clinically, women often present with nonspecific symptoms of vaginal discharge or low abdominal pain; this needs to be differentiated from vaginal disease, cervical disease, or both. Gonococcal and chlamydial infections are the most common cause of cervical disease. Vaginitis has a number of causes including trichomoniasis, bacterial vaginosis, and candidiasis. Because candidiasis is not a sexually transmitted infection and has very few long-term health effects, this will not be considered here for the sake of brevity.

Trichomonas

Trichomonas infection occurs in approximately three million women annually. The causative agent, *Trichomonas vaginalis*, is a flagellated protozoan. Signs and symptoms include a watery vaginal discharge, punctate hemorrhagic lesions on the cervix, and occasionally a frank cervicitis occurring in response to the vaginal infection. Symptoms are exacerbated during the menses because the organism can ingest hemoglobin and replication is increased during that time. Trichomonas syndromes in men have not been systematically described until recently,[142,143] because clinical practice was (and still is) presumptively to treat all male contacts of women with trichomoniasis. Trichomoniasis does not produce systemic disease in the host.

Diagnosis

Wet mount is the most inexpensive and widely used method for diagnosis of trichomoniasis. However, culture or newer DNA-based methods may be as much as 50% more sensitive, especially in women or men with asymptomatic infection. The development of new testing techniques has resulted in alternative sampling strategies. Traditional approaches to STD diagnosis in women necessitate a direct speculum examination, which is necessary to visualize the vaginal mucosa and cervix, and for sampling of the fornix. The availability of nucleic acid–based diagnostic technology for gonorrhea and chlamydia diagnosis prompted speculation that a speculum examination was not necessary and that a swab of the distal vaginal vault provided adequate specimen material. Studies by Schwebke et al[144] in an Alabama STD clinic and Blake et al[145] in a Baltimore adolescent clinic used culture techniques and demonstrated sensitivity of 85% to 90% compared with speculum examination; in an obstetric population, Witkin and colleagues evaluated 300 women and found that the sensitivity of a distal vaginal swab evaluated by PCR was greater than 93%.[146]

Treatment for trichomoniasis is metronidazole (2 g) as a single dose,[147] which is considered safe for pregnant women.[148,149] Metronidazole resistance is occasionally reported.[150]

Epidemiology

Despite the availability of better diagnostic tests, basic understanding of the epidemiology of trichomoniasis has not changed greatly. Trichomoniasis has characteristics of both an incident and prevalent disease; however, because of the large number of asymptomatic infections, determination of incidence is difficult. The CDC bases trend estimates on physician office visits,[151] but notes the unreliability of these figures. Nevertheless, large population-based studies of prenatal clinic attendees[152] and STD clinic attendees have continued to find high rates of trichomonas infection (ie, 10% to 15% of all pa-

tients) even when only the relatively insensitive traditional methods of diagnosis are used. In contrast, the infection was seen in only 2% to 3% of an unselected college student population.[153] Trichomonas has been associated with a number of complications, including premature rupture of membranes, and potential facilitation of HIV infection. In men, trichomonas infections often are asymptomatic, but they can occasionally be implicated in cases of chlamydia-negative nongonococcal urethritis. Finally, because of the high prevalence of this infection, trichomonas has been implicated as important in the management of rape victims. In a large Seattle study, trichomoniasis was diagnosed in 12% of rape victims[154]; however, the authors acknowledged the difficulty in differentiating incident infection caused by the assault from a potential prevalent preexisting infection.

In men, studies from different locales have confirmed the role of trichomonas in urethritis. The prevalence of *Trichomonas* organisms (asymptomatic and symptomatic) in Seattle STD clinic attendees was 11%[155]; in East African truck drivers, it was 6.0%[156]; in a San Francisco area STD clinic, it was 12%[157]; and in a Durban, South African clinic population, it was 19%.

For many years, trichomoniasis was considered to be a nuisance. Although it causes symptoms that even occasionally can be disabling, it causes neither upper tract nor systemic disease. In an immunocompromised host (such as in HIV-infected women), the organism load of *Trichomonas* organisms may be higher, but no systemic disease occurs in these patients.

Recent studies, however, have demonstrated that in pregnancy, trichomonal infection can be a contributing factor to premature rupture of membranes (PROM) and consequent perinatal morbidity and mortality. The Vaginal Infections in Pregnancy Study (VIPS) evaluated 13,816 pregnant women.[158] Trichomoniasis was found in 3%[159] of women, and it was associated with other clinical findings of vaginal infection, such as elevated pH, vaginal discharge, and cervical friability. These findings demonstrate the difficulty of independently assessing trichomoniasis as a risk factor apart from bacterial vaginosis and chlamydia. Trichomoniasis was also an independent risk factor for PROM in women who had intercourse more than once per week during pregnancy.[160]

Trichomoniasis has also been associated with the development of pelvic inflammatory disease. A case control study of high-risk women in Brooklyn, New York,[161] found that in those infected with chlamydia, coexistent trichomoniasis infection was a significant risk factor in the development of PID. The exact causative mechanism is unclear, but this finding is epidemiologically important because in many STD clinic settings, the prevalence of trichomoniasis in women with chlamydia or gonococcal infection can approach 25%.

Relationship to HIV Infection

Exudative STD infection, such as gonorrhea and chlamydia, has been conclusively linked to enhanced transmission of HIV.[162] In a prospective study conducted among prostitutes in Zaire, trichomoniasis was found to be highly prevalent, but the association with HIV seroconversion was not statistically significant (odds ratio 1.9; 95% CI 0.9–4.1). However, because of the high co-infection rates with other STDs, it is difficult in these studies to separate out trichomoniasis as an independent risk.

BACTERIAL VAGINOSIS

Bacterial vaginosis (BV) is a disorder that occurs as a result of ecologic disturbances among the vaginal flora.[163] The normal vaginal flora consists overwhelmingly of lactobacilli. As a result, the vaginal environment is acidic with a pH of less than 4.5. In bacterial vaginosis, alteration of the microflora occurs, with the population of lactobacilli replaced by gram-negative rods and anaerobes.[164] As a result, the pH increases above 4.5, often to 7 or higher. The clinical manifestations include vaginal odor, discharge, and the microscopic appearance of clue cells, which are

epithelial cells with numerous anaerobes bound to the surface creating a "ground-glass" appearance. A "fishy" odor is often present because of the production of amine compounds by the anaerobic bacteria. Bacterial vaginosis most frequently presents secondary to another infectious or a metabolic or iatrogenic event.

Diagnosis of BV is made on either evaluation of a vaginal smear gram stain,[165] demonstrating the characteristic alteration of the vaginal flora, or on clinical criteria. The clinical criteria are three of the following: homogeneous vaginal discharge, pH greater than 4.5, presence of an amine odor, and presence of clue cells.[166] Treatment of BV includes antimicrobials effective against anaerobes (eg, metronidazole or clindamycin), which enables re-establishment of the normal vaginal microflora. Recurrences are common.

Bacterial vaginosis occurs most commonly as a secondary disorder (Figure 20–8). The most common causes of secondary BVs include:

1. Alteration of vaginal microflora as a result of cervical infection and subsequent inflammation. In many of these cases, resolution of the primary cervical infection can result in resolution of the BV.

2. Alteration of vaginal microflora as a result of antibiotic use. Tetracyclines and other commonly used broad spectrum antibiotics are especially implicated in these disorders.

3. Direct instillation into the vagina of microbicides and douches. Douching is particularly associated with development of BV. Therefore, clinical counseling includes a specific recommendation not to douche. In fact, vaginal douching is not clinically recommended at any time.

Patients are seen who have primary bacterial vaginosis (ie, BV without any identifiable cause). BV in these patients does resolve with treatment; however, BV recurs frequently in this class of patients. The cause in most of these cases is unknown.

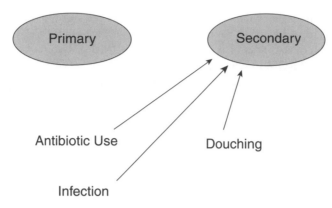

Figure 20–8 Bacterial vaginosis

The epidemiologic issues with BV are further complicated by the fact that BV occurs more frequently in sexually active women. However, correlative infectious conditions in the male partner have never been demonstrated. Sexual transmission of BV has been demonstrated to occur in lesbian patients. Treatment of bacterial vaginosis is fairly straightforward and involves specific antibiotic therapy against the anaerobic component of the BV pathogenic flora, allowing replacement with the normal lactobacilli.

Bacterial vaginosis has also been demonstrated to be a risk factor for premature rupture of membranes and premature delivery.[167–169] A large multicenter study found that, in a population of more than 10,000 women, the prevalence of BV was 16%. The adjusted odds ratio of BV and delivery of a preterm low birth weight infant was 1.4.[170] A follow-up study conducted by the same group found that treatment of BV in pregnant women reduced the BV-associated preterm risk by one half to two thirds.[171] BV was also demonstrated to be more common in black women, for reasons that are not completely clear.[172] After adjusting for maternal parity, age, education, insurance status, marital status, smoking, age at first intercourse, and number of male partners in the past year, the odds ratio for bacterial vaginosis in blacks compared with whites was 2.9. BV has also been associated with an increased incidence of postsurgical infections, including increased PID incidence after first trimester abortion,[173] and cellulitis after hysterectomy.[174] In addition, BV has recently been demonstrated to be a risk factor for HIV infection in women. This may be as a result of specific cultural practices, such as dry sexual intercourse.[175] However, further work is required in this area to conclusively define the issue.

PELVIC INFLAMMATORY DISEASE

Pelvic inflammatory disease[176,177] actually represents a constellation of syndromes, including endometritis, oophoritis, and pelvic peritonitis. PID is a poorly defined syndrome, in part because it is a soft tissue infection, affecting multiple organs, with no clearly defined diagnostic criteria.

The microbiology of upper urinary tract genital infection is complex.[178,179] Organisms that are isolated from the upper urinary tract, for example at laparoscopy or surgery, include *Neisseria gonorrhoeae, Chlamydia trachomatis,* organisms associated with the vaginal flora (eg, *Streptococcus* [group B], *Gardnerella, E. coli, Veilonella),* intraabdominal colonic organisms (eg, *Bacteroides),* and other anaerobes. The pathophysiologic progression[180] of PID is hypothesized to be a sexually transmitted lower genital tract (cervical) infection causing breakdown of the normal defense mechanisms, followed by ascent of bacteria into the uterus, fallopian tubes, and periovarian areas causing consequent inflammation (Figure 20–9).

Although sepsis can occur, mortality is rare in women with PID, probably because it is often a localized infection in an otherwise healthy age group. The tissue inflammation caused by PID often results in tubal scarring, which is the cause of the major sequelae of infertility and increased risk of ectopic pregnancy. The consequences of PID were elegantly shown by Westrom et al in a large cohort of Swedish women.[181,182] He diagnosed all cases of PID by laparoscopy (the "gold standard" diagnostic procedure) and followed them for over 25 years—from adolescence through the childbearing years. Findings in these

studies were 10% of women with one PID episode, 25% of those who had two episodes, and more than 60% of women with three episodes had tubal infertility. The relative risk of ectopic pregnancy for women with a history of PID was more than 10-fold higher when they were compared with women without an episode of PID.[183] Because these complications occur long after the initial disease process, the epidemics of infertility and ectopic pregnancy reflect the initial epidemic of gonorrhea or chlamydial infection after a substantial latency period. PID results in substantial economic costs in terms of direct medical costs, hospitalization costs related to the acute episode, and future costs related to infertility and ectopic pregnancy. Even after appropriately discounting the future costs, the cost of pelvic inflammatory disease in 1992 was an estimated $6 billion.

In the United States, an estimated 500,000 to 1,000,000 cases of PID occur annually[184] (Figure 20–10). Ascertainment of disease burden is difficult because the PID syndrome is not a reportable disease. Changes in the health care system have emphasized outpatient management of STDs. Therefore, although hospital discharges for PID since 1990 have dropped sharply, these data are unreliable because of the confounding caused by changing practice patterns.

Pelvic inflammatory disease is associated with several risk factors, including adolescence,[185] increased number of sexual partners, a previous episode of PID, use of an intrauterine device, and douching.[186] Clinical criteria traditionally used for diagnosis include two of three major criteria: lower abdominal pain, adnexal tenderness, or fever. Some have also added the presence of a lower genital tract infection (gonococcal or chlamydial cervicitis). Careful studies of clinical criteria, when compared with laparoscopy as the standard, found that the sensitivity and specificity of clinical criteria are 60% to 70% in expert hands.[187] Up to one fourth of PID cases may manifest no symptoms, especially when the disease is associated with chlamydia.[188] Therefore, many practitioners currently treat

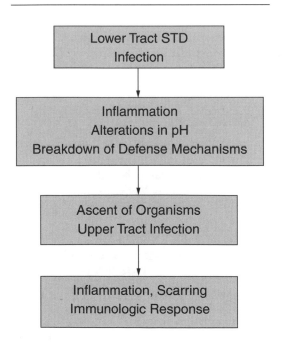

Figure 20–9 Pelvic inflammatory disease pathogenesis (STD, sexually transmitted diseases)

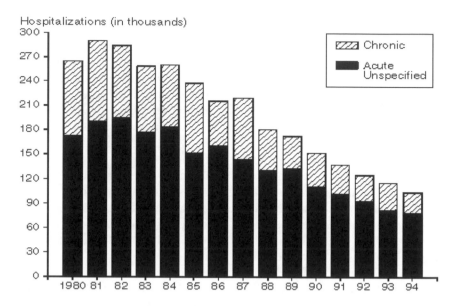

Figure 20–10 Pelvic inflammatory disease—hospitalizations of women aged 15–44 years: United States, 1980–1994. *Source:* Reprinted from National Hospital Discharge Survey (National Center for Health Statistics), Centers for Disease Control and Prevention.

women with mild cervical motion tenderness with regimens that are effective against PID, assuming that the benefit of preventing or curing early PID outweighs the increased cost of treatment, and potential side effects of antibiotics.[189]

Treatment strategies for PID are based on the underlying microbiology, which need to include antimicrobial coverage for *N. gonorrhoeae, C. trachomatis*, streptococci, gram-negative rods, and anaerobes. Treatment regimens, therefore, are complex[190,191] and beyond the scope of this chapter. Despite efforts to develop effective antimicrobial regimens, treatment efficacy has been difficult to assess. Most clinical treatment studies use clinical criteria to determine efficacy, despite the limitations of clinical diagnosis. Therefore, these studies are subject to both type I and type II statistical error. Furthermore, although the morbidity of PID is long term, few treatment studies have correlated effective anti-

microbial therapy with better long-term outcomes in terms of reduced incidence of infertility and ectopic pregnancy.

Treatment of acute PID is secondary prevention.[192] The consensus for primary prevention is that reducing gonococcal and chlamydial infections is the most effective approach. Screening interventions for chlamydia in the United States and in other countries[193] have demonstrated PID reductions of greater than 60%.

CONTROL OF SEXUALLY TRANSMITTED DISEASES AS AN HIV PREVENTION INTERVENTION

Epidemiologic Relationships

As a sexually transmitted disease, HIV transmission is facilitated by the same risk behaviors as those associated with the traditional STDs (eg, multiple sexual partners, sex with prostitutes, and drug-using sexual partners).[194] Because of these behavioral confounders, it has been difficult to establish a causal link between STDs and HIV infection. Cross-sectional and prospective studies in both the developed and developing worlds have firmly established that bacterial and viral STDs are biologic cofactors in facilitating HIV transmission. Multiple factors contribute to this biologic relationship, including:

1. Facilitated access to the vascular portal of entry. HIV has been cultured from the base of genital ulcers[195] in persons with coexistent genital ulcer disease and HIV infection. Similarly, mucosal inflammation caused by STDs, increased cervical friability[196] induced by STDs, or hormonal contraceptives may reduce the barriers to vascular entry.

2. Recruitment of target cells. STDs such as syphilis and chlamydia induce a lymphocytic response. Theoretically, recruitment of an increased number of CD4 target lymphocytes into an area exposed to HIV could facilitate infection.

3. Potentiation of HIV replication. Studies have demonstrated that HIV replication is potentiated by the presence of HSV (viral transactivation). Recent human challenge studies of gonorrhea in HIV-infected men demonstrated that gonococcal infection increases HIV shedding by 2 logs (100-fold increase).[197] These studies suggest that the presence of other STDs may increase the innoculum size beyond the threshold required for infectivity.

4. HIV subtype. HIV subtype C and E have been reported to preferentially infect Langerhan's epithelial cells, which are found on surfaces (eg, mucosal and skin). Subtype E has been found to predominate in areas where heterosexual transmission is common, such as in Southeast Asia and India. STDs, by disrupting the epithelial barrier, may facilitate contact with the Langerhan's target cells. However, other

investigators, using somewhat different methods, have not confirmed the initial report of increased affinity of HIV subtype E strains for cells. Whether different HIV-1 genotypes differ in their infectivity by sexual contact remains an open question.

Genital Ulcer Disease

Studies of HIV prevalence have demonstrated a three- to fivefold increased odds for HIV-positivity in a variety of patient populations with genital ulcer disease.[198] Initial studies, in gay men,[199] were conducted in the early 1980s. Genital ulcer disease became less of an issue in this population because of the precipitous decrease in STD incidence during that decade. In contrast, HIV transmission facilitated by genital ulcers is important, especially in developing countries, or in impoverished areas of developed countries. These populations included Baltimore syphilis patients,[200] homosexual men with genital ulcers,[199] and Kenyan STD clinic attendees in whom the majority of genital ulcer infections were caused by chancroid.[201,202] In the Nairobi studies, the cross-sectional HIV seroprevalence in persons with genital ulcers was 27% to 33%. In Baltimore, STD clinic patients with syphilis had HIV seroprevalence rates three to four times that of the general STD clinic population.[203,204] In a large survey of New York City STD clinic patients, HIV seroprevalence was found to be 16% in those with genital ulcers, whereas no epidemiologic relationship was demonstrated for nongenital ulcer disease.[205]

For genital herpes, establishing the relationship with HIV seroconversion requires reference-based serologic methods, because most HSV infections are asymptomatic. Early studies in blood donor populations[206] and STD clinic clients have established that serologic evidence of genital herpes[207] is associated with a two- to threefold increased odds ratio for HIV infection. Most prospective studies of genital ulcers and the risk for HIV infection have been performed in commercial sex workers (CSWs) or STD clients. In Kenya, where the population-based prevalence rate for persons aged 15 to 44 years is between 10% and 30%, the 6-month seroconversion rate for prostitutes with genital ulcers was 12%.[208] In India, the overall population-based incidence of HIV was more than twofold greater in CSWs. Prospectively, genital ulcer disease was associated with a sevenfold increased HIV seroconversion risk[209]; similar results were found in a large prospective study of Thai army recruits, which utilized history of a genital ulcer and seropositivity.[210] In the United States, a prospective study conducted among heterosexual patients in a Bronx STD clinic during a chancroid outbreak found that HIV seroconversion risk was threefold greater in men with a genital ulcer compared with those without genital ulcer disease.[99]

Gonorrhea and Chlamydia

Studies of gonococcal and chlamydial infection are complicated by the high prevalence and incidence of these infections.[211] The cross-sectional Nairobi prostitute studies suggested a twofold increased HIV risk among patients with chlamydia; however, this relationship was not stable in a multivariate analysis.[152,153] In Baltimore, a case control study of HIV seroconverters found a threefold increased risk in patients who had a diagnosis of gonorrhea at their last STD clinic visit prior to seroconversion.[212] Prospective studies in India[160] and Zaire[213] conclusively demonstrated an association between exudative STD and HIV seroconversion. In the Zaire study, prostitutes with chlamydia had a 4.6 relative risk of seroconversion; for those with gonorrhea, the relative risk was 3.6. However, both relationships were stable after controlling for other confounding variables. From a population perspective, gonorrhea and chlamydial infection may be more important risk factors because they can be associated with a higher attributable fraction of HIV seroconversion cases. For example, the Baltimore investigators,

whose population included a large number of intravenous drug users, concluded that the adjusted attributable fraction of HIV seroconversions related to coexistent gonococcal infection was 18%.

USE OF EPIDEMIOLOGIC MODELS TO GUIDE CONTROL EFFORTS

Epidemiologic models[214] for STD control are based on the May and Anderson concepts of microparasites. STDs form a unique subset, because exposure risk is not random, but is determined by exposure to new sexual partners. These sexual partner characteristics, or "mixing" patterns, become critically important. These models are based on the reproductive rate equation, $R_0 = \beta CD$, where β equals the transmission coefficient, C equals the turnover of partners, and D equals the duration of infection. As long as the reproductive rate remains above 1, the number of cases will be expected to increase; conversely, control efforts are directed toward decreasing either one or all of the constituent terms of the reproductive rate equation to drive the reproductive rate below 1.

Interventions specifically designed to decrease the transmission efficiency (β) include the use of barrier methods of contraception, microbicides, and condoms. Although most interventions reduce the transmission efficiency, public health epidemiologists need to be aware that occasionally, unanticipated effects can occur. For example, vaginal microbicides have been well documented to reduce the transmission efficiency of gonococcal and chlamydial infection; however, an increasing body of data suggests that vaginal microbicides may actually increase HIV transmission. Therefore, in a population with high HIV exposure potential, vaginal microbicides may not be appropriate. Nevertheless, continued research on the development and evaluation of safe and effective vaginal microbicides to prevent HIV is critically important.[226] Because these microbicides are under control of the women and can be inserted some time prior to intercourse, they have potential to be important in preventing transmission in some situations.[222] Similarly, hormonal contraceptives may also increase the potential for HIV transmission among women who are exposed. STDs similarly increased the transmission efficiency of HIV in most settings.

The variable C—the partner turnover—includes components related to the number of different partners to which an individual is exposed, thereby increasing the statistical risk of STD exposure, as well as the number of exposures with each partner (or dose). This variable is quite complex. From a simplistic standpoint, the most effective intervention would be to reduce this term to 0, which would negate the entire reproductive rate equation. This is the abstention model, which is impractical in most circumstances. Nevertheless, a reduction in the number of partner exposures through risk intervention, risk reduction, education, and counseling can have a substantial impact on the reproductive rate equation. Particularly effective use of these measures has been demonstrated recently in Thailand where reduction of high-risk exposures among Thai army recruits, both in terms of reducing partner exposures and increasing condom use rates, resulted in decreased STD incidence and HIV seroconversion.[236,237] From a qualitative standpoint, one criticism of this model has been that the quality of partners may be just as important as the quantity of partners. For example, commercial sex workers may be particularly high-risk partners in most settings for disease transmission and, therefore, qualitative factors need to be attached to the equation.

Reducing the duration of infection can also decrease the reproductive rate. Reducing the duration of infection is a practical option for curable diseases. Thus, it does not include the chronic viral diseases such as HIV, herpes simplex, and HPV. However, one could argue that antiviral medications, which reduce the load viral burden and shedding, actually have an important impact on the β term (transmission efficiency). Interventions that reduce infection duration, remove individuals from the infected pool, and reduce exposure opportunities for the population include population-based screening programs, effective treatment guidelines based on population base data, and partner notification. All of these interventions are driven by the goal to reduce the risks of exposure to asymptomatic infected individuals in the population.

Examples

STD Control as an HIV Intervention

The epidemiologic evidence suggests that control of STDs can reduce HIV seroincidence.[215] Because behavioral change is a long-term and incremental process, this option is increasingly attractive. A large population-based study in Tanzania has demonstrated that this can be a feasible approach.[216] In the Tanzanian study, STD clinical facilities were upgraded, and drug treatment regimens were improved to be in concordance with World Health Organization treatment guidelines.[217] In control communities, no changes were made. This intervention resulted in a 42% decrease in HIV seroconversions after 2 years, despite no change in sexual behavior patterns or condom use rates. Most of the decrease resulted from either decreased STD incidence or duration of STD infections. Another controlled trial of mass prophylaxis of STD with a combination of antibiotics given at 10-month intervals found no effect on HIV incidence, although the prevalence and incidence of treatable bacterial STDs were reduced significantly. In this population in the Rakai district of Uganda, the HIV prevalence and incidence were much higher than in Tanzania and the attributable risk of STDs for HIV incidence was lower than in the Tanzanian population.

Prevention Issues Specific to Women

Women are at higher risk for HIV and STD transmission because of both biologic and behavioral factors. During unprotected intercourse, women are potentially exposed to a higher inoculum through ejaculation than their male partner. Furthermore, the contact time between the mucosal surfaces and infectious secretions is longer for women exposed to an infected man than the reverse situation. Changes in the vaginal and cervical mucosa through inflammation or hormonally induced alterations can increase the tissue's friability and susceptibility to infection. Hormonal contraceptives have been epidemiologically associated with increased risk of HIV transmission,[218] which coincidentally causes a major policy dilemma in developing countries where overpopulation and the HIV epidemic coexist.

Nevertheless, women are at significant risk. In many sexual relationships, women may not be able to refuse sexual relations or require their male partner to use a condom because of either economic circumstance or fear of physical or emotional abuse.[219,220] For example, commercial sex workers may be at an economic disadvantage if the client's preference is for unprotected intercourse. These issues have intensified the need to develop female-controlled disease-prevention methods.

Female Condoms. Female condoms are one approach that has been approved in the United States since 1993. The female condom, which is inserted prior to intercourse, is a double-ring latex pouch with one ring adjacent to the cervix and the other to the introitus.[221] Evaluations of the device have been mixed. Cost is the major barrier to its increased use, with the per device cost ranging from $1 to $3 in the United States.

Vaginal Microbicides. Microbicides should demonstrate physical and chemical stability in the vaginal environment, allowing insertion some time before intercourse, should not interfere with sexual intercourse, and should also be inexpensive.[222] The ideal compound would be toxic to bacterial and viral pathogens and nontoxic to the host epithelium. Aside from the potential toxicity to host epithelium, another consideration is the potential effect on the commensal vaginal microflora, and the development of bacterial vaginosis and inflammation. To date, the available vaginal microbicides are chemical, water-soluble detergents that can solubilize the lipid membranes of bacteria and spermatozoa. Nonoxynol-9, which is the prototype, is effective against common bacterial STD pathogens.[223,224] However, studies in African prostitutes have demonstrated that nonoxynol-9 causes genital ulcer disease, which is associated with an increased risk of HIV seroconversion, most likely because of the chemical irritation of the vaginal mucosa.[225] Therefore, interest has increased in developing chemically stable, buffered, nonionic compounds with the potential for use as vaginal microbicide.[226]

INTERVENTIONS TO REDUCE THE RISK OF SEXUAL EXPOSURE THROUGH PROMOTING CONDOM USE

Condom Efficacy

Promoting condom use has been one of the central tenets of the HIV and STD risk-reduction strategy, both in the United States and abroad. Extensive programs have been developed to ensure the timely distribution of large numbers of condoms, and instructions for condom use have been part of the national STD guidelines since 1989.[227] Condoms are effective when used correctly and consistently. Studies of HIV discordant heterosexual couples in California[228] and Italy[229,230] have conclusively demonstrated that consistent condom use in controlled settings results in an approximately sevenfold decrease in HIV seroconversions. Condoms are also effective in reducing the risk of sexually transmitted diseases,[231] which further reduces the risk of HIV transmission.

Studies of condom use have focused on understanding the determinants and issues related to their use, especially considering the low consistent use rate reported in national surveys. Increased condom use is influenced by the appreciation of a perceived benefit (ie, STD/HIV prevention), peer group social norms, and exposure to sex education with specific instruction in condom use.[232–234] It is difficult to maintain the perceived benefit of prevention behaviors, such as consistent condom use, because prevention is effective when no adverse events occur. An absence of events is not as reinforcing as the self-reinforcing behaviors of other strategies such as commercial marketing. As with other sex education programs, promoting condom use has not been found to increase sexual activity in adolescents or to result in earlier sexual debut.[235] Effective condom promotion requires integration of public health and social marketing efforts. Probably the most intensive and successful effort has been implemented in Thailand, where the "100% Condom" program,[236] which has been implemented since 1991, includes intensive advertising, an infrastructure to purchase and distribute condoms, and linkages in promoting condoms with stakeholders, including the Army, provincial and municipality governments, and commercial sex workers. Recent large-scale reductions in HIV seroincidence in Thailand have been attributed, in part, to this program.[237] The Thai program provides a useful model of the development of an effective condom promotion and sexual risk-reduction campaign. The program includes open discussion of HIV prevention and condom promotion, mass media campaigns, and the active participation of a large variety of stakeholders, including the military, government, medical community, and even the brothels. This effective program's major accomplishment was to change the social norms across a broad spectrum of society to encourage condom use.

CORE GROUPS AND TARGETING

Besides the mathematical approaches, designing control strategies also requires assessing the impact or sociogeographic effects. STDs predominantly affect specific demographic subgroups. Within the broad population strata, STDs are often concentrated in areas where poverty and other limitations on health care access exist. This has resulted in development of the "core-group" concept.[238] The core groups are population subgroups disproportionately impacted by STDs, and which often act as the endemic reservoir of disease within a community.

These may be either sociologically or geographically defined. For example, in East Africa, the predominant core groups are long-distance truck drivers and commercial sex workers, whereas in the United States, often the direct link is to drug use.[239,240]

In the United States and Western Europe, core groups are often defined geographically as residents of defined core areas that typically are socioeconomically depressed. In the urban environment of the United States, core areas have been well documented for gonorrhea,[241–246] syphilis, and HIV. Within a core area, disease incidence can be 20 to 30 times that of surrounding areas. For example, in Baltimore we have identified discrete core areas wherein the reported gonorrhea rate in 1994 for persons aged 15 to 39 years was 6,821/100,000 for men and 4,341/100,000 for women,[247] and areas where primary and secondary syphilis incidence had similar disproportionate high rates (Figure 20–11). The geographic core concept appears to be most relevant to "incident STDs" such as gonorrhea, syphilis, and chancroid, but it is probably not as relevant for chronic viral STDs. At present, chlamydia has the characteristics of a chronic infection—with diffuse population-based prevalence patterns. However, with the institution of control programs, this will probably change.

The transmission efficiency of gonorrhea and syphilis through unprotected sexual exposure has been empirically estimated to be 30% to 50% per exposure, and treatment effectively breaks the transmission chain. Therefore, under most circumstances, introduction of gonorrhea into a community free of infection should not result in a sustained epidemic. Community-based models of STD transmission, therefore, postulate that core areas or epidemiologically defined core groups are critical to maintaining high rates of gonorrhea.[248,249] In these models, cores are characterized by a high transmission density,[250] an empiric function that is dependent on characteristics of the sexual network. In contrast to many other infectious diseases, STD transmission is dependent on behavior (ie, sexual intercourse).

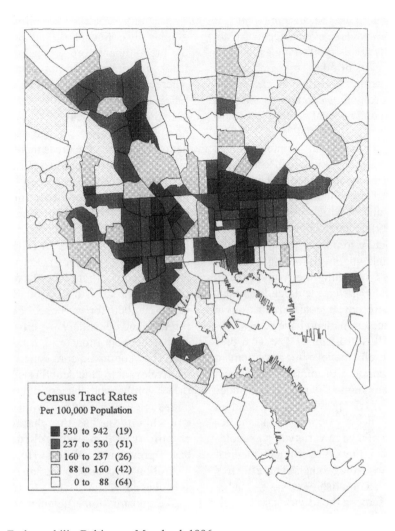

Census Tract Rates
Per 100,000 Population

■ 530 to 942 (19)
■ 237 to 530 (51)
▨ 160 to 237 (26)
□ 88 to 160 (42)
□ 0 to 88 (64)

Figure 20–11 Early syphilis, Baltimore, Maryland, 1996

STD transmission, therefore, is limited to sexual networks (ie, the interrelated sexual connections of a defined social group).[251–253]

Analyses of sexual networks provide a rational basis for defining transmissibility to susceptible sexual partners.[254] A sexual network is composed of the interrelated sexual connections of a defined social group. In a dense sexual network exist multiple pathways between sexual partners, leading to multiple sources for disease exposure.[255]

Based on the theory of core groups, two approaches to STD control are being studied—social networks and GIS-targeted screening.

Social Networks

Traditional STD intervention approaches have used partner notification as a major tool in control programs. As discussed, for diseases such as gonorrhea—with a short incubation period—or diseases with prolonged latency periods (asymptomatic infection) that are efficiently transmitted (eg, chlamydia), partner notification may not work. In contrast, syphilis has been traditionally controlled with partner notification using the rationale of the "critical period." As a control tool, however, partner notification has never been fully and formally evaluated. In settings wherein partners are not named (eg, in drug-related prostitution), the process fails.

New approaches have utilized understanding the social network (ie, sexual partners). These are individuals who are associated with the infected patient in a variety of everyday activities (not limited to sex partner) as opposed to traditional STD control efforts that attempt to identify the current sexual partner solely through case interviews. These approaches appear to be successful in identifying additional infected persons.

GIS Targeted Screening

Sexually transmitted diseases, especially syphilis and gonorrhea, are associated with a host of adverse socioeconomic indicators. In the United States, these are often correlated with residential housing patterns. In highly impacted areas, STD rates, evaluated by census tract, may be an order of magnitude higher than that of surrounding areas. For example, gonorrhea rates in adolescents in the inner-city areas of Baltimore, Washington, Miami, and similar settings can be as high as 10,000 to 15,000/100,000. In these densely populated, highly impacted areas, geographically directed screening interventions represent a potential control option.

CONCLUSION

Sexually transmitted diseases have a major impact, including direct medical costs, indirect medical costs, and facilitation of HIV infection. They are predominantly asymptomatic. Traditional intervention strategies for STDs have been oriented toward four goals:

1. Reducing the potential for exposure through both modifying risky behavior patterns and primary STD prevention.
2. Reducing the infected pool of individuals through screening programs.
3. Providing treatment-based regimens that are known to be effective.
4. Treating infected partners through contact notification.

REFERENCES

1. Eng TR, Butler WT. *The Hidden Epidemic—Confronting Sexually Transmitted Diseases.* Washington, DC: National Academy Press; 1997.

2. Brunham RC, Plummer FA. A general model of sexually transmitted disease epidemiology and its implications for control. *Med Clinics North Am.* 1990;74:1339–1352.

3. Centers for Disease Control and Prevention. *1996 Sexually Transmitted Disease Surveillance.* Washington, DC: US Government Printing Office; 1998.

4. Cates W Jr. Epidemiology and control of sexually transmitted disease in adolescents. In: Schydlower M, Shafer MA, eds. *AIDS and Other Sexually Transmitted Diseases.* Philadelphia: Hanly & Belfus; 1990:409–427.

5. Anderson RM. The transmission dynamics of sexually transmitted diseases: the behavioral component. In: Wasserheit JN, Aral SO, Holmes KK, et al, eds. *Research Issues in Human Behavioral and Sexually Transmitted Diseases in the AIDS Era.* Washington, DC: American Society for Microbiology; 1991.

6. Cates W Jr. Contraception, unintended pregnancies, and sexually transmitted diseases: why isn't a simple solution possible? *Am J Epidemiol.* 1996;143:311–318.

7. Hofferth SL, Kahn JR, Baldwin W. Premarital sexual activity among U.S. teenage women over the past three decades. *Fam Plann Prospect.* 1987;19:46–53.

8. Kost K, Forrest JD. American women's sexual behavioral and exposure to risk of sexually transmitted diseases. *Fam Plann Prospect.* 1992;24:244–254.

9. Potter LB, Anderson JE. Patterns of condom use and sexual behavior among never-married women. *Sex Transm Dis.* 1993;20:201–208.

10. Arvidson M, Kallings I, Nilsson S, Hellberg D, Mardh P-A. Risky behavior in women with history of casual travel sex. *Sex Transm Dis.* 1997;24:418–421.

11. Cooksey EC, Rindfuss RR, Guilkey DK. The initiation of adolescent sexual and contraceptive behavior during changing times. *J Health Soc Behav.* 1996;37(1):59–74.

12. Abma JC, Chandra A, Mosher WD, Peterson L, Piccinino L. Fertility, family planning, and women's health: New data from the 1995 National Survey of Family Growth. National Center for Health Statistics. *Vital Health Statistics.* 1997;23(19).

13. Centers for Disease Control and Prevention. Youth risk behavior surveillance—United States, 1997. *MMWR.* 1998;47:SS-3.

14. Wasserheit JN, Aral SO.The dynamic topology of sexually transmitted disease epidemics: implications for prevention strategies. *J Infect Dis.* 1996;174(Suppl 2): S201–S213.

15. Aral SO. The social context of syphilis persistence in the southeastern United States. *Sex Transm Dis.* 1996; 23(1):9–15.

16. Moses S, Manji F, Bradley JE, Nagelkerke NJ, Malisa MA, Plummer FA. Impact of user fees on attendance at a referral center for sexually transmitted diseases in Kenya. *Lancet.* 1992;22;340(8817):463–466.

17. Tichonova L. Epidemics of syphilis in the Russian federation: trends, origins, and priorities for control. *Lancet.* 1997;350:210.

18. Moses S, Muia E, Bradley JE, et al. Sexual behavior in Kenya: implications for sexually transmitted disease transmission and control. *Soc Sci Med.* 1994;39:1649–1656.

19. Nagelkerke NJ, Brunham RC, Moses S, Plummer FA. Estimating the effective rate of sex partner change from individuals with sexually transmitted diseases. *Sex Transm Dis.* 1994;21:226–230.

20. Gangakhedkar RR, Bentley ME, Divekar AD, et al. Spread of HIV infection in married monogamous women in India. *JAMA.* 1997;278:2090–2092.

21. Edlin BR, Irwin KL, Faruque S, et al. Intersecting epidemics—crack cocaine use and HIV infection among inner-city young adults. Multicenter Crack Cocaine and HIV Infection Study Team. *N Engl J Med.* 1994;331: 1422–1427.

22. Minkoff HL, McCalla S, Delke I, Stevens R, Salwen M, Feldman J. The relationship of cocaine use to syphilis and human immunodeficiency virus infections among inner city parturient women. *Am J Obstet Gynecol.* 1990;163:521–526.

23. Chirgwin K, DeHovitz JA, Dillon S, McCormack WM. HIV infection, genital ulcer disease, and crack cocaine use among patients attending a clinic for sexually transmitted diseases. *Am J Public Health.* 1991;81:1576–1579.

24. Telzak EE, Chiasson MA, Bevier PJ, Stoneburner RL, Castro KG, Jaffe HW. HIV-1 seroconversion in patients with and without genital ulcer disease. *Ann Intern Med.* 1993;119:1181–1186.

25. Zenilman JM. Ethnicity and sexually transmitted diseases. *Curr Opin Infect Dis (London).* 1998;11:47–52.

26. Centers for Disease Control and Prevention, Division of HIV/STD Prevention. *1996 Sexually Transmitted Disease Surveillance Report.* Atlanta: Centers for Disease Control and Prevention; 1997. Also available online at http://wonder.cdc.gov/rchtml/Convert/STD/ Title3600.html.

27. Hook EW III, Zenilman JM. Gonorrhea. In: Gorbach S, Bartlett JG, Blacklow N, eds. *Infectious Disease.* 2nd ed. Philadelphia: W.B. Saunders; 1998:969–974.

28. Sherrard J, Barlow D. Gonorrhea in men: clinical and diagnostic aspects. *Genitourin Med.* 1996;72:422–426.

29. McNagny SE, Parker RM, Zenilman JM, Lewis JS. Evaluation of urinary leukocyte esterase as a screening test for the detection of asymptomatic *Chlamydia trachomatis* and *Neisseria gonorrhoeae* in men. *J Infect Dis.* 1992;165:573–576.

30. Platt R, Rice PA, McCormack WM. Risk of acquiring gonorrhea and prevalence of abnormal adnexal findings among women recently exposed to gonorrhea. *JAMA.* 1983;250:3205–3209.

31. Wasserheit JN, Bell TA, Kiviat NB, et al. Microbial causes of proven pelvic inflammatory disease and efficacy of clindamycin and tobramycin. *Ann Intern Med.* 1986;104:187–193.

32. McCormack WM, Nowroozi K, Alpert G. Acute pelvic inflammatory disease: characteristics of patients with gonococcal and non-gonococcal infection and evaluation of their response to aqueous penicillin G and spectinomycin hydrochloride. *Sex Transm Dis.* 1977;4:125–131.

33. Bowie WR, Jones H. Acute pelvic inflammatory disease in outpatients: association with *Chlamydia trachomatis* and *Neisseria gonorrhoeae. Ann Intern Med.* 1981;95: 685–688.

34. Washington AE, Aral SO, Hanssen P-O, Grimes DA, Holmens KK. Assessing risk for pelvic inflammatory disease and its sequelae. *JAMA.* 1991;266:2581–2686.

35. Hillis SD, Joesoef R, Marchbanks PA, Wasserheit JN, Cates W Jr, Westrom L. Delayed care for pelvic inflammatory disease and a risk factor for impaired fertility. *Am J Obstet Gynecol.* 1993;168:1503–1509.

36. Washington AE, Katz P. Cost and payment source for pelvic inflammatory disease. *JAMA.* 1991;266:2565–2569.

37. Jaffe HW, Biddle JW, Johnson SR, Wiesner PJ. Infec-

tions due to penicillinase-producing *Neisseria gonorrhoeae* in the United States. *J Infect Dis.* 1981; 144:191–197.

38. Rolfs RT, Galaid EI, Zaidi AA. Pelvic inflammatory disease: trends in hospitalization and office visits: 1979 through 1988. *Am J Obstet Gynecol.* 1992;166:983–990.

39. Lebedeff DA, Hochman EB. Rectal gonorrhea in men: diagnosis and treatment. *Ann Intern Med.* 1980;92:463–466.

40. Centers for Disease Control. Declining rates of rectal and pharyngeal gonorrhea among males—New York City. *MMWR.* 1984;33:295–297.

41. Centers for Disease Control and Prevention. Gonorrhea among men who have sex with men—selected sexually transmitted disease clinics: 1993–1996. *MMWR.* 1997; 46:889–892.

42. Wiesner PJ, Tronca E, Bonin P, Pedersen AHB, Holmes KK. Clinical spectrum of pharyngeal gonococcal infection. *N Engl J Med.* 1973;288:181–185.

43. Hutt DM, Judson FN. Epidemiology and treatment of oropharyngeal gonorrhea. *Ann Intern Med.* 1986;104: 655–658.

44. Wise CM, Morris CR, Wasilauskas BL, Salzer WL. Gonococcal arthritis in an era of increasing penicillin resistance. *Arch Intern Med.* 1994;154:2690–3695.

45. O'Brien JP, Goldenberg DL, Rice PA. Disseminated gonococcal infection: a prospective analysis of 49 patients and a review of pathophysiology and immune mechanisms. *Medicine.* 1983;62:395–406.

46. Jackman JD, Glamann DB. Southwestern internal medicine conference: gonococcal endocarditis: twenty-five years experience. *Am J Med Sci.* 1991;301:221–230.

47. Harrison HR, English MG, Lee CK, Alexander ER. *Chlamydia trachomatis* infant pneumonitis. *N Engl J Med.* 1978;298:702–708.

48. Chaisilwattana P, Chuachoowong R, Siriwasin W, et al. Chlamydial and gonococcal cervicitis in HIV-seropositive and HIV-seronegative pregnant women in Bangkok. Prevalence, risk factors, and relation to perinatal HIV transmission. *Sex Transm Dis.* 1997;24:495–502.

49. Laga M, Plummer FA, Piot P, et al. Prophylaxis of gonococcal and chlamydial ophthalmia neonatorum. *N Engl J Med.* 1988;318:653–657.

50. Laga M, Plummer FA, Nzanze H, et al. Epidemiology of ophthalmia neonatorum in Kenya. *Lancet.* 1986;2: 1145–1149.

51. Ching S-F, Lee H, Hook E, Jacobs M, Zenilman J. Ligase chain reaction for detection of *Neisseria gonorrhoeae* in urogenital swabs. *J Clin Microbiol.* 1995;33: 3111–3114.

52. Smith KR, Ching S, Lee H, et al. Evaluation of ligase chain reaction for use with urine for identification of

Neisseria gonorrhoeae in females attending a sexually transmitted disease clinic. *J Clin Microbiol.* 1995;33: 455.

53. Zenilman JM. Surveys and urine STD diagnostic tests: a new paradigm for survey design and validity measurement [Editorial]. *Sex Transm Dis.* 1997;24:310–311.

54. Centers for Disease Control and Prevention. 1998 guidelines for treatment of sexually transmitted diseases. *MMWR.* 1998;47:RR-1.

55. Jaffe HW, Biddle JW, Thornsberry C, et. al. National gonorrhea therapy monitoring study: in vitro susceptibility and its correlation with treatment results. *N Engl J Med.* 1976;294:5–9.

56. Centers for Disease Control. Antibiotic-resistant strains of *Neisseria gonorrhoeae*—policy guidelines for detection, management and control. *MMWR.* 1987; 36(Suppl):5S.

57. Faruki H, Kohmescher RN, McKinney WP, Sparling PF. A community-based outbreak of infection with penicillin-resistant *Neisseria gonorrhoeae* not producing penicillinase (chromosomally-mediated resistance). *N Engl J Med.* 1985;313:607–611.

58. Knapp JS, Zenilman JM, Biddle JW, et al. Frequency and distribution of plasmid-mediated high level tetracycline resistant *Neisseria gonorrhoeae* (TRNG) in the United States. *J Infect Dis.* 1987;155:819–822.

59. Gordon SM, Carlyn CJ, Doyle IJ, et al. The emergence of *Neisseria gonorrhoeae* with decreased susceptibility to ciprofloxacin in Cleveland, Ohio. *Ann Intern Med.* 1996;125:465–470.

60. Moran JS, Levine WC. Drugs of choice for the treatment of uncomplicated gonococcal infection. *Clin Infect Dis.* 1995;20(Suppl):S47–S65.

61. Schwarcz SK, Zenilman JM, Knapp JS, et al. National surveillance of antimicrobial resistance in *Neisseria gonorrheae*. *JAMA.* 1990;264:1413–1417.

62. Cowan FM, French R, Johnson AM. The role and effectiveness of partner notification in STD control: a review. *Genitourin Med.* 1996;72:247–252.

63. Webster LA, Greenspan JR, Nakashima AK, Johnson RE. An evaluation of surveillance for *Chlamydia trachomatis* infections in the United States, 1987–1991. *MMWR.* 1993;42 (SS-3):21–27.

64. Centers for Disease Control and Prevention, Division of Sexually Transmitted Diseases. *1997 Annual Report.* Atlanta: Centers for Disease Control and Prevention; 1998.

65. Quinn TC, Zenilman JM, Rompalo AM. Sexually transmitted diseases—trends in the 1990s. *Adv Intern Med.* 1994;39:149–196.

66. Stamm WE, Hicks CB, Martin DH, et al. Azithromycin for empirical treatment of NGU syndrome in men. *JAMA.* 1995;274:545–549.

67. Romanowski B, Talbot H, Stadnyk M, Kowalchuk P, Bowie WR. Minocycline compared with doxycycline in the treatment of NGU and MPC. *Ann Intern Med.* 1993; 119:16–22.

68. McNagny SE, Parker RM, Zenilman JM, Lewis JS. Evaluation of urinary leukocyte esterase as a screening test for the detection of asymptomatic *Chlamydia trachomatis* and *Neisseria gonorrhoeae* in men. *J Infect Dis.* 1992;165:573–576.

69. Jaschek G, Gaydos CA, Welsh L, Quinn TC. Direct detection of *Chlamydia trachomatis* in urine specimens from symptomatic and asymptomatic men by using a rapid polymerase chain reaction assay. *J Clin Microbiol.* 1993;31:1209–1212.

70. Rietmeijer CAM, Judson FN, Boele van Hensbroek M, Ehret JM, Douglas JM. Unsuspected *Chlamydia trachomatis* infection in heterosexual men attending a sexually transmitted disease clinic: evaluation of risk factors and screening methods. *Sex Transm Dis.* 1991; 18:28–34.

71. Stamm WE, Holmes KK. *Chlamydia trachomatis* infections of the adult. In: Holmes KK, Mardh PA, Sparling PF, et al, eds. *Sexually Transmitted Diseases.* 2nd ed. New York: McGraw-Hill, Inc; 1990:181–193.

72. McCormack WM, Rosner B, McComb DE, Evrard JR, Zinner SH. Infection with *Chlamydia trachomatis* in female college students. *Am J Epidemiol.* 1985;121:107–115.

73. Johnson BA, Poses RM, Fortner CA, Meier FA, Dalton HP. Derivation and validation of a clinical diagnostic model for chlamydial cervical infection in university women. *JAMA.* 1990;264:3161–3165.

74. Jacobson D, Peralta L, Graham N, Zenilman J. Development of cervical ectopy: epidemiology and meta analysis of the relationship of ectopy and oral contraceptives to the risk of chlamydia infection. *Sex Transm Dis.* In press.

75. Cates W Jr, Wasserheit JN. Genital chlamydial infections: epidemiology and reproductive sequelae. *Am J Obstet Gynecol.* 1991;164:1771–1781.

76. World Health Organization Task Force on the Prevention and Management of Infertility. Tubal infertility: serologic relationship to past chlamydial and gonococcal infection. *Sex Transm Dis.* 1995;22:71–76.

77. Rompalo AM, Suchland RJ, Price CB, Stamm WE. Rapid diagnosis of *Chlamydia trachomatis* rectal infection by direct immunofluorescence staining. *J Infect Dis.* 1987;155:1075–1076.

78. Centers for Disease Control and Prevention. *Chlamydia trachomatis* genital infections—United States, 1995. *MMWR.* 1997;46:193–199.

79. Burstein GR, Gaydos CA, Diener-West M, Howell MR, Zenilman JM, Quinn TC. Incident *Chlamydia trachomatis* infections among inner city adolescent females. *JAMA.* 1998;280:521–526.

80. Gaydos CA, Howell MR, Pare B, et al. *Chlamydia trachomatis* infections in female military recruits. *N Engl J Med.* 1998;339:739–744.

81. Rosenbaum S. Negotiating the new health system: purchasing publicly accountable managed care. *Am J Prev Med.* 1998;14(Suppl 3):67–71.

82. Stamm WE, Kooutsky LA, Benedetti JK, Jourden JL, Brunham RC, Holmes KK. *Chlamydia trachomatis* infections in men. *Ann Intern Med.* 1984;100:47–51.

83. Chernesky MA, Lee H, Schachter J, et al. Diagnosis of *Chlamydia trachomatis* urethral infection in symptomatic and asymptomatic men by testing first-void urine in a ligase chain reaction assay. *J Infect Dis.* 1994;170: 1308–1311.

84. Schachter J, Moncada J, Whidden R, et al. Noninvasive tests for diagnosis of *Chlamydia trachomatis* infection: application of ligase chain reaction to first-catch specimens of women. *J Infect Dis.* 1995;172:1411–1414.

85. Addiss DG, Vaughn ML, Ludka D, Pfister J, Davis JP. Decreased prevalence of *Chlamydia trachomatis* infection associated with a selective screening program in family planning clinics in Wisconsin. *Sex Transm Dis.* 1993;20:28–35.

86. Addiss DG, Vaughn ML, Hillis SD, Ludka D, Amsterdam L, Davis JP. History and features of the Wisconsin *Chlamydia trachomatis* control program. *Fam Plann Perspect.* 1994;26:83–89.

87. Scholes D, Stergachis A, Heidrich F, Andrilla H, Holmes KK, Stamm WE. Prevention of pelvic inflammatory disease by screening for chlamydial infection. *N Engl J Med.* 1996;334:1362–1366.

88. Hook EW III, Marra CM. Acquired syphilis in adults. *N Engl J Med.* 1992;326:1062–1069.

89. Rolfs RT, Nakashima AK. Epidemiology of primary and secondary syphilis in the United States, 1981 through 1989. *JAMA.* 1990;264:1432–1437.

90. Thin RN. Early syphilis in the adult. In: Holmes KK, Mardh P-A, Sparling PF, Wiesner PJ, eds. *Sexually Transmitted Diseases* New York: McGraw-Hill; 1990: 711–716.

91. Lukehart SA, Hook EW III, Baker-Zander SA, Collier AC, Critchlow CW, Handsfield HH. Invasion of the central nervous system by *Treponema pallidum*: implications for diagnosis and treatment. *Ann Intern Med.* 1988;109:855–862.

92. Centers for Disease Control. Tertiary syphilis deaths— South Florida. *MMWR.* 1987;36:488–491.

93. Larsen SA, Steiner BM, Rudolph AH. Laboratory diagnosis and interpretation of tests for syphilis. *Clin Microbiol Rev.* 1995;8:1–21.

94. Quinn TC, Cannon RO, Glasser D, et al. The associa-

tion of syphilis with risk of human immunodeficiency virus infection in patients attending sexually transmitted disease clinics. *Arch Intern Med.* 1990;150:1297–1302.

95. Hutchinson CM, Hook EW III, Shepherd M, Verley J, Rompalo AM. Altered clinical presentation of early syphilis in patients with human immunodeficiency virus infection. *Ann Intern Med.* 1994;121:94–99.

96. Gourevitch MN, Selwyn PA, Davenny K, et al. Effects of HIV infection on the serologic manifestations and response to treatment of syphilis in intravenous drug users. *Ann Intern Med.* 1993;118:350–355.

97. Rolfs RT. Treatment of syphilis, 1993. *Clin Infect Dis.* 1995;20(Suppl 1):S23–S38.

98. Cowan FM, French R, Johnson AM. The role and effectiveness of partner notification in STD control: a review. *Genitourin Med.* 1996;72:247–252.

99. Andrus JK, Fleming DW, Harger DR, et al. Partner notification: can it control epidemic syphilis? *Ann Intern Med.* 1990;112:539–543.

100. Flood JM, Sarafian SK, Bolan GA, et al. Multistrain outbreak of chancroid in San Francisco, 1989–1991. *J Infect Dis.* 1993;167:1106–1111.

101. DiCarlo RP, Armentor BS, Martin DH. Chancroid epidemiology in New Orleans men. *J Infect Dis.* 1995; 176:446–452.

102. Schmid GP, Sanders LL, Blount JH, Alexander. Chancroid in the United States. *JAMA.* 1987;258:3265–3268.

103. King R, Gough J, Ronald A, et al. An immunohistochemical analysis of naturally occurring chancroid. *J Infect Dis.* 1996;174:427–430.

104. Centers for Disease Control and Prevention. Chancroid detected by polymerase chain reaction—Jackson, Mississippi, 1994–1995. *MMWR.* 1995;44:567–574.

105. Orle KA, Gates CA, Martin DH, Body BA, Weiss JB. Simultaneous PCR detection of *Hemophilus ducreyi, Treponema pallidum,* and herpes simplex virus types 1 and 2 from genital ulcers. *J Clin Microbiol.* 1996;34: 49–54.

106. Schulte JM, Schmid GP. Recommendations for treatment of chancroid, 1993. *Clin Infect Dis.* 1995; 20(Suppl 1):S39–S46.

107. Mertz GJ. Epidemiology of genital herpes infections. *Infect Dis Clin North Am.* 1993;7:825–839.

108. Corey L, Spear PG. Infections with herpes simplex viruses. *N Engl J Med.* 1986;314:686–691, 749–756.

109. Koutsky LA, Ashley RL, Holmes KK, et al. The frequency of unrecognized type 2 herpes simplex virus infection among women. *Sex Transm Dis.* 1990;17:90–94.

110. Corey L, Adams HG, Brown ZA, Holmes KK. Clinical course of genital herpes simplex virus infections in men and women. *Ann Intern Med.* 1983;98:973.

111. Langenberg A, Benedetti J, et al. Development of clinically recognizable genital lesions among women previously identified as having asymptomatic herpes simplex type 2 infection. *Ann Intern Med.* 1989;110: 882–887.

112. Wald A, Zeh J, Selke S, Ashley RL, Corey L. Virologic characteristics of subclinical and symptomatic genital herpes infections. *N Engl J Med.* 1995;333:770–775.

113. Augenbraun M, Feldman J, Chirgwin K, et al. Genital shedding of herpes simplex virus type 2 in HIV-seropositive women. *Ann Intern Med.* 1995;123:855–847.

114. Centers for Disease Control and Prevention, Division of Sexually Transmitted Diseases and HIV prevention. *Annual Report, 1995.* Atlanta: Centers for Disease Control and Prevention; 1996.

115. Johnson RE, Nahmias AJ, Magder LS, Lee FK, Brooks CA, Snowden CB. A seroepidemiologic survey of herpes simplex type 2 infection in the United States. *N Engl J Med.* 1989;321:7–12.

116. Fleming DT, McQuillan GM, Johnson RE, et al. Herpes simplex virus type 2 in the United States, 1976 to 1994. *N Engl J Med.* 1997;37:1105–1111.

117. Mertz GJ, Benedetti J, Ashley R, Selke SA, Corey L. Risk factors for the sexual transmission of genital herpes. *Ann Intern Med.* 1992;116:197–202.

118. Benedetti JK, Zeh J, Selke S, Corey L. Frequency and reactivation of nongenital lesions among patients with genital herpes simplex virus. *Am J Med.* 1995;98:237–242.

119. Ashley R, Cent A, Maggs V, Nahmias A, Corey L. Inability of enzyme immunoassays to discriminate between infections with herpes simplex virus types 1 and 2. *Ann Intern Med.* 1991;115:520–526.

120. Scott LL. Perinatal herpes: current status and obstetric management strategies. *Pediatr Infect Dis J.* 1995;14: 827–832.

121. Brown ZA, Vontver LA, Benedetti J, et al. Effects on infants of a first episode of genital herpes during pregnancy. *N Engl J Med.* 1987;317:1246–1251.

122. Mertz GJ, Loveless MO, Levin MJ, et al. Oral famciclovir for suppression of recurrent genital herpes simplex infection in women. *Arch Intern Med.* 1997; 157:343–349.

123. Langenberg AG, Burke RL, Adair SF, et al. Recombinant glycoprotein vaccine for herpes simplex virus type 2: safety and immunogenicity. *Ann Intern Med.* 1995;122:889–898.

124. Nelson KE, Eiumtrakul S, Celentano D, et al. The association of herpes simplex virus type 2 (HSV-2), *Haemophilus ducreyi,* and syphilis with HIV infection

in young men in northern Thailand. *J Acquir Immune Defic Syndr Hum Retrovirol.* 1997;16:293–300.

125. Koutsky L. Epidemiology of genital human papillomavirus infection. *Am J Med.* 1997;102:3–108.

126. Koutsky LA, Galloway DA, Holmes KK. Epidemiology of genital human papillomavirus infection. *Epidemiol Rev.* 1988;10:122–163.

127. Shah KV, Howley PM. Papillomaviruses. In: Fields BN, Knipe DM, eds. *Virology.* 2nd ed. New York: Raven Press; 1990:1651–1676.

128. Slattery ML, Overall JC Jr, Abbott TM, French TK, Robison LM, Gardner J. Sexual activity, contraception, genital infections, and cervical cancer: support for a sexually transmitted disease hypothesis. *Am J Epidemiol.* 1989;130:248–258.

129. Kiviat NB, Koutsky LA, Paavonen JA, et al. Prevalence of genital papillomavirus infection among women attending a college student health clinic or a sexually transmitted disease clinic. *J Infect Dis.* 1989; 159:293–302.

130. Bauer HM, Ting Y, Greer CE, et al. Genital human papillomavirus infection in female university students as determined by a PCR-based method. *JAMA.* 1991; 265:472–477.

131. Martinez J, Smith R, Farmer M, et al. High prevalence of genital tract papillomavirus infection in female adolescents. *Pediatrics.* 1988;82:604–608.

132. Hippelainen M, Syrjanen S, Hippelainen M, et al. Prevalence and risk factors of genital human papillomavirus (HPV) infections in healthy males: a study on Finnish conscripts. *Sex Transm Dis.* 1993;20:321–328.

133. Lorincz AT, Reid R, Jenson AB, Greenberg MD, Lancaster W, Kurman RJ. Human papillomavirus infection of the cervix: relative risk associations of 15 common anogenital types. *Obstet Gynecol.* 1992;79: 328–337.

134. Bosch FX, Manos MM, Munoz N, et al. Prevalence of human papillomavirus in cervical cancer: a worldwide perspective. *J Natl Cancer Inst.* 1995;87:796–802.

135. Koutsky LA, Holmes KK, Critchlow CW, et al. A cohort study of the risk of cervical intraepithelial neoplasia grade 2 or 3 in relation to papillomavirus infection. *N Engl J Med.* 1992;327:1272–1278.

136. Werness BA, Levine AJ, Howley PM. Association of human papillomavirus types 16 and 18 E6 proteins with p53. *Science.* 1990;248:76–79.

137. Tirelli U, Franceschi Silvia, Carbone, A. Current issues in cancer: malignant tumours in patients with HIV infection. *Br Med J.* 1994;308:1148–1153.

138. Daling JR, Sherman KJ, Hislop TG, et al. Cigarette smoking and the risk of anogenital cancer. *Am J Epidemiol.* 1992;135:180–189.

139. WHO Collaborative Study of Neoplasia and Steroid Contraceptives. Invasive squamous-cell cervical carcinoma and combined oral contraceptives: results from a multinational study. *Int J Cancer.* 1993;55:228–236.

140. Duncan ID, ed. *Guidelines for Clinical Practice and Programme Management.* Sheffield: NHSCSP Cervical Screening Programme; December 1997. MHSCSP Publication Number 8.

141. Chopra KF, Tyring SK. The impact of the human immunodeficiency virus on the human papillomavirus epidemic. *Arch Dermatol.* 1997;133:629–633.

142. Krieger JN, Jenny C, Verdon M, et al. Clinical manifestations of trichomoniasis in men. *Ann Intern Med.* 1993;118:844–849.

143. Krieger JN. Trichomoniasis in men: old issues and new data. *Sex Transm Dis.* 1995;22:83–96.

144. Schwebke JR, Morgan SC, Pinson GB. Validity of self-obtained vaginal specimens for diagnosis of trichomoniasis. *J Clin Microbiol.* 1997;35:1618–1619.

145. Blake DR, Duggan A, Quinn T, Zenilman JM, Joffe A. Sexually transmitted disease evaluation in young women—can it be done without a speculum? *Pediatrics.* 1998;102:939–944.

146. Witkin SS, Inglis SR, Polaneczky M. Detection of *Chlamydia trachomatis* and *Trichomonas vaginalis* by polymerase chain reaction in introital specimens from pregnant women. *Am J Obstet Gynecol.* 1996;175: 165–167.

147. Spence MR, Harwell TS, Davies MC, Smith JL. The minimum single oral metronidazole dose for treating trichomoniasis: a randomized, blinded study. *Obstet Gynecol.* 1997;89(5 Pt 1):699–703.

148. Burtin P, Taddio A, Ariburnu O, Einarson TR, Koren G. Safety of metronidazole in pregnancy: a meta-analysis. *Am J Obstet Gynecol.* 1995;172(2 Pt 1):525–529.

149. Schwebke JR. Metronidazole: utilization in the obstetric and gynecologic patient. *Sex Transm Dis.* 1995;22: 370–376.

150. Lossick JG, Muller M, Gorrell TE. In-vitro susceptibility and doses of metronidazole required for cure in cases of refractory vaginal trichomoniasis. *J Infect Dis.* 1986;153:958–955.

151. Centers for Disease Control and Prevention. *1996 STD Surveillance Statistics.* Atlanta: Centers for Disease Control and Prevention; 1997.

152. Cotch MF, Pastorek JG 2nd, Nugent RP, Yerg DE, Martin DH, Eschenbach DA. Demographic and behavioral predictors of *Trichomonas vaginalis* infection among pregnant women. The Vaginal Infections and Prematurity Study Group. *Obstet Gynecol.* 1991;78: 1087–1092.

153. McCormack WM, Evrard JR, Laughlin CF, et al. Sexu-

ally transmitted conditions among women college students. *Am J Obstet Gynecol.* 1981;139:130–133.

154. Jenny C, Hooton TM, Bowers A, et al. Sexually transmitted diseases in victims of rape. *N Engl J Med.* 1990;322:713–716.

155. Krieger JN, Jenny C, Verdon M, et al. Clinical manifestations of trichomoniasis in men. *Ann Intern Med.* 1993;118:844–849.

156. Jackson DJ, Rakwar JP, Chohan B, et al. Urethral infection in a workplace population of East African men: evaluation of strategies for screening and management. *J Infect Dis.* 1997;175:833–838.

157. Borchardt KA, al-Haraci S, Maida N. Prevalence of *Trichomonas vaginalis* in a male sexually transmitted disease clinic population by interview, wet mount microscopy, and the InPouch TV test. *Genitourin Med.* 1995;71:405–406.

158. Pastorek JG 2nd, Cotch MF, Martin DH, Eschenbach DA. Clinical and microbiological correlates of vaginal trichomoniasis during pregnancy. The Vaginal Infections and Prematurity Study Group. *Clin Infect Dis.* 1996;23:1075–1080.

159. Meis PJ, Goldenberg RL, Mercer B, et al. The preterm prediction study: significance of vaginal infections. *Am J Obstet Gynecol.* 1995;173:1231–1235.

160. Reid JS, Klebanoff MA. Sexual intercourse during pregnancy and preterm delivery: effects of vaginal microorganisms. The Vaginal Infections and Prematurity Study Group. *Am J Obstet Gynecol.* 1993;168(2):514–519.

161. Paisarntantiwong R, Brockmann S, Clarke L, Landesman S, Feldman J, Minkoff H. The relationship of vaginal trichomoniasis and pelvic inflammatory disease among women colonized with *Chlamydia trachomatis. Sex Transm Dis.* 1995;22:344–347.

162. Laga M, Manoka A, Kivuvu M, et al. Non-ulcerative sexually transmitted diseases as risk factors for HIV-1 transmission in women: results from a cohort study. *AIDS.* 1993;795–102.

163. Spiegel CA. Bacterial vaginosis. *Clin Microbiol Rev.* 1991;4:485–502.

164. Eschenbach DA, Hillier S, Critchlow C, Stevens C, DeRouen T, Holmes KK. Diagnosis and clinical manifestations of bacterial vaginosis. *Am J Obstet Gynecol.* 1988;158:819–828.

165. Spiegel CA, Amsel R, Holmes KK. Diagnosis of bacterial vaginosis by direct gram stain of vaginal fluid. *J Clin Microbiol.* 1983;18:170–177.

166. Amsel R, Totten PA, Spiegel CA, Chien KCS, Eschenbach D, Holmes KK. Nonspecific vaginitis. Diagnostic criteria and microbial and epidemiological associations. *Am J Med.* 1983;74:14–21.

167. Cotch MF, Pastorek JG 2nd, Nugent RP, et al. *Trichomonas vaginalis* associated with low birth weight and preterm delivery. *Sex Transm Dis.* 1997;24:353–360.

168. Silver HM, Sperling RS, St. Clair PJ, Gibbs RS. Evidence relating bacterial vaginosis to intraamniotic infection. *Am J Obstet Gynecol.* 1989;61:808–812.

169. Gravett MG, Nelson HP, DeRouen T, Critchlow C, Eschenbach DA, Holmes KK. Independent associations of bacterial vaginosis and *Chlamydia trachomatis* infections with adverse pregnancy outcome. *JAMA.* 1986;256:1899–1903.

170. Hillier SL, Nugent RP, Eschenbach DA, et al. Association between bacterial vaginosis and preterm delivery of a low birth weight infant. *N Engl J Med.* 1995;333:1737–1742.

171. Hauth JC, Goldenberg RL, Andrews WW, Dubard MB, Copper RL. Reduced incidence of preterm delivery with metronidazole and erythromycin in women with bacterial vaginosis. *N Engl J Med.* 1995;333:1732–1736.

172. Goldenberg RL, Klebanoff MA, Nugent R, Krohn MA, Hillier S, Andrews W. Bacterial colonization of the vagina during pregnancy in four ethnic groups. *Am J Obstet Gynecol.* 1996;174:1618–1621.

173. Larsson P-G, Platz-Christensen J-J, Thejls H, Forsum U, Pahlson C. Incidence of pelvic inflammatory disease after first-trimester abortion in women with bacterial vaginosis after treatment with metronidazole: a double-blind, randomized study. *Am J Obstet Gynecol.* 1992;166:100–103.

174. Soper DE, Bump RC, Hurt WG. Bacterial vaginosis and trichomoniasis vaginitis are risk factors for cuff cellulitis after abdominal hysterectomy. *Am J Obstet Gynecol.* 1990;163:1016–1023.

175. Sewankambo N, Gray RH, Wawer MJ, et al. HIV-1 infection associated with abnormal vaginal flora morphology and bacterial vaginosis. *Lancet.* 1997;350:546–550.

176. Cates W Jr, Rolfs RT Jr, Aral SO. Sexually transmitted diseases, pelvic inflammatory disease, and infertility: an epidemiologic update. *Epidemiol Rev.* 1990;12:199–220.

177. McCormack WM. Pelvic inflammatory disease. *N Engl J Med.* 1994;330:115–119.

178. Eschenbach DA, Buchanan TM, Pollock HM, et al. Polymicrobial etiology of acute pelvic inflammatory disease. *N Engl J Med.* 1975;293:166–171.

179. Wasserheit JN, Bell TA, Kiviat NB, et al. Microbial causes of proven pelvic inflammatory disease and efficacy of clindamycin and tobramycin. *Ann Intern Med.* 1986;104:187–193.

180. Wasserheit JN. Pelvic inflammatory disease and infertility. *Md Med J.* 1987;36:58–63.

181. Westrom L. Incidence, prevalence, and trends of acute pelvic inflammatory disease and its consequences in industrialized countries. *Am J Obstet Gynecol.* 1980; 138:880–892.

182. Westrom L, Joesoef R, Reynolds G, Hagdu A, Thompson SE. Pelvic inflammatory disease and fertility: a cohort study of 1,844 women with laparoscopically verified disease and 657 control women with normal laparoscopic results. *Sex Transm Dis.* 1992;19:185–192.

183. Chow JM, Yonekura ML, Richwald GA, Greenland S, Sweet RL, Schachter J. The association between *Chlamydia trachomatis* and ectopic pregnancy: a matched-pair, case-control study. *JAMA.* 1990;263: 3164–3167.

184. Rolfs RT, Galaid EI, Zaidi AA. Pelvic inflammatory disease: trends in hospitalizations and office visits, 1979 through 1988. *Am J Obstet Gynecol.* 1992;166: 983–990.

185. Bell TA, Holmes KK. Age-specific risks of syphilis, gonorrhea, and hospitalized pelvic inflammatory disease in sexually experienced U.S. women. *Sex Transm Dis.* 1984;11:291–295.

186. Wolner-Hanssen P, Eschenbach DA, Paavonen J, et al. Association between vaginal douching and acute pelvic inflammatory disease. *JAMA.* 1990;263:1936–1941.

187. Sellors J, Mahony J, Goldsmith C, et al. The accuracy of clinical findings and laparoscopy in pelvic inflammatory disease. *Am J Obstet Gynecol.* 1991;164:113–120.

188. Bowie WR, Jones H. Acute pelvic inflammatory disease in outpatients: association with *Chlamydia trachomatis* and *Neisseria gonorrhoeae. Ann Intern Med.* 1981;95:685–688.

189. Kahn JG, Walker CK, Washington AE, Landers DV, Sweet RL. Diagnosing pelvic inflammatory disease: a comprehensive analysis and considerations for developing a new model. *JAMA.* 1991;226:2594–2604.

190. Centers for Disease Control and Prevention. 1998 Sexually transmitted diseases treatment guidelines. *MMWR.* 1998;47:RR-1.

191. Centers for Disease Control and Prevention. Pelvic inflammatory disease: guidelines for prevention and management. *MMWR.* 1991;40(RR-5):1–25.

192. Washington AE, Cates W Jr, Wasserheit JN. Preventing pelvic inflammatory disease. *JAMA.* 1991;266: 2574–2580.

193. Kamwendo F, Foslin L, Bodin L, Danielsson D. Programmes to reduce pelvic inflammatory disease—the Swedish experience. *Lancet.* 1998;351(3S):25–28.

194. Wasserheit JN. Epidemiological synergy. *Sex Transm Dis.* 1992;19:61–77.

195. Kreiss JK, Coombs R, Plummer F, et al. Isolation of human immunodeficiency virus from genital ulcers in Nairobi prostitutes. *J Infect Dis.* 1989;160:380–384.

196. Kreiss J, Willerford DM, Hensel M, et al. Association between cervical inflammation and cervical shedding of human immunodeficiency virus DNA. *J Infect Dis.* 1994;170:1597–1601.

197. Moss GB, Overbaugh J, Welch M, et al. Human immunodeficiency virus DNA in urethral secretions in men: association with gonococcal urethritis and CD4 cell depletion. *J Infect Dis.* 1995;172:1469–1474.

198. Dickerson MC, Johnston J, Delea TE, White A, Andrews E. The causal role for genital ulcer disease as a risk factor for transmission of human immunodeficiency virus. *Sex Transm Dis.* 1996;23:429–439.

199. Stamm WE, Handsfield HH, Rompalo AM, Ashley RG, Roberts PL, Corey L. The association between genital ulcer disease and acquisition of HIV infection in homosexual men. *JAMA.* 1988;260:1429–1433.

200. Quinn TC, Cannon RO, Glasser D, et al. The association of syphilis with risk of human immunodeficiency virus in patients attending sexually transmitted disease clinics. *Arch Intern Med.* 1990;150:1297–1302.

201. Plourde PJ, Plummer FA, Pepin J. Human immunodeficiency virus type 1 infection in women attending a sexually transmitted disease clinic in Kenya. *J Infect Dis.* 1992;166:86–92.

202. Plummer FA, Simonsen JN, Cameron DW, et al. Cofactors in male-female sexual transmission of human immunodeficiency virus type 1. *J Infect Dis.* 1991;163: 233–239.

203. Hutchinson CM, Rompalo AM, Reichart CA, Hook EW III. Characteristics of patients with syphilis attending Baltimore STD clinics. *Arch Intern Med.* 1991; 151:511–516.

204. Quinn TC, Cannon RO, Glasser D, et al. The association of syphilis with risk of human immunodeficiency virus in patients attending sexually transmitted disease clinics. *Arch Intern Med.* 1990;150:1297–1302.

205. Torian LV, Weisfuse IB, Makki HA, Benson DA, DiCamillo LM, Toribo FE. Increasing HIV-1 seroprevalence associated with genital ulcer disease, New York City, 1990–1992. *AIDS.* 1995;9:177–181.

206. Holmberg SD, Stewart JA, Gerber AR, et al. Prior herpes simplex virus type 2 infection as a risk factor for HIV infection. *JAMA.* 1988;259:1048–1050.

207. Hook EW, Cannon RO, Nahmias AJ, et al. Herpes simplex infection as a risk factor for human immunodeficiency virus infection in heterosexuals. *J Infect Dis.* 1992;165:251–255.

208. Plourde PJ, Pepin J, Agoki E, et al. Human immunodeficiency virus type 1 seroconversion in women with genital ulcers. *J Infect Dis.* 1994;170:313–317.

209. Mehendale SM, Rodrigues JJ, Brookmeyer RS, et al. Incidence and predictors of human immunodeficiency virus type 1 serconversion in patients attending sexually transmitted disease clinics in India. *J Infect Dis*. 1995;172:1486–1491.

210. Celentano DD, Nelson KE, Suprasert S, et al. Risk factors for HIV-1 seroconversion among young men in northern Thailand. *JAMA*. 1996;275:122–127.

211. Weir SS, Feldblum PJ, Roddy RE, Zekeng L. Gonorrhea as a risk factor for HIV acquisition. *AIDS*. 1994;8:1605–1608.

212. Kassler WK, Zenilamn JM, Erickson B, Fox R, Peterman TA, Hook EW III. Seroconversion in patients attending sexually transmitted disease clinics. *AIDS*. 1994;8:351–355.

213. Laga M, Manoka A, Kivuvu M, et al. Non-ulcerative sexually transmitted diseases as risk factors for HIV-1 transmission in women: results from a cohort study. *AIDS*. 1993;7:95–102.

214. Garnett GP, Anderson RM. Sexually transmitted diseases and sexual behavior: insights from mathematical models. *J Infect Dis*. 1996;174(Suppl 2):150–161.

215. Royce RA, Sena A, Cates W Jr, Cohen MS. Sexual transmission of HIV. *N Engl J Med*. 1997;336:1072–1078.

216. Grosskurth H, Mosha F, Todd J, et al. Impact of improved sexually transmitted disease treatment on HIV infection in rural Tanzania: randomised controlled trial. *Lancet*. 1995;346:530–536.

217. Hayes R, Mosha F, Nicoll A, et al. A community trial of the impact of improved sexually transmitted disease treatment on the HIV epidemic in rural Tanzania: design. *AIDS*. 1995;9:919–926.

218. Marx PA, Spira AI, Getie A, et al. Progesterone implants enhance SIV vaginal transmission and early virus load. *Nat Med*. 1996;2:1084–1089.

219. Rothenberg KH, Paskey SJ. The risk of domestic violence and women with HIV infection: implications for partner notification, public policy, and the law. *Am J Public Health*. 1995;85:1569–1576.

220. Padian N. Prostitute women and AIDS: epidemiology. *AIDS*. 1988;2:413–419.

221. Leeper M. Preliminary evaluation of REALITY: a condom for women to wear. *AIDS Care*. 1990;2:287–290.

222. Stein ZA. HIV prevention: the need for methods women can use. *Am J Public Health*. 1990;80:460–462.

223. Niruthisard S, Roddy RE, Chutivongse S. Use of nonoxynol-9 and reduction in rate of gonococcal and chlamydial cervical infections. *Lancet*. 1992;339:1371–1375.

224. Louv WC, Austin H, Alexander WJ, Stango S, Cheeks J. A clinical trial of nonoxynol-9 for preventing gono-coccal and chlamydial infections. *J Infect Dis*. 1988;158:518–523.

225. Kreiss J, Ngugu E, Holmes K, Guinan ME, Stone KM, Peterson HB. Efficacy of nonoxynol-9 contraceptive sponge use in preventing heterosexual acquisition of HIV in Nairobi prostitutes. *JAMA*. 1991;268:477–482.

226. Paukels R, DeClercq E. Development of vaginal microbicides for the prevention of heterosexual transmission of HIV. *J Acquir Immune Defic Synd Hum Retrovirol*. 1996;11:211–221.

227. Centers for Disease Control. Sexually transmitted disease treatment guideline. *MMWR*. 1989;38(Suppl 8):1–43.

228. Padian NS, O'Brien TR, Chang Y, Glass S, Francis DP. Prevention of heterosexual transmission of human immunodeficiency virus through couple counseling. *J Acquir Immune Defic Synd Hum Retrovirol*. 1993;6:1043–1048.

229. Saracco A, Musicco M, Nicolosi A, et al. Man-to-woman sexual transmission of HIV: longitudinal study of 343 steady partners of infected men. *J Acquir Immune Defic Synd Hum Retrovirol*. 1993;6:497–502.

230. deVincenzi I. A longitudinal study of human immunodeficiency virus transmission by heterosexual partners. *N Engl J Med*. 1994;331:341–346.

231. Weller SC. A meta-analysis of condom effectiveness in reducing sexually transmitted HIV. *Soc Sci Med*. 1993;36.1635–1644.

232. Orr DP, Langefeld CD. Factors associated with condom use by sexually active male adolescents at risk for sexually transmitted disease. *Pediatrics*. 1993;91:873–879.

233. Cohen DA, Dent C, MacKinnon D, Hahn G. Condoms for men, not women—results of brief promotion programs. *Sex Transm Dis*. 1992;19:245–250.

234. Ku LC, Sonenstein FL, Pleck JH. The association of AIDS education and sex education with sexual behavior and condom use among teenage men. *Fam Plann Perspect*. 1992;24:100–106.

235. Sellers DE, McGraw SA, McKinlay JB. Does the promotion and distribution of condoms increase teen sexual activity? Evidence from an HIV prevention program for Latino youth. *Am J Public Health*. 1994;84:1952–1959.

236. Rojanapithayakorn W, Hanenberg R. The 100% condom program in Thailand. *AIDS*. 1996;10:1–7.

237. Nelson KE, Celentano DD, Eiumtrakol S, et al. Changes in sexual behavior and a decline in HIV infection among young men in Thailand. *N Engl J Med*. 1996;335:297–303.

238. Thomas JC, Tucker MJ. The development and use of the concept of a sexually transmitted disease core. *J Infect Dis*. 1996;174:S134–S143.

239. Bwayo J, Plummer F, Omari M, et al. Human immuno-deficiency virus infection in long-distance truck drivers in east Africa. *Arch Intern Med.* 1994;154:1391–1396.

240. Moses S, Plummer FA, Ngugi EN, Nagelkerke NJD, Anzala AO, Ndinya-Achola JO. Controlling HIV in Africa: effectiveness and cost of an intervention in a high-frequency STD transmitter core group. *AIDS.* 1991;5:407–411.

241. Rothenberg R. The geography of gonorrhea: empirical demonstration of core group transmission. *Am J Epidemiol.* 1983;117:688–693.

242. Zenilman JM, Bonner M, Sharp KL, Rabb J, Alexander R, and The Disease Intervention Staff of The Dade County Public Health Unit. Penicillinase-producing *Neisseria gonorrhoeae* in Dade County, Florida: evidence of core-group transmitters and the impact of illicit antibiotics. *Sex Transm Dis.* 1988;15: 45–50.

243. Rice R, Roberts P, Handsfield H, Holmes K. Socio-demographic distribution of gonorrhea incidence: implications for prevention and behavioral research. *Am J Public Health.* 1991;81:1252–1257.

244. Lacey CJN, Merrick DW, Bensley DC, Fairley I. Analysis of the sociodemography of gonorrhoea in Leeds, 1989–93. *Br Med J.* 1997;314:1715–1718.

245. Low N, Daker-White G, Barlow D, Pozniak AL. Gonorrhoea in inner London: results of a cross sectional study. *Br Med J.* 1997;314:1719–1723.

246. Ellen JM, Hessol NA, Kohn RP, Bolan GA. An investigation of geographic clustering of repeat cases of gonorrhea and chlamydial infection in San Francisco,

1989–1993: evidence for core groups. *J Infect Dis.* 1997;175:1519–1522.

247. Becker KM, Glass GG, Brathwaite W, Zenilman JM. The geographic epidemiology of gonorrhea in Baltimore using a geographic information system. *Am J Epidemiol.* 1998;147:709–716.

248. Yorke JA, Hethcote HW, Nold A. Dynamics and control of the transmission of gonorrhea. *Sex Transm Dis.* 1978;5:51–56.

249. Anderson RM, May RM. *Infectious Diseases of Humans—Dynamics and Control.* Oxford: Oxford University Press; 1992.

250. Rothenberg R, Potterat J. Temporal and social aspects of gonorrhea transmission: the force of infectivity. *Sex Transm Dis.* 1988;15:88–92.

251. Catania JA, Binson D, Stone V. Relationship of sexual mixing across age and ethnic groups to herpes simplex virus-2 among unmarried heterosexual adults with multiple partners. *Health Psychol.* 1996;15:362–370.

252. Potterat J, Rothenberg R, Woodhouse D, Muth J, Pratts C, Fogle J. Gonorrhea as a social disease. *Sex Transm Dis.* 1985;12:25–32.

253. Garnett GP, Anderson RM. Contact tracing and the estimation of sexual mixing patterns: the epidemiology of gonococcal infections. *Sex Transm Dis.* 1993;20: 181–191.

254. Rothenberg R, Narramore J. The relevance of social network concepts to sexually transmitted disease control. *Sex Transm Dis.* 1996;23:24–29.

255. Klovdahl AS, Potterat JJ, Woodhouse DE, Muth JB, Muth SQ, Darrow WW. Social networks and infectious disease: the Colorado Springs study. *Soc Sci Med.* 1994;38:79–88.

PART VI

Vectorborne and Parasite Diseases

CHAPTER 21

Lyme Disease

Diane E. Griffin

HISTORICAL INTRODUCTION

In 1975 a concerned mother in Old Lyme, Connecticut, reported to the Connecticut State Health Department that 12 children in her small town of 5,000 residents had an illness that had been diagnosed as juvenile rheumatoid arthritis. At approximately the same time, a mother from nearby East Haddam told physicians at the Yale Rheumatology Clinic in New Haven that an epidemic of arthritis was occurring in her family and neighbors. In response to this information, investigators established a system of surveillance in the communities east of the Connecticut River to identify all cases of "Lyme arthritis" to try and determine the cause of this new disease, suspected to be of infectious etiology (Figure 21–1). Fifty-one individuals (39 children and 12 adults) with similar symptoms of arthritis were identified. Of the 39 children, 17 lived on four country roads and, on those roads, 10% of children had the illness. Many families had more than one affected member.[1]

The disease these individuals described began with the sudden onset of pain and swelling in a knee or other large joint. The first attack of arthritis lasted about a week, but many individuals had recurrent attacks, usually involving large joints, with a similar distribution to that of the initial attack. More than half of those interviewed reported other flulike symptoms (e.g., headache, chills, fever, and malaise) suggestive of an infectious disease. In addition, 13 patients said that approximately a month before the signs of arthritis, they had noticed a red skin papule, which had developed into a large annular lesion with red margins and central clearing that continued to expand. This unique skin lesion was usually on an extremity; it was not painful, lasted 2 to 3 weeks, and was consistent with a previously described disease, erythema chronicum migrans (ECM). ECM, recognized primarily in Europe, had been associated with bites of the sheep tick *Ixodes ricinus*, but had not been associated with subsequent arthritis.[2] One patient remembered having been bitten by a tick at the site where the lesion developed. These data suggested that the disease often had manifestations other than, or in addition to, arthritis; it was probably caused by an infectious agent, likely to be arthropodborne; and it was potentially related to a disease previously described in Europe.[1]

CLINICAL PICTURE AND BIOLOGICAL INFORMATION

The Vector

Cases of the ECM skin rash occurred primarily in the summer (Figure 21–2), suggesting that the disease was seasonal and consistent with the possibility suggested by one of the original patients that it was tickborne. Therefore, in the summers of 1976 and 1977, ticks and patients in the areas around the Connecticut River were studied.[3–5] Forty-three new cases of Lyme dis-

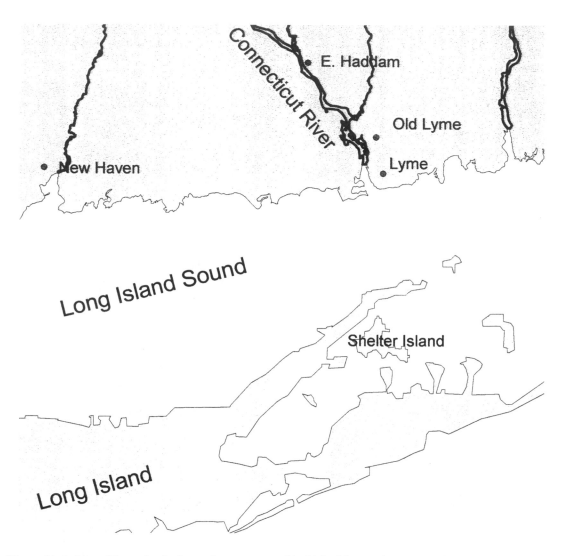

Figure 21–1 Map of the region in the northeastern part of the United States where Lyme disease was first recognized, the epidemiology of the disease was defined, and *Borrelia burgdorferi* was first isolated from *Ixodes scapularis* ticks.

ease were identified, mostly on the east side of the Connecticut River where the incidence was 2.8 cases per 1,000 residents compared with 0.1 cases per 1,000 residents on the west side of the river, an almost 30-fold difference. Of the 43 individuals, 9 (21%) remembered a tick bite at the site of the initial skin lesion within the 3 previous weeks. The tick was often described as "tiny." One individual had saved the tick and it

was identified as the deer tick *Ixodes scapularis* (Figure 21–3). Epidemiologic investigation (Table 21–1) revealed that the patients with Lyme disease had more cats and farm animals and had more often noted ticks on their pets and themselves than their neighbors without disease.[4]

Analysis of the ticks collected showed that *Ixodes scapularis* was much more abundant on the

Seasonal incidence of Lyme Disease USA, 1995

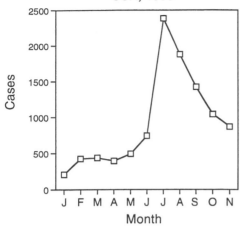

Figure 21–2 Seasonal incidence of erythema chronicum migrans

east than on the west side of the river. Immature *I. scapularis* were 13 times more abundant on white-footed mice (*Peromyscus leucopus*) and adult *I. scapularis* were 16 times more abundant on white-tailed deer (*Odocoileus virginianus*) in communities on the east side than the west side of the river (Table 21–2). Although no pathogen was isolated from the ticks or the people with Lyme disease, these data provided strong epidemiologic evidence for a tick-transmitted agent as the cause of Lyme disease.[5]

Ixodes scapularis, like most hard ticks, has a complicated life cycle that requires 2 years to complete and includes progression through the stages of egg, six-legged larval or seed tick, eight-legged immature nymph, and the eight-legged reproductively mature adult tick (Figure 21–4). At each stage, a blood meal is required

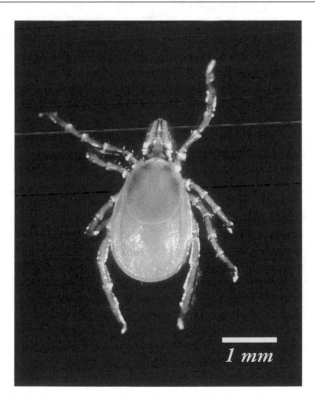

Figure 21–3 Adult female *Ixodes scapularis* tick collected in Maryland. Courtesy of Steve Dumler, Johns Hopkins University, Baltimore, Maryland.

Table 21–1 Risk Factors for Contracting Lyme Disease: Comparison of Patients with Their Neighbors, Connecticut, 1977

Risk Factor	Cases (%)	Neighbors (%)	Statistical Significance (P-value)
Male	53	44	ns
Rural environment	47	45	ns
Activities in woods	77	61	ns
Farm animals	26	11	<.05
Pets	86	81	ns
Cats	63	39	<.01
Ticks on pets	70	27	<.0001
Tick bites	44	25	<.05
Mosquito bites	72	70	ns

Source: Reprinted with permission from Steer, Broderick, and Malawista, Erythema Chronicum Migrans and Lyme Arthritis, *American Journal of Epidemiology*, Vol. 108, p. 317, © 1978, The Johns Hopkins University School of Hygiene and Public Health.

for morphogenesis and progression to the next stage. Adult ticks lay eggs in the early spring that hatch to become larvae. *Ixodes*, as do all tick species, walk to the end of grasses and tree leaves where they "quest," front legs waving in the air, until a suitable host brushes past them. Ticks do not fly, hop, drop, or jump to their next meal. The larvae feed once and then rest for the remainder of the year. The following spring nymphs emerge and feed once. The white-footed mouse, *Peromyscus leucopus*, is a primary host for immature *Ixodes*, but they also feed on other small mammals and birds, which can become infected with *Borrelia burgdorferi*. About half of all birds can be infected with *B. burgdorferi*; they and other mammals may be important reservoirs in some environments. In the southeastern United States, immature *Ixodes* feed on

Table 21–2 Numbers and Types of Ticks Collected from Various Sources East and West of the Connecticut River, 1997

Source	West			East		
	Number	Ixodes	Dermacentor	Number	Ixodes	Dermacentor
Humans	21	8	37	27	33	20
Dogs	26	2	78	16	27	96
Cats	10	12	17	4	3	5
White-footed mice	143	29	26	197	498	143
Other mammals	10	3	15	9	9	77
Dragging	0	0	0	1	8	43
Totals	210	54	173	254	578	384

Source: Reprinted with permission from Wallis, Kloter, and Main, Erythema Chronicum Migrans and Lyme Arthritis, *American Journal of Epidemiology*, Vol. 108, p. 325, © 1978, The Johns Hopkins University School of Hygiene and Public Health.

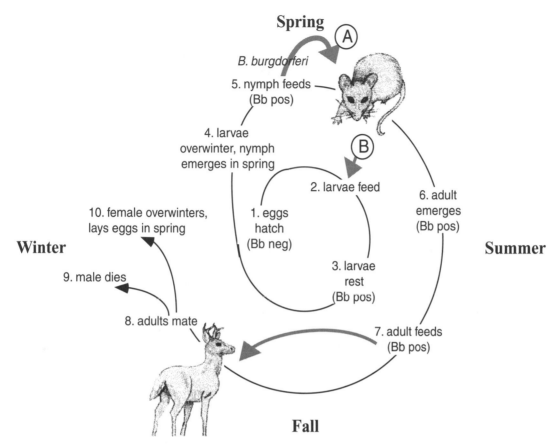

Figure 21–4 The life cycle of *Ixodes* ticks spans two years. In the first year, the eggs hatch (1) in spring and the six-legged larvae emerge, feeds once (2), and rests (3) for the remainder of the year. In the second spring, the eight-legged nymph emerges (4) and feeds once (5). The eight-legged adult emerges (6) in the summer and feeds once (7) before mating (8) in the fall. Male ticks die (9), females overwinter and lay their eggs (10) in the spring. *Borrelia burgdorferi* (*Bb*) is maintained in the tick population (A) by the transfer of the spirochete from nymphal ticks to the immature host, commonly the white-footed mouse (B), and then to the larval ticks. *Bb* vertical transmission is rare, so mice and ticks born in the spring are unlikely to carry *Bb*. In areas where the nymph feeds before the larvae *Bb* infection rates in the host and ticks are high (northeast United States). If the larvae feed before the nymph, they may feed on uninfected mice and the penetrance of *Bb* in the host and tick populations will drop (southeast United States). *Source:* Copyright © 1999, Carolyn Masters Williams.

lizards as well as mammals. Lizards are not competent carriers of *B. burgdorferi*.[6] Both nymphs and adults will feed on humans and can transmit Lyme disease.[7] After the nymph feeds, the adult emerges and feeds once in the summer or fall. Usually, adults feed on large mammals such as domestic pets, humans, and deer. Adults mate preferably on white-tailed deer, *Odocoileus virginianus*. The male tick dies, whereas the female overwinters and lays eggs the following spring.

Interstage and vertical transmission of *B. burgdorferi* is rare (<0.1%) so eggs are not commonly infected with *B. burgdorferi*.[6] The larvae may acquire the spirochete at the first feeding. The chance of the first host being infected is dependent on its being competent to carry *B. burgdorferi* and on its being exposed. Exposure is dependent on being previously bitten by an infected *Ixodes* tick. The white-footed mouse, for example, has as many as 10 litters of pups each year. As vertical transmission is rare, mice infected in the previous year will not pass their infection on to the next generation. Nymphal ticks that have emerged after the winter are responsible for transmitting *B. burgdorferi* to the next generation of mice. If nymphal forms of the tick emerge and feed before the larvae hatch, as is the case in the northern United States, host populations have a higher prevalence of infection than in the southern United States where larvae may hatch and feed before the nymphs. This order of feeding combined with feeding on *B. burgdorferi* incompetent hosts in the southeastern United States explains the high prevalence of *B. burgdorferi* in *Ixodes* from the northeastern (50%) as compared with the southeastern United States (1%).[6]

The distribution of *I. scapularis* is probably determined by the need for high humidity and availability of host species, particularly deer.[8] Populations of this tick are abundant in the northeastern and upper midwestern United States.[8]

The exact species of *Ixodes* tick associated with transmission of Lyme disease in the northeastern and midwestern United States remains a topic of discussion. The tick was originally identified as the northern form of *I. scapularis*,[4] then reclassified as a separate species, *I. dammini*, based on morphologic and ecologic characteristics. But more recently, because of mating compatibility and genetic similarity, the tick has been determined to be *I. scapularis*.[8-10] Both terms are found in the current and past literature. Related ticks, *I. pacificus*, the western black-legged tick, and *I. ricinus*, the sheep tick, are the primary vectors for Lyme disease along the Pacific coast of the United States[6,8] and in Europe, respectively.[8]

THE INFECTIOUS AGENT

Extensive searches for the etiologic agent of Lyme disease using a wide variety of culture techniques were unsuccessful. However, the agent was identified in the summer of 1981 when Willy Burgdorfer, a medical entomologist specializing in the study of ticks as vectors of infectious agents, was analyzing ticks from various parts of Long Island, New York. As part of his studies, he noted the presence of spirochetes in the midguts of most ticks collected on Shelter Island, a known focus of Lyme disease, which is located directly across Long Island Sound from the mouth of the Connecticut River (Figure 21–1). In an indirect immunofluorescent assay, these spirochetes were stained by sera from patients with Lyme disease, but not by sera from individuals without a history of Lyme disease,[11] suggesting an etiologic link to the disease. In retrospect, organisms morphologically characteristic of spirochetes had been associated with ECM in Europe in 1948,[12] but had not become accepted as indicative of the ECM infectious agent. Subsequently, the Lyme disease spirochete was isolated from the blood and tissues of patients with Lyme disease[13,14] and was identified as a new species of *Borrelia*, *Borrelia burgdorferi*.[15]

Borrelia species are spirochetal bacteria that are maintained in zoonotic cycles involving a diversity of wild mammals and birds as reservoirs. Ticks, primarily in the genus *Ixodes*, are the vectors. By definition, reservoir species are hosts that are commonly infected with an organism and remain infectious for the vector for prolonged periods of time. Vector competence describes the inherent ability of an arthropod to become infected with the organism and subsequently to transmit the infectious agent to a new vertebrate host. *Borrelia burgdorferi* has been isolated from the blood of white-footed mice, the epidemiologically implicated reservoir species and a preferred host of *I. scapularis* at early stages of the life cycle (Figure 21–4).[16] Further study has shown that larval ticks acquire *B. burgdorferi* when they feed on infected mice. Persistent infection is established in the tick and all subsequent stages of the vector remain infected. Infected nymphal ticks then transmit *B. burgdorferi* to uninfected mice. Therefore, all the data indicate that mice are the most important reservoir species for maintaining the invertebrate cycle of infection even though deer are important for the tick life cycle and can become infected.[7]

Borrelia species are motile, helical, gramnegative spirochetal bacteria. Their structure includes an inner membrane, an outer membrane, and periplasmic flagella. The outer membrane surface of the organism contains several lipoproteins. The primary outer surface lipoproteins (Osps) vary antigenically between strains and can undergo phase shifts as an important means of organism adaptation to growth in vertebrate and invertebrate hosts. OspA, which has at least seven distinct antigenic variants,[17] and OspB are encoded on a bicistronic operon and expressed on the surface of spirochetes within the midgut of unfed ticks. When infected nymphs take a blood meal, the *Borrelia* organisms begin to express OspC and cease expression of OspA (Figure 21–5). This switch is induced at least in part by the increase in temperature associated with taking a blood meal.[18–20] Infected ticks have several hundred *B. burgdorferi* in the gut lumen. When a blood meal is taken, the organisms begin to proliferate, increasing their numbers a hundred times. About 48 hours after engorgement, this expanded, OspC-expressing population of *Borrelia* begin to cross the gut epithelium into the hemocoelom and then enter the salivary glands. Appearance of *Borrelia* organisms in the salivary glands leads to transmission of organisms into, and infection of, the host on which the tick is feeding.[21] OspC is the primary surface antigen expressed by *Borrelia* organisms in vertebrate hosts.[18]

Although Lyme disease was first recognized in 1975, *B. burgdorferi* is not new to the United States. Museum ticks collected on Long Island in the 1940s were positive when examined recently by polymerase chain reaction (PCR) for *B. burgdorferi* DNA.[22] The case of a physician living in Wisconsin who developed ECM at the site of a tick bite was reported in 1970.[23] Three major sequence variants of 16S rRNA have now been distinguished and *B. burgdorferi sensu lato* has recently been divided into *B. burgdorferi sensu stricto*, *B. afzelii,* and *B. garinii*.[24] These strains appear to be associated with different clinical manifestations of infection.

THE DISEASE

Early Disease

Borrelia burgdorferi is introduced into the skin of a susceptible host by the saliva from an infected tick. The earliest manifestation of infection is usually an expanding skin lesion that appears within days to weeks at the site of the bite (Figure 21–6). The lesion starts as a red macule or papule. The later appearance of the lesion is characteristic of an ECM lesion with an erythematous border and a clearing center. *B. burgdorferi* can be isolated from this lesion,[22] and the region of erythema can continue to increase for many days and become very large. The lesion is usually warm, but not particularly painful or pruritic. This stage of Lyme disease is often accompanied by flulike symptoms including fever, chills, malaise, stiff neck, and headache. Even without treatment, these early signs and symptoms generally resolve within 3 to 4 weeks.[3] During this phase of the disease, *B. burgdorferi* can be isolated from the blood,[13,14] and it can be transmitted transplacentally from mother to fetus with potentially severe consequences for the fetus.[25,26]

Secondary Disease

The secondary phase of the disease, which usually occurs within 1 to 6 months after exposure, may be manifest by more generalized ECM lesions,[27] carditis,[28] or neurologic disease.[29] Dissemination to form multiple secondary annular skin lesions is usually accompanied by more intense systemic manifestations with severe lethargy, encephalopathy, myalgias, generalized lymphadenopathy, and splenomegaly.[27] A second type of skin eruption may also be seen, particularly in Europe, called lymphocytoma or lymphadenosis benign cutis. This condition con-

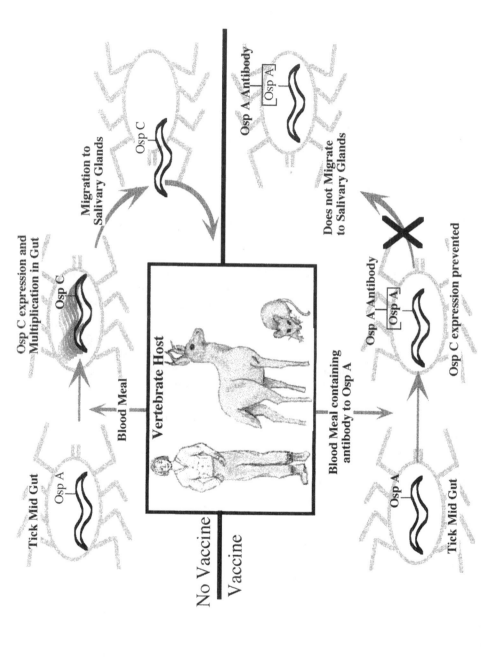

Figure 21–5 Schematic diagram of the changes in the expression of Osp proteins by *Borrelia burgdorferi* in infected ticks after taking a blood meal from an unvaccinated individual and an individual previously vaccinated against OspA. When the blood meal contains no OspA antibody, *B. burgdorferi* is induced to express OspC, multiply, and spread to the salivary gland of the tick which allows transmission to the host on which the tick is feeding. When the blood meal contains OspA antibody to *B. burgdorferi*, expression of OspC is inhibited, and neither multiplication nor spread to the salivary glands occurs. *Source:* Copyright © 1999, Carolyn Masters Williams.

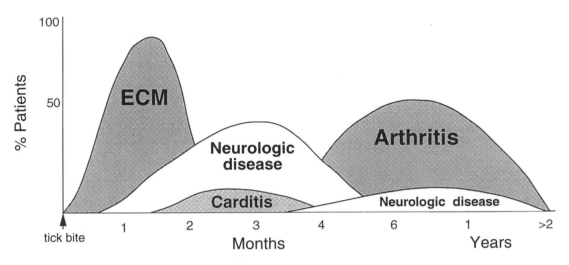

Figure 21–6 A schematic drawing of the clinical phases of Lyme disease indicating the approximate percentage of infected individuals who will develop the various manifestations of infection if left untreated. ECM, erythema chronicum migrans. *Source:* Copyright © Diane E. Griffin.

sists of a solitary red or violaceous lesion most commonly located on the ear lobe in children or on the nipple in adults. It can be accompanied by regional lymphadenopathy as well as other manifestations of Lyme disease. Carditis occurs in approximately 8% of untreated infected individuals and presents with palpitations associated with atrioventricular conduction abnormalities and occasionally S-T segment and T-wave changes on electrocardiogram. These signs and symptoms usually resolve within 6 weeks.[28]

Borrelia burgdorferi frequently invades the central nervous system (CNS)[30,31] and neurologic complications occur in 10% to15% of patients. These complications include meningitis, meningoencephalitis, cranial nerve palsies, and radiculitis.[29] Systemic symptoms can be present, but ECM and lymphadenopathy usually will resolve. However, neurologic disease can be the primary manifestation of Lyme borreliosis.[32] Meningitis is present in 80% of patients with neurologic disease at this stage, but it is often combined with other manifestations of neurologic involvement.[33] Approximately half of the patients with meningitis have some symptoms of encephalitis

(e.g., depressed consciousness, impaired concentration, seizures, ataxia, or behavioral abnormalities). The most characteristic neurologic abnormalities are cranial and peripheral neuropathies, most commonly Bell's palsy.[29,32–35]

Late Disease

The later stages of Lyme disease occur weeks to months after infection. The most common manifestation is arthritis, which can be monoarticular or oligoarticular; it occurs in approximately 60% of untreated patients. Large joints, particularly the knees, are most frequently affected, but occasionally small joints are involved as well. The arthritic attacks last weeks to months and can be recurrent over years.[36] *B. burgdorferi* can often be detected in synovial fluid aspirated from affected joints.[37]

Late Lyme disease also has a characteristic skin eruption, acrodermatitis chronica atrophicans, which is more commonly seen in Europe and associated with infection with *B. afzelii*. This chronic skin disease begins insidiously on the distal portions of the extremities with redness and swelling, followed by atrophy, and ultimately by loss of fingers and toes. The skin disease is associated with persistent infection, and it is often accompanied by joint deformities or polyneuropathy.[38]

Neurologic manifestations of late Lyme disease are less well defined; they include chronic progressive leukoencephalitis, which can resemble multiple sclerosis, generalized encephalopathy, and generalized polyneuropathy. These illnesses, which can begin many years after the primary infection, are often difficult to diagnose.[34,39,40]

DIAGNOSIS

The diagnosis of Lyme disease during the early phases of the disease is based primarily on the characteristic clinical presentation. The history of tick exposure is often helpful, although because of its small size, the tick bite may not have been recognized by the patient. Therefore, the season of the year and a history of living or vacationing in a known endemic area are also important information. The ECM rash is characteristic and sufficient for the diagnosis of primary disease. The clinical presentation of secondary disease, especially the combination of meningitis and cranial or peripheral neuropathy, should suggest Lyme disease as the leading diagnosis.[33] Culturing the organism is generally difficult and not appropriate for routine diagnosis.[41] *Borrelia* species DNA can be detected by PCR in synovial fluid, cerebrospinal fluid (CSF), and blood with varying levels of success. For instance, serum PCR was negative in all patients with ECM, synovial fluid PCR was positive in 85% of patients with Lyme disease arthritis, and CSF PCR was positive in 38% to 66% of those with acute neuroborreliosis.[30,31,37,41] Antibody to *B. burgdorferi* appears only weeks after infection and even *Borrelia*-specific IgM is often not present early in disease.[13,42] In untreated disease, antibody to the organism, as measured by enzyme immunoassay, is usually, but not always, present at the time of presentation with carditis, neurologic disease, or disseminated skin lesions.[13] In neurologic disease, antibody is usually also present in CSF.[43,44] Enzyme immunoassays using antigen consisting of purified periplasmic flagellin are more specific than those using whole cell sonicates of *B. burgdorferi*.[45] However, cross-reactivity of antibody with other bacteria, particularly other spirochetes, is still a problem.[45] The best results are obtained with a two-step approach that combines a flagellin enzyme immunoassay with a confirming immunoblot, a strategy similar to that used for serologic diagnosis of infection with human immunodeficiency virus.[46] Early treatment of the primary disease may reduce or abort the antibody response to the organism but not eliminate the late manifestations of infection, further complicating diagnosis.[13,47]

TREATMENT

The generally accepted treatment for primary disease is orally administered tetracycline, usually in the form of doxycycline, in adults and amoxicillin in pregnant women, lactating women, and young children.[48] Treatment is usually for 21 days. Erythromycin can be used as alternative therapy in patients allergic to tetracycline or penicillin. Treatment both shortens the course of ECM and reduces the incidence of later arthritis, carditis, and neurologic disease.[48–50]

Patients with minor cardiac (e.g., first degree atrioventricular block) or neurologic (e.g., Bell's palsy) involvement without other significant symptoms can be treated with the same regimen used for early disease. Those with more severe cardiac or neurologic disease or with arthritis should be treated with intravenous antibiotics, usually ceftriaxone.[51]

EPIDEMIOLOGY

Lyme disease is endemic in several areas of the United States, eastern and central Europe, and Russia.[52] The agent, *Borrelia burgdorferi,* is transmitted by *Ixodes* ticks, whose hosts are mice and deer. The nymphal forms of the ticks are pinhead-sized and are the most likely to bite humans. Both the incidence of Lyme disease and seropositivity as evidence of prior infection vary dramatically between geographic regions, which undoubtedly correlates with the prevalence of *Ixodes* ticks and the proportion of the ticks that are infected, as well as with the opportunity for human exposure to infected ticks.[53,54]

United States

Areas of the United States endemic for Lyme disease are the northeast, upper midwest, and the northern regions of the Pacific coast (Figure 21–7). However, physicians throughout the United States see cases of Lyme disease because of summertime vacation travel and occasional transmission in nonendemic areas.[55] Essentially, all cases of Lyme disease in the United States are caused by infection with *B. burgdorferi sensu stricto,*[17,24] although regional genetic heterogeneity exists within this group.[56] The ratio of apparent-to-inapparent infections is 1:1.[54] The vector for human infection in the northeast and midwest is *I. scapularis,* whereas the vector along the Pacific coast is *I. pacificus.* Transmission and early disease (ECM) occur primarily in the spring and early summer when ticks are most abundant and active (Figure 21–2). The incidence of Lyme disease has been steadily increasing since its recognition in 1975 (Figure 21–8) and the zones of relatively high incidence are expanding. In some areas, virtually 100% of the *Ixodes* ticks are infected with the Lyme disease *Borrelia* organisms. Lyme disease is currently the most common arthropodborne disease in the United States.[9]

The numbers of cases fluctuate from year to year. In the northeastern United States, this is likely to be linked to the fluctuating abundance of white-footed mice, a primary host for *I. scapularis* and the primary reservoir of *B. burgdorferi.* Acorns are an important food source for mice, and they are produced naturally in increased abundance every 2 to 5 years. Deer also eat the acorns. Another food source

for mice are the pupae of gypsy moths. Recent experimental studies have shown that defoliation by gypsy moths of oak forests in the eastern United States and the risk of Lyme disease are determined by local interactions between acorn abundance and the number of white-footed mice, moths, deer, and ticks.[57] Moth outbreaks are caused by reductions in mouse density that occur when no acorns are available, because moth pupae are more likely to survive. An increase in acorns increases the numbers of mice and the densities of *I. scapularis,* thereby predicting increased numbers of cases of Lyme disease.

On the Pacific coast, the transmission cycle for *B. burgdorferi* is different than it is on the Atlantic coast. Woodrats, rather than mice, are the primary reservoir hosts and *I. neotomae,* a non–human-biting tick, maintains *B. burgdorferi* in the enzootic cycle. The primary vector of *B. burgdorferi* to humans is *I. pacificus.* However, this tick feeds on a wide variety of hosts, but rarely on rodents such as the woodrat; thus, only 1% to 2% of these ticks become infected.[58]

Worldwide

The ECM skin lesion was first described in Sweden in 1909.[2] The distribution of the disease in Europe correlates with the distribution of *Ixodes ricinus,* the transmitting vector, and extends from north and central Europe into eastern Europe and Russia.[52,59] Strains of *Borrelia* organisms causing infection in Europe are much more varied than in the United States, and they include all three genospecies of *B. burgdorferi sensu lato: B. burgdorferi s.s., B. garinii,* and *B. afzelii.*[17,24]

In studies performed in southern Sweden, where 10% to 30% of ticks are infected, the highest rates of ECM were found to be among children aged 4 to 9 years and adults aged 60 to 74 years. No difference was seen in the incidence between males and females. In children, tick bites were more often about the head and neck than in adults, and bites in these regions increased the risk of neuroborreliosis.[60]

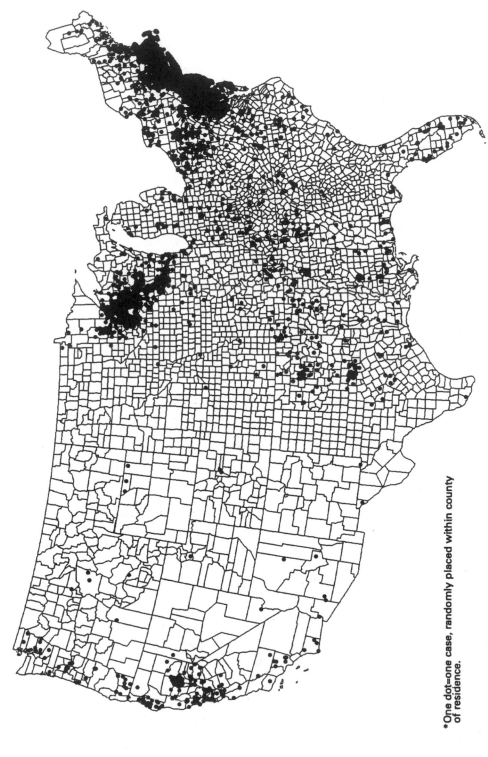

*One dot=one case, randomly placed within county of residence.

Figure 21–7 In 1997, a total of 12,801 cases of Lyme disease were reported by 46 states and the District of Columbia. The 10 states with the highest incidence of Lyme disease cases per 100,000 population were Connecticut, Rhode Island, New York, New Jersey, Pennsylvania, Delaware, Massachusetts, Wisconsin, Minnesota, and Maryland. These states accounted for 92% of the reported Lyme disease cases in 1997. *Source:* Reprinted from *Morbidity and Mortality Weekly Report*, Vol. 46, no. 54, 1998, Centers for Disease Control and Prevention.

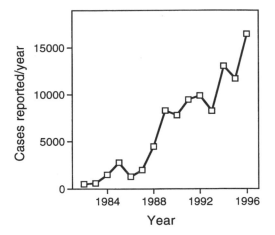

Figure 21–8 Reported cases of Lyme disease in the United States

EXPOSURE/RISK FACTORS

Because Lyme disease is transmitted by a tick vector, it is not surprising that persons living, working, or vacationing in a woodsy, rural environment are at increased risk.[53] The probability of contracting Lyme disease after a tick bite in an area of endemic disease ranges from 0.012 to 0.05.[61] Once exposed to an infected tick, the likelihood of transmission depends on how long the tick is attached. In mice, it has been shown that transmission of infection to the vertebrate host requires attachment for at least 36 hours.[62] The incidence of Lyme disease is significantly higher (20% vs 1.1%) if the duration of attachment is longer than 72 hours.[63] This observation is explained by the time needed for the *Borrelia* organism in the tick midgut to multiply, shift from expressing OspA to OspC, and migrate to the tick salivary glands for transmission (Figure 21–5).

CONTROL MEASURES

Prevention of a vectorborne zoonotic disease such as Lyme disease in humans can take the form of controlling the reservoir host species (mice), controlling the host species required for maintenance of the vector (deer), controlling the vector (ticks), preventing human exposure to the vector, and prophylaxis or immunization of humans against infection. Essentially all of these approaches have been or are being explored as mechanisms to prevent Lyme disease.

Control of host species has been attempted, but has not proved to be successful. *Peromyscus* populations fluctuate with food supply,[57] but abundance of acorns and other food in woodlands is not really amenable to human control measures. Deer populations have burgeoned in many regions; associated with increased *I. scapularis* populations and with increasing Lyme disease, deer are often blamed for this increase. One small study showed that a 70% reduction of the deer population had little impact on deer tick populations the next year,[64] and public resistance to deer control measures often exists.

Strategies for directly reducing the tick populations have been successful in limited areas. The most successful approach has been to scatter permethrin (an insecticide)–impregnated cotton balls over an area. These cotton balls are gathered up by white-footed mice and taken to their nests. Ticks residing on the mice are killed by the acaricide. This has resulted in up to a 95% reduction of *I. scapularis* populations in areas so treated. This approach, however, is expensive and impractical for large areas.

Preventing exposure to the vector is inexpensive and universally applicable. Wearing light clothing so ticks are visible, avoiding grass and shrubbery where questing ticks are likely to be waiting, applying insecticide, and limiting access to skin surfaces by wearing a long-sleeved shirt and long pants tucked into socks all decrease the likelihood of tick bite. Daily "tick checks" will result in removal of ticks before the 36 to 48 hours of attachment needed to transmit the Lyme disease agent.

Antibiotic prophylaxis after exposure to ticks has been studied by several investigators and no clear-cut recommendation has emerged. An analysis of cost-effectiveness concluded that empiric treatment is indicated for anyone with a tick bite if the probability of infection is greater than 0.036. By this formula, prophylaxis is not

---

The White-Footed Mouse

Published in 1957, long before the importance of the mouse would be recognized in the transmission of Lyme Disease, this description by Roger Caras predicts some of the difficulties faced in the control of Lyme disease:

- The mouse will build multiple nests, foiling attempts to line the nest with insecticide-impregnated cotton balls.
- There will be fluctuations in the number of mice, and thus fluctuations in the incidence of Lyme disease.
- Eradication of the mouse is unlikely.

Caras' text also reminds us that understanding the transmission of infectious diseases may take us far from the clinics, laboratories, and computer models in which epidemiologic research can become entrenched.

Their habitats range from the arid Southwest to the forests of New England. Despite the northern latitudes to which they have spread, none of them hibernate. They may nest in the ground or adapt one that they find. They are very clean about themselves, frequently washing and grooming, but they are very careless about their nests—so careless that they must often abandon a nest and construct another every few weeks.

The white-footed mouse is not a quiet animal and has many things to say to and about the world around him. He has various high-pitched squeaks, trills, and chitters for a variety of occasions, but he is most dramatic when he buzzes. His shrill buzz can last for five to ten seconds and can be heard up to fifty feet away. When really excited, he drums his forefeet in a wild fury.

The white-footed mice are not only nocturnal; they generally won't move around even on bright moonlit nights. For them, the dark world is the only safe one. The white-footed mouse is a very important link in the chain that connects the meat-eaters to the world of vegetable matter. Almost every animal that will eat meat (even just on occasion) hunts the white-footed mouse. Therefore, the mouse is always on guard. He survives as an individual by his wits (but usually doesn't get to see old age, however witty he may be) and as a species by his fecundity.

The population of white-footed mice in a given area runs in cycles. In the long-term cycle, the population will hit a peak every three or five years. On the short term, there are peak months. When white-footed mice are scarce, other animals suffer as the predators look elsewhere to meet their needs. Appetite is not cyclical.

Breeding can be year round if the winters are mild. Litter size varies from one to nine, with three or four being usual. A healthy female in an area where the food supply is good can deliver ten or eleven litters a year. Young born in the early Spring can breed before the first day of Summer. And so, prey as the predators might, there will always be more white-footed mice to carry on.

Source: Reprinted with permission from *North American Mammals, Fur-Bearing Animals of the United States and Canada*, Copyright © 1967, Roger G. Caras.

---

recommended in any region where the prevalence of infected ticks is less than 10%.[61] A trial of antimicrobial prophylaxis (amoxicillin for 10 days) concluded that even in highly endemic areas the risk of infection is so low that antimicrobial treatment is not routinely indicated because the number of adverse reactions to antibiotics was equivalent to the number of cases prevented.[65]

Vaccine

Efforts of many investigators are concentrated on the development of a vaccine. The target antigens have been the Osp proteins; however, these studies were initiated prior to delineation of the expression of different Osp proteins during the vertebrate and invertebrate *B. burgdorferi* replication cycles (Figure 21–5).

The current vaccine is based on inducing anti-body to OspA, the Osp expressed by *B. burg-dorferi* primarily in the infected tick. Vertebrate hosts infected by tick bite rarely produce anti-body to OspA and *Borrelia* organisms recovered from infected animals are not expressing OspA. However, OspA immunization does protect mice from *B. burgdorferi* infection.[66–69] Anti-body to OspA needs to be present at the time of infection, because if it is in the blood meal, it blocks spirochetal development in the infected tick, specifically midgut growth and salivary gland invasion, essential steps for transmission of *B. burgdorferi* from the vector to the host[19,67] (Figure 21–5). Thus, the OspA vaccine is a transmission-blocking Lyme disease vaccine. Early reports of efficacy trials of the OspA vac-cine in humans have been promising.

Two trials conducted in 1995 through 1996 have shown that vaccination with the OspA anti-gen is protective against Lyme disease. A third trial of the vaccine in 4,000 children (aged 4 years and older) is ongoing. Reports of the two trials are published in *The New England Journal of Medicine,* July 23, 1998.[70,71] In the trial con-ducted by Alan Steere and the Lyme Disease Vaccine Study Group,[70] 10,936 subjects (aged 15 to 70 years) were enrolled in a placebo-controlled clinical trial of a vaccine prepared with 30 µg of purified OspA antigen adsorbed to aluminum hydroxide (L-OspA with adjuvant, SmithKline Beecham, Collegeville, PA). In this trial, three immunizations were given at enroll-ment, 1 month, and 12 months. During the fol-lowing two Lyme disease transmission seasons, incident Lyme disease was evaluated in the two study arms. Table 21–3 shows the results of the trial. Results were presented for definite cases of Lyme disease, for those diagnosed clinically with supporting laboratory data, for asymptom-atic cases, and for those with no clinical symp-toms but laboratory confirmation of serocon-version. For those with definite disease, the study found a 49% vaccine efficacy in the first year (95% confidence interval [CI], 15% to 69%) after two immunizations, and a 76% vac-cine efficacy in the second year (95% CI, 58% to 86%) after three immunizations. The measured vaccine efficacy for preventing asymptomatic Lyme disease was 83% the first year, and 100% in the second year. In this study, antibody titer data were presented demonstrating an anamnes-tic response and a booster response, after the third injection. They were also able to demon-strate that antibody titer levels correlated with protection. Cases of Lyme disease among vac-cine recipients were found to have lower anti-body titers than those subjects who did not con-tract Lyme disease during the follow-up period.

The second study, by Leonard Sigal and the Recombinant Outer-Surface Protein A Lyme Disease Vaccine Study Consortium,[71] reported similar results with a non–adjuvant-adsorbed preparation of OspA (Pasteur Merieux Con-naught, Swiftwater, PA). For this trial, 10,305 subjects (aged 18 to 92 years) were enrolled to receive either two injections of a 30 µg prepara-tion of purified OspA antigen or an identically prepared saline placebo. Immunizations were performed at enrollment and 1 month later. In addition, 7,515 subjects received a third immu-nization, with either vaccine or placebo, 1 year after enrollment. The measured vaccine efficacy for definite cases was 68% (95% CI, 36% to 85%) in the first year of the study and 92% (95% CI, 69% to 97%) for those receiving three injec-tions in the second year of the study. Interest-ingly, the study measured zero vaccine efficacy in the second year for participants who did not receive the booster shot. Although the large con-fidence interval indicates an effect of the vac-cine, the study was unable to measure it. Both studies reported mild to moderate side effects in the vaccine recipients, including flulike symp-toms of chills, fever, and myalgias, but no severe or persistent consequences of vaccination were seen in either study.

Although the vaccine trials have demon-strated sufficient efficacy, concerns still remain about long-term side effects of vaccination. The adjuvant-adsorbed vaccine prepared by Smith-Kline Beecham has received "unanimous ap-proval" but "guarded endorsement" from the U.S. Food and Drug Administration (FDA). The

Table 21–3 Measured Vaccine Efficacy in Two Trials of OspA Recombinant Protein Vaccine

Study and Year	Vaccine Group No. Subjects (cases)	Placebo Group No. Subjects (cases)	Measured Vaccine Efficacy (95% CI*)
End of year one			
Sigal et al.[71]			
–Two injections	5156 (12)	5149 (37)	68 (37–85)
Steere et al.[70]			
–Two injections, definite Lyme	5469 (22)	5467 (43)	49 (15–69)
–Two injections, asymptomatic Lyme	5469 (2)	5467 (13)	83 (32–97)
Second year of study			
Sigal et al.[71]			
–Two injections	1379 (2)	1411 (5)	0 (0–60)
–Three injections	3745 (2)	3770 (26)	92 (69–97)
Steere et al.[70]			
–Three injections, definite Lyme	5469 (16)	5467 (66)	76 (58–86)
–Three injections, asymptomatic Lyme	5469 (0)	5467 (15)	100 (26–100)

*CI, confidence interval.

role of OspA antibodies in chronic Lyme disease–associated arthritis is at the root of this concern. OspA cellular and humoral responses are seen in patients with Lyme disease arthritis, but they are associated with arthritis that is resistant to treatment. Gross et al. have proposed that this may be due to molecular mimicry of the T-cell epitope of OspA and human leukocyte function–associated antigen 1 (hLFA-1).[72] Lyme disease arthritis, thus, appears to be the result of an autoimmune process where hLFA-1 is attacked by the patient's immune response to the OspA antigen. The inflammatory process of Lyme disease arthritis is most likely modulated by the cellular immune response, such as CD 8+ T cells. The vaccine, which induces humoral immunity,

B cells producing antibodies, may not produce the same autoimmune complications. To address these concerns, the FDA has charged the manufacturer to establish an active surveillance system to monitor adverse events for recipients of the Lyme disease vaccine. This enhanced system would be expected to collect better information regarding adverse outcomes than the passive reporting system used for most licensed vaccines. Chapter 10 has additional discussion of adverse event monitoring.

As it serves as a blocking antibody in the tick midgut, antibody to OspA transferred after infection is not protective. However, antibody to OspC correlates with recovery from infection, and passive transfer of this antibody to chronically infected immunodeficient mice leads to clearance of *B. burgdorferi* from blood and tissues.[56] It is possible that new vaccines will incorporate both OspA and OspC as immunogens.

CONCLUSION

Lyme disease in an example of a zoonotic disease. Its recent "emergence" into human populations is a product of human intrusion into an existing cycle of disease. In recent experiments, entomologists and molecular biologists have become archeologists, searching museums for specimens to test for *B. burgdorferi*. These analyses have shown that the spirochete has infected *Ixodes* ticks for decades and does not represent a new disease. Factors contributing to its emergence, instead, are changes in the host-vector environmental relationship. The environmental movement of the last 20 years has brought about increased attention to preservation of natural areas and increased occupation of suburban, semirural housing. Deer populations have burgeoned since they were almost eliminated from the United States at the turn of the century. As deer are fringe woodland dwellers, they have adapted well to the suburban environment. The increased availability of deer, as the preferred mating host, in turn, has allowed for an increase in the number of ticks. Humans intrude on the sylvan cycle of Lyme disease when they camp, hike, and otherwise enjoy the woodland area around them.

The epidemiologic questions surrounding the late complications of Lyme disease are difficult to answer. Which diseases are truly associated with Lyme is difficult to determine as the length of time between infection and disease makes causation difficult to prove. The establishment of long-term natural history experiments would be required to carefully document cases of Lyme disease and its sequellae. Understandably, such cohorts are expensive to construct and would not provide results for many years. The currently composed vaccine trials offer the opportunity for such research. However, because of the success of the vaccines, members of the placebo arm of the trials were offered vaccination. Presumably, the incidence of Lyme disease will be low in these cohorts.

The recently completed trials of the Lyme disease vaccine will possibly change the epidemiology of Lyme disease in the United States. However, questions about the safety of the vaccine will continue for many years. As the research is not complete regarding the role of OspA antibodies in Lyme disease, no definitive answers can be provided at this time. Although the efficacy of the vaccine has been demonstrated, its effectiveness (the ability of a vaccine to prevent disease as it is administered in the field) is unknown. The public's willingness to accept adverse events associated with vaccination will be dependent on their perception of the risk of Lyme disease.

REFERENCES

1. Steere AC, Malawista SE, Snydman DR. Lyme arthritis: an epidemic of oligoarticular arthritis in children and adults in three Connecticut communities. *Arthritis Rheum.* 1977;29:7–17.

2. Afzelius A. Erythema chronicum migrans. *Acta Dermatol Venereol.* 1921;2:120–125.

3. Steere AC, Malawista SE, Hardin JA, Ruddy S, Askenase PW, Andiman WA. Erythema chronicum migrans and Lyme arthritis. *Ann Intern Med.* 1977;86:685–698.

4. Steere AC, Broderick TF, Malawista SE. Erythema chronicum migrans and Lyme arthritis: epidemiologic evidence for a tick vector. *Am J Epidemiol.* 1978;108:312–321.

5. Wallis RC, Brown SE, Kloter KO, Main AJ. Erythema chronicum migrans and Lyme arthritis: field study of ticks. *Am J Epidemiol.* 1978;108:322–327.

6. Barbour AG, Fish D. The biological and social phenomenon of Lyme disease. *Science.* 1993;260:1610–1616.

7. Schulze TL, Bowen GS, Lakat MF, Parkin WE, Shisler JK. The role of adult *Ixodes dammini* (acari: ixodidae) in the transmission of Lyme disease in New Jersey, USA. *J Med Entomol.* 1985;22:88–93.

8. Lane RS, Piesman J, Burgdorfer W. Lyme borreliosis. *Annu Rev Entomol.* 1991;36:587–609.

9. Spach DH, Liles WC, Campbell GL, Quick RE, Anderson DE, Fritsche TR. Tick-borne diseases in the United States. *N Engl J Med.* 1993;329:936–947.

10. Oliver JH, Owsley MR, Hutcheson HJ, et al. Conspecificity of the ticks *Ixodes scapularis* and *I. dammini*. *J Med Entomol.* 1993;30:54–63.

11. Burgdorfer W, Barbour AG, Hayes SF, Benach JL, Grunwaldt E, Davis JP. Lyme disease—a tick borne spirochetosis? *Science.* 1982;216:1317–1319.

12. Lennhoff C. Spirochaetes in aetiologically obscure diseases. *Acta Dermatol Venereol.* 1948;28:295–324.

13. Steere AC, Grodzicki RL, Kornblatt AN, et al. The spirochetal etiology of Lyme disease. *N Engl J Med.* 1983; 308:733–740.

14. Benach JL, Bosler EM, Hanrahan JP, et al. Spirochetes isolated from the blood of two patients with Lyme disease. *N Engl J Med.* 1983;308:740–742.

15. Johnson RC, Schmid GP, Hyde FW, Steigerwalt AG, Brenner DJ. *Borrelia burgdorferi* sp. nov.: etiologic agent of Lyme disease. *Int J Syst Bacteriol.* 1984; 34:496–497.

16. Bosler EM, Coleman JL, Benach JL, Massay DA. Natural distribution of the *Ixodes dammini* spirochete. *Science.* 1993;220:321–322.

17. Wilske B, Preac-Mursic V, Gobel UB, et al. An OspA serotyping system for *Borrelia burgdorferi* based on reactivity with monoclonal antibodies and OspA sequence analysis. *J Clin Microbiol.* 1993;31:340–350.

18. deSilva AM, Fikrig E. Arthropod- and host-specific gene expression by *Borrelia burgdorferi*. *J Clin Invest.* 1996;99:377–379.

19. de Silva AM, Telford SR, Brunet LR, Barthold SW, Fikrig E. *Borrelia burgdorferi* OspA is an arthropod-specific transmission-blocking Lyme disease vaccine. *J Exp Med.* 1996;183:271–275.

20. Schwan TG, Piesman J, Golde WT, Dolan MC, Rosa PA. Induction of an outer surface protein on *Borrelia burgdorferi* during tick feeding. *Proc Natl Acad Sci USA.* 1995;92:2909–2913.

21. Ribeiro JMC, Mather TN, Piesman MJ, Spielman A. Dissemination and salivary delivery of Lyme disease spirochetes in vector ticks (acari: ixodidae). *J Med Entomol.* 1987;24:201–205.

22. Persing DH, Telford SM, Rys PN, et al. Detection of *Borrelia burgdorferi* DNA in museum specimens of *Ixodes dammini* ticks. *Science.* 1990;249:1420–1423.

23. Scrimenti RJ. Erythema chronicum migrans. *Arch Derm.* 1970;102:104–109.

24. Baranton G, Postic D, Saint Girons I, et al. Delineation of *Borrelia burgdorferi* sensu stricto, *Borrelia garinii* sp. nov., and group VS461 associated with Lyme borreliosis. *Int J Syst Bacteriol.* 1992;42:378–383.

25. Markowitz LE, Steere AC, Benach JL, Slade JD, Broome CV. Lyme disease during pregnancy. *JAMA.* 1986;255:3394–3396.

26. Ohlenbusch A, Matuschka F, Richter D, et al. Etiology of the acrodermatitis chronica atrophicans lesion in Lyme disease. *J Infect Dis.* 1996;174:421–423.

27. Steere AC, Bartenhagen NH, Craft JE. The early clinical manifestations of Lyme disease. *Ann Intern Med.* 1983; 99:76–82.

28. Steere AC, Batsford WP, Weinberg M, et al. Lyme carditis: cardiac abnormalities of Lyme disease. *Ann Intern Med.* 1980;93:8–16.

29. Reik L, Steere AC, Bartenhagen NH, Shope RE, Malawista SE. Neurologic abnormalities of Lyme disease. *Medicine.* 1979;58:281–294.

30. Nocton JJ, Bloom BJ, Rutledge BJ, Persing DH, Logigian Schmid EL, Steere AC. Detection of *Borrelia burgdorferi* DNA by polymerase chain reaction in cerebrospinal fluid in Lyme neuroborreliosis. *J Infect Dis.* 1996;174:623–627.

31. Luft BJ, Steinman CR, Neimark HC, et al. Invasion of the central nervous system by *Borrelia burgdorferi* in acute disseminated infection. *JAMA.* 1992;267:1364–1367.

32. Reik L, Burgdorfer W, Donaldson JO. Neurologic abnormalities in Lyme disease without erythema chronicum migrans. *Am J Med.* 1986;81:73–78.

33. Pachner AR, Steere AC. The triad of neurologic manifestations of Lyme disease: meningitis, cranial neuritis and radiculoneuritis. *Neurology.* 1985;35:47–53.

34. Reik L, Smith L, Khan A, Nelson W. Demyelinating encephalopathy in Lyme disease. *Neurology.* 1985; 32:1302–1305.

35. Schlesinger PA, Duray PH, Burke BA, Steere AC, Stillman MT. Maternal fetal transmission of the Lyme disease spirochete, *Borrelia burgdorferi*. *Ann Intern Med.* 1985;103:67–69.

36. Steere AC, Gibofsky A, Patarroyo ME, Winchester RJ, Hardin JA, Malawista SE. Chronic Lyme arthritis: clinical and immunogenetic differentiation from rheumatoid arthritis. *Ann Intern Med.* 1979;90:896–901.

37. Nocton JJ, Dressler F, Rutledge BJ, Rys PN, Persing DH, Steere AC. Detection of *Borrelia burgdorferi* DNA by polymerase chain reaction in synovial fluid from patients with Lyme arthritis. *N Engl J Med.* 1994;330:229–234.

38. Weber K, Schierz G, Wilske B, Preac-Mursic V. European erythema migrans disease and related disorders. *Yale J Biol Med.* 1984;57:463–471.

39. Halperin JJ, Volkman DJ, Wu P. Central nervous system abnormalities in Lyme neuroborreliosis. *Neurology.* 1991;41:1571–1582.

40. Logigian EL, Kaplan RF, Steere AC. Chronic neurologic manifestations of Lyme disease. *N Engl J Med.* 1990;323:1438–1444.

41. Wallach FR, Forni AL, Hariprashad J, et al. Circulating *Borrelia burgdorferi* in patients with acute Lyme disease: results of blood cultures and serum DNA analysis. *J Infect Dis.* 1993;68:1541–1543.

42. Berardi VP, Weeks KE, Steere AC. Serodiagnosis of early Lyme disease: analysis of IgM and IgG antibody responses by using an antibody-capture enzyme immunoassay. *J Infect Dis.* 1988;158:754–760.

43. Hansen K, Lebech A. Lyme neuroborreliosis: a new sensitive diagnostic assay for intrathecal synthesis of *Borrelia burgdorferi*–specific immunoglobulin G, A, and M. *Ann Neurol.* 1991;30:197–205.

44. Steere AC, Berardi VP, Weeks KE, Logigian EL, Ackerman R. Evaluation of the intrathecal antibody response to *Borrelia burgdorferi* as a diagnostic test for Lyme neuroborreliosis. *J Infect Dis.* 1990;161:1203–1209.

45. Karlsson M, Stiernstedt G, Granstrom M, Asbrink E, Wretlind B. Comparison of flagellum and sonicate antigens for serological diagnosis of Lyme borreliosis. *Eur J Clin Microbiol Infect Dis.* 1990;9:169–177.

46. Johnson BJ, Robbins KE, Bailey RE, et al. Serodiagnosis of Lyme disease: accuracy of a two-step approach using a flagella-based ELISA immunoblotting. *J Infect Dis.* 1996;174:346–353.

47. Halperin J, Krupp LB, Golightly MG, Volkman DJ. Lyme borreliosis-associated encephalopathy. *Neurology.* 1990;40:1340–1343.

48. Dattwyler RJ, Volkman DJ, Conaty SM, Platkin SP, Luft BJ. Amoxycillin plus probenecid versus doxycycline for treatment of erythema migrans borreliosis. *Lancet.* 1990;336:1404–1406.

49. Steere AC, Sigal LH, Rahn DW, Craft JE, DeSanna ET, Malawista SE. Treatment of the early manifestations of Lyme disease. *Ann Intern Med.* 1983;99:22–26.

50. Steere AC, Green J, Schoen RT. Successful parenteral penicillin therapy of established Lyme arthritis. *N Engl J Med.* 1985;312:869–874.

51. Dattwyler RJ, Volkman DJ, Halperin JJ, et al. Treatment of late Lyme borreliosis: randomized comparison of ceftriaxone and penicillin. *Lancet.* 1988;1:1191–1194.

52. Schmid GP. The global distribution of Lyme disease. *Rev Infect Dis.* 1985;7:41–50.

53. Gustafson R, Svenungsson B, Gardulf A, et al. Prevalence of tick-borne encephalitis and Lyme borreliosis in a defined Swedish population. *Scand J Infect Dis.* 1990; 22:297–306.

54. Steere AC, Taylor E, Wilson ML, Levine JF, Spielman A. Longitudinal assessment of the clinical and epidemiological features of Lyme disease in a defined population. *J Infect Dis.* 1986;154:295–300.

55. Oliver JH Jr, Chandler FW, Luttrell MP, et al. Isolation and transmission of the Lyme disease spirochete from the southeastern United States. *Proc Natl Acad Sci USA.* 1993;90:7371–7375.

56. Mathiesen DA, Oliver JH Jr, Kolbert CP, et al. Genetic heterogeneity of *Borrelia burgdorferi* in the United States. *J Infect Dis.* 1997;175:98–107.

57. Jones CG, Ostfeld RS, Richard MP, et al. Chain reactions linking acorns to gypsy moth outbreaks and Lyme disease risk. *Science.* 1998;279:1023–1026.

58. Brown RN, Lane RS. Lyme disease in California: a novel enzootic transmission cycle of *Borrelia burgdorferi. Science.* 1992;256:1439–1442.

59. Dekonenko EJ, Steere AC, Berardi VP, Kravchuk LN. Lyme borreliosis in the Soviet Union: a cooperative US-USSR report. *J Infect Dis.* 1988;158:748–753.

60. Berglund J, Eitrem R, Ornstein K, et al. An epidemiologic study of Lyme disease in southern Sweden. *N Engl J Med.* 1995;333:1319–1324.

61. Magid D, Schwartz B, Craft J, et al. Prevention of Lyme disease after tick bites: a cost-effective analysis. *N Engl J Med.* 1992;327:534–541.

62. Piesman J. Dynamics of *Borrelia burgdorferi* transmission by nymphal *Ixodes dammini* ticks. *J Infect Dis.* 1993;167:1082–1085.

63. Sood SK, Salzman MB, Johnson BJB, et al. Duration of tick attachment as a predictor of the risk of Lyme disease in an area in which Lyme disease is endemic. *J Infect Dis.* 1997;175:996–999.

64. Wilson ML, Levine JF, Spielman. Effect of deer reduction on abundance of the deer tick (*Ixodes dammini*). *Yale J Biol Med.* 1984;57:697–705.

65. Shapiro ED, Gerber MA, Holabird NB, et al. A controlled trial of antimicrobial prophylaxis for Lyme disease after deer-tick bites. *N Engl J Med.* 1992;327:1769–1773.

66. Luke CJ, Carner K, Liang X. An Osp A-based DNA vaccine protects mice against infection with *Borrelia burgdorferi. J Infect Dis.* 1997:175:91–97.

67. Telford SR, Kantor FS, Lobet Y, et al. Efficacy of human Lyme disease vaccine formulations in a mouse model. *J Infect Dis.* 1995;171:1368–1370.

68. Fikrig E, Barthold SW, Kantor FS, et al. Protection of mice against the Lyme disease agent by immunizing with recombinant OspA. *Science.* 1990;250:553–556.

69. Simon MM, Schaible UE, Wallich R, et al. A mouse model for *Borrelia burgdorferi* infection: approach to a vaccine against Lyme disease. *Immunol Today.* 1991; 12:11–16.

70. Steere AC, Sikand VK, Meurice F, et al. Vaccination against Lyme disease with recombinant *Borrelia burgdorferi* outer-surface lipoprotein A with adjuvant. Lyme Disease Vaccine Study Group. *N Engl J Med.* 1998; 339:209–215.

71. Sigal LH, Zahradnik JM, Lavin P, et al. A vaccine consisting of recombinant *Borrelia burgdorferi* outer-surface protein A to prevent Lyme disease. Recombinant Outer-Surface Protein A Lyme Disease Vaccine Study Consortium. *N Engl J Med.* 1998;339:216–222.

72. Gross DM, Forsthuber T, Tary-Lehmann M, et al. Identification of LFA-1 as a candidate autoantigen in treatment-resistant Lyme arthritis. *Science.* 1998;281:703.

CHAPTER 22

The Epidemiology and Control of Malaria

Richard H. Morrow

BACKGROUND, HISTORY, AND PUBLIC HEALTH IMPORTANCE

History of Malaria Control

Vertebrates, mosquitoes, and malaria have been interacting and evolving together for tens of thousands of years. Humans have been afflicted with malaria as long as there have been humans; documentation of what is certainly malaria dates back to 2700 B.C. in China, and malaria was featured in the writings of Homer, Aristotle, Plato, Socrates, Chaucer, Pepys, and Shakespeare.[1] It has been 100 years since the knowledge that malaria is caused by a protozoan parasite that infects red blood cells and is transmitted by mosquitoes from human to human became known. In 1902, Ronald Ross was awarded the Nobel Prize in Medicine for his work on malaria and its transmission cycle. Over the following several decades, major scientific advances were made in understanding the parasite, its cycles within anopheline mosquitoes, and its pathogenesis in humans.

The Greeks had known the relation of fever to swamps and low-lying water since the sixth century B.C. Advances in controlling mosquito breeding through drainage and environmental control were of key importance in the development of the Panama Canal and continued to be the major approach toward malaria control until after World War II. During World War II, two major biochemical/pharmaceutical advances in unrelated fields revolutionized malaria control and its treatment: Dichlorodiphenyltrichloroethane (DDT) as an insecticide was found to be highly effective against anopheline vectors, and chloroquine for treatment of individual patients replaced quinine as the principal antimalarial drug.

With these new tools, not only were ideas for reduction and control of malaria envisioned, but also the exciting prospect of total eradication of this horrendous disease began to be discussed. The fundamental notion involved the total elimination of all parasites of all human malaria species, principally by stopping the transmission by the vector from one human to the next. Residual spraying of DDT on the walls of households was the principal weapon to be employed and, in nearly all early trials, proved to be remarkably effective in killing those mosquitoes that had just enjoyed a blood meal from sleeping householders. The availability of chloroquine, a rapidly and uniformly curative with a wide margin of safety and very low cost, to treat anyone who might be infected from another area provided an additional tool that might help in areas of transition.

Following World War II, the newly formed World Health Organization (WHO) formulated a plan for worldwide malaria eradication at the 8th World Health Assembly in 1955. It was estimated that eradication using DDT residual spraying could be accomplished at a cost of less than 25 cents per person per year; the total cost for the first 5 years would be half a billion U.S. dollars.[2]

Plans were put into action in many areas of the world, and truly dramatic success was achieved in some regions. By 1958, the most inspirational, ambitious, complex, and costly health campaign ever undertaken was well underway.[3] Early campaign efforts in many countries in Europe, Asia, and Latin America were enormously successful. Indeed, in Malta, the anopheline vector was completely wiped out.[4] However, as time passed, there seemed to be little effect in many continental tropical countries of Asia and South America. In Africa, where malaria was by far of greatest importance, virtually nothing was even attempted. Unfortunately, with the great emphasis on logistics and organizational activities, there seemed a comparable de-emphasis on scientific research. Over a period extending for 20 years, virtually no innovative research about malaria was undertaken—the general opinion frequently and loudly expressed was, "We know what has to be done; let us get on with it!" An entire generation of researchers was lost to malaria.

Even by the mid-1960s, it was clear that eradication would fail. The complex logistical operational needs were too much for the weak infrastructures in most tropical countries; moreover, basic biologic developments emerged, including anopheline resistance to insecticides and parasite resistance to antimalarials.[5,6] The malaria eradication campaign came to be viewed as a major failure. In the wisdom of hindsight, it was a failure due to scientific arrogance and lack of foresight. In truth, however, large numbers of lives were saved in many countries, and major economic activities were spurred. Further, a major revolution in ideas about malaria control was fostered; gradually, it became clear that peaceful coexistence between humans and malaria parasites would have to be worked out.

Today, major advances have taken place in our understanding of the molecular biology of the malaria parasite and of the immunologic responses to it; in the development of diagnostic techniques, vector control methods, antimalarial drugs, and vaccines; and in trials of a variety of strategies for malaria control. Yet, despite these advances, a resurgence of severe malaria and an increased number of deaths, particularly in Africa, have taken place. Perhaps the term *resurgence* is not entirely apt as concerns Africa because malaria was never under any sort of control. Indeed, most African health officials did not rank malaria as a priority because the basic biologic factors of transmission were so intractable and because malaria was considered an inevitable and accepted part of life for the infants and children of the rural poor. Other serious problems, more amenable to control, were given priority. By the early 1980s, when primary health care programs aimed at diarrheal and respiratory diseases and diseases controllable through immunizations became increasingly effective in many African countries, the HIV/AIDS epidemic was rampant and fully occupied the attention of most health ministries and the International Agency-Donor communities. Only quite recently is malaria being viewed as a genuine priority in Africa; the recently initiated WHO "Roll Back Malaria" program exemplifies the renewed emphasis. Concerted action is yet to be taken, but at least there is now talk and the beginning of serious planning in some African countries. The starting point for this planning must be an in-depth understanding of the ecology, biology, and epidemiology of malaria as it exists in Africa.

Public Health Importance

The impact of malaria in human populations varies greatly in different parts of the world; wherever there is *Plasmodium falciparum*, there will be dire consequences. Although *Plasmodium vivax* malaria continues as a major cause of morbidity in parts of China, Southeast Asia, and Latin America, the overwhelming problems of malaria as a life-threatening disease continue to be in those countries with *P. falciparum* malaria, especially in Africa. Most of this discussion will focus on issues related to tropical Africa, where malaria is of greatest importance and where approaches to control have had the least success.

The public health significance of a disease depends on its incidence and resulting disability and mortality. These measures are particularly useful when known according to descriptive epidemiologic variables including person (age, sex, and other demographic variables, such as occupation, education, and social economic group); place (for example, urban and rural or particular geographical situations); and time (including seasonal or other cyclic variation or secular trends).

Incidence is usefully expressed in terms both of episodes per time period and of persons affected per time period. In many places where malaria is hypo- or mesoendemic, incidence in these terms has meaning and can be expressed as episodes per thousand persons per year or persons having episodes per thousand persons per year. In holoendemic areas, however, with an entomologic inoculation rate (EIR) ranging from dozens to hundreds of infectious bites per year per person, everyone is infected all the time and is being reinfected every few days. The very idea of incidence, or indeed of prevalence, has little meaning. The health status of an individual in these situations results from a balance between the parasite and the host defense systems. Clearance of parasites from the host occurs with reasonable certainty only when an individual is given an effective antimalarial drug; reinfection and, thus, a "new incident" case occurs as soon as the level of the antimalarial drug drops below the effective therapeutic level and the incubation time is allowed for the parasite.

The figure that from one to two million children die from malaria every year has remained the quoted estimate since first put out by WHO in the early 1950s.[7,8] Recently, estimates have varied more widely, ranging from a low of 856,000 total global deaths[9] to 1.5–2.7 million,[10] with 90% occurring in Africa. Whatever the estimate, the reality in Africa is that malaria is a major cause of mortality in infants and children and of disability in adults.

Recently, composite measures of disease burden in populations have been developed that combine the effects of disability and of mortality into a single indicator of healthy life loss that can be used to compare the relative importance of one disease with another.[11,12] In tropical Africa, malaria is the major cause of loss of healthy life, whether measured in disability-adjusted life years (DALYs), healthy life years (HeaLYs), or other nearly equivalent indicators. For example, in studies in Ghana, malaria was the leading cause of loss of healthy life and accounted for nearly 10% of discounted years of healthy life lost in the total population.[11,13]

THE BIOLOGY OF MALARIA PARASITES AND ANOPHELINE VECTORS

Malaria Parasites and Their Life Cycle

Four species of protozoan parasites of the genus *Plasmodium* infect humans: *P. falciparum, P. vivax, P. ovale*, and *P. malariae* (Table 22–1). Although *P. vivax* is the most widespread form of malaria infection in the world, *P. falciparum* causes the most severe disease and is responsible, by far, for most deaths and serious morbidity due to malaria.

The complex life cycle of the malaria parasite is given in Figure 22–1. The parasite undergoes three phases in the mosquito and two in the human host; at least a dozen separate steps have been defined in these transformations. The parasite is transmitted to humans by the sporozoite forms in the saliva of an infected female anopheline mosquito taking a blood meal. Sporozoites enter the venous blood system through the capillary bed, and, within a few seconds or a minute or two, those that avoid the defending reticuloendothelial (RE) system invade liver cells. Over the next 5–15 days, each sporozoite nucleus replicates thousands of times to develop into a hepatic schizont within the liver cells; when released from the swollen liver cells, each schizont splits into up to 40,000 daughter parasites, called *merozoites*. Merozoites attach to specific erythrocyte surface receptors (Duffy blood group antigen for *P. vivax*, glycophorin for *P. falciparum*[14]) and penetrate into the erythrocyte. Each intra-erythrocytic merozoite differentiates into a trophozoite that ingests human

Table 22–1 Malaria Parasites of Humans

Species	Intra-RBC Schizont Period	Type of RBC	Relapse (Hypnozoite)	Global Distribution
P. vivax	48 hours	Reticulocytes	Yes	Everywhere except tropical Africa
P. malariae	72 hours	Reticulocytes	No	Everywhere
P. ovale	48 hours	Older RBCs	Yes	Africa
P. falciparum	48 hours (±)	All	No	Tropical regions

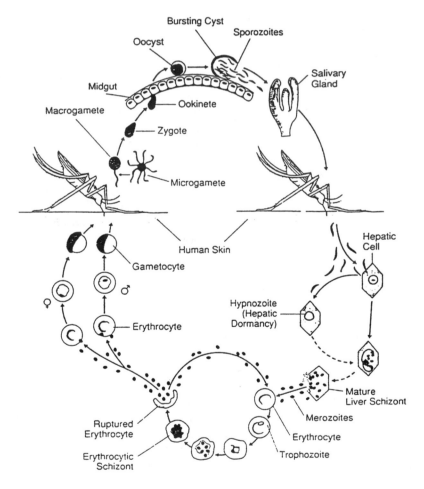

Figure 22–1 Life cycle of the malaria parasite. *Source:* Reproduced with permission. V. Nussenzweig and R.S. Nussenzweig. Progress Toward a Malaria Vaccine. HOSPITAL PRACTICE 1990;25(9):45. © 1990, The McGraw-Hill Companies. Illustration by Nancy Lou Riccio.

hemoglobin, enlarges and divides into 6–24 intra-erythrocytic merozoites, forming a schizont. The red cell swells and bursts, releasing the next batch of merozoites, which then attach and penetrate new erythrocytes to begin this cycle once again. Along with the liberation of the merozoites, the resultant hemolysis and release of "pyrogens" from infected red cells and the host response to these toxins correspond with clinical paroxysms of fever and chills; when synchronous, the simultaneous release from many red cells account for the periodicity of these symptoms in some patients. This second stage of asexual division takes about 48 hours for *P. falciparum, P. vivax,* and *P. ovale,* or 72 hours for *P. malariae.*[4] A single falciparum merozoite potentially can lead to 10 billion new parasites through these recurrent cycles.[1]

After a number of cycles within red cells, some merozoites differentiate into sexual forms called *gametocytes, macrogametocytes* (female), and *microgametocytes* (male), which are then available to be ingested by an anopheline mosquito during its next blood meal. Factors related to gametogenesis include the species of parasite, length of infection or number of intra-erythrocytic cycles, density of parasitemia, drug treatment, and age or immune status of the infected individuals.

Sporogonic Development

Once in the mosquito, the red cells are digested, freeing the gametocytes, which then begin sexual reproduction that leads to sporogonic development; the male and female gametes fuse, providing for genetic recombination, to form a zygote. Over the next 12–14 hours, the zygote elongates and forms into an ookinete, which then penetrates the wall of the mosquito's stomach to become an oocyst. During the next week or so the oocyst enlarges, forming more than 10,000 sporozoites. After the oocyst ruptures into the coelomic cavity of the mosquito, the sporozoites migrate to the anopheline salivary glands, ready to be injected back into the human host, thus completing the cycle.

These three phases of parasite development, from ingestion of gametocytes to when sporozoites in the salivary glands are poised for reinoculation into the human host, comprise the extrinsic cycle or sporogonic phase (within the vector outside the human host) and generally take from 7–12 days. The time required depends on the species of parasite and, in particular, the ambient temperature. For example, under optimal conditions, with temperature at 30° Centigrade, *P. falciparum* requires 9 days, but at 20°, it takes 23 days—a difference of 14 days for a temperature differential of 10°.[1,4] With an average life span for most anophelines of less than 3 weeks, it is clear that the ambient temperature is critical to transmission. Once infected with malaria, a female anopheline remains infected for life and transmits sporozoites with each blood meal taken.[4,15]

During this sporogonic development period, each female-male pair of gametocytes potentially can produce over 10,000 sporozoites for inoculation. Because dozens to thousands of gametocytes can be ingested with one blood meal, the potential exists for millions of sporozoites to be injected with one bite. Though such high inocula counts are not found, perhaps related to damage to the mosquito from heavy loads or insufficient nutrients/metabolites available to support such, limited studies of naturally infected mosquitoes have found sporozoite loads (the number of sporozoites in the salivary glands of an anopheline) from 10 to over 100,000 in *Anopheles gambiae* and *Anopheles funestus.*[16,17]

The assumption that sporozoites in the salivary gland are infectious remains uncertain in terms of a direct relation between sporozoite load and actual numbers of infective sporozoites delivered per bite. In vitro studies using experimentally infected mosquitoes have shown that most infected mosquitoes transmit fewer than 25 sporozoites per bite, but about 5% can transmit hundreds.[10] Epidemiologic studies comparing sporozoite rates (the proportion of anopheline females with sporozoites in their salivary glands) with infant infection have demonstrated that less than 20% of sporozoite inoculations result in infection.[18] However, great variation in the ratio of infant conversion rate (ICR) to the entomologic inoculation rate (EIR) has been found between places,[19] seasons,[20] and for evaluation of vector control.[21] Among other factors, antibodies ingested at the time of the bite may have a role in reducing infectivity. Human immunoglobulin G antibody has been found on sporozoites in 80% of infected anophelines, although its effect on sporozoite infectivity is not known.[22] In general, far lower numbers seem to be delivered than are found in the salivary glands; yet, some bites do transmit quite high numbers of infective sporozoites and, although speculative, it is possible that such high loads play a role in severe disease.

Biologic Differences among Malaria Species

There are important parasite species specific differences in this generic life cycle. With *P. vivax* and *P. ovale*, some sporozoites entering hepatic parenchymal cells do not immediately proceed to tissue schizogony but become uninuclear hypnozoites in the infected liver cell,[23] where they lie dormant for months to years. At some later time, they may differentiate into hepatic schizonts, leading to the cycle of erythrocytic schizogony and consequent relapse of symptoms. This biologic capability accounts for the relapses characteristic of *P. vivax* and *P. ovale*. Different strains of *P. vivax* from diverse areas of the world are known to have characteristic relapse patterns. Following acute infection with either *P. vivax* or *P. ovale*, patients are at risk for up to 3–4 years of having a relapse. There is no diagnostic test available to determine whether or not individuals have hepatic hypnozoites.

P. falciparum and *P. malariae* do not produce hypnozoites and, therefore, do not relapse following effective treatment, but untreated or inadequately treated infections with these parasites may cause persistent low-grade parasitemia, leading to recrudescent clinical disease.[24]

The different species of human malaria parasites have a particular affinity for particular erythrocytes. *P. vivax* and *P. ovale* parasites invade only the young reticulocytes; thus, the density of peripheral parasitemia in these infections rarely exceeds 3%. *P. malariae* is limited to older red cells, but *P. falciparum* infects erythrocytes of all ages and for this reason is able to produce high-density parasitemias with serious morbidity and high mortality.[4,15]

Aspects of the Molecular Biology of the Malaria Parasite

Although most research on the molecular biology of the malaria parasite has focused on the identification and cloning of genes that encode for essential antigens that might serve as targets for vaccine development, important advances in understanding other aspects of parasite biology have been made. Most work has been done with *P. falciparum*, which is the only human *Plasmodium* species so far cultured.

The most striking finding has been the great genetic diversity among *P. falciparum* parasite populations; the *falciparum genome* is highly variable, with heterogeneous phenotypic expression accounting for much of the highly successful evasion of host immune defense systems. In an early genetic analysis of dozens of *P. falciparum* isolates from three continents, all isolates were different from one another.[25] The common theme for nearly every characteristic of falciparum biology is also diversity: isoenzyme and electrophoretic patterns of the proteins from different isolates, drug resistance variation, morphologic expression, striking size differences in the 14 chromosomes of the genomes from different isolates, and antigenic variation.

The malaria genome is about 10 times more complex than that of a bacterium; an international collaboration to sequence the falciparum genome is well underway, and the sequencing is expected to be completed in the next couple of years.[6] Combined with other new technologic advances that aid in rapid identification of genes and their protein products, there will be a stronger basis not only for vaccines but also for rational drug design and the potential for identifying key parasite characteristics, such as drug resistance and, perhaps, parasite virulence. At present, there is scant evidence that severe disease is related to any specific parasite characteristic, but until recently, there have been only a limited number of possible markers available to consider. Because the underlying reasons for severe disease remain inadequately explained, the new potential for better understanding parasitic determinants of severe disease is promising.

Anopheline Mosquitoes and Their Life Cycle

The mosquito goes through four stages of growth during its life cycle, from egg to larva to pupa and to adult. Shortly after emerging as an adult and generally before the first blood meal, adult anopheline females mate; usually, they mate only once, then store the sperm, laying a total of 200–1,000 eggs in from 3 to 10 or 12 batches over their lifetimes.[4] The number of eggs produced depends on blood consumption from a vertebrate; each batch requires a fresh blood meal. After hatching, an anopheline larva feeds at the water's surface and develops over 5–15 days, transforming into the pupal stage; thereafter, it emerges within 2–4 days as an adult mosquito. The entire cycle requires a total of 7–20 days, depending on the anopheline species and the environmental conditions. Under favorable conditions of high humidity and moderate temperatures, female anophelines can survive at least a month—time enough for the parasite to develop after the first blood meal and for the mosquito to take another blood meal. This enables transmission of the parasite to a second human host and thereafter to others with each blood meal. Thus, after emerging, the female must survive for at least the 7–12 days of the extrinsic cycle before it can transmit; thereafter, it transmits with each blood meal, often taken every other day for the remainder of its life. Therefore, the longevity of the anopheline is critically important in determining the efficiency of transmission (see section on vectorial capacity, below).

Fifty to sixty species of the genus *Anopheles* are known to be capable of transmitting malaria to humans. Only the female anopheline requires blood meals to produce egg broods; therefore, it is only the female that is the vector for malaria. There is great variation in different species in their host feeding preferences, biting and resting habits, and in favored habitats for egg laying; knowledge of these variations in behavior is key to reducing transmission through vector control. Some anophelines feed on most any vertebrate, whereas others are very particular; a few take blood meals only from humans. Some bite humans only indoors; others may sometimes or even exclusively feed outdoors. Whether they rest indoors or outdoors after the meal is also critical in understanding transmission and effective approaches to control. Nearly all anophelines prefer clean water in which to breed, but some have very specific preferences for the aquatic environment in which to lay their eggs. For example, *Anopheles stephensi* can breed in tin cans and in confined water systems, whereas *Anopheles gambiae*, the most important vector in Africa, prefers small, open sunlit pools. In each ecologic area, an understanding of specific vector biology is essential for undertaking control measures.

Mosquitoes are able to seek out their host in response to a combination of chemical and physical stimuli, including carbon dioxide, certain body odors, warmth, and movement. Most anophelines feed at night, but some do so in late afternoon or early morning. During feeding, the mosquito injects salivary fluid containing enzymes into the subcutaneous tissue. These enzymes diffuse through the surrounding tissue and increase blood flow, facilitating both the blood meal and the transfer of sporozoites to the capillary bed area. Anophelines generally feed at night while the human is sleeping indoors; after feeding, the engorged female seeks a resting place on a nearby wall or in a secluded spot outdoors near the ground. They usually rest for several hours or until daylight before they seek refuge elsewhere. Some, however, bite outdoors, especially those that are forest dwellers, such as *Anopheles dirus*, and some that bite indoors, may fly outside to rest after their engorgement. Some species alter their behavior in the presence of DDT or other insecticides, becoming irritable in its presence and flying outside to rest.

In any particular ecologic area, the identification of potential vectors and those that are actually transmitting is the starting point for investigation of malaria transmission. The global distributions of malaria and the principal vectors for each area have been mapped and catalogued by Haworth.[26] However, as Haworth emphasized, there is enormous variation even within small geographic areas and relatively short periods of time. Further, there are major secular changes in the ecologic habitats nearly everywhere, brought on by such human activities as urbanization, deforestation, and irrigation.

A major problem concerning species identification is that of species complexes in which sibling groups, morphologically indistinguishable, are genetically distinct, having different cytogenetic characteristics. The sibling species may have quite different potential as vectors, with differences in susceptibility to malaria; resistance to insecticides; and even to host preference, biting, or resting habits. Much work has gone into methods for distinguishing among these sibling species, but so far, none are simple enough for routine field identification.

Field study methods had remained much the same for 25 years, but in the last few years, a range of new methods based on developments in immunology (eg, monoclonal antibodies) and molecular biology (eg, polymerase chain reaction) are leading to major changes in field methods. As these new tools become validated and standardized, further advances in understanding of the interacting ecologic, vector, host, and parasite factors should translate into improved approaches to control.[8] The factors that allow for the susceptibility of certain anopheline species to be parasitized by human *Plasmodia* species are not well understood and are presently being studied by a number of groups in the hope of selecting or developing genetically altered forms of anophelines that cannot transmit malaria but will replace those species that do.[27,28]

Vectorial Capacity and Entomologic Inoculation Rate

Understanding the dynamics of transmission is fundamental to understanding how best to reduce transmission through vector control measures. The EIR and vectorial capacity (VC) are two basic indices of malaria transmission. These measures are closely related, but it is important to know how they are derived and how they are used. Both are carried out and applied to a defined ecologic zone or geographic area, and both vary greatly in place and time.[19,21,29] The EIR is the number of infected bites that each person receives per night and is calculated by multiplying the human landing rate (HLR) by the sporozoite rate (SR). The HLR, previously termed the *human biting rate*, is obtained by capturing all mosquitoes that land on a person, the "bait," during the night and is expressed as the number of mosquitoes landing (bites) per night per person. The SR is determined by microscopic examination of dissected salivary glands to detect sporozoites in these captured mosquitoes, expressed as the ratio of infected anophelines to total collected. More recently, immunologic methods based on monoclonal antibodies have been developed to detect sporozoites in pools of the collected mosquitoes. Even with this advance, actually obtaining the HLR and the SR are difficult, tedious, and costly. However, they provide the only direct measure of malaria transmission.

Whereas the EIR provides a direct measure of the risk of human exposure to the bites of infected mosquitoes, the VC measures the daily rate of potentially infective contact, ie, the potential for malaria transmission, and is based solely on key vector parameters. The VC is the number of potentially infective contacts an individual human acquires, through the vector population, per unit time.[21,30] The formula for its calculation is:

$$VC = ma^2p^n/ - \log p$$

where *m* is the density of vectors in relation to humans (obtained by standardized sampling methods to give the number of female anophelines caught in a collection per person per night); a is the human biting habit (the proportion of blood meals taken from humans to the total number of blood meals taken from any animal) so that a person is bitten by ma vectors in 1 day; p is the daily survival probability of the vector; and n is the extrinsic incubation (or sporogonic) period of the vector measured in days so that a fraction p^n of the vectors survive the extrinsic incubation period. They still have an expectation of life of $1/-logp$ (the expectation of life is assumed to be independent of age); each of the surviving vectors bites a persons per day. In principle, the VC can predict the extent to which anopheline populations must be reduced in order to reduce transmission.

It is important to understand the nonlinear relation among these variables.[31] In Figure 22–2, the prevalence of parasitemia in the human population is charted against the average annual VC.[32] Note that, at low levels of VC, small increases result in a rapid rise in parasitemia prevalence rate; thereafter, a long plateau is reached, where large changes in the VC do not change the level of parasitemia. This is the circumstance in most of tropical Africa; in these areas, reduction of a 100- or even a 1,000-fold in the VC will not change the prevalence of malaria (although it may change the frequency and nature of severe malaria). For these reasons, malaria control for holoendemic areas, as in much of tropical Africa, must involve a "peaceful" coexistence, rather than an elimination of malaria.

Geographic Areas According to Intensity of Transmission

Traditionally, geographic areas have been classified into four broad categories, according

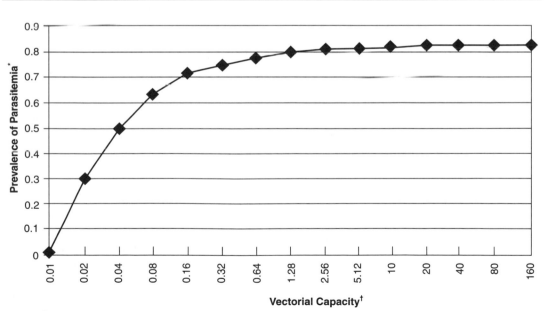

*Proportion of human population infected.
†Number of potentially infectious contacts per person per day.

Figure 22–2 Prevalence of parasitemia related to vectorial capacity. *Source:* Data from Garke Project Molineaux and Gramiccia, WHO, Geneva, 1980, p. 281.

to intensity of transmission and based on percentage of children aged 2–9 with enlarged spleens and malaria parasites,[33,34] as follows:

1. Holoendemic: areas of intense transmission with continuing high EIRs, where virtually everyone is infected with malaria parasites all the time. In older children and adults, detection of parasites may be very difficult because of high levels of immunity, but sufficient search will generally reveal the presence of parasites. Classification on the basis of children under age 10: spleen and parasitemia rates of over 75%.
2. Hyperendemic: regions with regular, often seasonal transmission but where the immunity in some of the population does not confer continuing protection at all times. Classification as above: spleen and parasite rate in children under age 10 from 50% to 75%.
3. Mesoendemic: areas that have malaria transmission fairly regularly but at much lower levels. The danger in these areas is occasional epidemics involving those with little immunity and resulting in fairly high mortality. In these areas, the under-10 children will have spleen and parasitemia rates ranging from 10% to 50%.
4. Hypoendemic: areas with limited malaria transmission and where the population will have little or no immunity. Spleen and parasitemia rates in the under-10 children will be less than 10%. These areas, too, can sometimes have severe malaria epidemics involving all age groups.

Further classification schemes have been devised in efforts to simplify the complexity of epidemiologic factors of malaria and to improve the targeting of strategies for malaria control. An expert group, brought together by WHO, used an epidemiologic approach based on principles of stratification in 1990 to define a set of eight major malaria paradigms intended to categorize typical transmission settings to facilitate discussion and more efficient planning of control efforts.[8,35] However, these, too, were oversimplifications and, in general, have not replaced the need to gather the detailed epidemiologic and entomologic data described above. Nevertheless, the basic notions are useful, and Exhibit 22–1 outlines the main paradigms developed by the expert group.[8] Most malaria situations can be characterized by one or a combination of these basic paradigms, which are helpful for characterizing the most appropriate control measures.

PATHOGENESIS IN INDIVIDUAL HUMANS

Infection and Disease

The distinction between infection and disease is particularly important in malaria. Infection with the malaria parasite does not necessarily result in disease, especially in highly endemic areas of the world (Figure 22–3), where much of the population is infected; children may have parasitemia prevalence rates of 50% or more and yet few will have symptoms.

Disease is the result of the combination of parasite multiplication and the host reaction to the parasite. The classic description of periodic shaking chills, severe fever, and drenching sweats every two or three days can be seen in nonimmune adults infected with *P. vivax* (every other day) or *P. malariae* (every third day). The symptoms in these cases result from the host response to synchronous lysis and release of pyrogens from infected red cells. However, with falciparum malaria, clinical manifestations, particularly in children, range from the totally asymptomatic to severe, overwhelming disease and rapid death. Children may present with drowsiness, coma, convulsions, or simply listlessness and fever with nonspecific symptoms. Abdominal cramping, cough and pulmonary symptoms, headaches, muscle pains, and varying levels of mental disorientation are common. Severe and complicated malaria due to falciparum malaria is a medical emergency.

Exhibit 22–1 Major Paradigms of Malaria Transmission

1. **Malaria of the Africa Savanna.** 80% of the world's malaria cases and 90% of the mortality occurs in Sub-Saharan Africa. The principal vectors are the *An. gambiae* complex, *An. funestus*, and *An. arabiensis*. All breed in abundance and are highly efficient transmitters of malaria. Because of extremely high inoculation rates, virtually all people become infected early in life and have high rates of infant and child mortality; the survivors gradually develop immunity sufficient to prevent death from malaria by the age of four or five. These areas can be further subdivided into those with perennial, continuing transmission throughout the year and those with seasonal peaks of heavy transmission during the rainy seasons, though with some transmission most all the time. Though holoendemic areas are commonly thought to be homogeneous, in fact, there are important time and space variations in microecology and in the transmission patterns.

2. **Forest Malaria** is common in many parts of the world, particularly in Southeast Asia and the Amazon basin of South America, where there are major human migrant intrusions into forest areas, due to economic pressures. These incursions include those specifically for timbering, gem and gold mining, and road construction, in addition to efforts to develop farms. In these areas, newcomers who enter the forest become heavily infected; frequently, they are older adolescents and adults. Forest mosquitoes, such as *An. dirus* generally have different habits from those in traditionally endemic areas; they are frequently outdoor biters and resters, and some bite during the day. Often, therefore, residual household insecticiding is not useful.

3. **Malaria associated with irrigated agriculture** occurs where breeding sites for the mosquitoes become established in the irrigation schemes, bringing together large populations of mosquitoes with large labor forces. This type occurs in cotton plantations in the Gezira in Sudan, irrigated rice cultivation in Sri Lanka, and sugar cane cultivation in South America and some parts of Africa. Engineering approaches to reduce breeding should be possible, but all too often, this has been considered too expensive and has not been done.

4. **Highland Fringe Malaria** occurs in populations settled at higher altitudes, such as the highland plateaus of Madagascar, in Papua New Guinea, Ethiopia, and parts of Kenya with irrigation and cultivation of crops at levels above 1,500 meters. Malaria is now seen to occur where it has never been before and is causing serious consequences in these areas.

5. **Desert Fringe and Oasis Malaria.** These areas have characteristics similar to that of the Highland Fringe Malaria.

6. **Urban Malaria.** There are two basic types of urban malaria: (a) that transmitted by vectors such as *An. stephensi* in South Asia, which have adapted to city water sources, such as wells, cisterns, and domestic containers and (b) in areas of shantytown encroachment into malarious areas, such as the semiurban African village-cities into African savanna or in settlements in the Amazon basin associated with gold mines. Larval control sometimes can be a useful option in these settings.

7 and 8. Other paradigms include those for **Plains Malaria** associated with traditional agriculture in South Asia and Central America and **Seashore Malaria**, which includes malaria on most small islands.

Host Response

Malaria, on a population basis, is the most intense stimulator of the human immune system known. Many biologic defense systems are activated in response to malaria infections, including the reticuloendothelial system with enhanced phagocytosis in the spleen, lymph nodes, and liver to remove altered RBCs and other debris, an intense activation of humoral defenses—indeed, humans can develop several grams per liter of immunoglobulin directed against ma-

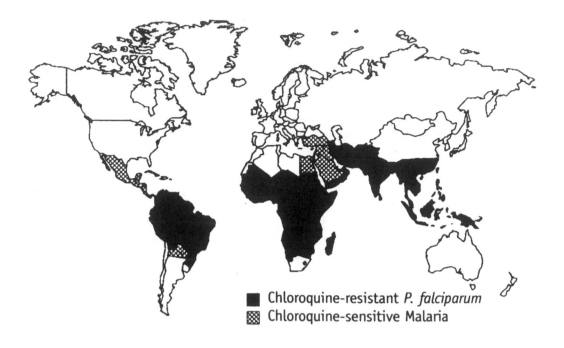

Figure 22–3 Malaria—endemic areas of the world. *Source:* Reprinted with permission from World Health Organization, World Malaria Situation in 1993, Part 1, *Weekly Epidemiological Record*, Vol. 71, No. 1, pp. 17–22, © 1996, World Health Organization.

laria—and a great range of cellular immune and cytokine cascade defenses. Some of these responses are protective; others contribute to the pathology (and often to both).

As humans, mosquitoes, and malaria parasites have evolved over time, many human genetic characteristics that provide partial protection against malaria have emerged. These genetic polymorphisms, mostly involving the red cell, the principal home for the parasite while in the human host, include structural variants in the β globin chain of hemoglobin, such as sickle-cell trait (hemoglobin S) and hemoglobins C and E; altered α and β chain production, leading to the α and β thalasemias (Mediterranean anemia); erythrocyte enzyme deficiencies, including glucose-6-phosphate dehydrogenase (G6PD); red cell cytoskeletal abnormalities, such as ovalocy-

tosis; and red cell membrane defects, such as Duffy blood group factor.[36–38] The mechanism that provides protection seems clear for sickle-cell trait—when red cells are invaded, they sickle and are preferentially removed by the RE system, thus reducing parasite density levels[39]— but have not been fully elucidated for other factors. Many genetic polymorphisms extract a heavy burden on the homozygous individual, eg, sickle cell disease (SS).

The pathogenesis of "big spleen disease" (tropical splenomegaly), which results from an excessive and inappropriate host response to malaria, is fairly common often in relatively nonimmune groups moving into areas of more intense transmission and is poorly understood. The disease starts in childhood, progressing through adolescence to young adulthood, with continuing severe anemia, high levels of IgM and antimalarial antibodies, a decrease in platelets and a huge spleen. Two lines of evidence indicate that this is directly the result of reaction to malaria: (1) those with sickle trait (SA) do not develop big spleen disease[40–42] and (2) individuals with tropical splenomegaly who take long-term antimalarial prophylaxis have gradual reduction in spleen size and anemia and return to normal health over many months.

Role of Protein, Iron, and Other Micronutrient Deficiencies in the Pathogenesis

The nutritional state of the human host influences the pathogenesis in both positive and negative ways. Protein-energy malnutrition (PEM) has long been thought to "protect" against serious clinical symptoms of malaria.[43] In a review of malaria pathology in West Africa, Edington found that children dying with marasmus or kwashiorkor rarely showed evidence of severe malaria.[44] Hendrickse reported that children with cerebral malaria were generally well nourished.[45] Experimental work in animals has confirmed that PEM reduces parasite density and clinical disease, and that increased protein intake is associated with increased parasitemia and death.[46,47] Several mechanisms probably influence these protective effects, but full elucidation is not in sight. At this time, clinicians must remain alert to possible recrudescence of malaria when treating marasmus or PEM.

Similarly, it has long been observed that infants with iron deficiency have less severe malaria than do those who are well nourished and that giving iron may increase severity.[43,48] These effects were examined in a recent meta-analysis of iron supplementation to children in malarious areas: Pooled analysis indicated small but significant increases in parasitemia, and small but not significant increases in splenomegaly and clinical attack rates in those given iron.[49] However, the risk of severe anemia was reduced by 50% and the authors found no reports of increases in severe malaria and concluded that, on balance, the value of iron supplementation far outweighed the minor intensification of malaria.

Deficiencies in a few other micronutrients are reported to ameliorate malaria infection under some circumstances. In animal models and some observational field studies, deficiencies of PABA, magnesium, pyridoxine, riboflavin, and vitamins C and E all seem to lead to reduced parasitemia (Anuraj Shankar and Sylvia Nan Crone, personal communication).

In contrast, vitamin A has a vital role in a host's capacity to combat malaria. Trials of vitamin A supplementation in preschool children in Papua New Guinea[50] and in Ghana[51] both indicate that vitamin A reduces malaria parasitemia and morbidity but may not affect severe malaria or mortality. In another randomized trial in Papua New Guinea, daily supplementation of preschool children with 10 mg zinc reduced malaria-attributable clinic attendance by 40% and had its greatest effect on attacks having high-density parasitemia (Shankar et al, manuscript in preparation). Along with evidence from animal studies, zinc deficiency, in contrast with vitamin A, may play a role in more severe malaria and possibly in malaria mortality.[52–54]

Deficiencies in folic acid, biotin, and pantothenic acid might also reduce host defenses against malaria and exacerbate infection and/or disease. Systematic work on these and other micronutrients is quite recent; their effects and clinical importance require much fuller explication. However, overall the studies of malaria and nutrition indicate that nutritional status plays a significant role in determining disease outcome.

Host–Parasite Interactions at the Cellular and Molecular Levels

Tracing the sequence of events for the merozoite to invade a red cell provides some appreciation of the complexity of host–parasite interactions. This initiating process of red cell infection requires at least four steps: the merozoite first attaches to the red cell surface membrane; then becomes reoriented to the surface membrane; consolidation of the binding follows; and, finally, the parasite penetrates through the red cell membrane into the interior. The parasite must provide one or more functional proteins for each step, and each protein displays antigens that may be targeted by the host's immune system. Many antigens do stimulate antibodies, and some show some correlation with protection.[55]

The antibody-dependent cellular inhibition (ADCI) of parasitic growth shows a fairly consistent correlation with protection in immune adults[56] and is effective in many different geographic areas. Hyperimmune sera from Senegal, Ivory Coast, and Laos produce similar inhibition of growth of parasites from The Gambia, Thailand, and Uganda.[57] ADCI is apparently an important component of the antimalarial immunity that can be passively transferred from immune adults to treat malaria infection in children.[58,59]

Infected red cells undergo complex changes, including the expression of protein aggregates, "knobs," on their surface.[6,60] These knobs are related to the capacity of infected red cells to adhere to endothelial cells lining capillaries and venules (cytoadherence) and cause microvascular obstruction and impaired delivery of oxygen and other vital metabolites. They also are responsible for rosetting, ie, the adherence of noninfected red cells to the infected cell, which also impedes microcirculation. Sequestering of parasites along capillary and venule beds prevents their elimination by the reticuloendothelial system and may aid parasite maturation by holding them in their preferred lower saturated oxygenated blood. This cytoadhesion in the internal capillary beds also accounts for the fact that peripheral parasitemia, as assessed by blood smear counts, greatly underestimates the total mass of parasitized red cells in *P. falciparum* infection. Cytoadherence to the capillary beds of the brain has long been associated with cerebral malaria.

In the human host, several ligands expressed on capillaries serve as receptors for attachment of infected erythrocytes. Mediators, such as tumor necrosis factor (TNF) released in the course of malaria infection, may activate some of these.

The parasite-encoded molecules that produce knobs and attach to these receptors have been identified. These knob proteins are highly variable in their antigenic expression and are products of highly variable genes, appropriately termed *var* genes. There are close to 150 different *var* genes, which occupy about 5% of the malaria genome.[6] Such a large genomic commitment to antigenic diversity for the protein responsible for cytoadherence is a good indicator of the key role that cytoadherence plays in the survival of *P. falciparum*.

Efforts have been made to relate specific phenotypic parasite characteristics, such as the capacity to stimulate release of cytokines, including TNF; the production of nitric oxide; and the cytoadherence and rosetting phenotypes (and their underlying genotypes) to the diversity of clinical events provoked by *P. falciparum* that lead to severe disease.[61–64] Although the rosetting phenotype has been reported as associated with cerebral malaria, no clear association has yet been found between any particular cytoadherance phenotype with cerebral malaria or other forms of severe malaria.[55,65]

In the field, there is great antigenic diversity within any given *P. falciparum* population, whether for populations within humans or within vectors.[66–68] No doubt contributing to the diversity of antigenic variability is frequent recombination within the vector, as evidenced by the finding of different alleles of the same locus within a single oocyst.[66,69]

Although there are some large scale differences geographically for a few parasite markers that remain stable over time, most antigenic markers demonstrate substantial time and place variation.[25,70,71] Studies of parasite antigen markers isolated from the same individuals over time have demonstrated diversity. In Senegal,[72] several parasite antigen markers were followed throughout a full set of seasons. During the dry season, with little or no transmission, each person continued with the same strain of *P. falciparum* (ie, the same set of parasite markers) and, generally, they continued without symptoms. During transmission season, however, isolates became diverse, with rapid turnover of strains within the individual. Symptomatic disease became common in children, and symptoms were always associated with a new strain. Only some of the new antigen marker patterns were associated with development of disease, and these were different in different children.

The Diversity of Falciparum Malaria Disease

As notions of eradication with its focus on parasites and vectors have faded, more research has been undertaken to define and understand clinical and epidemiologic features of malaria as a human disease. As a result, major advances have been made in differentiating distinctive forms of severe falciparum malaria disease and in understanding underlying pathogenic factors—inoculum size, differing "strains" of falciparum, differing immunologic responses, and various cofactors. This, in turn, contributed to an appreciation of distinctive epidemiologic features of different forms of clinical disease. A synthesis of new information from thorough clinical studies in diverse ecologic settings has led to new ideas about malaria disease and to new approaches to control that focus on reducing death and enhancing immune defenses, rather than reducing transmission as an end in itself. Such an approach requires an understanding of the relation of disease manifestations to intensity and constancy of transmission due to ecologic factors, genetic characteristics of the parasite, and genetic and acquired immune mechanisms in humans.

The first important clinical distinction to be made is between severe and nonsevere disease due to *P. falciparum*.[55] Severe malaria in children in holoendemic areas behaves as a disease different from nonsevere malaria. Although there may be value in differentiating various forms of nonsevere falciparum, this chapter will focus on the clearly distinctive features of the various forms of severe malaria, particularly those of cerebral malaria and of severe anemia with and without respiratory distress.[73–75]

Severe Malaria

P. falciparum disease is a major cause of death in children wherever there is a high intensity of infection. Recent results from community-based intervention studies[76,77] indicate that malaria may account for nearly half of the mortality rate of children younger than 5 years in holoendemic areas, rather than previous estimates of around 25% of those deaths.

In holoendemic areas, severe disease in children does not progress from mild or moderate illness; it strikes abruptly without warning. Mothers are frequently unable to get their infants and young children to a health center in time to provide treatment before the child dies, even when facilities with trained health workers are readily available. If they do manage to reach a hospital, many die within 24 hours of admission, despite treatment efforts.[78–80] In a trial of antimalarial prophylaxis in The Gambia, children under age five from families providing regular prophylaxis had much lower mortality than did those who depended on the use of well-staffed, nearby primary health care facilities.[81]

Rapid progression to severe disease is not characteristic in other areas of the globe with less intense transmission. In Southern Asia, malaria slowly progresses in severity over several days in both children and in adults and does so in both major types of severe disease that occur there: cerebral malaria, which has a median time of five days from onset to cerebral symptoms, and multiple organ dysfunction syndrome (MODS), which is somewhat slower in development, has a median time of eight days.[82] Early effective treatment before the onset of the severe phase is the key to reducing mortality in these circumstances; an option difficult to achieve with the fulminant African form. Although these slowly progressive types are also seen in Africa, they are distinctly less common in holoendemic areas than the rapid severe forms in children.

Clinical Patterns

The starting point for understanding the pathogenesis of severe malaria is a clear description of the clinical problem; yet few systematic clinical studies have reported the full spectrum of severe malaria. Recently, the Kenya Medical Institute unit at Kilifi at the coast of Kenya reported on 1,844 children admitted consecutively with malaria and diagnosed using the criteria of the WHO definition of severe malaria.[74,75,80] The results are summarized in Table 22–2.

It was particularly useful to focus on two life-threatening syndromes—those with neurologic deficit and those with respiratory distress—that are readily delineated clinically when the child is first seen. These provided greater prognostic value than that using the combined clinical and laboratory indicators used for the WHO definition.[75] A third important syndrome, though not so readily apparent clinically when first seen, is severe anemia. The roles of both hypoglycemia and metabolic acidosis in the pathogenesis of severe disease are clearly central. Hypoglycemia,

difficult to diagnose on clinical grounds alone, had a prevalence equivalent to that of respiratory distress and an even higher mortality. Hypoglycemia associated with cerebral malaria certainly contributed to the death of patients classified as unarousable coma and probably to those with acidosis.

Cerebral Malaria

The classical histopathologic picture of cerebral malaria is intense sequestration of infected cells in the cerebral microvasculature,[83] and clinically is associated with case-fatality ratios of from 10% to 50%.[8,84] Further careful clinical study indicates that cerebral malaria is heterogeneous and may include four overlapping syndromes with different pathogenic mechanisms. Four distinct groups of children fulfilling the WHO definition of cerebral malaria were distin-

Table 22–2 Prevalence of the Criteria Included in the WHO Definition of Severe Malaria in 1,844 Consecutive Admissions with a Primary Diagnosis of Malaria

	No. of Children Evaluated	Prevalence (%)	Mortality (%)
DEFINING CRITERION			
Unarousable coma	1,844	10.0	16.8
Severe malaria anemia	1,816	17.6	04.7
Respiratory distress*	1,833	13.7	13.9
Hypoglycemia	698	13.2	21.7
Circulatory collapse	1,844	00.4	71.4
Renal failure	1,844	00.1	0
Spontaneous bleeding	1,843	00.1	0
Repeated convulsions	1,842	18.3	06.8
Acidosis**	110	63.6	21.4
Hemoglobinuria	1,844	00.1	50.0
OTHER MANIFESTATIONS			
Impaired consciousness	1,844	08.2	06.0
Jaundice	1,806	04.7	11.9
Prostrate	1,571	12.2	05.2
Hyperpyrexia	1,842	10.6	01.6
Hyperparasitemia	110	08.9	04.3

* The original criteria specify pulmonary edema rather than respiratory distress.
** Blood-gas data were available for only a small subset. Respiratory distress is strongly associated with acidosis.

guished in the Kilifi study: (1) prolonged postictal state; (2) covert status epilepticus; (3) severe metabolic derangement (particularly with hypoglycemia and metabolic acidosis); and (4) children with a primary neurologic syndrome. Commonly, more than one of these situations coexist. A child may be acidotic, have hypoglycemia, and be in status epilepticus; recognition and proper management of all three, in addition to treatment of the malaria, is critical.[85,86] These distinctions are important for appropriate therapy, of course, but careful delineation also may help in defining underlying pathogenic factors.

Hypoglycemia is especially common in pediatric malaria. In Thailand, 23%[87] and in Malawi, 33%[88] of pediatric patients admitted for severe malaria had hypoglycemia; the outlook was grim for these patients. In the Malawi study, 37% with hypoglycemia died, and 26% were discharged with brain damage—many times higher than those diagnosed with cerebral malaria but with normal blood sugar levels. The combination of hypoglycemia with lactic acidosis, as described below, is particularly devastating.

Respiratory Distress

Pulmonary edema, often seen with adult respiratory distress syndrome (ARDS), is included in the WHO criteria for severe malaria and has long been recognized as a serious, frequently fatal complication of malaria in nonimmune adults.[74] Respiratory distress per se, however, does not appear in the original WHO criteria, nor is it emphasized in standard clinical textbooks. Signs of breathlessness were attributed to a combination of anemia and congestive cardiac failure. The term *respiratory distress* was considered a useful defining characteristic because, with minimum training, the clinical signs can be applied with good interobserver consistency.[89] As defined, respiratory distress also is an important prognostic marker in children with *P. falciparum* infections. In most cases, it reflects an underlying metabolic acidosis, usually associated with lactic acidemia. Hypovolemia and anemia are important underlying factors.

Although the Kilifi investigators listed four contributing factors for respiratory distress, including cardiac failure, coexistent pneumonia, direct sequestration of malaria parasites in the lungs, and increased central drive to respiration, in association with cerebral malaria; they found that respiratory distress was primarily associated with metabolic acidosis. The clinical signs of hyperventilation, driven by efforts to reduce CO_2, are highly sensitive and specific for the diagnosis of respiratory distress.[89] Acidosis results from several factors that increase lactase, including metabolic processes of the malaria parasite itself; reduced hepatic blood flow,[79] leading to reduced lactate clearance; high levels of cytokines that directly impair cellular metabolism and increase lactate production; and, finally, the major contributor is lactate production caused by reduced oxygen to the tissues. Metabolic acidosis plays a major role in the pathogenesis of severe disease, particularly in the overlap among different clinical syndromes.

Different manifestations of severe malarial morbidity arise from interaction of a limited number of pathogenic processes: red cell destruction, toxin-mediated activation of cytokine cascades, and infected cell sequestration in tissue microvascular beds. All lead to reduced tissue oxygenation as a unifying process in the pathogenesis of these major clinical syndromes of severe malaria.[86] Other severe but less common causes of malarial mortality include renal failure, pulmonary edema with adult respiratory distress syndrome, and disseminated intravascular coagulopathy (DIC).

Epidemiologic Features of Severe Malaria

Most descriptions of severe malaria disease in African children have focused on differentiating those with severe anemia from those with cerebral and neurologic involvement.[74,76,79,90] Clear epidemiologic differences parallel these distinctive clinical forms of severe malaria. As the intensity of transmission increases from one geographic area to another, the proportion of the population having severe malaria as compared to nonsevere shifts increasingly to younger age groups. Similarly, with increasing transmission, the proportion with asymptomatic malaria compared to those with symptoms is shifted to younger ages in the nonsevere malaria group. Thus, in the areas with the most intense transmission, severe malaria and death are restricted largely to children under age 5, and most clinical disease is seen in those under age 10.[55,90]

Within any one endemic area, the pattern of severe morbidity varies with age; severe anemia predominates in the youngest children with a median age of 15–24 months, whereas coma is more common in older children with a median age of 36–48 months. The shift in age may be related to a combination of increased challenge and more rapid development of immunity at higher levels of transmission.[75] Between endemic areas of differing levels of transmission intensity, there may be a marked difference in age distributions of children with severe malaria and in the relative importance of different clinical syndromes. For example, severe malaria usually presents as severe anemia and occurs at a younger age in Ifakara, where transmission is intense and the inoculation rate is over 100 infectious bites per year per person, as compared to Kilifi, where there is moderate transmission and an inoculation rate of less than 10, and where children with severe disease more commonly present with cerebral symptoms at an older age. Despite these differences, the overall incidence of severe disease in a cohort is about the same.[55,91,92] An additional factor that apparently affects the nature of severe malaria in a population is the constancy of transmission; an area of intense perennial transmission showed a higher incidence of severe anemia, whereas, in an area with intense seasonal transmission, there was a higher rate of cerebral malaria.[73]

Previous evidence that indicated a space-time clustering of severe malaria[93] has recently been strengthened in the Kilifi area through the use of a geographic information system and more sophisticated statistical analyses.[94] The same analyses were carried out for child deaths due to all causes, but no space-time clustering was found. The interpretation is that severe malaria occurs in localized microepidemics, but whether the space-time clustering of severe malaria is different from that which may occur with nonsevere malaria will be exceedingly difficult to discern because most episodes of nonsevere malaria are not reported in any consistent fashion. Certainly, there are marked local variations in transmission intensity in holoendemic areas, but whether these variations are related to the space-time clustering of severe malaria remains to be explored.

In areas of intense transmission, the prevalence and density of both asexual and gametocyte stages of *P. falciparum* reach a peak in early childhood and decline thereafter. Density of parasitemia declines before prevalence, and density of gametocytes declines before that of asexual stages. Density of asexual parasites at which symptoms appear increases in early life and declines thereafter,[95] indicating a separate immune response to toxic products of red cell rupture from that of the response to the parasites themselves. The antitoxic immunity builds rapidly with early infections but declines thereafter as effective immune responses to the parasites themselves slowly develop, directly reducing toxic products.[55,95]

Many questions remain about super infection, defined as infection on top of an already existing infection, common in holoendemic malaria areas with an EIR of dozens to hundreds each year. An important epidemiologic point is that the incidence of malarial disease, whether mild or severe, is limited to the period of transmission in areas of holoendemic seasonal malaria. Interpretation of this is that disease onset must require a recent inoculation.[96] Somehow, the newly inoculated parasite must differ from those parasites already present in that particular child. Quantitatively, there are more parasites already in the blood than will be released from the liver cells derived from the new batch of sporozoites. During the low transmission season, each child continues with the same parasite type and remains without symptoms, but during the high transmission season, parasite isolates are quite diverse, and there is rapid shifting of types within each child. Those that become symptomatic do so only with a new parasite type. Only some of the new types are associated with symptoms, but these types vary from child to child.[97]

There is some evidence that those with severe malaria have received no more inocula than have those with nonsevere malaria,[98] but much work remains to be done to relate number of sporozoites injected by individual inocula to clinical disease. Reports on the effectiveness of insecticide-impregnated bed nets indicate that the impact on mortality or on severe malaria is greater than the impact on nonsevere malaria; likewise, there is a greater reduction in clinical disease than in prevalence of asymptomatic parasitemia.[99]

In most child deaths in tropical Africa, malaria is a contributing factor, even though death may be attributed to another cause, such as diarrhea or pneumonia. When malaria is controlled in holoendemic areas, a major reduction in overall child mortality occurs, although previously much may have been attributed to other causes. To account for the frequency of sickle-cell trait (SA) in tropical Africa (ranging from 16% to 29% AS hemoglobin in adults), the historical case fatality rate that must be attributed to malaria is on the order of 10–20% of all children born with AA hemoglobin.[100] With application of the Hardy-Weinberg law, if 28% of the population has sickle trait and 72% is AA (assuming that children born with sickle-cell disease do not survive to adulthood—essentially true in West Africa until quite recently), then the S gene allele frequency in the adult gene pool would be 14%, as compared with 86% for the A. The selection coefficient for the AA genotype would then be $0.14/(1-0.14) = 0.1628$. The ratio of AS genotype individuals to AA for survivorship to adulthood would be $1/(1-0.1628) = 1.194$, which is equivalent to nearly a 20% excess death rate for those with AA before adulthood. Because the only advantage of AS over AA is that from severe malaria, the case fatality rate due to malaria in those with AA hemoglobin is 19.4%. The sharp age-specific rise in prevalence of sickle trait in West Africa from 20–24% in newborns to 26–29% in adults indicates the high survival value of AS hemoglobin, as compared with AA in this environment. This differential survival can be expressed as the ratio of proportion of AS in adults divided by that in newborns to the proportion of AA in adults divided by that in newborns. In the Garki study area with very high malaria transmission and sickle-trait rates, adults were 28.96% AS and 70.2% AA (0.84% were other, including those with AC and SC hemoglobin), whereas newborns were 23.6% AS and 73.78% AA (2.62% were other, including 2.1% SS and 0.5% AC), giving $3.86/2.99 = 1.29$; equivalent to a 29% case fatality rate in the AA because of malaria.[21]

Pregnant women in holo- and hyperendemic areas, particularly those with their first pregnancy, are at special risk for *P. falciparum* malaria, frequently developing severe anemia and sometimes death, even though the women had acquired a high level of immunity prior to their pregnancy.[101] Moreover, particularly with the first pregancy but to a lesser extent with the second and subsequent pregnancies, malaria may lead to growth retardation of the fetus, low birth weight, premature delivery, fetal death, and miscarriage.

Where severe anemia from malaria requires blood transfusion, the dangers of HIV and hepatitis B virus transmission are added risks to the consequences of malaria.

HUMAN FACTORS INFLUENCING MALARIA

Human factors, particularly at the population level but also at the individual, behavioral level, strongly influence the epidemiologic pattern of malaria and the efforts to control it. Agricultural development, population movement, and urbanization are important determinants of the pattern of malaria transmission. All control measures involve interplay of broad social, cultural, and economic factors.

Malaria has long been linked to farming practices. In Sub-Saharan Africa, the clearing of forest for crop production has led to increased breeding of *An. gambiae*, the most efficient vector of human malaria, which prefers sunlit, exposed pools of standing water to the full shade of tropical forest. The formation of small towns, dams, and irrigation schemes arising in concert with agricultural development in much of Africa has concentrated populations of humans and vectors in relatively confined areas near water supplies. Additionally, agricultural use of pesticides and fertilizers has been a major factor in development and spread of insecticide-resistant vectors. Thus, the very efforts to promote economic development and improve human conditions have increased the intensity of malaria transmission.

Population movements throughout Africa have contributed to an increased intensity of malaria transmission. Traditionally, in many parts of Africa, seasonal migration has been a part of life, with people moving from their village settlements to rural farms during the early months of the wet season when cultivation, planting, and weeding are carried out. Often, intensity of transmission is much higher in these areas than in their settled home villages, where water supplies are controlled. In a similar way, many pastoral Africans are exposed to higher transmission as they move their livestock between highlands and lowland pastures with the seasons.

Other reasons for population movement are related to population expansion, with movement into previously unoccupied and more marginally productive areas. The living and working conditions in these areas often result in greater exposure to malaria vectors. Africa has been especially afflicted with drought, famine, war, and political upheavals resulting in mass population displacement and refugee movements, all of which are frequently associated with increased malaria transmission. These groups frequently are poorly served by government health or malaria control programs and have less access to antimalarial and other aspects of health care. Disasters and conflicts, so prominent in Africa for decades, greatly contribute to the transmission of malaria and inhibition of antimalaria control efforts.

On the other hand, the major secular migrations to urban areas throughout Africa generally have little influence on malaria transmission. Although malaria in Africa is principally a rural rather than an urban disease problem, some anopheline species have come to be well adapted to city life. For example, *Anopheles arabiensis* has become a transmitter of malaria in many cities of Nigeria.[8] Generally, this vector is restricted to semi-urban slum areas, rather than the highly concentrated population areas in urban centers.

Although malaria can infect and cause severe disease in anybody, it is principally a disease of the poor and ignorant. Loss of healthy life due to malaria is much higher in poor rural areas of Africa than in the better-developed urban areas. Some notion of the difference in impact on different social groups can be seen in the studies by Oduntan[102] in Nigeria, who found that the sickle-trait rate among elite school children in Ibadan was under 20%, whereas, in school-aged children from rural areas and those not attending school, the AS rate was 26.3%. To account for this marked differential, the mortality rate due to malaria among those with AA hemoglobin in the poor must be many times greater than that in the elite, who would have had better nutrition and access to health services. If one assumes that, at birth, the distributions of AA, AS, and SS genotypes were the same and further assumes that none of the elite with AA died by school age, then 29.9% of those with AA in the nonelite segment would have died from malaria. However, with the strong tendency for social classes to intermarry, it is likely that the distributions would not have been the same and that at least some of this marked differential could be attributed to lower malaria mortality and less benefit from AS in the last generation or two among the elite. The interplay between environmental factors (malaria) and genetics (hemoglobin genotypes) ensures that sickle-trait rate will continue to be reduced among the better off, in whom the balanced polymorphism from selective protection for sickle-trait no longer holds. The dramatic differential in mortality from malaria by social class provides clear evidence that malaria control efforts should contribute to improved equity of health status.

Individual and community behavior are important factors influencing the population effects discussed above and are crucial in determining the success of malaria control. In Africa, there is great diversity in cultures and community structures. Understanding and acting in accord with the prevailing belief systems are essential; otherwise, these beliefs may serve as barriers to adoption of effective interventions. Health-seeking behavior, key for obtaining timely treatment, depends on understanding the need for treatment; thus, people's perceptions of malaria and its causes are very important. Even in communities that may have an appreciation of the importance of malaria and need to obtain appropriate treatment, the symptoms of cerebral malaria may be misunderstood because it produces convulsions and confusion. People frequently do not recognize these as signs for urgent treatment for malaria; indeed, such symptoms often are attributed to belief of supernatural causes, not something that modern medicine can affect.

Lack of understanding on the part of the people concerning what factors contribute to malaria is a barrier to the development of any antimalaria program that requires active cooperation, and, as is discussed in the section on control, virtually all approaches to control malaria do so require.

DIAGNOSIS

A definitive diagnosis of malaria infection is made by demonstration of malaria parasites in human tissue, usually in red cells. The standard technique is microscopic examination of a Giemsa stained thick and thin smear of blood on glass microscope slides; this technique will likely remain the gold standard for some time to come. Skilled technicians can not only determine the species of malaria, but also can obtain reliable quantitative estimates of the number of parasites (parasite density). The ability to detect

infections depends on the number of fields examined and the experience of the technician viewing the slide.

Although this approach continues as standard, there are problems of practical implementation and problems of interpretation. At the practical level, Giemsa-stained blood smears examined with standard light microscopes have been used for 70 years in every area in the world; millions of blood smears have been prepared and reliably examined by technicians with little or no formal education; and the cost of materials and equipment is modest. However, the work is tedious and requires continuous concentration; maintenance of the microscope and staining materials requires rigorous control; and training technicians and supervising their activities require discipline difficult to maintain. Economic advances in Africa have given a wider range of employment opportunities for those able to do this kind of work; turnover rates have become high, and salary levels have gone up. Quality control methods are essential, and approaches to maintain good morale among the technicians are critical.

The problems of interpretation of blood smears are twofold: First, peripheral smears may be falsely negative when there is infection under two circumstances: (a) In early stages of all malaria and in all stages of *P. falciparum*, parasites disappear from the peripheral blood during schizogony, so that few or no parasites may be seen in the peripheral blood smear, even when the capillary beds may be packed with sequestrated, infected red cells; and (b) in early infection, before red cells become infected, no practical way has been worked out to detect the hepatic phase of infection and, equivalently, hypnocytes of *P. vivax* and *P. ovale* cannot be detected.

Second, the peripheral smear may be "falsely" positive, in the sense that a blood smear from a febrile patient in an endemic area does not necessarily mean that the symptoms are due to malaria. Most school-aged children in holoendemic areas will have malaria parasites in the blood virtually all the time. Thus, there is no specific approach to diagnosing clinical disease in this situation. In highly endemic areas, patients are treated on the basis of clinical symptoms alone; usually, a clinician, quite appropriately, will give antimalarials to virtually any sick child. For research or special studies, criteria may be established for labeling a specific episode of fever as due to malaria, eg, any child with an axillary temperature greater than 38° plus a parasite density of more than 1% or approximated by 100 infected red cells per white cell.

Many efforts have been expended to develop other means for diagnosis that do not involve such demanding discipline and technical skills.[8] A variety of immunologic tests has been developed, and several have served important purposes. ELISA and RIA methods using a number of different antigens have proven reliable and reproducible but have little relevance to clinical diagnosis because antibodies do not reflect active disease. However, they have been used to assess effectiveness of population-based control measures. Several approaches that directly detect a variety of malaria antigens include those of antigen inhibition and competition, antigen capture, and several assay systems to detect soluble antigen.[103] Trials of a dipstick assay based on antigen capture of *P. falciparum* histidine-rich protein (HRP-II) antigen (ParaSight-F test) have shown promising sensitivity and specificity in several settings and the potential for parasite density estimates.[104,105]

DNA polymerase chain reaction as the basis for a diagnostic test offers great potential for diagnosis, including the determination of drug sensitivity. Thus far, the use of PCR has not been translated into a robust and reliable approach for use in clinical diagnosis in tertiary hospitals, let alone for use in the field. However, PCR genotyping is proving valuable in the analysis of malaria parasites in drug efficacy trials by distinguishing true recrudescences from new reinfections. It should also help in analyzing parasite populations during and after vaccine trials and, similarly, for changes in parasite populations resulting from vector control or environmental alterations.[106]

In Africa, the diagnosis of clinical malaria and the best drugs for treatment continue to depend on clinical suspicion and knowledge of the epidemiologic circumstances and known drug resistance in the particular area.

Determining Drug Resistance

Although other species of malaria have shown some drug resistance, the emergence of resistance by *P. falciparum* is by far the most important. Knowing the sensitivity to antimalarials is as important as the diagnosis of malaria itself, not only for treatment of individuals, but also to understand the spread and transmission of drug resistance. Ideally, a diagnostic test will be developed that is rapid, reliable, and inexpensive; PCR-based methods mentioned above show promise for such.

In vivo and *in vitro* test systems provide two complementary approaches to determine drug resistance of malaria parasites at present and are used to monitor the distribution and levels of drug resistance in particular geographic areas. This monitoring provides a basis for judging effective antimalarials for use in the area, but they afford little basis for certainty in any particular individual.

The WHO has developed a standard approach for *in vivo* testing in endemic areas:[107,108] A sample of infected patients is given the antimalarial drug according to an established regime; parasite density counts are performed at admission, at 24 hours, at 7 days, and optionally at 28 days. If the patient is improved and the parasite is not detectable at the end of 7 days (and still not detectable at 28 days), the parasite is considered sensitive to the drug. If there is clearance of parasites and clinical improvement at 7 days but recrudescence of parasitemia by 28 days, it is stage RI-resistant. If there is marked reduction but not complete clearance at 7 days, it is considered stage RII-resistant. If there is no evidence of response and the patient continues to get worse, it is considered to be fully resistant, RIII. The 7-day test is considerably simpler and avoids issues of reinfection; for the most part, this has become standard. There are several variations, but this remains the basic idea. An important limitation in interpreting the *in vivo* test is that those with a substantial immune response will improve, even if parasites are moderately resistant to the drug, and may well result in missing all but RIII levels of sensitivity. The test is performed on subjects regardless of age, parasite count, or previous therapy, but certainly should not be carried out in anyone seriously ill. Because the level of immunity will be higher in older children and adults in endemic areas, the usefulness of testing older age groups will be limited to detection of high levels of resistance.

In vitro testing of *P. falciparum*, the only species thus far cultured, is done with an *in vitro* culture system of red cells. Blood taken from a parasitemic individual is prepared for culture and incubated, along with increasing concentrations of antimalarial drug. The technique requires meticulous care and requires a fairly high level of parasitemia. When undertaken in experienced labs, the results are reproducible and provide an objective indicator of level of resistance independent of the host immune system.

Particularly for severe malaria in children that strikes with great rapidity, neither of these test systems is useful for making immediate decisions about what treatment should be provided for the individual patient.

TREATMENT OF MALARIA

The history of drugs used for treatment of malaria go back hundreds of years. In China, derivatives of the Qing-hao-su plant have been in use for centuries; in the early 1600s, Jesuit missionaries brought back to Europe cinchona bark used by Peruvian healers against fevers for generations. In 1820, the active ingredient was identified as an alkaloid, termed *quinine*,[1,4] the first highly active drug against a specific infection known to man. Quinine continues to be an important therapeutic agent, especially for drug-resistant falciparum malaria, but it has a relatively short shelf life and has more adverse reactions than does chloroquine.

Chloroquine, a 4-aminoquinoline initially synthesized in the late 1930s along with other candidate pharmaceuticals in Germany, was too toxic for use at the doses tried. During the war, the Allies captured some and found chloroquine to be highly effective against malaria.[1,8] Chloroquine is rapidly absorbed after oral administration, has a prolonged half-life of 33 days, and is active against asexual stages of all human species, except for strains of *P. falciparum* that have become resistant. Its mechanism of action remains unknown. After extensive use for over 40 years, much is known about its safety and toxicity. In appropriate doses, it is well tolerated, even when taken chronically for long periods: It is safe for young children and pregnant women. Although long-term, high-dose administration of chloroquine to patients with autoimmune disorders is associated with irreversible neuroretinitis, use at doses for prevention or treatment of malaria has not caused problems.[109] The only important adverse reaction is intense pruritis, reported almost uniquely but frequently by black Africans. Because of low toxicity, low cost, and effectiveness, chloroquine was the drug of choice to treat malaria for decades following World War II. Only after parasite resistance to chloroquine was demonstrated (see below) were serious efforts focused on developing alternative antimalarials.

A number of other antimalarial drugs have been developed, including other 4-aminoquinolines, such as amodiaquine, hydroxychloroquine, and other related drugs.[108,109] None have an advantage over chloroquine; all are more expensive; most provoke more adverse reactions; and now most have cross-drug resistance with chloroquine.

Pyrimethamine and proguanil, inhibitors of the enzyme dihydrofolate reductase that disrupts DNA synthesis, are active against *P. falciparum*, but resistance to both drugs has generally occurred quite rapidly. However, pyrimethamine used in combination with sulfonamides has a high therapeutic efficacy; a modest cost; and, until recently, relatively low rates of adverse reactions and drug resistance.

Sulfaxoxine-pyrimethamine (Fansidar), originally developed and promoted for its efficacy against chloroquine-resistant *P. falciparum* (though it is poorly active against *P. vivax*), has been widely used for treatment to replace chloroquine in areas of drug resistance. However, use of this combination for prophylaxis has been associated with severe and fatal adverse reactions, including cases of erythema multiforme, Stevens-Johnson syndrome, and toxic epidermal necrolysis due to the long-acting sulfonamide component. The risk may be as high as 1 in 6,000 users for prophylaxis. Also, increasing reports of Fansidar-resistant *P. falciparum* are further eroding its usefulness.[109]

Mefloquine, a synthetic 4-quinoline methanol structurally related to quinine and quinidine, has an unusually long half-life and is metabolized with great individual variability; it is now widely used for prophylaxis by visitors, particularly in Africa and other areas with chloroquine resistance. It is much more expensive and causes more adverse reactions than does chloroquine, with reports of occasional neurotoxic and even psychotic reactions with high doses and, uncommonly, it may potentiate dysrhythmias in persons on beta blockers.

Halofantrine is another new drug effective against chloroquine-resistant *P. falciparum*, but knowledge of its toxicity and long-term use is not yet established.

Artemisinin and related compounds have been derived from the Chinese herbal medicine, Qing-hao-su, in use for antifever therapy for centuries. Commercial production has recently been started, including a rapidly absorbed suppository formulation for young children; long-term studies have demonstrated a high degree of effectiveness with relatively low rates of adverse reactions.

Many antibiotics, including tetracycline and its longer-acting derivatives, doxycycline, clindamycin, chloramphenicol, and rifampicin, have a substantial antimalarial activity and can be used in combination with other drugs against drug-resistant malaria.

Primaquine, an 8-aminoquinoline drug, was developed, as was chloroquine, following the large screening program by the U.S. Army during World War II. It is unique, in that it has activity against all forms of the malaria parasite occurring in humans but has a much lower therapeutic efficacy ratio for blood stage forms than do the other antimalarials discussed above. Because of its effect on sporozoites and the hepatic forms, it can be used to prevent the establishment of infection in the liver (referred to as a *causal prophylaxis* in the literature) and to eliminate the hypnozoite stages of *P. vivax* and *P. ovale* that would lead to relapse of these species (antirelapse treatment), which is its most important use.[107,108] It is also effective in eliminating gametocytes and, thus, possibly could play a role in preventing the spread of drug-resistant strains. In theory, it might be used for reducing transmission, but issues of coverage, duration of activity, and adverse reactions all mitigate its use as a practical matter. Primaquine also specifically causes hemolysis in those with glucose-6-phosphate dehydrogenase (G6PD) deficiency that is common in Africans and those of African descent.

Epidemiology of Drug Resistance in Malaria

P. falciparum resistance to chloroquine was first reported in the late 1950s in South America in areas between Venezuela and Columbia and in Southeast Asia in the Thai-Cambodian and Thai-Burma border areas and spread to neighboring areas over the next several years.[107,108,110–113] Although it was nearly 20 years later that resistance was first demonstrated in Africa,[114] chloroquine-resistant malaria has now spread widely in Africa, as well. (See global map of chloroquine-resistant *P. falciparum*.) Further, starting in the very same geographic areas in Southeast Asia, *P. falciparum* has become resistant to other antimalarials, including mefloquine, halofantrine, pyrimethamine-sulfadoxine (Fansidar), and partially to quinine, even more rapidly than it did to chloroquine. Resistance to Fansidar is now widespread in Southeast Asia and South America, and there are increasingly frequent reports from Africa. Resistance to mefloquine and halofantrine have spread within Southeast Asia, but so far, there is little evidence of much resistance to these drugs in Africa.

The mechanisms of resistance, the factors that contribute to its spread, and the parasite genetics are incompletely understood. The basis for chloroquine resistance is related to the capacity of resistant *P. falciparum* strains to excrete chloroquine rapidly so that intracellular concentrations do not reach toxic levels.[109] The calcium channel-blocking drug verapamil inhibits this capacity for rapid excretion and, thus, has been found to restore sensitivity to chloroquine. This effect of verapamil has been found with all resistant parasite isolates, including those from Asia, South America, and Africa, consistent with the notion that there is one common mechanism for all strains with chloroquine resistance.

More is known about *P. falciparum* resistance to pyrimethamine than about that of any other drug. The resistance is due to specific point mutations in the dihydrofolate reductase (DHFR) enzyme of the parasite that changes the shape of its active site cavity.[115,116] At least five different point mutations have been identified and associated not only with in vitro resistance but also with clinical-epidemiologic resistance patterns. A PCR assay has been developed that can readily identify the mutations and is now being used to monitor the prevalence of pyrimethamine-resistant strains in the field.[117,118]

The relation between these mutations and resistance to Fansidar is complicated and incompletely understood. Despite a fairly high frequency of DHFR mutations in East Africa, *P. falciparum* continues to respond generally quite well to Fansidar.[109,119] Recently, mutations to dihydropteroate synthase (DHPS), the enzyme target for sulfadoxine, have been identified and are associated with *in vitro* resistance, and some epidemiologic evidence is consistent with their role in Fansidar resistance.[120]

Emergence of parasite resistance to chloroquine is generally attributed to two contributing factors in their use, common to the emergence of antimicrobial resistance in bacteria: the widespread use of the single drug, chloroquine, as well as treatment with suboptimal dosages of chloroquine. After emergence of resistance in one locale, the "resistant strain" is spread locally by selection of resistant parasites due to "drug pressure," then more distantly through vector and/or people movement, carrying the resistant strain.[107] However, some evidence indicates that these factors are insufficient to account fully for the spread of resistance, particularly that of the role of "drug pressure" as an important contributing factor. For example, chloroquine resistance was first detected in Zambia in the northeastern district of Isoka, where, at the time, there had never been much chloroquine available.

VACCINES AGAINST MALARIA

Prospects for a successful vaccine against malaria have been considered bright for a very long time; unfortunately, they have remained prospects and to date no vaccine has been demonstrated as effective and practical. The overwhelming evidence that humans develop strong protective response against malaria when repeatedly exposed to infection indicates that an effective vaccine should be possible. By age 6 virtually all children in holoendemic Africa have acquired substantial immunity: they are protected from severe and fatal malaria though they may have parasitemia and occasional bouts of fever. The population will have paid a high price for this protection, however, since under-five mortality from malaria is very high while the survivors are acquiring their immunity. Early studies by Ian McGregor et al[58] demonstrated that serum taken from immune adults in The Gambia could be used to treat young children in East Africa. In the early 1970s, David Clyde and others demonstrated that the injection of sporozoites from irradiated falciparum-infected mosquitoes provided protective immunity against challenges from falciparum malaria.[121,122]

In addition to the empirical evidence for an effective acquired human immune response, important advances have taken place in understanding basic immune mechanisms of defense, in the pathogenesis of malaria, and in approaches to vaccine sciences. Sub-unit vaccines composed of different parts of the malaria parasite, new methods for modifying parasite antigens, totally new approaches such as DNA vaccines and new adjuvants all give hope that the formidable impediments to malaria vaccine development will be overcome. Indeed since 1994 16 trials of vaccines in humans have been undertaken, mostly phase I and II, but still a great increase over the previous handful and more are in preparation.[123]

The many stages of the malaria parasite outlined in Figure 22–1 provide potential targets for immunization. Vaccine development has focused largely upon three main parasite stages: (1) the sporozoites (and more recently hepatic forms); (2) the asexual forms; and (3) the sexual forms.

Much effort has been put into sporozoite vaccine development because of the demonstrated immunity to sporozoites obtained from irradiated mosquitoes.[121,122] It was well appreciated there was little evidence of effective natural immune response to sporozoites, and it was acknowledged that the fleeting existence of sporozoites in blood made them a difficult target for an immune response. Nevertheless major efforts to develop a pre-erythrocytic vaccine have focused heavily on targeting the circumsporozoite (CS) protein, a major component of the surface of the sporozoite and a product of one of the first malaria genes to be cloned. It provided a target for both protective antibody and for cell-mediated immune responses. Clinical trials with early formulations were not promising, but further refinements have continued especially with improved adjuvants to enhance the cellular immune response. A new formulation is about to undergo clinical trials.[124] Other surface proteins have been targeted and indeed other sporozoite proteins and liver stage antigens are under investigation. Much has been learned through these efforts including a fuller appreciation of the substantial antigenic diversity of P. falci-

parum and of differences among species of malaria.[58,121,125–127]

Vaccines against asexual blood stages of P. falciparum would seem the most promising approach. Passive transfer of immunity has been shown with anti-merozoite immunoglobulin from West Africa given to East African patients.[58] However, P. falciparum undergoes great antigenic change with each new generation of merozoites: a set of antibodies directed against the first generation is ineffective against the next and the parasite presents a "moving target" to the host immune system. However, there appears to be a limited number of conserved surface antigens that occur against which a protective immunity can be built. Eventually surviving humans mobilize a sufficiently diverse set of antibodies that immunity to severe malaria is achieved. In holoendemic Africa, where the entomologic inoculation rate may be hundreds a year, protective immunity takes place over several years, representing thousands of inoculated parasites. The hope is to develop a vaccine that can induce similar levels of immunity in weeks or months, by age 6 months rather than by 6 years. Patarroyo and his colleagues developed a promising candidate with components directed against both pre-erythrocytic and asexual blood stages,[128,129] but this formulation has not proven to be effective in several large scale field trials.[130,131] Further work with formulations based upon this approach is going on by a number of groups.[123]

Finally there has been substantial work done on vaccines directed against the sexual stages of the malaria parasite, commonly termed "transmission blocking" vaccines. These represent a particularly interesting approach in that the vaccine would not protect the individual vaccinated but, rather, would reduce transmission from those who are infected to others, analogous to the use of residual insecticides in households. Demonstration of the effectiveness of such a vaccine is difficult since the effect of antibodies takes place in the mosquito after it takes blood meal from an immunized human. The test must demonstrate that a mosquito that would have become infectious from the bite does not do so. For example, mosquitoes are fed (either through xenodiagnosis or through membrane feeding) on immunized and on control humans, are followed through the sporogonic cycle, and then examined for the presence of oocysts and/or sporozoites. Thus major challenges involve development both of an effective vaccine and a test for the effectiveness of that vaccine. The potential usefulness of this kind of vaccine is discussed below.

APPROACHES TO CONTROL

The complexity of the malaria transmission cycle provides a wide variety of opportunities to stop or slow down transmission of parasites from man to vector to man. Historically, though based on the flawed theory of miasma, the major public health approach to malaria was the siting of communities away from low lying swamp areas to reduce vector contact. Today many approaches to malaria control are in use; appropriate selection depends on the ecologic and epidemiologic circumstances.

Broadly these approaches include a wide range of vector control methods and strategies for their use; antimalarial drugs and various strategies for their use; and, potentially, vaccines directed at various lifeforms of the parasite. For most strategies, detailed knowledge of the specific vector, specific parasite, and human economic, cultural, and social components are as vital for determining how best to intervene as are the specifics of the intervention tool itself. Control strategies that may be useful for Africa are outlined in Exhibit 22–2.

Vector Control Methods

The wide range of vector control methods is based upon attacking the mosquito in various parts of its life cycle: breeding site control, specific larvacide methods, adulticiding methods, and personal or household protection against adult biting.

Approaches focusing upon vector control have progressed beyond that of engineering and larvacide control to use of residual insecticiding

---

Exhibit 22–2 Control Strategies for Malaria in Africa

What can be done now:
- General infrastructure/institution improvement
- Role of vector control in areas with an EIR less than 100
  - Environmental improvements to reduce breeding
  - Impregnated bed nets
  - Personal protection
- Household use of antimalarial drugs for the under 5s
  - Monitoring for antimalarial resistance
- Improved immunization coverage, especially in remote areas, in anticipation of effective antimalarial vaccines

New tools to be developed:
- Vaccine development, especially asexual phase
- Drug development and acceleration of those in the pipeline
- Understanding of the molecular biology of the parasite
- Understanding of the sporogonic cycle to aid in reengineering of the anopheline
- Improved entomologic field methods for better understanding of microepidemiologic variation
- Understanding mechanisms of drug resistance and factors that contribute to its spread
- Better diagnostic tests that rapidly and inexpensively indicate drug resistance

of households, aerosol distribution of insecticides in some circumstances, the use of mosquito netting and screens, repellents of various types and most recently the development of insecticide impregnated bed nets.

Breeding Site and Larva Control

After the discovery of the role of mosquito vectors, efforts were directed toward elimination or reduction of vector breeding sites by swamp drainage and environmental control with engineering methods for water source reduction, water management with flushing and sluicing, covering of wells and other sources, vegetation clearing, and reforestation. DDT and other insecticides and specific larvacides have greatly added to breeding site control methods, particularly in urban settings. In addition to the engineering, mechanical, and chemical insecticide approaches, various biologic approaches including larva predators such as larvivarous fish and use of bacteria such as *B. thuriagensis*, which produce specific anti-larval toxins, are also in widespread use. Approaches to vector control through reduction of breeding sites continue to play a major role in malaria control strategies.

Adult Control

The use of DDT for household residual spraying had great impact on malaria control in many areas of the world, and its initial successes were principally responsible for the eradication efforts in the 1950s and 1960s. The conceptual foundation for eradication from use of residual insecticides was based upon anopheline resting behavior after engorgement with a blood meal as discussed earlier in this chapter. The effect is upon the mosquito that has already bitten; no protection is provided to those in the insecticided household, but rather to those whom these mosquitoes would later bite after becoming infected from the host. To reduce transmission virtually all households in the neighborhood must be sprayed. The effectiveness of this approach depends upon the biting and resting behavior of the mosquito and upon the willingness of the human population to have their households sprayed. Early campaign efforts to mobilize teams trained to spray insecticides within households and to obtain the cooperation of the house holders were undertaken in many countries in Europe, Asia, Latin America and enormous successes were obtained in a number of countries. Indeed, in Malta the anopheline vector was completely wiped out.[4]

Insecticide Impregnated Bed Nets

In the last ten years increasing experience with insecticide impregnated bed nets (IBNs) have shown reduction of transmission, clinical disease, and childhood mortality in at least three large controlled trials.[77,99,132,133] However, not all studies have demonstrated such positive benefits, and there is much controversy about the appropriate role of IBNs in control programs. An evaluation of a national program of impregnated bed nets under routine use, The Gambian National Impregnated Bed Net Programme, failed to provide evidence for any reduction in child mortality.[134] That IBNs can have an effect is without question; they are one more potentially valuable weapon to be included in working through an integrated approach to malaria control based upon epidemiologic, ecologic, and socioeconomic circumstances.

Personal and Household Protection

Repellents of various types, protective clothing, screening, bed nets, and other forms of personal protection against the bite of mosquitoes are all of importance and widely recommended, but aside from educational campaigns and exhortations this approach has never been viewed as a major component in malaria control programs.

Treatment Strategies

Depending upon the epidemiologic and ecologic situation of the malaria and the level of health services and community development, a variety of strategies for use of antimalarial drugs may be advantageous. In tropical Africa the principal approach to malaria control has been through the use of antimalarial drugs in passive case finding and treatment of those who present to clinics or pharmacies with symptoms of malaria.[135] Health workers in Africa are taught about the major symptoms of malaria and the need to treat it promptly with an appropriate antimalarial drug. Treatment of malaria in childhood is now accorded a prominent place in the Integrated Management of Childhood Illnesses (IMCI).[136] This important provider-oriented and facility-based approach focuses upon assessment and treatment of the major killing diseases of children and is being introduced widely into the poor countries of the world with assistance especially from WHO, UNICEF, USAID, and CDC.

Unfortunately, severe malaria kills children so rapidly that in most of Africa mothers cannot get their babies to facility-based treatment in time. Thus it is vital for a case treatment strategy to include community mobilization and education for families to understand the urgency to obtain treatment of their sick child. Recently plans were being formulated to extend the IMCI range of activities beyond the health facility to include critical family and community aspects.

A relatively untried strategy for timely provision of antimalarials is to train village-based mother coordinators to teach neighboring mothers to recognize symptoms of malaria in their children and to treat immediately at home. The mother coordinators, generally selected by their neighbors for this responsibility, also see to the distribution of antimalarials to be kept by the households. This approach now has been shown to be highly effective giving a major reduction in under-five mortality in a randomized trial in Northern Ethiopia at very low cost (Gebreyesus Kidane, personal communication, 1998).

Prophylaxis with antimalarials has been the standard and generally highly effective procedure for travelers and short-term residents of endemic areas. It has also been an effective approach for selected "captive" populations such as plantation workers or miners. From the public health viewpoint prophylaxis has also been shown to be highly beneficial in pregnancy, especially for first and second pregnancies.[137]

The role of prophylaxis for infants and young children is still not clear. In pilot studies in The Gambia prophylaxis was more effective than use of nearby primary health care facilities for treatment of children. The reason was that the rapid course of severe malaria did not give time for mothers to procure treatment.[99] There have been two major concerns about antimalarial prophylaxis: it might suppress development of an immune response and it might favor development of drug resistance, but there is little firm evidence for either. Even in tightly run prophylaxis programs there has been little retardation in development of immunologic defenses. Mathematical modeling could help to determine the proportion of the parasite population in a human population that would be affected by prophylaxis of under-two year olds and provide some indication of likelihood of adding to resistance development. The optimal age for reducing or stopping prophylaxis in children has not been established, but certainly before age 5 would seem reasonable for most areas. In many respects household treatment of possible malaria symptoms as discussed above would be virtually equivalent, would certainly not inhibit host defense mechanisms, would require less antimalarial distribution and would provide for a natural stopping age for use of antimalarials.

A major threat to either the approach to teach mothers to provide the antimalarial or the use of antimalarial for prophylaxis in the household is the increasing rate of chloroquine resistance. No other drug is as safe and as inexpensive as chloroquine; where chloroquine ceases to be useful, these strategies will have to be reexamined.

Progress in understanding drug resistance in malaria has been slow and much remains to be worked through. It seems likely that sexual reproduction within the vector plays an important role in the transfer and spread of resistance, but little work has focused on this aspect to date. Meanwhile several strategies may reduce or circumvent the effect of increasing drug resistance. Anti-malarial combinations can lessen the likelihood that single drug resistance emerges, particularly for new drugs such as the artemisimin derivatives (appreciating that such a strategy will increase costs and potential for increased adverse reactions); reinstitution of drugs such as chloroquine in areas where they have been out of use for some years; and of course continued drug development research for new drugs.

Strategies for Vaccine Use

Even after development of one or several vaccines, the most appropriate vaccine and the use of that vaccine will depend upon the epidemiologic situation. A sporozoite vaccine is designed to prevent initial infection from injected sporozoites. The vaccine has successfully prevented infection in animal studies, and complete protection against the challenge dose was achieved in humans immunized with sporozoites from irradiated mosquitoes.[121,122,126] A potential danger, however, is that if any sporozoite evades the defenses and penetrates a liver, a full blown malaria episode cell would follow. There is not sufficient experience thus far to know what the quantitative relationships between antibody and cellular immune response levels to magnitude of sporozoite challenges. An anti-sporozoite vaccine is likely to have a limited duration of protection and to have limited, if any, natural boosting; thus it should be useful for visitors to endemic areas, but perhaps not so effective for those living in endemic areas.

An asexual stage vaccine, however, would mimic that of natural immunity, and if used in children in holoendemic areas, perhaps only one or two immunizations in late infancy, after maternal antibodies had waned, would be sufficient. Then natural inoculations would provide the booster effect. In such a situation it would be counterproductive to reduce transmission since the transmission would be the method for vaccine boosting.

The use of vaccines directed against the sexual, gamete forms (the "transmission block-ing" vaccine) is more problematic: it might be useful as an additional control component in areas of relatively unstable malaria where other control measures are in place. It might be a particularly useful supplement to reduce spread of drug resistant parasites. Mathematical modeling could help in working through circumstances in which this type of vaccine would be advantageous. Its only use would be where malaria control efforts were focused on reduction or elimination of transmission; it would be counterproductive where the booster effect of natural infection is needed as with an asexual, blood form vaccine used to reduce the severity of infection rather than to reduce transmission.

Although this section has discussed approaches to control separately focused on vector control, antimalarial treatment or use of vaccines, most malaria control programs will need to use a combination of antimalarial measures tailored to fit the epidemiologic and ecologic circumstances.

THE FUTURE

The first priority for reducing the continuing, appallingly high mortality from malaria in Africa is to improve the use of currently available tools. To do so requires strengthened planning based upon detailed epidemiologic data combined with improved management and operational research capacity of the health system particularly that of primary health care and its support systems at the local community and district levels. It also will require basic human development improvements including strengthened infrastructural and institutional support for enhanced employment opportunities, strengthened women's groups, better access to microcredit, augmented community and family education, and better communication and transport systems. These general development improvements are needed because the strategies as elaborated above to achieve effective malaria control require understanding and concerted action at the household and community level. The fundamental institutional and profound structural reconstruction required to achieve these basic changes are only recently being acted upon in a handful of African countries. The sector wide action programs (SWAPs) in which all donors contribute to a common "basket" for which host country decision makers are responsible should assist in these changes when undertaken by countries with a sufficient technical and political competence to effectively use and account for the funding.[138] Globally the need for improved equity to generate the capacity for all countries and locales to make decisions for themselves not only must be recognized, but also the wealthy nations (and their voters) must be convinced that it is in their long-term interest.

Operational research to support improved planning and management, largely country and even locale specific, is needed if several of the most promising strategies indicated above are to be effective:

- approaches to the training of trainers for distribution and use of antimalarials by mothers in the household to treat their infants and children
- distribution, use, and continuing reimpregnation of insecticided bed nets
- continuing monitoring for drug resistance
- support for communities to work through their own approaches to take community actions to control malaria including reduction of vector habitats especially in areas with marginal or highly variable transmission
- continued improvement in immunization coverage particularly to the underserved populations in anticipation of an effective antimalarial vaccine

Certainly better tools are needed; research on nearly all aspects as outlined above should be valuable. The first research priority should be asexual phase vaccine development, especially now that health infrastructures in many African countries are sufficiently developed to deliver childhood vaccines to at least 75% of their population. Granted that there have been major tech-

nical impediments to the development of antimalarial vaccines as outlined above, the most important factor, until quite recently, is that global research agencies have put truly paltry sums to this effort. With the publication of *Investing in Health Research and Development* giving some sense of priority for global health research,[139] there was a renewal of interest in malaria vaccine research and funding for it in 1997–1998 was at least moderately increased. The new WHO "Roll Back Malaria" initiative is further evidence that malaria in Africa will be taken seriously.

Other major needs for research include the following:

- Continued efforts for drug development and acceleration of those that have long been in the pipeline. For example, antimalarial drugs derived from the Chinese wormwood plant, Artemisia annua, are only recently available in a limited number of countries after more than 20 years.
- Continued work to understand the molecular biology of the parasite, especially the metabolic pathways contributing to virulence that might be amenable to rational drug development; and that of the much neglected the sporogonic cycle, which may aid in efforts to reengineer anophelines as discussed below.
- Continued development of mathematical modeling done in direct concert with field investigations may facilitate a deeper understanding of the critical quantitative relationships involved in transmission control.
- Improved entomologic field methods for better understanding of micro-epidemiologic variation and for local anopheline control efforts.

A better understanding of the mechanisms underlying drug resistance and factors contributing to its spread will likely require a combination of the genetics, entomology, and epidemiology disciplines; simple, inexpensive, rapid, and robust diagnostic tests that would provide for quantification of parasite density and that would indicate drug sensitivity (or resistance) would be of great value.

Ideas about reengineering anophelines so that they do not adequately support the parasite through completion of the sporogonic cycle and yet maintain (or even improve upon) their competitive advantage in the field have received much attention as an imaginative new approach, but so far comparatively little funding. In the short run more basic research into the sporogonic cycle to better understand why some anopheline species support parasite development and others do not is needed. In the long run, however, reservations remain about the likelihood of success of this approach: species such as the *An. gambiae* complex have so effec-

tively evolved through the centuries in concert with the human *Plasmodia* species and have demonstrated such enormous capacity to rapidly adapt to a wide variety of changing conditions that successfully displacing them on continuing, sustainable basis would seem an unlikely bet.

Reduction of the continuing high mortality and morbidity from malaria in Africa will require both better use of current control measures—necessitating better epidemiologic and ecologic information for better planning; better management of control programs; and increased direct involvement of families and communities—and accelerated research toward vaccines, drugs, vector control approaches, and fundamental understanding of the parasite, vector, and human host as outlined above.

REFERENCES

1. Bruce-Chwatt LJ. History of malaria from prehistory to eradication. In: Wernsdorfer WH, McGregor I, eds. *Malaria: Principles and Practice of Malariology.* Edinburgh: Churchill Livingstone; 1988:1–69.

2. International Development Advisory Board. *Malaria Eradication: Report and Recommendations of the International Development Advisory Board.* Washington, DC: International Development Advisory Board; 1956.

3. World Health Organization Expert Committee on Malaria. *WHO Technical Report Series No. 357.* Geneva: World Health Organization; 1967.

4. Russell PF, et al. *Practical Malariology.* 2nd ed. New York: Oxford University Press; 1963:267–268.

5. World Health Organization. *Re-examination of the Global Strategy of Malaria Eradication.* A report by the Director-General to the 22nd World Health Assembly:1969.

6. Krishna S. Malaria. *Br Med J.* 1997;315:730–732.

7. World Health Organization. *Malaria Eradication from the Ninth Plenary Meeting.* Geneva: World Health Organization; 1955.

8. Oaks SC Jr, et al, eds. *Malaria: Obstacles and Opportunities.* Washington, DC: National Academy Press; 1991.

9. Murray CJL, Lopez AD, eds. *Global Comparative Assessments in the Health Sector.* Geneva: World Health Organization; 1994.

10. Beier JC. Malaria parasite development in mosquitoes. *Ann Rev Entomol.* 1998;43:519–543.

11. Ghana Health Assessment Project Team. A quantitative method of assessing the health impact of different diseases in less developed countries. *Int J Epidemiol.* 1981; 10:73–80.

12. Jamison DT, et al, eds. *Investing in Health. World Development Report, 1993.* New York: Oxford University Press, The World Bank; 1993.

13. Hyder AA, Rotlant G, Morrow RH. Measuring the burden of disease: healthy life years. *Am J Public Health.* 1998;88(2):196–202.

14. Miller LH, et al. The resistance factor to *Plasmodium vivax* in blacks: the Duffy blood-group genotype, *Fy-Fy. N Engl J Med.* 1976;295:302.

15. Garnham PCC. *Malaria Parasites and Other Hemosporidia.* Oxford, England: Blackwell Scientific Publications; 1966.

16. Beier JC, et al. Quantitation of malaria sporozoites in the salivary glands of wild Afrotropical Anopheles. *Med Vet Entomol.* 1991;5:63–70.

17. Pringle G. A quantitative study of naturally acquired malaria infections in *Anopheles gambiae* of East Africa. *Trans Roy Soc Trop Med Hyg.* 1966;60:626–632.

18. Pull JH, Grab B. *A Simple Epidemiological Model for Evaluating the Malaria Inoculation Rate and the Risk of Infection in Infants.* Geneva: World Health Organization; 1974:507–516.

19. MacDonald G. *The Epidemiology and Control of Malaria.* London: Oxford University Press; 1957.

20. Beadle C, McElroy PD, Oster CN. Impact of transmis-

sion intensity and age on *Plasmodium falciparum* density and associated fever implications for malaria vaccine trial design. *J Infect Dis.* 1955;172:1047–1054.

21. Molineaux L, Gramiccia G. *The Garki Project: Research on the Epidemiology and Control of Malaria in the Sudan Savanna of West Africa.* Geneva: World Health Organization; 1980.

22. Beier JC, et al. Effect of human circumsporozoite antibodies in *Plasmodium*-infected Anopheles (*Diptera: Cullicidae*). *J Med Entomol.* 1989;26:547–553.

23. Krotoski WA, et al. Demonstration of hypnozoites in sporozoite-transmitted *Plasmodium vivax* infection. *Am J Trop Med Hyg.* 1982;31:1291–1293.

24. Schwartz IK. Prevention of malaria. *Infect Dis Clin North Am.* 1992;6(2):313–331.

25. Creasey A, et al. Genetic diversity of *Plasmodium falciparum* shows geographic variation. *Am J Trop Med Hyg.* 1990;42:403.

26. Haworth J. The global distribution of malaria and the present control effort. In: Wernsdorfer WH, McGregor I, eds. *Malaria: Principles and Practice of Malariology.* Edinburgh: Churchill Livingstone; 1988.

27. Collins FH. Prospects for malaria control through genetic manipulation of its vectors. *Parasitol Today.* 1994; 10:370–371.

28. Crampton JM. Molecular studies of insect vectors of malaria. *Adv Parasitol.* 1994;31:1–31.

29. MacDonald G. The measurement of malaria transmission. *Proc Roy Soc Med.* 1955;48:295–301.

30. Garrett-Jones C. The human blood index of malaria vectors in relation to epidemiological assessment. *Bull WHO.* 1964;30:241–261.

31. Dye C, Lines JD, Curtis CF. A test of the malaria strain theory. *Parisitol Today.* 1996;12:88–89.

32. Dietz K, Molineaux L, Thomas A. A malaria model tested in African savanna. *Bull WHO.* 1974;50:347–357.

33. Metselaar D, van Thiel PM. Classification of malaria. *Trop Geogr Med.* 1959;11:157–161.

34. Molineaux L. The epidemiology of human malaria as an explanation of its distribution including some implications for its control. In: Wernsdorfer WH, McGregor I, eds. *Malaria: Principles and Practice of Malariology.* Edinburgh: Churchill Livingstone; 1988.

35. Najera JA. Malaria and the work of the WHO. *Bull WHO.* 1989;67(3):229–243.

36. Fleming AF, et al. Abnormal haemoglobins in the Sudan Savana of Nigeria. *Ann Trop Med Parasitol.* 1979; 73:161–172.

37. Weatherall DJ. Common genetic disorders of the red cell and the "malaria" hypothesis. *Ann Trop Med Parasitol.* 1987;81:539–548.

38. Miller LH. Impact of malaria on genetic polymorphism and genetic diseases in Africans and African-Americans. *Proc Natl Acad Sci.* 1994;91:2415–2419.

39. Luzatto L, Nwachuku-Jarret ES, Reddy S. Increased sickling of parasitised erythrocytes as mechanism of resistance against malaria in the sickle-cell trait. *Lancet.* 1970;1:319–321.

40. Bryceson AD, Fleming AF, Edington GM. Splenomegaly in northern Nigeria. *Acta Tropica.* 1976;33:185.

41. Fleming AF, Allan NC, Stenhous NS. Splenomegaly and sickle cell trait. *Lancet.* 1968;2:574–575.

42. Hamilton PJS, et al. Absence of sickle-cell trait in patients with tropical splenomegaly syndrome. *Lancet.* 1969;2:109.

43. Gilles HM. The development of malarial infection in breast-fed Gambian infants. *Ann Trop Med Parasitol.* 1957;51:58–72.

44. Edington GM. Pathology of malaria in West Africa. *Br Med J.* 1967;1:715–718.

45. Hendrickse RG. Interactions of nutrition and infection: experience in Nigeria, in nutrition and infection. In: Wolstenholme GEW, O'Connor M, eds. *Ciba Foundation Study Group 31.* London: Churchill Livingstone; 1967: 98–111.

46. Edirisinghe JS, Fern EB, Targett GAT. Resistance to super infection with *Plasmodium berghei* in rats fed a protein free diet. *Trans Roy Soc Trop Med Hyg.* 1982; 76:382–386.

47. Bakker NPM, et al. Attenuation of malaria infection, paralysis and lesions of the central nervous system by low protein diets in rats. *Acta Tropica.* 1992;50:285–293.

48. Smith AW, et al. The effects on malaria of treatment of iron-deficiency anaemia with oral iron in Gambian children. *Ann Trop Pediatr.* 1989;9:17–23.

49. Shankar AH, Stoltzfus RJ. A meta-analysis of controlled trials of iron supplementation to infants and children in malarious areas. 1998.

50. Shankar A, et al. Effect of vitamin A supplementation on morbidity due to *P. falciparum* in young children in Papua New Guinea: a randomized trial. *Lancet.* 1998; 17:354(9174):203–209.

51. Binka FN, et al. Vitamin A supplementation and childhood malaria in northern Ghana. *Am J Clin Nutr.* 1995; 61:853–859.

52. Bates CJ, et al. A trial of zinc-supplementation in young rural Gambian children. *Br J Nutr.* 1993;69:243–255.

53. Shankar AH, Kumar N, Scott AL. Zinc-deficiency exacerbates experimental malaria infection in mice. *FASEB J.* 1995;9:A4269.

54. Arif AJ, et al. Effect of zinc diet on xanthine oxidase activity of liver of mice infected with *Plasmodium berghei. Indian J Malariol.* 1997;24:59–61.

55. Molineaux L. *Plasmodium falciparum* malaria: some epidemiological implications of parasite and host diversity. *Ann Trop Med Parasitol.* 1996;90(4):379–393.

56. Drulihe P, Perignon JL. Mechanisms of defense against *Plasmodium falciparum* asexual blood stages in humans. *Immunol Lett.* 1994;41:115–120.

57. Khusmith S, Druilhe P. Antibody-dependent ingestion of *P. falciparum* merozoites by human blood monocytes. *Parasite Immunol.* 1983;5:357–368.

58. McGregor IA, Carington SP, Cohen S. Treatment of East African *P. falciparum* malaria with West African human gammaglobulin. *Trans Roy Soc Trop Med Hyg.* 1963;57:170–175.

59. Bouharoun-Tayoun H, et al. Antibodies that protect humans against *Plasmodium falciparum* blood stages do not on their own inhibit parasite growth and invasion in vitro, but act in cooperation with monocytes. *J Exp Med.* 1990;172:1633–1641.

60. Su XZ, et al. The large diverse gene family var encodes proteins involved in cytoadherence and antigenic variation of *Plasmodium falciparum* infected erythrocytes. *Cell.* 1995;82:89–100.

61. Allan RJ, et al. Strain variation in tumor necrosis factor induction by parasites from children with acute falciparum malaria. *Infect Immunol.* 1995;63:1173–1175.

62. Clark IA, Rockett KA. The cytokine theory of human cerebral malaria. *Parasitol Today.* 1994;10:410–412.

63. Clark IA, Rockett KA. Nitric oxide and parasitic disease. *Adv Parasitol.* 1996;371:1–56.

64. Gupta S, et al. Parasite virulence and disease patterns in *Plasmodium falciparum* malaria. *Proc Natl Acad Sci USA.* 1994;91:3715–3719.

65. Treutiger CJ, et al. Rosette formation in *Plasmodium falciparum* isolates and anti-rosette activity of sera from Gambians with cerebral or uncomplicated malaria. *Am J Trop Med Hyg.* 1992;46:503–510.

66. Babiker HA, et al. Random mating in a natural population of the malaria parasite *Plasmodium falciparum*. *Parasitology.* 1994;109:413–421.

67. Kwitatkowski D, Novak M. Periodic and chaotic host-parasite interactions in human malaria. *Proc Natl Acad Sci USA.* 1991;88:5111–5113.

68. McGuire W, et al. Variation in the TNF-alphapromoter region associated with susceptibility to cerebral malaria. *Nature.* 1994;371:508–511.

69. Hill WG, et al. Estimation of inbreeding coefficients from genotypic data on multiple alleles and application to estimation of clonality in malaria parasites. *Genet Res.* 1995;65:53–61.

70. Conway DJ, Greenwood BM, McBride JS. Longitudinal study of *Plasmodium falciparum* polymorphic antigens in a malaria-endemic population. *Infect Immun.* 1992; 60:1122–1127.

71. Forsyth KP, et al. Small area variation in prevalence of an S-antigen serotype of *Plasmodium falciparum* in villages of Madang, Papua New Guinea. *Am J Trop Med Hyg.* 1989;40:344–350.

72. Daubersies P, et al. PCR characterization of isolates from various endemic areas: diversity and turnover of *Plasmodium falciparum* populations are correlated with transmission. *Memorias do Instituto Oswaldo Cruz.* 1994;89(suppl 2):9–12.

73. Slutsker L, et al. In hospital morbidity and mortality due to malaria-associated severe anaemia in two areas of Malawi with different patterns of malaria infection. *Trans Roy Soc Trop Med Hyg.* 1994;88:548–551.

74. Warrell DA, Molyneux ME, Beales PF. Severe and complicated malaria. *Trans Roy Soc Trop Med Hyg.* 1990;84(suppl 2):1–65.

75. Marsh K, et al. The pathogenesis of severe malaria in African children. *Ann Trop Med Parasitol.* 1996; 90(4):396–402.

76. Greenwood B, Marsh K, Snow R. Why do some African children develop severe malaria? *Parasitol Today.* 1991;7:277–281.

77. Alonso PL, et al. The effect of insecticide-treated bed nets on mortality of Gambian children. *Lancet.* 1991; 337:1499–1502.

78. Brewster DR, Kwiatkowski D, White NJ. Neurological sequelae of cerebral malaria in children. *Lancet.* 1990; 336:1039–1043.

79. Molyneux ME, et al. Clinical features and prognostic indicators in pediatric cerebral malaria: a study of 131 comatose Malawian children. *Q J Med.* 1989;71:441–459.

80. Marsh K, et al. Indicators of life-threatening malaria in African children. *N Engl J Med.* 1995;322:1399–1404.

81. Greenwood BM, et al. Comparison of two strategies for control of malaria within a primary health care programme in The Gambia. *Lancet.* 1988;1:1121–1127.

82. Alles HK, Mendis KN, Carter R. Malaria mortality rates in South Asia and in Africa: implications for malaria control. *Parasitol Today.* 1998;14:369–375.

83. McPherson GG, et al. Human cerebral malaria: a quantitative ultrastructural analysis of parasitized erythrocyte sequestration. *Am J Pathol.* 1985;119:385–401.

84. Warrell D, Looareesuwan S, Warrell MJ, et al. Dexamethasone proves deleterious in cerebral malaria. *N Engl J Med.* 1982;306:313–319.

85. Waruiru CM, et al. Epileptic seizures and malaria in Kenyan children. *Trans Roy Soc Trop Med Hyg.* 1996; 90(2):152–155.

86. Marsh K, Snow RW. Host-parasite interaction and morbidity in malaria endemic areas. *Philos Trans R Soc Lond B Biol Sci.* 1997;352:1385–1394.

87. White NJ, et al. Severe hypoglycemia and hyperinsu-

linemia in falciparum malaria. *N Engl J Med.* 1983; 309:61–66.

88. Taylor TE, et al. Blood glucose levels in Malawian children before and during the administration of intravenous quinine for severe falciparum malaria. *N Engl J Med.* 1988;319:1040–1047.

89. English M, et al. Deep breathing reflects acidosis and is associated with poor prognosis in children with severe malaria and respiratory distress. *Am J Trop Med Hyg.* 1996;55:521–524.

90. Marsh K. Malaria—a neglected disease? *Parasitology.* 1992;104(suppl):s53–s69.

91. Snow RW, et al. Severe childhood malaria in two areas of markedly different falciparum transmission in East Africa. *Acta Tropica.* 1994;57:289–300.

92. Snow RW, Marsh K. Will reducing *Plasmodium falciparum* transmission alter malaria mortality among African children? *Parasitol Today.* 1995;11:188–190.

93. Snow RW, et al. Periodicity and space-time clustering of severe childhood malaria on the coast of Kenya. *Trans Roy Soc Trop Med Hyg.* 1993;87:386–390.

94. Armstrong Schellenberg JRM, et al. An analysis of the geographic distribution of severe malaria in children in the Kilifi District, Kenya. *Int J Epidemiol.* 1998; 27:323–329.

95. Smith T, et al. Relationships between *Plasmodium falciparum* infection and morbidity in a highly endemic area. *Parasitology.* 1994;109:539–549.

96. Greenwood BM, et al. Mortality and morbidity from malaria among children in a rural area of The Gambia, West Africa. *Trans Roy Soc Trop Med Hyg.* 1987; 81:478–486.

97. Lines J, Armstrong JRM. For a few parasites more: inoculum size, vector control and strain-specific immunity to malaria. *Parasitol Today.* 1992;8:381.

98. Adiamah JH, et al. Entomological risk factors for severe malaria in a peri-urban area of The Gambia. *Ann Trop Med Parasitol.* 1993;87:491–500.

99. Alonso PL, et al. A malaria control trial using insecticide-treated bed nets and targeted chemoprophylaxis in a rural area of The Gambia, West Africa. 6. The impact of the interventions on mortality and morbidity from malaria. *Trans Roy Soc Trop Med Hyg.* 1993;87(suppl 2):37–44.

100. Morrow RH. The application of a quantitative approach to the assessment of the relative importance of vector and soil transmitted diseases in Ghana. *Soc Sci Med.* 1984;19:1039–1049.

101. Brabin BJ. The risks and severity of malaria in pregnant women. In: *TDR/Applied Field Research in Malaria Reports*, no. 1. Geneva: World Health Organization; 1991.

102. Oduntan SO. The health of Nigerian children of school age (6–15 years). *Ann Trop Med Parasitol.* 1974; 68:129–143.

103. Khusmith S, et al. Two-site immuno-radiometric assay for detection of *Plasmodium falciparum* antigen in blood using monoclonal and polyclonal antibodies. *J Clin Microbiol.* 1987;25:1467–1471.

104. Shiff CJ, Premji Z, Minjas JN. The rapid manual ParaSight-F test. A new diagnostic tool for *P. falciparum* infection. *Trans Roy Soc Trop Med Hyg.* 1993;87:646–648.

105. Mharakurwa S, Manyame B, Shiff CJ. Trial of the ParaSight-F test for malaria diagnosis in the primary health care system, Zimbabwe. *Trop Med Int Health.* 1997;2:544–550.

106. Snounou G, Beck HP. The use of PCR genotyping in the assessment of recrudescence or reinfection after antimalarial drug treatment. *Parasitol Today.* 1998; 14:462–467.

107. Wernsdorfer WH. Epidemiology and drug resistance in malaria. *Acta Tropica.* 1994;56:143–156.

108. Bruce-Chwatt LJ, et al. Chemotherapy of malaria. In: *WHO Monograph Series*, no. 27. Geneva: World Health Organization; 1986.

109. Krogstad DJ. Malaria as a reemerging disease. *Epidemiol Rev.* 1996;18:77–79.

110. Harinasuta T, Migasen S, Boonag D. *UNESCO First Regional Symposium on Scientific Knowledge of Tropical Parasites.* Singapore: University of Singapore; 1962.

111. Thaithong S, et al. Clonal diversity in a single isolate of the malaria parasite *Plasmodium falciparum. Trans Roy Soc Trop Med Hyg.* 1984;78:242–245.

112. Maberti S. Desarollo de resistencia a la pirimetamima. Presentacion de 15 casos estudiados en Trujillo. *Med Trop Parasitol Med.* 1960;3:239–259.

113. Krogstad DJ, Herwaldt BL. Chemoprohylaxis and treatment of malaria. *N Engl J Med.* 1988;319:1538.

114. Campbell CC, et al. Chloroquine-resistant *Plasmodium falciparum* from East Africa. *Lancet.* 1979; 2:1151–1154.

115. Peterson DS, et al. Molecular basis of differential resistance to cycloguanil and pyrimethamine in *Plasmodium falciparum* malaria. *Proc Natl Acad Sci USA.* 1990;8:3018–3022.

116. Eldin de Pecoulas P, et al. *Plasmodium falciparum*: detection of antifolate resistance by mutation-specific restriction enzyme digestion. *Exp Parasitol.* 1995; 80:483–487.

117. Thaithong S, Beale GH, Chutmongkonkul M. Variability in drug susceptibility amongst clones and isolates of *Plasmodium falciparum. Trans Roy Soc Trop Med Hyg.* 1988;82:33–36.

118. Plowe CV, et al. Pyrimethamine and proguanil resis-

tance-conferring mutations in *Plasmodium falciparum* dihydrofolate reductase: polymerase chain reaction methods for surveillance in Africa. *Am J Trop Med Hyg.* 1995;52:565–568.

119. Ziba C, et al. Sustained efficacy of sulfadoxine-pyrimethamine as first-line treatment of malaria in under five Malawian children (Abstract 591). In: *Abstracts of the 44th Annual Meeting of the American Society of Tropical Medicine and Hygiene.* San Antonio, TX: Allen Press; 1995.

120. Plowe CV, et al. Mutations in *P. falciparum* dihydrofolate reductase and dihydropteroate synthase and epidemiologic patterns of pyrimethamine-sulfadoxine use and resistance. *J Infect Dis.* 1997;176:1590–1596.

121. Clyde DF, et al. Immunization of man against sporozoite-induced falciparum malaria. *Am J Med Sci.* 1973; 266:169–177.

122. Clyde DF, et al. Immunization of man against falciparum and vivax malaria by use of attenuated sporozoites. *Am J Trop Med Hyg.* 1975;24:397–401.

123. Engers HD, Godal T. Malaria vaccine development: current status. *Parasitol Today.* 1998;14:56–64.

124. Stoute JA, et al. A preliminary evaluation of a recombinant circumsporozoite protein vaccine against *Plasmodium falciparum* malaria. *N Engl J Med.* 1996;336:86–91.

125. Tsuji M, et al. CD4+ cytolytic T cell clone confers protection against murine malaria. *J Exp Med.* 1990; 172:1353–1357.

126. Nussenzweig R, et al. Protective immunity induced by the injection of X-irradiated sporosoites of *Plasmodium berghei. Nature.* 1967;216:160–162.

127. Hollingdale MR, et al. Non-CS pre-erythrocytic protective antigens. *Immunol Lett.* 1990;25:71–76.

128. Patarroyo ME, et al. A synthetic vaccine protects humans against challenge with asexual blood stages of *Plasmodium falciparum* malaria. *Nature.* 1988; 332:158–161.

129. Patarroyo ME, et al. Induction of protective immunity against experimental infection with malaria using synthetic peptides. *Nature.* 1987;328:629–632.

130. D'Alessandro U, et al. Efficacy trial of malaria vaccine SPf66 in Gambian infants. *Lancet.* 1995;346:462–467.

131. Nosten F, et al. Randomized double-blind placebo-controlled trial of SPf66 malaria vaccine in children in northwestern Thailand. SHOKLO SPf66 Malaria Vaccine Trial Group. *Lancet.* 1996;348:701–707.

132. Binka FN, et al. Impact of permethrin impregnated bed nets on child mortality in Kassena-Kankana district, Ghana: a randomized controlled trial. *Trop Med Health.* 1996;1:147–154.

133. Nevill CG, et al. Insecticide-treated bed nets reduce mortality and severe morbidity from malaria among children on the Kenyan coast. *Trop Med Int Health.* 1996;1:139–146.

134. D'Alessandro U, et al. The Gambian National Impregnated Bed Net Programme: evaluation of effectiveness by means of case-control studies. *Trans Roy Soc Trop Med Hyg.* 1997;91:638–642.

135. Buck AA, ed. *Proceedings of the Conference on Malaria in Africa: Practical Considerations on Malaria Vaccines and Clinical Trials.* Washington, DC: American Institute of Biological Sciences; 1986.

136. Gove S. Integrated management of childhood illness by outpatient health workers: technical basis and overview. In For the WHO Working Group on Guidelines for Integrated Management of the Sick Child. *Bull WHO.* 1997;75:7–24.

137. McGregor IA. Epidemiology, malaria and pregnancy. *Am J Trop Med Hyg.* 1984;33:517–525.

138. Cassels A. *A Guide to Sector-Wide Approaches for Health Development.* Geneva: World Health Organization; 1997.

139. Ad Hoc Committee on Health Research Relating to Future Intervention Options. *Investing in Health Research and Development.* Geneva: World Health Organization; 1996.

CHAPTER 23

Epidemiology of Helminth Infections

Clive Shiff

Parasitism is a way of life. Over evolutionary time the niche by which one species depends on another for subsistence has been elaborated in countless ways. Not only have parasitic species developed a means to adapt to existence in the gut, tissues, and within the cells of their hosts, these species also have evolved mechanisms to distribute their progeny so that they can readily find and be taken up by a new host. Parasites have adopted a variety of forms, some of which may appear grotesque. They have evolved stratagems to evade the immune defenses of their hosts; and they have coevolved with their hosts to the extent that they adapt to the behavior patterns of normal life and exploit these to enable them to migrate to other sources of hosts. All of these factors influence in some way the epidemiology of parasitic infections.

Transmission and acquisition of parasites by any naive host involves three factors: a source of infection or reservoir must be present from which the parental generation of the parasite radiates, a means of transmission must exist by which the parasite gains access to the host, and a susceptible host must be available. As these factors bear directly on the severity of parasitic infections and their importance in the communities of humans, they must be considered in any study on the epidemiology, health impact, and control of the infection. Parasites have evolved numerous strategies to be successful within their various hosts, but transmission essentially involves two types of cycle. The first is the *direct*

cycle where transmission is from person to person, usually through fecal waste in the environment. The second is the *indirect cycle,* which involves additional hosts or vectors that actively transfer the parasite from one host to another.

To demonstrate the complexity of this process, one example of each cycle will be discussed in detail. The direct cycle will be explained through consideration of the life cycle and epidemiology of hookworms. The indirect cycle will consider the complex epidemiology of schistosomes. The hookworms affecting humans belong to two species of nematode parasites, which produce similar infections, but because they are difficult to differentiate clinically and epidemiologically they usually are considered together. Transmission of these parasites depends on fecal contamination of the environment, absence of acceptable latrines, and a bare foot lifestyle. The schistosome parasite is a blood dwelling trematode that has a complex life cycle involving living in freshwater molluscs as well as the blood stream of its definitive host. The parasite has coevolved in tandem with its aquatic and human hosts producing a well-balanced association. However, the recent settling of human populations, with their need for water and their changing agricultural activities, as well as the burgeoning of these human populations, has increased the transmission of the parasite and, thus, has produced severe and debilitating infections. Therefore, overt disease caused by these parasites often results when the ecological

711

balances, to which the various populations have been adapted, have become unstable or have broken down, resulting in increasingly severe levels of infection.

HOOKWORM PARASITES OF HUMANS

Hookworms belong to the phylum *Nematoda*. Nematodes are tubular animals, diecious, with a definite body cavity in which the various organs are suspended. The gut is tubular, commencing in a complex oral region where the mouth and pharynx may have cutting teeth or plates, and the pharynx may be adapted for sucking and ingesting food. The body is covered with an outer cuticle, which is a complex structure consisting of several layers and which serves as a protective cover for the worms. The parasites are equipped only with longitudinal muscles, which accounts for the sinuous movements characteristic of the group. In parasitic nematodes the female is usually larger and packed with large ovaries and uterus. The males may exhibit complex external copulatory structures, which are characteristic of some species and which are used in identification. Eggs, which are usually characteristic for each species, are laid in large numbers; they may be embryonated or contain developing larvae. Usually the larval development takes several days and a first stage larva emerges. This stage is able to ingest food and will proceed through two molts to reach the L_3 stage, which in hookworms is infective; at this point larvae can no longer ingest food. The infective L_3 larva (called the *filariform* stage) is able to attach to and penetrate the skin of the next host by using proteolytic enzymes secreted in the apical area of the worm. Altogether, four larval molts occur before the adult develops, and it is always the third stage larva which is infectious.

Life Cycle

Two species of hookworm are known to infect humans: *Ancylostoma duodenale* and *Necator americanus*. The life cycles of these two parasites are similar and, thus, will be discussed to-gether (Figure 23–1). Embryonated eggs are passed in the feces of an infected person. In a suitable environment, one that is shady or dark, moist, and warm (22°C to 32°C), the eggs will hatch within 24 to 48 hours, releasing first stage larvae. These are not infective; they can ingest food, and will soon molt into second stage larvae after about 3 days. A second molt occurs after about 6 days and the resulting third stage larva is infectious—at the filariform stage. These larvae are unable to feed; however, under ideal conditions, they can survive and remain infectious for several weeks. Larvae invade by penetrating the skin between the toes or through the feet or ankles. However, they can also be transmitted through eating or handling unwashed, contaminated vegetables. Evidence also suggests that *A. duodenale* can be transmitted to suckling infants through milk. The filariform larvae secrete proteolytic enzymes that facilitate the penetration through the skin; they then enter the blood circulation and usually molt once more as they pass through the lungs. From the alveolar spaces, the larvae are coughed up in sputum, are swallowed, and thus gain entry to the human gut. The worms then reach the intestine where, as adults, they mate. They adhere to and lacerate the intestinal mucosa with their strong oral plates or teeth, they pump blood into the gut by means of the powerful muscular pharynx, and can continue to flush their gut with a stream of blood from the intestinal vessels they have penetrated. Thus, apart from consuming blood as a source of food, the parasites also cause considerable amounts of blood to be lost and voided in the feces of the host. Egg production commences 4 to 8 weeks after the initial infection and the worms can live approximately 3 years.

Epidemiology of Hookworm Infections

Hookworm infection is a worldwide problem that is most prevalent in warm, humid areas or environments. It is commonly found in the tropics, although it is also common in warm, wet areas of the temperate zones; it is frequently associated with anemia in the affected populations.

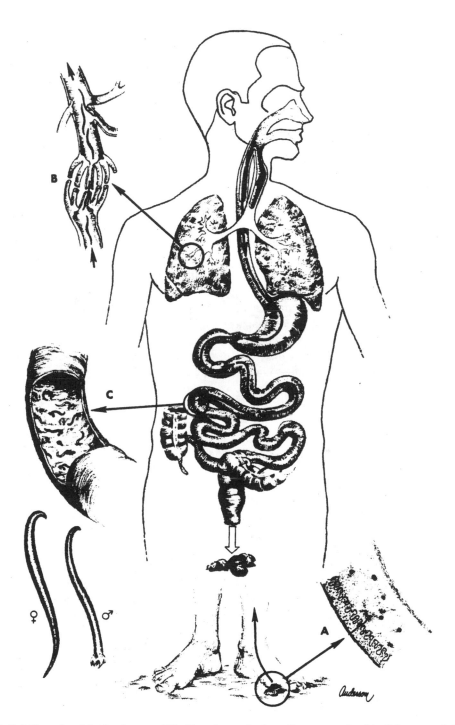

Figure 23–1 Life cycle of the hookworm. Filariform larvae in the soil penetrate the skin (**A**), are carried via the circulation to the lungs where they break out of the capillary bed into the alveolar spaces (**B**), then are swept up the bronchial tree, are swallowed, and become adult worms in the small intestine (**C**). *Source:* Reprinted with permission from Beck & Davis, *Medical Parasitology*, 3rd edition, p. 150, © 1981, W.B. Saunders Company.

Vulnerable populations are children, pregnant or lactating women, or women who menstruate heavily. The prevalence of geohelminth infections is age related, possibly because of immunologic factors or specific activities or behavior patterns related to age. The prevalence of hookworm is found to be lower among children aged under 5 years and it gradually increases with age; by age 8 years, a marked increase in prevalence occurs, which diminishes in later life. A clustering of infections is seen in certain children: Evidence shows that heavily or lightly infected children have a statistical predisposition to acquire similar infection intensities following deworming procedures if patterns of exposure have not changed.

The highest prevalence of hookworm infection is found in males, teenagers, and young adults, which may be related to occupational hazards. For example, tending crops such as in rice paddies where one must stand in the fields for many hours increases the exposure to hookworm and the likelihood of becoming infected. Other risk factors are associated with the extent of outdoor defecation, presence of defecation fields, and the type of soil, which should be loose and hold moisture well, thus providing a refuge for the infective larvae. Poor standard of living and sanitation are the major determinants of hookworm prevalence. Infection is usually higher in rural areas than in urban areas, and higher in people low on the socioeconomic scale. In parts of Europe and North America where hookworm was previously common, the infections have been all but eradicated because of improved access to effective sanitation and improved living conditions, including the wearing of shoes. Figure 23–2 shows a photograph of *Ancylostoma duodenale*.

Control Measures

No prophylactic drugs are available for hookworm infections, although iron therapy is useful in preventing serious nutritional depletion, especially in women and children. Mebendazole is often used to treat both hookworm and other geohelminth infections. Mass chemotherapy is effective in reducing the prevalence of all geohelminths, but the effects are short lived if no improvements are made in sanitation and health education. Considerable lack of knowledge exists about the transmission of intestinal parasites in many parts of the world. A study of mothers in urban slums in Sri Lanka demonstrated that 42% of mothers thought that parasites were acquired through eating sweets, 25% thought that they were transmitted through other children, and 25% did not know. None were aware of the relationship between contamination of soil with feces and transmission of the worms.[1] Kendall et al.[2] also mention that some societies consider that worms are normal symbiotes of the gut, which when mistreated (e.g., during a period of starvation or low food intake) can cause illness such as diarrhea.

One of the best measures an individual can take is wearing adequate footwear. This reduces the risk of infection, especially if worn in latrines, in the vicinity of human habitation, and during agricultural work. The appropriate use and maintenance of latrines also makes a difference. Hookworm eggs and larvae do not survive more than 1 or 2 months in soil, even under ideal conditions. Use of latrines helps reduce contamination of soil with the parasite and, therefore, this use also reduces transmission. Additionally, reducing the use of night soil as a fertilizer helps prevent the contamination of vegetables with parasites. Measures that can be used to prevent the transmission of all geohelminths include cleaning up stools of infants too young to use latrines; personal hygiene and care in preparing food, especially vegetables; the use of adequate footwear; and public education in elementary sanitation.

SCHISTOSOME PARASITES IN HUMANS

Three important species of schistosomes infect humans, with an additional two that occur in restricted areas. *Schistosoma haematobium* occurs primarily in Africa with extensions in the

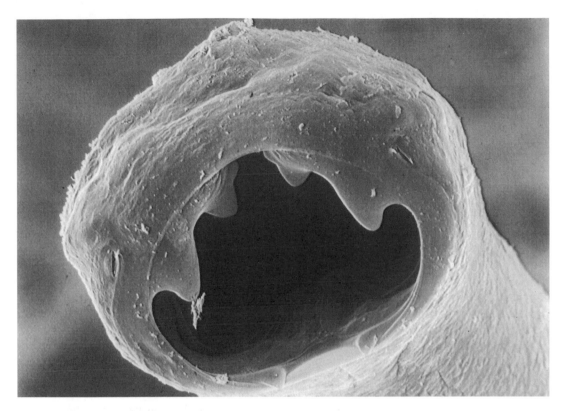

Figure 23–2 Photograph of *Ancylostoma duodenale*. Courtesy of Dr. G. Schad.

Middle East and western Asia. This species lives in the vesicular veins and capillaries of the bladder mucosa and causes the condition known as urinary schistosomiasis (bilharzia). *Schistosoma mansoni* occurs primarily in Africa, but also in the northern parts of South America (Brazil) and the Caribbean. Adults of this species normally live in the capillaries that drain the mesenteries; also sometimes found in the liver sinuses, they can produce the condition known as intestinal schistosomiasis (also known as intestinal bilharzia). *Schistosoma japonicum* occurs mainly in China and parts of Southeast Asia, particularly in the Philippines. This species, which occupies the same region of the body as *S. mansoni*, is a more virulent form of the parasite, and it frequently produces severe sequelae. The other species are *S. meekongi*, which is related to *S. japonicum,* found in Vietnam and adjoining territories, and *S. intercalatum*, which is related to *S. haematobium,* found in Cameroon and parts of West Africa. Because of their reliance on freshwater snails as aquatic intermediate hosts, the entire distribution of these parasites is associated with water resources in which the appropriate snail species are found.

Life Cycle

Adult schistosomes differ from typical trematode worms in their narrow, elongate shape and separate sexes. The male is the larger of the two, approximately 1.0 to 1.5 cm in length, with a cylindrical body folded to form a ventral gynecophoric canal in which the longer, slender female is embraced for most of the time. Both worms have two suckers, an oral sucker surrounding the mouth and a ventral sucker or acetabulum. The mouth leads into a blind gut that bifurcates along most of the length of the body. In the female, this is dark with hematin derived from the digestion of blood cells. The number of testes in the male, the length of the uterus, and the shape of the eggs in females are distinctive to the species.

Eggs are deposited in the fine capillaries of the organ where the worms are living. In vesicular schistosomiasis, this is the bladder; in the intestinal form, this is the intestinal mucosa. The eggs break through into the lumen of the bladder or gut, usually with a small amount of bleeding, and are passed to the exterior in the urine or feces. Many eggs do not break through the mucosa and remain in the tissue or are flushed into the liver where they form a nidus for granulomata to develop. In severe infections, these granulomata damage the affected organ. In some cases of ectopic egg deposition, severe long-term paraplegia can occur when the base of the spinal cord is involved.

If the schistosome eggs are deposited in freshwater, or in a place where they can be soon washed into the water, the cycle continues. The eggs hatch and a free-living, ciliated form, the miracidium, emerges. These miracidia use a number of environmental cues to seek out appropriate intermediate host snails. Miracidia move quite rapidly and can cover great distances in their search for snails. In some recent studies in Egypt, S. mansoni miracidia were shown commonly to infect snails 5 to 6 m distant, and some infected snails more than 20 m distant. The association is specific, and so only the correct species of mollusc will sustain the infection. The miracidia do not ingest food and so have an infective life limited to approximately 5 to 6 hours. During this time, they must find the appropriate snail. The miracidium attaches to the snail and secreting proteolytic enzymes penetrate into the tissues of the snail. The parasite then commences a process of asexual development. The miracidium enlarges into a mother sporocyst, a saclike organism that later buds off additional daughter sporocysts from layers of germinal epithelium. These daughter sporocysts migrate to the digestive gland of the snail where they grow and finally produce copious numbers of the next larval stage, the cercaria.

Cercariae emerge from infected snails in response to sunlight after a prepatent period of about 30 days, although this could be much longer in cool weather. Cercariae normally emerge around midmorning, and continue emerging from the snails throughout the day, although by afternoon the numbers soon decline. The cercariae are furcocercous (Figure 23–3) and move by vibrating the forked tail. Their main movement is up and down, vertical rather than horizontal, and their target is the skin of a nearby human being. They respond to appropriate skin lipids that stimulate the process of penetration, a process that must occur within 6 to 12 hours after emergence, as cercariae, too, have no means to ingest nutrient. When they commence penetration, cercariae secrete proteolytic enzymes, bore through the skin of the victim, then shed the tail, and, by contortions, penetrate into the subdermis, invade the lymphatic system, and move via the circulatory system to the lungs. In the lungs, the developing form, known as the schistosomulum, remains for a few days before continuing in the circulatory system to the liver. In the liver, the Schislosomula cercariae mature and move to the end organ system in pairs.

Epidemiology of Schistosomiasis

Reservoir of the Parasite Population

Of the various important species of schistosome that affect human populations, S. haematobium and S. mansoni are primarily anthropophilic. The reservoir is almost entirely confined to humans, although occasional episodes of transmission have been ascribed to other primates. With S. intercalatum, the picture is unclear; however, with S. japonicum and the related species, the parasites are found in a wide range of animals as well as the human population. The source of the reservoir fundamentally affects the epidemiology of schistosomiasis and will have an impact on attempts to control the disease.

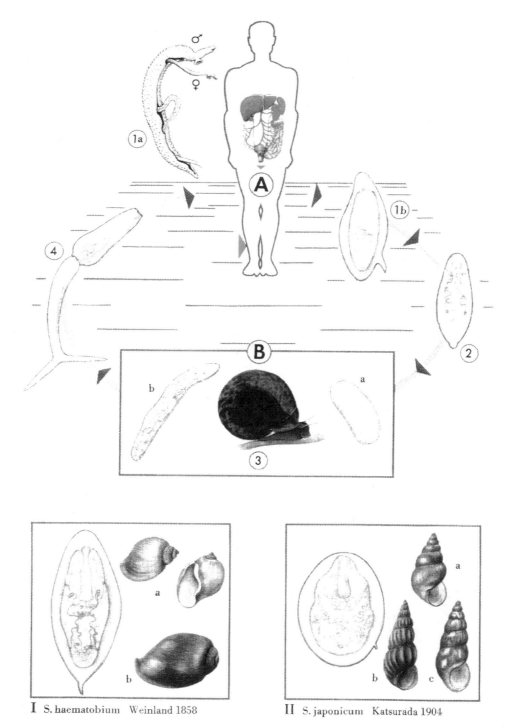

I s. haematobium Weinland 1858   II S. japonicum Katsurada 1904

Figure 23–3 Illustration of the schistosomes, miracidia, and cercariae life cycles. *Source:* Reprinted with permission from G. Pierkarski, *Medical Parasitology*, translation of *Medizinische Parasitologie in Tafeln*, 3, Aulage, © 1987, Springer-Verlag New York, Inc.

As with most other parasitic infections, schistosomes are overdispersed or aggregated in the reservoir population. That is, many hosts harbor few parasites, whereas a few hosts harbor many parasites with the distribution fitting the negative binomial. This aggregated distribution has been ascribed to numerous factors: the degree of individual susceptibility, patterns of exposure to transmission foci, age difference in susceptibility, and the development of acquired resistance to further infection. Each of these factors should be considered in the epidemiology of schistosomiasis.

Age Prevalence of Schistosomiasis

Examination of the prevalence of *Schistosoma* infection in any population living in an endemic region will show a typical distribution (Figure 23–4). The proportion of infected persons increases with age to a peak in childhood and adolescence. After the early 20s, age prevalence declines and in adult life it remains about one third as high as at the peak until old age when it declines further. The peak seen in these age prevalence curves is a factor of the endemicity or transmission rate (incidence) of infection, as can be seen in Figures 23–5 and 23–6, which show the pattern of infection in three regions of Zimbabwe wherein a high, medium, or low level of transmission occurs. These data clearly show how prevalence in the community is age specific and that it is strongly influenced by the transmission rate, which itself is a function of the amount of surface water in the area and the extent of human contact with the water.

Schistosomes are long-lived parasites. Estimations based on die-off of infections under conditions where snail control operations were carried out suggest a mean life of 5 to 6 years; in

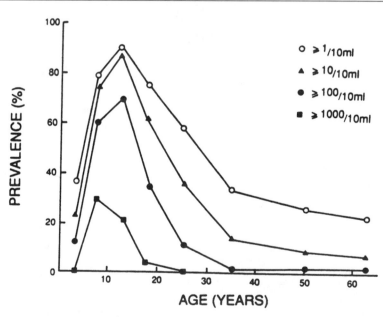

Figure 23–4 Prevalence and distribution of *Schistosome haematobium* egg output in relation to age in a Gambian community. *Source:* Reprinted with permission from H.A. Wilkens et al, The Significance of Proteinuria and Haematuria in Schistosoma Haematobium Infection, *Transactions of the Royal Society of Tropical Medicine and Hygiene*, Vol. 73, p. 75, © 1979, Royal Society of Tropical Medicine and Hygiene.

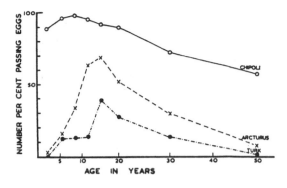

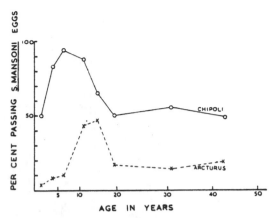

Figure 23–5 Prevalence of *Schistosome haematobium* infections in relation to age in three communities of Zimbabwe. *Source:* Reprinted with permission from V. de V. Clarke, The Influence of Acquired Resistance in the Epidemiology of Bilharziases, *Central African Journal of Medicine*, Vol. 12, No. 6, Supplement, p. 9, © 1966, Central African Journal of Medicine.

Figure 23–6 Prevalence of *Schistosome mansoni* infections in relation to age in two communities of Zimbabwe. *Source:* Reprinted with permission from V. de V. Clarke, The Influence of Acquired Resistance in the Epidemiology of Bilharziases, *Central African Journal of Medicine*, Vol. 12, No. 6, Supplement, p. 9, © 1966, Central African Journal of Medicine.

numerous instances, however, parasites have been found to live several decades. The decline in the level of infection seen in adults living in endemic areas may be related to acquired resistance induced by the current infection. This is a condition known as premunition, or acquisition of immunity in people subjected to infection by this parasite. Certainly, antibodies are produced by people, even those who no longer show evidence of infection by passage of parasite eggs in the excreta. Furthermore, treatment of the infection does not appear to annul this protection and the rate of acquisition of new infections among recently treated people, although high in children, declines abruptly in older children and adults (Figure 23–7). Recently, it has been suggested that the onset of puberty and the sexual maturation of the human host affect the ability of the parasite to invade. Numerous studies on human behavior and water contact have failed to show that this decline in prevalence in adults is a function of decreased water contact with age. When naive adults become infected with schistosomes, acute sequelae develop rapidly, which

suggests that sexual maturity plays little role in acquisition of infection.

Compiling of age prevalence curves of schistosome infection is necessary to determine the public health impact of the disease. Overall figures taken from a community as a whole might mask the severe impact the disease has on children. Furthermore, one must have some indication about the intensity (severity) of the infection. This can be obtained by estimating the intensity of infection or the associated worm burden. Actually, it is not possible to get an approximation of the number of worms infecting a patient; however, if the number of eggs passed in urine or feces is counted and expressed as a rate per 10 mL urine or gram of feces, then it is possible to predict where and in whom the most serious pathology may develop. Also, these estimates provide a good indication of the extent of the reservoir for the next generation of parasites. Egg burden in relation to age is clearly shown in Figure 23–7. In an intensive study in Zimbabwe, Clarke[3] translated this feature into a parameter he called the "infection potential." He showed

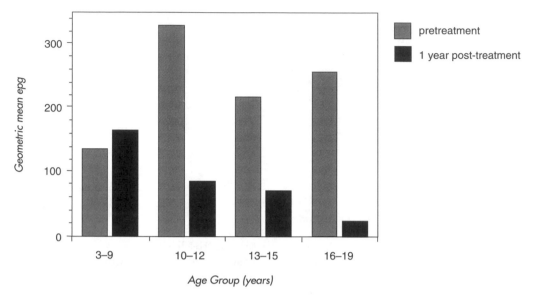

Figure 23–7 Geometric mean intensities of re-infection by age, one year after treatment of children in a high-transmission area (Mbugua et al in preparation). *Source:* Reprinted with permission from Butterworth et al, Immunity and Morbidity in Human Schistosomiasis, in *New Strategies in Parasitology*, K. P.W.J. McAdam, ed., p. 201, © W.B. Saunders Company.

that in high endemic areas, between 82% to 92% of *S. haematobium* eggs passed in a community were from children aged less than 12 years. The pattern with *S. mansoni* was similar, although in areas of lower prevalence, the egg load appeared to be more evenly distributed in the population. Studies in the Philippines and China indicated that age-related egg passage does not follow changes in prevalence as consistently as in *S. haematobium.*[4]

Transmission and the Role of the Intermediate Host

Knowing about the distribution of the intermediate host snails is a key to understanding the epidemiology of schistosomiasis. In all instances, the snails involved are freshwater gastropod molluscs; they are entirely aquatic, although they can survive dry periods in small number within mud refuges. They belong to the family *Planorbidae* and the genera *Biomphararia* (*S. mansoni*) and *Bulinus* (*S. haematobium*). In the *S. japonicum* cycle, the snails are prosobranchs, which have an operculum to close the main aperture of the snail; thus, they are amphibious and can survive periods of dryness and spend part of their life out of water. These snails are pioneering species with rapid rates of reproduction and they can reach huge numbers when conditions are ideal. They are detritus feeders and, hence, in their environment are seldom restricted by shortages of food. Although certain predacious animals consume snails, under natural conditions the predators have little impact on the snail populations. Snails are cold-blooded and reproduce more rapidly in summer than in winter. They lay eggs in small batches on plant surfaces, stones, or other objects, even plastic sheets floating in the water. Each snail can produce several hundred eggs a week. These eggs will hatch in about 7 days, and the emerging snails will mature in about 6 weeks. Snails surviving dry periods can repopulate ponds within a short time.

Factors Affecting Snail Infection Rates

Miracidia emerge from schistosome eggs passed into water, and they will detect and infect snails nearby. The process of development in the snails is temperature dependent and proceeds more rapidly in warmer weather. In Zimbabwe, it has been shown that the rising temperatures of spring will shorten the prepatent period, producing a heavy load of cercariae in the water in early summer. Patterns of snail population fluctuation and presence of infected snails in Egypt show peaks in spring and again in autumn. The intense heat of summer and the cold in winter negatively affect the snail populations as well as the number of infected snails. These factors produce a seasonal pattern to the risk of infection in endemic areas.[5]

The Susceptible Human

Transmission of schistosomes requires contact of a susceptible host with cercariae-infested water. Such contact with water can involve ritual ablution, domestic chores, agricultural activities, gardening or fishing, or even recreation and bathing. Occasionally an infection will occur from casual contact with water, even if the host is unaware of the contact. In most endemic areas, however, water contact is regular and systematic and part of a daily routine of life that entails a sustained exposure to the water and the risk of acquiring an infection when cercariae are present. It may be assumed that the longer the duration of contact, the heavier will be the worm burden, but this is not always the case because as people get older, the likelihood of re-infection diminishes, as discussed. The actual incidence of infection in a community is difficult to assess because in an endemic area a large proportion of the people will be infected and it is hard to assess acquisition of new infections. It is possible to treat a cohort of people and reexamine them after a period of time to assess the number of reacquired cases. However, because a strong immune response militates against re-infection, measurement of incidence in this way can only be done in young children who are still susceptible to re-infection. Recently, it has been shown that a circulating antigen can be detected in active cases, and this may make further epidemiologic studies easier to carry out. However, currently few data exist to assess the value of this test under field conditions.[6]

Schistosomiasis in the Community

Schistosome parasites have evolved a well-adapted association with their human hosts. This association has probably developed over evolutionary time, particularly because of a nomadic lifestyle. However, with the more recent development of agriculture and settling of the human population in village communities, infection severity has increased and the ill effects of the disease have become more noticeable. Where new dams have been constructed, where population movements have occurred bringing naive hosts into contact with the parasite, and where conditions have led to expansions of snail populations, the cycle of transmission has been exacerbated and the people have acquired disease. Thus, the public health problem of schistosomiasis is a product of perturbed ecological processes, and control of the disease needs to focus on reducing the increased contact between host, snail, and parasite. To do this, a careful consideration of all aspects of the complex life cycle and its various components must figure high in the development of control strategies.[7]

REVIEW OF OTHER GEOHELMINTHS

Worm Infections with Direct Life Cycles

A life cycle is considered direct when no intermediate host is involved and transmission is directly from one human host to another. The following species are transmitted directly, and they provide examples of direct cycles: *Strongy-*

loides stercoralis, Trichuris trichiura, Ascaris lumbricoides, and *Enterobius vermicularis.* Life cycles and brief notes on the epidemiology are discussed.

Strongyloidiasis:

The life cycle of *Strongyloides stercoralis* is similar to that of hookworm with some important modifications. Both a free-living cycle and a parasitic cycle exist. In the free-living cycle, larvae are passed in the feces of infected people. In the presence of waterlogged soil and abundant feces, the larvae mature into *rhabditiform* males and females. These are nonparasitic, noninfective form. With ideal conditions, the adults mate and produce several cycles of free-living worms; however, as food declines or the habitat desiccates, a filariform generation will develop, leading to a third stage—filariform larvae—which will remain on the fecal mass and penetrate through the skin of anyone contacting the larvae. The larvae circulate through the pulmonary alveolae, are coughed up, and migrate to the pharynx and finally to the intestine. They penetrate the mucosa in the duodenum and upper jejunum, molt twice, and become mature females in about 2 weeks. There are no parasitic males, so reproduction is parthenogenetic at this stage. The female is a delicate filariform worm 2 to 3 mm in length and 30 to 40 microns in width. Females produce an indeterminate number of embryonated eggs daily; these usually hatch in the mucosa and the larvae escape in the feces. Autoinfection can occur if the emerging first stage larvae molt twice internally and develop into the third filariform stage. These may re-invade the mucosa and proceed to re-establish a secondary infection. In immunocompromised hosts, this represents a severe stage of the infection.

With the advent of human immunodeficiency virus (HIV) infection and in cases of decreasing immunocompetence particularly associated with old age, cancer, or in patients receiving immunosuppressive drugs, strongyloidiasis has become increasingly important. In such people, dormant or new infections can disseminate and spread throughout the body. The infection is sporadic, particularly in communities where sanitation facilities are inadequate or defective.

Several species of *Strongyloides* occur in animals and the infection is known to be a zoonosis with reservoir populations in a variety of animals. This makes the infection difficult to control with chemotherapy alone. The best approach is treatment of positive cases together with emphasis on general use of latrines.

Trichuriasis (Human Whip Worm Infection)

Adults of *Trichuris trichiura* live attached to the wall of the cecum, and humans are the only source of infection. The adult worms have a large fleshy body and are attenuated in the anterior two thirds of the length, giving the picture of a whip. The mouth, at the distal end of the whip, is provided with a stylus and it is connected to a thin, capillarylike esophagus. This thin portion of the worm is insinuated into the mucosa of the cecum and large bowel, and it anchors the worms in place. The presence of the worms causes irritation, probably as a result of the feeding process which seems to involve tissue lysis by the parasite. The female is 35 to 50 mm in length with the male slightly smaller. Eggs are produced in situ and passed in the feces. These are characteristically barrel shaped and robust and are laid unembryonated. Development of the larvae takes about 3 weeks after which the eggs are infective. Eggs are not resistant to desiccation or bright sunlight. Transmission is most efficient in warm, humid, moist conditions and infection results from swallowing infective eggs. In areas of high endemicity, small children seem most vulnerable, and they can develop heavy infections, which may be caused by geophagy. *Trichuris* does not respond well to treatment, probably because its favored habitat is the lower bowel, a site difficult to reach with active drugs.

Ascariasis

Ascariasis is caused by *Ascaris lumbricoides,* the large round worm of humans. This is one of the world's most ubiquitous parasites and it has been recognized from ancient times. The adults, which are free living in the intestine, are very large; the female is 20 to 35 cm in length and 3 to 6 mm in diameter, and the male is slightly smaller. The severity of infection depends on the number of worms a patient carries; however, the worms produce prodigious amounts of eggs on a continuous basis—approximately 200,000 eggs per female can be passed in a daily stool. The eggs may be either fertile or infertile. Fertile eggs are encased in a thick shell consisting of three layers. The eggshell is remarkably stable and resistant to desiccation. It also prevents toxic substances from reaching the developing embryo. Thus, the eggs of *A. lumbricoides* can survive the rigors of sewage treatment and remain infective for many months, even years under ideal conditions.

The eggs produced unembryonated and as such are not infective. A period of development and two molts take place in the egg prior to it becoming infective. This takes place by ingestion, either in fecally contaminated food or in water, or even inhaled through dust. The larvae emerge in the intestine and immediately penetrate the gut epithelium and circulate through the blood system to the lungs where they may remain for 9 to 15 days. They are then coughed up and swallowed and finally return to the gut. In 8 to 10 weeks, worms are mature; if males and females are present, the females will start to produce fertile eggs.

Pinworm

Pinworm is caused by *Enterobius vermicularis*, a cosmopolitan parasite more common in temperate climates than in warmer areas, when less frequent bathing and infrequent washing of underclothes occurs. The worms are small nematodes, the male being somewhat smaller (2 to 5 mm in length and not more that 0.2 mm wide) than the female (2 to 13 mm long and up to 0.5 mm in diameter). The worms live in the cecum, appendix, and adjacent areas of the ascending colon. They occupy the mucous layer between the mucosa and the fecal matter. The gravid female becomes distended, and is packed with eggs. At this time, it migrates down the colon and out the anus. Normally, the eggs are deposited at one time, after which the female disintegrates. Eggs are not commonly laid in the bowel, although they are sometimes found in the feces. Usually, eggs are smeared over the perianal region and can best be seen and identified by the "scotch tape" test. For this test, a 6-cm length of clear scotch tape is placed over the anal area, pressed against the skin, and removed. The tape is then placed on a glass microscopic slide, with the tacky side to the glass. Eggs adhering to the adhesive can be seen by observing the glass slide under a low power microscope.

The eggs are elongate-ovoidal, distinctly compressed laterally, and flattened on one side; they measure 50 to 60 by 20 to 30 microns. The shell is relatively thick and colorless. The eggs embryonate and become infective a few hours after being laid. They are robust and resistant to disinfectants and drying, and may remain viable for up to 2 weeks. Eggs that are swallowed hatch when they reach the intestine, and the development to adult usually takes about 1 month.

The epidemiology is associated with contact between individuals usually living together or people who handle soiled clothing, particularly night clothes. Frequently, this occurs within families. Eggs are transferred from hand to mouth, particularly following scratching the perianal area after females have emerged and laid eggs, through inhalation of dust particles in bedrooms where an infected person may sleep, or similar person-to-person contact. Transmission is efficient and can lead to very severe infestations.

Control is a matter of treatment and prevention. As the eggs are resistant to disinfection, it is best to consider any contaminated area as infective for up to 2 weeks after treatment of any cases, and to maintain a high level of cleanliness and hygiene to prevent the cycle from restarting.

Examples of Worms with Indirect Cycles (including a Vectorborne Stage)

The parasites with indirect cycles belong to a group (or superfamily) of nematode worms called the *Filarioidea*. They live in the tissues or body cavity of a mammalian host and are transmitted by the bite of an arthropod vector. The females produce microfilariae, which are unique in that they are less differentiated than the first stage larvae of other nematodes. Highly motile and threadlike, they exist in the blood or subcutaneously in the mammalian host. The microfilariae in blood exhibit diurnal periodicity and are usually present in the peripheral circulation synchronized with the biting behavior of the insect vector. When taken up by an arthropod vector, they migrate through the gut wall into the hemocoel and then into the thoracic muscles of the insect. They proceed through two stages of development, finally reaching the third stage larva (L_3), which is infective and which invades a new mammalian host during the next blood meal. Seldom are more than two or three L_3 forms found in one mosquito.

Bancroftian Filariasis (Elephantiasis)

Elephantiasis is a condition caused by one of two parasites, *Wucheraria bancrofti*, which is widespread in most tropical areas, and *Brugia malayi*, which is an important human parasite in Southeast Asia and the Pacific Islands. In most of their distribution, both species exhibit nocturnal periodicity and microfilariae are in the peripheral circulation only at night.

The adults of these two species are threadlike and long; males are approximately 40 mm in length, whereas the females are approximately 100 mm in length. They are normally found coiled in lymph nodes in the inguinal region, although they can also occur in axillary nodes. Infiltration of plasma cells, macrophages, and eosinophils around the infected nodes occurs and eventually results in inflammation and swelling. In time the nodes become blocked and proximal lymphatic vessels become stenotic and obstructed, which leads to lymphedema and thickening of the subcutaneous tissue and eventually to elephantiasis. Approximately 8 to 12 months after an active infection is established, the worms become sexually mature and microfilariae appear in the blood and circulate in the

peripheral blood according to the diurnal periodicity described above. It appears from experimental work with animal models that the microfilariae can live as long as 200 days.

The epidemiology is very much associated with the local distribution of mosquito vectors. However, as several genera of mosquito can transmit microfilariae, the endemic areas are extensive. Peridomestic breeding places for culicine mosquitoes are becoming increasingly important, particularly in urban areas. Infection occurs in young people; however, because the vectors carry small numbers of infective parasites, it normally takes many years before noticeable sequelae of the infection occur.

Control of the disease depends on reducing the number of breeding sites of the vectors, particularly those in close proximity to houses. In areas where sewage treatment is inadequate and wastewater is allowed to stand in pools, and where effluent from domestic water usage occurs, mosquito populations abound and present serious problems. Control by various methods, such as vector control, reduction of potential mosquito breeding sites, the use of insect repellents, and extensive chemotherapy needs to be implemented. It has recently been shown that use of the drug ivermectin will reduce considerably the level of microfilaraemia and, in this way, restrict the reservoir of infection. A combination of these various approaches will likely be successful in reducing the prevalence of both these parasites.[8]

Onchocerca volvulus

Onchocerca volvulus is associated with the condition known as river blindness. The adults live in subcutaneous nodules where they lie in tangled masses of male and female worms. They reproduce by producing unsheathed microfilariae, which migrate through the skin intradermally. These forms are not found in the blood, but they frequently occur in the vitreous humor of the eye. The microfilariae are ingested during the process of feeding by blackflies (*Simulium* species), which breed in well-oxygenated, fast-flowing water, and are pests to people living near streams and rivers.

The microfilariae pass through two molts in the blackfly, and after about 6 to 8 days exist as L_3 forms in the thoracic muscles of the fly; finally they migrate to the mouth parts of the fly. At the next blood meal, the larvae leave the fly and penetrate the wound caused during the feed. Once in the skin of a new host, the larvae migrate to various parts of the body, penetrate through the subcutaneous tissue, molt further, and finally mature into adults. The prepatent period in humans is 3 to 15 months. The parasites reside in nodules, which may be in the deep fascia or in subcutaneous tissue. They are frequently palpable and can be removed surgically. The onchocercal nodules usually cause no symptoms, although they can be somewhat deforming. The main problems from the infection come from the long-lived microfilariae in the skin and eye. In chronic infections, a progressive loss of subcutaneous connective tissue occurs and the skin becomes loose and depigmented. Dermatitis and infiltration by lymphocytes can occur, adding to the irritation and disfigurement of the host.

Severe ocular pathology is frequently associated with savannah onchocerciasis transmitted by blackflies of the *Simulium damnosum* species group. Transmission in the forest environment can be intense and the prevalence of infection is high; however, blinding onchocerciasis is seen less frequently in people exposed to the forest dwelling species of blackflies.

The distribution of onchocerciasis is extensive in West and Central Africa, and stretching into East Africa, as far south as Malawi. It also exists in the Arabian peninsular, Yemen, Central America, and the northern part of South America. However, in the Americas, although ocular infiltration and damage occurs, little blindness is associated with the infection. To understand the epidemiology of onchocerciasis, it is important to know something about the vector. The blackfly belongs to the genus *Simulium*. Members of this genus, who are voracious blood feeders, are cosmopolitan in distribution. Both males and females take blood and they are worrisome nuisance pests associated with strong flowing water. Not all *Simulium* species carry *Onchocerca*. In Africa, the vectors belong to the *S. damnosum* complex and *S. neavei* group, whereas in South America, several anthropophilic species transmit the parasite.

The flies lay their eggs in water, preferably on rocks or emergent vegetation washed with fast-flowing, usually well-oxygenated water. The larval and pupal forms of the insect live on firm substrates immersed in the water where they feed on plankton and suspended particles. The adult flies do not normally venture far from their breeding sites, hence transmission of this parasite is associated with rivers. In parts of Africa, prior to the major control efforts of the Onchocerciasis Control Programme, villages near rivers and the associated lands were abandoned by peasant farmers who feared the infection.

Control of the disease has been based on a two-front attack using both chemical control of the vector and treatment of the infection among humans. Because of their restricted breeding habits, blackflies can be controlled by treating the rivers with specially formulated insecticides. The insecticide is adsorbed on clay particles suspended in the fast-flowing water and is selectively toxic to filter-feeding insects. This has been done for the past 20 years in a large part of West Africa, and it has been successful in reducing both the blackfly population and the transmission of *O. volvulus*. More recently, a drug (ivermectin), which eliminates the microfilariae from the skin of infected people for up to a year, has been used to augment the vector control efforts. Together, this work has reduced morbidity and blindness in a large section of the West African population. Because the drug does not kill adult worms, treatment has to be repeated every 12 months; however, methods to overcome this drawback are being developed and some hope exists that the infection will decline in importance as a public health problem.[9]

REFERENCES

1. De Silva NR, Chan MS, Bundy DA. Morbidity and mortality due to ascariasis: re-estimation and sensitivity analysis of global numbers at risk. *Trop Med Int Health.* 1997;2:519–528.

2. Kendall C, Foote D, Martorell R. Ethnomedicine and rehydration therapy: a case study of ethnomedical investigation and program planning. *Soc Sci Med.* 1984; 19:253–260.

3. Clarke V de V. The influence of acquired resistance in the epidemiology of bilharziasis. *Cent Afr J Med.* 1966; 12(Suppl 6):1–30.

4. Jordan P, Webbe G. Epidemiology: In: Jordan P, Webbe G, Sturrock RW, eds. *Human Schistosomiasis.* Oxford: CAB International; 1993:87–158.

5. Shiff CJ, Coutts WCC, Yiannakis C, et al. Seasonal patterns in the transmission of *Schistosoma haematobium* in Rhodesia. *Trans R Soc Trop Med Hyg.* 1974;73:375–380.

6. Ndhlovu P, Cadman H, Gunderson H, et al. Circulating anodic antigen levels in a Zimbabwe rural community endemic for *Schistosoma haematobium* using the magnetic beads antigen-capture enzyme linked immunoassay. *Am J Trop Med Hyg.* 1996;54:637–642.

7. Gryseels B. Human resistance to schistosome infections. *Parasitology Today.* 1994;10:380–384.

8. Nicholas L, Plichart C, Nguyen LN, Moulia-Pelat JP. Reduction of *Wucheraria bancrofti* adult worm circulating antigen after annual treatments of dethylcarbamazine combined with ivermectin in French Polynesia. *J Infect Dis.* 1997;175:489–492.

9. Molyneux DH, Davies JB. Onchocerciasis control: moving towards the millennium. *Parasitology Today.* 1997;13:418–425.

Index

I